Physiology and Anatomy

A homeostatic approach

Physiology and Anatomy

A homeostatic approach

Second edition

John Clancy BSc(Hons), PGCE
Nursing and Midwifery Research Unit,
University of East Anglia,
Norwich, UK

Andrew J McVicar BSc(Hons), PhD
School of Health Care Practice,
Anglia Polytechnic University,
Chelmsford, UK

Principal Nursing Adviser:
Christine Barrett BSc(Hons), RNT, RGN
Nursing Division School of Heath Studies,
University of Bradford,
Bradford, UK

A member of the Hodder Headline Group
LONDON · NEW YORK · NEW DELHI

First published in Great Britain in 1995 by
Arnold, a member of the Hodder Headline Group,
338 Euston Road, London NWI 3BH

http://www.arnoldpublishers.com

Distributed in the United States of America by
Oxford University Press, Inc.,
198 Madison Avenue, New York, NY 10016
Oxford is a registered trademark of Oxford University Press

Whilst the advice and information in this book is believed to be true and accurate at the date of going to press, neither the authors nor the publisher can accept any legal responsibility or liability for any errors or omissions that may be made. In particular (but without limiting the generality of the preceding disclaimer) every effort has been made to check drug dosages; however, it is still possible that errors have been missed. Furthermore, dosage schedules are constantly being revised and new side-effects recognized. For these reasons the reader is strongly urged to consult the drug companies' printed instructions before administering any of the drugs recommended in this book.

British Library Cataloguing in Publication Data
A catalogue record for this book is available from the British Library

Library of Congress Cataloging-in-Publication Data
A catalog record for this book is available from the Library of Congress

ISBN 0 340 76239 X

Commissioning Editor: Georgina Bentliff
Production Editor: Rada Radojicic
Production Controller: Iain McWilliams
Illustrators: Oxford Designers & Illustrators/Line Arts
Cover Design: Terry Griffiths

Typeset in 9.5/12 pt Minion by Scribe Design, Gillingham, Kent, UK
Printed and bound in Malta by Gutenberg Press

What do you think about this book? Or any other Arnold title?
Please send your comments to feedback.arnold@hodder.co.uk

Contents

Preface

Why *homeostasis?* The concept of homeostasis derived from engineering in which intrinsic control processes are used to enable systems to auto-regulate. The notion is one of a constant performance or environment, but in physiology such an interpretation is not strictly correct because there must be scope for adaptation to allow people to achieve developmental milestones, or to change performance level according to need. Homeostasis in the physiological sense therefore represents a dynamism that is central to human functioning. Nevertheless, the concept remains about control; few processes in the body occur by chance, and those that do promote corrective or adaptive responses. Control is necessary because people interact with their environment at social, spiritual, emotional, physical and chemical levels, which may act to induce such change within the body that conditions become suboptimal. Homeostasis therefore is the most important principle that underpins physiological processes.

Perfect regulation is unlikely. The tendency for change and the very dynamism of control processes means that parameters must vary, however slightly. For every parameter within the body there is a range of variation that could be considered 'normal' or optimal. This range may itself change with circumstances, for example when we perform exercise, or when a woman becomes pregnant, but there will still be control of that range. This book is concerned with the mechanisms that maintain parameters within their homeostatic range.

The education of health care professionals places an emphasis on producing students and staff knowledgeable about the holistic or physiological, psychological and sociological requirements of health. The integration of physiological functioning into this model has proved difficult in health care education, and the need to describe and explain body functioning in the context of an interactive framework prompted the writing of the first edition of this book, and several subsequent articles on the theme. The intention of the book was to utilize homeostasis as a framework to aid learning, provide an insight into the ways in which disturbances promote illness, and to help students appreciate the physiological basis of clinical practice.

This second edition builds on this successful format. The text has been reorganised and extended to provide a comprehensive explanation of how the body works. Regular information Boxes extend the discussion to identify how functions change with development, how failure of various aspects being discussed is responsible for ill-health, and also how health care intervenes in restoring wellbeing. The application of homeostatic principles to care is reinforced by inclusion of many examples of case studies, drawn from the four Branches of nursing care.

First and foremost, *Physiology and Anatomy: a homeostatic approach, second edition* is intended to be a student text. Many students find physiology a difficult discipline since it is based on facts as well as theories. As with any science there is a body of knowledge that has to be understood, but learning is not helped if a textbook contains only material that provides factual knowledge or reference material. This book takes a different approach from that provided by other texts on the subject because it provides a breadth of information that enables students to *understand* why certain processes must occur as they do. Homeostasis provides the framework for that understanding. Once the principle is grasped, the homeostatic processes that are involved in maintaining physiological function are often logical.

To facilitate learning, much of the book is organised according to the principles of homeostasis :

● *Section 1: An Introduction to the human body.* This section considers the construction of the human body, and what is meant by cell function. The basic principles of homeostasis are explored in depth.

● *Section 2: The need for regulation.* This section identifies the fundamentals of human functioning, including the composition of the body, metabolism and nutrition.

● *Section 3: Sensing change and co-ordinating responses.* This section explains how changes to the internal (and external) environment are identified, and how adaptive responses are enabled and co-ordinated.

● *Section 4: Effectors of homeostasis.* This section considers further systems of the body that are themselves capable of bringing about change, and so provide the means of correcting deficits or excesses.

Further Sections illustrate the application of homeostatic principles in relation to 'gene-environment' interactions, and to health care provision:

● *Section 5: Influences on homeostasis*. This section considers some of the vital interactive components that promote variation in the body.

● *Section 6: Homeostasis in action*. This section provides numerous examples of case studies that illustrate homeostatic principles in relation to health problems and health care interventions.

The book is completed by Appendices, which identify units of measurement and optimal values for various parameters.

Although each chapter of the book can be read individually, frequent cross-referencing with other chapters is used to highlight where the processes described integrate with those of other systems. However, the student is encouraged to first read Sections 1 and 2 since the principles and topics discussed and, in particular, the inclusion of a simple but unique feature, the homeostatic graph, are the foundations for what follows in the other chapters. Student exercises and review questions are provided throughout the book to encourage reflection on the material covered by the chapters and to facilitate learning. Answers to the review questions at the end of each chapter may be found on the Arnold web page, in the Anatomy and Physiology section.

Finally, we hope you enjoy and benefit from reading this book. Some of the revisions included in this new edition have arisen from comments made by readers of the last one. We would value comments on this edition too, otherwise how else could the next edition evolve!

John Clancy
Andrew J McVicar

Acknowledgements

For the production of this much enriched second edition of *Physiology and Anatomy: a homeostatic approach*, we have enjoyed the opportunity of collaborating with a group of dedicated and talented professionals. We are grateful to them all.

In particular our special thanks go to:

Christine Barrett at the University of Bradford for her advice on the nursing content, her editorial suggestions and her enthusiasm for the concept of the book. Many thanks for reading every word.

Anna Harris, midwifery lecturer, who provided various applications to midwifery to support nurses in their Midwifery placements.

Penny Goacher, a colleague at the University of East Anglia, who provided the challenging end-of-chapter Review Questions. We trust readers will attempt to answer these prior to looking up the answers on the Arnold Website: http://www.arnoldpublishers.com.htm

The contributors to the case studies. Their expertise in the four Branches of nursing has made the homeostatic graph come alive in all aspects of nursing care. Congratulations everyone. Most are lecturers of Nursing at UEA, others are former students who have (hopefully!) been inspired by our teaching: thanks go to you all.

Our employers, the University of East Anglia and Anglia Polytechnic University, for their support and help with resources.

Colleagues at both universities for their continued support, and for putting up with our moans and groans when we were working to deadlines.

The reviewers, whose excellent reviews and evaluative feedback have led directly to the production of this much improved second edition.

The Editorial and Production Teams at Arnold for their advice, support, enthusiasm, skill and investment in the second edition.

Each other for continued encouragement and staying power so that we have managed to complete several projects simultaneously, without having a nervous breakdown, so that we can now focus on developing our research careers.

Finally, this second edition would have been only a dream rather than a reality if it had not been for the numerous purchasers of the first one. Whoever you are, wherever you are, it really did make a difference.

This second edition is dedicated to our families:

Our partners Rachel Starling and Penny McVicar, for putting up with our working long and often unsociable hours, and baby Lauren, Clare and Lisa who have seen less of us as a result of our taking on an increased workload. Who knows they may be grateful of the rest!

Our very special parents Ann and Norman Clancy, and James and Mary McVicar

John Clancy
Andrew J McVicar, 2001

Section One

An introduction to the human body

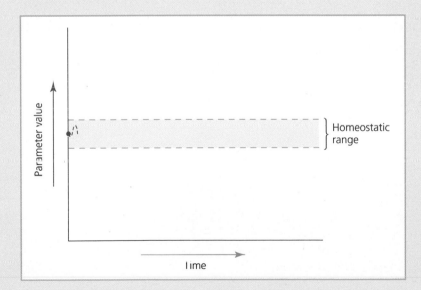

Chapter 1

Introduction to physiology and homeostasis

INTRODUCTION TO THE HUMAN BODY, ITS ORGANIZATION, AND THE HOMEOSTATIC BASIS OF BODY FUNCTIONS

You are about to begin the study of the human body. This book will enable you to learn how your body is organized structurally, and how it functions. The study of the human body involves several branches of science: biology, chemistry, physics, mathematics, psychology and sociology. Each contributes an understanding of how the body functions in health, during times of exercise, illness, pain, distress, trauma and surgery. Thus, an understanding each of these sciences to varying degrees, and how they link together, is of paramount importance to healthcare professionals, who need to view each patient as an individual. However, it must be stressed at the onset that human beings are biological organisms. We may live in highly sophisticated societies, and have very complex behaviours and different cognitive abilities, but healthcare professionals should not lose sight of the fact that ultimately our 'health' depends upon the functioning of biological structures.

The two branches of science covered in this book that will help you understand the human body are anatomy and physiology. Identifiable within these is the central concept referred to as homeostasis.

Definitions

Human anatomy refers to the study of the structure of the body. Physiology is concerned with the mechanisms of human bodily function. In this book you will see how the structure of the body is custom-built to perform particular functions in health (a sense of wellbeing). It follows, therefore, that abnormal structure leads to the abnormal functioning associated with ill-health. This structural and functional relationship is referred to by biologists as the 'principle of complementary'.

Homeostasis refers to the automatic, self-regulating processes necessary to maintain the 'normal' state of the body's environment, despite changes in the environment outside the body. Collectively, anatomical structure, physiological function and the maintenance of homeostasis enable the body to attain the basic needs necessary for health and a 'normal' life. This aspect is considered later in this chapter: before contemplating these basic needs, the reader should become familiar with how the body is organized.

Anatomical organization

The outside of the human body has a definite and recognizable shape. The inside has organs, which are located in specific positions relative to one another. The anatomical position of the body provides a reference point when studying or describing the position of body structures. This position is when the person stands erect, faces forward,

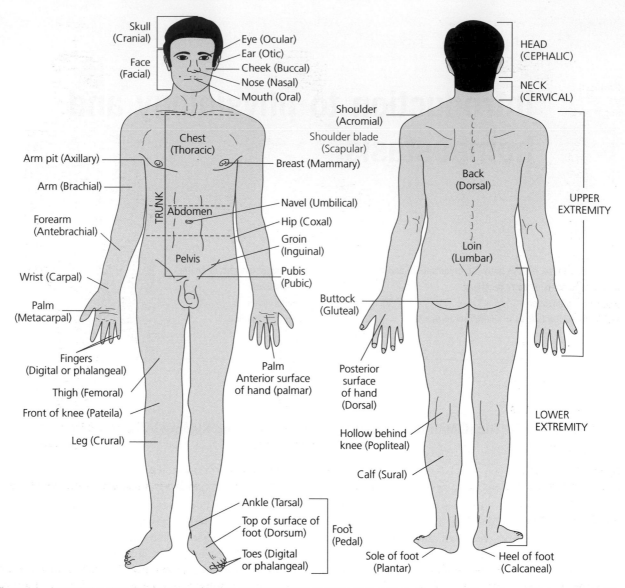

Figure 1.1 Anatomical position. The common names and anatomical terms (in brackets) are indicated for many of the regions of the human body. (a) Anterior view; (b) posterior view.

with arms at his/her side with palms facing forwards. For example, organs such as the heart are drawn according to this convention, such that features on, say, the left side appear on the right, as though the observer is looking into someone's chest.

A set of standard anatomical terms is used to describe each part of the body, the position of body structures, and their geographical relationships with each other. Many of these regional terms are illustrated in Figure 1.1. The main terms used relate to 'planes of the body', 'relative positioning of organs' and 'body cavity'.

Planes of the body

Body structures can be described in relation to three planes or imaginary lines – median (mid-sagittal), transverse

(horizontal) and coronal (frontal) – which run through the body (Figure 1.2). The median plane passes directly along the mid-line of the body, dividing the body into perfectly symmetrical right and left halves. The transverse plane passes horizontally through the body, dividing it into upper and lower portions. The coronal plane divides the body into front and back portions.

Terms of relative position

Directional terms are also used to describe the position of structures relative to each other (Figure 1.2). For example, 'anterior' and 'ventral' are used interchangeably and refer to the front surface of the body. They also have a broader meaning in the sense of a structure being closer to the front of the body. Examples are 'anterior

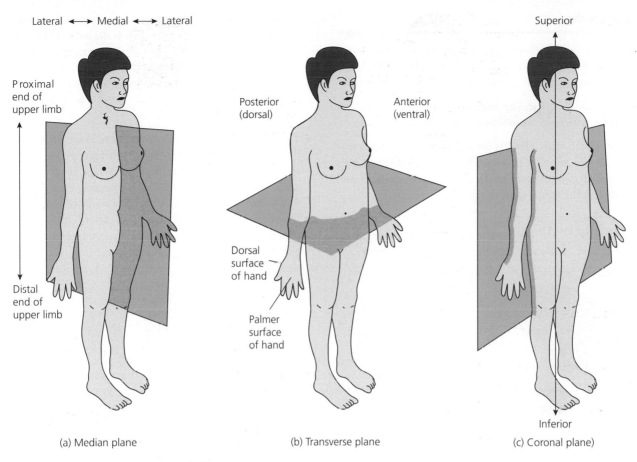

Lateral ←→ Medial ←→ Lateral

Proximal end of upper limb

Distal end of upper limb

(a) Median plane

Posterior (dorsal)

Anterior (ventral)

Dorsal surface of hand

Palmer surface of hand

(b) Transverse plane

Superior

Inferior

(c) Coronal plane)

Figure 1.2 Planes through the body. (a) Median (mid-sagittal) plane; (b) transverse plane; (c) coronal (frontal) plane.

Q. Which plane divides the body into (i) anterior and posterior parts; (ii) right and left parts that are mirror images of each other; and (iii) superior and inferior portions?

Q. Is the hip proximal or distal to the knee?

abdominal wall' or 'the heart is anterior to the spine'. In the same way, 'posterior' may refer to the back surface of the body, or it may mean a structure is nearer to the back of the body. Examples are 'the posterior surface of the arm' or the 'oesophagus (food pipe) is posterior to the heart'. 'Dorsal' is linked similarly to posterior. Likewise, 'medial' indicates that a structure is towards the mid-line of the body, whereas 'lateral' designates that a structure is away from the mid-line of the body. 'Proximal' indicates that the structure concerned is nearer the attached end of a limb, and thus the trunk of the body, whilst a 'distal' structure is further away from the attached end of a limb and/or the trunk. As an example, the shoulder is proximal to the elbow, whereas the elbow is distal to the shoulder.

In the clinical environment, healthcare professionals need to be familiar with these terms so they are all speaking the same language to avoid mistakes being made.

Initially, anatomical terminology may seem unfamiliar and difficult to understand. However, once you have mastered an understanding of basic words, including prefixes (the beginning of a word), roots (the main body of the word) and suffixes (the end of a word), you will discover the logical and helpful method in which structures are named. For example, once you understand that the prefix 'electro-' means electrical, the root 'cardiac' refers to the heart, and the suffix '-gram' means recording, then the meaning of the term 'electrocardiogram' becomes apparent.

Exercise

Use a biological dictionary to find out what the following terms mean: afferent, efferent, peripheral, deep, superficial, internal, external.

Exercise

Using Appendix C, try to learn 10 common prefixes and suffixes every weekday. When you are satisfied that you know most of the common prefixes and suffixes, learn 20 commonly used roots of the words. This will help you to understand the unfamiliar terminology associated with the clinical area.

Body cavities

The body can be divided into cavities produced by the bony skeleton (Figure 1.3). These cavities contain the internal organs (viscera). The main body cavities are:

- *The cranial cavity.* The bones of the skull enclose this cavity, which accommodates and protects the brain.

- *The spinal cavity.* This is formed by a hole (foramen = 'window') running through the vertebral column. This is called the vertebral canal, and it accommodates and protects the spinal cord.

- *The thoracic cavity.* This is the upper cavity of the trunk of the body. Its confines are the breastbone (sternum), ribs and associated intercostal muscles ('inter-' =

between, '-cost' = rib) and cartilage, vertebral column, diaphragm, and the structures below the neck. The cavity contains the windpipe (trachea), two lungs, the heart and its great vessels, the food pipe (oesophagus) and associated nerves, and lymphatic supply. The space between the lungs, occupied by the heart, is called the mediastinum.

- *The abdominal cavity.* This is the large lower portion of the trunk. It is confined by the diaphragm, pelvic cavity, spine, abdominal muscles, and lower ribs. It accommodates the organs concerned with digestion and absorption of nutrients, and other organs associated with these functions, i.e. the gall bladder, liver, spleen and pancreas. In addition, the kidneys, ureters and adrenal glands are also located in this region.

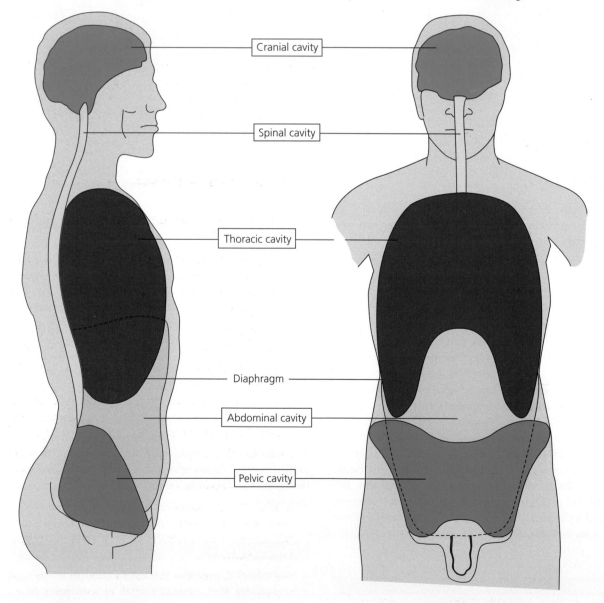

(a) Right lateral view   (b) Anterior view

Figure 1.3 Lateral and anterior views of the human body showing major cavities. (a) Right lateral view; (b) anterior view.
Q. What are the confines of the (i) thoracic cavity, (ii) abdominal cavity, and (iii) pelvic cavity?

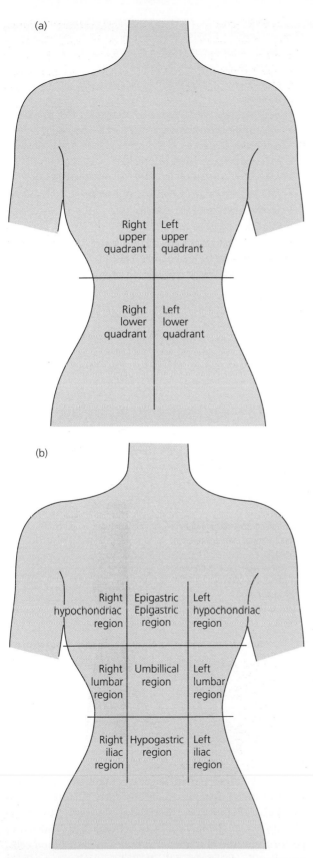

Figure 1.4 Anatomical subdivisions. (a) Quadrants of the abdomen. (b) The nine regions of the abdominal and pelvic regions.

Q. Which quadrant confines the stomach?

Q. Which region confines the appendix?

- *The pelvic cavity.* This is the lowest portion of the trunk, and is a continuation of the abdominal cavity. Its boundaries are the bony pelvis, sacrum and muscles of the pelvic floor. It contains the female reproductive structures, or some of the male reproductive structures (lower ureters, bladder and urethra). Other pelvic organs included the small intestine and the last part of the colon, the rectum and anal canal. It also includes the openings for the urethra, vagina and anus.

Blood vessels, lymphatic nodes and associated nerves are located in all the cavities. Sometimes it is necessary to be much more precise in locating organs of the body. A good example of this is the quadrants and the nine regions associated with the abdomen and pelvic areas (Figure 1.4). A surgeon requires such precision when a surgical incision has to be made.

The basic needs of the human body

The basic needs of the living body identified by biologists as the characteristics of life are:

1 *Feeding or nutrition.* This encompasses the intake of raw materials to maintain life processes such as growth, repair and the maintenance of a normal environment inside the body.

2 *Movement.* This is a characteristic in that people, or some parts of them, are capable of changing position.

3 *Respiration.* This refers to the processes concerned with the production of the energy necessary to maintain life processes and movement. In humans it involves breathing (external respiration) and the breakdown of food (internal respiration) inside the cells of the body.

4 *Excretion.* This is the removal from the body of waste products of chemical reactions, and excesses of certain dietary substances (e.g. water).

5 *Sensitivity and responsiveness.* These are the processes concerned with monitoring, detecting and responding to changes in the environment inside and outside the human body.

6 *Growth.* This generally implies an increase in size and complexity. It also includes repair of body parts, which have undergone damage or need to be replaced.

7 *Reproduction.* This is necessary for the continuation of the species.

BOX 1.1 SURFACE ANATOMICAL LANDMARKS

Surface anatomy is the study of external structures and their relation to deeper structures. For example, the breastbone (sternum) and parts of the ribs can be seen and felt (palpated) on the anterior aspects of the chest. These structures can be used as landmarks to identify regions of the heart and points on the chest at which certain heart sounds can be heard using a stethoscope (a process called auscultation). The normal 'lub-dup' sounds of the heart reflect normal structure and functioning of the heart valves. A deviation of this sound to the trained ear reflects abnormal structure and hence functioning.

Anatomical imaging involves the use of X-rays, ultrasound, computerized tomography (CT) scans, and other technologies to create pictures of internal structures. Both surface anatomy and anatomical imaging provide important information in diagnosing disease. Healthcare professionals will become familiar with such techniques during their training.

The following terms are used to apply anatomy and physiology to some specialties in medical science (you may need to look up the suffix '-ology'):

- *Allergy:* diagnosis and treatment of allergic conditions
- *Cardiology:* the heart and its diseases
- *Endocrinology:* glands that release hormones and hormone disorders
- *Gastroenterology:* the stomach and intestines and their disorders
- *Gynaecology:* disorders of the urinary tract and female reproductive organs
- *Haematology:* blood and blood disorders
- *Immunology:* mechanisms by which the body resists disease
- *Neurology:* the nervous system and its disorders
- *Obstetrics:* pregnancy and childbirth
- *Oncology:* study of cancer
- *Ophthalmology:* eye disorders
- *Otorhinolaryngology:* ear, nose and throat
- *Pathology:* diagnosis of disease based on changes in cells and tissues
- *Proctology:* disease of the colon, rectum and anus
- *Toxicology:* poisons
- *Urology:* disorders of the urinary tract and male reproductive organs

BOX 1.2 ACTIVITIES OF DAILY LIVING

To help nurses direct care to the basic needs of the body, Roper *et al.* in the 1980s devised a nursing model called the Activities of Daily Living (ADLs) (Table 1.1).

There is an underpinning assumption that the foundations of the earlier ADLs model postulated by Roper were adapted to the characteristics of life identified previously by biologists.

Human beings therefore are self-reproducing systems capable of growing and of maintaining their integrity by the expenditure of energy. They are, however, complex organisms, having cellular, tissue, organ and organ system levels of organization (Figure 1.5).

Table 1.1   Activities of Daily Living (ADLs) (after Roper *et al.*, 1990)

Breathing*
Eating and drinking*
Elimination*
Mobilizing*
Controlling body temperature
Maintaining a safe environment
Sleeping
Personal cleaning and dressing
Working and playing
Communication
Expressing sexuality*
Dying

*Based on basic needs of life. Others relate to further human needs.

LEVELS OF ORGANIZATION

Cellular level

The human body is composed of trillions of microscopic cells (see Chapter 2). Each cell is regarded as a basic unit of life, since it is the smallest component capable of performing most, if not all, of the characteristics of life (or basic needs). Cells can digest food, generate energy, move, respond to stimuli, grow, excrete and reproduce.

To support these activities, cells contain organelles that perform these specific functions (see Chapter 2). To facilitate cell function throughout the body, the body contains many distinct kinds of cells, each specialized to perform specific functions. Examples include blood cells, muscle cells, and bone cells. Each has a unique structure related to its function. Genes are the controllers of cellular functions, and these act indirectly through their role in enzyme production. Enzymes, therefore, are of funda-

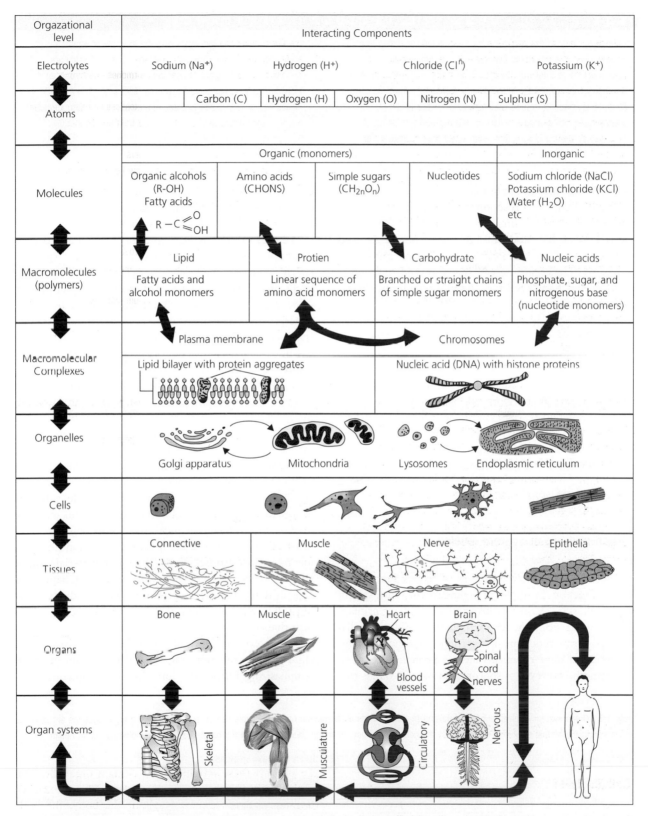

Figure 1.5 The hierarchy of organizational levels of the human organism indicates that specific interactions at each simpler level produce the more complex level above it.

BOX 1.3 ILLNESS – A CELLULAR IMBALANCE

Ultimately, every illness originates from a disturbance arising at a cellular level, and the interdependence of the components of the body means that a failure of one function leads to a deterioration of others. This is reflected in the diverse signs and symptoms of ill-health that require clinical intervention to restore health (or homeostasis). For example, a patient who has had a heart attack may display signs and symptoms that reflect poor functioning of the heart, lungs and kidneys. Using the example of nutrition mentioned in the main text, it is essential that the healthcare professional provides a diet appropriate to the requirements of the individual patient, i.e. a patient who is recovering from a minor illness has dietary needs to those of a patient who has undergone major trauma or surgery.

mental importance in the human body since they control the speed of chemical reactions so that they are compatible with a healthy life. Genes are thus commonly referred to as the 'code of life' (see Chapter 2), and enzymes as the 'key chemicals of life'. The chemical level of organization regarding cell structure and function is discussed in Chapter 5 under the umbrella term 'chemicals of life'.

Tissue level

A tissue is defined as a collection of similar cells and their component parts that perform specialized functions. There are many different types of tissues, so it follows that there must be different cell types that comprise these tissues. However, the entire body consist of just four primary tissues: epithelial or lining tissues, binding or connective tissues, muscular tissues, and nervous tissues. Chapter 2 discusses this level of organization.

Organ and organ system levels

An organ is an orderly grouping of tissues that give it discrete function. Examples of organs are the heart, spleen, ovary and skin. Most organs contain all four primary tissues. In the stomach, for example, the inside epithelial lining performs functions of secretion of gastric juice and absorption of some chemicals such as alcohol. The wall of the stomach, however, also contains muscle tissue (for contraction of the stomach) to help with the breakdown of food, nervous tissue (for regulation), and connective tissue (to bind the other tissues together).

An organ system is a group of organs that act together to perform a specific body function, e.g. the respiratory system maintains the levels of oxygen and carbon dioxide in the blood. These systems work with each other in a co-ordinated way to maintain the functions of the body. The concepts of tubular (hollow) organs and compact (parenchymal) organs are introduced in Chapter 2. The details associated with each organ are dealt with in their respective chapters, but the integration of organ function is important to note in this introductory chapter.

Each level of organization is instrumental in sustaining the functions of life for the human body. Table 1.2 illustrates each organ system's involvement in the regulation of the basic needs of the individual.

The basic needs are related to, and interdependent on, each other. For example, we must take in the raw materials of food and oxygen in order to provide sufficient energy to maintain normal body function. This energy is needed to support chemical reactions, such as those involved in growth and the muscle contraction necessary for movement. Consequently, these raw materials can be viewed as being the 'chemicals of life' (Chapter 5). Chemical reactions also produce waste products; these must be removed from the body to prevent cellular disturbances.

The interdependence of the basic needs means that a failure of one function leads to a deterioration of others (emphasizing further the 'principle of complementary').

Table 1.2 Organ system involvement in maintaining the basic needs of the human body. The table demonstrates that all the organ systems are involved in maintaining the normal environment needed by the cells of the body, to enable them to perform the basic needs of the individual during health

Basic need		Organ systems involved
Intake of raw material	Food	Digestive
	Oxygen	Respiratory
Internal transportation		Circulatory, lymphatic
Excretion		Urinary, respiratory, the skin
Sensitivity and irritability	Environment outside the body	Special senses, nervous, skeletomuscular
	Environment inside the body	Nervous, endocrine
Defence	Environment outside the body	Skin, special senses
	Environment inside the body	Immune, digestive, endocrine
Movement within the environment		Skeletal, muscular, nervous, special senses
Reproduction		Reproductive, endocrine

For example, malnutrition ('mal-' = bad or poor) results in the retardation of growth and development, lethargy, poor tissue maintenance, a reduced capacity to avoid infection, and a general failure to thrive.

In the context of this introductory chapter, it seems logical to establish the basis for optimum (ideal) biological functioning. The main topic reviewed in the remainder of this chapter is homeostasis.

HOMEOSTASIS: THE LINK WITH HEALTH AND ILL-HEALTH

An introduction to homeostatic control theory

The word 'homeostasis' translates as 'same standing', and is usually taken to indicate constancy or balance. Those students who have entered healthcare in recent years having taken courses that have had a significant human biology component are likely to have come across the term, since it is an important concept, especially in physiological studies.

The idea that a constancy of the internal environment of the human body is essential to life can be traced back to the views of the eminent French physiologist Claude Bernard, in the mid-nineteenth century. The turn of the twentieth century produced many important discoveries of how the body is regulated by hormonal and neural mechanisms.

In order to perform the basic functions of life successfully, there must be a 'consistency' within the body, and in particular in the environment inside cells, called the intracellular fluid ('intra-' = inside). The regulation of the composition and volume of fluids that surround cells, which collectively are called the extracellular fluids, helps to keep this environment constant. The main components of these fluids are discussed in detail in Chapter 6. Briefly, they are:

- *tissue fluid:* the fluid in which body cells are bathed. It acts as an intermediary between the cells and blood.

- *plasma:* the cell-free component of blood. Together with blood cells, it circulates through the heart and blood vessels, supplying nutritive materials to cells and removing waste products from them.

Two processes by which the composition of these fluids is kept constant are:

- the intake of raw materials;

- the removal (excretion) of waste products of chemical reactions, or of excesses of chemicals that cannot be stored, destroyed, or transferred to other substances inside the body.

Conventionally, homeostasis is considered to represent a balance or equilibrium between these two processes.

The modern view is that homeostasis is dependent upon an integration of physiological functions, since essentially all the organs of the body perform functions that help to maintain these constant conditions.

Organ systems, therefore, are homeostatic controllers that regulate the environment within cells throughout the body (Figure 1.6). This book concentrates on the homeostatic principles of human physiology, emphasizing in particular the role of each system in the maintenance of an optimal cellular environment (i.e. cellular homeostasis). It also discusses the influence of homeostatic control failure in producing some of the more common illnesses (i.e. homeostatic imbalances) that nurses and midwives are likely to encounter during their careers. In addition, the principles of healthcare intervention are mentioned in relation to the re-establishment of homeostasis and 'health' for the individual.

Homeostasis is usually considered to pertain to physiological or biochemical processes, and for the bulk of this text we will apply these principles. We also intend, however, where appropriate, particularly in relation to human development, stress, pain, and circadian rhythms, to discuss homeostasis pertaining to psychophysiological consistency within the body. Not separating the mind ('psychological') from bodily ('physiological') functions is important because the cells making up the human brain are no different in their basic characteristics from any

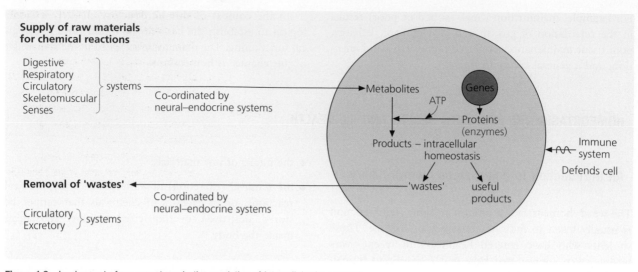

Figure 1.6 Involvement of organ systems in the regulation of intracellular homeostasis.
Q. Suggest why the following statements are used in physiology: (i) genes, 'the code of life'; (ii) enzymes, 'the key chemicals of life'.

other cells in the body. Thinking, emotions, behaviour and memories are all subjected to the same physical and chemical laws of other functions of the body. Thus, to understand health fully it is therefore necessary to be familiar with the psychophysiological processes that account for individual differences, as well as with the principles of homeostasis. In summary, individual differences are determined by a person's genes (i.e. nature), which are modified by environmental (i.e. nurture) factors. The person and his/her environment are therefore inseparable. Thus, it is necessary that the nature/nurture implications of a person's health and ill-health should be recognized since these interactions provide the foundations of healthcare (see Chapters 19–23).

Principles of homeostasis

Cannon, who introduced the term 'homeostasis' in 1932, defined it as 'a condition, which may vary, but remains relatively constant.' It was this definition, together with experience gained working alongside nurses and midwives using clinical laboratory values (Table 1.3), that inspired the authors to design the homeostatic graph (Figure 1.7). This is a simplified model to aid the understanding of a patient's physiological and biochemical parameters in health and disease.

Readers text are strongly recommended to familiarize themselves with this figure before dipping into other chapters, since variants of it and Figure 1.8 are used throughout this book as a model to explain:

- homeostatic principles;

- how components of homeostasis control function;

- how failure of components of control results in illness;

Table 1.3 Normal laboratory values for the development stages. Homeostatic ranges are guides for judging health and disease. This listing of normal ranges uses the measured or reasonable estimate of the central 90% of a normal distribution of values (see text for details). These adult ranges have proved to be clinically useful in hospital wards and clinics

Clinical chemistry	Normal adult values (homeostatic range)
Sodium	136–148 mmol/l
Potassium	3.8–5.0 mmol/l
Bicarbonate	24–32 mmol/l
Urea	2.6–6.5 mmol/l
Creatinine	60–120 mmol/l
Glucose	Random, 3.0–9.4 mmol/l
*CSF glucose	2.5–5.6 mmol/l
Total protein	62–82 g/l
Albumin	36–52 g/l
Globulin	20–37 g/l
Calcium	2.2–2.6 mmol/l
Transaminase	Up to 35 IU/l
pH	7.35–7.45
pCO_2	4.7–6.0 kPa
pO_2	11.3–14.0 kPa

*CSF, cerebrospinal fluid.

Q. Describe in scientific terms what is meant by the term 'normal range' when equated with the values expressed in clinical laboratory tables.

Exercise

Obtain from your clinical directorate a biochemistry ('U & Es') report and note the normal values.

- an individualized approach to care, in which healthcare interventions are used to re-establish homeostasis for the patient, or to provide palliative care to improve the quality of life for the dying patient.

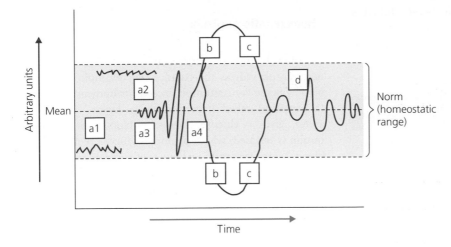

The homeostatic range

The variations in parameter values provide a range within which the parameter can be considered to be regulated. The fluctuation in parameter values within their normal (homeostatic) ranges provides the optimal condition in the body (see Table 1.3 and Figure 1.7). The range reflects:

- *the precision by which a parameter is regulated:* some parameters, such as body temperature, have a very narrow range (adult values = 36.2–37.7°C), whilst others, for example blood volume, have a relatively larger homeostatic range (male adult values = 52–83 ml/kg);

Exercise

Find out the meanings of the following units of measurement: °C and ml/kg.

- *individual variation of values within the population:* one person's normal range could fluctuate just above the minimum values of the range (Figure 1.7 (a1)), whilst another person's optimal range could fluctuate close to the maximum values (Figure 1.7 (a2)). It is also considered normal for some individuals to deviate on either side of the mean (or average) value (Figure 1.7 (a3)). To account for all individual variations within the population, it is also possible for some individuals to 'bounce' between the minimum, mean and maximum values (Figure 1.7 (a4));
- *variation of values within each person according to the changing metabolic demands:* it is quite usual for the maximum and minimum values of some parameters to vary within the individual as the person passes through the different developmental stages of the life span (see Table 1.3). The dotted lines associated with the maximum, mean and minimum values in Figure 1.7

indicate the dynamic nature of these values, i.e. for some parameters the maximum value may increase. It is generally well known, for example, that blood pressure increases with the age of a population, while most other parameter values decrease with adult age (e.g. muscle strength, visual acuity, see Chapter 20)

BOX 1.5 PREGNANCY AS AN ALTERED STATE OF HEALTH

Midwives often refer to pregnancy as an 'altered state of health'. That is, variations of the homeostatic values of physiological parameters are considered quite normal and necessary for the development of the unborn baby. For example, the hormones oestrogen and progesterone supersede levels experienced in the non-pregnant state. This is necessary if implantation and placentation are to ensure structural and functional development of the unborn baby. The new homeostatic range has adapted to the changing anatomical/physiological requirements associated with the developmental stage, pregnancy.

Variation within each person also occurs during times of illness (see case studies in Section 6, application boxes in Chapters 1–18, and Chapters 21 and 22). Variations also need to account for the changes associated with the individual's sleep–wake activities (circadian patterns, 'circa-' = about, '-dies' = day; see Chapter 23).

The maintenance of a constant arterial blood pressure is frequently cited in textbooks as an illustration of a homeostatic process at work. However, it is important that this pressure is increased naturally during exercise as it increases blood flow through the exercising muscle, ensuring that the oxygen supply to the muscle supports the increased demand. The elevation of blood pressure in exercise is itself a homeostatic adaptive process. It acts to provide the appropriate environment for the changing chemical needs of muscle, and this highlights the most important feature of homeostasis: physiological processes provide an *optimal* environment for bodily function. Whilst this may involve a near-constancy of some aspects of the environment (e.g. brain temperature), other functions may require a controlled change.

BOX 1.6 CLINICAL NORMAL AND ABNORMAL VALUES

In science, 'normal' means conforming to the usual pattern. The normal (homeostatic) range in statistical terms defines values of parameters expected for 95% of the population, e.g. the normal range of blood pH is 7.35–7.45 (Table 1.3). Statistically, this means that 95% of the population (i.e. 95 out of 100 people) has a pH that falls in this range. Thus, the homeostatic range of a parameter is useful in making judgement regarding the health status of an individual. It must, however, be emphasized that each person is unique, and those 5% of the population (i.e. 5 out of 100 people) naturally fall outside the normal range. These values reflect minor deviations from the homeostatic range, and are considered to be 'acceptable' in clinical practice, and so need no clinical adjustments. Alternatively, values that reflect sudden and large deviations from the homeostatic range are considered 'unacceptable'. This is referred to as a homeostatic 'imbalance' or 'disturbance', and healthcare intervention may be not only desirable but essential to sustain 'normality' for the patient.

Homeostasis, then, is about the provision of an internal environment that is optimal for cell function at any moment in time, despite the level of activity of the individual. Health occurs when bodily function is able to provide the appropriate environment. This usually entails an integration of the functioning of physiological systems, and its outcome is observed as physical wellbeing and psychological equilibrium. In order for homeostasis to be maintained, the body must have a means of detecting deviations (or changes) to homeostasis; assessing the magnitude of the deviation; and promoting an appropriate response to redress homeostasis (a process known as feedback). Feedback processes also provide the means of assessing the effectiveness of the response.

Receptors and control centres

The initial change in a physiological parameter is detected by sensory receptors, sometimes referred to as monitors or error detectors. The function of these receptors is to relay information about the disturbance to homeostatic control centres (analysers or interpreters). These centres interpret the change as being above or below the homeostatic range, and determine the magnitude of the change. As a result, they stimulate appropriate responses via effectors that bring about the correction of the imbalance in order to restore homeostasis. Once the parameter has been normalized, the response will cease (Figure 1.8(a) and (b)).

Homeostatic controls

Occasionally, only one homeostatic control mechanism is necessary to redress the balance. For example, when the blood glucose concentration exceeds its homeostatic range (a condition called hyperglycaemia; 'hyper-' = over or above, 'glyc-' = glucose, '-aemia' = blood), the hormone insulin is released, which promotes glucose removal from blood. More frequently, a number of controls are involved. For example, when blood acidity exceeds its homeostatic range (a condition referred to as an acidosis) three controls attempt to reduce the cidity values within the normal range:

- *Buffers.* These chemicals act to neutralize the excess acidity (see Chapter 6).

- *Respiratory mechanisms.* If the buffers are insufficient in removing the acidosis, then the rate and depth of breathing will increase in order to excrete more carbon dioxide, a potential source of acid in body fluids (see Chapter 14).

- *Urinary mechanisms.* If the increased rate and depth of breathing are insufficient to remove the acidosis, then the kidneys will produce a more acidic urine and so reduce the acidity of body fluids (see Chapter 15).

These corrective responses are time dependent; some respond quickly to the imbalance, but if they should fail to re-establish homeostasis this prompts other control mechanisms to correct the disturbance. The body therefore has short-term, intermediate and long-term homeostatic control mechanisms. In the above example, these are the buffers, respiratory and urinary mechanisms, respectively.

Exercise

Explain the homeostatic regulation of acidity in the blood.

Homeostatic feedback mechanisms

Negative feedback

Most homeostatic control mechanisms operate on the principle of negative feedback, i.e. when a homeostatic imbalance occurs, then in-built and self-adjusting mechanisms come into effect, which reverses the disturbance. The regulation of blood sugar demonstrates the principle of negative feedback control. An increase in blood glucose concentration above its homeostatic range sets into motion processes that reduce it. Conversely, a blood glucose concentration below its homeostatic range (hypogly-caemia) promotes processes that will increase it. In both

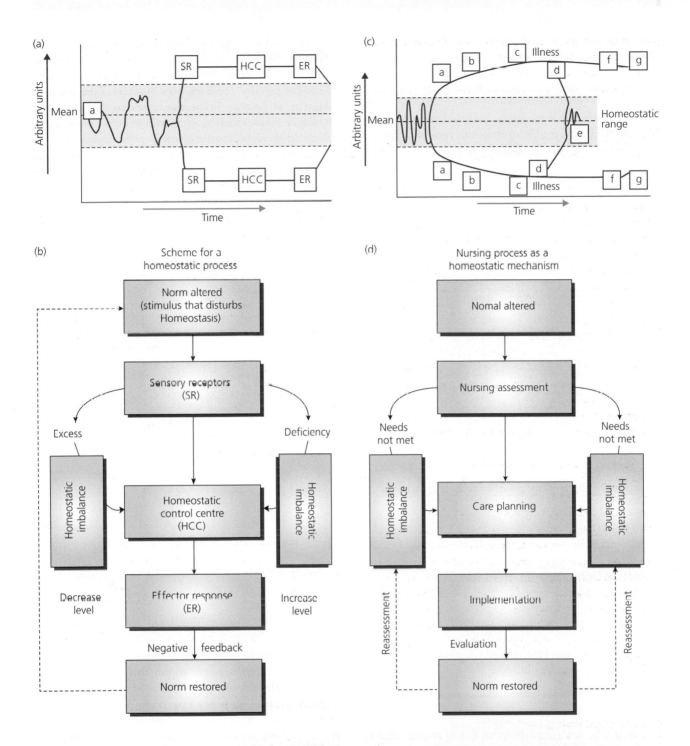

Figure 1.8 Homeostasis. Control, clinical intervention in illness, and nursing process. (a) and (b) General schemes demonstrating the roles of receptors, homeostatic control centres, and effectors via negative feedback in a control process. (a) Homeostatic dynamism reflecting individual variability. (SR) Receptors detect deviations from the homeostatic range. (HCC) Homeostatic control centres analyse the deviation and its magnitude of change. (ER) Effectors correct the imbalance.

(c) Clinical intervention following homeostatic control system failure. (a) Failure of receptors and/or short-term homeostatic control system and/or effectors in re-establishing homeostasis. (b) Failure of receptors and/or intermediate homeostatic control system in re-establishing homeostasis. (c) Failure of receptors and/or long-term homeostatic control system and/or effectors in re-establishing homeostasis. (d) Healthcare intervention to re-establish patient homeostasis. (e) Patient's re-established homeostatic status restored. (f) Palliative care improves quality of life without re-establishing homeostasis. (g) Death — an inability to survive the homeostatic imbalance.

Q. Describe the function of the components of homeostatic control when there is a deviation in a parameter being monitored.

(d) The nursing process as a homeostatic mechanism.

Q. 'Healthcare professionals may be described as external agents of homeostatic control.' Discuss.

situations, the result is the level of blood sugar is kept relatively constant over periods of time.

Positive feedback

There are times when promoting rather than negating a change of benefit. This is known as positive feedback. An example is observed during the menstrual cycle just before the release of the 'egg' (ovulation). The high levels of the hormone oestrogen at this part of the cycle reverse its normal inhibition on the hormone luteinizing hormone (LH); the positive feedback now stimulates the surge of LH. This is because LH is the hormone that promotes ovulation. Since positive feedback induces change, the effects tend to be transient; most physiological systems utilize negative feedback mechanisms as a means of maintaining stability. An inability to promote change when necessary can, however, cause a change in health. For example, a failure to produce the surge of the hormone that causes ovulation will result in sterility.

BOX 1.7 HOMEOSTATIC RANGE FLUCTUATIONS

The capacity to modify the homeostatic range is essential in certain circumstances (e.g. pregnancy, see box 1.5) and is of benefit in other situations (e.g. exercise). Variations in homeostatic ranges and in positive feedback responses provide flexibility to homeostatic processes. As in positive-feedback responses, many of the changes promoted by set-point alteration relate to a specific situation and are short lived. Some resettings are permanent, however, and so promote long-term change. These responses are vital to the process of human development during the individual's lifespan. They allow for growth, functional maturation during fetal development and childhood, puberty changes during adolescence, and changes associated with becoming an adult. However, losing this regulation is associated with old age. Thus, because of the dynamic nature of the parameters in health, the term 'homeostatic' (meaning 'same standing') may in the future be superseded by the more appropriate term 'homeodynamic' (meaning parameter variation). For the purpose of this text the former term is used.

HOMEOSTASIS AND ILL-HEALTH

If homeostasis provides a basis for health, then ill-health will arise when there is a failure of the components of the control processes involved (Figure 1.8 (c) and (d)). Imprecise control mechanisms include:

- receptors that fail to respond adequately to changes in the environment;

- homeostatic control centres that fail to analyse sensory information, and/or analyse the information incorrectly, and/or send incorrect information to the effector organs;

- effector organs that fail to respond to corrective directions from the control centres.

Failure to provide an optimal internal environment will cause further destabilization, and the integration of psychological and physiological (i.e. psychophysiological) functioning will become impaired. In this way, an environmentally induced change in the activities of one part of the body may have far-reaching consequences for whole body function. Thus, the authors encourage healthcare profes-sionals to take a transactional (or interactionist) view regarding the patient's condition (see Chapters 19–23).

All disorders are characterized by a primary disturbance of intracellular homeostasis within tissues somewhere in the body. The disease may be classed according to the primary disorder, such as a respiratory problem, a degenerative disorder, a tumour of a particular tissue, or as being due to immune system dysfunction or infection. However, all will have consequences for extracellular homeostasis, hence the functioning of cells and tissues other than those involved in the primary disturbance. Thus, healthcare may be directed at symptoms apparently removed from the primary problem, e.g. relieving constipation in a patient with a breast tumour.

Homeostatic principles in clinical practice

The signs and symptoms of an illness will be related to the homeostatic imbalances induced. For example, people with

Homeostatic principles are readily discerned within the stages of the nursing process (compare Figure 1.8 (b) and (d)).

- *Assessment and nursing diagnosis.* The assessment of the health deficit and the biological, psychological, social and spiritual needs of the individual correspond to the detection and assessment of change by the receptors of the homeostatic control mechanism.
- *Planning.* The planning of nursing care, based on the assessment and diagnosis stage, is comparable to the ways by which homeostatic controls analyse and determine the responses needed to correct the imbalance. Furthermore, just as the body has specific homeostatic controls for different parameters, the nurse needs to plan care according to the individual's needs. This can be illustrated using the simple example of dietary needs: a small amount of food, presented pleasantly, may be vital to encourage eating in the elderly patient who has a depressed appetite. On the other hand, an

energetic young patient will require a bulkier dietary intake, while a patient with a learning disability may need reminding of what and when to eat.

- *Implementation.* In the nursing process, implementation refers to putting into action the interventions planned in the previous stage. In a homeostatic perspective, this is analogous to the activation of effector organs to produce the appropriate response.
- *Evaluation.* The effectiveness of care is assessed in this stage, much as feedback processes provide a means of evaluating a psychophysiological response. For example, has the injection been given to prevent the patient's pain?
- *Reassessment.* The cyclical nature of the nursing process is emphasized by this stage, in which the patient is reassessed and new interventions considered if necessary. The dynamism of this process is also observed in homeostatic mechanisms described in this book; parameters fluctuate constantly within their normal ranges, and such changes must, therefore, be constantly reassessed.

diabetes are classed as type 1 or insulin-dependent diabetes mellitus (IDDM,) or as type 2 or non-insulin-dependent diabetes mellitus (NIDDM). Although not all people can be classified easily, as a general rule IDDM reflects a homeostatic failure of the gland cells to produce the hormone insulin, and NIDDM reflects an imbalance in the cells that respond to the insulin, or a failure to release sufficient quantities of the hormone from the gland. The signs and symptoms of diabetes mellitus, such as glucose in the urine (glucosuria), and vascular problems due to fat deposits in the blood vessels (atherosclerosis), reflect a common failure in both types of diabetes in blood sugar management.

Clinical intervention in illness and disease is concerned with correcting underlying problems, managing the symptoms, and enabling the patient to come to terms with the 'disorder'. In other words, clinical practice is concerned with restoring, as effectively as possible, the homeostatic status of the patient (Clancy and McVicar, 1996). Using the above example, people with IDDM are treated with insulin injections, whereas diet (and perhaps hypoglycaemic drugs, such as gliclazide, glipizide and metformin) controls the problem in people with NIDDM, since the levels of insulin may be comparable to the people without diabetes. By promoting normality, healthcare professionals are therefore acting as extrinsic homeostatic mechanisms. Some illnesses, however, such as terminal cancers, are not responsive to therapeutic intervention, and consequently the imbalance results in long-term malfunction and eventually death. The healthcare professional in these circumstances provides palliative care to improve the patient's quality of life (Figure 1.8 (c), part (f)). It is this connection of homeostasis to healthcare that promoted the writing of this book.

CONCLUSION

Homeostasis is a concept used throughout this book to explain how the internal environment is maintained at a level conducive to healthy functioning within the body compartments. Homeostatic control relies mainly upon negative feedback mechanisms that act to reverse imbalances and regulate parameters close to their optimal values. Prevention of parameter variation can be detrimental under some circumstances. The promotion of change via positive feedback mechanisms, or through resetting of homeostatic set points, is then of benefit. Failure of negative feedback processes, appropriate positive feedback responses, or set-point resetting, or a reduction in their efficiency, leads to illness.

Healthcare interventions are concerned largely with supplementing normal anatomical, biochemical and hence physiological processes in order to re-establish the homeostatic status of the individual. Homeostasis therefore provides a working framework for health, and nursing and midwifery care can be related directly to it. Such a scientific approach does not mean losing the sense of person. Rather, it presents a framework in which to view the health–ill-health continuum.

Summary

1 Humans are biological beings. The biological construction (anatomy and physiology) of the individual provides the basis for identifying how interactions with the external environment influence the psychophysiological health of the individual.

2 The maintenance of bodily functions regulates appropriate cellular activities, which are determined by enzymes, the products of gene expression.

3 The composition of the intracellular environment will influence the efficiency at which cells operate, and, accordingly, it is regulated so as to be optimal.

4 The concept of homeostasis helps to explain the importance to health of maintaining an optimal environment within which cells must function. 'Optimal' does not necessarily equate with constancy. It also relates to the control of change observed during daily activities of living, times of stress, illness, and postoperative recovery, and during the developmental phases of the lifespan.

5 Homeostatic control relies mainly upon negative feedback mechanisms that act to reverse changes and regulate parameters close to the optimal value.

6 Prevention of parameter variation can be detrimental under some circumstances. The promotion of change via positive feedback mechanisms or through a resetting of homeostatic set points is then of benefit.

7 Ill-health arises when there is a failure to maintain homeostatic functions, either at tissue or organ levels of organization. The interdependency of tissue functions means those homeostatic disturbances and associated signs and symptoms will also arise secondarily to the primary disorder.

8 Healthcare practices are related to homeostasis since they provide the extrinsic effectors that act to restore homeostasis in patient.

Review questions

1 Define homeostasis. What is its purpose?

2 Can you think of an example of how your body reacts to maintain homeostasis in your everyday life?

3 What can you do to help your body function efficiently? Think about your lifestyle. Could it be described as healthy? If not, which aspects could you (and are prepared to) address? Now think about patients in your care. Could their lifestyle be described as healthy? Which aspects could be improved and how could you, in your role as a health promoter, help?

4 What factors may affect the ability of the body to maintain homeostasis? Which factors can be avoided and which cannot?

REFERENCES

Cannon, W.B. (1932) *The Wisdom of the Body*. New York: Norton.

Clancy, J. and McVicar, A. (1996) Homeostasis. The key concept in physiological control. *British Journal of Theatre Nursing* **6**(2): 17–24.

Roper, N., Logan, W.W. and Tierney, A. (1990) *The Elements of Nursing*, 3rd edn. Edinburgh: Churchill Livingstone.

FURTHER READING

Clancy, J., McVicar, A.J. and Baird, N. (2001) *Fundamentals of Physiological Homeostasis for Perioperative Practitioners*. London: Routledge.

Hagedorm, M.I.E. and Gardner, S.L. (1999) Newborn Care: hypoglycemia in the newborn. Part I: Pathophysiology and nursing management. *Mother Baby Journal* **4**(1): 15–24.

Cell and tissue functions

The structure of the body can be described on four levels of organization: the chemical level (see Chapter 4), the cellular level and tissue level (described in this chapter), and the organ system levels (see Chapters 8–18).

As discussed in Chapter 1, human physiology is concerned with the 'correct' interdependent functioning of the organ systems, so throughout this book each system is considered as a 'homeostatic control system'. Each has a role to play in maintaining the equilibrium within cells, and hence tissues, organs and organ systems because of the interdependency of these different levels of organisations (Figure 1.5). For example, the respiratory system is concerned primarily with maintaining the homeostatic equilibrium of the gases oxygen and carbon dioxide in the blood. This is produced, principally, by way of breathing movements and gaseous exchange between the tiny air sacs in the lungs (called alveoli) and local blood vessels (called pulmonary capillaries). However, the system is ultimately concerned with ensuring that aerobic respiration ('aerobic' = presence of oxygen, 'respiration' = process of producing energy) by cells occurs within its homeostatic range, providing sufficient energy to drive chemical reactions within their normal physiological parameters. The respiratory system is also important in maintaining the acid–base balance of body fluids (see Chapter 6). Excessive acidity or alkalinity (basicity) threatens cell functions and life.

Organ systems cannot operate in isolation. Each works interdependently with others to ensure that the level of chemicals inside cells is maintained, enabling cells to perform the basic characteristics of life. Thus, the respiratory system supports all tissues and organs of the body, but also acts to maintain its component cells.

Exercise

Before continuing, you should be able to list the basic body needs (characteristics) of life. Refer to Chapter 1 if you are having trouble remembering.

BOX 2.1 THE IMPORTANCE OF CYTOLOGY IN HEALTH AND ILLNESS

Homeostasis is a concept applied by physiologists to explain how the internal environment is maintained conducive to healthy functioning, and how homeostatic imbalances, if uncorrected by the body, result in illness (see Chapter 1). A knowledge of the structure, function and needs of human cells in healthcare curricula is centred on understanding how tissue and organ dysfunction results in ill-health, and so provides the rationale for clinical intervention. For example, the condition obstructive respiratory disease induces hypoxaemia (insufficient oxygen in the blood) and hypercapnia (excess carbon dioxide in the blood), and may result in cell death (necrosis) in the patient. The body attempts to correct imbalances through natural homeostatic regulatory devices; in this example, it increases the rate and depth of breathing. A failure of regulatory devices to re-establish gaseous homeostasis makes healthcare intervention necessary to restore the 'health' of the individual.

The focus on cells makes it essential that cell activities are understood if the physiological bases of health and healthcare are to be appreciated. The concept of the cell as the 'basic unit of life' was introduced in the Chapter 1. In this chapter, the structure and function of the cell will be described in more detail.

CELLULAR LEVEL OF ORGANIZATION

The study of cells is called cytology ('cyt-' = cell, '-logy' = study). It investigates how cells are organized, i.e. the structure of cellular components, their role in intracellular homeostasis, how they are controlled, and cellular reproduction.

The cells are the basic building blocks, since the body is composed of them and their substances. Just as the body has organs to perform specialized homeostatic functions, cells have component parts called organelles ('little organs') that have specific homeostatic roles within the cell. Their structures are dependent upon the chemical components, such as proteins, lipids and lipoproteins, from which they are made. These structures in turn are dependent upon their constituent parts, i.e. amino acids, fatty acids, and lipids and proteins, respectively (Figure

> **BOX 2.2 THE CELL – THE BEGINNINGS OF LIFE**
>
> It is usually argued that human life begins as a single cell (zygote) that results from a fusion of the female's egg (ovum) and the male's sperm (see Chapter 18). The zygote undergoes cell division, giving rise ultimately to the trillions of cells that undergo differentiation and specialization into the tissues and organ systems of the human body.

1.5). These substances are thus referred to as being part of the 'chemical basis of life' (see Chapter 5) and ultimately come from the diet, hence the adage, 'We are what we eat.' This, of course, is not strictly correct, since

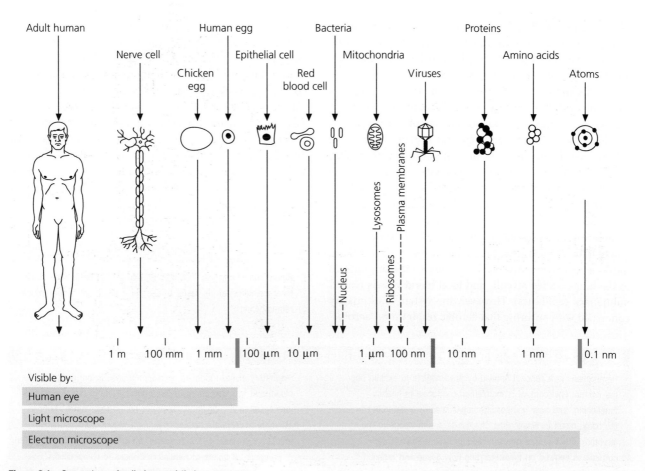

Figure 2.1 Comparison of cell sizes and their components.

m, metre; mm, millimetre; μm, micrometre; nm, nanometre. 1 m = 1000 mm; 1 mm = 1000 μm; 1 μm = 1000 nm.

we would be extremely overweight, and the food also has to be converted to a form that cells can use.

Overview of cellular anatomy and physiology

Cell size, shape and structure

Most cells are microscopic, with the average size ranging from 10 to 30 μm (micrometers, i.e. 10–30 thousandths of a millimetre) in diameter. The largest cell in the body is the female's ovum, which is approximately 500 μm in diameter and is just visible to the naked eye. The erythrocyte ('erythro-' = red, '-cyte' = cell) of blood is the smallest cell, being about 7.5 μm in diameter. The longest cell, which can measure up to 1 m in length, is the neuron ('neur-' = nerve), but even these are microscopically thin (Figure 2.1).

Exercise

Familiarize yourself with the following units. Those units less than 1 mm are not used widely outside science and so may be unfamiliar.

1 m (metre) = 100 cm (centimetres) = 1000 mm (millimetres) = 39.37 inches

1 cm = 10 mm = 0.39 inches

1 mm = 0.1 cm = 1000 μm (micrometers)

1 μm = 1000 nm (nanometres)

Cellular anatomy varies because cells perform different functions to maintain body homeostasis (Figure 2.2). A 'typical' or 'generalized' cell is shown in Figure 2.3. This is a composite of many types of cells, and will share features

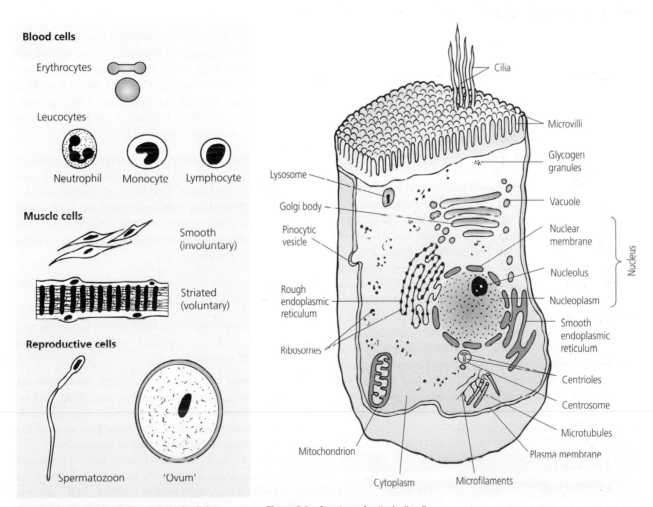

Figure 2.2 Types of cell. The variety of cellular structure reflects their different functions (principle of complementary structure and function).

Figure 2.3 Structure of a 'typical' cell.

with most cells within the body without being identical to any of them. Generally, cells have five principal parts:

1 *Cell membrane*. This is the outer boundary of the cell. It separates the intracellular ('intra-' = inside) and extracellular ('extra-' = outside) environments.

2 *Cytoplasm*. This is the ground material (or cellular fluid) between the nuclear and the cell membranes that suspends the cell's organelles and inclusions.

3 *Organelles*. These structural components have highly specialized intracellular roles that contribute to homeostasis within and outside the cell.

4 *Inclusions*. These include the secretory and storage chemicals of cells.

5 *Nucleus*. This contains the ground material (or nucleoplasm) that suspends the 'vehicles of heredity' (i.e. genes). These control cell division and chemical reactions (metabolism) and are, therefore, responsible for regulating intracellular homeostasis. Genes are comprised of deoxyribonucleic acid (DNA).

The homeostatic functions of these cellular components are summarized in Table 2.1, and are considered in detail in the next section.

CELLULAR ANATOMY AND PHYSIOLOGY

Cell membrane

The cell membrane (also known as the plasma membrane) provides a selective barrier between intracellular and extracellular compartments. Both compartments are aqueous (i.e. water based). The membrane therefore cannot be composed of water-soluble chemicals, since it would allow entry and exit of all water-soluble substances, and thus prevent the regulation of their intracellular and extracellular concentrations.

One of the earliest attempts at describing a generalized membrane substructure was by Danielli and Davson (1969). Their 'lipid bilayer model' referred to the plasma membrane as a 'unit' membrane, since all membrane-bound organelles have the same structure. The main biochemical components are lipids and proteins. Structurally, this model assumed that proteins were associated rigidly with a lipid bilayer. The 'fluid mosaic model', proposed by Singer and Nicolson (1972), followed this model. This model suggested a more dynamic structure in which proteins and other molecules could be inserted or removed according to need. The main lipids present are phospholipids and cholesterol. Phospholipids are polarized chemicals, having hydrophilic ('hydro-' = water, '-philic' = liking or attracting) and hydrophobic ('-phobic' = fearing or repellent) ends. Each phospholipid is positioned at right-angles to the cell membrane's surface. The hydrophilic heads are exposed to the fluid outside the cell (tissue fluid), and the hydrophobic tails are found inside the membrane, thus water or water-soluble substances cannot enter this region (Figure 2.4).

Exercise

Use a dictionary to define 'lipid', 'protein' and 'carbohydrate'.

According to the fluid mosaic model, the proteins embedded in the cell membrane are like 'icebergs floating in a sea of lipid'. Membrane proteins are broadly classed as integral and peripheral proteins. Integral proteins completely span the membrane, and peripheral proteins only partially span it. Membrane proteins have the following specialized functions:

● Some integral proteins have selective transport properties. They form 'pores' or channels extending through the membrane that allow the passage of water and specific electrolytes into and out of the cell without having to cross through the lipid layer. Other proteins form 'carriers', by which substances can be transported through the membrane (see later).

● Some peripheral proteins are 'markers' of specialized cells, hence are important in cell recognition and immunity (see Chapter 13). The cell membrane also contains carbohydrate chemicals that have been joined (conjugated) with proteins or lipids, called glycoproteins and glycolipids, respectively (Figure 2.4). These are also important in cell recognition.

● Some proteins act as receptor sites, or targets, for some hormones (see Chapter 9).

● Some proteins are enzymes, and hence are controllers of chemical (metabolic) reactions within, or associated with, the cell membrane.

The structural components of the cell membrane are thus of fundamental importance in sustaining cellular homeostasis, because of their interaction with chemicals inside and outside the cell, and because they provide the means of controlling entry and exit of substances.

The fluid mosaic model stresses that the plasma membrane is constantly changing its shape, since proteins and carbohydrates are mobile within and on the membrane lipids, and because portions of the membrane are continually being removed, recycled and replaced. Membranes also change their shape and surface area

Table 2.1 Role of cellular components in homeostasis

Component	Appearance	Description	Homeostatic functions
Plasma membrane	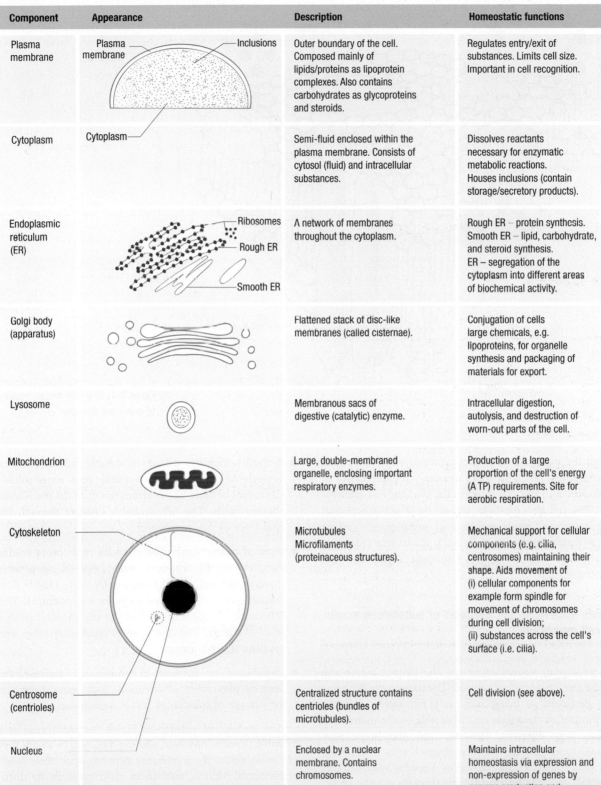	Outer boundary of the cell. Composed mainly of lipids/proteins as lipoprotein complexes. Also contains carbohydrates as glycoproteins and steroids.	Regulates entry/exit of substances. Limits cell size. Important in cell recognition.
Cytoplasm		Semi-fluid enclosed within the plasma membrane. Consists of cytosol (fluid) and intracellular substances.	Dissolves reactants necessary for enzymatic metabolic reactions. Houses inclusions (contain storage/secretory products).
Endoplasmic reticulum (ER)		A network of membranes throughout the cytoplasm.	Rough ER – protein synthesis. Smooth ER – lipid, carbohydrate, and steroid synthesis. ER – segregation of the cytoplasm into different areas of biochemical activity.
Golgi body (apparatus)		Flattened stack of disc-like membranes (called cisternae).	Conjugation of cells large chemicals, e.g. lipoproteins, for organelle synthesis and packaging of materials for export.
Lysosome		Membranous sacs of digestive (catalytic) enzyme.	Intracellular digestion, autolysis, and destruction of worn-out parts of the cell.
Mitochondrion		Large, double-membraned organelle, enclosing important respiratory enzymes.	Production of a large proportion of the cell's energy (A TP) requirements. Site for aerobic respiration.
Cytoskeleton		Microtubules Microfilaments (proteinaceous structures).	Mechanical support for cellular components (e.g. cilia, centrosomes) maintaining their shape. Aids movement of (i) cellular components for example form spindle for movement of chromosomes during cell division; (ii) substances across the cell's surface (i.e. cilia).
Centrosome (centrioles)		Centralized structure contains centrioles (bundles of microtubules).	Cell division (see above).
Nucleus		Enclosed by a nuclear membrane. Contains chromosomes.	Maintains intracellular homeostasis via expression and non-expression of genes by enzyme production and inhibition respectively. Contains store of hereditary information.

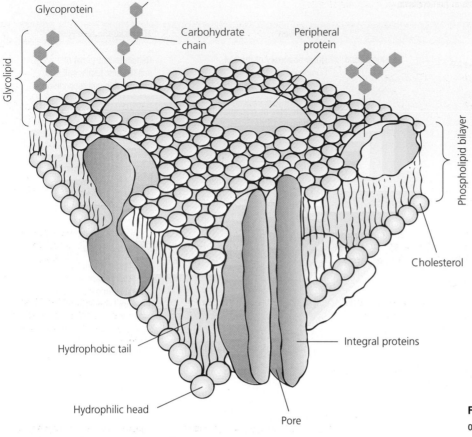

Glycoprotein

Carbohydrate chain

Peripheral protein

Glycolipid

Phospholipid bilayer

Cholesterol

Hydrophobic tail

Hydrophilic head

Pore

Integral proteins

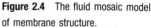

Figure 2.4 The fluid mosaic model of membrane structure.

during the processes of endocytosis and exocytosis. That is, normal cell functions make necessary the movement of substances into the cell to meet the demands of metabolism. The cell also needs to secrete those substances that are surplus, and waste products of metabolism. Various factors determine how rapidly such substances are transported, and their mode of transport across the cell membrane.

Factors influencing the transport of substances across the cell membrane

The passage of substances across the plasma membrane may be free, restricted or refused. The membrane is, therefore, described as being selectively permeable, and the distribution of chemicals on either side of the membrane is thus very different. However, the membrane may respond to varying environmental conditions, or intracellular homeostatic requirements, by allowing substances to enter and leave the cell by diffusing through it, or by crossing it by way of pores or carrier mechanisms. Factors affecting the passage of chemicals across the membrane are:

- *chemical size:* large chemicals enter and leave the cell more slowly than small chemicals;

- *chemical solubility:* oil or oil-soluble substances pass through the membrane more quickly than water-soluble substances because of the arrangement of the membrane phospholipids. The oils probably dissolve through the lipid layer of the membrane;

- *chemical charge:* uncharged particles enter more readily than electrically charged ones. Anions (negatively charged particles, e.g. chloride) enter more readily than cations (positively charged particles, e.g. sodium). This is because the outer surface of the membrane carries a positive charge, and like charges repel each other and opposite charges attract;

- *temperature:* an increase in temperature increases the random movement of chemicals and hence promotes the passage of substances across membranes.

The passage of substances across the membrane is a dynamic process, however, and the direction in which they can move across the membrane depends upon their mode of transport. That is, substances move passively by diffusion, or actively by active transport, pinocytosis or phagocytosis. All of these mechanisms play a role in ensuring that biochemical homeostasis in body fluids is maintained. The active and passive mechanisms involved in transporting substances across membranes are summarized in Table 2.2 and are explained further in the next section.

Table 2.2 Processes involved in movement of substances in and out of cells

Process	Description	Factors affecting rate	Examples in body
Passive processes	Substances move down their concentration gradients. No cell energy (ATP) required.		
Simple diffusion	Net movement of chemicals from regions of a high concentration to regions of a low concentration, until they are distributed evenly.	1 Size of chemical 2 Lipid solubility of chemical 3 Charge of chemical 4 Size of gradient 5 Surface area available	Movement of oxygen from lung to blood, from blood to tissue fluid, and from tissue fluid to cells. Vice versa for carbon dioxide.
Facilitated diffusion	Plasma membrane integral protein carriers allow passage through protein channels (Figure 2.5).	In addition to the above, availability of carrier	Movement of glucose and amino acids into all cells.
Osmosis	Water or solvent chemicals move from regions of a high concentration of water or solvent chemicals through a selectively permeable membrane (Figure 2.6).	1 Concentration gradients (i.e. osmotic pressure gradients) 2 Hydrostatic pressure (can act against osmosis)	Water moves into red blood cells from a hypotonic (weak; high water content) tissue fluid.
Filtration	Hydrostatic pressure forces water and small chemicals through selectively permeable membranes from areas of high pressure to areas of low pressure (see Chapter 9)	Amount of pressure, size of pores	Capillary exchange when blood pressure is greater than in tissue fluid. Ultrafiltration in the kidney nephron
Active processes	Cell energy (ATP) expenditure allows movement of substances against their concentration gradients.		
Active transport	Plasma membrane protein carriers transport ions, chemicals from regions of a low concentration to regions of a high concentration (Figure 2.7).	Availability of carrier chemicals, transported substance, and ATP	Sodium, potassium, magnesium, calcium in all cases.
Exocytosis	Cytoplasmic vesicles fuse with the plasma membrane and expel particles from the cell (Figure 2.9).	Availability of ATP	Neurotransmitter release and secretion of mucus.
Endocytosis	Membrane-bound vesicles enclose large chemicals, take them into the cytoplasm, and release them.		
1 Phagocytosis	'Cell eating'. Ingestion of solid particles. Phagosomes formed (Figure 2.8a).	Availability of ATP	Phagocytes (white blood cells) ingest foreign bodies (e.g. bacteria).
2 Pinocytosis	'Cell drinking'. Ingestion of fluid droplets and their dissolved substances. Pinosomes release contents into cytoplasm (Figure 2.8b).	Availability of ATP	Kidney cells take in nephron fluid containing amino acids.
3 Receptor-mediated endocytosis	Specific plasma membrane receptors bind with chemicals, forming ligands, and take them into the cell's cytoplasm via endosomes (Figure 2.8c)	Availability of ATP	Intestinal epithelial cells take up large molecules.

Q. List the passive and active homeostatic transport mechanisms of the cell.

HOMEOSTATIC MECHANISMS BY WHICH SUBSTANCES ARE TRANSPORTED ACROSS THE CELL MEMBRANE

Passive processes

Diffusion

Diffusion is the passage of chemicals from regions of high (strong) concentration to regions of low (weak) concentration of that substance, resulting eventually in its uniform (equal) distribution. Diffusion also acts as a transport mechanism within the cell. For a common domestic example of diffusion, let us consider making a diluted orange drink. If we put water into the tumbler first, and then add the concentrated orange juice, the orange particles diffuse outwards from their point of entry. Initially the colour is lighter further away from the juice's entry point. Later the orange solution has a uniform colour, since the orange chemicals have moved down their concentration gradient until an even distribution is achieved. In considering the diffusion of chemicals across a membrane, the process can be subdivided into that of simple diffusion, and that of facilitated diffusion because of the restricted nature of the membrane for some substances.

Simple diffusion

Small, uncharged, lipid-soluble substances pass readily across the cell membrane. Diffusion of these chemicals is in both directions, occurring between the intracellular and extracellular compartments. The net passage of the substance depends upon the direction of the concentration gradient. For example, the movement of oxygen from blood to intracellular fluid is necessary to produce energy from the breakdown of food. The movement of carbon dioxide is in the reverse direction to prevent its accumulation inside the cell. Such diffusion movements will be essential since changes in the rate could be disastrous for metabolism and hence for the maintenance of intracellular homeostasis.

Other substances that undergo diffusion include:

- lipid-soluble materials, such as steroid hormones, oestrogens and progesterones;

- small charged particles that are not lipid soluble, e.g. sodium (Na^+), potassium (K^+) and chloride (Cl^-) but that can diffuse through the membrane through channels provided by integral proteins within it;

- chemicals such as urea, ethanol and water that have a weak charge polarity. Urea and ethanol are fat soluble, and so diffuse through the lipid part of the membrane. Water moves across membranes by osmosis (a special form of diffusion).

Rate of diffusion

Diffusion across the cell membrane is quicker when the following conditions occur:

- A greater surface area is available. In certain areas of the body, the surface area of cells is increased by the presence of finger-like processes called villi and microvilli (see Chapters 10 and 15).

- There is a greater permeability of the membrane to specific substances. For example, the resting membrane of nerve cells is approximately 20 times more permeable to potassium compared with sodium. Consequently, potassium exit from the cell is more rapid than sodium's entry. The concentration gradients for potassium and sodium are sustained by an intracellular pump mechanism, called the sodium/potassium ATPase pump (see Chapter 8). Nevertheless, the constant leak of potassium is responsible for the positive electrical charge on the surface of the cell membrane.

- Increased concentration gradients.

BOX 2.3 VILLI AND MICROVILLI

The development of villi and microvilli could be regarded as an evolutionary adaptation by multicellular organisms to ensure a greater rate of absorption of digested foods to maintain their increased metabolic demands.

Facilitated diffusion

Facilitated diffusion is a quicker mechanism than simple diffusion. The process involves carrier chemicals, usually integral proteins, in the membrane. Carriers transport relatively large chemicals (e.g. glucose and amino acids) across the membrane, thus releasing these substances into the cytoplasm (Figure 2.5).

Rate of facilitated diffusion

Besides those factors noted above that increase the rate of simple diffusion, another important factor in controlling the rate of facilitated diffusion is the amount and availability of carrier chemicals. Some carrier-mediated mechanisms are influenced by hormonal actions. For example, insulin is a hormone (i.e. a chemical messenger) that lowers blood glucose and is secreted when the glucose concentration is above its homeostatic range. Insulin enhances the carrier mechanism of glucose, and so facilitates the diffusion of glucose into its target tissues, thereby increasing its utilization inside the cell. The homeostatic regulation of blood glucose concentration is described in detail in Chapter 9.

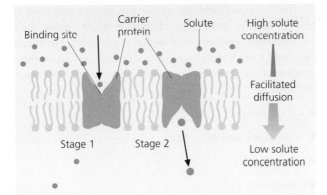

Figure 2.5 Model of facilitated diffusion. A solute chemical (e.g. glucose) is transported across the cell membrane by a carrier protein. Stage 1: carrier chemical binds with the solute, which then changes its shape (stage 2), so that a channel is opened and the solute can pass into the cell's cytoplasm. The process does not utilize energy; solute chemicals pass down a concentration gradient.

BOX 2.4 REHYDRATION THERAPY: A FACILITATED PROCESS

The administration of the solution made up of 1 tablespoon sugar and 1 tablespoon salt added to 1 litre water (known as rehydration therapy) is an example of facilitated diffusion in action. The sugar facilitates the absorption of salt, hence speeding up diffusion.

Osmosis

Osmosis is the flow of solvent (in most circumstances, water) across a selectively permeable membrane from a dilute to a more concentrated solution. Osmosis is thus a special case of diffusion. Membranes provide little resistance to the movement of water. Therefore, providing that the dissolved substance (the solute) cannot pass through the plasma membrane, then the net effect of osmosis is that more water will move to areas of lower solvent concentrations (i.e. higher solute concentration) than in the opposite direction (Figure 2.6). This continues until the pressure of the increasing volume of the solution on one side of the membrane counterbalances the movement.

The osmotic pressure of a solution therefore is the force required to stop the net flow of water across a selectively permeable membrane when the membrane separates solutions of different concentrations. The plasma membrane maintains different fluid compositions inside the cell relative to outside it. However, there is usually no osmotic pressure difference, as osmosis will be determined by the osmotic potential of the solute composition of the fluids. Changes in the total concentration on one side of the membrane can occur, however, if that of an individual

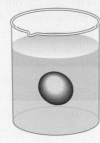

(a)

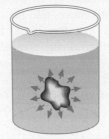

(b)

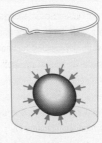

(c)

Figure 2.6 Osmosis and red blood cells. (a) Isotonic solution. The concentration of solute/solvent chemicals is the same in the solution surrounding the cell as in the cell. The net movement of water is zero. (b) Hypertonic solution. The concentration of solute chemicals is greater, hence concentration of water chemicals is lower, in the solution compared with inside the cell. The net movement of water is out of the cell (dehydration). The cell shrinks (crenation) and may die if the solution is extremely hypertonic. (c) Hypotonic solution. The concentration of solute chemicals is lower, hence concentration of water chemicals is greater, in solution compared with the inside of the cell. The net movement of water is into the cell, causing the cell to swell. The cell may burst (lysis) if the solution is extremely hypotonic.
Q. Explain why osmosis is referred to as a special case of diffusion.

solute alters, which will subject the membrane to osmotic effects. It is important, therefore, that cells have relatively constant internal and external osmotic pressures to maintain intracellular and extracellular water balance. This principle can be demonstrated by suspending erythrocytes (red blood cells) in a solution, such as 0.9% sodium chloride, which is isotonic ('iso-' = equal, '-tonic' = pressure, strength) to the intracellular fluid. In such an environment there will be random movement of water into and out of cells, but with the absence of an osmotic gradient the volume moved in either direction will be equal. Consequently, there will be no net movement, and the cell volume is unchanged (Figure 2.6(a)).

When extracellular environments are hypertonic ('hyper-' = strong, above normal), however, water moves out of the cell by osmosis and causes a decrease in cell volume, with the membrane becoming wrinkled or crenated (Figure 2.6(b)). This process occurs in the homeostatic imbalance of dehydration. Alternatively, when extracellular environments are hypotonic ('hypo-' = weak, below normal), water moves into the cell by osmosis and causes an increase in cell volume. If the extracellular environments are sufficiently hypotonic (i.e. diluted), water continues to enter until the intracellular pressure exerted on the cell membrane causes the cell to lyse or burst. The lysis of erythrocytes is termed 'haemolysis' (Figure 2.6(c)).

BOX 2.5 INTRAVENOUS INFUSION OF NORMAL SALINE

Cells must maintain their isotonic interdependence, otherwise changes in fluid balance, and the resultant effects on solute concentrations, will disturb intracellular homeostasis. Fluids administered intravenously for clinical reasons are normally isotonic to prevent intracellular fluid imbalance. A common fluid used in clinical practice is 'normal' (isotonic) saline (approximately 0.9%, which means that 0.9 g NaCl is dissolved in every 100 ml water) administered as an infusion (see Chapter 6).

Filtration

The filtration process forces small chemicals through pores within the membranes of small blood vessels (called capillaries) with the aid of water (or hydrostatic) pressure. Movement is from regions of high to low hydrostatic pressures. Chemicals such as proteins in blood are too large to pass through the filter pores, and so remain within the vessel. Details of the capillary exchange mechanism, and the filtration process in the kidney, are described in Chapters 12 and 15, respectively.

Active processes

Active processes require energy expenditure. The energy is released from an energy storage chemical called adenosine triphosphate (ATP) produced from the breakdown of food inside the cell. The energy is liberated from ATP breakdown (catabolism), i.e.

$$ATP \leftrightarrow ADP + P + energy$$

The difference between active and passive processes is that in passive processes, chemicals move down their concentration gradient, and in active processes, chemicals can move from low to high concentration (i.e. against their concentration gradients or 'uphill'). Active processes include:

- active transport
- endocytosis and exocytosis
- phagocytosis
- pinocytosis
- receptor-mediated endocytosis.

Active transport

Active transport involves transporting substances across the plasma membrane, usually by integral proteins using the energy released from ATP breakdown as its driving force (Figure 2.7). Active transport carriers are often referred to as 'pumps'. The most cited example in the human body is the sodium/potassium ATPase pump. ATPase is an enzyme that releases energy from ATP. This active pump compensates for the diffusion exchange of sodium and potassium, and so maintains their extracellular and intracellular concentrations. A calcium pump exists in muscle cells (see Chapter 17). Other substances transported by active transport include amino acids, some simple sugars, iron, hydrogen and iodine.

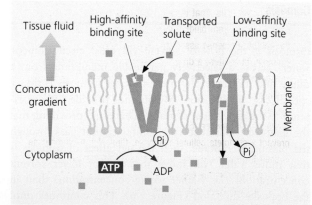

Figure 2.7 Active transport. Phosphorylation of carrier chemicals increases their affinity for the specific solute to be transported. Removal of the phosphate from the carrier decreases its affinity for the solute, and it is passed into the cytoplasm. Note use of energy (and phosphate) from ATP, which permits transport of solute against diffusion gradient.

Endocytosis and exocytosis

These active processes transport large chemicals (collectively called macrochemicals; 'macro-' = large), such as proteins and lipids, and small amounts of fluid into or out of certain cells. Endocytosis involves enclosing the material to be ingested inside a portion of the plasma membrane to form a small vesicle, and then bringing the substance into the cell ('endo-' = inside). The reverse of this process, exocytosis ('exo-' = outside), is an important mechanism by which cells secrete substances. For example, digestive cells secrete enzymes, endocrine cells secrete hormones, sweat gland cells secrete sweat, and nerve cells secrete neurotransmitter secretions using exocytosis.

Exocytosis is an important transport mechanism for all cells. It is necessary for the elimination of waste products of metabolism, and for the removal of surplus chemicals that cannot be stored, destroyed or transferred into other materials that the cell can use. The cellular organelle known as the Golgi body is important in exocytosis, and is described later.

Endocytosis and exocytosis are therefore instrumental in maintaining intracellular and extracellular homeostatic ranges of metabolites.

Phagocytosis

This is a form of endocytosis. Phagocytosis literally means 'cell eating', and begins when the cell membrane encircles the particle to be ingested by membrane distensions called pseudopodia ('pseudo-' = false, '-podia' = arms). The membrane then folds inwards to form a vesicle called a phagosome, which leaves the plasma membrane and enters the cytoplasm. The contents of the phagosome then undergo digestion by enzymes collectively called lysozymes (Figure 2.8(a)). An example is the white blood cells, which have a defensive role to ingest foreign particles such as bacteria that have entered the body (see Chapter 13).

BOX 2.6 DRUG INTERACTION AT A CELLULAR LEVEL

Drugs alter cellular function by targeting membrane or intracellular receptors, carrier chemicals, chemical pumps or enzymes.

- *Receptors.* Some drugs can deceive membrane receptors since they have a similar shape to the natural ligands. Agonistic drugs, such as the painkiller diamorphine, cause the cells to act in the same way as they would with the body's natural ligand, endorphin. That is, it operates on the same receptor sites as the body's painkillers (see Figure 21.6 for site of action). Lipid-soluble agonists, e.g. corticosteroids, enter the cell and bind to intracellular receptors, thereby altering cellular function by changing gene activity and hence enzyme synthesis. That is, this type of drug can stop the natural ligand from binding to the receptors, thus inhibiting the cellular response associated with such binding. For example, tamoxifen, a drug used in the treatment of breast cancer, operates in this manner by preventing oestrogen binding to its receptors. Drugs classified as partial agonists operate as agonists or antagonists depending on the predominant chemical conditions in the body. They usually prevent a complete cellular response. Clinically, hyaluronidase is used to render the tissues more easily permeable to injected fluids, and is especially useful in some old people since they will have lost receptors as a consequence of the ageing process.
- *Carrier chemicals.* Drugs can inhibit carrier functioning, e.g. the tricyclic antidepressants such as clomipramine prevent the uptake of certain neurotransmitters associated with depression (see Chapter 8, and the case study of a man with depression in Section 6). Frusemide, a diuretic (used to increase urine production), prevents the movement of ions in the kidney tubule (see Chapter 15). Drugs can also enhance carrier efficiency, e.g. amphetamines (commonly known as 'speed') enter cells to instigate the secretion of noradrenaline in the brain. Noradrenaline is responsible for the effects (heightened awareness, loss of appetite, etc.) of using speed.

- *Pump mechanisms.* Local anaesthetics, such as lignocaine and procaine, block the pain impulse by maintaining the activity of the sodium/potassium ATPase pump activity in the pain fibres (see Chapter 21). Calcium antagonists, such as nifedipine, are used in the treatment of angina and hypertension, since they dilate the blood vessels and stop the entry of calcium into the heart cells. Calcium is the trigger for muscle contraction, so inhibiting its entry into the muscle cells of the blood vessels causes their relaxation, which decreases blood pressure. See Chapter 17 for details of calcium action in muscle, and the case studies of the young woman with secondary hypertension and of the man with chest pain in Section 6. Calcium agonists, such as digitalis, strengthen the heartbeat, and are given to patients with heart failure. Digitalis causes a slight increase in calcium inside the muscle cells of the heart, and so enhances the force of contraction and strengthens the heartbeat.
- *Enzymes.* Some drugs inhibit normal enzyme action. For example, paracetamol is given to provide relief from certain types of pain. This drug inhibits the enzyme prostaglandin synthetase, thereby inhibiting the production and secretion of prostaglandin, the most potent pain-producing substance in the body. Other forms of pain relief, such as transcutaneous nerve stimulation, acupuncture, massage, imagery, relaxation and even placebo therapies, also operate at a cellular level. You should be able to understand the site of cellular action of these methods of pain relief after reading Chapter 21.
- Some viruses (e.g. human immunodeficiency virus, HIV) enter the cell by attaching to specific receptors on certain white blood cells (see Chapter 13, and the case study of the young man with symptomatic HIV/AIDS in Section 6).

It is frequently argued that the above section is concerned more appropriately with medical therapy. However, the authors would argue that healthcare professionals such as nurse and midwives are required to have such a specific scientific knowledge base if an 'holistic' approach to healthcare is to be provided.

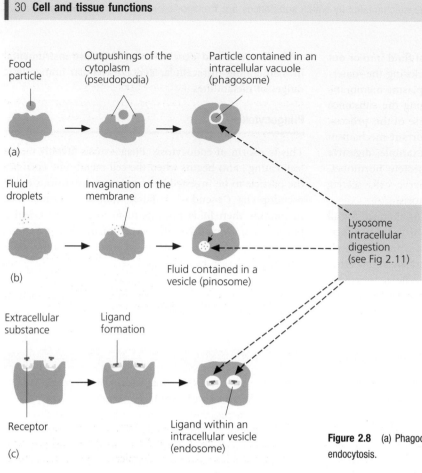

Food
particle

Outpushings of the
cytoplasm
(pseudopodia)

Particle contained in an
intracellular vacuole
(phagosome)

(a)

Fluid
droplets

Invagination of the
membrane

Fluid contained in a
vesicle (pinosome)

(b)

Lysosome
intracellular
digestion
(see Fig 2.11)

Extracellular
substance

Ligand
formation

Receptor

Ligand within an
intracellular vesicle
(endosome)

(c)

Figure 2.8 (a) Phagocytosis. (b) Pinocytosis. (c) Receptor-mediated endocytosis.

Pinocytosis

Another from of endocytosis, pinocytosis literally means 'cell drinking'. In this process, tiny droplets of fluid and their dissolved components stick to the plasma membrane, which then invaginates to form a vesicle called a pinosome. This structure separates from the membrane and enters the cytoplasm, and the pinosome contents may then undergo lysozymal digestion (Figure 2.8(b)).

Receptor-mediated endocytosis

This mechanism involves plasma membrane receptors that recognize and bind to specific extracellular chemicals to form complexes called ligands. This area of the plasma membrane then invaginates to form a cytoplasmic vesicle called an endosome. The receptors separate from the ligand structures within the cytoplasm, and are returned to the cell membrane. The ingested chemicals may be broken down by lysozymes (Figure 2.8(c)), but may also influence cell functions. For example, the hormone thyroxine enters the cell by this process.

Transport across the placenta

Transport across the selectively permeable placenta is via passive and active processes.

Passive transport

Most substances pass through the placenta by passive transport – either simple or facilitated diffusion. Both

BOX 2.7 HORMONAL CHEMISTRY DICTATES THEIR INTERACTIONS AT A CELLULAR LEVEL AND TRANSPORT ACROSS THE PLACENTA

Endocrinology is the study of hormonal action. Hormones are chemical messengers in the body that act to co-ordinate (in association with the neural messages) all body activities to ensure bodily homeostasis. During embryological development, some of the immature endocrine cells specialize to produce hormones that belong to the protein family of chemicals, whereas others specialize to produce steroid hormones. The chemistry of the hormone dictates the way in which it affects cell metabolism. Protein-based hormones, such as insulin, act on membrane receptors, whereas steroid-based hormones, such as oestrogen, dissolve through the membrane lipid layer and therefore affect metabolism inside the cell.

types of passive diffusion can only take place 'downhill', i.e. along an electrochemical gradient. Simple diffusion depends on a difference in concentrations of substances, such as oxygen, in the maternal and fetal blood. The speed of transfer varies on the gradient and properties of the substance as well as on the resistance of the membrane.

Facilitated diffusion depends on a concentration difference, but the facilitated diffusion of certain substances, such as glucose, is aided by a carrier protein. These large proteins in the cell membranes speed up the rate of transfer.

Active transport

Active transport is required against an electrochemical gradient, and energy expenditure is required by the placenta in order for transport to take place 'uphill'. Pinocytosis is used for the transport of even more complex molecules. Material, for example iron, makes contact with the syncytiotrophoblast, which then invaginates to surround it, thus forming a vesicle that discharges its contents onto the fetal side. Iron is found in both the fetal and maternal blood either unbound or bound to transferrin, a protein. Iron concentrations in the fetus are two to three times higher than in the mother. An example of transfer by pinocytosis is of unbound iron through the placenta.

Exercise

Take a breather from your studies. Then reflect on your understanding of the following transport mechanisms used by the cell to control the entry and exit of chemicals to maintain intracellular homeostasis: diffusion, osmosis, active transport, phagocytosis and pinocytosis.

CELL ORGANELLES

Organelles have specific roles to play in maintaining the homeostasis of the cell. Their structure helps to maintain the basic needs of the cell. For convenience, they are considered individually in this section, but it should be remembered that they function interdependently, just as organ systems work interdependently to maintain the homeostasis of the body.

Exercise

Re-familiarize yourself with the basic needs of the body (see Table 1.2), because these needs are met by the organelles of the cell.

Endoplasmic reticulum

The endoplasmic reticulum (ER) is a membrane system that forms an extensive parallel network of cavities called cisternae. Structure and extent vary from cell to cell depending upon the activity of the cell. ER functions associated with cellular homeostasis are:

- The ER provides passageways through which materials are transported within the cell. The organelle makes definite connections with the nuclear and plasma membranes, and thus may be a link between these two structures, and between adjacent cells (Figure 2.9).

- The ER segregates the cytoplasm into areas of different biochemical activity.

- The ER increases the surface area available for a variety of enzymatic reactions.

- The cisternae of the ER act as temporary storage sites for specific chemicals, such as lipids, proteins and glycogen (a carbohydrate storage chemical), which have been produced by the cell.

There are two types of ER, classified according to whether the membrane is associated with ribosomes (small structures concerned with protein synthesis). Both types are often continuous with one another and are interchangeable depending upon the metabolic requirements of the cell.

Rough endoplasmic reticulum

Rough (granular) ER is studded with ribosomes on its outer surface. Ribosomes are involved in protein synthesis, therefore rough ER is found in all cells since enzymes belong to the protein family of chemicals. Enzymes are necessary to all cells because they catalyse (speed up) chemical reactions, ensuring that the rate of metabolism is compatible with life processes. The rough ER is an extremely important organelle that contributes to maintenance of intracellular homeostasis. It is more abundant in cells that are most actively engaged in protein synthesis, e.g. those that produce hormones and those that produce digestive enzymes.

BOX 2.8 CARCINOGENS AFFECT RIBOSOMAL FUNCTIONING

Some carcinogens (chemicals that produce cancer) detach ribosomes from the ER, resulting in unusual sites of enzymatic activity, thereby changing the protein synthetic activities of the cell.

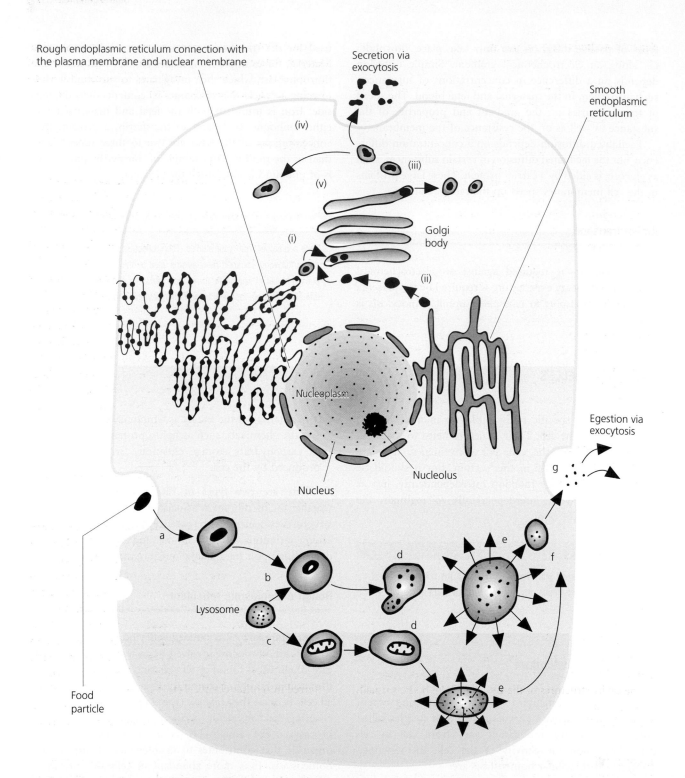

Figure 2.9 The homeostatic roles of the lysosome, Golgi body and the endoplasmic reticulum. Lysosome: (a) phagosome produced from phagocytosis; (b) lysosome moves toward phagosome; (c) lysosome moves toward 'worn-out' organelle, e.g. mitochondrion; (d) intracellular digestion of particle and organelle; (e) useful products of this hydrolytic breakdown absorbed into the cytoplasm; (f) vacuole contains useless (residual) products of this hydrolytic breakdown; (g) exocytosis (egestion) of the residual products.

Golgi body: (i) protein from rough endoplasmic reticulum; (ii) lipid from smooth endoplasmic reticulum; (iii) conjugated lipoprotein complex in vacuole from Golgi body; (iv) conjugated lipoprotein complex secreted from cell; (v) conjugated lipoprotein complex utilized in cellular metabolism (e.g. production of organelle membrane).

Q. Give a reason why the following statements are used in physiology: (i) cell, the 'basic unit of life'; (ii) enzymes and ATP, the 'key chemicals of life'; (iii) Golgi body, the 'packaging factory of the cell'; (iv) lysosomes, the 'suicide bags of the cell'; (v) genes, the 'vehicles of heredity'.

Smooth endoplasmic reticulum

The smooth (agranular) ER is smooth in appearance due to the absence of ribosomes. The smooth ER is concerned with the synthesis of non-protein substances, which vary from cell to cell. For example, the smooth ER of the adrenal glands and testes produces steroid hormones, whilst in liver cells cholesterol may be synthesized. The smooth ER of muscle cells is involved in calcium storage (remember calcium is the important trigger for muscle contraction). In addition, the smooth ER of liver cells is important in detoxifying potentially harmful substances, such as drugs and carcinogens.

BOX 2.9 DRUGS AFFECT SMOOTH ENDOPLASMIC RETICULUM FUNCTIONING

Barbiturates (a group of drugs that reduce the activity of the central nervous system) are classified according to their pharmacological actions. Some are general anaesthetics (e.g. thiopentone sodium), and others have hypnotic and sedative actions (e.g. phenobarbitone). Other drugs have tranquillizing properties (e.g. diazepam). All these drugs increase the amount of smooth ER, and influence the activity of its enzymes. Some of these enzymes in turn inactivate the effects of barbiturates, which results in barbiturate tolerance and the need for increased dosages of these drugs for them to exert their effects.

Golgi complex

The Golgi complex (also known as the Golgi body or Golgi apparatus) is found in all cells except erythrocytes. It is structurally and functionally connected to the ER and consists of four to eight flattened membranous sacs, similar to the smooth ER except that the sacs resemble a stack of dinner plates. The sacs are called cisternae, as they are part of the cavity structures of the ER. The Golgi body is usually located near to the nucleus, facing the plasma membrane, from which the contents of the cisternae may be discharged.

Homeostatic roles of the Golgi complex

The principal roles of the complex are to process, sort and deliver chemicals – mainly proteins but also lipids and carbohydrates – to various parts of the cell that need them. In addition, it is responsible for the packaging of secretory products before exocytosis. Thus secretory cells, such as neurotransmitter secreting neurons (see Chapter 8), that produce digestive enzymes (see Chapter 10), and endocrine cells of the pancreas (see Chapter 9), have an abundance of Golgi complexes.

Some Golgi vesicles remain inside the cytoplasm to perform intracellular roles, such as the regeneration of membranes of organelles and their enzymes so as to replace damaged ones (Figure 2.9).

Lysosomes

These organelles originate from the Golgi body. Lysosomes have a thicker membrane than the rest of the organelles because they contain approximately 40 different 'digestive' enzymes, which must be isolated from the rest of the cell. These are capable of breaking down all the chemical components of the cell, such as the nucleic acids (by enzymes called nucleases), lipids (lipases), proteins (proteases), and carbohydrates (carbohydrases). Collectively, the enzymes are called lysozymes. These enzymes, like most proteins, are synthesized in the rough ER and are transported to the Golgi body for processing into lysosomal vesicles after leaving the Golgi body (Figure 2.9). Lysosomes are found in most cells, especially in those tissues that experience rapid changes, such as liver cells (see Chapter 10), spleen cells, white blood cells (see Chapter 11), and bone cells (see Chapter 3).

Homeostatic roles of lysosomes

Lysosome functions include:

- *intracellular digestion:* any substance that has been ingested by phagocytosis or pinocytosis is taken into the cytoplasm in a membrane-lined vesicle (phagosome or pinosome). The vesicle coalesces with lysosomes, and lysozymes are released into the sac and break down the substance, mainly into substances that the cell can use. These useful products are absorbed into the cytoplasm and may be (i) added to the pool of these chemicals in the cell, if required, to maintain their homeostatic ranges; (ii) stored in more complex forms; or (iii) transferred into other chemicals that can be used. The residue materials that cannot be used are secreted from the cell to prevent a surplus homeostatic imbalance occurring (Figure 2.9);

- *destruction of worn-out parts of the cell:* defective or damaged organelles are treated in the same manner as above so as not to compromise intracellular homeostasis (Figure 2.9). Sometimes the organelle is referred to as the 'digestive body' or 'dissolving body' of the cell because of these breakdown activities;

- *autolysis:* for most tissues, cell death during our lifetime is inevitable. Cell death is associated with the release of lysozymes into the cytoplasm, and this 'self-destruction' mechanism (called autolysis) accounts for the rapid deterioration of many cells following their death. Some cell materials, such as the protein keratin, found in hair and nails, persist after the death of the cell. Dead cells must be replaced to sustain the structural and functional integrity of the human body. It also ensures that some material (such as the membrane's lipoproteins, enzymes, etc.) from the dead cells can be re-utilized into the general metabolism. The lifespan of cells varies enormously – perhaps this is related to the autolytic

activity of their lysosomes. Some cells, such as those of the skin and those lining the gut, have a very quick turnover rate, perhaps just a day or two. Red blood cells live for between 100 and 120 days, while nerve cells may persist through an individual's life. Autolysis therefore has a role in maintaining homeostatic levels of chemicals in the body. Lysosomes are often called the 'suicide bags' of the cell because of this autolytic function.

Mitochondria

The size, shape and number of mitochondria vary from cell to cell depending upon their level and type of activity. Different cell types, however, show the same basic mitochondria structure of a double-membraned organelle (Figure 2.10(a)). The smooth outer membrane encloses the mitochondria contents, and the inner membrane is arranged in a series of shelf-like projections, almost at right-angles to the longitudinal axis of this comparatively large organelle. The function of these folds (called cristae) is to increase the surface area for the enzymatic reactions involved in cellular respiration (Figure 2.10(b)).

Homeostatic role of mitochondria

Mitochondria are concerned with aerobic respiration, i.e. the energy-producing process involving the breakdown

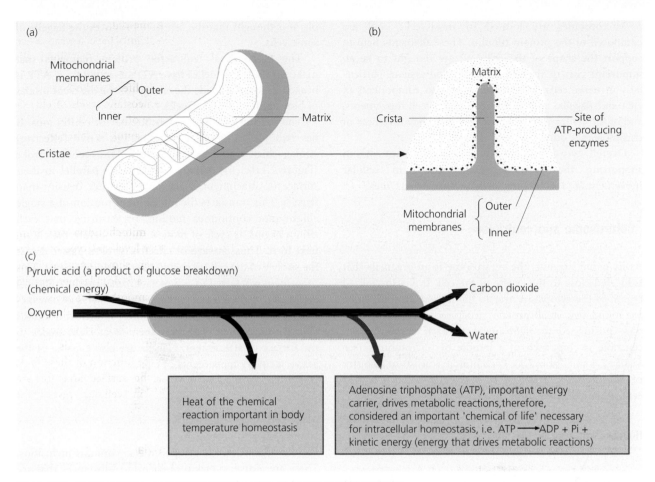

Figure 2.10 (a) Mitochondrion. (b) Magnified view of a crista. (c) Internal (aerobic) respiration.
Q. Suggest why the mitochondria is referred to as the 'power house of the cell'.

of fuel (food) chemicals in the presence of oxygen. Some of the energy produced is stored as chemical-bond energy in ATP. This bond energy is simply released as required by the breakdown of ATP (Figure 2.10(c)). Owing to their energy-producing function, mitochondria are often referred to as the 'power houses of the cell'. They provide about 78% of the cell's energy, the remaining 22% coming from reactions occurring in the cytoplasm (see Chapter 4). Energy from respiration is also liberated as heat. Thus, respiration is an important contributor to the homeostatic regulation of body temperature within the body (see Chapter 16). Carbon dioxide and water are also products of respiration, and are important in controlling the acid/base balance of body fluids.

Cytoskeleton

Within the cytoplasm of most cells, there are various-sized filaments that form a flexible framework known as the cytoskeleton. There are four types of filaments: microfilaments (the thinnest), intermediate filaments, thick filaments, and microtubules (the thickest) (see Figure 2.3).

Homeostatic roles of the cytoskeleton

Microfilaments are composed of a contractile protein called actin. This substance provides mechanical support for various cell structures, and is thought to be responsible for many cell movements.

Intermediate filaments consist of proteins that vary depending upon the cell type, e.g. keratin is found in epithelial cells (i.e. cells that line organs) and neurofilaments are found in nerve cells. These filaments help maintain the shape of the cell and the spatial organization of organelles.

Thick fibres are found only in muscle cells. They consist of the contractile protein myosin. Actin fibres are also found in muscle cells, where they interact with myosin in a sliding mechanism that forms the basis for muscle contraction (see Chapter 17). Non-filament myosin is found in most cells, however, where its function is to produce local forces and movement.

Microtubules are located in most cells, and are composed of the protein tubulin. These filaments help to support the shape of the cell, and are thought to be an important part of the cell's transporting system, particularly in nerve cells. Microtubules are also components of cilia and flagella, and so are involved in cell movements, and of the centriole, which is involved in the movement of chromosomes during cellular division.

Overall, cytoskeletal structures have important roles in supporting the position of organelles, in cellular movement, and as binding sites for specific enzymes.

Centrosome and centrioles

As its name suggests, the centrosome is an organelle that is located close to the centre of the cell. It is a specialized region of the cytoplasm near to the nucleus, within which are found two small protein structures called the centrioles, positioned at right-angles to each another. Each centriole is composed of a bundle of microtubules (see Figure 2.3 and Table 2.1). Each bundle consists of a cluster of microtubules, arranged in a circular pattern, with a central pair isolated from the rest.

Homeostatic role of the centrioles

During cell division, the centrioles move to the opposite sides (poles) of the cell and produce a system of microtubules, called the spindle, which radiates to the equator of the cell. Chromosomes become attached to the spindle's equator before migrating to the poles of the cell, seemingly connected to the microtubules (see later). Failure to form a spindle prevents normal cell replication (see Box 2.18).

Cilia and flagella

These are fundamentally similar structures, differing only in size and their modes of action. The more numerous cilia are generally shorter, often cover the whole surface of the cell, and generally are used for moving fluids along channels or ducts. The larger flagella are often found singly, or in small groups, and generally are used to move the whole cell, e.g. sperm cell (Figure 2.11(c)(i)).

Both organelles, together with microvilli, are extensions of the plasma membrane. They contain microtubules along their length, and in cross-section they show the 9+2 pattern (Figure 2.11(b)(i)). That is, there are nine groups of two tubules arranged in a circle, plus an isolated pair in the centre of the circle. At the base of these organelles is the basal body. This controls the activity of the organelle, and is probably important in their formation. Below the basal body there is a structure similar to that of the centri-ole; it is thought that the centriole produces the flagella of some cells.

The longitudinal contractile protein filaments that make up these organelles have ATPase activity, i.e. ATP is broken down to provide the energy for the different modes of beating of cilia and flagella.

The beating of cilia is intermittent, not continuous. It has two phases or strokes, called the active (effective) stroke, which produces movement, and the recovery stroke (Figure 2.11(c)(ii)). Ciliary movement is parallel to their surface of attachment. Cilia have a greater density than flagella. This translates the intermittent motion of a single cilium into continuous motion, by ensuring that each cilium begins its cycle of motion slightly before the cilium next to it. Thus, a wave of effective strokes passes across the surface of the cell (like wind over a field of wheat). This movement is referred to as a metachromal rhythm. Flagella are longer, and each can contain several waves of contraction at any one time. They therefore produce continuous effective movement. The movement is at right-angles to the surface of attachment. Flagella are also capable of the active-recovery movements of cilia.

Cytoplasmic inclusions

Besides organelles, the cytoplasm also contains inclusions. These are a diverse group of chemical substances that are usually food or stored products of metabolism. Thus, inclusions are not permanent cytoplasmic components, as they are continually being destroyed and replaced. Examples of inclusions, and their homeostatic roles, are:

- *melanin*, a pigment present in the outer layer of skin (epidermis). Increasing the deposits of melanin causes tanning of the skin, and occurs as an adaptive protection mechanism against the sun's ultraviolet radiation. The pigment is also found in the hair and the eyes;

- *haemoglobin*, a pigment present in erythrocytes. The principal role of haemoglobin is to transport oxygen in the blood (see Chapter 14). It also transports carbon dioxide to help regulate acid/base balance of body fluids (see Chapter 6);

- *glycogen*, a storage carbohydrate found in liver and skeletal muscle cells. It is produced from glucose whenever the homeostatic range of blood glucose is superseded;

- *lipids*, stored in adipocytes ('adip-' = fat) whenever the homeostatic ranges of the constituent chemicals, fatty acids and glycerol, in blood have been superseded;

- *mucus*, produced in secretory cells that line some organs. Its functions are to lubricate the cells (epithelia) lining these organs, and to contribute to the external defence mechanisms of the body. For example, the mucus produced by the lining of the respiratory system has a

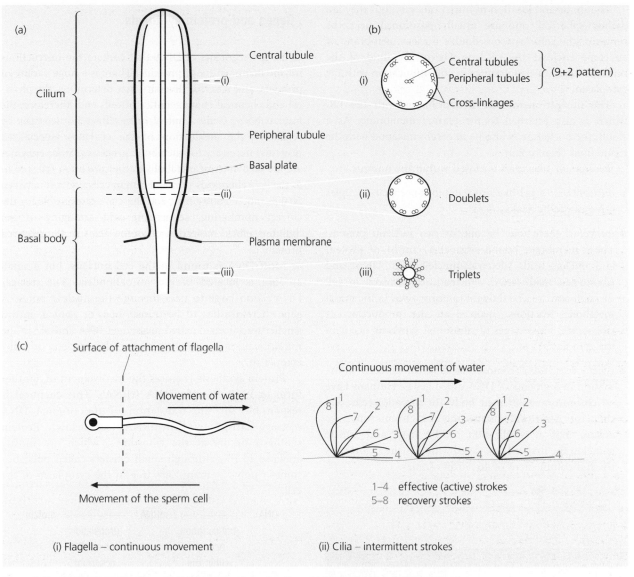

(a)

Cilium

Basal body

Central tubule

Peripheral tubule

Basal plate

Plasma membrane

(i)

(ii)

(iii)

(b)

(i)   Central tubules
       Peripheral tubules   } (9+2 pattern)
       Cross-linkages

(ii)   Doublets

(iii)   Triplets

(c)

Surface of attachment of flagella

Movement of water

Movement of the sperm cell

(i) Flagella – continuous movement

Continuous movement of water

1–4   effective (active) strokes
5–8   recovery strokes

(ii) Cilia – intermittent strokes

Figure 2.11   (a) Structure of a cilium. (b) Transverse sections of a cilium. (c) Mode of action of cilia and flagella.

Q. How are cilia, flagella and centrioles related to one another?

Q. Give examples of where you would find ciliated cells. Name the male's flagellated cell.

protective function against atmospheric microbes that have entered the airways.

Nucleus

Most cells possess one nucleus. The nucleus is the homeo-static control centre for cellular operations. It has two principal roles:

- To store heredity information (genes), and to transfer this information from one generation of cells to the next, and from one family generation to the next.

- To maintain intracellular homeostasis by directing metabolic reactions. It does this by expressing specific genes in order for the cell to synthesize appropriate enzymes that ensure that the chemicals inside the cell are within their normal ranges.

BOX 2.12 ERYTHROCYTE STORAGE BANKS

Mature erythrocytes lack a nucleus and hence genetic material, therefore they cannot duplicate or produce enzymes. They have a low rate of metabolism and so remain functional in blood storage banks.

The shape and location of nuclei can vary, but they are mainly spherical, and are usually positioned near the centre of the cell. A porous double nuclear membrane or envelope encloses the nucleus. Hence the fluid of the nucleus, called nucleoplasm, is in communication with the cytoplasm.

The nuclear membrane is continuous with the ER, which is also attached to the plasma membrane. As a result, the nucleus may also be in communication with the tissue fluid (Figure 2.9).

Prominent structures enclosed within the nucleus are:

- *nucleoplasm:* a gel-like ground substance that occupies most of the nucleus;

- *nucleolus:* there may be one or two nucleoli present. These membrane-bound organelles consist of protein and nucleic acids (deoxyribonucleic acid, DNA, and ribonucleic acid, RNA). Nucleoli are involved in cell division and are also thought to be involved in the initial metabolic reactions involved in the production of ribosomes. Final stages of ribosomal synthesis occur in the cytoplasm;

- *genetic material:* chromosomes store the heredity information in segments of DNA called genes. Humans have 46 chromosomes in their body (or somatic) cells. Sex cells (or gametes) contain only 23 chromosomes to ensure that at fertilization of the male and female gametes, the first cell associated with life (the zygote) has the full complement of 46 chromosomes.

BOX 2.13 GENES – THE LINK WITH METABOLISM AND ILLNESS

The nucleus of each human cell, except gametes, contains the chromosomes that comprise our genetic make-up (genotype) that encodes the observable and measurable characteristics (phenotypes) that we inherit from our biological parents. These phenotypic characteristics emerge during embryological development as the genes on the chromosomes are expressed to control metabolism of the cell. It is still uncertain how genes are expressed in humans to enable cells to differentiate into a diverse range with specialized functions (skeletal, digestive, renal, etc.) and at a specific time of embryological development (see Figure 20.3).

Chromosomes contain the necessary information to maintain homeostasis of all cells, and hence the functional equilibrium of tissues, organs and organ systems. Interference of this information by cells being infected by viruses, or altered by carcinogens or ultraviolet and ionizing radiation may lead to homeostatic imbalances, resulting in the malfunctioning of organ systems.

Genes and protein synthesis

Genes are segments of DNA that contain the instructions for the manufacture of proteins. There is a huge variety of proteins, and it is this diversity that determines the physical and chemical characteristics of cells and, therefore, the human body. Genes control intracellular homeostasis by regulating the production of the enzymes (specialized proteins) necessary for metabolic processes. Since enzymes are the mediators of metabolism, they are often referred to as the 'key chemicals of life'. Human cells contain between 50 000 and 100 000 genes, and these are responsible for the correct numbering, sequencing and arranging of the 'building block' molecules of amino acids in the required protein.

Most DNA is found in the cell nucleus, but a small amount is located in the mitochondria. The nuclear DNA is too large to pass through the nuclear pores. A gene therefore has to be transcribed, or copied, into a smaller nucleic acid called messenger RNA (mRNA). The mRNA can move freely between the nucleus and the cytoplasm.

Protein synthesis requires the involvement of another form of RNA, transfer RNA (tRNA). This chemical is responsible for the translation of the original DNA message carried by the mRNA (see below). Protein synthesis occurs at the ribosomes, which are mostly attached to ER, although small clusters called polyribosomes ('poly-' = many) are free in the cytoplasm of the cell.

DNA ⟶ mRNA ⟶ protein
(transcription occurs within the nucleus) (translation involves tRNA, occurs at ribosomal level)

Structure of DNA

In 1953, Watson and Crick were awarded the Nobel Prize for the discovery that genes were composed of the chemical DNA, which in turn was composed of relatively few types of molecules called nucleotides. DNA consists of two polynucleotide chains (i.e. each consisting of many nucleotides) coiled around each another as a double helix (Figure 2.12(a)). Each nucleotide consists of (Figure 2.12(b)).

1 one of the four organic bases: adenine (A), guanine (G), cytosine (C) or thymine (T);

2 sugar (deoxyribose, hence the name deoxyribonucleic acid);

3 phosphate.

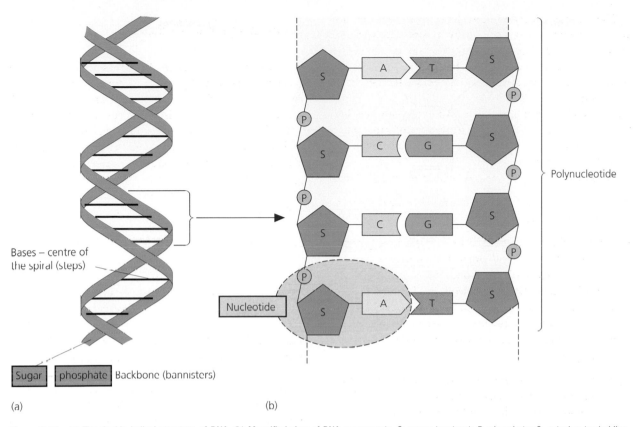

Figure 2.12 (a) The double-helical structure of DNA. (b) Magnified view of DNA components. S, sugar (pentose); P, phosphate; C, cytosine (pyrimidine base); T, thymine (pyrimidine base); A, adenine (purine base); G, guanine (purine base).

The two strands of DNA are arranged so that one is complementary to the other through specific base pairing. Adenine of one strand pairs specifically with thymine in the other strand, and cytosine always pairs with guanine (Figures 2.12(b) and 12.13(a)).

A sequence of just three of these base pairs provides the code for an amino acid. Since mRNA is a copy of only one of the strands of DNA, only the three bases on this strand form that code. This group of three bases is referred to as a triplet (or codon), and the sequencing of triplets along a portion of DNA that code for a particular protein is termed a gene (Figure 2.14(a)). Smaller genes code for polypeptides, which are the subunits of proteins. A typical gene, however, contains a sequence of approximately 20 000 base pairs, although there is considerable variability between genes. The segment of copied DNA is called the cistron.

Proteins are made up of a large number of amino acids. There are 20 different amino acids available and, since the four bases can be arranged in 64 different triplet combinations ($4 \times 4 \times 4 = 64$), some triplets must code for the same amino acid (Table 2.3). For example, the triplets CCA, CCG and CCC all code for the amino acid, glycine.

BOX 2.14 EVOLUTION AND GENE THERAPIES

The genetic 'blueprint' or code in this triplet form is used by all organisms and always relates to the same amino acids. It is the metabolism of these amino acids that varies between different organisms, leading to their diversity. This commonality supports the view that all organisms evolved from a common ancestry. This helps to explain why viruses can replicate in human cells by incorporating their nucleic acid into our own. Gene therapies under development largely depend upon this process as a mean of inserting genes into defective cells (Lea, 1997; Munro, 1999).

Structure of RNA

RNA consists of a single polynucleotide strand. Each nucleotide within this strand is composed of:

1 one of the four organic bases: adenine (A), guanine (G), cytosine (C) or uracil (U) (uracil replaces the thymine of DNA, but has a similar structure);

2 sugar (ribose, hence the name 'ribonucleic acid', see Figure 2.13(b));

3 phosphate.

(a)   **Purines**   **Pyrimidines**

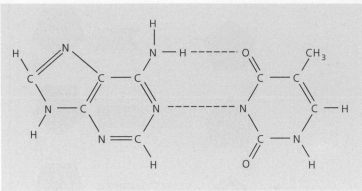

Adenine   Thymine

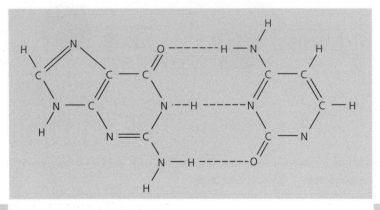

Guanine   Cytosine

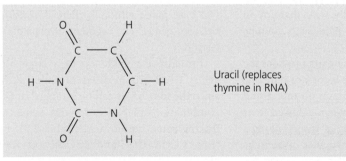

Uracil (replaces thymine in RNA)

(b)

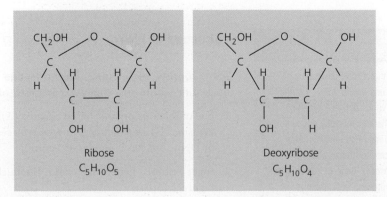

Ribose
$C_5H_{10}O_5$

Deoxyribose
$C_5H_{10}O_4$

Figure 2.13   (a) Organic base structure. (b) Sugars associated with the nucleic acids.

(a)

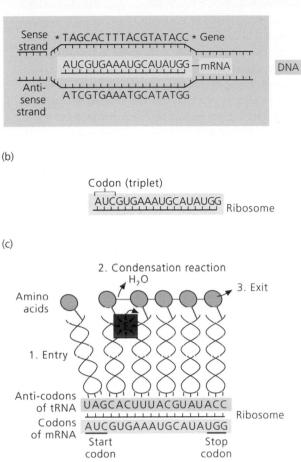

(b)

Codon (triplet)

AUCGUGAAAUGCAUAUGG Ribosome

(c)

Figure 2.14 Protein synthesis. (a) Transcription. mRNA synthesis alongside DNA strand in the nucleus. Note the gene is comprised of the triplets from *—* on the sense strand. (b) mRNA passes out of the nucleus to become attached to ribosomes. (c) Translation. Transfer RNA (tRNA) brings the amino acids to the ribosome. E, energy from catabolism of ATP (ADP + P$_i$ + energy. Note that tRNA anticodons are the original triplets on the sense strand of DNA, which code for the specific amino acids.

Q. With the aid of this diagram, explain how proteins are synthesized using the following terms: DNA, mRNA, tRNA, codons, sense strand, anti-sense strand, cistrons, anticodons, transcription, translation, amino acids, proteins, nucleus, ribosomes, polyribosomes, endoplasmic reticulum, cytoplasm, peptide bonds, energy and ATP.

Transcription of the gene code

Transcription is the first stage in protein synthesis; it occurs in the nucleus. The process involves copying the sequence of bases encoded in the DNA chemical into the sequenced nucleotides of mRNA using the enzyme RNA polymerase. The single strand of nucleotides in RNA differs from DNA in that it contains the organic base uracil rather than thymine found in DNA, but the two chemicals are very similar. Consequently, during transcription the adenine of DNA is complementary for uracil.

Table 2.3 The mRNA codons for amino acids

UUU } phe	UCU }	UAU } tyr	UGU } cys
UUC }	UCC } ser	UAC }	UGC }
UUA } leu	UCA }	UAA } 'stop'	UGA 'stop'
UUG }	UCG }	UAG }	UGG trp
CUU }	CCU }	CAU } his	CGU }
CUC } leu	CCC } pro	CAC }	CGC } arg
CUA }	CCA }	CAA } gln	CGA }
CUG }	CCG }	CAG }	CGG }
AUU }	ACU }	AAU } asn	AGU } ser
AUC } ile	ACC } thr	AAC }	AGC }
AUA }	ACA }	AAA } lys	AGA } arg
AUG met	ACG }	AAG }	AGG }
GUU }	GCU }	GAU } asp	GGU }
GUC } val	GCC } ala	GAC }	GGC } gly
GUA }	GCA }	GAA } glu	GGA }
GUG }	GCG }	GAG }	GGG }

ala, alanine; arg, arginine; asn, asparagine; asp, aspartic acid; cys, cysteine; gln, glutamine; glu, glutamic acid; gly, glycine; his, histidine; ile, isoleucine; leu, leucine; lys, lysine; met, methionine; phe, phenylalanine; pro, proline; ser, serine; thr, threonine; trp, trytophan; tyr, tyrosine; val, valine.

Q. Identify the potential mRNA codons that code for the tripeptide comprised of the following amino acids: alanine, histidine, valine and tyrosine.

Q. List the corresponding DNA triplets that code for this codon and tRNA anticodon.

For example, a DNA template with the base sequence of TAG, CAC, TTT, ACG, TAT, ACC would be transcribed into the complementary strand of RNA as AUC, GUG, AAA, UGC, AUA, UGG (see Figure 2.14(a)). Apart from the insertion of uracil, this sequencing is identical to the complementary strand of DNA.

The template strand of DNA that is copied is called the sense strand, and the one not being transcribed is the anti-sense stand, since it complements the sense strand.

Translation

Once mRNA has been transcribed from DNA, the DNA reassumes its double-helical structure. The mRNA leaves the nucleus to become attached to the ribosome (Figure 2.14 (b) and (c)), and its genetic message is translated. Translation occurs in a number of steps:

1 The process begins when the 'front' end of mRNA has attached itself to a ribosome and begins to move across it (Figure 2.14(c)). In doing so, the ribosome decodes the message by reading the triplets (codons). The first codon acts as a 'start' code; subsequent codons code for specific amino acids.

2 Transfer RNA (tRNA) chemicals in the cytoplasm are anticodons that are a complementary match for the codons on mRNA. Each tRNA chemical combines with a

BOX 2.15 NEONATAL SCREENING IDENTIFIES MUTATIONS

Sickle cell anaemia is a life-threatening condition instigated by a change of just one DNA base paring. This results in an abnormal gene. The change in base sequencing is called a genetic mutation, and it is responsible for the signs and symptoms of multiple organ system imbalances in the individual (see Chapter 20). Lees *et al.* (2001) suggested that early treatment (before symptoms develop) can improve both morbidity and mortality. Screening for the condition in the neonatal period would enable early diagnosis and therefore early treatment. Phenylketonuria (PKU) is another disease in which a genetic mutation has occurred. The presence of this abnormal gene means that people with PKU cannot produce an enzyme called phenyl hydroxylase, which is essential for converting the amino acid phenylalanine into tyrosine. Consequently, phenylalanine accumulates in the blood, tissues and central nervous system, resulting in brain damage leading to diminished mental development. Newborns are screened for PKU by the neonatal screening test (previously called the Guthrie heel-prick blood test). Babies identified as having PKU must be given a phenylalanine-free diet to protect against the effects of the condition (Poustie and Rutler, 2001). This neonatal test also screens for hypothyroidism and cystic fibrosis.

specific amino acid in the cytoplasm and adds it to the growing chain on the ribosome, according to the sequencing required by the arrangement of codons on the mRNA. For example, the mRNA codon for the amino acid glycine is GGU, GGC, GGA or GGG, and the respective anticodons are CCA, CCG, CCU and CCC (Table 2.3). The tRNA that carries glycine from the cytoplasm for incorporation into the growing protein will have one of these anticodons; it will bond only to glycine and to no other amino acid. Note that tRNA anticodons are analogous to the original DNA triplets (except that tRNA has uracil in place of thymine). The term 'initiation' refers to the process of positioning the first amino acid at the appropriate mRNA codon site on the ribosome.

3 Following initiation, elongation of the amino acid chain begins with the mRNA moving across the ribosome, one codon at a time. The codon is read by the ribosome, and the corresponding tRNA anticodon brings the specific amino acid and joins it to the previous one. A bond is formed between adjacent amino acids, using energy liberated from ATP catabolism. Further amino acids are added until a terminal 'stop' codon that stops the process is formed (Figure 2.14(c)). In this way, a polypeptide ('poly-' = many) is produced. Post-translational processing will incorporate this into a final protein molecule.

GENES AND CELL DIVISION

All cells originate from the division of the zygote. Cell division, an important basic characteristic of life, is necessary to maintain cellular homeostasis. It ensures that:

1 the genetic material (the 'blueprint' for homeostatic function) is transmitted from one cell to another, and from one generation to the next;

2 the development of the organism through cell differentiation and specialization occurs;

3 growth of organisms takes place in specific stages of human development, e.g. neonate to infant to young child;

4 dying, diseased, worn-out and damaged cells are replaced to maintain the structural integrity of the human body, hence ensuring adequate organ system functioning;

5 optimal cell size is not exceeded, since this would lead to intracellular homeostatic imbalances.

BOX 2.16 AGEING AND HOMEOSTASIS

Ageing is a normal process associated with a progressive alteration of the body's homeostatic adaptive responses. In part, ageing is caused by a decrease in cell numbers, resulting in atrophy of organ systems and hence physiological and psychological functional decline. Historically, the medical specialty that deals with medical problems is geriatrics, and the nursing care associated with these patients is referred to as 'care of the elderly' or, more recently, 'care of the older person'.

Optimal cell size depends on an ideal surface area/volume ratio being achieved, since surface area relates to entry and exit of substances, and volume relates to utilization of the substances. The surface area is the cell's available plasma membrane. This regulates the entry and exit of substances and, therefore, accommodates intracellular requirements. As cells grow, the surface area increases at a slower rate when compared with the change in cell volume. This is because the surface area increases with the square of the cell radius, whereas the volume increases with the cube of the radius. If the plasma membrane cannot support the increase in volume, then intracellular imbalances will occur, i.e. there will be insufficient nutrients available and a build-up of waste products of chemical reactions will occur. Cells therefore probably have in-built mechanisms (perhaps a gene or genes) that register the point at which cellular function is impaired and causes cell division to preserve the homeostatic status of cells. The components of homeostasis are involved, i.e. intracellular receptors detect the impairment and send the information to the homeostatic control of the cell (gene). The gene produces the enzyme DNA polymerase, which causes cell division to sustain the surface area/volume ratio compatible for preserving homeostatic function.

There are two types of cell division: somatic (body) cell division (mitosis), and reproductive cell division (meiosis). In each case, the dividing 'parent' cells produce 'daughter' cells.

Mitosis

Mitosis ensures that the daughter cells have the same number of chromosomes (hence genes) and identical DNA as the parent cell. For this to occur, the DNA of the parent cell must first be duplicated so that one copy can be passed into each daughter cell. Mitosis is therefore sometimes referred to as duplication division. The occurrence of mitosis completes one cell cycle and initiates the next one.

The cell cycle

The cell cycle is the sequence of events by which a cell duplicates its contents and divides into two (Figure 2.15(a)). The cell cycle consists of two major stages: the interphase, during which a cell is not dividing, and the mitotic stage, during which the cell is dividing (Figure 2.15(b)).

Interphase

The cell does most of its growing in preparation for cell division during the interphase. It is *not* a 'resting' stage, as described in some textbooks. The interphase has presumably been referred to as the resting stage because a physical characteristic of the phase is the absence of visible chromosomes. DNA appears as a thread-like mass of material within the cell nucleus, and is referred to as chromatin. There are three distinctive phases to the interphase: G1, S and G2 (Figure 2.15(b)); 'S' stands for 'synthesis' of DNA, and 'G' stands for 'gaps' in DNA synthesis.

The G1 phase occurs immediately following the mitotic phase (i.e. after a new cell has been produced). During G1, the cell is actively duplicating its organelles and other cellular components, but not its DNA. The centrosome begins to replicate in this phase, but does not end until G2.

The S phase occurs between the G1 and G2 phases. During the S phase, the DNA replicates to ensure that the daughter cells formed will have identical genetic material to the parent cell. During DNA replication, its helical structure partly uncoils, and the two strands separate where hydrogen bonds connect the base pairings (Figure 2.16). Each exposed base (known as the template nucleotide) picks up a complementary base nucleotide (with its associated sugar and phosphate). Uncoiling and complementary base pairing continue until each of the two original DNA strands is joined

---

BOX 2.17 THE CELL CYCLE AND CHROMOSOMAL DAMAGE

A 'typical' body cell with a cell cycle time of 25 h has a G1 phase lasting 5–10 h, an S phase of 6–8 h, and a G2 phase of 3–6 h. The duration of these phases is quite variable according to the ability of the specialized cells to repair, regenerate and divide (see Figure 11.11). Some specialized cells (e.g. most nerve cells) remain in the G1 phase for a very long time, and may never divide again. These are said to be in the G0 state (Figure 2.15(b)). However, most cells enter the S phase and thus are committed to cell division. Division is limited in skeletal muscle cells and neurons after specialization because of their complexity.

Although DNA duplication should conserve the genetic make-up of a cell, errors can occur during mitosis, with the consequence that daughter cells may exhibit chromosomal abnormalities such as additional chromosomes. Depending on the extent of the abnormality, such errors during cell division in the adult may not affect bodily function because this reflects the net effect of many

thousands of cells. An accumulation of errors with age may, however, contribute to declining function with age, or even to the incidence of certain diseases such as cancers. In the embryo and fetus, however, when cells are specializing, differentiating and growing, errors in cell division can have a pronounced influence on tissue development and function.

An extra chromosome present in the zygote is called a trisomy ('tri-' = three, '-somy' = bodies). Trisomy may have a devastating effect, since all the cells derived from the zygote will have an extra chromosome (hence extra genes), causing the signs and symptoms that are used to diagnose the syndrome. The best known example is trisomy 21, previously known as Down's syndrome, in which the trisomy occurs as an error during meiosis of the female gametes (hence the condition is known as a maternal syndrome). (See the case study of a man with Down's syndrome in Section 6).

(a)

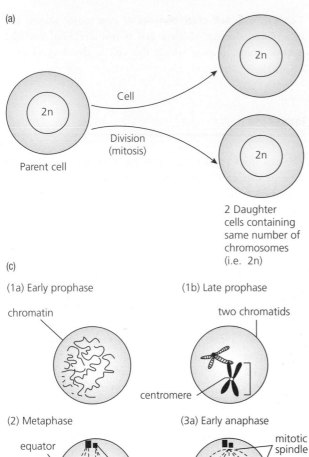

Parent cell

Cell Division (mitosis)

2 Daughter cells containing same number of chromosomes (i.e. 2n)

(b)

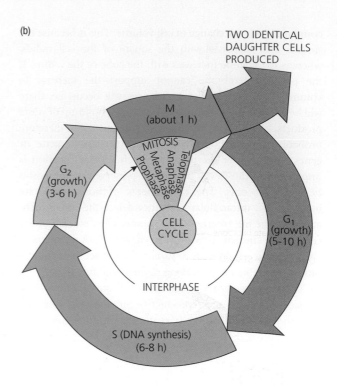

TWO IDENTICAL DAUGHTER CELLS PRODUCED

(c)

(1a) Early prophase

chromatin

(1b) Late prophase

two chromatids

centromere

(2) Metaphase

equator

centrioles

(3a) Early anaphase

mitotic spindle

(3b) Anaphase

(4) Telophase

cleavage furrow

Figure 2.15 (a) Cell division. Simple scheme demonstrating that the dividing parent cell produces two identical daughter cells with the same number of chromosomes. (b) Stages and phases associated with the cell cycle.
(c) Diagrammatic representation of the various phases of the mitotic stage of cell division (the cell goes progressively through the phases 1–4). *Prophase:* chromatin shortens and coils into chromosomes (chromatids), nucleoli and nuclear membrane become less distinctive, and centrioles separate and move to the opposite poles of the cell. The mitotic spindle appears. *Metaphase:* centromeres of chromatid pairs line up on the cell's equator to form the chromosomal microtubules and attach to centrioles. *Anaphase:* centromeres divide, and identical chromosomes move to opposite ends of the cell. *Telophase:* nuclear membrane reappears and encloses chromosomes, chromosomes resume chromatin form, nucleoli reappear, mitotic spindle disappears, and centrioles duplicate. Cleavage furrow forms around equatorial plane, progressing inwards, and separates the cytoplasm into two separate and equal portions.

completely to a newly formed complementary DNA strand. The original DNA has now become two identical DNA molecules.

During the G2 phase, the cell continues to grow, and enzymes and other proteins are synthesized in preparation for cell division: before mitosis can begin, the cell needs to double its mass and contents. The replication of the centrosome is completed in this stage. Once a cell has completed the G2 phase, the mitotic stage begins.

Mitotic stage

This stage lasts for about 1 h. It consists of nuclear division (mitosis), i.e. when the nucleus and its chromosomes divide, and cytoplasmic division (cytogenesis). These events are visible underneath a microscope.

Biologists divide mitosis into four phases: prophase, metaphase, anaphase and telophase. See Figure 2.15(c) for a summary of the events associated with each stage.

Figure 2.16 Replication of DNA.

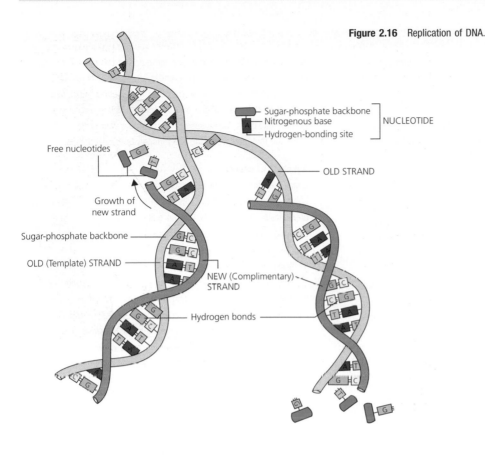

Sugar-phosphate backbone
Nitrogenous base } NUCLEOTIDE
Hydrogen-bonding site

Free nucleotides

OLD STRAND

Growth of new strand

Sugar-phosphate backbone

OLD (Template) STRAND

NEW (Complimentary) STRAND

Hydrogen bonds

Meiosis

Meiosis is referred to as 'reduction division', since it ensures that the daughter cells have only half of the chromosome complement, i.e. the cells will have only 23 chromosomes (the haploid number, 'hapl-'= half) in contrast to the 46 chromosomes (the diploid number, 'dipl ' = double) of the parent cell. Reduction division occurs in the male and female sex organs (gonads) during the production of the male and female sex cells (gametes; spermatozoa and ova, respectively) (see Chapter 18). Meiosis is necessary so that the 'normal' chromosomal number is restored in the zygote after fertilization, but it has major implications for inheritance (see Chapter 20).

The role of genes in cell homeostasis

Many cellular reactions occur in specialized organelles and distinctive areas of the cytoplasm. All metabolic activities directly involve enzymes, and thus are controlled indirectly by the nuclear DNA, since genes are responsible for enzyme synthesis. The availability of enzymes therefore controls biochemical/physiological and psychological activities to ensure homeostasis. The chemical nature of these reactions means, however, that regulating the availability of raw materials (reactants or substrates) and/or products provides

another means of controlling metabolic activities. For example, if we restrict the oxygen supply to cells, ATP levels decrease, even though there may be adequate levels of glucose for cell respiration to occur. A decrease in ATP will affect cellular metabolism generally, since it is involved in many chemical reactions. If the levels of oxygen are restored, then (providing glucose levels are adequate) ATP levels will be restored and normal cellular activity will be resumed.

How are genes controlled?

Whilst enzymes provide the link between genes and metabolic activity, the question arises as to how gene activity is expressed at the appropriate time. Various models of control have been proposed. These are based mainly on work with bacteria, and they suggest ways by which genes (DNA) control enzyme synthesis in response to the presence of substrates (reactants), end products, and/or external regulatory mechanisms. We will discuss only one model here, since it is outside the scope of this book to explore the variety of models that exists.

The Operon theory of genetic expression

One way to maintain the steady state (i.e. intracellular homeostasis) is to modulate enzyme production according

BOX 2.18 TUMOURS AND CANCER

All disorders involve a disturbance of cell function somewhere within the body. Many examples are provided throughout this book; this section will concentrate only on disorders of cell division.

A tumour is a swelling produced by an abnormally accelerated period of growth and reproduction of cells (called neoplasm). Tumours are classified as benign or malignant. Benign (non-cancerous) tumour cells are localized and encapsulated. These cells develop singly, or occasionally in small groups, and usually pose no threat to life. They are deemed safe as long as the tumour does not produce symptoms through pressure on vital tissues or become unsightly. Only a small percentage of benign tumours lead to 'secondary' growths (or metastases). These are referred to as 'innocent' tumours and may not be removed. If the size or position of the tumour, however, impairs tissue or organ function, then surgical removal is required. This procedure is straightforward since benign tumours are encapsulated. Post-surgery, there is no danger of secondary tumours and little chance of recurrence.

Malignant (cancerous) tumour cells leave the original tumour site and infiltrate other tissues and organs. This spread (metastasis) is dangerous and difficult to control. This is because at their new sites metastatic cells divide mitotically and produce secondary tumours that will affect the functional capacity of the newly affected tissues or organs.

The term 'cancer' refers to a variety of illnesses, many of which are characterized by the appearance of tumours. Cancers are classified according to the type of tissue involved:

● *Carcinoma:* malignancy of epithelial cells. Epithelial cells line hollow tubes and organs throughout the body.
● *Leukaemia:* malignancy of certain white blood cells.
● *Sarcoma:* malignancy of other body cells.

The functions of cancer cells differ from normal cells. They are abnormally large or small, and many have chromosomal abnormalities. Cell division is accelerated, and changes in function are largely irreversible. As the number of cancer cells increases, organ function becomes abnormal, and homeostatic imbalances associated with that system and the interdependent organ systems become apparent. Also, cancer cells compete with normal cells for nutrients, thus compromising the function of localized cells.

Aetiology of cancer

Cancer research has yet to demonstrate fully why cancer cells behave in the way they do. Nevertheless, much is known about the predisposing factors (Table 2.4). In addition, many environmental carcinogens have been identified, including plant poisons, microbial and animal toxins, tar (benzpyrene) in cigarette smoke, food additives, and deficiencies of vital nutrients such as vitamin A.

Specificity is also observed, since most carcinogens affect only those cells capable of responding to them, and very few carcinogens, such as radiation, affect cells generally throughout the body. In general, cells normally capable of rapid division record a high incidence of cancer, since they are more likely to respond to chemical or radiation carcinogens. Consequently, the incidence of epithelial tissue and stem cell (immature cells prone to rapid division) cancers are very high, whilst the rates of muscle and nervous tissue cancers are comparatively low.

Principles of correction

Because of the incurable nature of some cancers, prevention is paramount and this obviously involves avoiding exposure to known carcinogens. Should a tumour grow, however, then the odds of survival are markedly increased if the cancer is detected early, especially before it undergoes metastasis. Treatment of malignant tumours must be accomplished by one of the following:

● *Killing the cancer cells.* The treatment for early accessible tumours is surgical removal, accompanied by dissection of the related lymph glands, which may contain some migrating cancer

Table 2.4 Summary of 'cancer inducers'

Hereditary predisposition
Inherited characteristics make the individual more susceptible. Approximately 19 forms of inherited cancers have been identified to date.

Radiation exposure
The governmental health safety standards protect against harmful levels of carcinogenic substances. The problem is that not all the environmental 'pollutants' have been tested for their potential carcinogenicity.

Sex
Certain cancers are frequently associated with one particular sex. For example, breast cancer is more common in females.

Carcinogen/mutagen factors
Many carcinogens are mutagens, since they cause chromosomal changes, e.g. insecticides.

Chronic tissue damage
Injuries, instead of repairing or regenerating the cells affected, can produce cancer cells. For example, skin cancers due to overexposure to UV radiation (sunlight).

Age
Gene activity changes throughout life, and thus one's susceptibility to certain cancers changes. For example, colonic cancers are more common in people over 40.

Viruses
There are increasing numbers of viruses being linked to certain cancers, e.g. the papilloma virus that is responsible for cervical cancer.

cells. Deep X-ray radiation (radiotherapy), heating or freezing of cells are particularly effective treatments before metastasis. Radiotherapy prevents cell division by using ionizing radiation to break down the chemicals in chromatin and the cytoplasm. Radiation can be directed specifically at the tumour, but other parts of the patient's (and therapist's) body must be protected. The lead aprons worn in X-ray departments protect against these damaging particles.

- *Preventing replication of cancer cells*. Cytotoxic drugs (chemotherapy) kill cancerous tissue by preventing mitotic divisions (Moran, 2000). For example, the drugs vinblastine and vincristine prevent mitotic activity of the cancer cells by blocking the assembly of the mitotic spindle. The problem is that these drugs are nonspecific in their effects. Consequently other mitotically active cells, such as those of the gastrointestinal

tract, bone marrow and hair, are affected, which explains the side effects of these drugs, including sore mouth, gastrointestinal tract disturbances, anaemia and hair loss.

The most effective therapies often involve a combination of procedures, e.g. radiation plus chemotherapy, or surgery followed by radiation plus chemotherapy.

At present, tumour cells cannot be poisoned without harming healthy cells. Immunotherapy involves administering substances that enable the immune system to recognize and attack just the cancerous cells, and recent advances in 'designer' drugs also raise the possibility of specific treatments in the future.

For further information, see the case study of a woman with breast cancer in Section 6, and the articles by McCaughan and Thompson (2000) and Hinds and Moyer (1997).

---

to the changing environment inside the cell. For example, when the concentration of the end product of a reaction is above its homeostatic range, enzymes involved in its production could be inhibited and so prevent further increase. The converse is true for an excess of reactants (Figure 2.17), i.e. enzymes are produced to remove the

excess. The Operon theory attempts to explain the regulation of enzyme synthesis.

Jacob and Monod (1961), the proposers of the Operon theory, worked with the bacterium *Escherichia coli* (*E. coli*). They reported that they could produce two enzymes on demand if the cultured medium of *E. coli* was changed

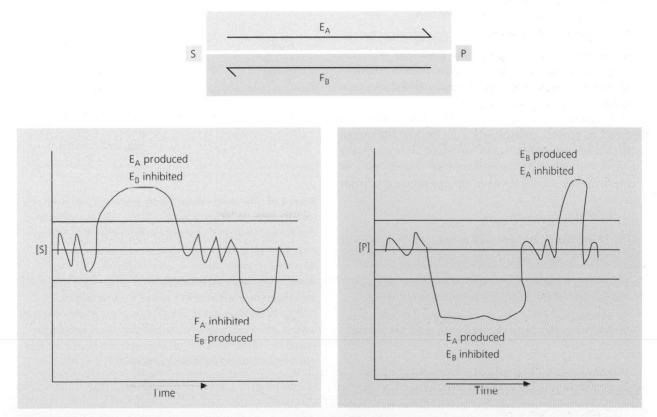

Figure 2.17 Intracellular metabolic homeostasis via enzyme production and inhibition. The reaction goes to the right when there is excess substrate (S) and a deficiency of the product (P). This is controlled by producing or activating enzyme A (E_A), and by stopping the production of, or deactivating, enzyme B (E_B). The reaction goes to the left when there is an excess of P and a deficiency of S. This is controlled by producing or activating E_B, and by stopping the production of, or deactivating, E_A. The reaction stops when the homeostatic ranges of both S and P are achieved.

from the monosaccharide glucose to a disaccharide, lactose, made of glucose and galactose. When grown on a glucose medium, *E. coli* was able to use glucose directly in cellular respiration (Figure 2.18(a)). When grown on a lactose medium, however, the following enzymes were produced:

- *Permease:* produced to make the membrane more permeable (hence the enzyme's name) to lactose, which is a larger chemical than glucose. Remember, large molecules move across the cell membrane at a slower rate than small molecules.

- *Beta-galactosidase:* produced to convert lactose into its constituents, glucose and galactose (Figure 2.18(b)).

Jacob and Monod explained enzyme production, or induction, by way of the Operon theory. They argued that there was a linear segment of DNA called the Operon that controlled enzyme (protein) synthesis. In this case, the Operon was composed of three genes – two structural and one operator (or promoter):

- *Structural gene:* contains the code necessary for the production of the enzyme. In this case, two structural genes are involved: the permease gene and the (Beta-galactosidase gene.

- *Operator gene:* controls the transcription of the structural gene necessary for protein synthesis.

Another gene called the regulator (or repressor) gene is involved in Operon activity. This gene codes for the production of a regulatory or repressor protein (enzyme) that regulates the activity of other genes within the Operon (Figure 2.18(c)).

The genes and their transcribed proteins therefore interact to provide control over the Operon. The overall effects of this interaction are to 'switch on', or express, the structural gene when needed, and to 'switch off', or repress, the structural gene when enzyme production is not needed.

When an enzyme is required, e.g. when there is an excess of the substrate (reactant), the structural gene is expressed to reduce the substrate level to within its homeostatic range (Figure 2.17). Enzyme synthesis may be repressed, e.g. when there is an excess of the product, or when there is a low level of the substrate specific for that particular enzyme. Using the example above, when *E. coli*

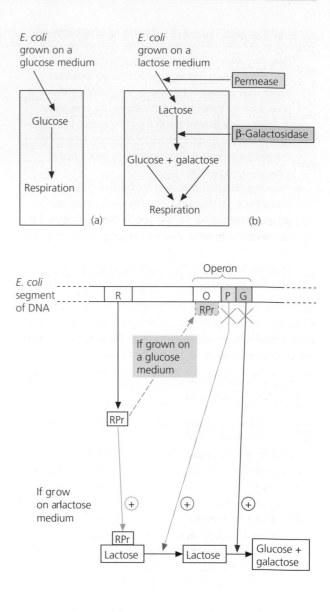

Figure 2.18 The Jacob—Monod Operon theory. (a) *E. coli* grown on a glucose medium. (b) *E. coli* grown on a lactose medium. (c) Enzyme induction and inhibition. R, repressor (or regulator gene); O, operator gene; P, permease; G, β-galactosidase genes (structural genes); RPr, repressor (or regulator) protein; +, enzyme induction; X, enzyme inhibition. Summary: enzyme induction when grown on a lactose medium, enzyme inhibition when grown on a glucose medium.
Q. *Using the principles applied to the Operon theory, describe how (i) the levels of intracellular metabolites are controlled; (ii) cell specialization occurs; (iii) overexposure to UV light may cause skin cancers; (iv) drugs may be used to correct homeostatic imbalances.*

is grown on a glucose medium, there is no suitable substrate (i.e. lactose), so there is no need to express the permease or Beta-galactosidase structural genes. Consequently, the repressor protein blocks the operator and so represses transcription of the structural gene. This repression prevents the wasteful production of enzymes, a factor that is important in controlling intracellular homeostatic levels of enzymes.

Conversely, when *E. coli* is grown on a lactose medium, permease is produced to allow faster movement of lactose into the cell (a build-up of the substrate thus occurs). It then becomes necessary to express the Beta-galactosidase gene to enzymatically convert lactose into its constituent monosaccharides (Figure 2.18 (b) and (c)).

Gene expression: the link with intracellular homeostasis, health, ill-health and development

Enzyme induction and inhibition are directly responsible for maintaining intracellular homeostasis. According to the Operon theory, enzyme production involves the activation of the operator gene necessary for synthesis of that enzyme. As outlined earlier, enzyme synthesis may be promoted by the following situations:

1 The availability of the enzyme is below its homeostatic range (see Figure 1.7).

BOX 2.20 HYPOTHYROIDISM

A failure to increase enzyme production will result in deficient substrate utilization. For example, in hypothyroidism there is a deficiency of thyroid hormone production. This deficiency means that the synthesis of enzymes involved in the conversion of glucose into energy is compromised, since thyroxine controls the rate of enzyme production. Cell metabolism is therefore depressed, resulting in symptoms such as apathy, slow thought processes, and a slowed pulse rate.

2 The substrate (metabolite) is beyond its homeostatic range. The excess material must be removed, using further enzymes to remove the homeostatic imbalance. For example, in health excesses may be removed in various ways:

- The substance may be stored in a related form, e.g. excess intracellular glucose is stored as glycogen by the production of the enzyme glycogen synthetase.

- The substance may be converted into another form, e.g. non-essential amino acids (i.e. not essential as a dietary requirement) may be transferred or transaminated into other non-essential amino acids if needed, i.e. if their homeostatic levels are compromised. Alternatively, the excess essential amino acids (essential as a dietary requirement) may be broken down or deaminated into energy-producing chemicals (keto acids) and urea. Keto acids are fed into the cellular respiratory pathway; urea is a metabolic waste product that is usually excreted. Transamination and deamination processes are instigated by the synthesis of enzymes known as transaminases and deaminases, respectively.

BOX 2.21 PHENYLKETONURIA

If the substrate is beyond its homeostatic range, its utilization must be increased to remove the homeostatic imbalance. Failure to remove the imbalance of surplus substrate can have severe consequences. Phenylketonuria (PKU) is such an example. You should already be able to name the substrate that is in excess with this condition. See box 2.15, and the case study of the boy with PKU in Section 6.

Toxic substances (e.g. alcohol), administered substances (e.g. drugs) and circulating substances (e.g. hormones) are converted to less active forms or are destroyed. Failure to produce the enzymes involved will result in prolonged activities of these substances. This is one of the complications of cirrhosis of the liver, in which liver function is severely disrupted. Transamination and deamination occur in the liver. A raised serum transaminase level is indicative of liver disorders.

3 'Old' or defective organelles must be broken down, and new organelles must replace the loss, to ensure intracellular homeostasis. The metabolic reactions involved require enzymatic synthesis and action.

4 Ultimately, a patient's illness (homeostatic imbalance) is a result of an environmentally induced gene expression or repression. Healthcare interventions seek to redress the patient's homeostasis. Interventions operate at a cellular level either directly by switching genes on or off, or indirectly by modulating gene expression, thus affecting enzyme synthesis or their activities (see box 2.6).

BOX 2.22 CELL SPECIALIZATION: A MATTER OF GENE EXPRESSION

The expression or repression of genes can also explain cell differentiation and specialization that occurs during the different development stages of human life. Each developmental stage has specific anatomical, physiological and psychological characteristics. The development of such characteristics involves the functioning, or non-functioning, of enzyme systems by way of gene expression and repression respectively. An individual's genes, or genotype, therefore determine the biophysical and biochemical characteristics, or phenotype, of the individual (see Chapter 20).

5 The subjective perceptions of pain, stress, and the 'time' inside your body (circadian rhythms) also involves gene–enzyme interactions.

Gene expression is vital to the integrity of metabolic activity in cells. Loss of genes by deletion or mutation will produce significant alterations to cell metabolism, some of which may be sufficient to induce a disease state (see Chapter 20). Most disorders that arise from the inheritance of single defective genes have now been identified; most are evident at birth. The most common example in the UK is cystic fibrosis (CF). In up to 90% of patients with CF, pancreatic insufficiency necessitates the use of pancreatic enzyme replacement therapy, but there are concerns about the self-administration of inappropriately high dosages of enzymes (Basketter et al., 2000).

Recent years have also provided increasing evidence for genetic involvement in diseases of adulthood. These disorders seem likely to involve mutations in many genes, or altered gene expression, but the promoting mechanisms are incompletely understood. Some mutations may be inherited, whilst others are accumulated during life. For example, colorectal cancer tends to occur in middle to late adulthood, and its incidence is greatest in countries with high socioeconomic standards. The onset of colorectal cancer is related to prolonged contact between the faecal mass and colon mucosa. A diet low in dietary fibre and high in fats increases the risk of developing the cancer because of the accumulation of substances made by colonic bacteria that mutate DNA. The development of colorectal cancer appears to result from genetic deletions from various chromosomes (Department of Health, 1995). Clearly, an individual who inherits some of these deletions will be at increased risk of accumulating the remaining deletions during life. This helps to explain the occurrence of cancer primarily as a disease of adulthood. Some genes seem to be more crucial in this than others, e.g. people who inherit an altered dominant gene on chromosome 5 exhibit familial adenomatous polyposis coli. These people have a high incidence of polyps within the colon, and are more likely to develop colorectal cancer at an earlier age then those people who do not have the gene.

Note the role of diet and lifestyle in this disorder. The aetiology of the cancer is one of gene inheritance (i.e. nature) combined with environmental influences on genes and gene expression (i.e. nurture). The recognition of environmental modification of genes and/or gene expression will result in health education in the not-too-distant future for the prevention of many common disorders, including heart disease and insulin-independent diabetes mellitus (Department of Health, 1995). Information obtained from the Human Genome Project initiated in 1990 and targeted for completion in the year 2005. This project has implications for nursing research, and healthcare and nursing practice. It will substantially revise our understanding of disease susceptibility and causation from a nature–nurture perspective. Additional genetic tests will develop and gene therapies will be explored (Munro, 1999).

TISSUES AND TISSUE FUNCTION

A tissue is defined as a collection of similar cells and their component parts that perform specialized homeostatic functions. The entire body is composed of only four primary tissue types – epithelial tissues, connective tissues, muscular tissues and nervous tissues – each having many subtypes with different roles.

The study of tissues is called histology ('histo-' = tissue). Histology is concerned with the broader patterns of cellular organization, the structure of tissues, and how this structure is important in determining the tissue's homeostatic functions in the organization of the whole person. Tissues are a good example of the complementary interplay between structure (anatomy) and function (physiology).

Each cell type differentiates during embryonic development from the three embryonic germ layers (endoderm, mesoderm and ectoderm; see Chapter 20). The expression and non-expression of developmental genes (see the earlier discussion on the Operon theory) control the process of specialization, e.g. a muscle cell is formed by the expression of genes concerned with the structural and functional development of this cell type, and by the non-expression of other developmental genes such as blood cell genes. Functional specialization is necessary, as each cell type has an important homeostatic role to play in the person. There is a 'division of labour', so that the individual can carry out the characteristics of life described in Chapter 1. For example, muscle tissues enable the individual to carry out movement (see Chapter 17), skeletal tissue supports the body, glandular tissues act as secretory cells that release enzymes or hormones, and vascular tissues are involved in the defence of the body. Once they have specialized, some cells lose their ability to perform other functions. For example, the mature red blood cell is concerned with the transport and exchange of respiratory gases, but as a result of this specialization it loses its capacity to divide, since it has no nucleus or nuclear components. Nerve and muscle cells generally also lose this replication function once they become specialized, with the consequence that if such tissues are damaged they are capable of only limited regeneration.

The body also contains a number of membranes formed from epithelial cells supported by connective tissue. This chapter is concerned with epithelial and connective tissues, and the types of membrane found in the body. Nervous tissue, skeletal muscle tissue, muscle tissue types, and specialized connective tissues, such as bone and the vascular (blood) tissues, are described in later chapters.

Epithelial tissues

There are three types of epithelia:

● simple epithelia, which are just one cell thick;

● compound epithelia, which are more than one cell thick;

● glandular epithelia, which produce the secretions of the body.

All are derived from the embryonic germ layers, and since they have different structures, they have different functions.

Homeostatic functions of epithelia

● *Protection:* simple (to a limited extent) and compound epithelia protect the underlying tissues from pathogenic invasion, desiccation (drying out), and harmful environmental factors, such as ultraviolet radiation.

● *Transport:* simple epithelia have important roles in controlling the transport of substances across membranous surfaces.

● *Lining:* simple, compound and glandular epithelia line internal cavities and tubes of the body, such as the respiratory and digestive tracts.

● *Secretory:* glandular epithelia are responsible for producing a variety of substances (sebum, sweat, tears, etc.) that have particular homeostatic functions, e.g. the production and secretion of sweat are important thermoregulatory mechanisms (see Chapter 16).

Epithelial tissues consist of flat sheets of cells. All epithelia have a basement membrane, i.e. a thin layer of 'cementing' material on the underside of the tissue that holds the cells together.

Simple epithelia

Simple (covering and lining) epithelial cells are arranged as a single layer. These tissues are located in areas where they can carry out their roles of absorption or filtration, e.g. the respiratory surfaces of the lung.

Pavement epithelia

Figure 2.19(a) is a surface view of pavement (squamous) epithelia cells; it shows how these cells are connected together via interdigitating junctions, giving the border a crazy-pavement-like appearance. The side view in Figure 2.19(b) demonstrates that this tissue is made up of very thin, flat cells. Squamous epithelia are not found in areas where there is wear and tear, but will be located in areas that are adapted for the homeostatic functions of rapid diffusion, osmosis and filtration, e.g. in the alveoli of the lungs, the double-membranous Bowman's capsule of the kidney nephrons, the internal lining of the blood vessels and the inner surface of the heart, the lining of lymphatic capillaries, and the serous membranes of the body. These epithelia generally have fluid on one side and blood vessels on the other, so transport can occur between the two. They permit frictionless flow of fluids across their surfaces.

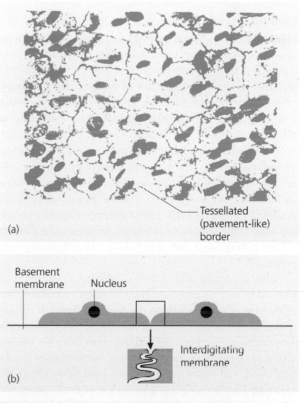

Figure 2.19 Squamous (pavement) epithelium. (a) Surface view; (b) side view.

Cuboidal epithelia

Figure 2.20 is a side view of a cuboidal epithelium; it shows the cubic shape of the cells. These cells are slightly thicker than the pavement tissues, but they are still thin enough for substances to pass through them. This type of tissue is typically concerned with absorption and secretory functions, and are found in, for example, the thyroid gland, sweat glands, germinating layer of the epidermis of the skin, anterior surface of the lens of the eye, surface of the ovaries, and the proximal tubules of the kidneys. In these tubules, the epithelium bears microvilli, which increase the surface area for absorption of water. The nuclei of both squamous and cuboidal epithelia are centralized, and are either round or oval in shape.

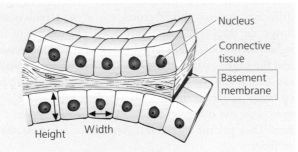

Figure 2.20   Side view of cuboidal epithelium.

Columnar epithelia

Figure 2.21(a) is a side view of a columnar epithelium; it shows that these cells are taller or thicker than cuboidal cells. The nuclei are oval, and are situated near the base of the cell. Examples of location are the lining of the digestive tract from the small intestine to the anus, and the lining of the gall bladder. The functions of columnar epithelia are varied. They provide a smooth area over which food can pass without friction, protect underlying tissues, and aid food absorption (i.e. the cells in the ileum possess microvilli that increases their surface area; Figure 2.21(b)). Some intestinal cells are modified columnar cells, called goblet or mucus-secreting cells; their secretions lubricate or moisturize food to aid its passage and the physical and chemical digestive processes.

Some columnar and cuboidal cells have cilia on their free surfaces (Figure 2.21(c)), which facilitate the movement of materials along the duct. Examples of ciliated epithelia are the linings of the airways, where ciliated cells move inhaled dust particles and microbes from the trachea and areas beyond to the oesophagus, so that they can be swallowed; and the lining of the Fallopian tubes, where the cells move the female gamete to the site of fertilization, and the zygote and developing embryo to the site of implantation.

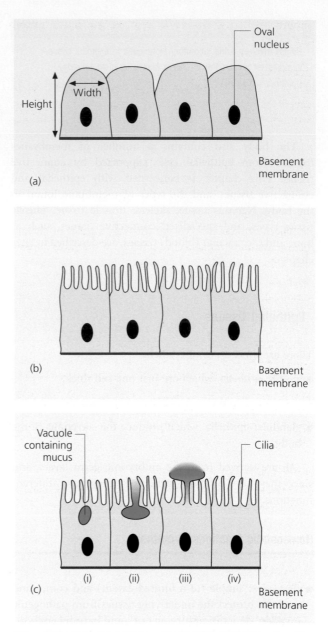

Figure 2.21   Columnar epithelium. (a) Side view. (b) Bearing microvilli. (c) Containing goblet cells bearing cilia: (i) goblet cell producing vacuole of mucus; (ii) vacuole moves towards the surface of the epithelium, which bears the cilia; (iii) secretion of mucus across the surface of the epithelium; (iv) process.

Compound epithelia

Compound (or stratified) epithelial tissue consists of two or more layers of cells. Only the basal layer lies in contact with a basement membrane. Cells of the other layers are derived from this layer. Compound epithelia are found wherever mechanical stresses are present, e.g. at the surface of the skin. One of their functions is to protect underlying tissues; others produce secretions, e.g. those lining the mouth and the anus. Stratified epithelia are named according to the shape of the surface cells.

Stratified squamous epithelia

These epithelia are found wherever mechanical stresses are severe. The basal cuboidal, or columnar cells are in contact with the basement membrane, and are actively dividing.

Exercise

Identify the type of cell division associated with basal cells.

The new daughter cells go through a series of changes before attaining the squamous shape of the most superficial cells. These cells are sloughed off during times of friction. Locations include the lining of the mouth, tongue, oesophagus and vagina, i.e. wet areas that are subjected to wear and tear.

Keratinized stratified squamous epithelia

This is a particular form of squamous epithelium in which the cells contain the waterproofing protein keratin. This enhances the barrier properties of the tissue, making it resistant to friction and aiding the prevention of pathogenic invasion. The epidermis of the skin is an example of this type of epithelium.

Stratified cuboidal epithelium

The role of this tissue is mainly protective. It is located in sweat glands, the pharynx and the epiglottis.

Stratified columnar epithelia

The functions of this tissue are protection and secretion. It is located in the male urethra, and in the lactiferous ducts of the mammary glands.

Transitional epithelia

This is usually made of three or four layers of cells, and is a tissue capable of being stretched. Before stretching, it has a cuboidal shape; when stretched, the cells have a squamous appearance (Figure 2.22). Its expansion properties help prevent rupture of the organ in which it is found, e.g. the lining of the urinary bladder.

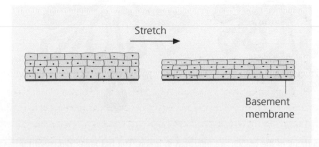

Figure 2.22 Side view of transitional epithelium.

Pseudo-stratified epithelium

This tissue appears to be an epithelium of several layers of columnar or cuboidal cells. It is, in fact, a simple epithelium as all the cells have direct contact with the basement membrane (Figure 2.23). Examples of location are the lining of the larger excretory ducts of many glands, and parts of the Eustachian tube, which connects the middle ear with the throat (or pharynx).

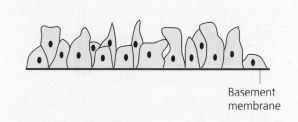

Basement membrane

Figure 2.23 Side view of pseudo-stratified epithelium.
Q. How are epithelial tissues classified?
Q. Where would you expect to find the following tissues: (i) simple cubical epithelium with microvilli; (ii) simple squamous epithelium; (iii) pseudo-stratified epithelium; (iv) transitional epithelium?

Glandular epithelia

This type of epithelium secretes various substances from glandular cells, which either cover a lining epithelium or lie deep in a covering epithelium. The production and secretion of substances requires energy expenditure, therefore the cells have a high mitochondria content. In addition, they usually have an abundance of endoplasmic reticulum and Golgi apparatus, which are responsible for the production and packaging of the secretions.

Glands are classified as either exocrine or endocrine. Their embryological development is summarized in Figure 2.24.

Exocrine glands

Exocrine glands secrete their substances into ducts (either as simple or compound exocrine glands) or directly on to a free surface (Figure 2.25). Secretions from exocrine glands, which are watery, are referred to as serous secretions. In contras, mucus glands produce viscous (mucous) secretions.

Most glands in the body are exocrine, including:

● *sweat glands*: secrete sweat or perspire to cool the skin. Sweat also contains excretory products such as urea (see Chapter 16);

● *digestive glands*: the secretions from these glands break down food materials, providing blood and hence body cells with their nutrient requirements (see Chapter 10);

- *ceruminous glands:* secrete earwax (cerumen), which adheres to atmospheric dust particles and microbes that have entered the outer ear canal, thus preventing their entry into the delicate organs of the inner ear (see Chapter 7);

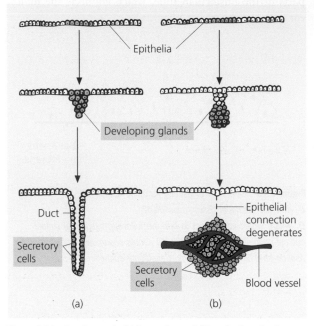

Figure 2.24 Development of (a) exocrine and (b) endocrine glands.

- *lachrymal glands:* moisturize and cleanse the surface of the eye by secreting tears. They also contain antibodies, thus act as an external defence mechanism (see Chapters 7 and 13).

Exocrine glands are classified according to the complexity of their ducts, e.g. simple or compound glands, the shape of their secretory structure, e.g. simple or compound tubular (Figure 2.25), or how the gland releases its secretion (Figure 2.26). The mode of secretion is referred to as holocrine, apocrine or merocrine:

- *Holocrine ('holos-' = entire) glands.* Secretion from these glands occurs after the entire cell has become packed with secretions causing them finally to lyse or burst, thus releasing these secretions (Figure 2.26(a)). Future secretions from this tissue depend upon the lysed cell being replaced by the mitotic division of stem cells. An example is the skin's sebaceous (oil) gland cells.

- *Apocrine ('apo-' = off) glands.* The secretory products accumulate at the margin of the cell's membrane (Figure 2.26(b)). This portion, together with the surrounding cytoplasm, pinches off from the rest of the cell to form the secretion. Further secretions require a period of anabolic reconstruction of the secretory products. An example is the mammary (lactiferous) glands.

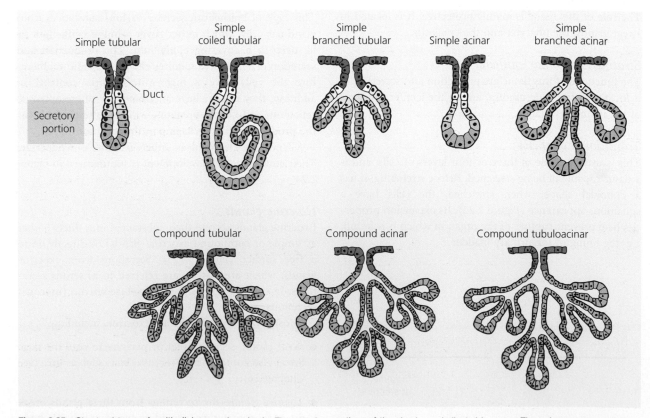

Figure 2.25 Structural types of multicellular exocrine glands. The secretory portions of the glands are indicated in green. The red areas represent the ducts of the glands.

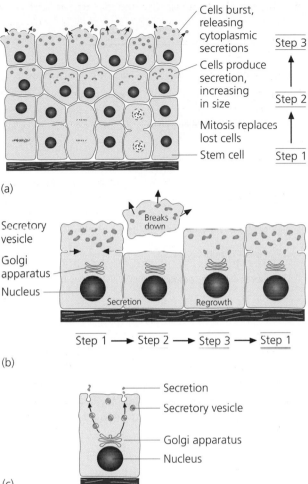

(a)

(b)

(c)

Figure 2.26 Mechanisms of glandular secretion. (a) Holocrine secretion occurs when superficial gland cells break apart. (b) Apocrine secretion involves the loss of cytoplasm. Inclusions, secretory vesicles and other cytoplasmic components may be shed in the process. (c) In merocrine secretion, secretory vesicles are discharged at the surface of the gland cell through exocytosis.

Q. How do apocrine, merocrine, and holocrine glands differ from each another?

- *Merocrine ('meros-' = part) glands.* These cells provide their secretory products in vesicles, which are then exocytosed (Figure 2.26(c)). Salivary glands are examples of merocrine tissue.

Endocrine glands

Endocrine glands do not have ducts, and therefore are sometimes referred to as ductless glands. These glands secrete their products (i.e. hormones) directly into the circulatory system, which takes them to a site of action in their target tissues. The endocrine system, together with the nervous system, co-ordinates all bodily activities in order to provide overall homeostatic functions. The main endocrine glands are considered in Chapter 9.

Mixed glands

Mixed glands contain a mixture of exocrine and endocrine glandular tissue. The pancreas is an example, secreting a variety of hormones (see Chapter 9) from its endocrine glandular tissue and a host of digestive enzymes (see Chapter 10) from its exocrine tissue. The male gonads, the testes, are another example.

Exercise

Refer to Chapter 18 to identify the exocrine and endocrine secretions of the testes.

Connective tissues

Connective tissues are the most common tissue type in the body. Their general functions are to:

- protect the delicate organs that they surround;
- provide a structural framework for the body;
- support and bind other interconnecting tissue types within organs;
- transport substances from one region to another;
- protect against potential pathogenic invaders;
- store energy reserves.

The binding and supportive connective tissues are highly vascular. An exception is cartilaginous connective tissues, which are avascular ('a-' = absence), and as a consequence repair is not perfect following damage. These various tissues have distinct diverse appearances, but all have three common characteristics: they all possess a fluid, jelly-like or solid ground substance called a matrix, various cell types responsible for secretion of the matrix, and various protein fibres.

Connective tissues can be subdivided into the 'true' (proper) connective tissues, and those that are specialized for particular functions (Figure 2.27).

True connective tissues

These contain a viscous matrix and two types of cell:

- *Fixed (immobile) cells.* Some of these cells have homeo-static repair functions (e.g. stem cells, fibroblasts or fibrocytes), whereas others have homeostatic defence functions (e.g. macrophages) or storage functions (e.g. adipocytes, melanocytes).
- *Wandering cells.* These cells have varying properties. Mobile defence cells (e.g. macrophages, mast cells) go to sites of injury, and produce and release substances such

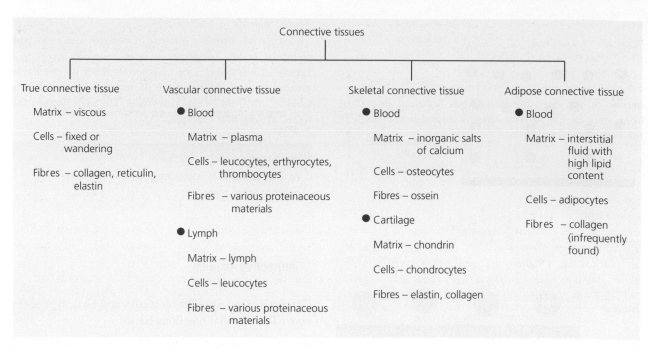

Figure 2.27 Connective tissue classification.

as histamine and heparin at the site, which have local circulatory effects. T- and B-lymphocytes are wandering cells responsible for the cellular and humoral immune responses (see Chapter 13).

Three different kinds of protein fibres are associated with connective tissues. Collagen fibres are long, straight, stiff and strong, and provide tensile strength. Reticular fibres, made of reticulin, are interwoven between the collagen fibres, adding flexibility to the properties provided by the collagen. Elastic fibres, made of elastin, are branched and stretchable, and give the tissue some elastic properties.

There are four types of true connective tissue: white fibrous tissue, yellow elastic tissue, loose areolar connective tissue, and adipose connective tissue (Figure 2.28).

White fibrous tissue

This tissue may also be termed dense collagen tissue because of the large numbers of these closely packed fibres. There is less matrix associated with this tissue compared with loose connective tissue. The fibres are produced by types of fibrocytes located between the fibres, and are usually arranged in parallel bundles. The tissue appears

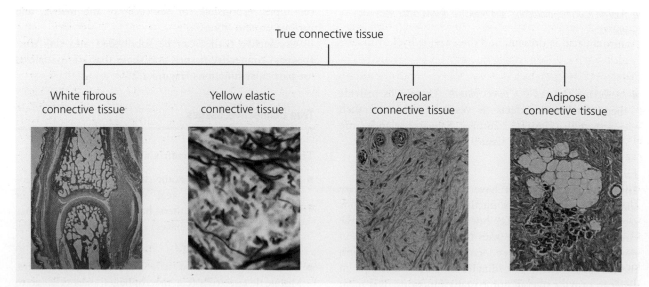

Figure 2.28 True connective tissue classification.

white or silvery, and is tough but pliable. It is found in tendons, which attach muscles to bone, and in ligaments, which strengthen joints between bones.

Less frequently, the fibres are arranged in an irregular fashion. These tissues form the fascia of muscles, the dermis of the skin, the periosteum (external lining) of bone, and the supportive capsules around organs such as the kidneys and testes.

Yellow elastic tissue

This connective tissue is composed of elastin fibres produced by another type of fibrocyte. These fibres make a loose branching network, and are capable of stretching and returning to their original position. Much more matrix is present than in white fibrous tissue. Examples of location are in those ligaments that must provide more elasticity than collagen ligaments, the trachea, bronchial tubes, true vocal cords, lungs, and the walls of arteries.

Loose areolar connective tissue

This tissue contains the three different types of connective tissue fibres – collagen, elastin and reticulin – and thus has the properties of all three. Cell types present depend upon location, but include macrophages, plasma cells (antibody-producing cells derived from B-lymphocytes), melanocytes (melanin-producing cells), and adipocytes (fat-storing cells). Consequently, this tissue has defence, protective and energy-storage homeostatic functions. Loose connective tissue is found throughout the body. Examples are the mucus membranes, the outer layers of blood vessels and nerves, the choroid layer of the eye, the covering of muscles, the mesenteries of the gut, and the subcutaneous layer of the skin.

The collagen fibres of the subcutaneous layer of the skin firmly fix the skin to the muscle underneath, although the elastin fibres allow some stretching of the skin and allow the skin to recoil immediately, whilst the reticulin fibres add flexibility. A thick viscous matrix of hyaluronic acid is present, and the enzyme hyaluronidase (which breaks down hyaluronic acid) may be added to hypodermic injections, as this changes the constitution of the matrix into a water consistency and so aids the transportation of drugs, reduces tension, and eases the pain of injection. Some bacteria, macrophages and sperm cells also utilize this enzyme to increase their penetrative capacity.

Adipose connective tissue

This tissue is concerned with the storage of fat. It contains large, fat-containing cells, or adipocytes, but has little matrix and few fibres. It is located subcutaneously (as the fat of the skin) around vital organs, such as the kidneys, at the base and the surface of the heart, and in the marrow of long bones. Its homeostatic functions are the storage and provision of energy (mobilized fatty acids

> ## BOX 2.26 LIPOSUCTION
>
> Suction lipectomy, or liposuction, is the removal of subcutaneous fat ('lipo-' = fat, '-ectomy' = removal of) from certain areas of the body, such as the buttocks, thighs, breast and abdomen. This treatment results in only temporary removal of fat, however, and is not used to treat obesity. It is usually performed for cosmetic reasons.

can be utilized by the mitochondria of most cells), insulation to reduce heat loss, and protection of organs against injury.

Other types of connective tissues are skeletal connective tissue (see Chapter 3) and vascular (blood) connective tissue (see Chapter 11).

Epithelial membranes

Epithelial membranes are not to be confused with epithelial tissue: they are a combination of an epithelium and its underlying connective tissue. They can be subdivided into serous membranes, mucous membranes and cutaneous membranes. Synovial membranes are also found around skeletal joints, but these are not epithelial membranes as they have no epithelia; instead, they are composed of loose connective tissue, elastic fibres, and fat. Synovial joints are considered in detail in Chapter 3.

Serous membranes

Serous membranes (or serosa) cover the surface of organs and consist of a loose connective tissue and a layer of mesothelium, which is an epithelial layer of cells similar to simple squamous epithelium. They are single-membranous structures, but they fold back on themselves, leaving a small space between the 'outer' and 'inner' portions; they therefore appear as a double membrane. The inner, or visceral, membrane covers the surface of the organ, and the outer or parietal layer attaches it to the wall of the cavity in which the organ lies (e.g. the visceral/parietal pleurae around the lungs and the visceral/parietal pericardia around the heart). The peritoneum, which lines the abdominal and pelvic organs, and body wall, is the largest serous membrane in the body.

Mucous membranes

Unlike serosa membranes, mucous membranes (or mucosa) line cavities that open directly to the exterior, i.e. the digestive, respiratory and reproductive tracts. The mucosa has an epithelial layer that secretes mucus. The functions of mucus are to prevent cavities from drying out, to prevent dust and potential pathogenic organisms from passing down the airways, and to lubricate food in the digestive tract so as to ease the passage through the tract and to aid the processes of digestion and absorption.

The structure of the membrane varies according to location and function. For example, in the oesophagus and the anal canal the epithelial layer is stratified, as there is much wear and tear. In the intestine, a simple columnar epithelium aids the absorption of nutrients.

Finally, the cutaneous membrane (skin) is a complex structure involving a variety of tissues. Its anatomy and function are considered in detail in Chapter 16.

Exercise

Distinguish between serous and mucous membranes.

ORGANS

An organ is an orderly grouping of tissues with a discrete function. Organs can be tubular (hollow) or compact (parenchymal).

Tubular organs

During embryological development, the body may be visualized as a large tube containing several inner tubes, such as the respiratory system, cardiovascular system, digestive system, reproductive system, and urinary system. Each of these internal tubes has various functions, but structurally they are very similar to each other in that they are all formed of layers of tissues superimposed on one another in a specific way.

Each tubular organ has three basic layers:

- an inner lining tissue, or epithelium, and its underlying binding or connective tissue;

- a middle layer, consisting of alternating layers of muscle and connective tissue;

- an external layer, consisting of connected tissue and an epithelium.

Compact organs

Compact organs may be large, e.g. the liver, or small, e.g. the ovaries. Compact organs also have a common structure. A connective tissue capsule usually encloses the organ. If the organ is suspended in a body cavity, e.g. the thoracic cavity, it will be surrounded by a serous membrane. One side of the organ has a thicker area of connective tissue that penetrates the organ, forming the hilus. Compact organs have an extensive framework of connected tissue, or stroma. Strands of connected tissue, called septae (or trabeculae), extend into the organ from the capsule and hilus, sometimes dividing the organ into complete sections called lobules. Compact organs consist of functional cells (parenchymal) that predominantly occur in masses, chords, strands or tubules, depending on the specific organ. Parenchyma may be divided into functional distinctive regions, such as an outer cortex and an inner or deeper medulla.

ORGAN SYSTEMS

An organ system is a group of organs that perform a specific body function, e.g. the respiratory system maintains the levels of oxygen and carbon dioxide in the blood. The major organ systems of the human body are summarized in Table 1.2. These systems work in a co-ordinated way to maintain the homeostatic functions of the body. The details associated with each organ are dealt with in their respective chapters.

Summary

1 A cell is the basic unit of life, the smallest component capable of performing the basic characteristics of life.

2 Enzymes and ATP are the key chemicals of life. Enzymes regulate the rate of metabolic reactions so that they are compatible with life. ATP provides the energy to drive metabolism.

3 Cells vary in size, shape and function. The shape of a cell is related closely to its function, a phenomenon referred to as the principle of complementary structure and function.

4 Intracellular homeostasis is vital to the health of the individual, owing to the interdependency of the body's component parts.

5 Each organ system is an indirect homeostatic regulator of cellular metabolism.

6 The cell's passive and active transporting mechanisms are homeostatic control processes, since they help to determine the concentration of intracellular metabolites so that the characteristics of life can be performed.

7 Cellular components – organelles – have precise homeostatic functions that are essential in maintaining intracellular homeostasis.

8 The control of organelle function depends on the production of enzymes, the synthesis of which is genetically controlled and environmentally modified, perhaps according to the principles underpinning the Operon theory.

9 Homeostatic failures may result from: inborn or inherited errors of metabolism (see Chapter 20); inappropriate numbers of chromosomes (see Chapter 20); the effects of environmental agents, e.g. overexposure to UV radiation can produce skin cancer; and the ageing process (see Chapter 20).

10 Clinical intervention is often based upon correcting the genetic failure. This can be direct, e.g. chemotherapy or genetic engineering, or indirect, e.g. through medical or surgical intervention, or by adapting one's lifestyle to avoid harmful environmental agents.

11 Tissues perform specialized homeostatic functions essential for the maintenance of overall body homeostasis.

12 There are four principal tissues: epithelial, connective, nervous and muscle tissues. Membranes are composites of epithelial and connective tissue.

13 The principal tissues are classified according to the number of cell layers they possess, their structure and their function.

14 The principle of complementary structure and function predestines the tissue's location. Epithelial tissues, for example, may possess specialized structures such as microvilli, which increase their surface area – these are present in areas concerned with absorption.

15 Glandular epithelia may be simple or multicellular. Their secretions are defined as apocrine, holocrine or merocrine according to how they are released from the cell.

16 Connective tissues possess cells and their products, i.e. fibres and a matrix. They are classified according to the fibre distribution (loose or dense), and usually by the type of fibre they possess (elastin, reticulin and collagen). The exception is adipose connective tissue, which is named after its specialized fat-storage cells, adipocytes.

17 Membranes may be serous, mucous, cutaneous or synovial, the latter being the only membrane that does not contain an epithelium and so is not an epithelial membrane.

Review questions

1 Cells come in many shapes and sizes but have certain features in common. Draw a diagram of a typical cell, and label each structure.

2 Discuss the functions of the following: (i) nucleus, (ii) nuclear membrane, (iii) nucleoplasm, (iv) nucleoli, (v) chromatin, (vi) centrosome, (vii) mitochondria, (viii) cytoplasm, (ix) endoplasmic reticulum, (x) Golgi apparatus, (xi) ribosomes and (xii) lysosomes.

3 Draw a diagram of the plasma membrane. Why can it be described as selectively permeable? Does this mean all harmful substances are not able to gain access to the cell?

4 Define these terms: (i) passive transport, (ii) diffusion, (iii) facilitated diffusion, (iv) osmosis, (v) filtration, (vi) active transport, (vii) bulk transport, (viii) anabolism and (ix) catabolism.

5 Drugs act at cell level. How does a drug know which cells to target?

6 How do drugs reach target cells?

7 How do drugs achieve their effects?

8 Try and answer questions 5–7 for drugs you are using yourself or in your practice.

REFERENCES

Basketter, H.M., Sharples, L. and Bilton, D. (2000) Knowledge of pancreatic enzyme supplementation in adult cystic fibrosis (CF) patients. *Journal of Human Nutrition and Dietetics* **13**(5): 353–61.

Danielli and Davson (1969) cited in Davson, H. (1970) *A Textbook of General Physiology*, 4th edn. Edinburgh: Churchill Livingstone.

Department of Health (1995) The genetics of common diseases. A second report to the NHS Central Research and Development Committee on the new genetics. London: Department of Health Publications.

Hinds, C. and Moyer, A. (1997) Support as experienced by patients with cancer during radiotherapy treatments. *Journal of Advanced Nursing* **26**(2): 371–9.

Jacob, F. and Monod, J. (1961) Genetic regulatory mechanisms in the synthesis of proteins. *Journal of Molecular Biology* **3**(5): 318–56.

Lea, D.H. (1997) Gene therapy: current and future implications for oncology nursing practice. *Seminars in Oncology Nursing* **13**(2): 115–22.

Lees, C.M., Davies, S. and Dezateux, C. (2001) Neonatal screening for sickle cell disease. The Cochrane Library, Issue 1. Oxford: Update Software.

McCaughan, F.M. and Thompson, K.A. (2000) Information needs of cancer patients receiving chemotherapy at a day-case unit in Northern Ireland. *Journal of Clinical Nursing* **9**(6): 851–8.

Moran, P. (2000) Cellular effects of cancer chemotherapy administration. *Journal of Intravenous Nursing* **23**(1): 44–51.

Munro, C.L. (1999) Implications for nursing of the Human Genome Project. *Neonatal Network* **18**(3): 7–12.

Poustie, V.J. and Rutler, P. (2001) Dietary interventions for phenylketonuria. The Cochrane Library, Issue 1. Oxford: Update Software.

Singer, S.J. and Nicolson, G.L. (1972) The fluid mosaic model of the structure of the cell membranes. *Science* **175**(18 February): 720–31.

Watson, J.D. and Crick, F.H.C. (1953) Molecular structure of nucleic acids: a structure for deoxypentose nucleic acids. *Nature* **171**: 737. [The original description of the DNA helix.]

FURTHER READING

Beery, T.A. (2000) The evolving role of genetics in the diagnosis and management of heart disease. *Nursing Clinics of North America* **35**(4): 963–73.

Koch, R.K. (1999) Issues in newborn screening for phenylketonuria. *American Family Physician* **60**(5): 1462–6.

Merelle M.E., Nagelkerke, A.F., Lees, C.M. and Dezateux, C. (2001) Newborn screening for cystic fibrosis. The Cochrane Library, Issue 1. Oxford: Update Software.

Chapter 3

The skeleton

INTRODUCTION

The skeleton and its associated muscles support the body against gravity. This system is usually considered as the skeletomuscular system, but the skeleton is an organ system in its own right, and this chapter is concerned with its role in body support. However, this is only one of the roles performed by bone. Other roles include:

- *Strength and protection.* The presence of bone makes the body resilient to impact, whilst the bony 'box' of the skull and the cage-like structure of the ribs provide protection for vital underlying organs.

- *Calcium phosphate store.* The body contains a relatively large amount of calcium phosphate, the bulk of which is found in bone mineral. The skeleton therefore acts as a reservoir of calcium and phosphate ions that can be accessed by the body if the blood becomes deficient in them, or that can be added to if there is excess in blood.

- *Synthesis of blood cells.* Although not strictly speaking a role of bone, this is a role of the skeleton. Bone marrow provides the main site of blood cell production in adults.

The latter two processes are explored elsewhere in this book. This chapter is concerned with the ways in which bone structure and the skeleton provide support and protection for the body. The chapter therefore describes the structure of bone, and the construction of the skeleton and its joints, and also highlights aspects of skeletal structure that facilitate the maintenance of an upright posture and the absorption of stresses during movement.

ANATOMY AND PHYSIOLOGY OF BONE

Structure of bone

A common image of the skeleton is of a collection of oddly shaped, dry, dead bones. Whilst there is no doubt that bones are strangely shaped, the reality is that our skeleton is comprised of a dynamic living tissue that is continually remodelled throughout life.

Essentially, bone is comprised of a connective tissue. This means that it consists of a matrix of protein (collagen and others, including a special bone protein called ossein) that is secreted by specialized cells. Its supportive strength comes from the deposition of mineral (a mixture of calcium phosphate and calcium carbonate called hydroxyapatite) in the matrix, but the matrix conveys a certain degree of flexibility to bones.

Although they are strong, bones are also comparatively light; this is facilitated by the presence of internal spongy bone tissue (called cancellous bone or trabecular bone), and by cavities. The cavities may be filled with marrow tissue, adipose tissue, or even air in the facial sinuses. The main strength of bone, however, arises from an outer layer of dense mineralized tissue called compact bone.

Compact bone

Compact bone is the very hard and dense material that people normally associate with bone. Close examination of a cross-section reveals it to have a complex structure. It consists of minute cylindrical structures (less than 0.5 mm in diameter) called osteons or Haversian systems (Figure 3.1). Osteons are comprised of concentric layers, or lamellae, of bone that enclose a central, or Haversian, canal. This canal runs along the axis of the bone, and conveys blood vessels, lymphatic vessels and neurons into the bone tissue of the osteon. Side canals radiate into the lamellae, enabling blood to perfuse much of the compact bone structure. Other smaller channels, called canaliculi, branch from the side canals. These are too small to permit the passage of blood vessels, and are filled with tissue fluid. Expansions of the canaliculi (called lacunae) contain the bone cells (or osteocytes; 'osteo-' = bone). Nutrients must diffuse from vessels within the side canals, along the canaliculi to the osteocytes.

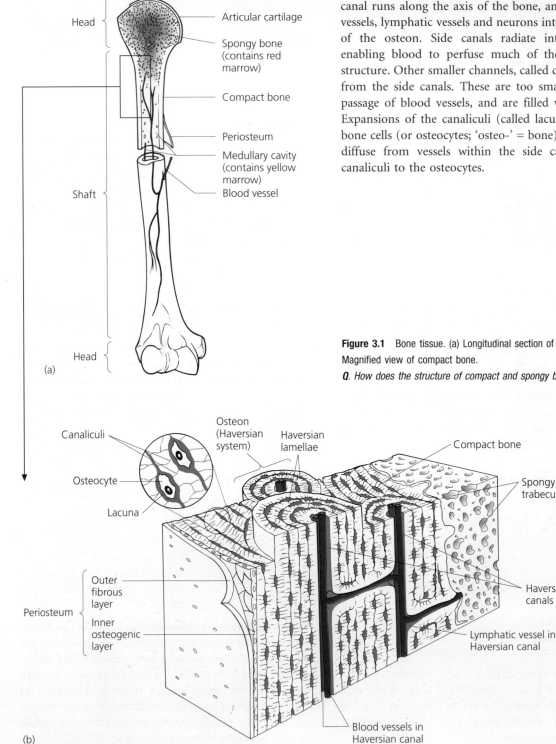

Figure 3.1 Bone tissue. (a) Longitudinal section of a long bone. (b) Magnified view of compact bone.

Q. How does the structure of compact and spongy bone differ?

Infections of bone can be blood-borne (see Box 3.8) or, more commonly, they can arise in open or compound fractures where there is tissue injury. Bone infections may lead to the formation of a fluid-filled area of necrotic tissue called an abscess. An abscess is a swelling that contains pus, i.e. detritus from dead cells and perhaps microorganisms. Abscesses are problematic even in soft tissues, but at least these tissues provide the possibility of drainage without causing too much structural damage. Abscesses in bone are more difficult to treat:

● Bone abscesses are very painful. Soft tissues expand to accommodate the accumulation of pus, but the hard structure of bone prevents this, so pressure builds up.

● Draining an abscess will often necessitate damaging the bone in order to gain access to the area.

● The absence of a blood supply through the canaliculi means that microorganisms present within the lacuni are not easily accessed by the immune system cells. Similarly, the delivery of blood-borne agents such as antibodies will be less effective. For this reason, bone infections will be treated aggressively with high doses of antibiotics.

The loss of bone may be extensive, and lead to a prolonged period of immobility. This also has implications for the patient (see Box 3.5).

The blood vessels in bone originate from the outer covering of bone, which is a fibrous membrane called the periosteum (see below). The layer of compact bone is usually perforated at points by nutrient foramina (nutrient 'windows') that permit blood vessels to enter and drain the tissue. Branches of these vessels not only provide blood for cells within the compact bone, but also supply the underlying spongy bone and the marrow within the bone cavity.

Trabecular bone

Trabecular (cancellous or spongy) bone consists of a meshwork of calcified 'beams' called trabeculae (Figure 3.1) that give it the appearance of a sponge. The meshwork is rigid and is constructed along the lines of greatest pressure exerted on the bone. These minute 'archways' and 'beams' provide considerable strength. The spaces within the meshwork help to reduce bone weight.

Osteoporosis

In osteoporosis, the bone retains its general structure, but its strength is reduced as a consequence of loss of bone mass (Rosen, 2000). Spongy bone seems to be most affected, but the site of loss can be local or more general. The loss of bone mineral is normal during the lifespan, commencing when we are in our 40s. As mineral is lost, the antigravity support of bone is compromised, which brings with it a substantial increase in the risk of fracture and loss of mobility. Compression fractures of the vertebrae, and fractures of the neck of femur, are frequent consequences of the loss of bone strength (Leslie, 2000).

Osteoporosis is a common problem in older people. It occurs in both men and women, but its consequences are more frequently observed in women. This is because men generally have stronger (i.e. more calcified) bones than women, and because the hormonal changes that occur around the menopause accelerate mineral loss in women. Sex steroid hormones influence bone mineralization during puberty, which seems to be important in maintaining bone density. The withdrawal of oestrogen after the menopause makes women particularly vulnerable to osteoporosis, and the incidence of fractures is much higher in elderly women than in age-matched men. Health education is aimed at encouraging people to maintain as high a bone density as possible in earlier years through physical activity and adequate diet. The former is a direct reference to the effects that physical stress has on the activities of bone cells.

Osteomalacia

This is a rare condition in Western countries. Its cause is usually a deficiency of vitamin D. This vitamin (now thought of as a hormone) has a vital role in maintaining the calcium ion concentration in blood plasma through its promotion of calcium uptake from the bowel (see Chapter 9). A lack of vitamin D means that less calcium is available for bone mineralization. Osteomalacia differs from osteoporosis in that the bone maintains a relatively normal protein matrix, so the ratio of mineral to protein declines, making the bones softer and less supportive. This may not necessarily be due to inadequate dietary intake of the vitamin (or a synthesized source; inactive vitamin D is also made in the skin from a precursor); it could also occur as a consequence of malabsorption of the vitamin, or through a failure of the liver to activate it. The problem may also be secondary to certain tumours that secrete parathyroid hormone and so promote excessive calcium resorption from bone (Chapter 9).

The consequences of having a poorly supportive skeleton is illustrated in children who have the related condition rickets, in which the increased pliancy of the bones results in a bowing of the long bones of the legs due to the effects of gravity.

Bone marrow

Bone marrow occupies the spaces within trabecular bone and a cavity at the centre of the bone. It is a connective tissue but, unlike the surrounding bone, it is soft. Protein fibres support adipose (fat) cells and cells involved in the synthesis of blood cells. All marrow is red at birth, and the colour reflects the synthesis of red blood cells (and white, in lower numbers) that occurs there. In adults, red marrow becomes restricted to the ends of the long bones, the vertebrae, and the flat bones of the skull, pelvis, sternum and clavicle. Elsewhere, adipose tissue dominates, and the marrow becomes 'yellow' and fatty and plays little role in the production of blood cells.

BOX 3.3 FAT EMBOLISM

The yellow marrow that predominates in many bones can be problematic following bone trauma or surgery. This is because bone damage may result in fat leakage into the circulation. As a consequence, the arrival of fat globules in the coronary circulation, cerebral circulation or lung can act as emboli, and so obstruct the vessels. This may be fatal for the patient.

Periosteum

The periosteum ('peri-' = surround) is a sleeve of tough, dense, connective tissue that covers the surface of bone. The outer layer is continuous with the tendons, which attach muscle to bone, and the ligaments, which reinforce skeletal joints, so it makes a strong junction. Some fibres penetrate into the compact bone, which not only reinforces the structure but also helps to transfer forces from the moving muscles into the bone itself. The inner layer of the periosteum contains osteogenic cells, which can transform into bone cells ('-genic' = creation).

Endosteum

This is a layer of osteogenic cells that lines the canals within bone and the bone cavities. The transformation of these cells into active bone cells (see below) has an important role in bone remodelling and repair.

Bone cells

There are various types of bone cells, classified according to their role in bone:

- *Osteocytes* are the main cells of fully developed bone. They maintain the protein/mineral matrix. Many are trapped within the lacunae of compact bone.

- *Osteoblasts* produce new bone. They are responsible for calcium deposition, and will lay down new bone following injury.

- *Osteoclasts* are capable of removing mineral from the protein matrix. They are especially responsible for bone resorption during bone remodelling (see below).

- *Osteogenic cells* are found in the periosteum and endosteum. They are stem cells capable of differentiating into osteoblasts or osteoclasts during times of mechanical stress or following injury.

Bone growth

The process of bone growth is illustrated by the changes observed in a long bone such as the femur. At birth, such 'bones' are in fact largely made of cartilage (Figure 3.2). There are, however, two areas in which mineralization of the bone (ossification) is occurring: the shaft of the bone, and the ends, or epiphyses (singular = epiphysis) of the bone. The benefit of having a structure that is largely cartilaginous is that it can grow much more rapidly than one that is ossified. The disadvantage is that the 'bone' is poorly weight bearing until much of the shaft has been ossified. In an older child, the shaft is largely bone, but the epiphysis continues to be cartilaginous, except in the centre, where mineralization is still occurring, which facilitates continued growth.

Between the epiphysis and the bony shaft is an area of rapid growth called the epiphysial plate. Here cartilage-producing cells are arranged in columns that extend from the epiphysis into the shaft. The cells at the epiphysial end of these columns are reproducing rapidly. Below these, the cells are maturing, and below these cells they are becoming encased in mineral by osteoblasts. Osteoclasts will also be active, helping to extend the marrow cavity as the shaft grows in length. Thus, mineralization of the shaft is in a process of 'catch-up' with the cartilage of the epiphysial plate.

Bone diameter also increases as bone grows in length. This is caused by the activity of osteoblasts, which lay down layers of new bone beneath the periosteum.

Bone remodelling

Although it is heavily mineralized, bone continues to be altered throughout life:

- Calcium salts are deposited or removed as required by the body, e.g. in the regulation of plasma calcium ion concentration.

- There is selective deposition of mineral, which results in the changes in bone shape that are observed during growth.

- 'Old' bone is renewed, and injured bone is replaced.

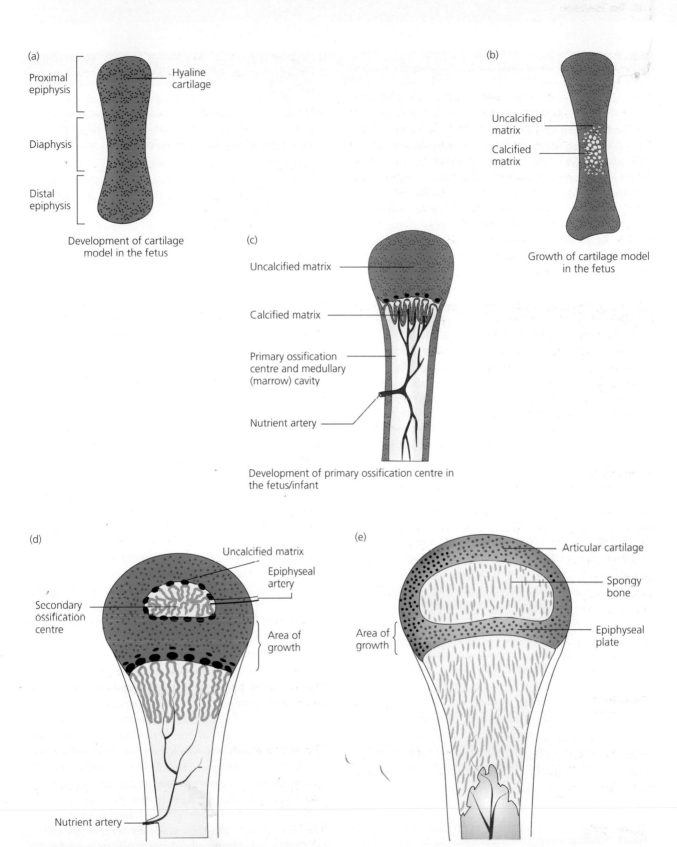

(a)

Proximal epiphysis

Diaphysis

Distal epiphysis

Hyaline cartilage

Development of cartilage model in the fetus

(b)

Uncalcified matrix

Calcified matrix

Growth of cartilage model in the fetus

(c)

Uncalcified matrix

Calcified matrix

Primary ossification centre and medullary (marrow) cavity

Nutrient artery

Development of primary ossification centre in the fetus/infant

(d)

Uncalcified matrix

Epiphyseal artery

Secondary ossification centre

Area of growth

Nutrient artery

Development of secondary ossification centre in epiphysis during childhood

(e)

Articular cartilage

Spongy bone

Epiphyseal plate

Area of growth

Formation of articular cartilage and epiphyseal plate during childhood

Figure 3.2 Bone growth at the epiphysial plate. A change in length is shown. Note how the rate of growth can be sustained only through the growth of cartilage, with ossification occurring behind. (a) Development of cartilage model in the fetus. (b) Growth of cartilage model in the fetus. (c) Development of primary ossification centre in the fetus/infant. (d) Development of secondary ossification centre in the epiphysis during childhood. (e) Formation of articular cartilage and epiphysial plate during childhood.

BOX 3.4. DEVELOPMENT: BONE GROWTH AND GROWTH PATTERNS

The rapid rate of growth that occurs during childhood occurs largely because of the activity of growth hormone, which stimulates the epiphysial plate to produce more cartilage. During puberty, the growth rate speeds up further because of the stimulatory action of sex steroids. These hormones, however, are also ultimately responsible for causing bone growth to cease. Thus, not only do they stimulate the epiphysial plate, but they also promote ossification within the shaft and within the mineralizing centre of the epiphysis. Eventually, the rate of ossification outstrips that of new cartilage growth, and the epiphysis becomes ossified and continuous with the shaft. The only remaining sign of the cartilage is a lining of the tip of the bone, as part of the anatomy of the skeletal joint.

The general pattern of body growth is similar between individuals, although there is variation in the ages at which patterns change. There are slight sex differences in growth rate, with girls tending to grow faster during middle childhood years, but boys exceeding girls during later childhood. Both sexes exhibit a pronounced increase in limb length relative to trunk length, and a broadening of the shoulders, chest and trunk.

Growth charts are used to document growth rates in children. Variation between children is acknowledged, but the charts allow for this by providing the expected range for both boys and girls. They must be used with caution, however, in multi-ethnic populations since such standardized charts do not allow for cultural variations. The monitoring of growth rates is usually performed within community-based care; in particular, it is one of the roles of the community nurse.

Q. Standardized growth charts utilize percentiles. What does this mean?

The latter two processes involve the removal of mineral from one part of the bone and deposition in another. Resorption of mineral normally precedes deposition, so osteoclasts are active for a period then followed by osteoblast activity.

Physical stress placed on bone is an important stimulus to promote such bone remodelling, with calcium deposition in the 'stressed' areas being favoured. This process ensures maximum strength at the most load-bearing points within the skeleton, such as the femur head. The process is more effective in young adults than in older people because the activity of these bone cells is greatest in young people and slows during middle age. Nevertheless, the osteoclasts and osteoblasts continually act to renew bone throughout life.

Bone, then, is a dynamic tissue, yet the control of bone density and shape is little understood. Certainly the hormones parathyroid hormone, calcitonin and vitamin D have an influence on bone mineral, but their release and actions relate to the homeostatic control of plasma calcium concentration (see Chapter 9) and not to modelling and remodelling of bone. Growth hormone and the sex steroids also have an influence during childhood and puberty, but much remains to be discovered.

Bone healing

Fractures or breaks in bone are caused when the forces applied exceed the capacity of the bone to resist them. This may result from accidental application of excessive physical stress on a bone, but it can also arise during normal activity if bone density and/or flexibility are severely compromised, e.g. in osteoporosis. The different types of fracture are shown in Figure 3.3.

The main processes involved in wound healing were explained in Chapter 2. Healing of bone follows the usual pattern, but there are some subtle differences, since body support depends upon a strong skeletal structure. The tissue is actually very good at reorganising itself, partly because mechanisms are in place that provide continual remodelling. Wound healing simply has to step up these mechanisms.

The fracture and resulting inflammatory response will activate macrophages and other leucocytes, which instigate debris removal, activation of fibrocytes, and granulation as part of the normal healing process. The main difference in bone healing is that the new bone matrix will have to be laid down and mineralized, and the entire structure reorganized, so that compact bone and spongy bone is formed. Thus, the activities of bone cells must be promoted so that bone structure is returned to how it was before the fracture.

This is achieved by a change in the activity of osteogenic cells. Osteogenic cells in the periosteum/endosteum are converted to osteoblasts, which then begin to produce new bone in the fracture area. The role of these cells is usually to form a hardened mass around the fracture site, called a callus. This provides strength to the fracture area, and enables the bone to be brought back into (tentative) use. Osteoclast activity will then gradually remove the callus, and further osteoblasts will redeposit calcium according to the required bone shape and structure. The bone will eventually regain its full structure, although the process may take several months for completion. Once a bone has basically healed after injury, the patient should be encouraged to undertake light exercise, because this promotes an increase in bone density.

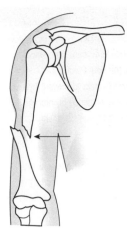

(a) Open fracture/displaced i.e. skin broken and fragments separated.

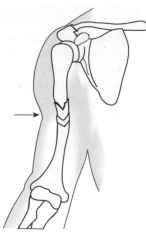

(b) Comminuted fracture i.e. bonebroken in 2 or more places. Fragmented.

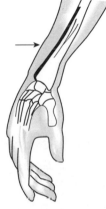

(c) Greenstick fracture i.e. fracture extends only part way through the bone Usually in children.

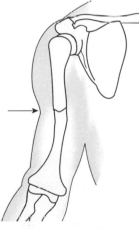

(d) Impacted fracture.

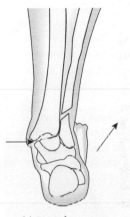

(e) Pott's fracture

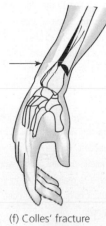

(f) Colles' fracture

Direction of fracture		
Type of fracture	Features	
Transverse	Across the bone	
Oblique	At an oblique angle to the longitudinal axis of the bone	
Spiral	Fracture forms spiral ëtwistí encircling bone; produced by rotatory force	
Linear	Parallel to the longitudinal axis of the bone	

Accordingtodeformingforce		
Type of fracture	Features	
Compression	Adjacent cancellous bones compacted; usually heals rapidly due to minimal soft tissue in jury caused by deforming force	
Avulsion	Bone pulled apart; ligaments remain intact	
Stress	Undisplaced microfracture caused by repetitive stress.	

Figure 3.3 Types of bone fracture.

Q. Name the osteocytes involved in bone healing.

BOX 3.5 CONSEQUENCES OF BONE TRAUMA

The supportive role of bone frequently cannot be utilized following bone trauma, especially of those bones that help to support the body against gravity. Immobility has the following risks:

- *Joint stiffness and contractures.* This could reflect muscle contracture or possible fibrosis of the joint capsule. Physiotherapy and the maintenance of limb movement are essential to prevent this complication, which has led to the concept of 'passive exercise'. Although exercise cannot really be considered to be passive, this term reflects the use of extrinsic manipulation of the limb to flex and extend the joint (see Box 17.8).
- *Deep vein thrombosis.* Blood clotting is promoted if blood flow is compromised, either because of localized hypoxia or because trauma has stimulated it. Immobility increases the risk of thrombosis in the legs because the use of muscle to return blood to the heart is compromised and so blood flow is poor. Limb pain, especially during muscle use, may be an indicator of thrombosis, particularly if it is accompanied by tenderness and swelling. Deep breathing and limb exercise will facilitate returning the blood to the heart, as will compression stockings (which reduce the capacity of the limb veins). Early mobilization will also help to reduce the risk.

- *Decubitus ulcers (pressure sores).* Immobility can restrict blood flow to the skin and induce hypoxia (poor tissue oxygenation), since weight compresses the tissue against the bed. Frequent repositioning or using a ripple mattress will help to prevent hypoxia. Good skin hygiene will help to reduce the incidence of infection, and will also facilitate regular assessment of skin condition.

Other possible complications of bone trauma are:

- *Fat embolism.* The release of fats from adipose tissue within yellow bone marrow may lead to blockage within coronary or pulmonary vessels, producing symptoms such as tachycardia or hypoxia.
- *Necrosis of bone.* Bone cells, especially those within compact bone, receive little or no blood, even in good health. They depend upon diffusion of nutrients from vessels within the vicinity. Bone trauma can remove blood flow completely, leading to cell death. Decisions on mobilizing must take into account the possibility of bone necrosis, since pressure applied to the wound could compromise blood supply further still.
- *Infection.* This is of particular concern if the skin has been broken. Pain, swelling, pus and pyrexia are indicators. Bone infections are difficult to treat once they become established because of the poor blood supply to bone cells.

BOX 3.6 MANAGEMENT OF FRACTURES

There is no single plan for the management of fractures, since the severity of injury, involvement of soft tissue, and age of the patient are all variables. The objectives of management are to:

- use manipulation and/or traction to regain the correct position/alignment of the bones, and to restore bone fragments to their normal position;
- immobilize as necessary (see below);
- observe for the presence of neuropathy, or respiratory or mental distress (perhaps indicative of fat emboli; see Box 3.3), or of shock (due to bleeding);
- rehabilitate using mobility/load-bearing exercises (see Box 17.8).

Immobilizing

Immobilizing usually uses plaster casting, fixation of the fracture with a metal pin or plate, or traction. External fixation devices may also be used. Casts are made from layers of bandage impregnated with plaster, resin or fibreglass. They are used to immobilize a joint, and to hold bone fragments in alignment. The type of cast used depends upon the joint to be fixated. Care includes observing for signs of nerve or circulatory problems, such as cool extremities, pain, discoloration, tingling/numbness, weak pulse, paralysis and necrosis.

Where bone fragmentation is extensive, the pieces may be held together with internal fixation. The pins etc. will often be removed

as healing progresses, or they may be left in situ either because removal is not feasible or in order to strengthen the resulting new bone.

Traction (and casting, pins etc.) aids realignment of broken bones and ensures immobilization of the joint/body part. Traction is used in complex situations where there is patient immobility. Not only does it immobilize a joint, it also encourages blood supply/healing in the damaged area, and helps to prevent contractures from developing. In skin traction, force (i.e. weights) is applied to the skin, e.g. via a foam rubber strip. In skeletal traction, force is applied directly to the skeleton via pins or wires implanted at strategic points. In each case, the amount of force applied will require monitoring and perhaps adjusting, and skin care will be important. With skeletal traction, care must also be taken to prevent infection around the inserted pins (Mellett, 1998).

External fixation devices are useful to support a complex fracture where fragment movement is possible even with casting or traction. The devices are especially useful if there is an open wound, as they permit wound care. Such devices may also be used to realign bones in young children with congenital abnormalities. In this case, the devices encourage appropriate growth.

Bone shape and external features

Bones are found in various shapes and sizes, according to function, but some generalizations can be made:

- *Long bones*. Bone length is greater than bone width. Long bones are found in the limbs. They provide a wide scope for body movement, but also help to absorb the stresses of body weight.

- *Short bones*. These bones are of nearly equal width and length. They are generally not strong, but produce flexible structures, such as the wrist and ankle.

- *Flat bones*. These are thin, plate-like bones. Their roles are to provide protection, e.g. the skull, and to provide an extensive surface area for the attachment of large muscles, e.g. the shoulder blade or scapula.

- *Irregular bones*. These are bones with complex shapes that are related to their functions, e.g. the bones of the vertebral column.

- *Sesamoid bones*. These bones strengthen tendons. The kneecap, or patella, is the main example.

Bones also have many irregular external features, arising from the need for muscle/ligament attachment, articulating joints between bones, and (sometimes) the passage of blood vessels, nerves and lymphatic vessels:

- Protrusions that serve primarily for muscle attachment are referred to as processes, tubercles (tuberosities) or trochanters.

- Condyles are protrusions that form an articulating surface and so have a smooth area lined, in life, with joint cartilage.

- Some bones, particularly the flat bones, are strengthened by ridges of bone called crests or spines.

- In some bones, the passage of vessels/nerves is facilitated by a notch or groove on the bone.

ANATOMY OF THE SKELETON

Axial skeleton

The skeleton is comprised of 206 bones. It can be divided into the axial and the appendicular skeletons.

The axial skeleton consists of the skull, vertebral column (backbone), ribs and sternum (breastbone), and the hyoid bone, i.e. the bones that form the vertical axis of the body (Figure 3.4).

The skull

The skull consists of 8 cranial bones and 14 facial bones. The cranium forms a bony 'box' that surrounds and protects the brain. The bones are smooth on the outside but uneven internally as a consequence of brain shape and the presence of blood vessels. Vessels and nerves gain access to the cranial cavity via openings in the skull; for example, the spinal cord enters via the foramen magnum at the base of the skull (Figure 3.5). The cerebral lobes and the cerebellum of the brain produce three distinct bulges, called fossae, on the bones of the cranium.

The facial bones provide attachment for facial muscles, form the mandible (lower jaw), protect cavities such as those of the nose, eyes and sinuses, and form the palate of the mouth. The nomenclature of facial bones is complex, sometimes referring to associated tissues (e.g. the nasolachrymal ducts, which conduct tears from the eye

orbit to the nasopharynx, and pass through the lachrymal bones of the orbit), but usually referring to the classical names of facial anatomy (e.g. the zygomatic bones form the prominences of the cheeks or zygoma).

The major bones of the skull are shown in Figure 3.5. Most of the joints between them are fixed, i.e. held tightly by cartilage and dense connective tissue, and do not perform any kind of movement. These are the sutures of the cranium, and the fused joints between many facial bones. Cranial sutures do not form fully until some time after birth.

BOX 3.7 THE FETAL SKULL

Head size at birth is large relative to that of the trunk (Figure 3.6). At birth, the brain weighs about 25% of its final adult weight. The brain grows rapidly; this is facilitated by the incomplete jointing of cranial bones, which results in the presence in the infant of membrane-covered spaces called fontanelles. Most fontanelles close during the first few months, but the anterior fontanelle is not closed fully for 18–24 months. The actual joints, or sutures, do not form until after 5 years of age, by which time growth of the brain and cranium has slowed considerably.

In contrast to the fixed joints of the skull, the mandibular joint between the mandible and the temporal bone of the cranium allows a wide range of movement: mouth opening, closing, protrusion, retraction and side-to-side movement. The range of articulation is essential because it aids food chewing, and communication through facial expression.

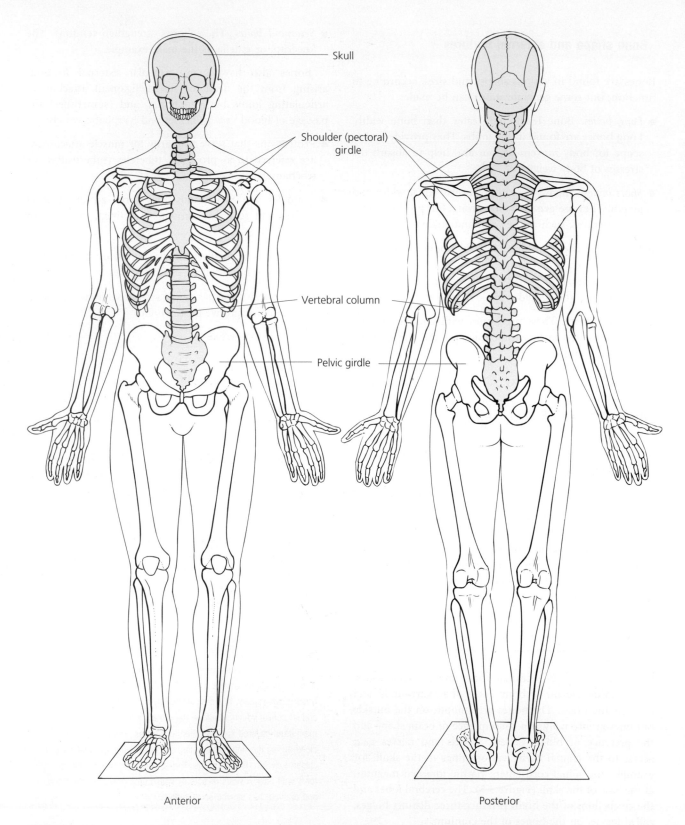

Skull

Shoulder (pectoral) girdle

Vertebral column

Pelvic girdle

Anterior

Posterior

Figure 3.4 The two major divisions of the skeletal system: the axial and appendicular skeletons. The axial skeleton is highlighted.

Q. List the bones associated with each division of the skeletal system.

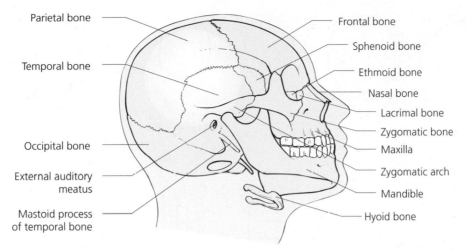

Parietal bone

Frontal bone

Temporal bone

Sphenoid bone

Ethmoid bone

Nasal bone

Lacrimal bone

Zygomatic bone

Occipital bone

Maxilla

External auditory
meatus

Zygomatic arch

Mandible

Mastoid process
of temporal bone

Hyoid bone

(a)

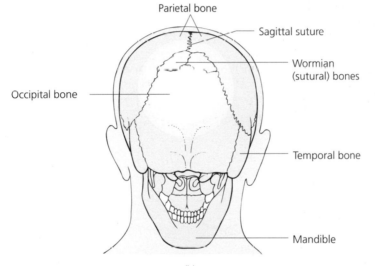

Parietal bone

Sagittal suture

Wormian
(sutural) bones

Occipital bone

Temporal bone

Mandible

(b)

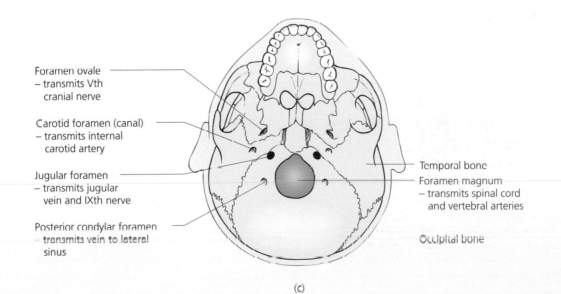

Foramen ovale
– transmits Vth
cranial nerve

Carotid foramen (canal)
– transmits internal
carotid artery

Jugular foramen
– transmits jugular
vein and IXth nerve

Temporal bone

Foramen magnum
– transmits spinal cord
and vertebral arteries

Posterior condylar foramen
– transmits vein to lateral
sinus

Occipital bone

(c)

Figure 3.5 The principal bones of the adult skull. (a) Lateral view; (b) posterior view; (c) inferior view (this also includes the larger foramina features).

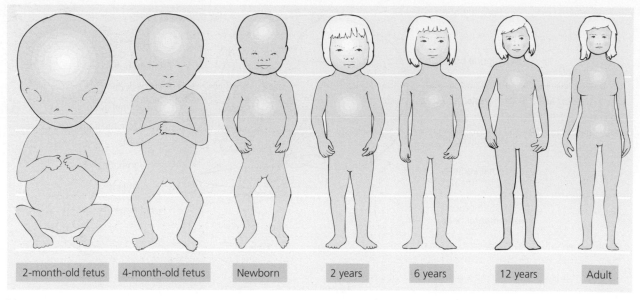

2-month-old fetus | 4-month-old fetus | Newborn | 2 years | 6 years | 12 years | Adult

(a)

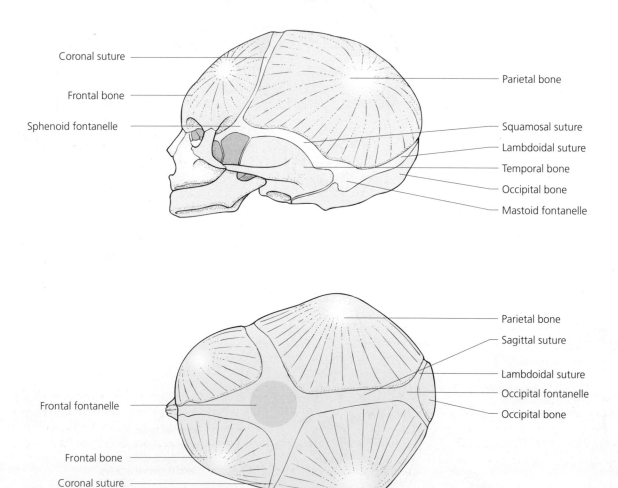

Coronal suture

Frontal bone

Sphenoid fontanelle

Parietal bone

Squamosal suture

Lambdoidal suture

Temporal bone

Occipital bone

Mastoid fontanelle

Parietal bone

Sagittal suture

Lambdoidal suture

Occipital fontanelle

Occipital bone

Frontal fontanelle

Frontal bone

Coronal suture

(b)

Figure 3.6 The fetal skull. (a) Fetal skull size relative to the trunk. (b) The skull of an infant in detail: side view and view from above.

Q. How does the fetal skull differ from that of an adult (shown in Figure 3.5)?

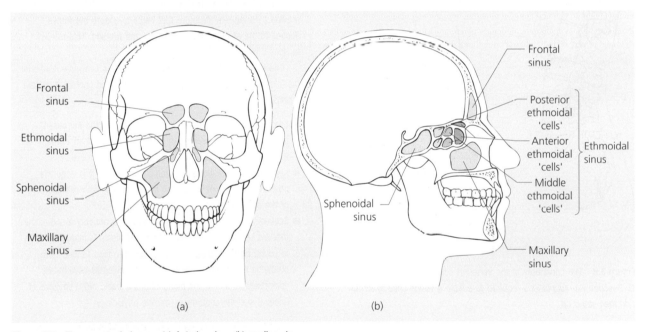

Figure 3.7 The paranasal sinuses. (a) Anterior view; (b) median view.
Q. Are the frontal sinuses medial or lateral to the maxillary sinuses?

The sinuses are air-filled cavities within the frontal, maxillary, ethmoid and sphenoid facial bones (Figure 3.7). The cavities help to lighten the bone, and their association with the nose gives resonance to the voice. Secretions into the sinuses drain into the nasal cavities.

The vertebral column

The vertebral column supports the upright or bipedal posture of the body, and protects the spinal cord, but provides flexibility of movement. Individual vertebral joints provide only limited movement and are very supportive, but the column has a high degree of flexibility in bending forwards; sideways and backward movements are limited. This flexibility is provided by the column, which consists of 33 individual bones (Figure 3.8):

- seven cervical (i.e. of the neck);
- twelve thoracic (i.e. of the upper trunk, or thorax);
- five lumbar (i.e. of the lower trunk);
- five sacral (i.e. of the sacrum, a component of the pelvis);
- four coccygeal (i.e. of the coccyx or 'tail').

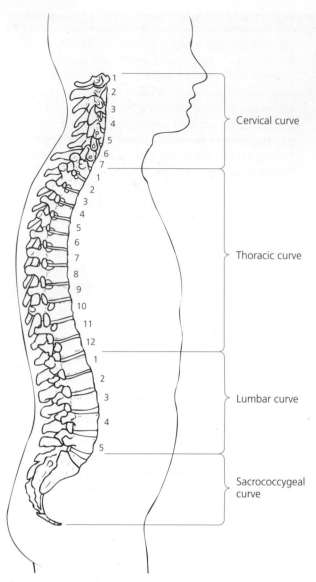

Cervical curve

Thoracic curve

Lumbar curve

Sacrococcygeal curve

Figure 3.8 The curvatures of the vertebral column.

Q. Describe the adaptations required to enable a young child to sit up and then stand up.

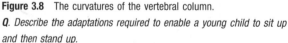

The individual bones of the sacrum and coccyx are usually fused together, although the coccyx articulates with the sacrum.

A large central cavity within the cervical, thoracic and lumbar bones, called the vertebral foramen (foramen = window), accommodates the spinal cord, whilst spaces between adjacent bones, called the intervertebral foramina, allow access for blood vessels and spinal nerves (Figure 3.9(d)).

The cervical, thoracic and lumbar vertebrae show differences in size and proportions, but the structures generally are similar (Figure 3.9). The main variation is in the first two cervical bones. These bones (abbreviated C1 and C2) are modified to form a joint with the base of the skull. C1 (the atlas) has articulating surfaces on the upper aspect, which allow forward and backward movements of

---

BOX 3.9 CURVATURE OF THE VERTEBRAL COLUMN

The vertebral column has a distinct S-shape in side view (Figure 3.8). The curvatures are referred to as the cervical, thoracic, lumbar and sacrococcygeal curvatures according to the position in the vertebral column. They result from contraction of the muscles of the back and a tightening of ligaments.

Although babies are born with thoracic and sacrococcygeal curvatures, the cervical and lumbar curvatures develop later. The development of the cervical curvature after about 3 months is necessary if the head is to be held erect, whilst development of the lumbar curvature during the later part of the first year is necessary if the baby is to sit up and eventually stand.

The vertebral curvatures also help to ensure that the body's centre of gravity (i.e. the point in the body through which most of the weight acts) lies over the pelvis when we are standing. The lumbar curve is especially important in this respect, and its curvature may increase if weight distribution in the body alters, e.g. during pregnancy. The curvatures of the vertebral column also provide a spring-like structure that helps to absorb the forces applied to the skeleton during walking and running. This role is facilitated by the intervertebral discs.

The influence of gravity on spinal curvatures is apparent where there is persistent asymmetry of muscle tone and posture (Lonstein 1999):

● Lordosis is an exaggerated lumbar curvature. The increased lumbar curvature observed in pregnant women is an example of a temporary lordosis.

● Kyphosis is an exaggerated thoracic curvature. It is generally observed in older people, often in association with osteoporosis of the spinal column.

● Scoliosis is a lateral curvature. It is most commonly found in the thoracic region of the spinal column. Scoliosis is frequently seen in young children, especially girls, and can lead to long-term problems if left untreated. Its presence indicates asymmetric contraction of the lateral muscles of the back, often because of unequal skeletal anatomy or muscle physiology.

Physiotherapy can be used effectively to treat abnormal spinal curvatures, especially in children. There are also surgical procedures that can be used to stabilize the spinal column, including fusing vertebrae using bone grafts, or using spinal implants such as metallic rods and screws.

---

the head. C2 (the axis) has an upper vertical process, the odontoid process, which projects from the body of the bone into the modified vertebral foramen of the atlas, allowing rotational movement of the head. Each of the remaining bones in these sections of the vertebral column has a 'body' and three bony processes:

● The main body, or centrum, of a vertebral bone provides strength and acts as a shock absorber during postural changes. The size and shape of the centrum varies with

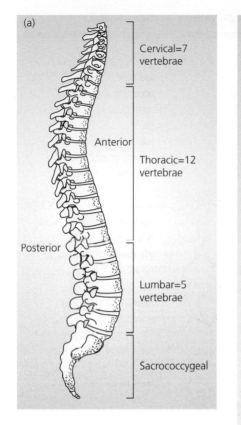

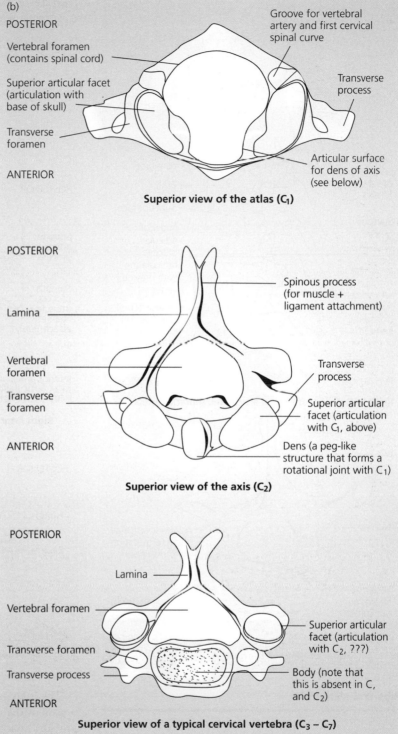

Figure 3.9 (a) Location of the vertebrae; (b) cervical vertebrae (superior views).

Q. How many vertebrae are there in each region of the vertebral column?

position in the vertebral column. The largest centrum is found in the lumbar vertebrae (Figure 3.9(d)), since the lower back is close to the centre of gravity of the body on standing and reinforcement is necessary here. The centrum of a vertebral bone is separated from its neighbour by an intervertebral disc comprised of an outer fibrocartilage layer and an inner semi-solid core. The discs contribute to vertebral column flexibility, and also help to absorb shocks during movement.

● Two lateral processes articulate with their neighbours and provide some muscle and ligament attachment points.

● The spinous process on the posterior of the bone also provides attachment for muscles and ligaments.

Thoracic vertebrae also have articular surfaces, which form joints with the ribs. Between them, the three processes and the connecting bars of bone form a structure called the vertebral arch (which arches over the spinal cord).

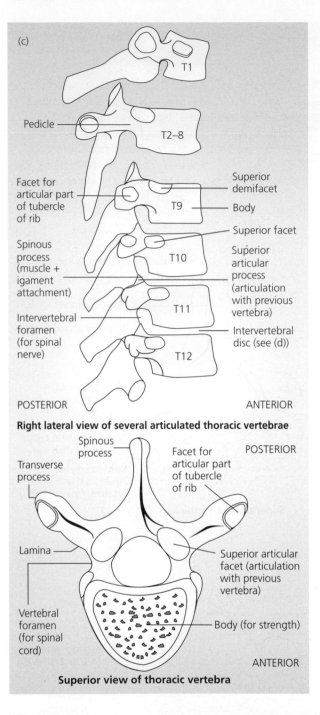

(c)

T1

Pedicle

T2–8

Facet for articular part of tubercle of rib

Superior demifacet

T9

Body

Superior facet

Spinous process (muscle + ligament attachment)

T10

Superior articular process (articulation with previous vertebra)

Intervertebral foramen (for spinal nerve)

T11

Intervertebral disc (see (d))

T12

POSTERIOR

ANTERIOR

Right lateral view of several articulated thoracic vertebrae

Spinous process

Transverse process

Facet for articular part of tubercle of rib

POSTERIOR

Lamina

Superior articular facet (articulation with previous vertebra)

Vertebral foramen (for spinal cord)

Body (for strength)

ANTERIOR

Superior view of thoracic vertebra

Figure 3.9 (c) thoracic vertebrae; (d) lumbar vertebrae.
Q. How many vertebrae are there in each region of the vertebral column?

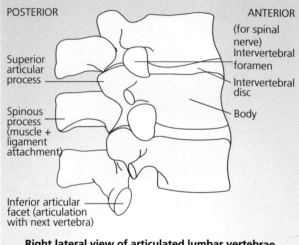

(d)

POSTERIOR

ANTERIOR

Superior articular process

(for spinal nerve) Intervertebral foramen

Intervertebral disc

Spinous process (muscle + ligament attachment)

Body

Inferior articular facet (articulation with next vertebra)

Right lateral view of articulated lumbar vertebrae

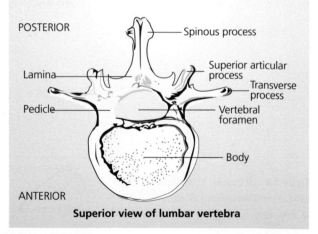

POSTERIOR

Spinous process

Superior articular process

Lamina

Transverse process

Pedicle

Vertebral foramen

Body

ANTERIOR

Superior view of lumbar vertebra

Ribs and sternum

The sternum is a flat, dagger-shaped bone situated in the anterior midline of the chest (Figure 3.10). There are three parts: the manubrium, the body and the xiphisternum; these articulate and facilitate chest expansion during breathing. The xiphisternum provides attachments for some abdominal muscles and for the diaphragm. It is cartilaginous until well into adulthood, when it ossifies. The manubrium and body have pairs of articular surfaces that form joints with the rib bones. The manubrium also articulates with the clavicle (collarbone).

The ribcage provides protection for the underlying organs of the chest (lungs, heart, and associated vessels), provides attachment for postural and respiratory muscles, and helps support the shoulder girdle of bones.

Seven pairs of ribs articulate directly with the sternum via cartilage (Figure 3.10). These are referred to as 'true' ribs. Five pairs are 'false' ribs, since they are not attached directly to the sternum. Three pairs of false ribs are attached to the costal cartilage of the last true rib. Two pairs of false ribs have no sternal attachment; these are the 'floating' ribs attached to the last of the previous false ribs. The floating ribs extend far enough down the back to provide some protection for the kidneys.

There are three general causes of back pain: muscle/ligament strain, disc problems and vertebral problems. Muscle strains and ligament strains occur when muscles are overstretched, or when a joint is moved forcibly against its natural direction of movement. Muscle problems are discussed in Chapter 17, but it is worth noting here that the increased lumbar curve that is observed in pregnancy places additional stresses on the ligaments of the vertebral column and is largely responsible for the lower back pain that is frequently experienced during pregnancy.

Should the tough outer layer of a vertebral disc rupture, then the viscous core distends through the fissure and exerts pressure on nearby spinal nerves, or irritates the meninges, producing pain. This is a 'slipped' or prolapsed disc. Disc degeneration may also be observed. This seems to be age linked, but its cause is poorly understood.

Vertebral problems include spondylolysis, spondylolisthesis, spinal stenosis, and spondylitis. In spondylolysis, there is a structural weakening of the vertebral arch of the vertebral bone, leading to increased risk of the facets of vertebrae moving forward through the occurrence of 'microfractures'. This problem is usually hereditary. Spondylolisthesis is a slipping forward of one vertebra over another. If severe, surgery will be required. Spinal stenosis occurs when a nerve root, or several roots, become entrapped. It is usually an acquired problem, and may require decompression treatment. Inflammation specifically of the vertebral joints is called spondylitis, and ossification of the joint tissue is referred to as *ankylosing* spondylitis. Both conditions reduce vertebral flexibility and restrict mobility.

People working in environments in which they regularly lift heavy loads are especially at risk of developing chronic back pain. This is an important consideration when using lifting and handling methods in nursing (Worthington, 2000).

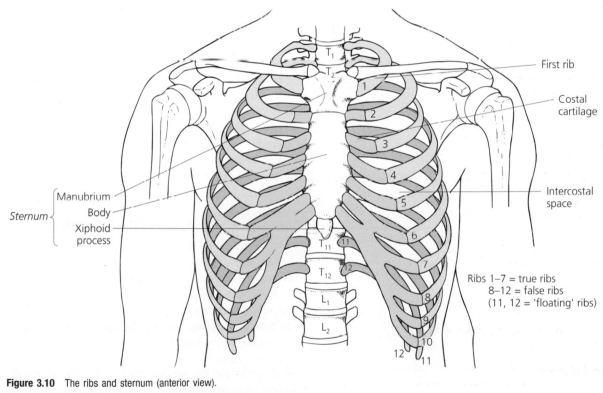

Figure 3.10 The ribs and sternum (anterior view).
Q. Why are ribs classified as true, false or floating?

Hyoid

The hyoid is a U-shaped bone found at the base of the tongue (Figure 3.5(a)). It does not articulate with any other bone or cartilage, but forms an attachment for several muscles involved in chewing and swallowing.

Appendicular skeleton

The appendicular skeleton consists of the limb bones and the bones of the limb girdles. It is so called because these bones are 'appended' onto the axial skeleton (Figure 3.4).

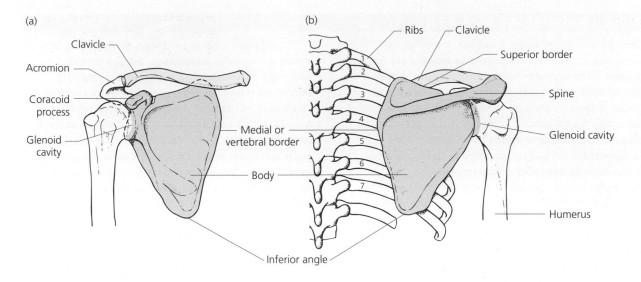

(a)

Clavicle
Acromion
Coracoid process
Glenoid cavity

(b)

Ribs — Clavicle
Superior border
Spine
Glenoid cavity
Humerus
Medial or vertebral border
Body
Inferior angle

(c)

Acromion
Coracoid process
Forms 'socket' of shoulder joint
Glenoid cavity

Figure 3.11 The pectoral girdle and shoulder joint. (a) Anterior view; (b) posterior view; (c) the scapula in lateral view.

Q. Name the bones of the pectoral girdle.

Q. Why is it easier to dislocate the shoulder rather than the pelvis?

The scapulae are large, flat, triangular bones. The blade is strengthened by a ridge or spine on its posterior surface. Although large, the blade articulates at just one end, with the clavicle and humerus of the arm, and much of it is held in place by many muscle attachments and ligaments. Its structure and mode of attachment facilitate the rotational movement of the shoulder.

Exercise

Neither the clavicle nor scapula has a direct connection with the vertebral column. The bones are held in place largely by muscles and ligaments, coupled with the joint between the slender clavicle and the sternum. Such an arrangement means the shoulder has a high mobility – the scapula slides over the posterior surface of the ribs as the joint is rotated – but is relatively poorly weight bearing. Compare the diagram of the shoulder in Figure 3.11 with that of the pelvis in Figure 3.13. Note the powerful skeletal structure of the pelvis compared with that of the shoulder, and note the massive muscle attachment areas provided by the pelvis.

Shoulder, arm and hand

The shoulder or pectoral girdle consists of the two collar-bones (clavicles) and shoulder blades (scapulae) (Figure 3.11). The clavicle is a slender bone that articulates with the sternum at one end and the scapula at the other. The clavicles provide a site for muscle attachment, and help to brace the shoulder.

The bones of the arm consist of the humerus of the upper arm, and the ulna and radius of the forearm. The humerus is a long bone that articulates with the scapula at the shoulder and with the radius and ulna at the elbow (Figure 3.12). The joint with the scapula is a ball-and-socket joint (see later) that provides a wide range of movement. At its distal end, at the elbow, the humerus is flattened to form articular surfaces with the ulna and radius. The bone is strengthened at this point by condyles,

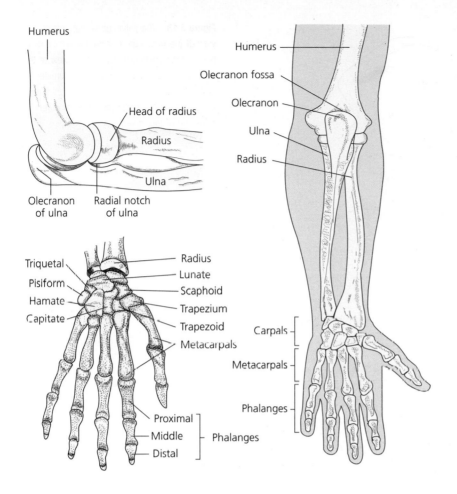

Figure 3.12 The bones of the right forearm (radius and ulna, with detail) and hand.

Q. Is the radial pulse palpated on the medial or lateral aspect of the wrist?

one of which (the medial epicondyle) is crossed by the ulnar nerve. It is this nerve that is pinched against the humerus (i.e. the funny bone) when the elbow is knocked.

The radius of the forearm is found on the outer, or lateral, side, whilst the ulna is found on the inner forearm, or medial side. The radius is the more substantial of the two. The two bones are held together along their length by connective tissue.

The two bones of the forearm produce a complex system of joints that enable the mobility of the forearm. The ulna forms a hinge joint (see later) with the humerus, which permits the elbow to be flexed. The end of the ulna is extended as the olecranon process, which forms the 'elbow bone' and helps to prevent overextension of the arm when the elbow is straightened (Figure 3.12). The radius forms a pivotal joint with the humerus, which allows the forearm to rotate. Note, however, that the radius rotates around the ulna; the hinge joint of the latter cannot rotate. Both bones form joints (called elipsoidal joints; see later) with the carpal bones of the wrist, thus allowing a high degree of flexibility of the wrist, but the radius forms a more substantial wrist joint than does the ulna.

The wrist bones are called carpals. There are eight in each wrist (Figure 3.12). The carpals are short bones arranged roughly in two rows, and connected by ligaments.

The first row articulates with the radius and ulna, and the other articulates with the five metacarpal bones of the palm. The latter articulate with the finger bones, or phalanges. There are three phalanges in each finger, and two in the thumb. The ellipsoidal joints between the phalanges facilitate the hand-grip movement.

Pelvis, leg and foot

The pelvic or hip girdle is the site of the body's centre of gravity. Not surprisingly, it is an extremely robust structure. It is strengthened by fusion of its composite bones and by inflexible joints with the vertebral column (Figure 3.13). The bones also provide large attachment areas for the major postural muscles of the back, buttocks, and thigh. Such substantial attachments are essential because the muscles must act to prevent flexing of the hips due to the effects of gravity.

The pelvic girdle consists of two large 'innominate' bones and the sacral bones of the vertebral column. The innominate bones are each comprised of three individual bones, called the ilium, ischium and pubis, which have fused together to form a strong bowl-shaped structure (Figure 3.13). The junction of the three bones near the lower aspect of the pelvis forms a deep depression called

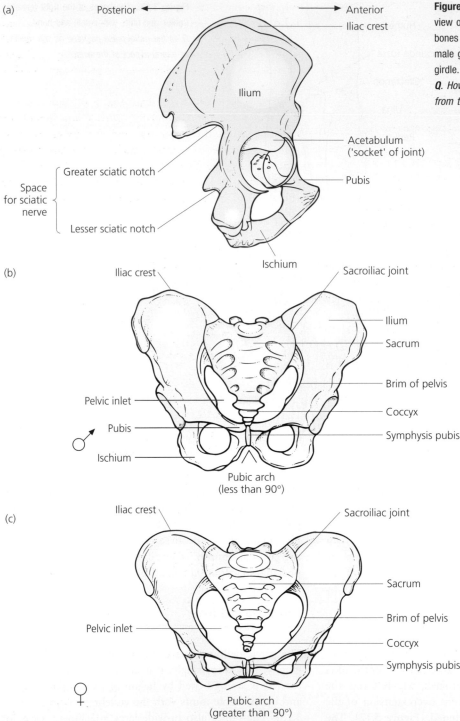

(a)

Posterior ← → Anterior

Iliac crest

Ilium

Acetabulum ('socket' of joint)

Greater sciatic notch

Space for sciatic nerve

Lesser sciatic notch

Pubis

Ischium

Figure 3.13 The pelvic girdle. (a) Lateral view of the right side to show the component bones and acetabulum; (b) anterior view of the male girdle; (c) anterior view of the female girdle.

Q. How does the female pelvic girdle differ from that of the male?

(b)

Iliac crest

Sacroiliac joint

Ilium

Sacrum

Brim of pelvis

Pelvic inlet

Coccyx

Pubis

Symphysis pubis

Ischium

Pubic arch (less than 90°)

(c)

Iliac crest

Sacroiliac joint

Sacrum

Brim of pelvis

Pelvic inlet

Coccyx

Symphysis pubis

Pubic arch (greater than 90°)

the acetabulum, which acts as a receptacle for the head of the thigh bone or femur.

The ilium is the largest of the three bones, and it is the crest of this bone that can be palpated at the hip. The ilium is a large, flattened bone, strengthened by bony ridges or spines, that forms attachments with the large postural muscles of the thigh and buttock. It is joined to the sacrum by ligaments and connective tissue, and movement is very restricted. The ischium is also a substantial bone, and supports the weight of the body when sitting. The pubis

extends to the front of the lower abdomen; the right and left pubic bones unite at the symphysis pubis. The bowl-shaped structure provided by these bones protects the organs of the lower abdomen, including the reproductive tract.

The femur is a strong, long bone that articulates at the hip and the knee. The large, rounded head of the femur forms a ball-and-socket joint with the acetabulum of the hip, which provides a large degree of rotational and abductional movement. The femur has a distinctive inner curvature not thrown widely out of position during walking, thus helping to maintain balance. The femur curvature also provides a spring-like action, which enables it to absorb some of the forces applied to it during walking. This helps to reduce the jarring effect on the pelvis and vertebral column.

Bony protrusions at the knee end of the femur (called the medial and lateral condyles) provide attachments for the muscles of the lower leg, and also make the joint substantial. The processes articulate with the kneecap (patella) and the tibia of the lower leg. The patella is secured in position by extensive cartilages and ligaments (Figures 3.15 and 3.19). The knee not only has to be strong

(Figure 3.14). In women, the wider pelvis necessitates an even more pronounced curvature because the acetabulum is even further from the body midline than it is in men. When standing, the curvature brings the knee joint, shinbones and foot close to the vertical axis of the body, and therefore almost in line with the centre of gravity. This facilitates weight bearing, and also means that the centre of gravity is

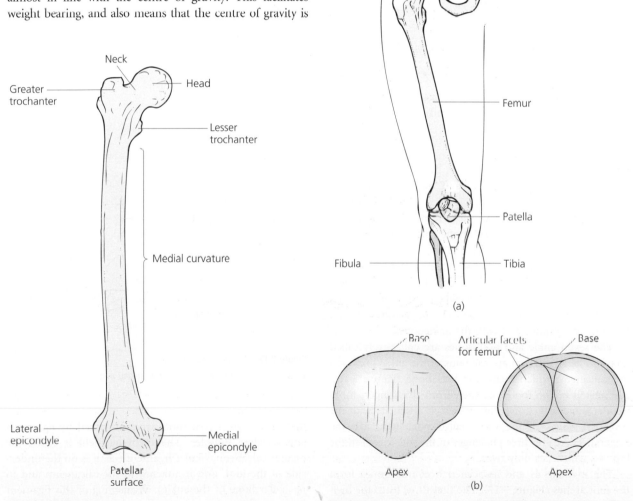

Figure 3.14 The femur.

Q. How do the ball-and-socket joints of the pelvis and shoulder compare?

Figure 3.15 The bones of the upper leg and kneecap (patella). (a) The femur, anterior view; (b) the right patella: left, anterior view; right, posterior view.

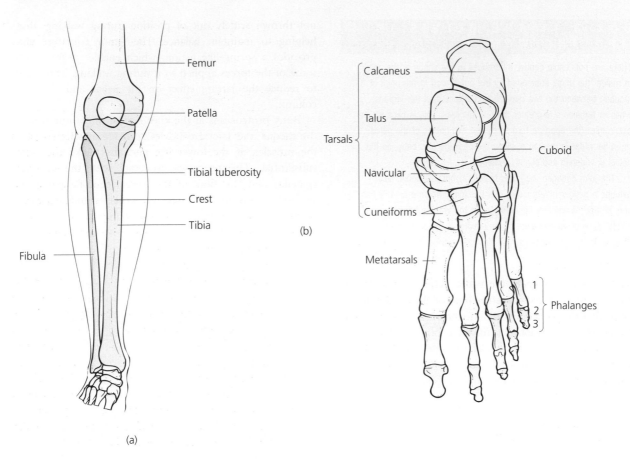

Figure 3.16 The bones of the lower leg and foot. (a) The tibia and fibula, anterior view; (b) the foot.

Q. Compare the bone structure of the foot with that of the hand (Figure 3.12).

to support the weight of the body, but must also receive and withstand forces applied to it during squatting or kneeling.

The two bones of the lower leg are called the tibia and fibula. The tibia forms the shinbone (the prominent crest running along the front of the bone can easily be palpated), and articulates with the femur at the knee and with the bones of the ankle (Figure 3.16). The fibula is a more slender bone (it is not weight bearing, but it does provide some muscle attachments), and articulates with the tibia at the knee and with the anklebones.

The seven ankle and heel bones are collectively called tarsals. The largest two are the talus of the ankle joint and the calcaneus, which forms the heel bone (Figure 3.16). The instep of the foot is formed from five longer, more slender bones called metatarsals, which articulate with the proximal bones of the toes (called phalanges, like the fingers). There are three phalanges in the toe, except in the big toe, which has only two.

The metatarsals and associated heel/anklebones form the foot arches (Figure 3.17). The first three form the high arch, called the medial longitudinal arch, on the inside of the foot, while metatarsals IV and V form the lower arch, called the lateral longitudinal arch, on the outside of the

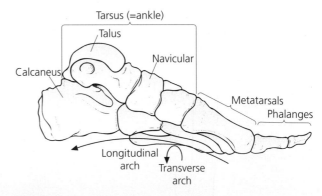

Figure 3.17 The arches of the foot.

Q. What happens to the foot arches on taking a step?

foot. The arched structures are maintained by ligaments and attached muscles. The main ligament is called the plantar calcaneonavicular ligament (i.e. it is on the under-side of the foot, and it attaches to the calcaneum and to navicular bone of the ankle). Weakening of this ligament leads to a failure to maintain the relative positions of these bones and therefore of the high arch, and causes a 'fallen arch' or 'flat foot'.

The foot skeleton during standing and walking

On standing, the body weight is exerted on each ankle, and then distributed between the heel bone (calcaneus) and the metatarsal bones. The relatively large size of the calcaneus was noted earlier. Its shape helps give it strength, and also provides a site of attachment for the large calf muscles via the Achilles tendon. The articulation between the tibia/fibula bones of the lower leg and the main bone of the ankle (the talus) is most stable in the standing position or, especially, when the foot is flexed in the crouching position. Extending the foot causes the articulation to occur with the narrower part of the talus; this is a weaker arrangement and reduces the stability of the joint when standing on tip-toe.

During walking, the strength of the calcaneus enables it to withstand the initial impact with the ground. The body weight is then distributed quickly to the lateral border of the foot along the metatarsals, and eventually across the heads of the metatarsals to the head of the first metatarsal bone at the base of the big toe (the 'ball' of the foot). By this time, the heel will have left the ground. Running increases the forces applied, and the distal heads of the metatarsals distribute the weight more evenly. The roles of the toes during walking/running are to provide stability at the point of contact with the ground, and to impart a forward thrust that facilitates the movement.

The role of the arches is to absorb the forces applied to the foot, especially during walking/running. Thus, they flatten slightly during impact of the foot on the ground and, being highly elastic, release the energy again as they spring back into shape once the foot is lifted. In this way, momentum is imparted onto the movement, raising the energy-efficiency of the process. The arches also help to prevent blood vessels and nerves in the foot from being crushed.

> **Exercise**
>
> Compare the bones of the arm and hand with those of the leg and foot. Note the similarity in terms of bone number and arrangement, but note also how they are adapted to accommodate the respective limb function.

Joints

Strictly speaking, a joint is simply the point of contact between bones or between cartilage and bone. Its presence, therefore, does not always imply movement, although many joints do move. Joints are divided into three categories:

- Joints between bones that provide little or no movement are called *fixed joints*.

- Joints between bone and cartilage are called *cartilaginous joints*.

- Joints that allow movement are called *synovial joints*, and the various types of these joints give the body a wide diversity of movement.

Fixed and cartilaginous joints

Fixed joints include the sutures of the skull, in which a thin layer of dense fibrous connective tissue unites the bones (during life, some sutures are replaced by bone so that there is complete fusion); the joint between the shafts of the ulna and radius of the forearm; and the joint between the tibia and fibula near the ankle. The latter two joints provide stability at points of stress; these joints have more loose and elastic connective tissue than is found in sutures, which helps the joints to absorb the shock of movement.

Cartilaginous joints include the symphysis pubis between the anterior surfaces of the pubis bones of the pelvic girdle, and the discs between the bodies of vertebrae. They differ from fixed joints in that the fibrocartilage present makes the joint slightly more moveable. Such flexibility enables the symphysis to move slightly during birth, and the vertebral column to be flexible and to absorb forces during walking. The joint between the cartilaginous tip of a growing bone, called the epiphysis, and the underlying bone matrix is also a cartilaginous joint, although the presence of bone mineral makes this joint fixed.

Synovial joints

Synovial joints are characterized by the presence of a joint cavity (Figure 3.18). The cavity contains synovial fluid, enclosed within a tough fibrous capsule. The fluid is viscous because of the presence of hyaluronic acid (a normal constituent of cartilage), and is secreted from the

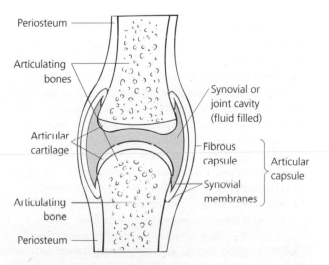

Figure 3.18 A general synovial joint.
Q. What other types of skeletal joint are there?

Inflammatory conditions of synovial joints are referred to collectively as arthritis ('arthro-' = jointed). *Osteoarthritis* is a degenerative (but non-inflammatory in its cause) condition of synovial joints. The causes can be secondary to joint trauma/stress or congenital factors, or can be idiopathic (primary). Idiopathic causes are more common, and seem to be linked to ageing. The disorder involves the breakdown of cartilage by enzymes, which results in the flaking, cracking and eventual loss of joint cartilage. As the cartilage thins, there is frictional contact between bones, which causes bone erosion and induces pain. The problem may be exacerbated over time by calcification of the joint capsule and production of bony outgrowths called osteophytes. Joint flexibility may then be very much reduced.

Rheumatoid arthritis (or rheumatoid disease) is an autoimmune disorder of connective tissue, and is primarily an inflammatory disease of the joint capsule, articular cartilage and ligaments. There is joint deformity, swelling and pain. The cause of the response is obscure, probably with a combination of factors involved, such as genetic propensity, and hormonal and reproductive factors.

In extensive damage, correction of a degenerated joint may involve reconstruction of the joint structure (called arthroplasty) using bone grafts and implants. Total joint replacement with artificial joints may be necessary in advanced inflammatory disease.

---

blood plasma. The role of synovial fluid is to provide lubrication, and to provide nutrients for cartilage cells within the joint. An important property of the fluid is that the viscosity reduces as the joint is used, thus increasing the lubricant effects during exercise, much as oil does in a car engine. Phagocytic cells within the fluid keep the joint free of debris.

The capsule consists of a tough, but flexible, outer layer of dense connective tissue that unites the articulating bones and helps prevent dislocation. Some of the connective tissue fibres of the capsule are arranged in parallel bundles, which are oriented to provide maximal strength to the joint. Such bundles are called ligaments. The inner layer of the capsule consists of loose connective tissue, elastin, and adipose tissue. This is the synovial membrane (which secretes the synovial fluid).

The joint surface of the articulating bones is smoothed by a covering of hyaline cartilage. Additional cartilaginous discs (or menisci) may be present to ensure a tight fit between joint surfaces of very different shapes, e.g. within the knee (Figure 3.19).

Although the general structure of synovial joints is similar, there are wide variations in the movement they facilitate. Various subtypes of joint are recognized (Figure 3.20):

- *Ball and socket*. This consists of a ball-shaped surface of one bone fitted into the cup-like socket of another. The advantage of this type of joint is that it permits movement in three planes, including rotation. Examples are the shoulder and hip joints, although the need to maintain posture against gravity means that the hip has less freedom of movement than the shoulder.

- *Hinge*. The convex surface of one bone fits into the concave surface of another. This structure provides movement in one plane only. Examples are the elbow, knee and ankle.

- *Pivot joint*. A protrusion from one bone articulates within a ring (partly bone, partly ligament) structure on another. The joint provides rotational movement. Examples include the joint between the first two vertebrae (atlas and axis), which allows rotation of the head, and the joint

Joints subjected to physical stresses must be reinforced if they are not to be dislocated. Those joints that have to support the body weight are reinforced with substantial ligaments and cartilage, and are associated with powerful muscles. For example, the structure of the knee joint (which is actually an aggregate of three joints) is shown in Figure 3.19. Note the presence of extensive ligaments and muscle tendons, and also how the orientation of the fibres of these connective tissues stabilizes the joint. Cruciate ligaments ('crux-' = cross) within the joint capsule between the tibia and the femur help to reduce any twisting motion of the knee.

A sprain is an injury to ligaments produced by a wrenching or twisting movement. There is rapid swelling, which worsens with time, and severe pain on movement of the joint. Treatment includes:

- a cold compress applied intermittently for up to 36 h to suppress pain and swelling; analgesia;
- if necessary, elevation of the affected limb to help reduce swelling;
- mild heat later to improve blood flow and so promote wound healing;
- immobilization of the joint, usually by splint or elastic dressing;
- teaching the patient to regain use of the joint only gradually, with rest periods.

The joint should also be observed for signs of continuing problems, e.g. bone necrosis through poor blood supply, or instability that may make repeat dislocation likely.

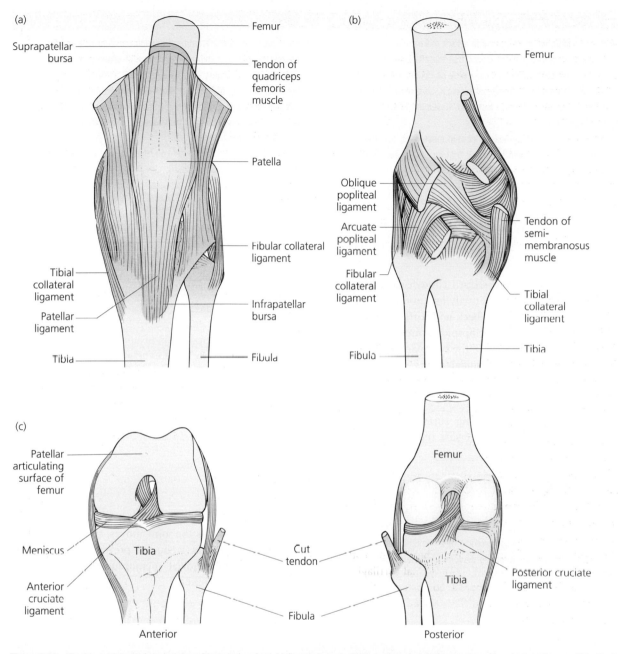

Figure 3.19 The knee joint. (a) Anterior view; (b) posterior view; (c) flexed views to illustrate the cruciate ligaments and menisci cartilages within the joint.

Q. What is a menisectomy?

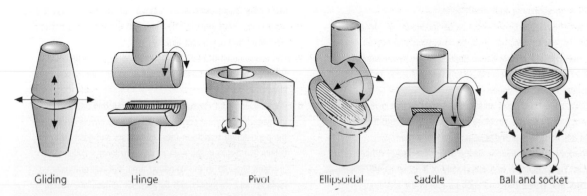

Figure 3.20 Subtypes of synovial joints and their movements.

Dislocation occurs when the bones in a joint move from their normal position, with the consequence that the articular surfaces are no longer in contact. The problem may be congenital, if a joint has not fully formed or matured; pathological, as a result of joint degeneration; or traumatic, due to forced movement in an inappropriate plane.

There is joint deformity, loss of normal movement, and pain. Dislocation also carries with it the risk that blood vessels may have been damaged. Treatment includes analgesia, X-ray to assess the extent of damage, realignment of the joint, and immobilization. Surgery may be required if damage is extensive, involving suturing of the torn ligaments and (in the knee) possibly removal of part of a damaged meniscus cartilage. This procedure is often performed using an arthroscope to visualize the interior of the joint capsule.

between the proximal ends of the ulna and radius of the forearm, which allows rotation of the forearm and hence of the hands.

- *Ellipsoidal joints.* An oval-shaped condyle on one bone articulates with an elliptical cavity on another. The joint permits up-and-down and back-and-forth movements. Saddle joints are modified ellipsoidal joints that allow a greater range of movement in the two planes. Unlike the ball-and-socket joint, ellipsoidal joints do not allow rotation. An example is the joint between the radius and the carpal bones of the wrist.

- *Gliding joints.* The articulating surfaces are flat and permit movement from side to side and back and forth.

Although twisting and rotation might be expected to be possible by this structure, they are normally prevented by ligaments, or by adjacent bones. Examples are those between the carpals of the hand, between the tarsals of the foot, between the sternum and clavicle, and between the scapula and clavicle.

Exercise

Place the tips of your fingers over the joints identified as examples in this section on synovial joints. Can you feel how the skeletal structures are moving according to the differing joint structures?

These are painful inflammatory problems, typically produced by excessive use of a joint, or compression of the joint area. Intervention is to encourage resting the joint until the problem subsides.

Bursae

In places where the skin, tendons or muscles rub on the surface of the bone as the joint moves, small sacs of fluid called bursae (singular = bursa) prevent friction. These sacs are made of synovial membrane, and the fluid is similar to synovial fluid.

Summary

1 Bone tissue is a type of connective tissue, mineralized to give it a supporting role. A bone is composed of compact bone and cancellous (or spongy or trabecular) bone.

2 Compact bone is a hard, dense tissue composed of cylindrical structures called osteons, in which blood vessels and nerves are located within a central canal. Bone cells are found within fluid-filled pockets called lacunae, into which nutrients must diffuse from the central canals.

3 Cancellous bone consists of small arches of bone that give it a spongy appearance. The structure is still supportive, but it also lightens the bone and provides spaces for bone marrow.

4 Bone marrow is red or yellow. Redness is related to blood cell synthesis. Yellow marrow consists mainly of adipose tissue.

5 The shape of a bones depends upon its role in the skeleton, e.g. the major limb bones are long and relatively narrow.

6 The mineral matrix of bone is secreted by specialized cells called osteoblasts. The process continues throughout life as other cells called osteoclasts remove mineral and release it into body fluids. Bone mineral therefore reflects a balance between osteoblast and osteoclast activity.

7 The laying down of new bone mineral is called ossification. It is most apparent as cartilage is replaced as bone grows in length.

8 Bone healing also involves ossification, but this time not of cartilage. Cells in the connective tissue that covers bone (i.e. the periosteum) transform into osteoblasts and ossify the connective tissue in the area of injury to form a callus. This provides strength to the damaged area, but will gradually be replaced as osteoblasts and osteoclasts remodel the tissue.

9 The skeleton consists of axial and appendicular components.

10 The axial component is comprised of the skull, hyoid, sternum, ribs and vertebrae.

11 The appendicular component is comprised of the shoulder and pelvic girdles, arms and legs, and hands and feet.

12 The skeleton provides support for the body, but also has features, such as curvatures, that enable it to absorb physical stresses associated with standing and walking.

13 Joints are a feature of the skeleton. Some are immovable; others, called synovial joints, facilitate movement according to their structure and the activities of associated muscles.

14 Synovial joints are reinforced with ligaments and muscle tendons, especially where they have to support the body against gravity.

15 Synovial joints are found in a variety of forms according to the movement they facilitate.

Review questions

1 What are the functions of bones?

2 What are bones comprised of? What do osteoblasts and osteoclasts do?

3 Differentiate between cartilage and bone. Which has the best blood supply? How does this affect healing rates of these tissues?

4 What type of physical activity strengthens bones? How does body mass index affect bone strength?

5 Why does osteoporosis affect mainly postmenopausal women?

6 Which dietary components affect bone health?

7 Outline the stages of bone healing. What factors will influence this process?

8 Why is mobilization of patients encouraged? Which members of the multidisciplinary team will be involved?

REFERENCES

Leslie, M. (2000) Issues in the nursing management of osteoporosis. *Nursing Clinics of North America* **35**(1): 189–97.

Lonstein, J.E. (1999) Congenital spinal deformities: scoliosis, kyphosis and lordosis. *Orthopaedic Clinics of North America* **30**(3): 387–405.

Mellett, S. (1998) Care of the orthopaedic patient on traction. *Nursing Times* **94**(22): 52–4.

Rosen, C.J. (2000) Pathophysiology of osteoporosis. *Clinics in Laboratory Medicine* **20**(3): 455–68.

Worthington, K. (2000) Health and safety. Watch your back. *American Journal of Nursing* **100**(9): 96.

Section Two

The need for regulation

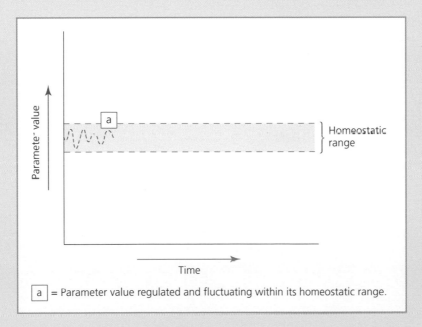

a = Parameter value regulated and fluctuating within its homeostatic range.

Chapter 4

Chemical reactions in cells: metabolism

Basic chemistry
Metabolism: a general overview

Cellular respiration
Further reading

'Metabolism' describes the complex array of chemical reactions that take place during the day-to-day activities of cells. In essence, metabolism is the basis of cell function. Understanding the processes involved helps to identify the needs of cells and hence the necessity for the systemic functions of the body to meet those needs. The reactions taking place inside cells will depend on the chemical environment within the cell (intracellular homeostasis), which in turn will require the delivery of the reactants and an appropriate extracellular environment.

The term 'metabolism' is generic. It is divided into reactions in which new molecules are synthesized by joining together atoms and molecules, and those in which molecules are broken down into smaller constituent units.

'Anabolism' is a general term for synthetic processes, and 'catabolism' is a term applied to the breaking-up processes.

In order to understand this material, it is important first to gain an awareness of how molecules arise from the combination of constituent atoms. Accordingly, the next section provides an explanation of the fundamental aspects of chemistry.

Exercise

At this point, it might be useful to refer back to Chapter 1 and remind yourself of the integration of physiological function required to maintain cellular homeostasis.

BASIC CHEMISTRY

All living and non-living things consist of matter in gaseous, liquid or solid form. All matter is made up of a limited number of chemical elements combined together in ways that ultimately produce the huge diversity of substances that make up the natural world. Chemistry is essentially about the properties and behaviours of these elements and their combinations. In biology, the main interest is in the chemistry of living matter, which is referred to as biochemistry.

Elements

Chemical elements are the basic building units of matter. They are substances that cannot be broken down into simpler substances by ordinary chemical reactions. Ninety-two different elements occur naturally, but a dozen or so others that are too unstable to occur naturally are known to science. Elements are designated abbreviations or symbols, mostly based on the first one or two letters of the name of the element. This may, however, refer to the classical name, which can add to the confusion. Examples of symbols of elements abundant in the body are C (carbon), O (oxygen), H (hydrogen), N (nitrogen), Na (sodium; classical name, natrium), K (potassium; classical name, kalium), Ca (calcium), P (phosphorus) and Fe (iron; classical name, ferrium).

The diversity of cell structure and function is made possible because many chemical elements may be combined with others to form myriad different substances, the properties of which result in the extensive range of chemical reactions that occur from moment to moment within a cell.

Atoms

Each element consists of units called atoms. The atoms of one element will be different from those of other elements. Needless to say, atoms are minute; the smallest are less than 0.000 000 01 cm in diameter, and even the largest are only about 0.000 000 05 cm in diameter. Some natural substances, such as diamond (a form of carbon) and gold (symbol Au), may be comprised almost entirely of one kind of element. Usually, however, matter consists of two or more different elements combined together in various proportions.

There are two main features to the structure of an atom: the nucleus and its 'cloud' of surrounding particles called electrons (Figure 4.1). Physicists have identified a number of different particles and subparticles within the nucleus; the major ones are neutrons and protons, which are comparatively large and heavy compared with electrons. Protons and electrons are electrically charged: by convention, protons carry a positive charge, and electrons a negative charge.

Atoms of an element will have the same number of protons and electrons, and so will be electrically neutral overall (since the number of positive particles equals the number of negative ones). All atoms of one element will have identical numbers of protons and electrons, whilst atoms of different elements contain different numbers of protons in their nuclei. For example, hydrogen atoms, which are the smallest atoms, have only one proton and one electron, whereas uranium atoms, which are the largest naturally occurring atoms, have 92 of each. The number of protons in an atom's nucleus is called its atomic number; this is depicted in the Periodic Table of elements as the number above the symbol for each element (Figure 4.2).

The mass (i.e. weight) of an atom reflects the number of protons and neutrons present; electrons are so small that their mass is insignificant in comparison. The atomic mass is shown in the Periodic Table as the number below each element, and is related to that of the smallest and lightest element hydrogen, which is given a standardized mass of 1. Thus, oxygen, with an atomic mass of 16, is 16 times heavier than hydrogen, so 1 g hydrogen contains the same number of atoms as 16 g oxygen.

Although atoms of one element have the same number of protons, it is possible for their nuclei to have different numbers of neutrons. This does not influence the chemical activity of the atom, but it does slightly alter the mass. Atoms of a single element with different numbers of neutrons are called isotopes.

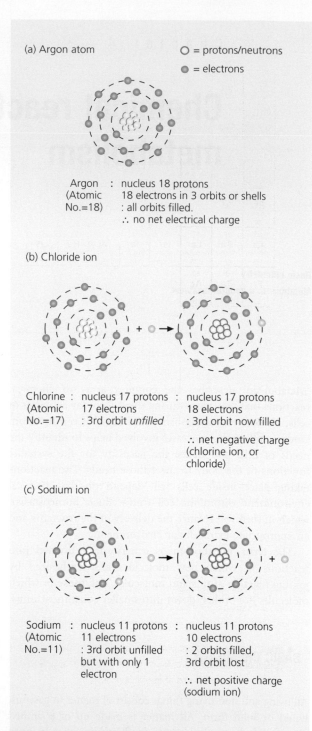

Figure 4.1 Schematic representation of atoms and ions. (a) An argon atom depicted as an example of an 'inert' element. Notice how the electron orbits around the nucleus contain a full complement of electrons. (b) A chlorine atom. The outer electron orbit is unfilled; in gaining an additional electron, the orbit is now filled but the excess electron causes the 'atom' to become negatively charged. This is now a chloride ion. (c) A sodium atom must lose an electron to ensure that the outer electron orbit is full, thus giving the 'atom' a positive charge; this is a sodium ion.

Q. Where would the additional electron come from that the chlorine atom requires to form the chloride ion?

I	II												III	IV	V	VI	VII	
							1 **H** Hydrogen 1											2 **He** Helium 4
3 **Li** Lithium 7	4 **Be** Beryllium 9												5 **B** Boron 11	6 **C** Carbon 12	7 **N** Nitrogen 14	8 **O** Oxygen 16	9 **F** Flourine 19	10 **Ne** Neon 20
11 **Na** Sodium 23	12 **Mg** Magnesium 24												13 **Al** Aluminium 27	14 **Si** Silicon 28	15 **P** Phosphorus 31	16 **S** Sulphur 32	17 **Cl** Chlorine 35.5	18 **Ar** Argon 40
19 **K** Potassium 39	20 **Ca** Calcium 40	21 **Sc** Scandium 45	22 **Ti** Titenium 48	23 **V** Vanadium 51	24 **Cr** Chromium 52	25 **Mn** Manganese 55	26 **Fe** Iron 56	27 **Co** Cobalt 59	28 **Ni** Nickel 59	29 **Cu** Copper 63.5	30 **Zn** Zinc 65		31 **Ga** Gallium 70	32 **Ge** Germanium 72.5	33 **As** Arsenic 75	34 **Se** Selenium 79	35 **Br** Bromine 80	36 **Kr** Krypton 84
37 **Rb** Rubidium 86	38 **Sr** Strontium 88	39 **Y** Yttrium 89	40 **Zr** Zirconium 91	41 **Nb** Niobium 93	42 **Mo** Molybdenum 96	43 **Tc** Techetium (99)*	44 **Ru** Ruthenium 101	45 **Rh** Rhodium 103	46 **Pd** Palladium 106	47 **Ag** Silver 108	48 **Cd** Cadmium 112		49 **In** Indium 115	50 **Sn** Tin 119	51 **Sb** Antimony 122	52 **Te** Tellurium 128	53 **I** Iodine 127	54 **Xe** Xenon 131
55 **Cs** Caesium 133	56 **Ba** Barium 137	57 **La** Lanthanum 139	72 **Hf** Hafnium 178.5	73 **Ta** Tantalum 184	74 **W** Tungsten 184	75 **Re** Rhenium 186	76 **Os** Osmium 190	77 **Ir** Iridium 192	78 **Pt** Platinum 195	79 **Au** Gold 197	80 **Hg** Mercury 201		81 **Tl** Thallium 204	82 **Pb** Lead 207	83 **Bi** Bismuth 209	84 **Po** Polonium (210)	85 **At** Astatin (210)	86 **Rn** Radon (222)
87 **Fr** Fraicium (223)	88 **Ra** Radium (226)	89 **Ac** Actinium (226)																

58 **Ce** Cerium 140	59 **Pr** Praseodymium 141	60 **Nd** Neodymium 144	61 **Pm** Promethium (145)*	62 **Sm** Samarium 150	63 **Eu** Europium 152	64 **Gd** Gadolinium 157	65 **Tb** Terbium 159	66 **Dy** Dysprosium 162.5	67 **Ho** Holmium 165	68 **Er** Erbium 167	69 **Tm** Thullium 169	70 **Yb** Ytttterbium 173	71 **Lu** Lutetium 175
90 **Th** Thorium 232	91 **Pa** Protactin 231	92 **U** Uranium 238	93 **Np** Neptunium (237)*	94 **Pu** Plutonium (242)*	95 **Am** Americium (243)*	96 **Cm** Curium (247)*	97 **Bk** Berkalium (249)*	98 **Cf** Californium (251)*	99 **Es** Einsteinium (254)*	100 **Fe** Fermium (253)*	101 **Md** Mendelivium (256)*	102 **No** Nobelium (254)*	103 **Lw** Lawrencium (257)*

*The relative atomic mass of an element whose isotopic composition is variable is shown in parenthesis. Elements marked with * are those which do not occur naturally on earth.*

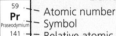

59 — Atomic number
Pr — Symbol
Praseodymium
141 — Relative atomic mass

Figure 4.2 The Periodic Table of elements. Ninety-nine per cent of the human body is comprised of those elements highlighted.

Q. Carbon, hydrogen, oxygen and nitrogen are the most prevalent elements in the body, and hence in our diets. In which dietary constituents would you expect to find these elements?

BOX 4.1 RADIOISOTOPES IN PRACTICE

Radioisotopes have a number of implications for medicine:

- Iodine is a normal constituent of thyroid hormones, and the uptake of a radioisotope of iodine by the gland is frequently used to assess production of thyroid hormones.

- If the energy of the radiation is large enough, then the impact of radiated particles with other atomic nuclei can be used to displace some of their nuclear particles. This is the basis of treating cancer by radiotherapy, the principle of which is to change the chemical structure of the genetic material of tumour cells and so destroy them.

- In more recent developments, imaging the activity of parts of the brain has become possible by administering the sugar glucose that has been produced so that it contains a radioisotope of carbon.

Conversely, excessive irradiation of normal cells can also make them cancerous as gene changes cause a loss of control of cell division.

Radioisotopes

Some isotopes become unstable, with the result that the nucleus fragments and neutrons are emitted as 'radiation'. Such isotopes are called radioisotopes. For example, carbon atoms (atomic number 6) usually have six protons and six neutrons (i.e. the atomic mass is 6+6 = 12). Another form of carbon exists that has eight neutrons in its nucleus (i.e. the atomic mass is now 6+8 = 14). This form of carbon is referred to as carbon-14 to distinguish it from carbon-12. Both forms are chemically identical, but the atomic nuclei of carbon-14 are less stable and emit the excess neutrons as radiation, causing them to change to the more stable carbon-12.

Electrolytes

Although atoms are electrically neutral, some may lose or gain electrons and so disturb the balance between positive and negative charges. The loss of electrons gives an atom a net positive charge, since the protons will now be in excess of the electrons, whilst a gain of electrons gives it a net negative charge as the number of electrons will now exceed the number of protons. The presence of an electrical charge means that a solution of ions will carry an electric current, and so another term for ions is electrolytes: this is the term used most widely in clinical practice. Negatively and positively charged ions are called anions and cations, respectively, because when an electric current is passed through a solution, they move to the electrodes called the anode and cathode, respectively.

Exercise

Obtain a blood analysis card from the haematology department or your GP surgery, and note the range of ions that may be tested for. In particular, note the units of measurement. Refer to Appendix A to determine what these units mean.

Ions occur when atoms lose or gain electrons, which produces an imbalance in electrical charge. Such an imbalance could also arise if an atom loses or gains protons – so why doesn't this occur? To answer this, refer to the text explanation relating to the structure of atoms.

Ions arise in those elements in which the electrons are not distributed evenly around the nucleus of the atom. Electrons spin in a series of orbits around the nucleus, which for convenience can be visualized as a series of concentric circles (Figure 4.1(a)). The orbits equate to energy levels or 'shells', the stability of which is determined by the number of electrons present. Each orbit has a maximum number of electrons that it can contain: the first orbit holds a maximum of two electrons, the second orbit eight, and the third eight (in smaller atoms) or up to 18 (in large atoms). The chemical properties of an atom relate to the tendency for the outermost orbit to move towards being full of electrons, as then it is stable. In an ion, the orbit has gained electrons to fill the outer orbit, or has lost electrons to remove that orbit entirely thus making the (full) preceding one the new outer orbit.

For example, chlorine (Cl) atoms have the atomic number 17, and so normally have 17 protons and 17 electrons. This means that the third electron orbit will contain only seven electrons (2+8+7; Figure 4.1(b)). For maximum stability, the outer orbit might be removed by loss of all seven electrons, but it is easier for the orbit to be filled by accepting one more electron. This will produce an 'atom' with 17 protons and 18 electrons, giving it a net negative charge: this is the chlorine (or chloride, as it is usually called) ion. The additional electron will have been obtained from another atom.

In contrast, sodium (atomic number 11) normally has 11 electrons, with just one in its outer orbit (2+8+1; Figure 4.1(c)). To achieve maximum stability, the atom would need either to acquire another seven electrons to fill the outer orbit, or to lose the one it already has and so lose that orbit completely. Losing the single electron represents the easiest means, and this leaves the ion with 11 protons and 10 electrons, and hence a positive charge. The lost electron could contribute to another ion, e.g. the chloride ion mentioned above. The loss of an electron by a sodium atom and the gain of that electron by a chlorine atom enables the formation of sodium chloride (NaCl, table salt).

Atoms of some elements, such as helium (He), neon (Ne) and argon (Ar), have just the right number of electrons to fill their orbits and therefore do not have to lose or gain electrons for stability. These are called inert elements; they do not usually take part in chemical reactions. This makes the gas helium useful in clinical evaluations of lung function as it can be inhaled without physiological consequences.

The concentrations of ions dissolved in our body fluids must be controlled closely because the presence of an electrical charge makes ions chemically active, and so they have important physiological actions. Some ions, such as those of zinc (Zn^{2+}) and aluminium (Al^{3+}), are found in such low concentrations that they are referred to as trace elements. However, their presence is essential for certain enzymes to function normally, and they may be extremely toxic when in excess. Their regulation remains poorly understood.

Exercise

Refer to the text to explain why sodium ions have one electrical charge, zinc ions two, and aluminium ions three. Why are these ions positively charged rather than negative?

Acids, bases and buffers

Acids

Hydrogen has the smallest atoms of all elements, having just one proton and one electron. To achieve stability the atom needs to gain an additional electron to fill the orbit, or to lose the electron it has and so become just a proton. The former case is achieved when the atom shares electrons with another atom, e.g. with oxygen to form water (see next section). The latter case occurs when the atom donates its electron to another atom, which then becomes an ion. For example, if hydrogen chloride gas (symbol HCl) is dissolved in water, it dissociates into its constituent ions:

$$HCl \iff H^+ + Cl^-$$

Hydrogen $\iff$ Hydrogen + Chloride
chloride   ions   ions

A chemical that produces hydrogen ions when it dissolves in water is called an acid. In this example, HCl dissolved in water forms hydrochloric acid. The arrows indicate that the reaction is reversible, i.e. the ions can recombine to form hydrogen chloride. However, hydrochloric acid dissociates very readily, so at any given moment the solution will be comprised almost entirely of hydrogen and chloride ions. This tendency of hydrochloric acid to be almost fully dissociated makes it a strong acid.

In contrast, some acids do not break down very easily. For example, if carbon dioxide is combined with water, carbonic acid is produced; this may also dissociate into its constituent ions:

$$H_2CO_3 \Leftrightarrow H^+ + HCO_3^-$$

Carbonic $\Leftrightarrow$ Hydrogen + Bicarbonate
acid   ions   ions

Again, the arrows indicate that the reaction is reversible, but in this example the acid does not dissociate very readily, so at any given time the concentration of hydrogen ions in the solution will be low. This is a weak acid. Nevertheless, some hydrogen ions will be present and it is these that give, for example, the tang to fizzy (carbonated) drinks.

You may have noticed from the above equations that acids also release other (negatively charged) ions. This helps to explain why there is a relatively high concentration of bicarbonate ions (from carbonic acid) in blood plasma. The high concentration of bicarbonate ions emphasizes the relative importance of carbon dioxide as a source of acidity in body fluids.

Bases and buffers

Hydrogen ions are extremely reactive. One of their most detrimental actions in biological systems is to combine with proteins, thus altering cellular function and disturbing homeostasis. Their concentration must be regulated in order to avoid the major cellular dysfunction that would result from the presence of too many hydrogen ions (see Chapter 15 for further details). One obvious mechanism would be to chemically combine the ions with another substance, and so remove them as ions from the solution; substances that will do this are called bases. However, if the resultant combination is unstable it will usually break down again, leaving most of the hydrogen ions still in solution. To effectively remove the hydrogen ions from solution requires bases that do not form unstable combinations. These bases are then referred to as buffers; the process is called buffering. To illustrate buffering, we can use the same examples as above.

The chloride ions produced when hydrochloric acid dissociates will be bases, as this is a reversible reaction. These chloride ions, however, will be ineffective at buffering because of the strong tendency for the reformed hydrochloric acid to dissociate: if more hydrogen ions are added to the solution, they will combine with chloride, but the resultant acid dissociates again immediately, so most of the hydrogen ions will remain free. The acidity of the solution will therefore increase.

The bicarbonate ions produced when carbonic acid dissociates will also be bases, since the reaction is reversible. Addition of hydrogen ions to the solution will promote the reaction to form carbonic acid. As we have seen, this is a weak acid and slow to separate into its constituent ions, so at any given time few of the added hydrogen ions will be free in the solution. The added hydrogen ions will therefore have little effect on the acidity of the solution. Bicarbonate ions, then, are effective buffers. Other important buffers in body fluids include phosphate ions and some proteins (including haemoglobin in red blood cells).

Buffers, then, maintain a near-constancy of the acidity of a solution by preventing an increase in the concentration of 'free' hydrogen ions (Figure 4.3). However, the buffering action entails hydrogen ions combining with the base ions and so removes the base chemical as well. Continued addition of hydrogen ions will eventually deplete the base. At this point, the 'buffering capacity' of

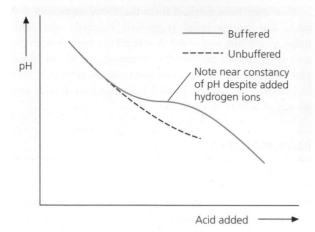

Figure 4.3 Influence on pH of adding acid (i.e. hydrogen ions) to either a solution that is unbuffered (dotted line) or one that contains a buffer chemical (solid line). Notice the plateau region where pH is held almost constant by the buffer.

Q. *The near-constancy of pH in the plateau region indicates that the added hydrogen ions have not affected the acidity of the solution. What has happened to them?*

the solution will have been exceeded, and so the acidity will start to increase as further hydrogen ions begin to remain free in solution. The addition of more buffer will help to prevent this and is the basis of one of the homeostatic mechanisms which come into play when the acidity of body fluids is disturbed (see Application Box 4.3, and also Chapter 15: The kidneys and urinary tract, for details).

BOX 4.3 RAISING THE BUFFERING CAPACITY OF BODY FLUIDS

Bicarbonate ions can be administered in order to improve the buffering capacity of body fluids. For example, antacid preparations for indigestion typically consist of bicarbonate in some form and will buffer gastric acid and so prevent the acidity from rising further. If sufficient bicarbonate is ingested, then the buffering becomes even more effective and the hydrogen ion concentration will begin to decrease and may even be neutralized.

In severe respiratory disorders or renal failure, the capacity of the body to excrete carbon dioxide or hydrogen ions, respectively, is decreased, leading to accumulation of acid within the body fluids. As the buffering capacity of the blood is exceeded, the patient will be diagnosed as having an acidosis. If this is severe, bicarbonate infusions may be used to counteract the increased acidity.

Units of acidity

The ion concentrations in solutions are normally given using the units of millimoles per litre (mmol/l; see Appendix A). Hydrogen ion concentration may be given this way,

but the buffering of body fluids is so effective that even smaller units are used (e.g. nanomoles per litre, nmol/l, where 1 million nanomoles = 1 millimole). In practice, these very low concentrations are usually converted into another unit called the pH value. This is determined using a pH meter. pH is a scale from 1 to 14 in which a value of 7 is neutral:

$$1 \text{———} 7 \text{———} 14$$

Strong Acidic (increased acid concentration, i.e. H^+>base)	Weak	Weak	Strong Alkaline (increased base concentration, i.e. base>H^+)
		Neutral (H^+ = base)	

The neutral point of pH 7 relates to a situation in which hydrogen and alkali ions are equal; this is the pH of pure water (H_2O; separates weakly into H^+ and OH^- ions). Values below pH 7 are acidic and represent an increased concentration of hydrogen ions, and values above pH 7 represent increasing alkalinity, hence decreasing concentrations of hydrogen ions. The relationship between pH and hydrogen ion concentration is identified in Box 4.4.

BOX 4.4 pH AND HYDROGEN ION CONCENTRATION

The pH of blood averages 7.4 in health, although any value between 7.35 and 7.45 is considered normal. Thus, blood is slightly alkaline. A pH of 7.4 represents a concentration of hydrogen ions of 40 nmol/l, which is slightly less than that of water (i.e. the weak dissociation of water into H^+ and OH^- ions produces an H^+ concentration of 100 nmol/l).

Decreased pH values reflect an increased hydrogen ion concentration, and increased pH represents a decreased hydrogen ion concentration. The pH scale is an example of a logarithmic scale: a change in one pH unit represents a 10-fold change in hydrogen ion concentration. Thus, pH 8 represents a hydrogen ion concentration of one-tenth that at neutral pH 7, whilst a pH of 6 represents a 10-fold increase. Acidity in the stomach is about pH 3 during digestion, which represents a concentration of hydrogen ions of 1 million nmol/l(i.e. 1 mmol/l). To put this into context, pH 3 represents a 25 000-fold increase in hydrogen ion concentration than is present in blood at pH 7.4, yet the pH has changed by only 4.4 units. This relationship between pH and hydrogen ion concentration must be kept in mind when interpreting blood analysis data.

Molecules and compounds

When two or more atoms combine in a chemical reaction, the resultant substance is a molecule. If the molecule

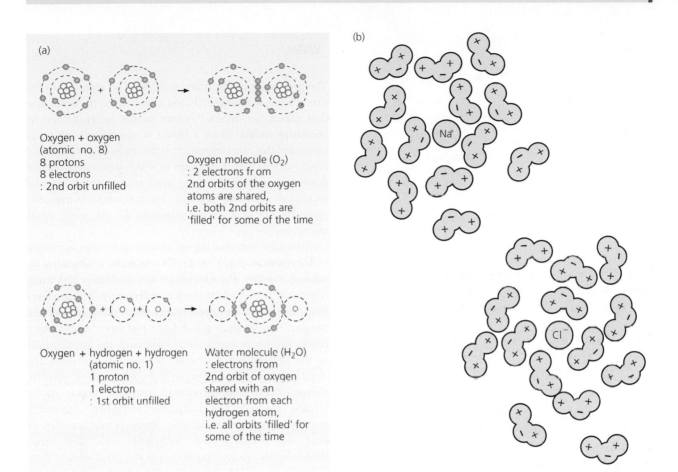

(a)

Oxygen + oxygen
(atomic no. 8)
8 protons
8 electrons
: 2nd orbit unfilled

Oxygen molecule (O_2)
: 2 electrons from
2nd orbits of the oxygen
atoms are shared,
i.e. both 2nd orbits are
'filled' for some of the time

Oxygen + hydrogen + hydrogen
(atomic no. 1)
1 proton
1 electron
: 1st orbit unfilled

Water molecule (H_2O)
: electrons from
2nd orbit of oxygen
shared with an
electron from each
hydrogen atom,
i.e. all orbits 'filled' for
some of the time

(b)

Figure 4.4 Bonding between atoms. (a) An oxygen atom can form a covalent bond with another oxygen atom to form an oxygen molecule (i.e. O_2), or with two hydrogen atoms to form a molecule of water (H_2O). (b) The uneven distribution of electrical charge within a water molecule means that the molecule can act as a solvent of atoms/molecules that also have a charge. This is how, for example, table salt (sodium chloride) dissolves in water.

contains atoms of different elements, it may be referred to as a compound, although the term 'molecule' tends to be used generically.

Take, for example, an atom of oxygen (atomic number 8), which has a total of eight electrons, six of which are in its outer orbit (2+6; see Figure 4.4(a)). For maximum stability an oxygen atom therefore must gain two electrons in order to fill the outer orbit. In this instance the atom does not usually become an ion; instead, it shares electrons with another atom, such as another oxygen atom. In this way, there will be brief moments in which the atom will have a full complement of electrons, as some of those of the second atom spin around it; similarly the second atom will sometimes also have a full complement. The time spent without a full complement is negligible, so in effect the two atoms have attained stability. This combination of atoms by sharing electrons is called a covalent bond.

The oxygen atom could, of course, share electrons with atoms of other elements; Figure 4.4(a) also shows an oxygen atom sharing electrons with two hydrogen atoms. Hydrogen (atomic number 1) has only one electron in its outer orbit (remember that this is the first orbit, and can

maximally hold two electrons), and by sharing electrons with oxygen the hydrogen atoms will also each 'gain' the extra electron they need for stability. Such covalent bonds are essential to life – they are relatively easy to form, but they are stable and not expensive in terms of the energy required.

In these examples, the molecule consisting of two oxygen atoms is given the symbol O_2 – the subscript number denotes the presence of two atoms; this is the form in which oxygen is found in the atmosphere. The molecule or compound consisting of an oxygen atom and two hydrogen atoms is given the symbol H_2O, i.e. water. Note how the change in constituents changes the properties of the substance.

Oxygen and water molecules are relatively simple as they involve just a few atoms. Some atoms have a capacity to share many more electrons, and so more complex molecules are possible. For example, a carbon atom (atomic number 6) has four electrons in its outer orbit (2+4; Figure 4.5). To 'gain' the four electrons it requires to fill the outer orbit, a carbon atom may, for example, share electrons with four hydrogen atoms to produce the molecule CH_4 (methane), or it may share electrons with

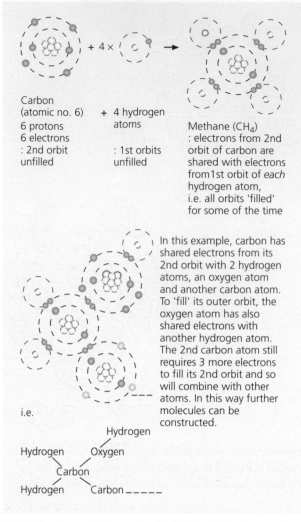

Carbon
(atomic no. 6)
6 protons
6 electrons
: 2nd orbit
unfilled

+ 4 hydrogen
atoms

: 1st orbits
unfilled

Methane (CH_4)
: electrons from 2nd
orbit of carbon are
shared with electrons
from1st orbit of *each*
hydrogen atom,
i.e. all orbits 'filled'
for some of the time

In this example, carbon has
shared electrons from its
2nd orbit with 2 hydrogen
atoms, an oxygen atom
and another carbon atom.
To 'fill' its outer orbit, the
oxygen atom has also
shared electrons with
another hydrogen atom.
The 2nd carbon atom still
requires 3 more electrons
to fill its 2nd orbit and so
will combine with other
atoms. In this way further
molecules can be
constructed.

i.e.

Hydrogen

Hydrogen   Oxygen

Carbon

Hydrogen   Carbon _ _ _ _ _

Figure 4.5   The versatility of carbon: the building of simple or complex organic molecules.

Q. Look closely at the diagram of the carbon atom. How many electrons does it have in its outer orbit? How many can it contain when full? How many electrons could it share with other atoms?

another carbon atom (Figure 4.5). This latter carbon atom may, of course, combine with yet more atoms to gain the additional three electrons it now requires for stability, and so the process may continue. Potentially, such molecules may involve hundreds of atoms, and they are said to be macromolecules ('macro-' = large); there are many examples of these in cells, e.g. carbohydrates, proteins and fats.

The capacity of carbon atoms to combine with so many other atoms makes it a particularly versatile element. It is perhaps not surprising, therefore, to find that carbon-based compounds form the chemical basis of all living organisms. The chemistry of carbon and its compounds is referred to as organic chemistry to distinguish it from the chemistry of other elements (called inorganic chemistry).

Water

The properties of water are considered so essential to life that scientists assume that life is only likely to occur (on this planet or others) where water is available. Its chemistry makes water a liquid at normal air temperatures, and this is an important factor in its role. As a liquid it provides us with a medium in which substances may be dissolved, and hence transported around the body and within cells, and one in which chemical reactions may take place. Its role as a solvent relates to the properties of its molecules.

Although the sharing of electrons by the hydrogen and oxygen atoms, (Figure 4.4), is numerically ideal to achieve stability, the oxygen atomic nucleus is very large compared with that of the hydrogen atoms. This means that the shared electrons spend more time around the oxygen nucleus than around the hydrogen nuclei. As a result, the water molecule is polarized: the oxygen pole of the molecule has a weak negative charge from the electrons, and the hydrogen pole has a weak positive charge. These charges enable hydrogen bonds to be formed through the attraction to other electrically charged ions and molecules; there is no transfer of electrons between the hydrogen and this other ion/molecule, so hydrogen bonds are even weaker than covalent bonds. Hydrogen bonding explains why water is such a good solvent (Figure 4.4(b)), and hence why body fluids can contain so many different ions (see Chapter 6). In contrast, substances such as lipids that do not carry a charge are poorly soluble in water. In this way, the lipid-based cell membrane forms an effective barrier between the aqueous environments inside and outside cells, which enables cells to maintain a composition of fluid inside them that is quite different to that of the fluids outside.

Hydrogen bonds within cells

Whilst hydrogen bonds explain the solvent properties of water, within cells they also have other roles. This is because the small size of hydrogen atoms relative to other atoms will often also cause polarization in these molecules, leaving the hydrogen atoms with a weak positive charge and other constituent atoms with negative charges. Hydrogen bonds therefore form between various molecules in cells, but because they are weak they are easily broken, and so require very little energy. For example, hydrogen bonding between the constituent molecules of DNA helps to hold the two chains of the DNA molecule together. The two chains must be separated during the processes of DNA replication or RNA transcription (see Chapter 2), and the presence of hydrogen bonds means that this is done easily and efficiently.

METABOLISM: A GENERAL OVERVIEW

As we have seen, anabolic processes in metabolism involve the formation of chemical bonds (predominantly covalent bonds) between atoms or molecules, and so require the constituent atoms or molecules (i.e. the reaction substrates) to be present in adequate amounts, together with sufficient energy for the bonds to be made (Figure 4.6). The energy and the substrates required are produced when chemical bonds in other substances are broken, i.e. by catabolism. Within cells, the appropriate catabolic and anabolic reactions must proceed in an appropriate way, and at a rate conducive to the demands placed on the cell; this is ensured by the presence of chemicals called enzymes.

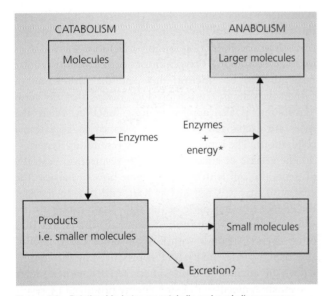

Figure 4.6 Relationship between catabolic and anabolic processes. Some products of catabolism (and perhaps anabolism) may not be useful to cells, and so will be removed from the cell and excreted.

*The energy required for anabolism will be provided by the catabolism of 'fuels', e.g. glucose molecules.

Enzymes

Enzymes are catalysts: they accelerate a specific chemical reaction but do not actually take part in it themselves and so are not changed by it. By promoting a specific reaction, perhaps just one of thousands of reactions occurring within a cell, the rate at which that reaction proceeds is increased. This may be vital if that biochemical process is to be compatible with life.

In chemical terms, enzymes are polypeptides or proteins (proteins are made of polypeptides combined together), i.e. they are large molecules comprised of lots of amino acids. Cells produce a huge variety of enzymes, and the nomenclature for them used by biochemists and clinicians can be bewildering. Some enzymes have generic names according to the chemical group on which they act, e.g. a protease is an enzyme that breaks down proteins. The name of an enzyme can be more specific, e.g. sucrase is an enzyme that breaks down sucrose into its constituent simple sugar units of glucose and fructose. Sometimes, an enzyme is named after its chemical action, e.g. a dehydrogenase enzyme is one that dehydrogenates (i.e. removes a hydrogen atom from) a molecule, whilst a hydroxylase enzyme adds a hydroxyl group (-OH) to the molecule.

Note that enzyme names usually end in the suffix '-ase'. An enzyme may also contain a non-protein cofactor without which it will not function. These cofactors may be ions, such as calcium and magnesium, or complex molecules called coenzymes, such as some B-group vitamins.

Exercise

Carry out a literature search on wound treatment methods. Identify how enzymes may be used in wound cleaning and healing.

The interactions between substrate and enzyme are illustrated in Figure 4.7. In this example, an enzyme E is attached to compound A to form an enzyme–substrate complex. The three-dimensional structure of the enzyme molecule means that only substance A will fit into it. In this example, the enzyme's action promotes the separation of the compound into two of its constituent compounds, B and C.

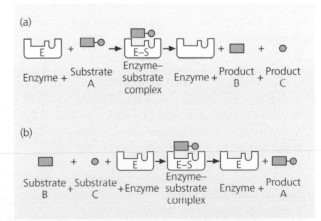

Figure 4.7 Enzyme–substrate reactions. Note how a single enzyme can promote the production of products from a certain substrate, but can also promote reformation of the substrate from those same products.

Q. What determines whether the enzyme will form products or substrate?

BOX 4.5 ENZYME SPECIFICITY: CARDIAC AND LIVER ENZYMES

The 'lock and key' idea suggests that the enzyme (the 'lock') accepts a molecule that has a complementary shape (the 'key'). These principles apply to various chemical interactions within the body, e.g. in the combination of an antibody with an antigen during an immune response, or in the combination of a hormone or a drug with a receptor on a cell membrane. The common factor here is the specificity of the interaction.

Enzymes produced by a cell are normally for the cell's own use. In addition to those enzymes common to processes in all cells, there will also be enzymes that relate to the role of that particular cell type. Enzymes may become detectable in blood if the cells are damaged; those that are specific to the cell type may then be isolated and used for diagnostic purposes. For example, the appearance in blood of the enzymes lactic dehydrogenase (LDH) hydroxybutyrate dehydrogenase (HBD), glutamate oxaloacetate transaminase (GOT) and glutamate pyruvate transaminase (GPT) is an indicator of myocardial infarction or liver damage.

It is clear from Figure 4.7 that substances B and C could also fit individually into the enzyme shape. The enzyme might then promote bonding between them, and hence reform substance A, i.e. enzymes promote reversibility of reactions. The question therefore arises as to which substance(s) a cell would produce using this enzyme: A or (B + C)? Generally this is determined by how much of A or (B + C) is present, since the predominant substrate is more likely to gain access to the enzyme's active site. Thus if A is in excess of (B + C), then A is more likely to attach to the enzyme. This is referred to as competitive binding, and has a number of applications (see Box 4.6).

If the utilization of B and C is increased in a cell, then the rate of their production will increase accordingly since there will be even fewer of these molecules to compete with A for the binding sites on the enzyme. In this way, the increased utilization of B and C is matched by increased production, and so cell homeostasis is maintained.

From this discussion, it should be obvious that a lack of a particular enzyme will prevent a certain reaction from occurring, whilst a surfeit of the enzyme could cause the reaction to proceed too quickly. The control of the enzyme is achieved by regulating its synthesis or by interfering with its availability. Other enzymes will also be involved in these processes, and this is a classic example of the interrelationships that operate in living organisms and contribute to homeostasis.

Energy production by cells: cellular respiration and ATP

We noted earlier how breaking chemical bonds provides the source of energy for cell processes. This is the process referred to as cellular respiration (sometimes referred to as internal respiration). Oxygen must be available for cellular respiration to be efficient; this, and the production of carbon dioxide as a waste product, means that the term 'respiration' is also applied to lung function, where the gases are exchanged (sometimes referred to as external respiration). The lungs comprise the respiratory system.

The release of energy by cellular respiration basically presents the cell with two problems: how to harness the energy so that it is not lost as heat, and how to transfer the energy to other parts of the cell. These problems are solved by the incorporation of (some of) the energy into other chemical bonds within a substance called adenosine triphosphate (ATP). ATP is produced by the combination of adenosine diphosphate (ADP) with another phosphate molecule (P) using energy produced by respiration. Thus:

$$ADP + P + energy \rightarrow ATP$$

The bond in ATP is readily broken again, provided that an enzyme called ATPase is present. This enzyme is found

BOX 4.6 COMPETITIVE BINDING

Competitive binding will apply wherever substances have to compete for a spot on a protein. An example is the action of the enzyme carbonic anhydrase found in red blood cells. In the tissues, this enzyme promotes the formation of bicarbonate ions from carbon dioxide, which is present in relatively high concentration. Within the lungs, the carbon dioxide concentration falls as the gas is excreted. Competitive binding then favours the conversion of bicarbonate ions to more of the gas, which can then also be excreted.

In another example, phenylketonuria (PKU) is an inherited condition in which the amino acid phenylalanine is not fully utilized. As a consequence, the concentration of phenylalanine in the blood rises, and it begins to compete more effectively for the protein-carrier process that transports amino acids into the brain. Thus, the developing brain of a child, which has a large demand for all types of amino acid, can become deprived as uptake is now dominated by phenylalanine transport. Intervention is aimed at reducing the phenylalanine concentration by restricting its presence in the diet. Control has to be instigated early: PKU is normally tested for by midwives within 7–10 days of birth (see also the case study of a man with phenylketonuria in Section 6).

Some drugs also utilize competitive binding. They compete for binding sites of hormones or other biological chemicals such as neurotransmitters, and in doing so prevent the actions of that chemical, i.e. they are antagonistic drugs.

in structures throughout the cell, and releases energy from ATP so that it can be utilized:

$$ATP \rightarrow ADP + P + energy$$

Harnessing energy initially as ATP is essential if the energy of respiration is to be made available for other reactions in the cell. The levels of ATP within a cell must therefore be maintained for normal cellular function, and increased if the metabolic demands of a cell increase (e.g. in a skeletal muscle cell during exercise). Cellular respiration therefore is equated with the metabolic rate of the cell.

Cellular respiration utilizes a battery of enzymes primarily to release energy from the chemical bonds within glucose molecules. A single molecule of glucose generates a net 38 molecules of ATP. The first eight of these are produced in the cell cytoplasm by reactions that do not use oxygen; this is referred to as anaerobic respiration ('an-' = without, 'aer-' = air). The remaining 30 ATP molecules are produced using oxygen in a process referred to as aerobic respiration, which takes place within the mitochondria of the cell.

As most of the ATP produced by respiration involves utilizing oxygen, measuring the amount of oxygen a person uses per minute provides a measure of the metabolic rate of their entire body.

Metabolism and body temperature

The efficiency by which energy from respiration is harnessed is less than 50%, and further energy is lost when it is released from ATP and utilized. Overall, efficiency is normally only of the order of 20–25%, and even athletic training will not raise this by more than just a few per cent. In other words,

> ### BOX 4.7 METABOLIC RATE
>
> In considering an individual's metabolic rate, it is necessary to consider two aspects: the basal metabolic rate (BMR) and the increment due to activity. The BMR relates to the basic processes that keep us alive, including cell division during tissue repair, growth in children, and growth in pregnant women. The BMR varies between individuals primarily due to differences in gender, age and body size, so it is normally expressed as a standardized value. Clinically, the BMR becomes an important consideration in metabolic disorders such as hyperthyroidism ('hyper-' = greater than normal), in which an excessive production of thyroid hormones raises the rate above the normal range. The BMR is also elevated in individuals with fever through the resetting of the set point for body temperature, and after surgery or trauma through the activities of the hormone cortisol.
>
> The increment in metabolic rate due to activity will clearly relate to physical activities, but will also include mental activities and even the increased metabolism observed after eating a meal. Physical activity level makes the most important contribution and so is a factor in dietary recommendations (see Chapter 5).

some 75% or so of the energy released in respiration is lost as heat. Much of this must be dissipated from cells, because excess heat denatures the structure of enzymes and so would affect the rate of chemical reactions. Not all heat is immediately lost from the body, however, since maintaining a core temperature of about 37°C is necessary if metabolic processes in essential organs are to occur at an optimal rate. Some of the heat produced by metabolism therefore is utilized to maintain this core temperature. The role of metabolism in relation to temperature homeostasis is explored further in Chapter 16 (The skin).

CELLULAR RESPIRATION

Aerobic respiration

Aerobic metabolism of glucose

You should read this section in conjunction with Figure 4.8.

Glucose is a relatively large molecule, insoluble in lipids and unable to diffuse directly into the cell. It enters cells through facilitated diffusion, via carrier proteins that 'flip' the sugar across the cell membrane. The molecule is then converted by a series of enzyme-driven reactions to a substance called pyruvate. This process occurs within the cytoplasm and is an anaerobic stage (i.e. it occurs in the absence of oxygen; see later) that generates eight molecules of ATP from one molecule of glucose. The pyruvate then

> ### BOX 4.8 ORAL GLUCOSE/ ELECTROLYTE THERAPY
>
> The means by which glucose enters into cells is an example of facilitated diffusion (see Chapter 2). The process is made more efficient by utilizing the concentration gradient for sodium, which is greater than that of glucose, to drive the carriage. To do this, sodium ions must also combine with the carrier protein. Glucose uptake by cells of the small intestine operates in the same way, and this is one reason why electrolytes are incorporated into oral rehydration solutions used to counteract the consequences of diarrhoea

enters the cell's mitochondria, where it is converted using another enzyme into a substance called acetyl coenzyme A, which enters another complex series of enzymatically controlled reactions called the tricarboxylic acid cycle (the

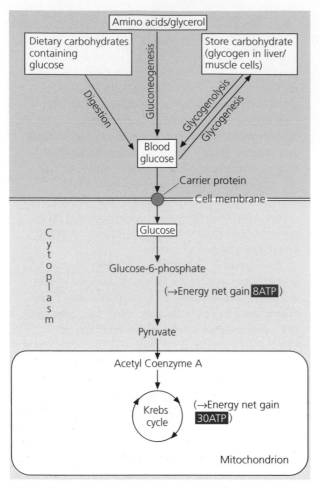

Figure 4.8 Glucose metabolism (or 'cellular respiration'). Note that this is a very simplified diagram of the processes involved. Once glucose has entered a cell, it undergoes many conversions promoted by numerous enzymes. The ATP that is produced in the cytoplasm does not require oxygen (i.e. this is anaerobic respiration). The ATP produced in the mitochondria occurs in a process that utilizes oxygen (i.e. this is aerobic respiration). Each molecule of glucose generates a net 38 molecules of ATP. Overall the equation for the reaction is written as $C_6H_{12}O_6 + 6O_2 \rightarrow 6CO_2 + 6H_2O$.

Q. How many molecules of ATP are gained from a molecule of glucose by anaerobic and aerobic respiration? Which of these processes is the most efficient?

Q. Can you define 'gluconeogenesis', 'glycogenolysis' and 'glycogenesis'?

TCA or Krebs cycle). This cycle of reactions is important because the stepwise reactions release energy in a slow, controlled fashion, which makes the harnessing of the energy as ATP much more efficient, hence the 30 molecules of ATP per molecule of glucose in this aerobic (i.e. utilizing oxygen) part of the process.

One feature of the aerobic process is that electrons are released from atoms by the TCA cycle of events, and these are then transferred along a series of further chemicals found in the membranes of mitochondria. This is the stage of the process that requires oxygen, and it is the main source of energy release and harnessing. The chemicals concerned are

called cytochromes (also referred to as the electron transport chain). One important cytochrome is derived from the B vitamin niacin, so this must be present in our diet.

The aerobic metabolism of glucose via the TCA cycle produces waste products (CO_2 and H_2O), the excesses of which are removed from the body via the lungs/kidneys. Homeostatic regulation of the functioning of these organs ensures that the removal is sufficient to prevent a build-up of these wastes (see Chapters 14 and 15).

Aerobic metabolism of fatty acids and amino acids

You should read this section in conjunction with Figure 4.9.

In addition to producing energy from glucose, cells also have the enzymes necessary for the respiration of fatty acids

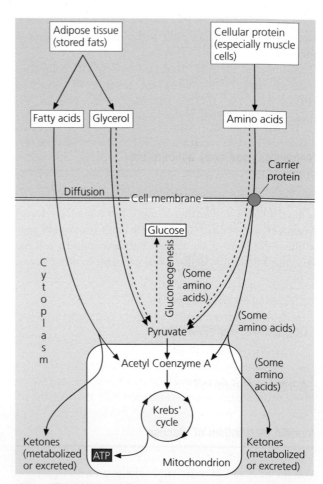

4.9 Aerobic metabolism of fats and proteins. Note that certain amino acids, and glycerol from fats, may be converted to pyruvate and so may be used to generate new glucose molecules (= gluconeogenesis). Note also that the metabolism also produces ketones as by-products, unlike the carbon dioxide and water produced by glucose metabolism (see Figure 4.8).

Q. When might gluconeogenesis be useful to us?

Q. Undernourishment, or altered metabolism in diabetes mellitus, tends to favour the metabolism of fats and proteins. The excessive amount of ketones produced may then become a problem. Why?

(from fat) and certain amino acids (from protein). Some fatty acid metabolism occurs continuously alongside that of glucose, and may account for about one-third of energy production, but it is more pronounced when carbohydrate intake and stores are low; this is the basis of promoting weight loss by dieting. Amino acids contribute about 15% to the basal metabolic rate, but this proportion will also be increased if carbohydrate intake is low, and if fat stores have been depleted, leading to the loss of muscle protein.

Within cells, the fatty acids or amino acids are converted into the intermediary substance acetyl coenzyme A identified earlier in the metabolism of glucose. In this way they can enter the TCA cycle. Some amino acids, and the glycerol released from the breakdown of stored fats, may be converted to pyruvate, and so may also enter the TCA cycle; alternatively, they may be converted to glucose

for use elsewhere in the body, since the processes that convert glucose to pyruvate are reversible.

This complex interplay of the use of metabolic fuels is useful for two reasons:

- Glucose, fatty acids, glycerol and some amino acids can all be converted to acetyl coenzyme A, and so all are sources of energy via the TCA cycle in mitochondria. Under normal circumstances, therefore, it is highly unlikely that cells will be starved of metabolic fuels.

- The capacity of cells to convert glycerol or some amino acids to glucose means that the availability of glucose can be increased to support tissue repair in damaged tissues, or to support muscles during exercise. The process of producing glucose from non-carbohydrate sources is referred to as gluconeogenesis ('creation of new glucose'); it is stimulated by the hormones cortisol (in wound healing) and adrenaline (in exercise).

Once it has entered the TCA cycle, acetyl coenzyme A will lead to the production of carbon dioxide and water, as noted in the metabolism of glucose. However, converting fatty acids and amino acids to acetyl coenzyme A also produces substances called ketones. These may be excreted in urine, or may be reused by some tissues for energy, e.g. cardiac muscle, but there is a limit to the effectiveness of such processes. The extent of the increased fatty acid and amino acid metabolism that is observed in poorly controlled diabetes mellitus means that ketone production is greatly increased. The ketones are detectable as a pear-drop smell on the person's breath, known as ketosis. The ketones may also appear in blood as ketoacids; if these are produced in excess of what can be removed from the body in urine, they will induce acidosis (excessive acidity), meaning that there are excess hydrogen ions in body fluids, which disrupt cell functioning. Acidosis is a potentially life-threatening situation and it must be corrected.

Anaerobic metabolism

Although most energy (and hence ATP) that is produced by cells involves the use of oxygen, we have also noted that some ATP production occurs within the cytoplasm, in the absence of oxygen. Such anaerobic metabolism is less efficient than aerobic metabolism, in that it generates only eight ATP molecules (out of a total of 38) per molecule of glucose. The ATP generated in this way is nevertheless an important contribution, but it is insufficient on its own to sustain cell functioning for very long. In addition, the process produces lactic acid. This is highly toxic to cells, and so has to be removed or at least deactivated. Lactic acid is taken up from blood by the liver, where it is detoxified by a process that requires oxygen.

During sharp bursts of exercise, or exercise that is prolonged and severe, the oxygen supply to muscles may not be sufficient to maintain aerobic respiration. Oxygen will initially be unloaded from the pigment myoglobin found within some muscle fibres, but once this source is depleted anaerobic metabolism will play a more significant role. The consequential build-up of lactic acid must be metabolized after exercise has finished, and the deoxygenated myoglobin must be replenished with oxygen. The metabolism of lactic acid after exercise, and the reloading of myoglobin, means that oxygen consumption will have to be greater than is usual at rest – this extra is called the 'oxygen debt', and explains why people breathe heavily after exercise, even though they have stopped the activity.

Controlling metabolism

Metabolism is determined by a number of factors, not least the supply of substrates to cells, the entry of substrates into cell structures, and the production/activities of appropriate enzymes that will catalyse reactions. The means of control are therefore varied. Hormones control much of the metabolism, but it should be noted that any physiological disorder, not just hormonal, will have consequences for metabolism somewhere within the body. Thus, disorders of metabolism arise because of the inability of a cell to perform essential biochemical activities. Normally this means a problem in delivering the necessary substrates or in their utilization, and restoring these is the main goal for many care practices. Future practice is also likely to include manipulating substrate use, through altering the availability of enzymes.

Some hormones are considered specifically as mediators of metabolism because they influence directly the concentrations of fuel molecules in blood, or their utilization by cells. This section focuses on the actions of these hormones, the disorders related to which are classed in clinical circles as disorders of metabolism.

The hormones insulin and glucagon are instrumental in regulating the glucose content of blood and its utilization by cells. Glucagon elevates blood glucose concentration if

---

BOX 4.11 METABOLISM IN DIABETES MELLITUS

Normal ranges for 'fasting' glucose concentration in blood plasma: newborn, 2.2–3.3 mmol/l (at 1 day); child, 3.3–5.5 mmol/l; adult, 3.9–5.8 mmol/l.

Diabetes mellitus produces medium- and long-term symptoms related to an increased blood glucose concentration arising from inadequate production of, or responses to, the hormone insulin. The medium term relates to the increased production of urine and the risk of urinary tract infections as a consequence of the presence of glucose in the urine (glycosuria). The presence of ketosis is also likely to occur at or around this time, i.e. the concentration of ketones in blood will increase as lipid metabolism is raised and the pear-drop odour of acetone, a type of ketone, will be noticeable on the person's breath. In addition, there is a continuous risk that inadequate dietary and insulin control may result in episodes when blood glucose concentration is too low (hypoglycaemia; 'hypo-' = less than normal, 'glyc-' = glucose, '-aemia' = of the blood). Brain cells in particular are sensitive to this, and behavioural changes including aggression may be observed; the problem may even progress to coma and perhaps death.

Hyperglycaemia ('hyper-' = greater than normal) in diabetes also influences cell function, particularly of sensory nerve cells and cells in the walls of small blood vessels. Long-term control is aimed at facilitating glucose utilization by cells, thus reducing the occurrence of hyperglycaemia, and the production of ketoacids from ketones. Long-term problems are related largely to the slow deterioration of nerve cell function and the microcirculation, particularly in the feet, kidneys and eyes, arising from the actions of glucose on these tissues. The rise in fatty acid concentrations in blood also increases the risk of heart disease.

The risks of coma and damage to tissues have resulted in aggressive therapeutic approaches to control blood glucose concentrations. Much of this, however, involves a self-care regime, and patient education is therefore essential. One of the difficulties associated with diabetes care is that people will often report feeling well – the damage arising from the increased glucose is insidious – and lapses in control may occur as a consequence. In addition, imposing rigorous control may also be perceived by the individual as being too demanding, and of placing unacceptable restrictions on their lifestyle.

it is at risk of falling below the homeostatic range (e.g. between meals, or during stressful episodes such as serious illness or major surgery). It does so by mobilizing glucose from glycogen stores, and by promoting the generation of glucose from fatty acids and amino acids. This latter process is also promoted in times of stress by the actions of adrenaline and cortisol, which provide additional metabolic support by mobilizing glucose, fatty acids and amino acids, and so increase their input into cell respiration. Examples of this are seen in the stress response described in Chapter 22.

Insulin, on the other hand, promotes glucose uptake by cells when blood glucose concentration is increased following a meal that contains carbohydrate. Glucose utilization will therefore increase (which is why we feel warm after a large meal), but in the liver the uptake of glucose will also lead to the production of a glucose store (glycogen), or even to its conversion to fatty acids and perhaps amino acids. Insulin is the only hormone that acts to reduce

blood glucose concentration, and a failure to produce insulin, or a failure of cells to respond to it, results in the condition diabetes mellitus, characterized by a persistent increase in blood glucose concentration (hyperglycaemia; see Box 4.11).

Growth hormone also modulates the mobilization of metabolic fuels, primarily amino acids and fatty acids. Deficiency of growth hormone in children causes dwarfism, as the growth rate of tissues is suppressed, and excess causes giantism. Attention to growth patterns during childhood will usually identify problems arising from a disordered production of growth hormone. Excess growth hormone in adults promotes excessive skeletal growth, leading to acromegaly. Normal activities of growth hormone also include a diabetogenic action, as it inhibits some of the actions of insulin. Chronically high levels of the hormone exacerbate this action, and will eventually cause insulin production to decrease. There is also an increased risk of tissue problems, e.g. in cardiac functioning.

BOX 4.12 METABOLISM AND OBESITY

Fatty acids make a substantial contribution to cellular respiration, and it is noted in Chapter 5 just how useful fat stores are to us. Obesity represents excessive fat storage and is a health risk for the following reasons:

● The emphasis on fat means that there is usually hyperlipidaemia. This raises the risk of lipid deposits (or atheroma) in blood vessels, and hence of coronary heart disease, hypertension and stroke.
● The excessive body weight makes it harder for muscles to move the body, raising the effort required. The stress placed on the heart to maintain circulation even under normal circumstances is therefore increased.
● Obesity is often associated with a resistance to the actions of the hormone insulin, raising blood glucose concentrations. It is thought that this effect predisposes the person to insulin-independent diabetes mellitus.

Obesity represents an imbalance in which either the person is predisposed to storing (and synthesizing) fat, or there is a level of energy utilization (i.e. activity) that is inadequate for the level of fat intake. In the latter, this illustrates the biological importance of energy stores: the body does not excrete excess metabolic fuels, but stores them in case of lack of food. Sedentary lifestyles are of concern in the developed world, and are thought to be an important factor in the increasing incidence of obesity in the UK.

Predisposition to obesity is also likely in some individuals. Recent interest has focused on the genes involved in the production and actions of adipose hormones called leptins. Their elevation in blood with obesity has led to suggestions that they may be involved in the genesis of this condition. A strain of obese mouse that has a defect in leptin function is known; these mice respond well to injections of the hormone. However, most common forms of human obesity are not related to the specific gene defect that is observed in this mouse, so the role of leptins in obesity, though likely, remains unclear.

BOX 4.13 METABOLIC RESPONSES TO SURGERY

Surgery promotes metabolic responses that represent a resetting of homeostatic means as a consequence of the release of metabolic hormones in response to the surgical trauma (including pain). Their actions to promote metabolism are those associated with a 'stress' response. As such, these hormones should be viewed as an adaptive process to the situation that helps to promote survival. Readers should refer to Chapter 22, since this explains the release of metabolic hormones in relation to stress theory.

The hormones involved are adrenaline, cortisol and growth hormone. They promote the breakdown of glycogen and fat stores, and so mobilize glucose and fatty acids. A raised blood glucose concentration (or hyperglycaemia) is observed that favours the

functioning of tissues, especially the brain. Many tissues will also generate energy from the released fatty acids. The significance of increased mobilization of metabolic fuels is that cell division and tissue growth and repair are facilitated.

The availability of metabolic fuel is also facilitated by glucose synthesis, prompted by the actions of cortisol to induce protein breakdown and the conversion of the amino acids to glucose by the liver. Protein synthesis is also decreased, exacerbating the reduction in protein, and muscle loss may be observed. The persistence of protein depletion may hinder long-term wound healing, and may have implications for the general welfare of patients.

Thyroid hormones have a particular role as regulators of the basal metabolic rate, rather than as mediators of fuel availability. A deficiency in their production or actions can have profound effects on child development, especially mental development. In adults, a deficiency of thyroid hormones (hypothyroidism) leads to a depressed basal metabolic rate, with symptoms of lethargy, fatigue and feeling cold. The pulse rate is also slowed as cardiac metabolism is reduced. Hyperthyroidism, in which excess thyroid hormones are produced, has the opposite effects – increased basal metabolic rate, hyperactivity, feeling hot, and a rapid pulse rate.

Recent research has also identified a group of hormones called leptins that appear to be involved in regulating fat metabolism. Leptins are produced by adipose tissue and are thought to act within the hypothalamus to promote a reduction in food intake, and feeling of satiety (see Box 4.12).

Summary

1 Metabolism encompasses those chemical reactions that lead to synthesis (i.e. anabolism) or breakdown (i.e. catabolism) of substances by cells.

2 Atoms of elements provide the basic units of which chemical molecules are comprised.

3 Ions, or electrolytes, are formed when atoms lose or gain electrons in order to improve the stability of their atomic structure. These are positively or negatively charged according to whether they lose or gain electrons. The presence of an electrical charge makes ions chemically and physiologically active. Ions are constituents of body fluids.

4 Molecules are formed when two or more atoms bond together. This may entail electrical attraction (e.g. hydrogen bonds) or sharing electrons (i.e. covalent bonds). Both types of bond are relatively easy to form. Covalent bonds in particular are involved in anabolism and catabolism. Forming bonds in anabolic processes requires an input of energy, so metabolic rate equates with the energy production by cells to facilitate this.

5 Acids are chemicals that produce hydrogen ions when they dissolve in water. Bases are those that may combine with hydrogen ions to reform the acid substance. Weak acids do not readily produce hydrogen ions, and in this instance the bases that promote their formation are effective at removing hydrogen ions from body fluids. This is referred to as buffering.

6 Acidity is measured as pH units.

7 Enzymes are proteins that act as catalysts to promote anabolism or catabolism according to the relative availability of substrates (this is referred to as competitive binding). Their role depends upon their precise three-dimensional structure arising from the sequence of amino acids of which they are composed. This sequence is determined by DNA, and hence explains how genes determine cell structure and functions.

8 Cellular respiration describes the processes by which enzymes cause the release of energy by breaking molecular bonds. Respiration provides an intermediary chemical, ATP, which transfers energy from these energy-producing processes to all areas of the cell for utilization.

9 Glucose is the main substrate for respiration. One molecule of glucose generates 38 molecules of ATP. Eight of these molecules are produced in the cytoplasm by processes that do not require oxygen; this is referred to as anaerobic respiration. The remaining 30 molecules of ATP are produced within mitochondria by aerobic respiration, i.e. using oxygen.

10 Aerobic respiration of glucose entails a gradual change to the glucose molecule and the harnessing of energy as it is released. One of the substances produced during this process is called pyruvate; this can also be produced by cells using fatty acids and some amino acids. In this way, cells can utilize these fuels in addition to glucose.

11 Aerobic respiration of glucose generates carbon dioxide and water as waste substances. Carbon dioxide is a source of acid and so must be excreted via the lungs.

12 Aerobic metabolism of fatty acids and amino acids generates ketones, a source of ketoacids. These must be removed by the kidneys and liver.

13 Anaerobic processes generate lactic acid. This is removed by the liver and kidneys.

Review questions

1 The subject of biochemistry is vast, and it can be confusing to work out which areas of knowledge you will require for practice. You will need to recognize certain elements and their chemical symbols, and how they bond together to form compounds or molecules. Familiarize yourself with these terms: element, atom, ion, molecule and compound.

2 Elements you should become familiar with due to their physiological importance include oxygen, hydrogen, sodium, chlorine, potassium and carbon. There are other important elements of physiological significance whose chemical symbols are as follows: Ca, I, Fe, Mg, N, P and S. Look up and identify the elements listed. Memorize these chemical symbols, as they will be referred to frequently in clinical practice. Define the terms hypokalaemia, hyponatraemia, hypercalcaemia and hypercapnia. How would these affect cellular homeostasis?

3 Chemicals can combine to form molecules or compounds. These include the substances we recognize in our daily lives such as proteins, fats, carbohydrates and water. Which macronutrients contain nitrogen?

FURTHER READING

Texts on metabolism and biochemistry abound. Readers might find the following useful in relation to some of the specific points raised in this chapter regarding metabolism in surgery, diabetes mellitus and obesity.

Clancy, J., McVicar, A. and Baird, N. (2002) Chapter 7 Anaesthesia, stress and surgery, in: *Fundamentals of Physiology for Perioperative Practitioners*. London: Routledge.

Lean, M. (1998) *Clinical Handbook of Weight Management*. London: Martin Dunitz.

Williams, G. and Pickup, J.C. (1999) *Handbook of Diabetes*, 2nd edn. Oxford: Blackwell Science.

Chapter 5

Nutrients and nutrition

Introduction
The chemicals of life, and their dietary sources
References

IINTRODUCTION

Our diet should provide all of the chemicals that are necessary for cell metabolism, for the production of cell structures, and for the body fluids within and outside cells. In recognition of this a German philosopher, Ludwig Feuerbach (1804–1872), once quipped '*Man ist was man isst*' ('one is what one eats'). Though not technically correct, this is an appropriate play on words and the quip is not far from the truth.

This chapter considers the main constituents of cells and their sources from our diets.

BOX 5.1 THE NURSE'S ROLE IN PROMOTING AN ADEQUATE DIET

Whilst this chapter is concerned with the biological aspects of the diet, it should be remembered that eating is also a social phenomenon. Practitioners must be aware of aspects related to this, in addition to the importance of eating a balanced diet. Some issues to be considered are:

- the individual's need for independence, if possible;
- either privacy or social communication while eating may be preferred;
- ward routines may disturb eating behaviours;
- individuals have distinct dietary habits;
- specific groups have specific dietary needs, e.g. cultural aspects or developmental stage;
- age and gender influence the preferred diet;

- positioning and use of utensils may be influencing factors for patients who require help with eating;
- sick people may have poor appetites: observe the amounts eaten and look for signs of undernutrition;
- poor mouth care may affect eating behaviours;
- financial constraints may prevent the eating of an ideal diet, so dietary recommendations must be flexible enough to be cost effective for the individual;
- a working knowledge of the functioning of the gastrointestinal tract should improve the understanding of dietary factors in individuals with disordered functions.

Some of these activities will be supported by involvement of a multiprofessional team, especially a dietician.

THE CHEMICALS OF LIFE, AND THEIR DIETARY SOURCES

A balanced diet

Approximately 95% of the mass of the human body is comprised of the elements carbon, hydrogen, oxygen and nitrogen in various combinations to form carbohydrates, proteins, fats and water. Another 4% (mainly bone) is made up of phosphorus and calcium, whilst the remaining 1% consists of about 18 other elements, such as potassium and sodium. Our diets should contain the same elements, but will also have to support the energy requirements of cells, and contain fibre to aid the function of the gut in digesting food. Digestion is essential, because many of the foods we eat contain the elements in complex molecules that have to be reduced to simpler ones if they are to be absorbed into the body.

Health organizations make recommendations regarding the intake of almost all nutrients. Recommended intakes are calculated from their rates of utilization, storage or excretion, and are continually under review. The aim of such nutrition standards is to ensure that everyone receives sufficient amounts of each nutrient. Accordingly, a number of indices (collectively called Dietary Reference Values; Department of Health, 1991) have been developed. The most widely used one in the food industry is the recommended daily allowance (RDA), which is based on estimated average requirements. The difficulty with setting standards is that the needs of the body change according to the individual's age and stage of development. The situation is complicated further because there are individual differences in the rates at which nutrients are absorbed from the gut. Thus, someone who absorbs a nutrient at half the rate of another individual must eat twice as much to obtain the same amount (Figure 5.1).

Whilst the amounts of nutrients required may vary between people, there is no uncertainty as to the types of nutrient required. The principal components of a healthy diet are:

- carbohydrates (other than fibre)
- proteins
- lipids (including fats)
- energy (not a chemical, but considered a dietary constituent)
- fibre (mainly forms of carbohydrate)
- vitamins
- minerals
- nucleic acids
- water.

In terms of bulk, most of our food intake consists of carbohydrates, proteins and fat, but all of the constituents listed above are necessary for the maintenance of growth

BOX 5.2 ENTERAL AND PARENTERAL NUTRITION

The normal means of feeding is not always possible in various disorders, so food must be delivered directly into the digestive system (enteral nutrition) or into the circulatory system (parenteral nutrition).

Enteral feeding entails the delivery of foodstuffs in a semi-liquid state into the stomach, or possibly even the intestine, using a tube that has been inserted via the oesophagus (Guenter et al., 1997). This is clearly an unpleasant procedure for a patient, and may not always be effective if bowel dysfunction prevents digestion and/or absorption of nutrients.

In parenteral feeding (Reilly, 1998), sterile food solutions are administered intravenously via a catheter placed in a convenient vein. Parenteral nutrition supplies protein, carbohydrate, fat, electrolytes, minerals and water, i.e. the range of constituents of a normal diet other than nucleic acids and fibre. Parenteral feeds are available in a range of compositions or formulae, and can be made up in pharmacy according to dietetic advice if necessary. The intention is to maintain organ function and fluid/electrolyte balance until enteral or oral feeding becomes possible.

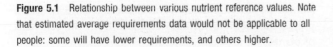

Figure 5.1 Relationship between various nutrient reference values. Note that estimated average requirements data would not be applicable to all people: some will have lower requirements, and others higher.

and health. It is important that individuals have the appropriate amount of each nutrient type; this is referred to as a balanced diet. From a practitioner's viewpoint, it is important to understand what constitutes a balanced diet and also to recognize how a person's illness, or perhaps surgery, may result in recommended changes to their diet. Such changes will depend upon the diagnosis and the severity of the problem. Health trusts and hospitals employ dieticians to advise on nutrition and so help individuals with their particular diets. The dietician, therefore, is an integral member of the health team.

The nutrients

Carbohydrates

Carbohydrates contain atoms of carbon ('carbo-'), hydrogen ('hydr-') and oxygen (indicated by '-ate'), and include substances such as sugars, starch and fibre. Carbohydrates have various functions in cells:

● They are the primary energy source in cells.

● They may be incorporated into, or combined with, other molecules.

● They may have roles in membrane functions, or may be structural components of those membranes.

● They may act as energy reserves.

Carbohydrates, then, are very versatile, and some may even be converted into other essential substances, such as the constituents of proteins and lipids, and so supplement these.

Monosaccharides, disaccharides and polysaccharides.

Carbohydrates may be divided into three main groups: monosaccharides, disaccharides and polysaccharides. Their names often end in the suffix '-ose'. Monosaccharides ('mono-' = single; 'saccharide' = sugar) are simple sugars that contain three to seven carbon atoms in their molecules; they are highly soluble in water. Biologically important examples are pentoses ('pent-' = five; the molecule contains five carbon atoms) and hexoses ('hex-' = six; the molecule contains six carbon atoms). For example, the pentose sugar ribose is a constituent of nucleic acids (hence *ribo*nucleic acid), e.g. DNA, and the hexose sugar glucose is the most important source of energy in cells.

Disaccharides ('di-' = two) consist of two monosaccharides joined together. Sucrose (cane or table sugar) is a common example, and is formed by combination of the monosaccharides glucose and fructose. Other examples include lactose (milk sugar). which is a combination of glucose and galactose, and maltose (malt sugar), which is a combination of two glucose molecules (Figure 5.2(a)).

Polysaccharides ('poly-' = many) consist of numerous monosaccharides joined together, and may be very large molecules. Unlike mono- and disaccharides, they are usually poorly soluble in water, and so form important components of cell membranes. Glycogen is a polysaccharide made from numerous glucose units that forms a convenient means of storing glucose in our cells, especially in the liver and in skeletal muscle. Starch is the equivalent storage polysaccharide in plants. Dietary fibre is also a polysaccharide, and includes cellulose from the cell walls of plants.

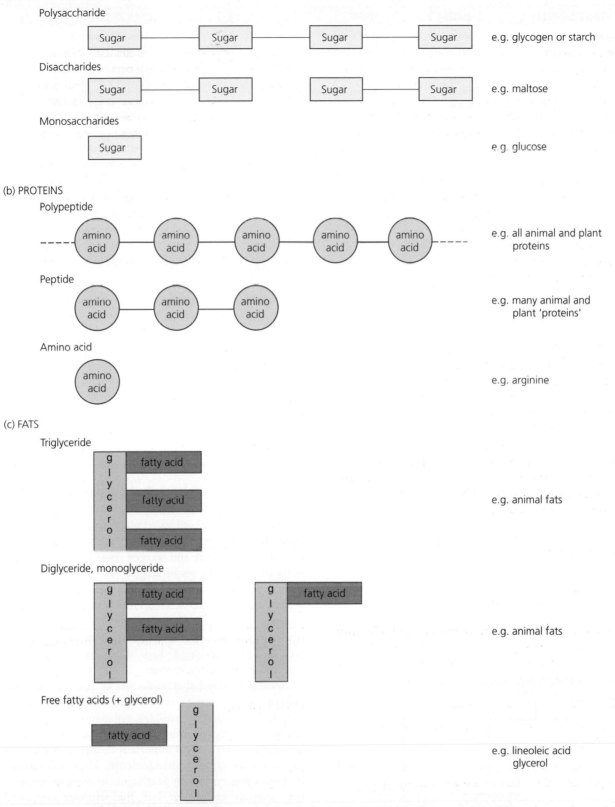

(a) CARBOHYDRATE

Polysaccharide

Sugar — Sugar — Sugar — Sugar   e.g. glycogen or starch

Disaccharides

Sugar — Sugar   Sugar — Sugar   e.g. maltose

Monosaccharides

Sugar   e.g. glucose

(b) PROTEINS

Polypeptide

amino acid — amino acid — amino acid — amino acid — amino acid   e.g. all animal and plant proteins

Peptide

amino acid — amino acid — amino acid   e.g. many animal and plant 'proteins'

Amino acid

amino acid   e.g. arginine

(c) FATS

Triglyceride

glycerol | fatty acid | fatty acid | fatty acid   e.g. animal fats

Diglyceride, monoglyceride

glycerol | fatty acid | fatty acid   glycerol | fatty acid   e.g. animal fats

Free fatty acids (+ glycerol)

fatty acid   glycerol   e.g. lineoleic acid glycerol

Figure 5.2 Outline of the structure of the main food groups. (a) Polysaccharides; (b) polypeptides (proteins); (c) fats (a form of lipid). Note how each is an example of a macromolecule ('macro-' = large), but each has distinctive molecular subunits (simple sugars, amino acids and fatty acids, respectively) that form the 'building blocks' of the macromolecules.

Q. What are the constituent elements of sugars, amino acids and fatty acids?

Table 5.1 Common carbohydrate constituents (excluding fibre) of a Western diet

Carbohydrate class	Examples	Source	Products
Polysaccharides	Starch	Plant tissues	Digested to glucose
	Glycogen	Animal tissues, especially liver	Digested to glucose
Disaccharides	Sucrose	Sugar cane/beet	Digested to glucose and fructose
	Maltose	'Malted' foods (from starch)	Digested to glucose
	Lactose	Milk	Digested to glucose and galactose
Monosaccharides	Glucose	Fruits, honey, vegetables	Absorbed and utilized as glucose
	Fructose	Fruits, honey, vegetables	Absorbed and utilized as fructose or converted to glucose
	Galactose	Digestion product of lactose	Converted to glucose in liver
Sugar alcohols	Sorbitol	Fruits, and manufactured from glucose	Converted to fructose in liver
	Inositol	Cereal brans, and manufactured from glucose	Inositol is inert

Dietary carbohydrates

Carbohydrates are widespread in nature and are important energy stores in organisms. The glycogen content of animal tissues is generally low, so most of our dietary carbohydrate is derived from foods based on plant tissues. On average, starch comprises 60% or more of the carbohydrate in our diet, and is found in large quantities in the stems, roots, tubers and seeds of plants.

Starch and glycogen, together with disaccharides such as sucrose from sugar cane and sugar beet, and lactose from milk, are digested to their simple monosaccharide constituents (Table 5.1). Note the predominance of glucose – this is our most important 'fuel', and even fructose and galactose may be converted to glucose in the liver. Other carbohydrates in food may already be in the forms of monosaccharides, e.g. glucose syrups prepared from starch, and fructose from fruits and vegetables. As monosaccharides, sugars can be absorbed from the bowel and utilized.

In dietary terms, the sucrose obtained from plant sources is called an extrinsic sugar because it is not a component of cell walls (Figure 5.3). Similarly, the complex of sugars found in honey, and the lactose in milk, are also extrinsic sugars. Those carbohydrates that do form important structural components of cells of our foods are called intrinsic sugars; they include fructose and glucose found in fruits and vegetables. Extrinsic sugars have been linked to dental decay, so intrinsic sugars are considered to be the better dietary form.

Proteins

Proteins (and smaller molecules called peptides) are major constituents of cellular structures. They form enzymes, plasma proteins, and cell secretions such as hormones and antibodies. Like carbohydrates, they are comprised largely of carbon, hydrogen and oxygen, but they also contain nitrogen atoms. Atoms of sulphur and phosphorus may also be present. The basic building units of proteins are amino acids (Figure 5.2(b)), which are also complex molecules. There are 20 naturally occurring amino acids. Chains of several, or perhaps several hundred, amino acids are called polypeptides; linkage of two or more polypeptide chains produces a protein.

Bearing in mind that molecules of polypeptides and proteins may be up to several hundred amino acids in length, the number of possible combinations and permutations of the types of amino acids is colossal. The sequencing of the amino acids is important because it determines the final shape of the protein molecule. Thus, cells initially synthesize proteins simply as straight chains of amino acids (the primary structure), but the structure may coil (secondary structure) and bend (tertiary structure) as further bonds are made between component amino acids (Figure 5.4). There is, therefore, tremendous scope for variety in protein size and 3-dimensional shape, and this is particularly important considering the role that protein

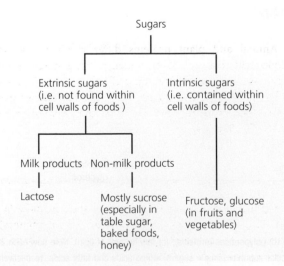

Figure 5.3 Classification of dietary sugars.

Q. Which type of sugar is the most detrimental to teeth?

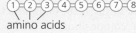

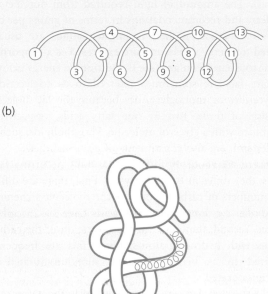

Figure 5.4 Primary, secondary and tertiary structure of proteins. (a) Primary structure: an amino acid chain determined by the genetic code of the cell. (b) Secondary structure produced by folding and coiling of the amino acid chain. (c) Tertiary structure: a three-dimensional structure produced by further coiling and folding. Note that (b) and (c) arise from interactions between certain amino acids in the primary structure, producing a final structure that is characteristic and specific to that protein. *Q*. *Why is the three-dimensional shape of a protein important?*

shape plays in the specific actions of enzymes, identified in Chapter 4 (Chemical reactions in cells. Metabolism).

Amino acids are normally utilized intact, but some may be broken down further, e.g. to produce energy. In this instance, the nitrogen within them cannot be reused and is excreted from the body in urine as a constituent of urea. To maintain nitrogen homeostasis, the intake of nitrogen (as protein) must therefore be equal to these losses (see Figure 6.1(b)), so protein intake must be relatively high to maintain health.

Dietary proteins

Protein foods may be in the form of animal or vegetable protein. In an average Western diet, about one-third of dietary protein comes from plant sources and two-thirds from animal sources. The main animal sources are meat and fish (i.e. from muscle) and dairy products. The main plant sources are seeds, including cereals, peas, beans and nuts. Root vegetables are usually deficient in protein, although potatoes contain significant amounts. Green vegetables are not a rich source of protein.

BOX 5.4 PROTEIN DEFICIENCY

Kwashiorkor is an example of protein deficiency; it is very rare in the UK. When it is seen, it is more likely to involve a child since children need relatively large intakes of protein to maintain normal growth. Kwashiorkor has a complex array of symptoms, some of which have also been related to inadequate vitamin and mineral intake. Muscle wasting, growth failure, and a general failure to thrive are characteristic. A deficiency in plasma protein concentration (referred to as hypoproteinaemia) is also observed, contributing to the development of oedema.

Deficiencies in specific amino acids are also possible, and in the UK are more likely than protein depletion per se. Vegetarians are particularly at risk: beans are deficient in those amino acids, such as cysteine, that contain sulphur, but wheat is a rich source of these; wheat is deficient in the amino acid lysine, but some beans are rich in this. Wheat and beans therefore contain complementary proteins, which, if eaten together, will provide adequate amounts of these particular amino acids.

Digestion of food in the bowel (see Chapter 10) releases the constituent amino acids from protein; they are then absorbed and utilized. While some amino acids can also be synthesized within the liver from others by a process called transamination, there are 10 (12 in infants) amino acids that cannot be made. These are the essential amino acids, and must be obtained from our diet:

arginine
histidine
isoleucine
leucine
lysine
methionine
phenylalanine
threonine
tryptophan
valine

Animal and plant proteins differ in their essential amino acid contents. Most animal proteins have the full range of amino acids, including all of the essential ones, and so are complete proteins, but vegetable proteins may not contain adequate amounts of all the essential amino acids. (See Box 5.4)

Lipids

The group of substances referred to as lipids includes fats and oils, cholesterol (a component of cell membranes), steroid hormones and prostaglandins (both chemical messengers within the body).

Like carbohydrates, lipids are composed of carbon, hydrogen, and oxygen, but they have a very different molecular structure and most are insoluble in water. This has physiological implications, e.g. in the digestion of dietary lipids by the gut, and in the carriage of lipids by the circulatory system, where they are made soluble by combining them with protein to make a complex molecule called a lipoprotein.

The basic constituents of lipids are molecules called fatty acids. Fats consist of up to three fatty acids combined with a molecule of glycerol (Figure 5.2(c)). Fats are important energy stores in the body; they contain more than twice the chemical energy of a comparable amount of carbohydrate. The higher energy content of fats compared with carbohydrates is very useful. Most of our energy reserves are stored as fat, so a person who is overweight by, say, 8 kg due to excess fat would be 16 kg overweight if the equivalent energy storage had been as carbohydrate! Cell utilization of the energy produced by fat catabolism is highly inefficient, however, and fats normally provide only a supplementary source of energy, carbohydrates being the main source.

Cholesterol is another biologically important lipid that is used to make cell membranes, steroid hormones and prostaglandins (see Box 5.5). It is a modified fatty acid, referred to as a phospholipid because it also contains a phosphate molecule within its structure.

Dietary lipids

Most lipids in our diet are in the form of animal fats and vegetable oils (similar in composition to fats, but with slight differences that make them liquid at normal temperatures). The amount of lipid required from our diets is unclear, and recommendations in terms of grams per day cannot be made. Rather, recommendations are usually related to energy needs, and are expressed as a proportion of the total energy intake (see the section on energy below). Dietary fats are sometimes referred to as triglycerides, diglycerides or monoglycerides because the fat molecule consists of three, two or one fatty acids, respectively, combined with a glycerol molecule. Phospholipids, such as cholesterol, are also constituents of a normal diet.

There are about 40 different naturally occurring fatty acids; they differ in two main ways. First, there are different numbers of carbon atoms in the molecule's chemical backbone, e.g. long-chain fatty acids have 14–25 carbon atoms. Second, they differ in the saturation of the carbon atoms with hydrogen atoms, hence fats are frequently referred to as being saturated, monounsaturated or polyunsaturated.

Unsaturated fats are those in which the fatty acids contain carbon atoms combined with fewer than the maximum of four other atoms, i.e. a carbon atom must

BOX 5.5 CHOLESTEROL

Normal ranges for (total) cholesterol concentration in blood: child, 3.11–5.18 mmol/l; adult, 3.63–8.03 mmol/l (note this range exceeds the recommended upper limit; see below).

Cholesterol is the basic ingredient of cell membranes, and a precursor for the synthesis of steroid hormones. Although it is essential to health, plasma concentrations of cholesterol above 5.2 μmol/l are associated with an increased risk of cardiovascular disease (Lindsay and Gaw, 1997). Some authorities suggest that it is important to also consider which form the cholesterol is in. To be transported in blood, lipids are normally combined with another molecule (usually a protein to make a lipoprotein) in order to make them soluble. A high concentration of cholesterol as low-density lipoprotein (LDLP) is thought to predispose to the formation of fatty plaques within blood vessels, because it is in this form that the lipid is deposited in the tissues. Excess lipid is then removed from the tissues as high-density lipoprotein (HDLP), which returns to the liver where the excess is broken down or passed into bile.

An ideal ratio of HDLP to LDLP in blood is 2:1, i.e. it favours removal of excess cholesterol from tissues. Factors that reduce LDLP have been recognized, but it is also suggested that means of raising HDLP should also be explored (Safeer and Cornell, 2000). Factors that promote a favourable ratio are:

- *oestrogens:* women have an advantage up to the menopause, but incidence of heart disease rises rapidly after menopause, at least partly because of increased formation of atheroma;

- *exercise:* active people have a better lipid profile.

Negative factors are:

- *lack of exercise:* causes a fall in HDLP and hence a fall in the HDLP : LDLP ratio;
- *smoking:* causes a decrease in HDLP;
- *excessive cholesterol in the diet:* increases LDLP concentrations;
- *excessive saturated fat in the diet:* promotes high concentrations of LDLP, as saturated fat is converted to cholesterol in the liver;
- *familial hypercholesterolaemia:* an inherited condition in which a gene mutation prevents uptake of excess cholesterol by the liver, and hence prevents metabolism of excess lipid.

Dietary cholesterol is not necessarily an indicator of the likely level in blood, because our liver can convert saturated fatty acids to cholesterol. This is the reason why dietary recommendations are that both cholesterol and saturated fat content of the diet should be limited. Soluble fibre in the diet reduces the uptake of cholesterol from the bowel, and so helps to reduce blood cholesterol (see the section on fibre below). Cholesterol levels in blood may also be reduced using cholesterol-lowering drugs. For example, the most effective drugs that lower LDLP in blood are statins. These inhibit cholesterol synthesis by the liver. However, cholesterol-lowering drugs may have unpleasant side effects, and so are usually recommended only when the hypercholesterolaemia is resistant to dietary control.

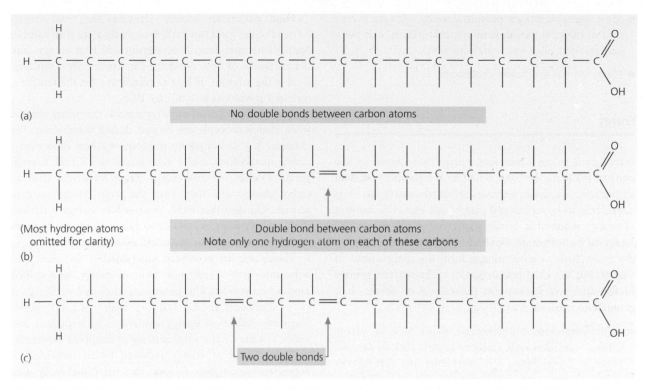

Figure 5.5 (a) Structure of a saturated fatty acid (e.g. palmitic acid). (b) Structure of an unsaturated fatty acid (e.g. oleic acid). (c) Structure of a polyunsaturated fatty acid (e.g. linoleic acid).

Q Which form of fatty acid is considered to carry a health risk because it may be used to synthesize cholesterol?

share two of its electrons with just one other atom; this is called a double (covalent) bond (Figure 5.5 (b) and (c)). Potentially, this bond may be opened to incorporate another atom into the molecule, which is why it is considered to be unsaturated within the fat. Monounsaturated fats contain fatty acids with just one unsaturated carbon atom; several atoms will be unsaturated in polyunsaturated fats. Saturated fats are those in which none of the constituent fatty acids contain double bonds between carbon and other atoms (Figure 5.5(a)). All forms provide energy, but saturated fats are considered to be less desirable because they are in a form that can be utilized by the liver to make cholesterol.

Of the variety of polyunsaturated fatty acids, only three are considered essential for life: linoleic acid, linolenic acid and arachidonic acid. Essential fatty acids are used in a variety of ways by the body. One of the most important is the synthesis of a group of chemical messengers called prostaglandins, which provide local modulation of the activities of many tissues, and mediate pain production when there is tissue damage. Of the three, it is most important that we obtain linoleic acid from our diets since the other two can be synthesized from other fatty acids by the liver (note that this is different from essential amino acids, all of which must be present in the diet). Foods vary in their content of linoleic acid; sunflower oil, corn oil, nuts and wheat germ are rich sources. Synthetic fatty or oily foods, e.g. margarine, often contain added essential fatty acids.

The fat content of foods varies depending upon the source:

- Beef, lamb and pork are rich sources of fats, even when visible fat is removed.

- The white meat of poultry is low in fat, but duck and goose may contain as much fat as beef.

- Animal fats may be saturated or unsaturated, and the cholesterol content varies: egg yolk and dairy fats are high in cholesterol.

- Fat in fresh fish varies according to species. Cod and haddock have low fat contents, while that of mackerel is quite high.

- The fat in fish is usually unsaturated, and the cholesterol content is normally low.

- Most vegetable fats are polyunsaturated, with the exception of olive oil (which is monounsaturated), and palm and coconut oils (which are saturated).

- Plants do not synthesize cholesterol.

Energy

Although it is not a nutrient, energy is required by the body to maintain the basal activities of cells and to sustain an increase in those activities when necessary, so it is considered to be an integral part of our diet. The amount of energy required is usually expressed in relation to the intake of carbohydrate, lipid and protein, since these are the main 'fuels'. Carbohydrates form the main source of energy, but the ideal proportion of carbohydrate, relative to fats and protein, remains the subject of debate. It is generally considered that:

- carbohydrates should comprise about 50% of energy intake. Since non-milk extrinsic sugars, such as sucrose, promote dental caries, it is considered that only 10% of energy requirements (i.e. about one-fifth of total carbohydrate intake) should come from this source;

- dietary fats should contribute about 35% of our energy needs, but the type of fatty acid present must also be taken into account. Only 10% of energy should be supplied by saturated fatty acids, because of their association with cholesterol deposition in blood vessels;

- dietary protein provides about 15% of energy needs.

Food packaging usually identifies the total energy content of the food, and still frequently gives it in calories (cal). Remember that these are units of heat energy, and not measures of how good the food tastes! By definition, 1 cal is the amount of heat required to raise the temperature of 1 g water (i.e. 1 ml) by 1°C.

The calorific value of a food represents the energy released when chemical bonds are broken during metabolism. For example, 1 g carbohydrate produces 4.1 kcal (kilocalorie) during metabolism, and 1 g fat produces 9.2 kcal. Clearly, fats are a richer source of energy, weight for weight, than are carbohydrates, and they form the main energy store in animals. On the other hand, most cellular energy is derived from carbohydrate metabolism, hence there is a greater dietary requirement for carbohydrate than fats.

The calorie has now been superseded by the joule. This is because heat is only one form of energy, so a calorie cannot be considered to be an empirical unit of energy. 1 cal is equivalent to 4.2 J (i.e. 1 kcal = 4.2 kJ). Foods frequently still show energy content in both calories and joules, but the calorie value is likely to disappear eventually.

The amount of energy required by an individual is dependent upon two factors: the basal metabolic rate (BMR) that cells exhibit in terms of basic functioning, cell division, etc., and the individual's physical activity level (PAL). As the name implies, the BMR is the overall energy utilization when the body is totally at rest and no additional influences such as a recent meal or exercise are imposed. The PAL is a factor used to convert the BMR to an energy intake recommendation:

BMR × PAL = estimated average requirement for energy.

BOX 5.6 MONITORING PROTEIN CATABOLISM

Protein normally forms only a small resource for energy production. However, protein utilization is increased when there is a deficit of alternative sources, e.g. in starvation or uncontrolled diabetes mellitus, or when metabolism is stimulated in favour of mobilizing amino acids, e.g. following surgery, when amino acids are required for wound healing. Under these circumstances, the concentrations in urine of urea (a waste product of amino acid metabolism in the liver) and 3-methylhistidine may be used as measures of protein catabolism. 3-Methylhistidine is a product of the breakdown of muscle protein, so its presence in urine is indicative of diminishing muscle protein.

BOX 5.7 WEIGHT-LOSS DIETS AND SLIMMING

While some people may have a genetic propensity to obesity (see Box 4.12), for most people being overweight means that there has been, for some time, an imbalance between energy intake and energy expenditure. Surveys suggest that many people in the UK frequently impose diets on themselves, sometimes involving support organizations but often as individuals. Pharmacies and health shops sell dietary aids in abundance. Many of these operate on the principle of bulk – the product absorbs water and fills up the stomach, reducing appetite. Others are constructed carefully with the intention of encouraging fat metabolism, but supporting it with carbohydrate metabolism as well. Other dietary constituents, such as vitamins, are also accounted for.

Most importantly, it is essential to reduce energy intake so that energy consumption is now in excess of energy intake (Jebb and Moore, 1999). Diets seek to reduce energy intake, sometimes very rapidly, but this usually leaves the individual feeling very hungry, so compliance with the diet becomes burdensome and more likely to fall. Most authorities advocate moderate control of dietary energy intake, but with an increase in physical activity as well.

Some drugs promote either a reduction in hunger and/or a feeling of satiety, and so help to reduce food intake. New preparations are likely to appear in the not-too-distant future – a drug that will promote rapid weight loss with minimal effort will be a sure money spinner.

For example, an adult male who partakes in little physical activity at work or during leisure time will have a PAL of 1.4. Thus, if the BMR is 7300 kJ/day (1740 kcal/day), then:

Energy required = 7300 × 1.4 = 10 200 kJ (2430 kcal) per day.

For men with high levels of activity, the PAL will be 1.9. Thus:

Energy required = 7300 × 1.9 = 13 900 kJ (3300 kcal) per day.

PAL values are slightly different in women. With moderate activity levels, the PAL is 1.6 for women and 1.7 for men, and with high levels of activity, the PAL is 1.8 for women and 1.9 for men.

Fibre

Dietary fibre is mainly the carbohydrate component of ingested plant material that cannot be digested fully. Strictly speaking, fibre is not a nutrient because it does not contribute to body chemistry, but it is nevertheless an important dietary constituent (see Box 5.8).

Some fibre does dissolve in water. Although it is not digested in the conventional way, it is broken down partially in the colon by bacteria, producing gas, water and fatty acids (note that these fatty acids are not components of the original carbohydrate molecule, but are produced from the carbohydrate by bacteria in the gut). This kind of fibre is called soluble fibre, and includes hemicellulose, pectin and gum. Dry beans, oat bran, and cabbage-type vegetables are rich sources of soluble fibre. Uncooked, insoluble fibre, such as cellulose, will not dissolve in water or fats, and is largely unchanged in the bowel. Cereal bran is an important source of insoluble fibre.

Vitamins

The name 'vitamin' is a shortened version of 'vitamine', i.e. types of chemicals called amines that are vital for life. It is now known that not all vitamins are amines. Most vitamins cannot be synthesized by cells, and so must be present in the diet, although vitamins are required in only small quantities to sustain growth and metabolism. Some vitamins are coenzymes, i.e. they work in conjunction with certain enzymes.

There are 13 vitamins known to be essential for life. Their nomenclature is very confusing, reflecting the history of their discovery. Most were named according to the order of discovery, i.e. A, B, C, etc., but the one that was identified as vitamin B was later found to consist of a group of substances, each with individual actions, so numbers (B_1, B_2, etc.) were introduced. Matters were also complicated when some vitamins were found to have existing names (e.g. vitamin B_3 is nicotinic acid or niacin), whilst others were later found not to be true vitamins at all and so were deleted from the series (e.g. there are no vitamins B_4 or G).

Vitamins are also classified according to whether they are soluble in water or fat. Thus, vitamins A, D, E and K are classed as fat-soluble vitamins, whilst vitamins of the B complex and vitamin C are classed as water-soluble vitamins. Fat-soluble vitamins require the presence of fatty acids in the bowel for their absorption, and may also be stored in the body to a limited degree. Water-soluble vitamins are excreted rapidly, and so are not stored.

As shown in Tables 5.2 and 5.3, vitamins have a wide range of functions, and are found in a variety of foodstuffs.

BOX 5.8 BENEFICIAL EFFECTS OF DIETARY FIBRE

Dietary fibre is thought to have a number of beneficial effects (Blackwood *et al.*, 2000):

- Fibre in the colon will absorb water and so increase the water content of faecal stools, making them easier to pass, and so helping to prevent constipation and complications such as haemorrhoids (piles).
- Fibre promotes muscle movements of the gut (peristalsis; see Chapter 10), and so reduces the time required for faecal matter to pass through it. This reduces the time available for microorganisms to produce deoxycholate, a known carcinogen, from bile salts secreted into the gut from the gall bladder. It is suggested that dietary fibre therefore helps to reduce the risk of bowel cancer, although recent evidence suggests that fibre alone does not reduce the risk markedly.
- Soluble fibre interferes with the absorption of fatty acids and bile salts, which are produced from cholesterol, leading to further cholesterol and fatty acid utilization in the body, so helping to reduce blood lipid concentrations and helping to reduce the risk of atheroma plaques forming within blood vessels.

BOX 5.9 VITAMIN EXCESS AND DEFICIENCY

Small amounts of just some of the vitamins we eat are stored in the body. Fat-soluble vitamins are stored in fat (adipose) tissue and in the liver, but few of the water-soluble vitamins is stored, with the exception of vitamin B_{12}. The stores are not normally extensive, although the liver contains sufficient vitamin B_{12} for a 2–3-year supply! Vitamin deficiencies, rather than excesses, are more likely to occur, but are avoidable with a balanced diet. Their consequences are identified in Tables 5.2 and 5.3.

Avoiding vitamin deficiency by taking supplements is currently popular, but recommended doses should be adhered to, since vitamin excess, especially of fat-soluble vitamins, can raise stores to toxic levels. For example, excess vitamin D promotes excessive uptake of calcium from the gut, leading to deposition of calcium in soft tissues, and excess vitamin A can cause liver damage. Such large build-ups of vitamins are unlikely from normal dietary intakes, but are possible if vitamin preparations are taken.

Table 5.2 Fat-soluble vitamins

Vitamin	Source	Storage in body	Homeostatic functions	Effects of deficiency	Effects of excess
A	Liver, green leafy vegetables Synthesized in gut from β-carotene	In liver	Maintain epithelia Provide visual pigment Bone/teeth growth	Atrophy of epithelia, e.g. dry skin and cornea, increased susceptibility to respiratory/urinary/digestive tract infection, skin sores 'Night blindness' Slow bone/tooth growth	Anorexia, dry skin, sparse hair, raised intracranial pressure in children; blurred vision, enlarged liver in adults
D	Synthesized as provitamin D_3 in skin using UV light. Also in fish liver, fish oils, egg yolk, milk	Slight at most	Absorption of calcium and phosphate from gut	Demineralization of bone (rickets in children, osteomalacia in adults)	Excess calcium absorption from gut. Calcium deposition in soft tissues
E	Nuts, wheatgerm, seed oils, green leafy vegetables	In liver, adipose tissue and muscle	Inhibits catabolism of membrane lipids Promotes wound healing and neural function	Abnormal organelle/ plasma membranes. Oxidation of polyunsaturated fatty acids	Toxic build-up unlikely
K	Produced by intestinal bacteria. Also in spinach, cauliflower, cabbage and liver	In liver and spleen	Synthesis of blood clotting factors	Delayed blood clotting	Haemolysis and increased bilirubin in blood in children; Otherwise toxic build-up unlikely

Mineral salts

Mineral salts such as sodium chloride (table salt) and sodium bicarbonate (baking powder) dissociate into their constituent ions when dissolved in water. Minerals generally are found dissolved in body fluids, and so are not stored to any degree. Body fluids contain a variety of ions, and changes in this ionic environment can have adverse effects on cell function (Table 5.4). The concentrations of most ions in body fluids therefore must be regulated if homeostasis is to be maintained (see Chapters 6 and 15).

Minerals are also important structural constituents (but not in a storage capacity, except for calcium and iron). For example, sulphur is an essential constituent of many proteins (it is found in certain amino acids such as cysteine), iron is a constituent of the blood pigment haemoglobin, and calcium and phosphorus are constituents of bone. Some minerals, e.g. copper,

selenium, zinc, aluminium, iodide and fluoride, are required in such small amounts that they are considered to be trace elements, but they still have important roles. For example, iodine is a constituent of thyroid hormones, fluoride is a component of bone and tooth minerals, and zinc and selenium are important enzyme cofactors.

Nucleic acids

Nucleic acids form the genetic material of cells and provide the 'blueprint' for protein synthesis, including enzymes and proteins that control cell functions. There are two types of nucleic acid: deoxyribonucleic acid (DNA) and ribonucleic acid (RNA). Both are very large molecules, being comprised of a backbone of ribose and phosphate molecules, to which are attached sequences of molecules called purines and pyrimidines (often referred to as 'bases',

BOX 5.10 MINERAL EXCESS AND DEFICIENCY

Since most minerals are not stored in the body, deficiency may arise if dietary intake does not match mineral excretion. Most minerals are abundant in foodstuffs, and most people could actually readily reduce their mineral intake, especially of sodium chloride. Deficiencies are more likely to arise in trace minerals; dietary supplements are widely available for these. Excessive intake of those minerals that are stored can be detrimental, however.

Minerals may be toxic if stores are excessive. For example, excessive iodine has toxic effects on the thyroid gland (causing thyrotoxicosis), and excessive iron is a cause of poisoning in young children. Excessive fluoride causes mottled teeth and porous, brittle bones.

Table 5.3 Water-soluble vitamins

Vitamin	Source	Storage in body	Homeostatic functions	Effects of deficiency	Effects of excess
B₁ (thiamin)	Whole grain, eggs, pork, liver, yeast	Not stored	Coenzyme in carbohydrate metabolism Essential for acetylcholine (neurotransmitter) synthesis	Build-up of pyruvic/lactic acids Energy deficient Partial paralysis of digestive tract/skeletal muscle (i.e. beri-beri) Degeneration of myelin sheath (polyneuritis)	Toxic build-up unlikely
B₂ (riboflavin)	Small quantities produced by gut bacteria Also in yeast, liver, beef, lamb, eggs, whole grain, peas, peanuts	Not stored	Component of coenzymes in carbohydrate and protein metabolism, especially in eye, blood, skin, intestinal mucosa	Blurred vision, cataracts Lesions of intestinal mucosa Dermatitis Anaemia	Toxic build-up unlikely
B₃ (niacin or nicotin-amide)	Yeast, meats, liver, fish, whole grain, peas, beans Also synthesized from amino acid tryptophan	Not stored	Component of coenzyme NAD in intracellular respiration Assists breakdown of cholesterol	Hard, rough, blackish skin Dermatitis, diarrhoea (pellagra) Psychological disturbance	Burning sensation in hands/face, cardiac arrhythmias, increased glycogen utilization
B₆ (pyri-doxine)	Salmon, yeast, tomatoes, maize, spinach, whole grain, liver, yoghurt Some synthesized by gut bacteria	In liver and muscle	Coenzyme in fat and amino acid metabolism	Dermatosis of eye, nose, mouth Nausea Retarded growth	Toxic build-up unlikely
B₁₂ (cyano-cobalamin)	Liver, kidney, milk, eggs, cheese, meats Not found in vegetables Requires intrinsic factor from stomach for absorption	In liver	Coenzyme for haemoglobin synthesis and amino acid metabolism	Pernicious anaemia Nerve axon degeneration	Toxic build-up unlikely
Folate (folic acid, folacin)	Synthesized by gut bacteria Also in green leafy vegetables and liver	Not stored	Synthesis of nucleotides Red/white blood cell production	Macrocytic anaemia due to abnormally large red blood cells	Toxic build-up unlikely
Panto-thenic acid	Liver, kidney, yeast, cereals, green vegetables	In liver and kidney	Constituent of coenzyme A in carbohydrate metabolism, gluconeogenesis and steroid synthesis	Fatigue Muscle spasms Lack of some steroid hormones	Toxic build-up unlikely
Biotin	Synthesized by gut bacteria Also yeast, liver, egg, yolk, kidney	Not stored	Component of coenzymes for pyruvic acid utilization in cellular respiration	Mental depression. Muscular pain Dermatitis Fatigue Nausea	Toxic build-up unlikely
C (ascorbic acid)	Citrus fruits, tomatoes, green vegetables	A little in plasma	Promotes protein metabolism Promotes formation of connective tissue Detoxifier Promotes wound healing	Retardation of growth Poor connective tissue repair/growth (scurvy), including swollen gums, tooth loosening, fragile blood vessels Poor wound healing	Not toxic Note: no evidence for effect to prevent infection

but not to be confused with those chemicals involved in acid/base regulation in the body).

As cells die, some of their nucleic acid constituents will be reused, but some are broken down to the waste substance uric acid. The constituents required by cells to synthesize nucleic acids must therefore be obtained in part from the nucleic acids ingested in our diets, following their digestion and absorption in the gut. Fortunately, the

Table 5.4 Dietary sources of selected minerals, and their functions

Mineral	Source	Function	Effects of deficiency
Calcium	Milk, egg yolk, shellfish, green leafy vegetables	Formation of bones/teeth Blood clotting, muscle contraction Muscle/nerve action potentials Endo- and exocytosis Cell division	Loss of bone density, e.g. osteomalacia/ rickets
Phosphorus	Milk, meat, fish, poultry, nuts	Formation of bones/teeth Buffer chemical Muscle contraction/nerve activity Component of ATP, DNA, RNA and many enzymes	Deficiency rare
Potassium	Widespread; 'Lo-salt'	Action potential of muscle/nerve cells	Neuromuscular depression
Sodium	Widespread; table salt	Major osmotic solute of extracellular fluids Action potential of muscle/nerve cells	Hypovolaemia
Chlorine (chloride)	Non-processed foods; usually found with sodium, e.g. table salt	Involved in acid–base balance Major osmotic solute of extracellular fluids Formation of gastric acid	Deficiency usually occurs with sodium
Magnesium	Beans, peanuts, bananas	Constituent of many coenzymes Role in bone formation and muscle/nerve cell functions	Muscle weakness Convulsions Hypertension
Trace minerals Iron	Widespread but especially meats, liver, beans, fruits, nuts, legumes	Component of haemoglobin Component of chemicals involved in cell respiration	Anaemia
Iodine (iodide)	Seafood, cod-liver oil, iodized table salt	Component of thyroid hormones	Thyroid hormone deficiency (induces thyroid goitre)
Fluorine (fluoride)	Tea, coffee, fluoridated water	Component of bones/teeth	Decreased bone/teeth density
Zinc	Widespread, but especially meats	Component of some enzymes Promotes normal growth, spermatogenesis Involved in taste and appetite	Dermatitis Growth retardation Diarrhoea
Copper	Eggs, wholewheat flour, liver, fish, spinach	Haemoglobin synthesis Component of some enzymes, or acts as cofactor	Retarded growth Cerebral degeneration
Chromium	Yeast, beer, beef	Involved in insulin synthesis Maintains HDL concentrations in plasma	Rare – may be involved with diabetes mellitus

structure of nucleic acids is similar in all organisms, so these are readily available in foods. However, processed foods tend to be low in nucleic acids.

Water

Water is familiar to us in our everyday life, and makes up a substantial proportion of our body volume, but it would be wrong to regard it as being a simple space filler in our tissues. We noted in Chapter 4 that water molecules are polarized, i.e. the oxygen part of the molecule carries a very weak negative charge, and the hydrogen pole carries a weak positive charge. These properties are sufficient to make water an excellent solvent for other charged particles, e.g. ions, and also help to hold larger molecules together by bonds that cells are able to break very easily.

Some 60% of our body weight (range 50–70% depending upon the proportion of fat) results from water. The water is distributed in a precise and regulated way (see

Chapter 6), and determines the volumes and, to a certain extent, the solute concentrations of the various body fluids. It is also a component of many metabolic reactions. Water is constantly lost from the body and must be replenished from our diets. Most water is ingested in the fluids we drink, but even the driest of foods contain a significant amount of water; e.g. cereal grains are comprised of about 10% water by weight.

Lifespan influences on recommended daily intakes of nutrients

This section provides only an overview. Further details are available from guidelines published by the UK Department of Health (1991; 1997; 1998).

Newborn to infant

There are two nutritional considerations during this period of life: the requirements of the nursing mother, and those of the baby, who is entirely dependent at this time. Human milk is highly varied in composition, and changes even between feeds. In general, 100 g breast milk provides about 290 kJ (70 kcal) energy. The average breastfeeding woman produces 700 ml milk per day, so the energy cost to the mother during lactation will be of the order of 2000 kJ (500 kcal) per day. Some of this energy is supplied from fat deposits stored by the mother during pregnancy, but much must be supplied by the mother's diet. The energy costs will also increase with time, as the growth of the baby accelerates. In proportionate terms, the energy needs of the baby during the first 6 months of life are higher than at any other time of life (Figure 5.6).

The infant will double its birth weight during the first year of life, and nutritional requirements will change periodically. Provision of all nutrients remains important, but particularly important nutrients during this time are protein (for growth), iron (for blood), vitamin D (to promote calcium uptake by the gut), calcium and fluoride (for bone and teeth development, even before teeth have erupted). If breastfeeding, the mother must increase her intake of these nutrients. The dietary needs for iron usually increase only after the first 5–6 months, as the baby's stores are normally quite high at birth.

Not all infants are breastfed initially, and infant formulas are treated to modify their composition. Although nutritionally adequate, these formulas will be deficient in other constituents of breast milk, especially antibodies. Cow's milk is an unsuitable alternative (see Box 5.11).

Babies are developmentally unready for solid food until about 4 months of age, although cultural practices may mean babies are weaned before or after this (Coutts, 2000). In particular, babies have difficulty in moving food to the back of the mouth for swallowing and in digesting cereals. Delay in weaning runs the risk of inducing protein deficiency as the growth of the baby accelerates. It is also important to note that infants are less able to synthesize amino acids in their livers than older children and adults, and that there are 12 essential amino acids, not 10, in this age group.

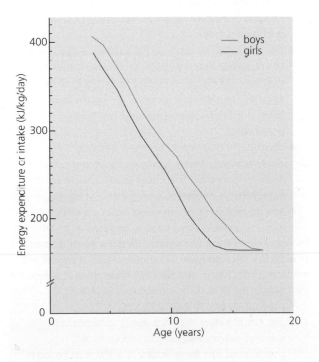

Figure 5.6 Energy requirements standardized for body weight in boys and girls up to the age of 18 years.

BOX 5.11 BREAST MILK VERSUS COWS' MILK

Substituting cows' milk for breast milk is not recommended because:

- there is less lactose in cows' milk;
- the protein of cows' milk, mainly casein, is harder to digest (although human milk also contains a little casein);
- the absorption of iron from breast milk is considerably more efficient than from cows' milk;
- cow's milk contains more sodium, which places a greater demand on the infants' kidneys to excrete the load;
- the range of free amino acids contained in breast milk is beneficial (infants need 12 essential amino acids, instead of the 10 that adults need);
- the vitamin content of cows' milk is very different from that of breast milk;
- the baby may respond to allergens present in cow's milk.

Infant formulas are used widely as substitutes for breast milk. The UK Department of Health (1996) has published guidelines on these.

Growing child, adolescent, and young adult

Growth during childhood accelerates as the child enters puberty. This is therefore a critical period for nutrition, and recommended intakes of all nutrients increase sharply. For example, protein intake might increase almost three-fold between the ages of 3 and 14 years. Energy requirements relative to body size are much higher in children and adolescents than in adults in order to support the rate of growth and the high levels of physical activity exhibited by this group (Figure 5.6). The energy intake might almost double between 3 and 14 years of age.

Adults 23–50 years

Growth effectively ends at the age of 19–22 years, and nutrition then largely becomes a case of maintenance. Energy requirements of this age group are particularly influenced by levels of physical activity, but on average are about 8 000 KJ (1900 kcal) per day in women and 10 500 KJ (2500 kcal) per day in men.

Pregnancy

The diet of the pregnant woman must clearly support the increased tissue mass produced by an increased uterus size, the fetus and placenta, an expanded blood volume, and extra fat deposits, and also must maintain the increased metabolic activity related to that increased mass (see Box 5.12). The third trimester is particularly important in this respect: additional energy intake of about 800 kJ (200 kcal) per day is most important during this period.

Adults 50–75 years

The ageing process is most noticeable after about the age of 50 years, when physical activity may decline, basal metabolism diminishes, digestive activity is reduced, secretions (e.g. of saliva) are less pronounced, perceptions of taste and smell change, and lifestyles alter. However, nutrient requirements are generally the same as at 30 years, except that less energy is needed.

Adults 75+ years

Most people over 75 years show a decrease in activity levels compared with a 50–60-year-old, although there are wide variations. Basal metabolic rate is appreciably decreased above 75 years; appetite therefore diminishes, which can have implications for nutritional homeostasis (see Box 5.13).

BOX 5.12 NUTRITIONAL REQUIREMENTS IN PREGNANCY

Most nutritional requirements are increased during pregnancy, but these can often be obtained through a well-balanced diet. The following should be given specific attention:

- *Carbohydrates.* In line with fetal growth, carbohydrate requirement increases during pregnancy. To reduce the risk of maternal tooth decay, it is better to obtain the extra carbohydrates from polysaccharides, i.e. from bread, potatoes and rice rather than from 'extrinsic' sugars in sweets, cakes, etc.
- *Proteins.* Requirement for protein increases during pregnancy and lactation. A total of 39 g/day is required during pregnancy (compared with about 36 g/day in a non-pregnant adult woman), and 46 g/day during lactation. However, excessive intake may impair fetal growth, and dietary intake in the UK is usually sufficient.
- *Lipids.* Lipid requirement increases slightly during pregnancy, but dietary intake in the UK is usually sufficient.
- *Fibre.* The requirement for fibre increases during pregnancy in order to aid maternal bowel functions. The RDA is 30 g, but note that too much fibre can inhibit absorption of iron from food.
- *Vitamin A.* The RDA in pregnancy rise from about 2000 to 2500 IU (international units; see Appendix A), but the use of vitamin

supplements should be avoided as high levels have been found to influence birth defects.

- *Folic acid.* Deficiency of folic acid (a B vitamin) is associated with neural tube defects (NTDs) in embryos (see Chapter 20). A supplement (0.4 mg/day) is therefore recommended before and during the first trimester of pregnancy. If there is a previous history of NTD, then daily supplementation of 5 mg is recommended.
- *Vitamin E.* The requirement increases in pregnancy to help prevent premature delivery, spontaneous abortion and stillbirth. However, dietary intake in the UK is usually sufficient, and supplements are recommended only for those at high risk.
- *Iron.* The requirement for iron increases during pregnancy, but routine supplements are no longer recommended in the UK since dietary intake (and maternal storage) is usually sufficient.
- *Calcium.* The requirement for calcium increases in pregnancy. It is thought to help prevent premature labour. However, dietary intake in the UK is usually sufficient, and supplements are recommended only for those at high risk.
- *Zinc.* This is the most important mineral for successful pregnancy outcome. Requirements increase by 30% in pregnancy and 40% during lactation. The RDA is 20 mg, but in the UK this is usually met by dietary intake.

BOX 5.13 NUTRITIONAL BALANCE IN OLDER PEOPLE

Appetite at all ages normally equates with the energy needs of the body. Thirst centres within the hypothalamus of the brain influence water intake, and sodium receptors, also in the hypothalamus, induce a 'salt' appetite in which salty foods are eaten in preference. However, the regulation of the intake of most individual nutrients, such as vitamins, is coarse and imprecise. Food requirements, and hence appetite, generally diminish over the age of 75 years as metabolism slows, but there is a risk that the low food intakes observed in inactive elderly people may not provide adequate amounts of other nutrients for health (Department of Health, 1992).

It is especially important that food is presented in a palatable and appetizing way, and that the food eaten is of adequate quality. Sadly, institutions often fail to meet these criteria, and carers should be aware of what food, if any, is eaten by elderly people at home, in the community and in hospital.

Summary

1 Nutrients provide the substrates for all body structures, and the constituents of body fluids.

2 A balanced diet contains adequate daily amounts of all nutrients.

3 Carbohydrates include complex polysaccharides, smaller disaccharides, and simple sugars (monosaccharides). Dietary carbohydrates are digested to their monosaccharide components, of which glucose is the most prevalent.

4 Proteins are composed of amino acids. Some amino acids, having been ingested as proteins, may be converted to different ones within the liver, but there are 10 (12 in infants) amino acids that cannot be synthesized in the body: these are essential amino acids, and must be present in the diet.

5 Lipids are composed of fatty acids, perhaps modified or combined with glycerol to form glycerides or fats. Fatty acids are saturated or have degrees of unsaturation, i.e. their chemical structure has bonds that can be opened to accept other atoms or molecules.

6 Saturated fatty acids may be converted within the liver to cholesterol, an example of a modified lipid. This is an important lipid in the body, but potentially can have detrimental effects on blood vessels.

7 Energy is considered to be a nutrient. On average, 50% of energy intake should be as carbohydrates, 35% as lipids, and 15% as protein. Energy requirements relate to the basal metabolic rate and to physical activity levels.

8 Fibre is not digested in the conventional way, if at all. It has beneficial effects on the bowel.

9 Vitamins are a complex group of chemicals central to living processes that have a range of functions. Small quantities of each are required. Some are fat soluble, others water soluble. Fat-soluble vitamins may be stored to a limited degree; this makes toxic levels a possibility, although unlikely with normal diets. Vitamin deficiency is more likely to be a problem.

10 Minerals range from those that are very abundant to those that are trace elements. Most are not stored to any degree, so a regular intake is necessary. This means that trace element deficiency is possible.

11 Nucleic acids, i.e. DNA and RNA, must be synthesized by dividing cells. While components are reusable, some are metabolized, so nucleic acids must be present in the diet. Growth requires additional nucleic acid.

12 Water is often taken for granted, but it is a vital component of body chemistry as a solvent and as a determinant of volume.

13 Nutrient requirements change during life, primarily as a consequence of growth during childhood and declining metabolic rates in later adulthood. Pregnancy and lactation have further implications for maternal dietary requirements.

Review questions

1 What are the components of a balanced diet? How does the body utilize these components?

2 Why should the practitioner assess nutritional status? What factors are assessed?

3 How is body mass index (BMI) measured? What are the limitations for using this measurement? How may physical activity affect BMI?

4 Which groups of people may be at risk of nutritional deficiency? What are the specific problems for each of these groups?

5 How do nutritional requirements alter with age? How does the diet alter across age groups? (Consider in utero, neonatal, infant, childhood, adolescence, adulthood and old age).

6 What are the consequences of undernutrition and overeating?

7 What is obesity? What are the health risks associated with obesity? How does physical activity help maintain a healthy weight?

8 Alcohol is calorie rich but nutrient poor. Bearing this in mind, how may alcoholism affect nutritional status?

9 How does abnormality, illness or injury affect nutritional status? Define dysphagia.

10 Think about your own diet. Would you describe it as healthy? What drives you to eat the foods you do?

REFERENCES

Blackwood, A.D., Salter, J., Dettmar, P.W. and Chaplin, M.F. (2000) Dietary fibre, physicochemical properties and their relationship to health. *Journal of the Royal Society of Health* **120**(4): 242–7.

Coutts, A. (2000) Nutrition and the life cycle 2: infancy and weaning. *British Journal of Nursing* **9**(21): 2205–16.

Crombie, N. (1999) Obesity management. *Nursing Standard* **13**(47): 43–6.

Department of Health (1991) *Dietary Reference Values for Food Energy and Nutrients for the UK*. London: HMSO.

Department of Health (1992) *The Nutrition of Elderly People*. London: HMSO.

Department of Health (1996) *Guidelines on the Nutritional Assessment of Infant Formulas*. London: HMSO.

Department of Health (1997) *Healthy Diets for Infants and Young Children: a guide for health professionals*. London: HMSO.

Department of Health (1998) *National Diet and Nutrition Survey: people aged 65 years and over*. London: HMSO.

Guenter, P., Jones, S. and Ericson, M.(1997) Enteral nutrition therapy. *Nursing Clinics of North America* **32**(4): 651–68.

Jebb ,S.A. and Moore, M.S. (1999) Contribution of a sedentary lifestyle and inactivity to the etiology of overweight and obesity. Current evidence and research issues. *Medical Science, Sports and Exercise* **31**(11 suppl): S534–41.

Lindsay, G.M. and Gaw, A. (1997) *Coronary Heart Disease Prevention: a handbook for the health care team*. New York: Churchill Livingston.

Reilly, H. (1998) Nutrition. Parenteral nutrition: an overview of current practice. *British Journal of Nursing* **7**(8): 461–7.

Safeer, R.S. and Cornell, M.O. (2000) The emerging role of HDL cholesterol. Is it time to focus more energy on raising high density lipoprotein levels? *Postgraduate Medicine* **108**(7): 87–90.

Serpell, L., Treasure, J., Teasdale, J. and Sullovan, V. (1999) Anorexia nervosa: friend or foe? *International Journal of Eating Disorders* **25**(2): 577–86.

Thomas, D. (1999) An unhealthy obsession with body image. *Practice Nurse* **17**(4): 252–5.

Wiedeman, M.W. and Pryor, T.L. (2000) Body dissatisfaction, bulimia, and depression among women: the mediating role of drive for thinness. *International Journal of Eating Disorders* **27**(1): 90–95.

Body fluids

IINTRODUCTION

It is important that the chemical environment in which biochemical reactions take place in cells is optimal if the reactions are to progress efficiently. Water and the substances dissolved in it, which together make up the body fluids, provide such an environment. Minerals are amongst the most abundant constituents of body fluids; this chapter describes the principal minerals present, and their roles in cellular function, and introduces the ways in which body fluid composition and volume are regulated. Further details of body fluid homeostasis can be found in a later chapter in relation to kidney functioning (see Chapter 16).

> **Exercise**
>
> The physiology of body fluids is that of water and electrolytes. Before proceeding, you may find it helpful to first revisit the sections on atoms, electrolytes and water in Chapter 4.

BODY FLUID COMPARTMENTS

The adult body contains some 40–45 l water (Figure 6.1), equivalent to about two-thirds of our body weight. Approximately 25 l of this is found inside cells (and thus is referred to as intracellular fluid), and the remaining 18 l or so comprises the extracellular fluid ('extra-' = outside). Extracellular fluid is subdivided into:

● *interstitial or tissue fluid:* the component that bathes our cells; approximately 12 l in volume;

● *blood plasma:* approximately 3 l in volume; the blood cells come under the intracellular compartment;

● *transcellular fluids ('trans-' = across):* specialized fluids secreted by epithelia into distinct spaces, e.g. synovial fluid into skeletal joints; 1–3 l in total volume.

All of our body fluids contain various types of ions. The physiological activities of the main ions found within these compartments are discussed in the next sections.

Extracellular fluids

Blood plasma and interstitial fluid

Cellular function requires substances to be transported to and from the cells, but although the microscopic vessels or capillaries within tissues may be close to cells, they remain separated from them by the interstitial (tissue) fluid that bathes them. Reliance on simple diffusion to allow

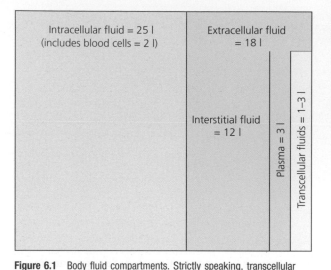

Figure 6.1 Body fluid compartments. Strictly speaking, transcellular fluids are part of the extracellular compartment, but they have compositions very different to that of plasma and interstitial fluid, and so are usually considered separately.

Q. Give four examples of transcellular fluids.

BOX 6.1 FLUID COMPARTMENTS IN INFANTS

Infants have a higher percentage of total body water in comparison to older children and adults. In addition, the daily exchange of extracellular fluid through secretion and reabsorption occurring within the gastrointestinal tract is relatively much higher, and may be equivalent to as much as 45% of total body weight per day. Such differences in infant are attributed to relative differences in body and organ sizes, and the immaturity of physiological processes concerned with fluid balance. As a consequence, impairment of fluid intake can rapidly alter the level of hydration, e.g. in persistent vomiting.

adequate exchange of substances through the interstitial fluid between cells and blood plasma would not be efficient. A better system is utilized in which the substances are actually 'carried' by fluid movement to the vicinity of cell membranes.

This is achieved by the passage of water, with its dissolved solutes, out of the plasma and into the interstitium, and thence back into the plasma again. Thus the two fluids are continuous, so the ionic compositions of blood plasma and interstitial fluid are almost identical (Table 6.1). A requirement for the movement of fluid in this way is that the capillaries are highly permeable to water and solutes. The permeability is not so great, however, to allow large molecules, such as proteins, to enter the interstitium

in significant amounts. The main difference between the composition of plasma and interstitial fluid is that plasma has a considerably higher protein concentration. The dynamics of the capillary exchange process are explained later.

The main ions found in plasma and interstitial fluid are sodium, potassium, calcium, chloride, bicarbonate and phosphate. Sodium and chloride are the most abundant (Table 6.1), while potassium, calcium and phosphate ions are present in relatively low concentrations. About half the calcium present in the extracellular fluid is chemically bound to proteins and so will not influence cell function directly. However, the concentration of the remainder dissolved in the fluid, and therefore ionized, may change rapidly should calcium be released from the bound component. The binding of calcium to plasma protein is influenced by the acidity of the blood, and the release of bound calcium does not normally occur because the acidity is closely controlled at a pH of about 7.4. This pH value means that the hydrogen ion concentration in blood plasma is extremely low (see Box 4.4), and this has arisen

Table 6.1 Concentrations of main ionic constituents of intracellular and extracellular fluids

| Constituent | Extracellular fluid | | Intracellular fluid |
	Plasma (mmol/l)	Interstitial fluid (mmol/l)	Skeletal muscle cell (mmol/l)
Cations			
Sodium (Na^+)	142	145*	12
Potassium (K^+)	4.3	4.4	150
Calcium (Ca^{2+})	1.2**	1.2**	4
Anions			
Chloride (Cl^-)	104	117*	4
Bicarbonate (HCO_3^-)	24	27*	12
Phosphate (HPO_4^{2-}, $H_2PO_3^-$)	2	2	40
Proteins (g)	70	Approximately 0	25
pH	7.4	7.4	7.0

*Slight differences in plasma result from negative charge on plasma proteins.
**Ionized calcium. Total calcium concentration in plasma is about twice this.

B O X   6 . 2   A R T E R I O S C L E R O S I S

Arteriosclerosis is a 'hardening' of the arteries that arises through scarring and calcification. It is irreversible, and is a causative factor in high blood pressure (hypertension) and thrombosis (presence in a vessel of a blood clot that occludes, or partially occludes, the vessel). The aetiology of the problem is multifactorial (see Chapter 12), but one of the risk factors is the local concentration of calcium and phosphate ions. It is of note here that many calcium salts have a relatively low solubility in water, a

factor that aids deposition in bone. This is easily demonstrated by observing the deposits found in kettles and central heating systems in hard water areas. In plasma and interstitial fluid, the concentration of calcium ions and associated ions, such as those of hydrogen phosphate (HPO_4^{2-}), is close to that at which the salts will start to precipitate out of solution. Close regulation of the low concentrations of these ions is therefore desirable to prevent deposits occurring.

largely because the hydrogen ions produced by metabolism are buffered by ions especially bicarbonate ions. Table 6.1 shows that the concentration of bicarbonate ions is relatively high in plasma and interstitial fluid, although nowhere near that of sodium or chloride. Phosphate ions are another buffer chemical in the extracellular fluid, but the concentrations of this in plasma and interstitial fluid are very low (see Box 6.2).

Transcellular fluids

The transcellular fluids are separated from blood plasma by a continuous layer of cells (i.e. an epithelium), and are produced as secretions of those cells. They include the specialized fluids found in the brain and spinal cord (cerebrospinal fluid, CSF), in parts of the stomach (gastric fluid), and in the eyes (intraocular fluid), and also secretions such as saliva, pancreatic and intestinal juices, semen, cervical fluid and sweat. The total volume of transcellular fluid

is variable, particularly because of changes in the secretion of bowel fluids, but in general it amounts to about 1–3 l.

The composition of transcellular fluids may be kept near constant, as in the cerebrospinal fluid, or may vary according to the circumstances at the time, as in gastric fluid. The solutes found in these fluids are of the same types as found in other extracellular fluids, but their respective concentrations are different from those of the blood plasma and the interstitial fluid (compare Tables 6.1 and 6.2). This is because the cells that secrete them exert some control on the composition of the resultant fluid.

Intracellular fluids

Since cells have widely differing functions, it is not surprising that there is variation in the composition of the intracellular fluid between tissues. Some generalizations can be made, however, and the composition of fluid from muscle cells, as shown in Table 6.1, gives a general impression.

B O X   6 . 3   T H I R D   C O M P A R T M E N T   S Y N D R O M E

The body has two major fluid compartments – the extracellular and intracellular fluids. Third compartment syndrome occurs if the volume of fluid in a location suddenly becomes excessive. The additional fluid derives from the blood plasma and tissue fluids and so promotes a redistribution of these fluids, leading potentially to circulatory collapse.

The commonest causes of this syndrome are surgery and peritonitis. Surgery can cause a cessation of gastrointestinal activity, including peristaltic contractions. Fluid secretion in the stomach and duodenum (of which much is reabsorbed again later

in the intestines) continues, but without peristalsis it does not pass along the bowel to the absorptive sites. Consequently, the fluid content of the bowel may become excessive.

Peritonitis can cause the syndrome because the peritoneum membrane that lines the abdomen becomes much more permeable to fluids and proteins, leading to an accumulation of fluid within the abdomen, referred to as peritoneal oedema, or ascites. As with the bowel fluids, the accumulation of peritoneal fluid can occur quite quickly, hence the (apparent) occurrence of a significant 'third compartment'.

Table 6.2 Mean ionic concentrations of some transcellular fluids

Fluid	Na+ (mmol/l)	K+ (mmol/l)	Cl− (mmol/l)	HCO₃− (mmol/l)	pH
Saliva	33	20	34	0	6.6
Gastric juice	60	9	84	0	3.0
Bile	149	5	101	45	8.0
Pancreatic juice	141	5	77	92	7.7
Cerebrospinal fluid	141	3	127	23	7.5
Sweat	45	5	58	0	5.2

Intracellular and extracellular fluids are separated by the cell membrane, which is not fully permeable to solutes. Indeed, the permeability to many solutes is 'selective', a consequence of which is that intracellular fluids have a very different composition from that of the interstitial fluid that bathes the cells. The situation is complicated by the presence in cell membranes of ion-transporting processes, such as the sodium/potassium exchange pump (see Chapter 2), which actively transports sodium ions from the intracellular fluid and releases them into the extracellular fluid and transports potassium in the opposite direction. Thus, intracellular fluids contain high concentrations of potassium but relatively low concentrations of sodium (Table 6.1); generally, this is the opposite situation to that found in the extracellular fluids.

Calcium ions take part in many reactions within the cell, e.g. by acting as cofactors that aid the actions of certain enzymes. It may seem surprising, therefore, that intracellular concentrations of calcium ions are similar or even lower than they are outside the cell (Table 6.1). However, the availability of calcium ions is a factor in the control of many biochemical reactions, e.g. in muscle contraction (see Chapter 17). To control availability, a large proportion of the calcium content of a cell will be bound to proteins and released as required. The total calcium content (ionized and bound) of cells, therefore, will be more than the ionized component indicates.

Phosphate is abundant within cells, whilst bicarbonate ion concentration is considerably lower than that found in extracellular fluids. These ions act as buffers, an important role considering the continual production of hydrogen ions by metabolism. Phosphate ions are also an integral part of cellular metabolic processes. For example, phosphate-based compounds such as ATP act as energy transporters within the cell (see Chapter 4).

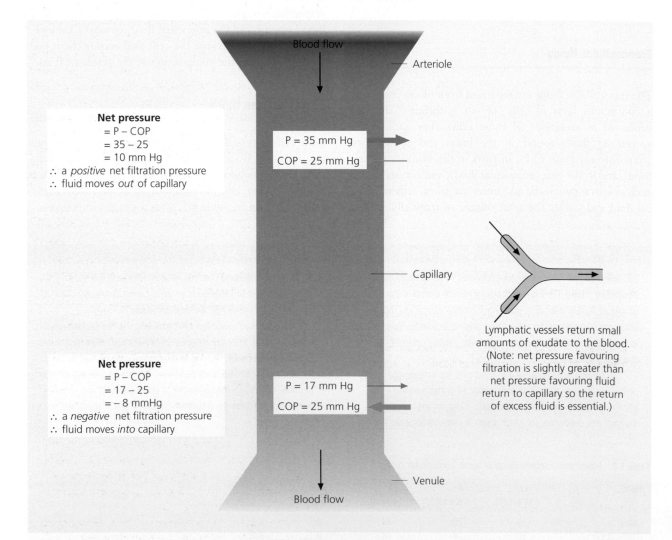

Net pressure
= P − COP
= 35 − 25
= 10 mm Hg
∴ a *positive* net filtration pressure
∴ fluid moves *out* of capillary

P = 35 mm Hg
COP = 25 mm Hg

Net pressure
= P − COP
= 17 − 25
= − 8 mmHg
∴ a *negative* net filtration pressure
∴ fluid moves *into* capillary

P = 17 mm Hg
COP = 25 mm Hg

Blood flow

Arteriole

Capillary

Lymphatic vessels return small amounts of exudate to the blood. (Note: net pressure favouring filtration is slightly greater than net pressure favouring fluid return to capillary so the return of excess fluid is essential.)

Venule

Blood flow

Figure 6.2 Fluid exchange between plasma and interstitial fluid across the capillary wall. The net movement of fluid into or out of the capillary will depend largely on the difference between the pressure favouring outward movement (the hydrostatic or blood pressure in the capillary, P) and that favouring inward movement (the osmotic pressure due to plasma proteins, called the colloid osmotic pressure, COP).

Q. Why don't the electrolytes in plasma contribute to the osmotic pressure component of capillary exchange?

Movement of water and solutes within and between compartments

Movement within compartments

Fluid compartments are not static, and water, with its constituents, is constantly on the move. Within the intracellular compartment, fluid movement occurs as 'cytoplasmic streaming' as a consequence of a combination of random motion of molecules, small diffusion gradients, and small thermal gradients. This flowing of the fluid helps to move substances around the cell, a process that is more efficient than if diffusion alone was the only mechanism.

Within the extracellular compartment, fluid movement is a combination of bulk flow and the exchange between the blood plasma and the interstitial fluid.

Bulk flow

As the term implies, bulk flow is the movement of material en masse from one point to another. Obvious examples are the muscular movement of bowel contents, which propels foodstuffs and fluids through the digestive tract, and the flow of blood through the cardiovascular system. Bulk flow provides the means of transporting substances on a large scale and in the shortest possible time.

Exchange between the plasma and interstitium

An exchange of fluids and solutes between the plasma and the interstitial fluid is essential in order to transfer substances from the plasma through the interstitial fluid to the cells at a rate that is conducive to normal cell function. The exchange of fluid occurs in tissues, where capillary blood vessels come into the proximity of cells. Capillary exchange occurs as a result of:

- having the wall of the capillary fully permeable to water and most solutes, although not to most large molecules such as proteins;

- the interplay of physical forces that promote such movements.

The forces involved in capillary exchange are illustrated in Figure 6.2. Basically, the relatively high hydrostatic (i.e. fluid) pressure within the capillary tends to force fluid out into the interstitial fluid; this force is opposed by osmosis (specifically referred to as the colloid osmotic pressure or oncotic pressure) induced by the plasma proteins that are retained in the capillary. At the arterial end of the capillary, the net pressure favours movement of water out of the blood vessel. However, this loss of fluid means that the hydrostatic pressure diminishes along the capillary. Thus, towards the venous end of the vessel, a point will be reached when the colloid osmotic pressure now exceeds the hydrostatic pressure, and so water (and solutes) will then be drawn back into the vessel. As a result, there is virtually no difference in the volume of blood that enters a tissue in an artery and that which leaves it in a vein.

The importance of plasma protein concentration in this process is clear. In reality, small quantities of protein penetrate the interstitium, and this slight alteration in the

---

BOX 6.4 OEDEMA

Read this box in association with Figure 6.2. Oedema is an accumulation of fluid in the interstitial compartment as the consequence of a disturbance in the capillary exchange of fluids. It may result from a number of causes:

- Elevated capillary hydrostatic pressure as a consequence of dilation of blood vessels entering the tissue, as occurs in inflammation or during hot weather; increased back pressure from veins, as occurs in congestive heart failure; or (in legs) as a consequence of gravity following standing for a long while, especially if the valves of leg veins are ineffectual.
- Decreased colloid osmotic pressure (due to hypoproteinaemia) as a consequence of loss of plasma proteins via the urine, reduced synthesis of plasma proteins, as occurs in various liver conditions or in malnutrition, or plasma dilution resulting from fluid overload.
- Blocked drainage of interstitial fluid by lymphatic vessels, perhaps caused by a tumour or by parasitic organisms.

Oedema may form:

- peripherally, either locally or generalized. Local oedema might be gravitational (e.g. in the ankle), or due to obstruction of tissue drainage during surgery, or due to the positioning of an immobile patient. Generalized oedema is more likely to involve an elevated central venous pressure (e.g. in congestive heart failure) or hypoproteinaemia (e.g. due to urinary loss of protein in nephrotic syndrome);
- in the abdomen (peritoneal oedema, or ascites) as a consequence of increased fluid secretion across the peritoneum (e.g. in liver failure, where the reduced circulation of blood through the liver raises the pressure in the hepatic portal vein);
- in the lungs (pulmonary oedema) as a consequence of increased secretion of fluid out of the pulmonary capillaries (e.g. elevated pulmonary capillary pressure as a consequence of left-sided heart failure).

Although treatment must aim to correct the underlying cause, relief may be provided simply by utilizing gravity to reduce the capillary hydrostatic pressure. This may involve sitting the person up to help relieve pulmonary oedema, tilting the bed, or suspending limbs, depending upon the site of the oedema.

Diuretic drugs may be also be used to promote urinary sodium and water excretion, and thus to reduce extracellular fluid volume and oedema. Alternatively, treatment may be aimed at reversing a reduced plasma protein concentration by the infusion of plasma extracts or synthetic protein.

balance of forces acting across the capillary wall results in a small net loss of fluid from the plasma. These proteins, and the accumulated interstitial fluid, are returned to the circulatory system via the lymphatic system (see Chapter 13).

Movement between intracellular and extracellular compartments

In Chapter 2, we described how water may pass through a selectively permeable membrane, such as the cell membrane, by osmosis. Thus, movement of water across the cell membrane will occur if the solution on one side of the membrane has a higher solute concentration than the solution on the other side. There are a number of solutes present in body fluids, including various ions and substances such as glucose, proteins and urea, so the potential osmotic effects of these fluids are determined by

the net effect of the concentration gradients of these individual solutes. The term normally used to denote the osmotic potential of a solution is *osmolality*, which is measured by the effect that solutes have to depress the freezing point of water (see Appendix A). Note, however, that the osmolality gives no information as to the variety or types of solute present, or of their individual concentrations, only their net effect (see Box 6.5).

Since water moves so easily across cell membranes, it is unlikely that a difference of osmotic potential between intracellular and extracellular fluids will last for long because equilibration will occur and make the total osmotic potential of the two compartments similar. One consequence of this is that should dehydration increase the solute concentration, and hence the osmolality, of the extracellular fluid, this will osmotically remove water from cells and result in cellular dehydration. This disrupts cell functions, as a near-constant intracellular environment is necessary (see Box 6.6).

BOX 6.5 OSMOTIC PRESSURE, OSMOTIC POTENTIAL, AND OSMOLALITY

Osmotic pressure relates to the idea that water movement across a selectively permeable membrane can be prevented if a pressure is applied to the opposite side of the membrane. The amount of pressure to be applied will be related directly to the extent of osmosis, which enables scientists to quantify the osmosis. Osmotic potential is a qualitative term that is usually used when solutions are compared, e.g. normal saline (see later) is considered as having the same osmotic potential as body fluids, even though their compositions are different.

Osmolality converts osmotic potential (and osmotic pressure) into a value based on the ability of solutes to lower the freezing point of water. Normal body fluids are said to have an osmolality of about 285 mosmol/l (milliosmoles per litre). The measurement enables comparisons to be made more readily than by using osmotic pressure. The concept of osmotic pressure is most important in relation to fluid exchange across a blood capillary (Figure 6.2), since here blood pressure is counteracted by the osmotic pressure exerted by the plasma proteins.

BOX 6.6 DEHYDRATION AND OVERHYDRATION

Dehydration results in a concentrating of the extracellular and intracellular fluids, and a reduction in cell volume. Obvious external signs are a dry oral mucosa and 'hollowing' of tissue around the eyes, and a loss of skin turgor. If oral rehydration is not possible, then enteral or parenteral therapy must be applied. Caution must be taken not to rehydrate too quickly, as there is a danger of causing too rapid an influx of water into the cells, thus inducing overhydration. Overhydration of cells should not be confused with

oedema, since it results in an increase in cell volume, whereas oedema is an accumulation of extracellular fluid.

Dehydration and overhydration usually affect the whole body and hence the function of all cells, but symptoms of neurological dysfunction are initially the most noticeable, with the affected person experiencing headaches or, if the imbalance is more severe, lethargy, personality changes, mental confusion, or even coma and death.

ACTIONS OF WATER AND ELECTROLYTES, AND PRINCIPLES OF BODY FLUID HOMEOSTASIS

Water and ions are continually added to our body fluids through our diets. Most ions ingested in our foods are absorbed from the bowel regardless of whether we are deficient in them. Our diets normally contain more than adequate amounts of the major ions, and the ionic constitution of our body fluids is determined mainly by the rate at which they are excreted, especially in the urine. In order

to regulate the ionic contents of the body fluids, the rate of addition and the rate of excretion must be kept equal, i.e. we must remain in a state of ionic balance, a classic example of homeostasis.

Fluctuations in body fluid composition occur when there is a mismatch between intake and excretion. Such fluctuations are more likely to occur in those fluids that

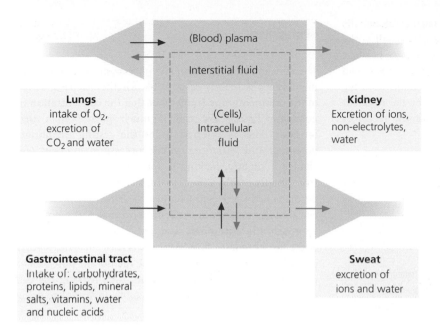

Figure 6.3 Schematic diagram of the exchanges of water and solutes between fluid compartments and the external environment. Note that it is the composition of blood plasma that is most susceptible to rapid change, and that interstitial fluid and hence intracellular fluid will be influenced indirectly by those changes.

exchange substances with our external environment, i.e. the extracellular fluid (Figure 6.3). The homeostatic mechanisms that regulate body fluid composition are stimulated by such changes. The detection of change in the extracellular fluid involves receptor cells, and the regulatory response results from the effects that such changes have on these specialized cells. Body fluid homeostasis is discussed further in Chapter 16, when kidney function is described in detail, but it is useful at this point to consider the actions of the constituents of body fluids and how they relate to those processes.

Water

As noted previously, water is the solvent in which most of the chemical reactions that comprise metabolism take place. Clearly, the concentrations of solutes dissolved in the water will change according to the rate of addition and removal of those solutes, but they can also be altered by adding or removing water since this will dilute or concentrate the fluids (and will also alter their volume). Changes in water balance could be expected to alter cell functions, and thus water homeostasis is essential.

The body is normally able to regulate water balance very effectively. For example, dehydration will induce an increase in the total solute concentration of plasma and interstitial fluid, which will cause the movement of water out of cells by osmosis, thereby concentrating the intracellular fluid. This causes receptor cells (called 'osmoreceptors'; see Chapter 16) to initiate changes in water intake and excretion by influencing our perception of thirst and promoting a reduction in urine volume. Overhydration will have opposite effects on the osmotic pressure of plasma: it will suppress thirst and promote the production of a large volume of dilute urine, the

intention being to remove excess water and restore the balance state.

Sodium and chloride

Sodium (Na^+) and chloride (Cl^-) ions are the most abundant electrolytes in extracellular fluid, and are usually considered together. They have two areas of activity.

1 The ions influence cell membrane processes, e.g. sodium ions aid the carriage of large molecules, such as glucose and amino acids, into the cells. In order to do this, sodium and the substance concerned both combine with the same protein carrier molecule in the cell membrane, and the concentration gradient for sodium causes diffusion into the cell. Chloride ions, being negatively charged, may interfere with the movement of positive ions. For example, in parts of the central nervous system, chloride ions may suppress the electrical changes that occur when the nerve cells are stimulated by interfering with the diffusion of sodium or potassium ions. This promotes 'inhibition' of nerve transmission (see Chapter 8).

2 Being so abundant, these ions are the main contributors to the osmotic potential of extracellular fluid, and so have a role in the distribution by osmosis of water between the extra- and intracellular compartments.

The means of controlling sodium chloride balance relates to the osmotic activities of the ions. An increased sodium chloride intake (e.g. salty food) will raise the sodium chloride concentration of extracellular fluid, promote osmosis from cells and cause thirst, and so lead to increased water retention and water intake, i.e. the responses are those that are normally associated with dehydration (see above).

However, unlike the control of water balance alone, the changes here are induced by the intake of the salt – the person may already have been in a state of water balance, and so the volume change induced by the responses would be in excess of normal. The excretion of sodium (and the excess water) by the kidneys is stimulated by the resultant increase in blood volume, detected by stretch receptors located within the circulatory system.

BOX 6.7 HYPERNATRAEMIA AND HYPONATRAEMIA

Normal ranges for sodium concentration in blood plasma: newborn, 139–146 mmol/l; infant, 139–146 mmol/l; child, 138–145 mmol/l; adult, 136–146 mmol/l.

Hypernatraemia ('hyper-' =greater than normal, 'natrium' = sodium, '-aemia' = of blood) occurs when blood sodium concentration is persistently greater than normal values. It usually results from an inability to regulate sodium concentration, e.g. in renal failure, or from dehydration. Hyponatraemia ('hypo-' = less than normal) often reflects excessive hydration of the extracellular fluids, but it can also arise if there is excessive loss of the ion, e.g. vomiting.

Therapy must relate to the underlying cause, including whether there is a change in water balance. This will usually entail assessment of how salt and water input and output compare.

BOX 6.8 HYPERKALAEMIA AND HYPOKALAEMIA

Normal ranges for potassium concentration in blood plasma: newborn, 3.9–5.9 mmol/l; infant, 4.1–5.3 mmol/l; child, 3.4–4.7 mmol/l; adult, 3.5–5.1 mmol/l.

When blood potassium concentrations are increased to above the normal range, this is referred to as hyperkalaemia ('kalium' = potassium). Although some adaptation by cells is possible, the elevated potassium may cause nerves and muscles to become overexcited, most noticeable as an increased heart rate and poor rhythm. Hyperkalaemia may be caused by an inability to excrete potassium adequately, e.g. in renal failure or a dysfunctional adrenal gland. Excessive hyperkalaemia can cause death.

Hypokalaemia will have the opposite effect, making heart cells more difficult to excite, leading to a decreased pulse rate. Hypokalaemia can be induced by excessive use of diuretic drugs that promote potassium excretion, or by a dysfunctional adrenal gland. Regular observations of pulse rates are important in these settings.

Therapy for hyperkalaemia includes treating underlying factors such as acidosis in which hydrogen ions enter cells and are exchanged for potassium ions, and improving excretion of the ion, e.g. by use of oral or rectal ion-exchange resins. Treatment for hypokalaemia will usually entail oral potassium supplements. Potassium infusions are normally only used when essential because of the potential for overinfusion leading to hyperkalaemia.

Potassium

The concentration gradient for potassium (K^+) across cell membranes is mainly responsible for the electrical status of the cell membrane (remember that the concentration of potassium inside the cell is much greater than that outside). This is referred to as the resting membrane potential, and variations in the potassium gradient will change it slightly, making it approach or deviate further from the threshold value at which nerve and muscle cells becomes activated (see Chapter 8). Thus, an increase in extracellular potassium concentration makes the potential approach the threshold, and so makes the membrane easier to stimulate. Similarly, a decrease in extracellular potassium concentration causes the membrane potential to deviate further from the threshold, thus making the cell more difficult, perhaps even impossible, to stimulate using physiological stimuli.

Since the plasma potassium ion concentration can have this profound effect on excitable cells, it is not surprising that the plasma concentration is monitored directly, and that an increase in concentration alters the excretion of potassium in urine.

Calcium

Calcium (Ca^{2+}) has two major areas of activity. Calcium ions have important intracellular actions. Various hormones stimulate the release of calcium ions from stores within target cells; these ions then promote the actions of certain enzymes in the cell. In muscle cells, calcium ions are necessary for the contractile process (see Chapter 17). Smooth and cardiac muscle cells have little calcium storage, so it is necessary for these cells to take up calcium ions from the extracellular fluid. Following contraction, these cells pump the ions back out again. Drugs classed as calcium antagonists interfere with this process and help to prolong muscle contraction in the heart.

The threshold membrane potential at which excitable cells are stimulated is also influenced by the calcium ion concentration of extracellular fluids. For example, a reduction in calcium ion concentration reduces the threshold, with the result that the cell is more easily stimulated.

The pronounced effects that calcium ions exert on excitable cells means the calcium ion concentration of extracellular fluid is monitored directly. Responses to a change in plasma calcium ion concentration are complex, as calcium balance involves the level of transfer between plasma and bone, the rate of uptake from the bowel, and the rate of excretion in the urine (see Figure 9.11).

BOX 6.9 HYPERCALCAEMIA AND HYPOCALCAEMIA

Normal range for (ionized) calcium concentration in blood plasma: newborn, 1.07–1.27 mmol/l; infant/child/adult, 1.12–1.23 mmol/l.

Hypercalcaemia is a persistent elevation of blood calcium concentration above the normal range. It occurs usually as a consequence of a failure of regulating the transfer of the ion into and out of bone (usually because of a hormone imbalance, especially of parathyroid hormone), or because of excessive acidity in blood (which releases calcium from that bound to plasma protein). The short-term consequence is a reduction in the activity of nerve and muscle cells, e.g. constipation arising from diminished bowel movements may be observed.

Hypocalcaemia may arise because of inadequate uptake from the bowel, excessive transfer to bone, or excessive renal losses. The problem is frequently due to hormone deficiency, but it may also be induced by alkalosis due to sudden depletion of hydrogen ion concentration in blood, e.g. in excessive breathing during anxiety (which removes too much carbon dioxide, a source of acidity). Muscle spasms may be observed as nerve and muscle cells become overexcitable, e.g. carpopedal spasm (of the hand) is an observation frequently seen in anxiety-induced hypocalcaemia.

Therapy for hypercalcaemia involves treating the underlying cause, but it may also entail promoting the loss of calcium in urine by enhancing renal losses, e.g. by using saline infusion to promote urine production and electrolyte loss. Treatment for hypocalcaemia may be by oral supplement, but calcium gluconate infusion may be used in severe cases.

BOX 6.10 BICARBONATE ION RESPONSE TO ACIDOSIS

Normal range for bicarbonate concentration in (arterial) blood plasma: newborn/infant/child/adult, 21–28 mmol/l.
Normal range for bicarbonate concentration in (venous) blood plasma: newborn/infant/child/adult = 22–29 mmol/l (note slightly higher range for venous blood, since bicarbonate is generated from carbon dioxide in tissues).

Blood bicarbonate ion concentration may be elevated as part of a compensatory response of the kidneys to an acidosis, e.g. when lung function is poor and carbon dioxide retention is observed. This change is to be expected and helps to buffer the extra acidity.

The term 'base excess' is used by doctors to estimate the extent of the compensatory response to an acidosis. Carbon dioxide generates bicarbonate as well as hydrogen ions (see Chapter 4), so carbon dioxide retention elevates plasma bicarbonate concentration in addition to promoting an acidosis. The analysis of a blood sample takes this generation of bicarbonate into account and provides a base excess value to indicate how much additional bicarbonate has been retained by the kidneys. This value is important because bicarbonate ions may also be administered as part of the therapy to reduce an acidosis, and the base excess makes it more likely that overcorrection may occur.

In extreme circumstances, more bicarbonate may be infused to reduce the acidity, but this carries the risk of inducing an alkalosis due to overinfusion. A slower elevation of blood bicarbonate may be induced if an infusate that contains lactate is administered, as this is converted to bicarbonate by the liver. Citrate – an anticoagulant used for storing blood   is also converted to bicarbonate in the liver, and excessive blood transfusion can induce a slight elevation in blood bicarbonate, and hence induce an alkalosis (see Box 6.11).

Bicarbonate and phosphate

As discussed earlier, and in more detail in Chapter 4, bicarbonate (HCO_3^-) and phosphate (HPO_4^{2-}) ions are important buffer chemicals in body fluids that help cell enzymes to operate at an optimum rate. An excess or deficiency of buffers will therefore affect enzyme efficiency by altering the concentration of hydrogen ions present (i.e. the pH). The concentration of bicarbonate ions in blood plasma is regulated by responses to acidity changes (see Box 6.10) through alterations in its production (from carbon dioxide) and excretion (as carbon dioxide in the lungs, and as bicarbonate in urine).

Phosphate ions, when combined with calcium ions, also form the main mineral component of bone. There is, therefore, a continual process of release and uptake of phosphate to and from the extracellular fluid, as bone is resorbed and reformed. It is therefore not surprising that regulation of the concentration of phosphate ions in blood plasma is linked to the control of calcium. It is controlled in particular by changes in phosphate excretion in urine.

Hydrogen

Although these ions are present in only very small concentrations, the importance of hydrogen ions in pathology makes it worthy of mention here. Hydrogen ions have a potent damaging effect on protein structure and function, so their concentration must be regulated very closely. The concentration of hydrogen ion is monitored directly. Increased acidity stimulates the removal of carbon dioxide, a source of acidity, via the lungs. Alternatively, an increased acidity of blood passing through the kidneys promotes the urinary excretion of hydrogen ions. By a related mechanism, the kidney may also alter the buffering capacity of plasma by changing the excretion bicarbonate ions (see Box 6.10).

BOX 6.11 ACIDOSIS AND ALKALOSIS

Normal ranges for acidity of arterial blood: newborn (full-term) at birth, pH 7.11–7.36 (H^+ = 43–77 nmol/l); newborn (full-term) at 1 day, pH 7.29–7.45 (H^+ = 35–51 nmol/l); infant/child/adult, pH 7.35–7.45 (H^+ = 35–44 nmol/l).

We have encountered the terms 'acidosis' and 'alkalosis' at various points in this chapter. It is important to distinguish between the two. Acidosis is a set of signs and symptoms (headache, blurred vision, fatigue, weakness, possibly tremors and delirium) arising from an excess of hydrogen ions in body fluids, thus making them more acidic (pH value less than 7.35). This is usually as a result of:

● carbon dioxide retention (respiratory acidosis);
● excessive metabolic acid production (metabolic acidosis; the precise name depends upon the cause, e.g. ketoacidosis in

diabetes mellitus, lactic acidosis in anaerobic metabolism);
● inadequate excretion of hydrogen ions, e.g. in renal failure (also usually referred to as metabolic acidosis).

Similarly, alkalosis is a set of signs and symptoms (weakness, muscle cramps, dizziness, carpopedal spasm, paraesthesia) arising from insufficient hydrogen ions in body fluids, thus making them more alkaline than they should be (pH value greater than 7.45). This is usually as a consequence of:

● inadequate generation of acids;
● excessive retention of buffer chemicals.

Alkalosis is caused by the reverse of those factors identified for acidosis.

USE OF INFUSATES IN PRACTICE TO SUPPORT BODY FLUID COMPARTMENTS

The infusates used to support body fluids can be divided into colloids, crystalloids, and blood cell preparations. Blood cell preparations are not considered here; their uses are self-explanatory, and are noted in Chapter 11. This section also gives only an overview of the common infusates, primarily to relate their use to the discussion in this chapter. Practice issues surrounding the delivery of intravenous infusates are discussed by Workman (1999).

Colloidal infusates: plasma expanders

A colloid is a substance that forms a viscous consistency with water. Colloidal infusates may be of protein (e.g. gelatin) or carbohydrate (e.g. dextran). Both types can be used to replace plasma protein when it is very deficient, which will restore to normal the osmotic pressure due to colloids in plasma. This helps to restore fluid exchange in

BOX 6.12 INTRAVENOUS THERAPY

Access to the vascular compartment must be made aseptically to prevent the introduction of infectious agents. The access is normally through:

● peripheral venepuncture, in which a needle is inserted through the skin into a superficial vein, often in the hand or arm, and connected to a catheter tubing. A butterfly needle is often used, since the flanges can be taped to the skin to keep the needle in situ. The purpose of the catheter is to facilitate regular blood sampling, infuse a medication, commence fluid therapy, or administer radio-opaque/radioactive material;
● insertion of a large-bore catheter into a major vein, normally a subclavian vein, internal jugular vein or femoral vein. Such catheters enable the measurement of central venous pressure or the delivery of large volumes of fluids or viscous fluids, as used in total parenteral nutrition.

Infusates may be administered using a bag/drip-feed method, in which gravity and blood flow at the needle tip encourage the

addition of fluid to blood at the needle tip, or via a pump (syringe driver).

Complications (see Workman, 1999) may arise from:

● *phlebitis:* a redness and swelling of skin at the site of venepuncture. Irritation or pain is usually present. The inflammation represents a defence response to infection, the chemicals being delivered into the vein, or the needle/catheter material. Apart from being unpleasant for the patient, phlebitis also raises the risk of blood clotting (thrombophlebitis) at the needle tip sufficiently to cause an embolus;
● *extravasation:* occurs if the needle tip exits through the wall of the vein, leading to infusate delivery into the surrounding tissue, resulting in swelling (i.e. oedema) and pallor as blood flow to the area is compromised;
● *blockage:* either at the tip of the needle (protein deposition, blood clot, or compression of tissue against it) or through a kink in the catheter tubing.

Table 6.3 Composition of crystalloid infusates

	Na$^+$ (mmol/l)	Cl$^-$ (mmol/l)	K$^+$ (mmol/l)	Ca^{2+} (mmol/l)	Lactate (mmol/l)
5% dextrose	0	0	0	0	0
0.9% saline	153	153	0	0	0
Hartmann's (lactated Ringer) solution	131	111	5	2	29

the tissues whilst the production of plasma proteins recovers. The role of colloid infusions, therefore, is to support the plasma subcompartment of the extracellular fluids. Protein infusions are more effective than dextrans, but they carry the risk of inducing an immune response.

Crystalloid infusates

These infusates dissolve in water and are used to support the extracellular and/or intracellular fluids. Various crystalloid infusates are used in practice (Table 6.3):

- *Saline (sodium chloride solution).* Sodium chloride is found predominantly within the extracellular fluid, so this infusate largely supports that compartment. The most widely used saline is normal or isotonic saline (0.9% sodium chloride solution; i.e. 0.9 g per 100 ml). This has an osmotic pressure similar to that of body fluids, so water in the infusion will not move into cells in any quantity. In some circumstances, hypertonic saline may be used (e.g. 2.5% sodium chloride solution) to raise the osmotic pressure of extracellular fluids and hence cause the withdrawal of water out of cells by osmosis.

- *Dextrose.* This is a solution of glucose. It is usually administered as an isotonic solution (5%; i.e. 5 g per 100 ml), and so might not be expected to promote water movement in or out of cells. However, unlike saline, the glucose will be taken up by cells and utilized, effectively

leaving water behind. The loss of solute means that water can now pass into cells by osmosis, thus helping to hydrate the intracellular fluid.

- *Dextrose/saline.* This combines the advantages of both saline and dextrose. Cell hydration is promoted, but the saline component also helps to ensure that some of the infusion remains within the extracellular compartment.

- *Hartmann's solution.* This provides a more comprehensive support for extracellular fluid than saline alone. It is sometimes referred to as a lactated Ringer solution. A Ringer solution is one that has an electrolyte composition that matches closely extracellular fluid: Hartmann's solution approximates to human extracellular fluid, except that it contains lactate rather than bicarbonate ions. The lactate ions are converted to bicarbonate by the liver, so bicarbonate is added to blood, but at a much slower rate than if it was in the infusate. This helps to reduce the likelihood of bicarbonate overload.

- *Potassium.* Potassium chloride solution may be infused to increase the potassium concentration in blood plasma. However, infusion runs the risk of inducing potassium overload if it is administered too quickly, so this infusate is not used widely in general settings. If it is required, potassium support is usually provided by Hartmann's solution or by potassium in combination with saline or glucose, in which the potassium concentration is close to the normal values for extracellular fluid.

BOX 6.13 ISOTONIC, HYPERTONIC AND HYPOTONIC INFUSATES

Isotonic infusates

Despite their different compositions, normal saline, 5% dextrose solution, and Hartmann's solution have the same osmotic effect on a selectively permeable membrane. Remember that osmosis relates to a concentration gradient, and does not change with individual types of solute. These three solutions have the same overall solute concentration and thus have the same osmotic properties. The osmotic potential of these solutions is the same as that of the body fluids. Cells suspended in any of these solutions will not show a change in their state of hydration, at least not initially (dextrose is the exception, as cell hydration will gradually increase when the glucose is utilized). Thus, the three solutions noted here are said to be isotonic ('iso-' = same) to body fluids.

Hypertonic infusates

These solutions have an osmotic potential that is greater than that of body fluids. Thus, cells suspended in them will shrink as water is lost by osmosis. Such infusates are not used as widely as isotonic solutions, but they do have a value in practice where there is excessive intracellular hydration, or to promote water movement from a transcellular fluid.

Hypotonic infusates

Hypotonic infusates are used rarely because they have an osmotic potential less than that of body fluids and so cells will take in water rapidly by osmosis, resulting in cell swelling, and even lysis. 5% dextrose solution provides a means of slowly improving cell hydration, and so reduces the risks of cell swelling, and is a preferred means of promoting cell hydration.

Summary

1 Body fluids are subdivided into the extracellular and intracellular compartments.

2 The extracellular fluid is comprised of blood plasma, the interstitial fluid and transcellular fluids. Transcellular fluids are secreted by specialized epithelia, and therefore have a different ionic composition from that of the rest of the extracellular fluid.

3 Blood plasma and interstitial fluid have very similar compositions because interstitial fluid is continually being formed from plasma, and returned to it, in the capillary beds of tissues. Pores in the blood vessels are sufficiently large to allow passage of water and the majority of solutes, except plasma proteins.

4 Normal cell function, appropriate for the tissue in which it is found, requires the rigorous regulation of all the processes that take place. Ions play a central role in determining cell function, and part of homeostatic regulation requires a control of the intracellular ionic environment.

5 Intracellular fluids and the interstitial fluid are separated by the cell membrane. The properties of this lipid membrane enable cells to have different ionic compositions to the surrounding fluid.

6 Although the maintenance of cell membrane functions helps to regulate intracellular fluid composition, the intracellular environment and the cellular volume are also influenced by the extracellular fluid composition. The regulation of extracellular fluid composition and volume helps to stabilize cell membrane activities, and is also necessary to ensure that chemical processes occurring in this fluid also progress efficiently.

7 An important aspect of water and ionic regulation is that a balance between input and output (excretion) is maintained. Much of the regulatory process involves the control of urinary excretion of ions and water. Detection of an imbalance involves specialized receptors that respond to aspects specific to the actions of the electrolyte concerned.

8 Disturbances in fluid and electrolyte balance are commonplace, both in day-to-day living (relatively minor, since diets and homeostatic changes in renal function rapidly correct the imbalance) and clinically (potentially severe).

9 Clinical therapies frequently entail the infusion of fluids to support body fluid volume and composition.

10 Infusates include blood cells, plasma, crystalloids (e.g. saline or glucose) and colloids (to support plasma volume). There is a variety of crystalloid infusates; the choice is determined by the disturbance and, in particular, the fluid compartment that requires most support.

Review questions

1 Our bodies contain a high percentage of water. Find out the proportion of our weight attributable to water. How does this proportion vary throughout life? Which patient groups are at increased risk of dehydration?

2 Rapid weight fluctuations may be due to excessive fluid gain or loss. What is the rationale for regular weighing of some patients?

3 Monitoring of fluid balance may be necessary with some patients. Consider ways in which fluids may gain entry to and exit from the body.

4 Sweating is an important thermoregulatory mechanism. How could you assess fluid loss via this route for a feverish patient?

REFERENCES

Workman, B. (1999) Peripheral intravenous therapy management. *Nursing Standard* **14**(4): 53–62.

Section Three

Sensing change and co-ordinating responses

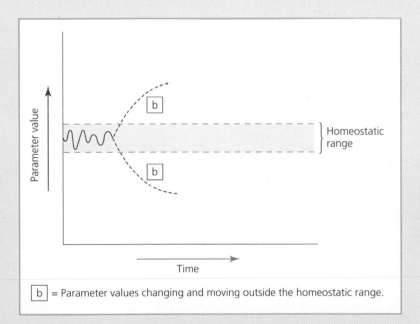

b = Parameter values changing and moving outside the homeostatic range.

Chapter 7

The senses

INTRODUCTION

If homeostasis is to be effective, then the body must be able to detect changes in the internal and external environments in order to produce an appropriate corrective or adaptive response. In other words, there must be a sensory system that is able to detect the diverse range of stimuli that impact on the body, and effector systems that can produce a breadth of responses necessary to ensure that the internal environment remains optimal.

Exercise

You may find it useful to refer back to Chapter 1 to clarify why homeostasis includes both corrective and adaptive responses.

Sense or perception?

Strictly speaking, our 'senses' are the faculties by which the body receives information regarding its internal and external environments. Note, however, that a 'sense' does not necessarily equate with 'sensation' or 'perception', since these terms refer to our capacity to be consciously aware of a change to some aspect of our environment. Having a conscious awareness of a stimulus is frequently not essential, so our senses do not always convey perception. Thus, being continually aware of what is happening to body fluid composition, blood pressure or body temperature would

BOX 7.1 CONSCIOUSNESS

Arousal, say from sleep, commences when neural activity from the brainstem 'wakes up' the rest of the brain, especially the cerebral cortex (see Chapter 8). Consciousness, however, implies something beyond this – a capacity of the brain to make us 'aware'. The fundamental need for neurological interpretation of sensory information if an individual is to be 'conscious' has implications during surgery when consciousness and arousal are inhibited by general anaesthesia (Oulette and Oulette, 1998) or brain injury (Price and Burns, 1999).

From a sensory viewpoint, consciousness means that we can consciously perceive our environment and interpret it in a meaningful way. How this interpretation of sensory information occurs continues to elude science, and provides a distinction between physiology and psychology. The use of radioactively labelled markers, such as

glucose, is now providing insight into the neurological changes that accompany 'thinking', but how a pattern of neural activity is translated into a mental image remains unknown.

What is clear is that memory and sociocultural factors have important roles in the construction of mental images, sounds, speech, writing, etc. Such involvement helps to explain why there is such subjectivity in interpretation (e.g. see Chapters 21 and 22), and why this can have such an impact on health and healthcare.

Coma appears to represent a failure of consciousness. Comatose individuals show no apparent recognition of sensory input (although input from, say, the lungs that does not entail 'awareness' may still be operative). Interestingly, triggering memory through the use of familiar sounds or voices has sometimes been successful in reversing the coma.

not be practical, except when changes are extreme. On the other hand, a sense such as pain must be perceived to provide us with the information that tissues have been damaged or are threatened.

Our senses require the presence of specialized cells or cell structures collectively referred to as receptors. These are found throughout the body, and range in structure from complex cells, such as those of the retina of the eye, to simple surface molecules, such as those found on the cell membrane within synapses at nerve cell junctions and cells that are the targets for hormones. The functions of various surface chemicals have been described in other chapters. This chapter is intended to supplement the chapters on neural and endocrine co-ordination and will therefore concentrate on those receptors that promote activity in sensory nerve cells.

Understanding the functions and roles of the senses is clearly important if the self-regulating processes involved in homeostasis are to be appreciated. Many senses are

identified in the chapters on effector systems (Section 3) because of their involvement in regulating them. This chapter therefore explains only some of the general principles involved, and the classification used, but does not explore the physiology of these senses any further. Much of the chapter encompasses those senses referred to as the 'special senses', the functions of which relate mainly to the monitoring of the external environment.

BOX 7.2 THE SENSES IN HOLISTIC PRINCIPLES OF HEALTH

The task of incorporating physiological processes into a framework based on holistic principles of health can, at times, present a challenge. This is especially the case when attempting to place systemic functioning into the context of psychosocial interaction. Understanding the senses can provide insights into the holistic nature of health (and healthcare) since it is our senses that provide us with the image of our world. This image is constructed by the brain according to the information it receives, but if we consider those

senses that are 'translated' into a mental, conscious perception, then the image will also be influenced by the context in which it was received. Our senses provide the links with our environment, especially the social environment, so the contextualization of stimuli, based on experiences, is an important aspect of subjectivity and individuality. Recognizing this provides the means by which the psychosocial and physical aspects of health can be integrated and applied to individualized care (see Chapter 21 onwards).

RECEPTORS AND THEIR ROLES

Sense receptors and sensory modalities

The sensing of environmental change normally requires the presence of specialized receptor cells that are sensitive to a specific stimulus. For example, dehydration causes a rise in the osmotic pressure of plasma, which is detected by cells that are sensitive to the change in volume of fluid within them. Dehydration is unlikely to be a localized occurrence – in this example, the detected change would be indicative of an alteration in body fluid osmotic pressure throughout the body. The receptors therefore need to be located only in an appropriate position; osmotic receptors are located within the hypothalamus, close to the pituitary gland, which secretes the hormone responsible for altering kidney function when we are dehydrated. In contrast, sensing touch at the fingertips conveys absolutely no information, for example, of what is happening to our feet. Touch receptors therefore must be distributed about the body.

The specific type of stimulus detected by a receptor is called its modality, e.g. touch, pressure and temperature. Many of our receptors are unimodal ('-modal' = mode or kind), i.e. they are so specific that they are able to detect an individual modality, such as osmotic pressure, and their responses therefore relate only to the intensity of stimulation. Other receptors are polymodal, and can detect different types of stimuli, although these will still relate to the same homeostatic role of the receptor. For example:

- vision involves the detection of the intensity of light (brightness) and its wavelength (colour);

- hearing involves the detection of sound intensity (loudness) and frequency (tone);

- smell and taste involve the detection of chemical intensity (concentration) and type (e.g. pungent, floral or acrid smells, and sweet, sour or salty tastes).

Polymodal receptors provide us with our 'special' senses. The complexity of these is such that the receptors are organized into anatomical features recognizable as sense organs – the eyes, ears, nose and tongue. Pain is also polymodal, in that it has qualities of both intensity and type (throbbing, aching, stabbing, sharp); some texts include this as a special sense, although there are no specific sense 'organs' for pain. In recognition of the particular relevance of pain to healthcare professions, this 'sense' has been placed into a separate chapter (Chapter 21), and we will give it only a brief mention here.

The special senses are useful in another important way. In being stimulated by change, most receptors can only provide information of the occurrence of an event. For example, touch indicates contact, whilst the stimulation of osmotic receptors mentioned earlier indicates that a change in water balance has occurred. However, receptors for vision, hearing and smell all provide information on circumstances or changes that are operative some distance from the body, which enables an assessment to be made as to their likely impact on the body before the event. Similarly, perceiving an unpleasant taste allows us to reject a substance that could perhaps be injurious to the body, while pain provides us with a warning that further tissue damage will ensue unless we respond. In these ways, our special senses provide a 'predictive' facility that enables us to take steps if necessary to either prevent a disturbance in homeostasis, or at least to minimize it, or perhaps even to encourage it if it is likely to be desirable.

General characteristics of receptors

Transduction

Receptors are transducers: they convert energy present within the stimulus (e.g. heat or light) into electrical energy by altering the electrical properties of the cell membrane of the receptor. This is achieved by an alteration in the distribution of electrolytes between the intracellular and extracellular fluids. Thus, receptor cells and other excitable cells, such as nerve and muscle cells, have the capacity to change the permeability of their membranes to certain ions (usually sodium or potassium), leading to their movement into or out of the cell. The distribution of ions normally produces a voltage difference (called an electrical potential) across even an unstimulated cell membrane, with the inside of the cell being negative with respect to the outside. The process of transduction, therefore, requires the generation of small changes in this electrical potential. Such changes are called generator potentials, and their rate of production relates to the degree of stimulation.

If the summated generator potentials meet or exceed a threshold level, this will trigger events within the receptor cell. These may, for example, promote the release of a hormone such as oxytocin from the posterior pituitary gland, or generate in associated sensory nerve cells the

electrical changes that are referred to as action potentials. The threshold level for a specific stimulus determines the sensitivity of the receptor, and hence is a factor in the efficiency of homeostatic control. Thus, receptors will have a low threshold in the homeostatic regulation of those parameters that have narrow homeostatic ranges.

Receptor fields

Sensory receptors may be discrete cells (e.g. in the retina of the eye) or nerve endings (e.g. touch receptors in the skin). Those that are nerve endings may be branched extensively and extend over an area called a receptor field. Some receptor fields are large, others small. The smaller the field, the greater our ability to 'place' the stimulus (Figure 7.1). For example, the points of a pair of compasses applied to the fingertips can be discerned as two distinct points, even when they are only about 1.5 mm apart. This is because the fingertips have a high receptor density with small receptor fields in which the stimulus is detected by more than one receptor even when the points are close together. On the back, however, the two points are discerned separately only when they are some 35–40 mm apart. This is because the receptor density is less, and the field for each receptor is large, so when the two points are close together they stimulate just one receptor and cannot be discerned as two stimuli.

Adaptation

Receptors of many senses exhibit a decreasing sensitivity in response to continued stimulation, even though the stimulus is still present. Touch is a typical example: life would be very unpleasant if we were to be constantly aware of contact with our clothes, with chairs, with the ground, or with spectacles, etc. In these instances, once the stimulus has been received, and perhaps acted upon, it becomes more important to detect a new change rather than to remain aware of the 'safe' old one. Thus, these types of

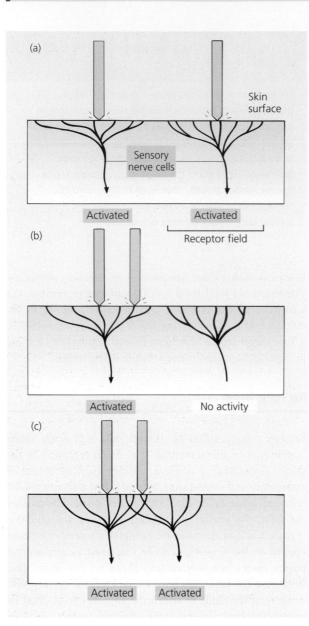

Figure 7.1 Two-point discrimination. (a) The two points are in contact with two receptor fields, and so will be detected by each of the two nerve cells. (b) The points are too close together to be discriminated, as both are in contact with the same receptor field, and hence the same nerve cells. (c) The overlapping receptor fields help to discriminate two points, even when the contacts are close together, as both nerve cells are activated but one possibly more than the other.

Q. Give an example where two-point discrimination is (i) excellent and (ii) poor?

receptors adapt to the stimulus and can respond again if the stimulus changes.

Receptors may be 'slowly adapting' (known as tonic) or 'rapidly adapting' (phasic). Tonic receptors tend to be those that provide information regarding relatively steady states of the body, such as blood composition and body position. Rapidly adapting receptors are important if states can change rapidly, since they may convey moment-to-

moment information regarding changes in the stimulus. For example, receptors in our skeletal joints provide information not only that the joint has been flexed but also how rapidly it was flexed (i.e. its velocity) and whether that velocity changed (i.e. accelerated). This is essential if movement is to be controlled (see Chapter 17).

Types of receptor

Receptors are sometimes referred to according to their location. This is usually a collective term, however, and does not distinguish receptor type. For example, cutaneous receptors are those found in the skin, whilst visceroreceptors are those found in the viscera (i.e. internal organs of the body). A more usual means of classification relates to the kind of stimulus the receptors detect:

Mechanoreceptors

Mechanoreceptors are sensitive to mechanical deformation and include receptors of touch, pressure, vibration and stretch. They are relatively simple in structure, consisting of the terminals of sensory nerve cells, which are either 'free' or encapsulated. Mechanoreceptors include:

● *Merkel's discs:* disc-like arrangements of 'free' nerve terminals in contact with epidermal cells in the skin that respond to touch;

● *Meissner's capsules:* egg-shaped structures in the dermis of the skin containing nerve terminals that respond to touch;

● *Pacinian corpuscles:* oval structures distinguished by their concentric onion-like layers of connective tissue. Nerve terminals are found within the layers. They are pressure receptors, and are located in deep subcutaneous tissues, submucosa tissue, tissue around joints, and mammary glands;

● *root hair plexus:* 'free' nerve endings are wrapped around the base of a hair root and respond to deformation induced by movement of the hair shaft when it is touched;

● *proprioreceptors:* group of receptors involved in the control of posture and movement ('proprio-' = position). *Muscle spindles* are stretch receptors that contain nerve endings in contact with modified skeletal muscle fibres. They respond to changes in muscle length and play a crucial role in the control of muscle contraction (see Chapter 17). *Golgi tendon organs* are stretch receptors within the tendons that monitor the tension induced when the attached muscle contracts. They seem to have a protective role and cause muscle contraction to cease (i.e. 'give way') suddenly if the tension threatens injury. *Joint receptors* provide information about the position of the joint and about how rapidly

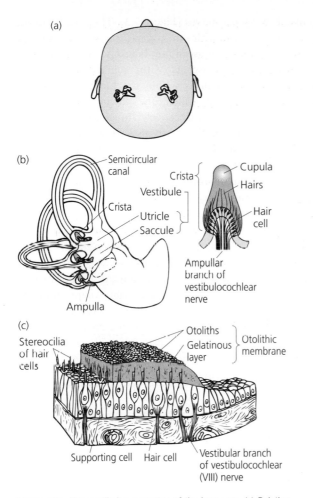

Figure 7.2 The vestibular apparatus of the inner ear. (a) Relative position within the head. (b) Vestibular structures: utricle, saccule and semicircular canals. An enlarged crista is shown. (c) Details of the utricle and saccule.

Q. Why are the receptor cells often referred to as 'hair cells'?

the position is changing during movement. They consist of nerve endings associated with connective tissue within the joint. The *vestibular apparatus* of the inner ear includes three semicircular canals attached to a distended structure called the vestibule (Figure 7.2). The base of each canal connects with the vestibule via a distended region called an ampulla, within which are found the receptor cells, the hair-like cilia of which are embedded in a gel projection called the cupula. Movement of the head causes fluid to flow within the canals, which deflects the cupulae and so stimulates the receptor cells, thus providing information that the head has moved. The vestibule itself contains two sac-like areas called the utricle and saccule (Figure 7.2), both of which also contain receptor cells. These also have hair-like cilia projecting into a membrane; on the surface of this gel-like membrane lie small crystals of calcium carbonate called otoliths ('oto-' = ear, '-lith' = stone), which slide over the surface of the membrane when the head is moved. This distorts the projections of the receptor cells and stimulates them;

- *auditory receptors:* these are described later, but basically they respond to a distortion produced by pressure waves in the fluid of the inner ear.

Thermoreceptors

Thermoreceptors are 'free' nerve endings that have properties that enable them to respond to fluctuations in temperature. There are 'hot' and 'cold' receptors that respond to different temperature ranges, although the ranges overlap. Together, they provide information over a range of skin temperatures.

Chemoreceptors

Chemoreceptors are sensitive to changes in the concentration of chemicals within the body fluids. This is a diverse range of receptors. Examples are those that monitor the hydrogen ion concentration or the glucose concentration in blood plasma. Such receptor cells usually carry surface chemicals that will interact specifically with the substance to be monitored. When activated, these sensory cells either promote electrical activity in associated nerve cells, as in the detection of increased blood acidity by the carotid bodies, or promote the release of a hormone, as in the release of aldosterone from the adrenal gland when blood potassium is elevated. Taste and smell (described later) are also examples of chemoreceptors.

Nocireceptors

Nocireceptors (or nociceptors) are responsive to noxious stimuli. They are usually referred to in relation to pain. Nociceptors are probably free nerve endings, some of which at least are sensitive to chemicals released from damaged cells in the vicinity. Others appear to be those of other senses, such as touch or temperature, which convey an unpleasant sensation when stimulated excessively.

Photoreceptors

Photoreceptors are sensitive to light. Details of these receptor types and how they are stimulated are given later.

Interpretation of receptor activity

Overview

Electrical activity generated by receptors associated with the nervous system is conducted via sensory nerve cells to the central nervous system. Much of the activity eventually arrives in the brain for integration, co-ordination and, if appropriate, to convey conscious perception of the stimulus. The pathways along which sensory information travels is generally as follows:

Receptor → Thalamus of brain → Cerebral cortex
(relay centre) (sensory association area; interpretation)

This plan is very simplistic, however, and pathways may involve other parts of the brain before activity enters the thalamus. Similarly, information may be transmitted to parts of the brain other than the cerebral cortex, such as the cerebellum (involved in movement control; see Chapter 17), and may not always involve transmission through the thalamus, although this usually is the case. Processing may not even involve the brain at all, with the information being integrated by the spinal cord.

Sensory pathways

Sensory activity from peripheral receptors enters the dorsal horn of grey matter within the spinal cord via the dorsal roots of the spinal nerves (Figure 7.3). There, some of the nerve cells synapse with others that ascend the cord to the brain. Some of these ascending neurons are found in the lateral and anterior aspects of the spinal cord, and pass directly to the thalamus within the brain. Accordingly, these pathways are called the lateral and anterior spinothalamic tracts, respectively. In general, the lateral tract conveys information from nociceptors and thermoreceptors, while the anterior tracts carry information from touch and pressure receptors in the skin. A feature of these tracts is that the neurons within the cord that are stimulated by incoming sensory nerve cells actually cross over to the other side of the cord before passing to the thalamus. In this way, information from receptors on one side of the body passes to the opposite side of the brain.

In contrast, those sensory fibres that carry activity from touch receptors in deeper tissues, and from proprioreceptors (especially those in joints), do not synapse immediately within the cord. Instead they ascend the spinal cord, passing up the posterior aspects of the cord (Figure 7.3; note that the sensory fibre of a single neuron from the toes must therefore have a length of up to 1.5–2 m). Accordingly, these pathways involve posterior spinothalamic tracts; these are actually observable as surface features on

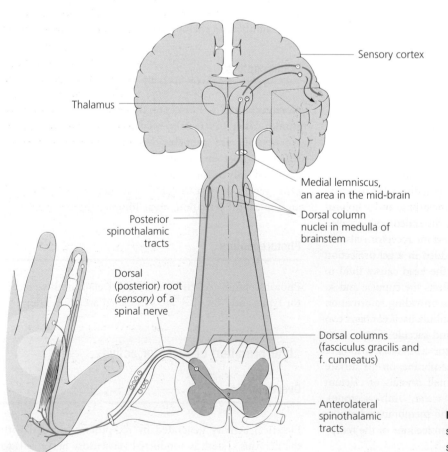

Figure 7.3 Routes of transmission from sensory receptors to the sensory cortex: the spinothalamic tracts.

the cord, and are called dorsal columns. The neurons eventually synapse with aggregates of nerve cells within the brainstem, called the dorsal column nuclei, the fibres of which then cross over to the other side and pass to the thalamus. As with the other spinothalamic tracts, the crossing over of neurons within the brainstem means that the left side of the brain receives information from the right side of the body, and vice versa.

Proprioreceptor activity from muscles may also ascend via the posterior spinocerebellar tract (which therefore lies in a posterior aspect, and passes to the cerebellum at the back of the brain) of the spinal cord. The role of these receptors and the cerebellum in relation to the control of posture and movement are discussed in Chapter 17.

The special senses of vision, hearing, smell and taste are in the head, so electrical activity does not pass via the spinal cord but goes direct into the brain tissue via cranial nerves. The activity passes either directly to the thalamus, and then to the cerebral cortex, or passes via other parts of the brain particularly within the brainstem and hypothalamus, and so may miss out the thalamus entirely.

> **Exercise**
>
> Find the sections on the thalamus, cerebral cortex and cerebellum in Chapter 8 and familiarize yourself with their position within the brain, and their roles.

THE SPECIAL SENSES

This section considers in detail the anatomy and physiology associated with the 'special' senses of vision, hearing, taste and smell. The predictive element of the special senses was described earlier and has obvious advantages in the course and planning of actions, the consequences of which are that the internal environment is more likely to be optimal if threatening situations can be avoided. The special senses facilitate our capacity to operate in the range of environments with which we come into contact each day, and help us to maintain independence of our actions. In so doing, it could also be said that these senses play a role in our social and psychological wellbeing, in addition to the maintenance of physiological homeostasis.

Vision

Overview

Vision requires the detection of light, the properties of which include brightness (intensity) and colour (wavelength). The receptor cells of the eye contain chemicals – known as visual pigments – that absorb light and consequently break it down into component molecules. It is this process that activates the cell membrane, which in turn stimulates action potentials in associated sensory nerve cells. The pigment chemical then reforms.

The ratio of undissociated to dissociated pigment provides a means of monitoring light intensity, while having different pigments that respond optimally to certain wavelengths conveys a means of detecting colour. Light receptors therefore respond to electromagnetic stimuli, but only within the relatively narrow range of wavelengths determined by the pigments present. This is why we cannot see light at the extreme ends of the electromagnetic spectrum, i.e. infrared (IR) and ultraviolet (UV) light.

General anatomy of the eye

The eye is basically a sense organ that focuses light waves onto the receptor cells, but it also has the capacity to adjust the amount of light incident on the receptor region. Its anatomy is related to these functions.

The eye is approximately spherical, with a white-coloured fibrous protective and supportive layer called the sclera. At the front of the eye, the sclera becomes the delicate and transparent cornea. A thin layer of modified skin – the conjunctiva – extends from the eyelids to the sclera surrounding the cornea (Figure 7.4(a)), which helps to protect the lining within the socket. Laterally, the sclera is attached to the bone of the orbit of the skull by six extrinsic muscles that produce lateral and vertical movement of the eye upon contraction or relaxation. The muscles are controlled by the oculomotor and trochlear nerves (cranial

> **BOX 7.4 STRABISMUS AND NYSTAGMUS**
>
> Strabismus is a condition in which the eye drifts from position when the gaze is focused on an object. Often referred to as 'lazy eye', it arises because of an imbalance in control of the ocular muscles. The eye must be trained by, at times, covering the normal eye and thus making the 'lazy' eye dominate the vision.
>
> Nystagmus is a rhythmic movement of the eyes, producing a flickering effect. It may be caused by an incorrect conditioning of this reflex, in which case it is usually present from childhood. However, nystagmus can also suggest the occurrence of neurological disturbance or drug abuse.
>
> A similar flickering can be stimulated by a sudden change in the stimulation of the vestibular apparatus of the ear (called a vestibular-ocular reflex) that is thought to operate when the head is turned suddenly.

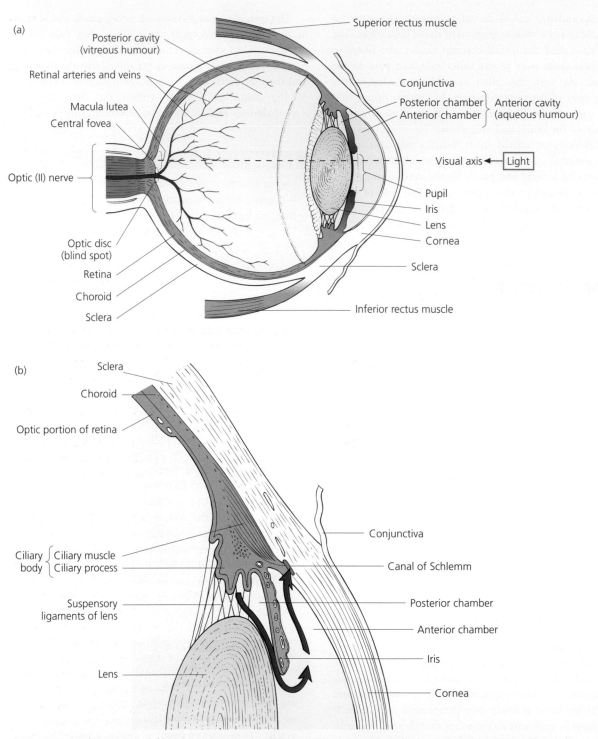

Figure 7.4 (a) General features and visual axis of the eye. (b) Enlargement to show detail of the iris, ciliary body, and the circulation of the aqueous humour.

Q. *What is glaucoma?*

nerves III and IV; see Figure 8.5). At the back of the eye, the sheath of the optic nerve fuses with the sclera.

Lubrication of the sclera and, in particular, the cornea is provided by secretions from the lachrymal (tear) gland found at the top outer area of each eye. Secretions drain into the nasal cavity via the lachrymal duct, which origi-

nates at the inner corner of each eye. Tears also provide a means of irrigating the eye when an irritant is present.

Below the sclera lies a vascular layer called the choroid, which provides the sclera with nutrients. The choroid extends from the rear of the eye to the ciliary body, which in turn forms the iris (Figure 7.4(b)). The lens is suspended from the ciliary body by the suspensory ligaments, and the ciliary body also contains smooth muscle cells capable of altering the shape of the lens. Lying within the choroid are parasympathetic and sympathetic

nerve fibres that control lens shape and also enter the iris to alter the aperture as appropriate.

The inner coat of much of the eye consists of the light-sensitive retina. This extends from the ciliary body around

BOX 7.5 CONJUNCTIVITIS

Conjunctivitis is an inflammation of the conjunctiva caused by an infection or by the presence of irritants (Mead, 2000). Antibiotic creams may be administered. Eyewashes might also be used, although the possibility of cross-infection to other people, or to the other eye, means that they must be used with caution.

BOX 7.6 OBSERVING THE RETINA

Observing the retinal blood vessels, using an ophthalmoscope, is an important clinical aid in the diagnosis of, for example, cerebral hypertension. This is because any distension of a blood vessel produced by a higher-than-normal blood pressure within the eye will compress any vessels passing immediately below it. Such compressions can be observed. Diabetes mellitus also has an adverse effect on retinal blood vessels. Early signs of deterioration can be detected by observing the vessels.

Use of the ophthalmoscope entails shining a thin beam of light into the eye and peering through a lens arrangement that allows an image of the retina to be seen. The practitioner usually must hold the ophthalmoscope very close to the eye, a disconcerting experience for some people.

The pupillary constriction that would be anticipated by use of the light, and that would prevent observation of the retina, is prevented by the use of a drug, such as atropine, that blocks the parasympathetic nerve endings responsible for causing the contraction of the pupil. Atropine is administered in eye drops a short time before the investigation. Unfortunately, the effect lasts for a few hours, so patients should avoid bright lights for a few hours and, ideally, should be escorted home.

The lens of the eye divides the eyeball into two fluid-filled compartments (Figure 7.4(a)). The anterior compartment contains aqueous humour, which is a thin, watery fluid that is constantly being formed by the ciliary body and then reabsorbed by the canal of Schlemm at the base of the ciliary body (Figure 7.4b). This circulation of fluid is important because the humour supplies the nutritive needs of the cornea and iris. The compartment behind the lens is filled with vitreous humour (literally 'glass-like'), a colourless fluid that is made jelly-like by the presence of small amounts of mucoprotein. This is the largest compartment; the fluid, once formed, cannot be replaced, even if lost by injury.

BOX 7.7 EYE SURGERY

Techniques for eye surgery have advanced considerably in recent years, especially with the advent of laser treatments.

Corneal transplantation

The cornea does not have blood vessels, which is very useful from the point of view of corneal transplants, since immune cells do not gain access and tissue rejection presents less of a problem than elsewhere in the body. The surgery does result in the loss of some aqueous humour, but this will be replaced as more is secreted from the ciliary body.

Glaucoma

If the rate of secretion of aqueous humour exceeds that of its resorption, then an increased humour pressure will result, called glaucoma. The cornea then bulges, resulting in blurred vision, especially around the edges of the image. The elevated pressure in the anterior chamber is also transmitted to the vitreous humour, which then crushes the retinal blood vessels. Blindness may result if it is untreated. Treatment is aimed at improving fluid drainage through the canal of Schlemm, either by surgery or by the pharmacological contraction of iris sphincter muscles to release the occluded duct. Alternatively, a trabeculectomy may be performed, in which a valve is placed within the sclera behind the upper eyelid, which allows drainage of excess fluid.

Cataracts

A cataract is a lens that has lost its transparency due to biochemical changes within it. This will prevent the transmission of light, resulting in blindness. Correction of total vision loss is often by removal of the lens, whilst leaving the membrane at the back of the lens intact, so that the vitreous humour is preserved, followed by implantation of an artificial lens (Fischel and Lipton, 1996). The preferred method is phacoemulsification, in which a small diamond-tipped blade is inserted through the edge of the cornea to allow access of other microequipment. The anterior capsule of the lens is removed, and the lens is disintegrated using ultrasound or laser ablation. A flexible lens is then inserted and secured. This method enables insertion of an artificial lens without the need for an extensive incision (and sutures) to the cornea. It is a rapid technique that does not usually entail a stay in hospital (Linebarger et al., 1999).

Detached retina

This is a separation of part of the retina, often as a result of eye trauma that has caused a deformation of the eyeball. Laser therapy is used to reattach the separated tissue. Scarring may cause loss of some retinal cells but, as with the blind spot, the brain can use vision from the other eye to compensate for this.

the inner surface of the rear of the eye. It is in the retina that the light receptor cells – the rods and cones – are found. The retina also has its own nerve cells associated with the receptor cells, which aid in processing the information before it is passed into the optic nerve. The receptors are considered in more detail below. Two features worth mentioning here, however, are that the inner surface of the retina contains the blood vessels that maintain the layer, and that the exit point of the optic nerve (called the optic disc) is devoid of receptors, and so is called the blind spot. Thus, light must pass through the vessels before detection by most of the retinal receptors, and the light ideally must not be incident on the optic disc. Not surprisingly, the blind spot is off-centre and incident light largely avoids it. In addition, the light from an object that does fall onto the blind spot in one eye will fall elsewhere on the retina of the other eye. In this way, the brain can compare the images from both eyes and remove any perception of a blind spot.

Light enters the eye through the cornea, passes through the lens, and ultimately arrives at the receptor cells of the retina. Although widespread in the retina, the receptor cells are particularly dense at the 'yellow spot' or fovea, an area in line behind the lens that is devoid of blood vessels. The fovea is packed with cone receptors, which convey colour vision, although small numbers of these will also be found in other areas of the retina. Some rods will also be present in the fovea, but they are mainly found outside it. Thus, the image of whatever is the centre of our attention is focused onto the fovea for high definition, colour analysis and clarity, but peripheral images can still be discerned though in less detail.

The foveal cones are only 2–3 µm in diameter, which means that the difference in angle of light incident on the fovea to stimulate a single cone cell, but not an adjacent one, is only about one-hundredth of a degree. This means that light from small variations in appearance of an object will fall on different receptor cells, thus enabling us to distinguish the detail. The ability to discern detail is called visual acuity.

The iris aperture, the lens and the cornea provide a breadth of vision that is referred to as the visual field. The curvature of the cornea enables us to see beyond 180 degrees; with two eyes looking directly ahead, the visual field is of the order of 210 degrees. Although objects at the perimeter of such a wide field of view may not be observed in detail, any movement is detected easily. In fact, movement within the visual field is an extremely potent stimulus that causes a reflex movement of the eyes so that the moving object can be scrutinized to determine whether we should be interested in it. The control of eye movement is described later.

Exercise

The importance to us of directing our gaze at movements within the visual field is readily observed. Notice that however deep a conversation you are engaged in, something moving unexpectedly within your field of view causes an unconscious, albeit usually momentary, glance at it.

Physiology of vision

The light from an object that has attracted our attention must be focused if its image is to be formed at the fovea. In other words, light rays are bent or refracted on entering the eye so that they fall onto that particular part of the retina. Vision, therefore, can be considered to involve four stages:

1 refraction of light waves onto the receptor cells;

2 transformation of light energy into electrical energy;

3 interpretation of electrical signals generated in the eye;

4 control of the amount, or intensity, of the light, so that this is appropriate and does not under- or overstimulate the receptor cells.

Light refraction

Light rays are refracted when they pass from one medium into another, e.g. from air to water. Most of the refractive power of the eye is in the cornea as light passes through its cells, and little further refraction occurs through the humours. The lens usually provides the final focusing of light onto the retina. The lens is basically a concentric series of transparent layers of lens fibre (i.e. proteins) enclosed within a transparent capsule. The curvature of the lens capsule is flexible, and may be distorted by contraction or relaxation of the muscle cells of the ciliary bodies to which the lens is attached. This in turn alters the focal length of the lens and therefore its capacity to refract light rays.

The degree to which light must be refracted depends upon the angle at which the light rays are incident on the eye. If the light is from a near object, it must be refracted greatly to bring it into focus on the retina, while light from a distant object requires less refraction (Figure 7.5): the lens is said to accommodate. At about age 40-45 years, the close focusing or accommodating ability of the lens begins to decline as its structure and biochemistry changes.

BOX 7.8 MEASURING VISUAL ACUITY

In practice, acuity is measured by the reading of letters of different sizes, called Snellen tests. These include rows of letters that should be visible to an observer at certain distances away. The letters are designed so that their height will subtend an angle incident on the eye of one-twelfth of a degree if it is read at the appropriate distance. Thus, a person standing 6 m (20 feet) away should be able to read the appropriate row of letters: this is called 6/6 (20/20) vision. In contrast, a person who has to stand 6 m away to read letters that should normally be readable from a distance of 18 m has 6/18 vision, i.e. they have an acuity defect.

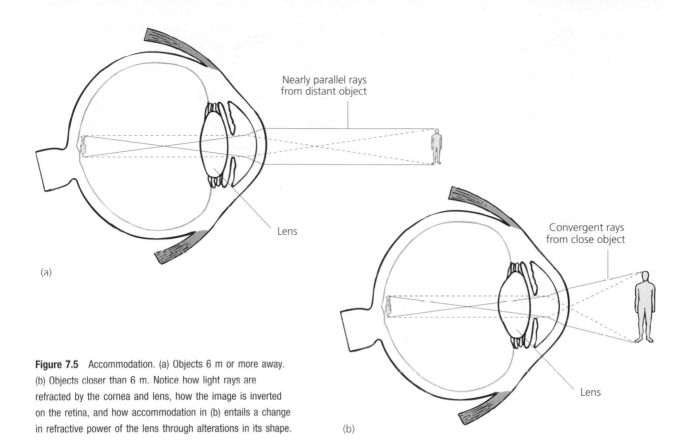

Figure 7.5 Accommodation. (a) Objects 6 m or more away. (b) Objects closer than 6 m. Notice how light rays are refracted by the cornea and lens, how the image is inverted on the retina, and how accommodation in (b) entails a change in refractive power of the lens through alterations in its shape.

BOX 7.9 BLURRED VISION

Blurred or distorted vision results from a failure of the refraction of light rays to focus an image on the retina. A thickened lens or elongated eyeball will cause the image to be focused at a point in front of the retina, a condition called myopia or near-sightedness (Figure 7.6(a)). A long, slimmer lens, or a shortened eyeball or poor accommodation ability, such as occurs with age, may cause the focal point to fall behind the retina, a condition called hypermetropia or long-sightedness (far-sightedness) (Figure 7.6(b)).

An irregular curvature of the lens or cornea will disturb the focusing of central and peripheral aspects of an image; this is called astigmatism (Figure 7.6(c)). The capacity for a lens to accommodate to near objects diminishes with age, producing an inability to focus on near objects, or presbyopia.

All of these disorders are correctable with appropriate spectacle lenses. For example, a convex spectacle lens will cause convergence of light rays before they are incident on the cornea, which will correct a refractory deficiency as in long-sightedness (Figure 7.6(b)). Similarly, a concave lens will cause divergence of light rays to correct excessive refraction produced by the eye, as in short-sightedness (Figure 7.6(a)).

Blurred vision can also arise if there is a loss of lens transparency through a change in its structure (a cataract; see Box 7.7).

Activation of the retinal receptor cells

Figure 7.7 shows a section through the retina. It appears to be inverted in that the receptor cells lie below the associated nerve cells and, for much of the retina below, the blood vessels. Such barriers are of little consequence, because light is a powerful energy source, although acuity is aided by the lack of vessels in the fovea.

The receptor cells can be subdivided into those sensitive to wavelengths of light within the visible colour range (the cones) and those that are most sensitive to low light intensities and do not convey colour (the rods). A typical rod cell is shown in Figure 7.8. It contains the usual cell organelles but also contains light-sensitive pigment. This pigment, called rhodopsin, is comprised of two molecules, retinene (a derivative of vitamin A) and opsin. Light promotes the breakdown of rhodopsin into its constituents, which depolarizes the receptor cell membrane and produces action potentials. The two substances then recombine to reform the pigment, which is then available to respond to light again.

The sensitivity of rod cells to light is determined by the amount of undissociated rhodopsin relative to dissociated pigment. In bright light, at any given time most of the pigment is dissociated because it breaks down immediately upon reforming, which reduces its sensitivity. In contrast, much of the pigment is undissociated in poor light; the

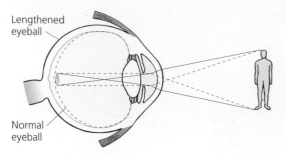

(a) Near-sighted (myopic) eye, uncorrected

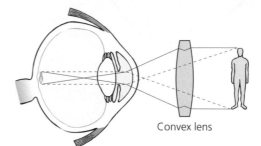

Near-sighted (myopic) eye, corrected

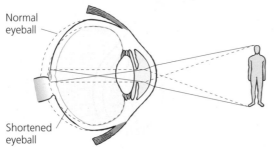

(b) Far-sighted (hypermetropic) eye, uncorrected

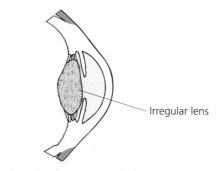

Far-sighted (hypermetropic) eye, corrected

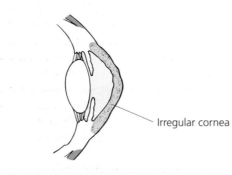

(c) Astigmatism from an irregular cornea

Astigmatism from an irregular lens

Figure 7.6 (a) Near-sighted vision and its correction. (b) Far-sighted vision and its correction. (c) Astigmatism, in which the sharp focusing of an image is compromised by a scattering of light rays by an irregular cornea or lens.

Q. When is a spectacle lens said to be (i) convex and (ii) concave? Which type of lens is used in short-sightedness?

availability of the pigment makes the eye most sensitive in dim light. Thus, if a person enters a dark room from a bright one, sensitivity increases substantially during the first few minutes as pigment reforms. Sensitivity increases further during the next 20 min or so, but only monochromatic vision will be possible since the cones require much greater light intensities to function. This increased sensitivity when light is poor is called visual adaptation, and allows us to gain some vision even when there is very little light available. Of course, if the same person then re-entered a brightly-lit room, the effect would be dazzling, as rhodopsin would dissociate in large quantities, producing an overwhelming stimulation of the retina. Eventually, adaptation would again occur as a new balance of dissociated to undissociated pigment becomes established and vision is restored.

Cones behave in a similar fashion to rods, but they contain slightly different pigments called visual purples. These exhibit peak sensitivity to light wavelengths corresponding to violet/blue, bluish green/yellow and orange/red (Figure 7.9); they are known as blue, green or red cones, respectively. Generally, they are most sensitive to the wavelengths that make up white light, which is a combination of blue, green and red light (as shown by a rainbow). The human eye cannot discern infrared and ultraviolet light unless aids are used.

Available evidence suggests that colour vision depends upon what proportions of blue, green and red cones are stimulated. This trichromatic theory does not explain why we are able to distinguish metallic colours, or brown, but to see the full range of visible colours does require the correct proportions of the three types of cone to be

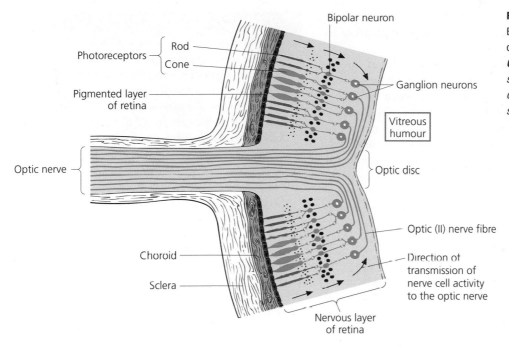

Figure 7.7 The retina. Blood vessels have been omitted for clarity.
Q. Why is the retina sometimes said to be upside down in terms of its structure?

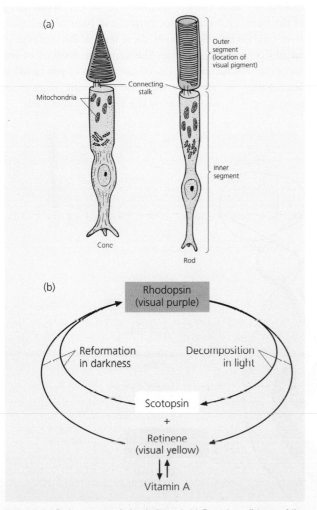

Figure 7.8 Rods, cones and visual pigment. (a) Receptor cell types of the retina. (b) The behaviour of visual pigment (rhodopsin) in light and dark. See text for explanation.

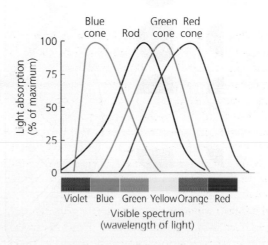

Figure 7.9 Light absorption by rods and cones.
Q. How might the cones enable us to see yellow?

present. It is also clear that people who are deficient in particular cones have a colour 'blindness' appropriate to the deficit (Box 7.10).

Generator potentials of the rods and cones at threshold or above will promote depolarization of the sensory nerve cells that they synapse with. The retina contains a complex arrangement of interacting nerve cells that have been given various names (Figure 7.7(a)). The main type are the bipolar cells, which synapse with horizontal cells and ganglion cells before action potentials are conducted into the optic nerve and thence to the brain. This interaction between various nerve cells means that some processing of the information occurs before the action potentials even leave the eye.

Interpretation of the visual signals

Electrical activity passes from the retina to the optic nerve (cranial nerve II; see Figure 8.5) and then to the brain. Activity from the left side of the retina of each eye passes to the right side of the brain, and vice versa (Figure 7.10). The cross-over of neural pathways from the left and right sides of the retinae occurs at the optic chiasma, a structure that lies just anterior to the pituitary gland at the base of the brain. The significance of cross-over is that it enables a comparison of the data from each eye, which helps us to perceive depth in the visual world. After cross-over, the bundles of nerve cells pass to a part of the thalamus called the dorsal lateral geniculate body, but remain packed

tightly into discrete nerves. Lesions of these parts of the pathway cause a profound loss of vision (Figure 7.10). After the thalamus, the neural pathways diverge, so electrical activity from the retina eventually arrives at various parts of the brain for processing.

The visual perceptional areas of the brain are comprised of virtually all of the occipital lobe of the cerebrum, parts of the frontal/parietal motor cortex, and parts of the brainstem (see Chapter 8 to clarify these terms). Recognition of an object probably involves the cognitive analysis of the topographical features of the object, e.g. its edges, based at least partly on memory but also involving degrees of reasoning. The mechanism of the latter is still unclear.

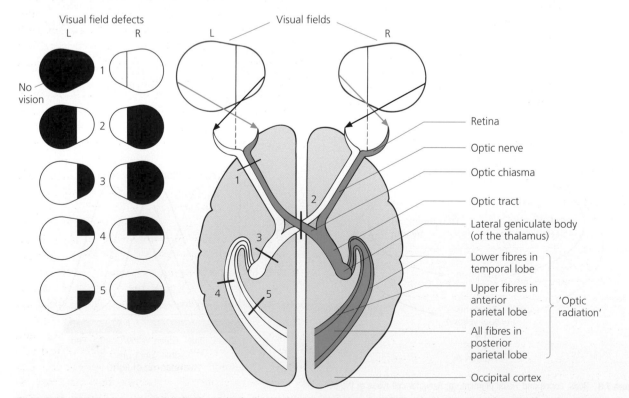

Figure 7.10 Visual pathways and the effects of lesions at various points producing visual field defects. Note that information from the right side of each eye passes to the right side of the brain, that from the left, to the left side of the brain.

Other parts of the brain that receive sensory input from the eye provide additional information and/or influence behaviour. They include:

- the *suprachiasmatic nucleus* (i.e. it lies above the optic chiasma) of the hypothalamus, which is thought to control the sleep/wake circadian rhythmicity in response to light cues (see Chapter 23);

- the *accessory optic nuclei* and *superior colliculi* of the brainstem, which are involved in controlling eye movement;

- the *pretectum* areas of the brainstem (see Chapter 8), which are involved in controlling pupil diameter.

Control of the intensity of light entering the eye

We described earlier how retinal receptor cells are able to adapt to differences in light intensity and how this is an important homeostatic response that enables us to maintain vision in both poor and bright light. The efficiency of the process is influenced by the amount of light entering the eye: in poor light, the adaptation will be restricted by very low light levels, and in bright light the process will be limited by excessive light. Adaptation, therefore, is facilitated by admitting as much light as possible under poorly illuminated conditions, and by restricting the entry of light under bright conditions.

Upon entering the eye, light must pass through the pupil of the iris. As well as containing pigmented cells, this also contains antagonistic smooth muscle cells arranged in a radial and circular fashion. As the name suggests, radial cells extend from the centrally located pupil to the periphery of the iris, and the circularly arranged cells extend circumferentially around the pupil. In bright light, parasympathetic nerve activity stimulates contraction of the circular muscle cells, and relaxes the radial ones, resulting in a constriction of the pupil. In dim light, sympathetic nerve activity contracts the radial cells, and relaxes the circular ones, resulting in pupil dilation. The aperture of the pupil can therefore be altered according to the light conditions. The process works as a reflex, and so occurs automatically and very rapidly. The reflexes operate via parts of the brainstem.

The influence of sympathetic activity in dilating the pupil may also play a role in the 'fight, flight and fright' response in the alarm stage of the general adaptation syndrome (see Chapter 22). This is because pupil dilation increases the illumination of peripheral areas of the retina, and may even expand the visual field. Visual perception will therefore be heightened under threatening (or exciting) circumstances.

Control of eye movement

The physiology of vision also includes the control of eye position in relation to focusing on near or distant objects, and in relation to following a moving object. Thus, if attention is switched from a distant to a near object, the eyes must converge so that the image of the object still lands on the fovea of each eye (Figure 7.11(a)). Continual assessment of the position of the image ensures that it is kept on the fovea. As the object moves toward the eyes, so the image is returned to the fovea by further convergence, even to the extent of causing the eyes to be 'crossed'. The neurological processing that is necessary to control these movements takes about one-fifth of a second. To put this into context, the last visual fixation that a batsman has on a cricket ball travelling at 160 km/h will be when the ball is still more than 10 m away from him! The delay has implications when we are following a rapidly moving object, e.g. when driving a car.

At other times, we may wish to focus on an object that is moving across the visual field. Movement within the visual field is a potent stimulus to attract attention, and the eyes will usually focus reflexly on an unexpected moving object (Figure 7.11(b)), and perhaps track it as it moves across the visual field. This 'visual pursuit' of a moving object is a complicated process and involves 'programming' by the brain of the direction and speed of movement. Provided that the movement is not too rapid, tracking is very smooth (Figure 7.11(c)). If the movement is rapid, however, the eyes must carry out extremely quick catching-up movements, which means that for a fraction of a second the object is not exactly where the brain perceives it to be! These rapid eye movements are called saccades (Figure 7.11(d)); similar movements, without the 'programming', are also performed in, for example, scanning a piece of text or a painting. They are amongst the fastest movements that the body is capable of producing, but they may be problematic if the programming is delayed (see Box 7.13).

BOX 7.12 PUPIL DIAMETER AS A MEANS OF ASSESSMENT

It is important in healthcare to understand how pupil diameter is controlled. Pupil dilation will occur in response to sympathetic activity during times of heightened excitement and agitation, and will also be observed if a patient is in danger of entering circulatory shock as sympathetic stimulation is enhanced then

States of depressed mental function, especially in drug overdose, make the reflex response to light sluggish or even absent. Stimulation of the retina with a light pen will then not produce a normal reflex constriction of the pupil. Similarly, a patient with a brainstem trauma may not respond normally to the light pen. The autonomic reflex involves neurological structures within the brainstem for its co-ordination. For this reason, pupil response to light stimulation is a part of the assessment of brainstem trauma or even 'brain death'.

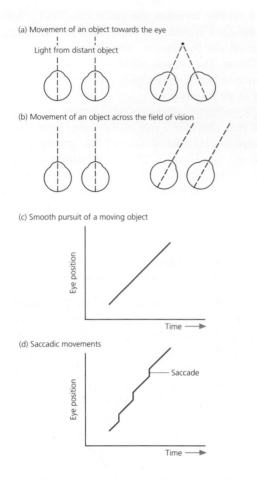

(a) Movement of an object towards the eye

Light from distant object

(b) Movement of an object across the field of vision

(c) Smooth pursuit of a moving object

Eye position

Time

(d) Saccadic movements

Eye position

Saccade

Time

Figure 7.11 (a) Convergence movement of the eyes to maintain an image on both retinae when an object moves towards the eyes. (b) Pursuit movement of the eyes to maintain images on both retinae when an object moves across the visual field. (c) Tracking diagram for pursuit movement. The straight line indicates 'smooth' pursuit. (d) Tracking diagram for pursuit movement when an object is moving quickly. Saccadic ('jumping') movements must be used to enable the eyes to catch up with the position of the object.

BOX 7.13 ALCOHOL AND VISION

Excessive alcohol slows down the integration involved in the processing of movement of an object in the visual field. Convergence movements are slowed, making it difficult to judge distances, thus making stopping distances much longer when driving. If following an object across the field, the individual typically will have to perform saccades to keep up, even at relatively slow rates of movement. However, saccades are only effective if the brain can register the new position. The delay introduced by alcohol means that by the time the saccade is accomplished, the object has moved on again. In other words, the object is not exactly where the brain thinks it is, leading to poor judgement.

Hearing

Overview

Sound is the perception of small pressure waves generated in air or water by a vibrating object, e.g. the vocal cords of the larynx. The vibrations set up alternate compressions and decompressions of the air; the number of compressions per second (or cycles per second; 1 cycle/s = 1 Hertz or Hz) gives the sound its frequency, which is perceived as pitch. The amplitude of the compressions gives sound its intensity or loudness. Sound intensity is measured in decibels (dB): rustling leaves have an intensity of 15 dB, and conversation 45 dB. The ear is very sensitive; normally it can detect intensities almost as low as 0 dB and frequencies over a range of 20–20 000 Hz. A sound intensity of 115–120 dB produces pain within the ear, and persistent exposure to 90–100 dB can cause permanent hearing damage.

Sound intensity and frequency are complex modalities, but some generalizations can be made regarding the basis of their detection. The pressure waves that make up sound are conducted through the ear and generate pressure waves of the same frequencies within the fluid-filled inner ear (cochlea). Here, the receptor cells are distorted by the movements that are induced by the pressure waves. The pattern of distortion seems to be important in conveying information regarding sound intensity and frequency. The receptors of hearing are therefore a type of mechanoreceptor.

General anatomy of the ear, and physiology of hearing

The ear is divided into three component parts: the external, middle and inner ears (Figure 7.12). The visible external ear (pinna) is deeply folded, which introduces minor perturbations in the sound pressure waves and helps in locating its source. Comparison of signals from both ears also facilitates the location of sound. The aperture of the external ear penetrates the skull via the auditory meatus (external auditory canal), which terminates at the eardrum (tympanic membrane). This membrane is under a degree of tension, and vibrates at the same frequencies as those of sound pressure waves incident upon it. Earwax (cerumen) helps to maintain the health of the skin within the external auditory canal, and to collect particles from the air, thus protecting the eardrum. Hairs also help to filter particles. Excessive production of wax can impair hearing, especially if it becomes impacted on the eardrum (see Chapter 16).

The vibrating membrane sets up similar vibrations in the transmission system of the middle ear, which is comprised of three small bones or ossicles called the malleus, incus and stapes within an air-filled chamber

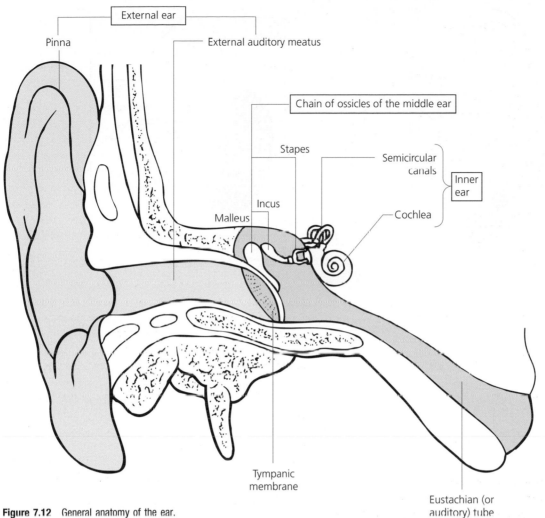

Figure 7.12 General anatomy of the ear.

(Figure 7.13(a)). The presence of a middle ear conveys four major advantages:

- The force of vibration is greatly increased in the ossicles, which is essential as the tympanic membrane is considerably larger than the aperture of the inner ear, and also because the inner ear is fluid filled and so requires more energy to cause movements of the fluid.

- The middle ear chamber connects directly with the nasopharynx (the cavity at the back of the nose) via the Eustachian (auditory) tube. Thus, any major change in external air pressure can be applied quickly to the middle ear by opening the aperture of the auditory tubes in the nasopharynx through swallowing. In this way, the pressure on either side of the tympanic membrane can be equilibrated and prevent 'ballooning' of the eardrum. Although this protects the membrane from damage, it will not protect against very sudden changes in air pressure, such as in an explosion, which can cause the membrane to perforate.

- The middle ear chamber provides a means of dissipating the sound pressure waves after they have traversed

the inner ear, thus making the receptor cells receptive again to further stimulation.

- The transmission of vibrations along the chain of ossicles means that if our external environment is extremely noisy, then excessive amplitudes of vibration can be reduced by altering the contact between the bones and the tympanic membrane and inner ear. This is achieved by the contraction of small muscles (called the tensor tympani and the stapedius) that pull the malleus bone away from the tympanic membrane, and the stapes bone away from the aperture to the inner ear. This mechanism is a reflex response, and is analogous to the reduction of pupil diameter observed when the eye is exposed to bright light, in that excessive stimulation is prevented from entering the receptor area – another example of homeostatic adaptation. The slight delay in adaptation may make loud sound almost deafening on initial exposure; similarly, moving from a noisy environment into a quiet one initially makes hearing difficult.

The stapes bone, the final link in the chain of ossicles, has a flattened surface that makes contact with the

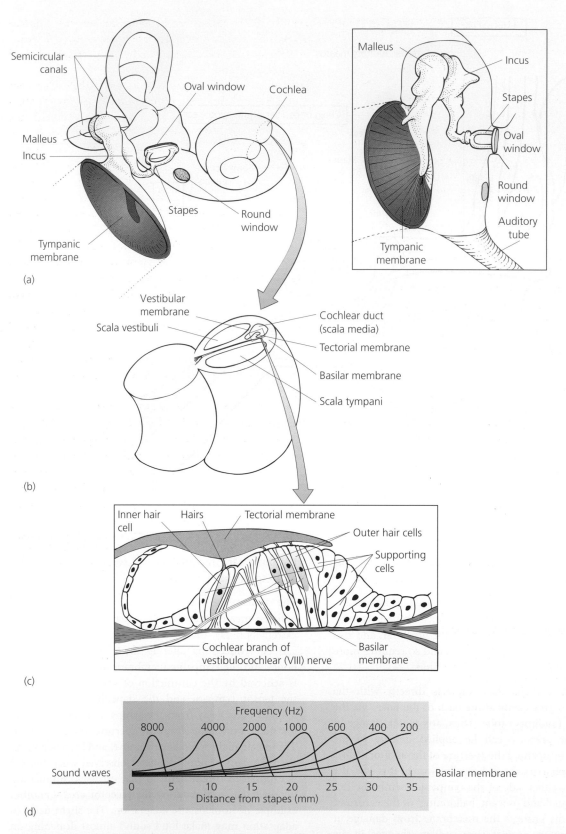

Figure 7.13 Structures involved in hearing. (a) Anatomy of the middle and inner ear. (b) General structure of the cochlea. (c) Detail of the anatomy of the cochlea to show the hearing receptors and associated structures (the organ of Corti). (d) The role of vibrations of the basilar membrane in the cochlea to provide initial frequency discrimination of sound waves. Low-frequency sounds are most effective at a distance from where sound enters the cochlea at the stapes, and high-frequency sounds are most effective close to the stapes.

Q. How do sound waves pass from the air to the basilar membrane?

The auditory tube may allow bacteria from the nasopharynx to enter the middle ear, causing inflammation, a condition called otitis media (Berry, 2000). Young children are especially at risk because of the relatively short length of the tube. Antimicrobial drugs may prevent further progress of infection.

The accumulation of pus and inflammatory effusion in the middle ear interferes with the functioning of the ossicles, reducing clarity of hearing, and the pressure exerted on the inner ear produces tinnitus. This is known as otitis media with effusion, commonly called glue ear. Antimicrobial drugs may be prescribed for this, but the presence of effusion also means that rupture of the tympanic membrane as a consequence of pressure in the middle ear, or the spread of infection to the inner ear, are risks. Because of this, clinicians may recommend the insertion of a small tube, or grommet, through the tympanic membrane to relieve the pressure produced by the build-up, although the value of grommets has been questioned and they are less popular today than they were in the past (Thompson, 2000). The grommet is removed once the infection has been cleared using antibiotics, and the middle ear has cleared of pus.

membrane that occludes the aperture to the inner ear. This aperture, called the oval window or fenestra ovalis, provides access to the fluid-filled cochlea in which the receptor cells are found, so vibration is transferred from the ossicles to the cochlear fluid. Pressure waves generated within the fluid are eventually dissipated into the middle ear via another membrane-enclosed aperture called the

round window or fenestra rotunda. The inner ear contains a number of structures: the cochlea involved in hearing, and the components of the vestibular apparatus involved in balance.

The cochlea is shaped like a snail's shell. The coils increase the surface area of the receptor membrane within them. Figure 7.13(b) shows a cross-section through the cochlea. This figure shows how the cochlea is divided into three fluid-filled compartments called the scala media, scala vestibuli and scala tympani. The fluid inside the scala media is referred to as endolymph ('endo-' =inner); it bathes the receptors and associated structures (see below). The fluid in the scala vestibuli and scala tympani is referred to as perilymph ('peri-' = surrounding). The names of the fluids help to reinforce how the cochlea operates. Basically, sound waves are transmitted from the oval window into the endolymph of the scala media, where they stimulate the receptor cells. The pressure then has to be dissipated, which is achieved by the passage of the pressure waves into the perilymph of the scala vestibuli, and then into the other chamber, the scala tympani, via a small hole at the tip of the cochlea. The pressure waves are then transmitted from this compartment into the middle ear via the round window.

The receptors in the scala media must be stimulated by the pressure waves as they pass through the endolymph. Figure 7.13(c) shows a cross-section through the compartment. The structure shown is clearly very complex, but it can generally be described as one in which the receptor cells 'sit' on a membrane, called the basilar membrane, with their hair-like cilia projecting into a gel-like matrix,

Clinically, an initial hearing test involves assessment of the intensity 'threshold' of sounds across a range of frequencies. An audiogram can then be produced that, when compared with norms, indicates any loss of hearing at given wavelengths (Figure 7.14). Tones generated via headphones are conducted to the inner ear by the usual route, but tones can also be conducted via bones of the skull. Conduction of sound through bone (by applying the tone to the mastoid process behind the ear) bypasses the middle ear, and any hearing defect can then be narrowed down to an inner- or middle-ear deficit. Hearing difficulties may also arise, of course, through errors in the interpretation by the brain of signals arriving from the ear.

Disruption of the conduction pathway of the middle ear is called conduction deafness. Inner-ear problems include the effects of excessive endolymph pressing down on the basilar membrane. Recent developments in microtechnology have seen the testing of cochlear implants, electrodes connected to a transducer behind the ear that stimulate the cochlear nerve directly. Impairment of cochlear nerve function causes nerve deafness. Nerve deafness frequently disturbs the vestibular apparatus of the inner ear, producing further symptoms of vertigo and nausea. Collectively, this is called labyrinthine disease. More commonly, this results

from infection of the inner ear, trauma, local arteriosclerosis, allergy or ageing.

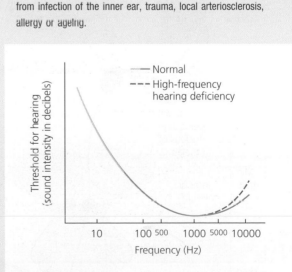

Figure 7.14 Audiogram to detect the range of frequencies that may be heard, and the sensitivity of hearing.
Q. Where do you think the range of frequencies for the human voice might lie on this graph?

the tectorial membrane. Vibrations in the endolymph cause the basilar membrane to be deflected and a wave of oscillations to pass along it. The hair projections of the receptor cells are distorted; it is this that results in the generation of action potentials in the sensory nerve endings.

The conduction of sound waves through water is highly efficient. Low-frequency sounds travel easier than high-frequency ones. Evidence suggests that low-frequency components of sounds produce greatest oscillation of the basilar membrane towards the apex of the cochlea, whilst high-frequency sounds stimulate the earlier sections. This is illustrated in Figure 7.13(d). In this way, the basilar membrane provides the first stage in enabling the ear to differentiate sound frequencies. The amplitude of vibration of the membrane seems to provide information about the intensity of the sound waves. Thus, as with vision, some processing of the stimulus is provided by the sensory organ itself. The full process is extremely complex, however, and is beyond the bounds of this book.

The sensitivity of the cochlea depends upon the frequency of the sound waves. Although the ear can detect frequencies between 20 and 20 000 Hz, it is most sensitive to the range of frequencies associated with human speech (1000–4000 Hz).

Interpretation of auditory signals

Sensory nerve fibres from the receptors in the cochlea pass via the cochlear fibre bundles of the vestibulocochlear nerve (cranial nerve VIII; sometimes called the auditory or acoustic nerve; see Figure 8.5) to the cochlear nuclei of the brainstem (Figure 7.15). Here, they synapse with other nerve fibres, which subsequently synapse with other neurons within various nuclei of the brainstem, including the inferior colliculi, before passing to a part of the thalamus

BOX 7.16 TINNITUS

Tinnitus is a persistent ringing sound in the ears. It is a symptom, rather than an actual condition. It seems to be present when the production of excessive endolymph depresses the basilar membrane. Ménière's syndrome and inner ear infection both promote tinnitus, but it is observed in a number of other disorders, and it is often poorly understood. Treatment depends upon cause (Kaltenbach, 2000), but may include destruction of tissue using ultrasound, a reduction in endolymph secretion through the use of diuretics, local vasodilatation using an elevated blood CO_2 content, or, in extreme cases, surgical intervention.

Figure 7.15 Sensory pathway from the cochlea to the relevant part of the sensory cortex (auditory cortex).

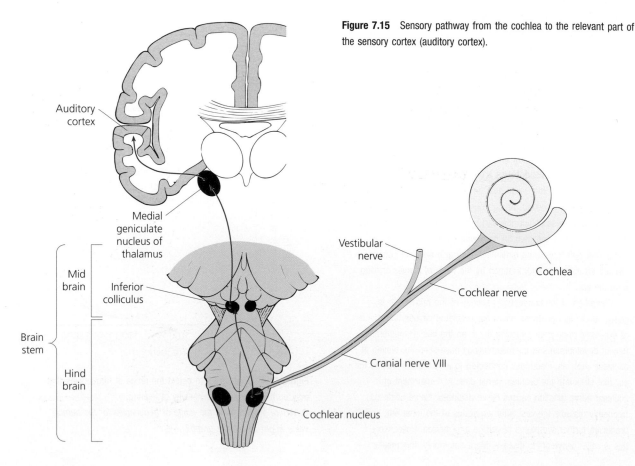

called the medial geniculate body (see Chapter 8 to clarify these terms). Neurons then carry the signal to the auditory area of the cortex of the temporal lobes of the cerebrum. Sensory nerve fibres from each ear interact within the brain, and each temporal lobe actually receives input from both ears, so damage to one temporal lobe normally has minimal effects on hearing. A further pathway within the brainstem also carries information to the reticular formation, a structure that has various functions, including involvement in the sleep/wake cycle. Thus, sound is an effective waking stimulus, even from deep sleep.

Taste and smell

Overview

Taste and smell receptors are highly specialized chemoreceptors. As with other chemical senses, they are stimulated when molecules interact with other molecules on the surface of the receptor cells. Unlike other chemoreceptors, however, these receptors respond to an enormous range of molecules. Before detection, the molecules must first be dissolved in water, which is provided by saliva and nasal secretions. The two senses are not mutually exclusive, and stimulation of the olfactory receptors of the nose is an important aspect of taste, even though taste is looked upon as being a feature of the oral cavity.

Exercise

Put on a blindfold and place a nose-clip over your nostrils. Ask a friend to place a piece of apple or onion in your mouth without telling you what it actually is. Can you tell what the piece is, and the difference between the two? Repeat the test, but this time ask your friend to inform you whether you are eating apple or onion. Now can you tell the difference between them? Explain your findings.

Sensory anatomy of the tongue, and physiology of taste

Taste (gustation) is sensed by receptors present in 'buds' on the surface of the tongue, epiglottis, pharynx and palate. Each bud consists of four types of cell, some of which are chemoreceptors, others being responsible for nutritive support (Figure 7.16(a)). There are some 10 000 taste buds on the tongue alone, clustered together in papillae. Each papilla may contain up to five taste buds called

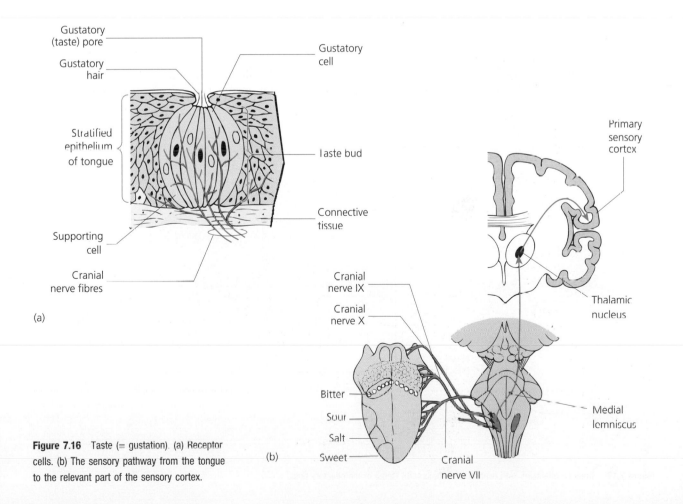

Figure 7.16 Taste (= gustation). (a) Receptor cells. (b) The sensory pathway from the tongue to the relevant part of the sensory cortex.

fungiform papillae (so-called because of their shape), or up to 100 buds called vallate papillae. Smaller filiform papillae are also present, but these contain few if any taste buds.

Four basic tastes have been identified: sweet, sour, bitter and salt. The taste buds responsible for these modalities are arranged in particular areas of the tongue (Figure 7.16(b)), but all four are 'tasted' to various degrees by the receptors of the palate, epiglottis and pharynx. Tastes such as 'sweet' are obviously desirable, as they imply a rich calorific value of the food present in the mouth. Bitter tastes may be offensive, and if extreme the food may be rejected as potentially toxic. Salt and acidic foods may or may not be considered desirable. For example, salt depletion of the body fluids stimulates a 'salt', appetite and salty foods may then be chosen in preference to others.

The four kinds of taste buds do not appear to differ in terms of their cell structures. The ways in which the molecules generate action potentials in associated sensory nerve cells is still debatable. Different cell membrane or metabolic pathways are presumably involved, which may explain why substances such as the dipeptide lysyltaurine tastes salty yet clearly does not contain sodium chloride, and why lead salts taste sweet yet do not contain sugars. Further phenomena that illustrate the complexity of taste are that a protein modifier called miraculin will make acidic substances taste sweet, and that genetic variation means that only a proportion of people can taste the substance phenylthiocarbamide (PTC).

Interpretation of taste

Activity from the anterior two-thirds of the tongue passes via the facial nerve (cranial nerve VII) to the brainstem (Figure 7.16(b)). The glossopharyngeal nerve (cranial nerve IX) conveys activity from the posterior third. Fibres from the pharynx, epiglottis and palate pass to the brainstem via the vagus nerve (cranial nerve X; see Figure 8.5). Within the brainstem, all inputs pass to a collection of nerve cells within the medulla oblongata (the nucleus of the tractus solitarius) from which fibres pass to specific areas of the thalamus. They then synapse with other neurons that pass to the cortex of the parietal lobe.

Sensory anatomy and physiology of smell

The sense of smell (olfaction) depends upon receptors in the mucous membrane of the nasal epithelium, a 5-cm^2 area in the roof of the nasal cavity. The presence of two nostrils helps in the determination of the direction from which a smell originates, because they introduce a slight delay in the stimulation of one part of the olfactory epithelium relative to the other. There are some 10–20 million receptor cells, which are modified nerve cells, in the nose (with other supportive or secretory cells). The nerve endings are expanded into olfactory rods, from which cilia project into the bathing fluid layer and molecules dissolved within the mucus interact with surface molecules in the cilia membrane (Figure 7.17). Proteins present within the fluid are thought to facilitate the presentation of odour molecules to the receptors.

Odour-producing molecules are generally small, but odour depends more on molecular configuration than size. The olfactory cells are particularly sensitive at detecting characteristic odours, and humans can distinguish up to 4000 different odours. However, the detection of intensity of particular odours is not so well developed. How such a

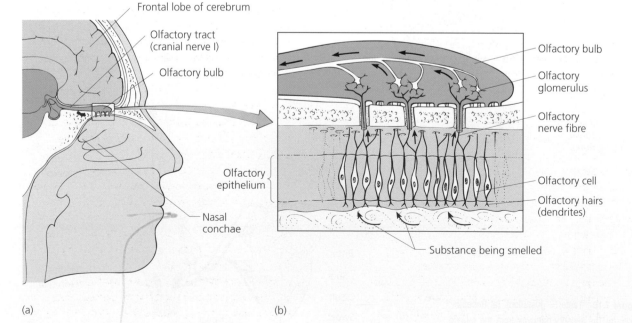

(a)   (b)

Figure 7.17 Smell (= olfaction). (a) Location of receptors. (b) Detail of the olfactory bulb.

diverse range of odours can be detected is unknown, but it is unlikely to depend simply upon a similar range of complementary receptor molecules (i.e. by a 'lock and key' process). For example, the chemicals camphor and hexachlorethane smell identical, but they are very different molecules with different chemical properties.

Attempts to classify smell modalities have suggested that odours can be separated into seven types: putrid, musky, floral, pungent, peppermint, ethereal and camphoraceous. A combination of these is suggested to produce the range of odour perceptions of which we are capable. The diversity of odours goes beyond the limits of these modalities, however, and to call these 'primary' odours would be misleading. Pain fibres also originate in the olfactory epithelium, and are stimulated by irritative characteristics of odours, e.g. peppermint and chlorine. Sneezing and tear secretion are induced reflexly after stimulation of these fibres; these are clearly defensive mechanisms against a perceived noxious vapour.

Adaptation to a stimulus is also noticeable with smell, and may apply to a single odour within a collection of odours, the 'thresholds' for other odours being unchanged. Adaptation allows us to remain within a particular environment without constantly perceiving a particular dominant odour, unless it is noxious. The mechanism is unknown, but it probably involves modulation of receptor function and central processing.

Interpretation of olfactory signals

Sensory fibres from olfactory receptors terminate in the olfactory bulb, a distended terminal of the olfactory nerve (cranial nerve I; see Figure 8.5), where they synapse with other neurons in the olfactory glomeruli (Figure 7.17). These form synapses with other neurons within the vicinity, before neural activity passes via the olfactory nerve to various structures within the limbic system (see Chapter 8), including an area of the cerebral cortex. Smell appears to be unique amongst the senses, in that sensory neural activity does not relay via the thalamus in the brain.

Initial processing of the activity probably occurs in the olfactory glomeruli, but final processing occurs in the primary olfactory cortex located in the temporal lobe of the cerebrum. Pathways linking the limbic system with the hypothalamus provide the input to hypothalamic 'drive' centres associated with odours, e.g. autonomic arousal and sexual arousal.

Summary

1   The homeostatic control of physiological systems and cellular function is dependent upon the facility to 'sense' changes in all aspects of the internal environment, and also of many elements of the external environment.

2   Senses depend upon receptor cells that have specializations, usually of the cell membrane, that enable them to respond to specific parameters. Some senses are polymodal in that they can detect more than one quality of a stimulus. These are the special senses of vision, hearing, taste, smell (and pain).

3   Receptors are transducers, i.e. they can take a particular stimulus (light, sound, etc.) and convert it into electrochemical nerve impulses.

4   The generation of nerve impulses increases with intensity of stimulation, but a threshold must be exceeded before a nerve impulse is transmitted from the receptor.

5   Information from peripheral senses passes to the brain via tracts within the spinal cord. Numerous relays may be involved, but almost all pass through the thalamus of the brain on the way to the sensory areas of the cerebral cortex.

6   The eye is a sense organ that causes light rays to be focused onto receptors of the retina. Biochemical features of the receptors allow us to perceive light of different wavelengths (colour) as well as intensity.

7   Information from the retinal receptors passes via the thalamus to various components of the brain, particularly the visual cortex of the occipital cerebral lobe. Processing produces vision, and is also important in controlling eye movement.

8   The ear consists of external, middle and inner structures, the latter including organs of hearing and of balance. Transmission of sound to the fluid-filled inner ear occurs via small ossicles within the air-filled middle ear.

9   Pressure waves induced in the cochlea of the inner ear are converted into electrochemical signals that provide both intensity and frequency information. Electrochemical activity passes to various parts of the brain, but especially to the auditory cortex of the temporal lobes.

10 Taste and smell result from stimulation of chemoreceptors of the tongue and nasal cavities. Although involving an interaction between receptor molecules present on the receptor cell membranes and food or odour molecules, the process is more complex than a simple 'lock-and-key' mechanism. The actual mechanism is not understood, but it enables us to detect a wide variety of different molecules.

11 Information from the nose and tongue passes to various structures within the brain. Apart from the cerebral cortex, other important olfactory processing areas include structures of the limbic system.

Review questions

The eyes

1 The eyes contain sensory receptors called photoreceptors. What kind of stimulus will activate photoreceptors?

2 Where are the receptors located?

3 There are two types of photoreceptors: rods and cones. Which type respond to bright light and colour? What happens in colour blindness?

4 What prevents the eyeball from collapsing?

5 All cells require a supply of oxygen and nutrients. How do the lens and cornea (both transparent structures) obtain their supplies?

6 Retinopathy is a common complication of diabetes. Why does this occur?

7 Light from close objects enters the eye at a more acute angle than light from distant objects. How does the eye manage to cope with this and make sense of the information it receives?

8 How does the eye cope with differing intensities of light?

9 What is the difference between refraction and reflection?

10 What and where is the fovea?

The ears

11 The ear is an important structure not only as the organ of hearing but also for maintaining balance. Hearing problems can occur at any age, in any patient group. The ear is divided into different regions: inner, middle and outer. Match the following structures to the appropriate region: external auditory meatus, auditory tube, semi-circular canals, ossicles, oval window, cochlea, perilymph and tympanic membrane.

12 Describe how sound vibrations are converted into impulses that can be conveyed to the brain. Which nerve carries this information?

13 Explain the role of the external ear in 'collecting' sound. Why do people with hearing difficulties cup their hand around their ear in order to hear better?

14 How do the vibrations of the ear drum (tympanum) created by sound waves reach the inner ear? Name the structures that are involved in this process. Why does glue ear cause hearing loss?

15 What is the function of the auditory tube? (Think about your ears popping when you fly or travel through tunnels at high speed.). Why do throat infections often end up in the ears?

16 The inner ear converts vibrations into nerve impulses. How is this achieved?

17 How do we (i) locate the source of sound; (ii) identify its pitch; (iii) distinguish between loud and quiet sounds?

18 Draw a labelled diagram of the semi-circular canals. Explain how these help us to maintain balance even with our eyes closed.

19 What do decibels (dB) measure? What dB rating is considered to be hazardous to hearing? When may this occur?

20 What are the major health problems of the ear? Suggest the nurse's role in their prevention/management. Identify the patient group most likely to be affected.

REFERENCES

Berry, P. (2000) Otitis media in children: diagnosis, treatment and prevention. *Postgraduate Medicine* **107**(3): 239–41.

Fischel, J.D. and Lipton, J.R. (1996) Cataract surgery and recent advances: a review. *Nursing Standard* **10**(41): 39–43.

Kaltenbach, J.A. (2000) Neurophysiologic mechanisms of tinnitus. *Journal of the American Academy of Audiology* **11**(3): 125–37.

Linebarger, E.J., Hardten, D.R., Shah, G.K. and Lindstrom, R.L. (1999) Phacoemulsification and modern cataract surgery. *Survey of Ophthalmology* **44**(2): 123–47.

Mead, M. (2000) Procedures for Practice Nurses. The illness conjunctivitis. *Practice Nurse* **19**(5): 215–16.

Oulette, S.M. and Oulette, R.G. (1998) Monitoring for intraoperative awareness: what's new? *Current Reviews for Perianaesthesia Nurses* **20**(10): 107–13.

Price, D. and Burns, B. (1999) Brain injuries. *Emergency Medical Services* **28**(6): 65–70.

Thompson, J. (2000) Clinical update. Otitis media with effusion. *Community Practitioner* **73**(8): 728–9.

Chapter 8

The nervous system

INTRODUCTION

Chapter 1 emphasized how the processes that promote physiological homeostasis involve recognition that a parameter has changed, and an initiation of an appropriate corrective response. Chapter 7 noted that the change is detected by specialized receptor cells that are often either modified nerve cells or cells associated with nerve cells. Co-ordination of the homeostatic response to such change is often mediated by further nerve cells, by promoting a change in the functioning of the particular target cells and tissues. Nerves provide an anatomical link with the tissues, which means that the neural network throughout the body is extensive and complex. Of even more complex anatomy are the brain and spinal cord, as these must interpret sensory data and produce an appropriate neural output to tissues. The different elements that constitute the anatomy of the nervous system, and their physiology, are described in this chapter.

This is a difficult topic and readers should read the following overview section carefully before tackling the later sections, since this highlights some general features of the nervous system.

OVERVIEW

Nerves and nerve cells

What is a nerve?

It is important to make a distinction between nerves and nerve cells. Nerves form an extensive network of conducting pathways, which spread throughout the body and provide a means of rapid communication between parts of the body. A cross-section through a nerve shows that it consists of a tough protective covering of connective tissue, called the epineurium ('epi-' = upon, '-neurium' = neural matter) in the form of a tube, and numerous bundles of sectioned nerve cells within the tube (Figure 8.1). The bundles of nerve cells are separated from others by more connective tissue, called the perineurium ('peri-' = surround), and by blood vessels. The latter send out fine capillary branches that enter the bundles to supply the nerve cells with nutrients. Each nerve cell is surrounded by a further, delicate, connective tissue layer, called the endoneurium.

Nerves, then, are conduits for collections of nerve cells, or more precisely the long processes of these nerve cells

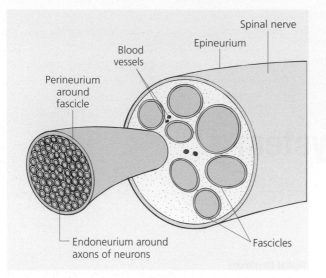

Figure 8.1 Section through a peripheral nerve.

Q. The epineurium, perineurium and endoneurium are examples of connective tissue. What are the characteristics of this kind of tissue?

BOX 8.1 LOSS OF NERVE SUPPLY TO A TISSUE

A single nerve may contain thousands of nerve fibres (cells) that connect more than one tissue with the brain/spinal cord. For example, the femoral nerve (found in the thigh; the name relates to the thighbone, called the femur) contains nerve cells that connect with the muscles of the leg, the bone and joints of the limb, and the blood vessels and skin of the limb. Nerve trauma, therefore, will influence all of the tissues innervated by that nerve.

Regeneration of nerve connections is possible after trauma but success depends upon two factors:

- Are severed ends of nerve cells able to remake contact? The partial restoration of senses observed in the skin of reconnected hands or feet suggest that this can occur.
- Can surviving nerve fibres (assuming that the nerve trauma has left some of the nerve intact) branch to connect with cells that have lost their nerve connections? There is evidence that this may occur, with nerve cells sending out connections to cells, e.g. muscle cells, in the vicinity.

Reforming connections probably involves the secretion locally of chemical nerve growth factors, in conjunction with chemical attractants. Some of these chemicals have been identified, and may also be involved in the outgrowth of nerves toward their target tissues in the embryo/fetus. These substances have potentially important clinical applications, e.g. in stimulating the regeneration of spinal cord after spinal trauma.

---

referred to as nerve fibres, bundled together rather like wires in an electrical cable. Some of these fibres pass along the nerve from the brain/spinal cord to the tissues, and some pass from tissues to the brain/spinal cord. The diameter of the nerve is determined by how many nerve fibres are present within it, thus it changes along its length as nerve fibres enter or exit it as it passes through tissues. This usually means that a nerve is thickest close to its connection with the brain or spinal cord.

Nerve nomenclature

Nerves are frequently named according to from whence they originated or to which tissue they supply. For example, the pelvic nerves contain nerve cells that pass to/from the pelvic region, while the optic nerve originates in the eye. Unfortunately, the nomenclature is not always so obvious. The names of many nerves derive from Latin or Greek, and may refer to features other than sources or targets. For example, the name of the vagus nerve comes from the Latin for 'wandering', and refers to the extent to which this nerve extends throughout the thorax and abdomen of the body. Branches from the vagus innervate a variety of organs, so naming the nerve according to source or target is not feasible.

Nerve nomenclature is therefore complex. Specific nerves are mentioned elsewhere in this book where relevant, but will only be named in this chapter if appropriate to the discussion or as examples.

Structure of nerve cells

Nerve cells are commonly referred to as neurons. Conduction across the distances between tissues and the brain/spinal cord is facilitated by the neurons being long, up to 1.5 m or more. It is the elongated sections of a neuron that comprise the nerve fibre and may be observed if a nerve is sectioned. In contrast, the processing of information within the brain or spinal cord usually involves neurons that are short and that interact with many neighbouring nerve cells. All neurons contain cell organelles, such as a nucleus and mitochondria, but these are largely localized to a distended portion called the cell body.

Efferent neurons

Those nerve cells that extend from the brain or spinal cord and pass to tissues elsewhere in the body are collectively said to be efferent ('eff-' = away from) neurons. These neurons will ultimately change tissue functions and so are also referred to as motor neurons. The cell body of such cells is located at one end of the neuron, either within the spinal cord itself or within intermediate neural structures called ganglia (singular = ganglion) that may be some distance from the spinal cord (but will themselves connect with the cord). The elongated section of the nerve cell that makes up the nerve fibre of an efferent neuron is the axon (Figure 8.2).

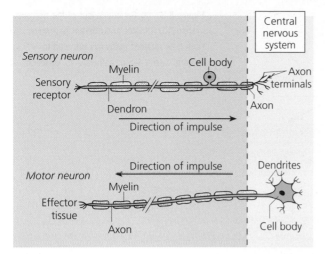

Figure 8.2 Sensory and motor neurons within the nervous system. Note that a single peripheral nerve contains both sensory (afferent) and motor (efferent) neurons, i.e. they are mixed nerves.

The cell bodies of efferent neurons have extremely fine branching processes called dendrites ('dendron' = Greek for 'tree'). These are important because it is via these processes that the nerve cell is able to receive electrical inputs from other nerve cells in the vicinity. The end of the axon within the target tissue will also normally terminate in fine branching processes. These are referred to simply as axon terminals; they conduct impulses from the axon towards cells within the vicinity.

Afferent neurons
Those nerve cells that carry impulses from sensory receptors within the tissues to the brain/spinal cord are collectively called afferent ('aff-' = towards) neurons. Afferent neurons are also called sensory neurons, because the information they convey usually originates at sensory receptors. In these neurons, the cell body is found as an offshoot from the fibre. For most of these cells, this is usually close to where they enter the spinal cord (Figure 8.2), and the large number of cell bodies present produces a distension of the nerve at this point. This is called a spinal ganglion, or dorsal root ganglion (so called because these afferent cells enter the posterior or dorsal aspect of the spinal cord).

The elongated fibre of the cell that extends from the sensory receptor to the cell body is called the dendron, and that from the cell body to the spinal cord the axon. Thus, the dendron conducts nerve impulses towards the cell body, and the axon conducts impulses away. In efferent cells described above, the cell body is situated at one end of the cell, so there is no dendron, only an axon. However, efferent cells do have dendrites, i.e. small branching features that conduct impulses towards the cell body.

The axon terminals of a sensory nerve cell form junctions with dendrites of other neurons within the spinal cord.

Myelin and Schwann cells
To increase the rate of conduction of electrical impulses by nerve cells, their dendrons and axons are frequently (but not always) covered with an insulating fatty material called myelin (Figure 8.2). Myelin is secreted by non-neural cells called Schwann cells that are associated closely with the neurons and that lay down the myelin in concentric layers around the nerve fibre. Nerve conduction is considered later, but it is important to note here that myelin never forms a complete sheath along a nerve cell. Gaps called nodes of Ranvier are essential because myelin is not a complete insulator and electrical current must be regenerated from time to time, which requires access to tissue fluid by the cell membrane.

The synapse
Actual physical contact between cells is not usually present, although the gap is generally only about 20 nm (i.e. 20 millionths of a millimetre) wide. The whole structure at the end of the dendrite or axon terminal, including the gap, is called a synapse; this plays a central role in determining whether nerve impulses are transmitted from one neuron to the next. The process is mediated by a chemical released from the terminals called a neurotransmitter. Synaptic function, with examples of how it can influence nerve transmission, is described later.

Organization of the nervous system

The discussion so far has highlighted that some nerve cells pass to and from tissues of the body, and the brain/spinal cord, and that neural processing takes place in the latter. Accordingly, the nervous system can be divided into two broad anatomical components: the *peripheral nervous system* (PNS), which conducts impulses to and from tissues, and the *central nervous system* (CNS), in which processing of information occurs (Figure 8.3).

Organization of the peripheral nervous system

The organization of peripheral nerves can be subdivided according to the functional aspects and the tissues served (Figure 8.3): *autonomic nerves* mediate those changes in tissue functions that are generally involuntary, and co-ordinate the functions of most organs in the body; *somatic nerves* promote the contraction of voluntary muscles, and in particular mediate the control of posture and movement.

The roles of the autonomic and somatic branches sometimes overlap in the control of the body. For example, breathing involves contraction of the diaphragm and intercostal muscles, which is mediated by somatic nerves, but autonomic nerves influence airway resistance. Similarly, the contraction or relaxation of the urinary bladder is an

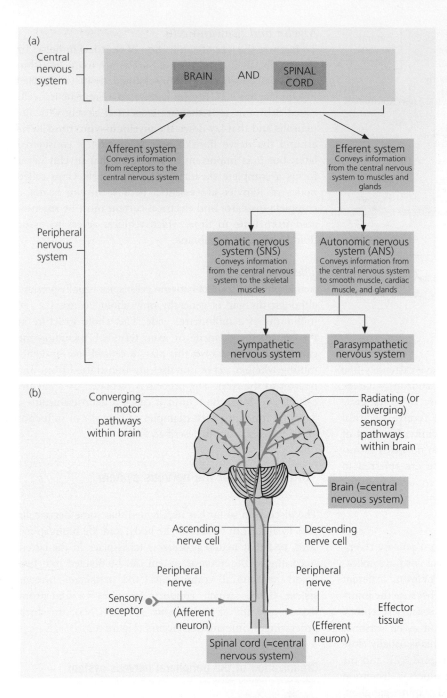

autonomic function, but normal bladder emptying also requires voluntary relaxation of the external sphincter muscles of the pelvic floor.

In certain cases, autonomic function may even be voluntarily overridden. For example, the ability to empty an unfilled urinary bladder voluntarily is achieved by exercising voluntary control of the autonomic nerves involved. Similarly, stress relaxation techniques also demonstrate limited conscious control of the resting heart rate, which is a parameter under the involuntary control of the autonomic nervous system.

The role of autonomic nerves in controlling organ functioning, and hence homeostasis, is considered in more detail later. The role of somatic nerves in mediating muscle

contraction is considered in Chapter 17 in relation to the skeletomuscular system and posture maintenance.

Exercise

Record your own pulse whilst consciously trying to relax yourself. Can you notice a slowing of the pulse? You may need to keep practising.

If you have been following the text, you should now be appreciating just how confusing the terminology related to the nervous system can be! It might be worth reviewing this by considering the following summary:

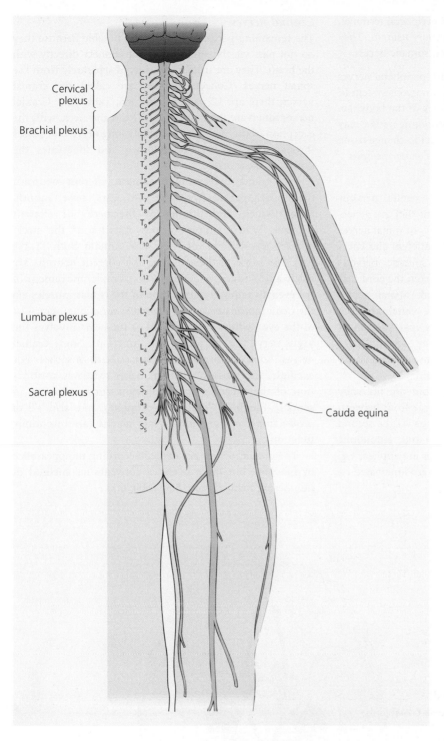

Figure 8.4 General organization of spinal nerves and the somatic nervous system (plexus = aggregation of nerves or neurons). C, cervical; T, thoracic; L, lumbar; S, sacral. Numbers refer to vertebrae within the respective parts of the vertebral column.
Q. How many thoracic spinal nerves are there?
Q. What is the 'cauda equina'?

Labels on figure:
Cervical plexus
Brachial plexus
Lumbar plexus
Sacral plexus
Cauda equina

C₁ C₂ C₃ C₄ C₅ C₆ C₇ C₈ T₁ T₂ T₃ T₄ T₅ T₆ T₇ T₈ T₉ T₁₀ T₁₁ T₁₂ L₁ L₂ L₃ L₄ L₅ S₁ S₂ S₃ S₄ S₅

- The *central nervous system* is comprised of the brain and spinal cord, which co-ordinate sensory information transmitted from the tissues of the body and promote an appropriate nerve activity to the tissues.

- The *peripheral nervous system* is a collective term for the system of nerves, and associated structures called ganglia, that transmit impulses either to the central nervous system, or from it to the tissues.

- The *somatic nerves*, which are a branch of the peripheral nervous system, are those nerves that convey impulses to and from skeletal muscle.

- The *autonomic nerves*, which are a branch of the peripheral nervous system, are those nerves that convey impulses to and from the organs of the body.

- *Afferent neurons* are nerve cells within peripheral nerves that convey impulses to the central nervous system. These will normally have receptors at their peripheral terminal, and so may also be referred to as *sensory neurons*. They may be found in both autonomic and somatic nerves.

● *Efferent neurons* are nerve cells within peripheral nerves that convey impulses from the central nervous system to tissues (skeletal muscle or other tissues of the body, i.e. distinction between somatic and autonomic nerves may not be made). Because these neurons act to change tissue functions, they are often referred to as *motor neurons*.

Spinal nerves

Most peripheral nerves enter or exit the central nervous system via the spinal cord, at which point they are generally called spinal nerves. There are 31 pairs of spinal nerves (Figure 8.4). Each spinal nerve contains afferent and efferent neurons of the autonomic and somatic nervous systems, and it is only at some distance from the cord that the two branches can be distinguished. Spinal nerves enter/exit the spinal cord between the vertebrae, at a distance from the brain. Clearly the spinal cord must contain neural pathways of both the somatic and autonomic systems, which will conduct the neural activity to and from appropriate parts of the brain.

Spinal nerves do not have names, but are normally referred to by the position of the vertebrae from between which they extend, e.g. thoracic 2 emerges via the second thoracic vertebra. Once the somatic and autonomic branches have separated, however, names are applied, e.g. the intercostal muscles of the chest wall are innervated by the intercostal nerves.

Cranial nerves

The remaining peripheral nerves are notable because they do not pass via the spinal cord but connect directly with the brain. They are usually considered separately from the spinal nerves. Collectively they are called the cranial nerves; there are 12 pairs (Figure 8.5; Table 8.1). Cranial nerves innervate the tissues of the head and neck, with the exception of the vagus, an extremely long nerve that passes through the thorax and abdomen and innervates the organs of these areas.

The cranial nerves may contain afferent neurons, mainly originating from the eyes, ears, nose, mouth, facial tissues, and arteries of the neck, or efferent neurons, which supply various muscles of the neck, salivary glands, etc., or they may contain both (Table 8.1). For some of these nerves, the efferent neurons are solely autonomic or somatic. For example, movement of the eyeballs requires stimulation of the ocular muscles via the oculomotor nerve (i.e. a somatic function; 'oculo-' = of the eye), whilst basal control of the heart involves the vagus nerve (i.e. an autonomic function). Some cranial nerves, however, contain neurons of both branches. For example, the glossopharyngeal nerve mediates contraction of the muscles of the pharynx for swallowing (a somatic function; 'glossus' = tongue) and also saliva production from certain salivary glands (an autonomic function).

The cranial nerves are named according to appearance or function, but there is also a conventional method of numbering them (Figure 8.5; Table 8.1).

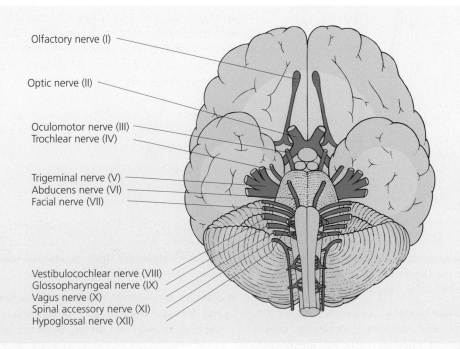

Olfactory nerve (I)
Optic nerve (II)
Oculomotor nerve (III)
Trochlear nerve (IV)
Trigeminal nerve (V)
Abducens nerve (VI)
Facial nerve (VII)
Vestibulocochlear nerve (VIII)
Glossopharyngeal nerve (IX)
Vagus nerve (X)
Spinal accessory nerve (XI)
Hypoglossal nerve (XII)

Figure 8.5 The cranial nerves and their origins in the brain.
Q. How many cranial nerves are there?

Table 8.1 Functions of the cranial nerves

Cranial nerve	Homeostatic function	Tissues innervated
Olfactory (I)	Sensory	From olfactory epithelium of the nose
Optic (II)	Sensory	From retinal cells of the eye
Oculomotor (III)	Motor	To the rectus muscles (inferior, superior, medial) and inferior oblique muscles that move the eyes
		To the upper lip area
Trochlear (IV)	Motor	To the superior oblique muscle of the eye
Trigeminal (V)	Ophthalmic sensory	From areas around the orbits of the eyes, nasal cavity, forehead, upper eyelids, and eyebrows
Maxillary	Sensory	From the lower eyelids, upper lip, upper gums and teeth, mucous lining of the palate, and the skin of the face
Mandibular	Mixed	Sensory from the skin of the jaw, lower gums and teeth, and lower lip
		Motor to the muscles of mastication, and the floor of the mouth
Abducens (VI)	Motor	To the rectus muscles (lateral) that move the eyes
Facial (VII)	Mixed	Sensory from taste receptors (anterior two-thirds of tongue)
		Motor to muscles of facial expression; includes visceral efferents (autonomic nervous system) to the submandibular and sublingual salivary glands, and tear glands
Vestibulocochlear (VIII)		
Vestibular	Sensory	From the vestibular apparatus (balance organs) of the inner ear
Cochlear	Sensory	From hearing receptors of the cochlea of the inner ear
Glossopharyngeal (IX)	Mixed	Sensory from the pharynx, tonsils, and posterior third of tongue; includes visceral afferents (autonomic nervous system) from carotid arteries and aortic arch
		Motor to pharynx (i.e. swallowing movements), and visceral efferents (autonomic nervous system) to parotid salivary glands
Vagus (X)	Mixed	Sensory from the pharynx, larynx and oesophagus, and visceral afferents (autonomic nervous system) from the thorax and abdomen
		Motor to the larynx, pharynx and soft palate (swallowing movements), and visceral efferents (autonomic nervous system) to viscera of the thorax and abdomen
Accessory (XI)		
Cranial	Motor	To the pharynx, larynx and soft palate (swallowing movements)
Spinal	Motor	To the sternocleidomastoid and trapezius muscles of the neck
Hypoglossal (XII)	Motor	To the musculature of the tongue

Q. Which nerves are involved in swallowing movements?

Organization of the central nervous system

The general anatomy of neurons of the brain and spinal cord is similar to that of peripheral neurons in that they consist of a cell body with fibre-like structures (dendrons and axons), and branching terminals (dendrites and axon terminals). Likewise, synapses permit interactions to occur between cells. Estimates of the number of cells that each brain cell interacts with suggest that a single neuron may be associated directly with tens of thousands of other brain cells. The brain contains some 100 000 million (i.e. 100 billion) neurons, and the potential 'circuitry' is therefore unimaginably extensive.

The central nervous system also contains non-neural cells called neuroglial cells. Estimates suggest that neuroglial cells outnumber neurons by as many as 10 to 1, so they comprise much of the brain mass. Neuroglial cells can be subdivided according to their position and function, as outlined in Table 8.2. Schwann cells, which we mentioned earlier, are a type of neuroglial cell.

Neural organization of the spinal cord
In general, the neurons of the cord may be considered under three categories:

- neurons whose fibres pass up the cord to the brain, and so form afferent, or ascending, pathways;

BOX 8.2 THE BRAIN AS A 'STABLE' TISSUE

We are probably born with all of the central nervous system neurons that we will have in life. Brain growth and development during childhood therefore involves neuronal growth, the forming of connections, or synapses, between neurons with appropriate others, and the growth of neuroglial tissue (i.e. non-neural support cells).

The complexity of neural connections within the brain means that cell division would make it unlikely that the brain circuitry

could be maintained. It appears that neurons remain with us for the duration of our lives. Some may die, although current thinking is that ageing does not have a pronounced effect on neuronal numbers but can have a profound effect on the maintenance of synapses. The lack of cell division activity means that this stable tissue does not readily form tumours. Most brain tumours arise from the more reproductively active glial cells, hence the term 'glioma' used for this kind of tumour.

Table 8.2 Neuroglial cells

Type of cells	Description	Homeostatic function
Central nervous system Astrocytes ('astro-' = star, '-cyte' = cell)	Star-shaped cells with numerous processes Protoplasmic astrocytes found in grey matter of the CNS; fibrous astrocytes found in white matter	Twine around nerve cells to form supporting network in brain and spinal cord; attach neurons to their blood vessels
Oligodendrocytes ('oligo-' = few, 'dendro-' = tree)	Resemble astrocytes in some ways, but processes are fewer and shorter	Give support by forming semi-rigid connective tissue rows between neurons in brain and spinal cord Produce myelin sheath around neurons of the CNS
Microglia ('micro-' = small, '-glia' = glue)	Small cells with few processes derived from monocytes Normally stationary, but may migrate to site of injury Also called brain macrophages	Engulf and destroy microbes and cellular debris
Ependyma (= upper garment)	Epithelial cells arranged in a single layer Range in shape from squamous to columnar Many are ciliated	Form a continuous epithelial lining for the ventricles of the brain (spaces that form and circulate cerebrospinal fluid) and the central canal of the spinal cord
Peripheral nervous system Neurolemmocytes (Schwann cells)	Flattened cells located along the nerve fibres Cells encircle the axon many times to form a series of concentric rings Inner layers contain myelin	Produce insulating sheath of myelin around nerve fibres, to enhance conduction velocity of impulses along the axon

Q. Which type of neuroglial cell produces myelin for peripheral nerve cells, and which type produces myelin for nerve cells within the central nervous system?

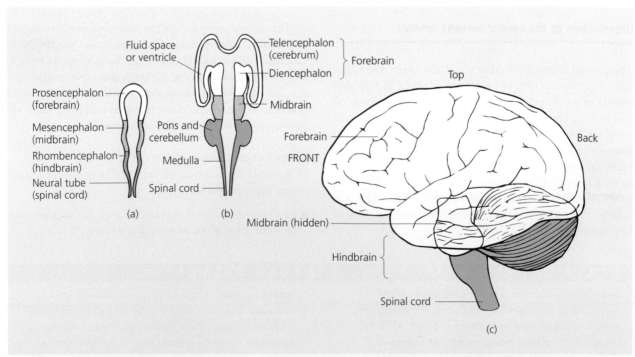

Figure 8.6 Outline of brain development. (a) Commencement of development of the head end of the neural tube in the embryo. (b) Further development of the three main components of the brain structure. The forebrain and the hindbrain in particular have enlarged in relative terms. (c) Side view of the final brain. Note how the orientation of the forebrain has changed relative to the mid- and hindbrain, and that much of these latter are now enclosed by the forebrain. See Box 8.3 for explanation

- neurons whose fibres pass down the cord from the brain, and so form efferent or descending pathways;

- neurons that provide connections between various ascending and descending neurons, called interneurons ('inter-' = between).

The axons of ascending and descending neurons pass along the periphery of the cord. In cross-section, the insulative layer of myelin on many of these neurons makes these areas appear white, hence this area is referred to as the 'white matter' of the spinal cord. The cell bodies of these neurons, however, are found more centrally in the cord, and the absence of myelin around the cell bodies makes this area appear darker (hence 'grey matter'; this is, in fact, an inaccurate term because the tissue appears grey only at post mortem – in life it is pink).

Neural organization of the brain

Superficially, the brain can be observed to consist of a number of structures relating to the forebrain and hindbrain; the midbrain is not visible (see Box 8.3 for an explanation of these terms). Many of the external features of the brain are dominated by the highly convoluted cerebrum of the forebrain (Figure 8.7(a)). The two halves of the cerebrum are referred to as cerebral hemispheres, and their separation is indicated clearly by a deep cleft called the longitudinal fissure. The outer surface of the cerebral hemispheres is referred to as the cerebral cortex ('cortex' = (tree) bark), which is composed of grey matter due to the presence of huge numbers of nerve cell bodies that are not myelinated. The ridges of the convolutions are called gyri (singular = gyrus), while the indentations

between the ridges are called sulci (singular = sulcus). The convolutions increase the surface area of the cerebrum (to about 0.2 m^2 in an adult); this is of note because the cerebral cortex is an important processing area, so the convolutions enable more of this processing tissue to be contained within the skull.

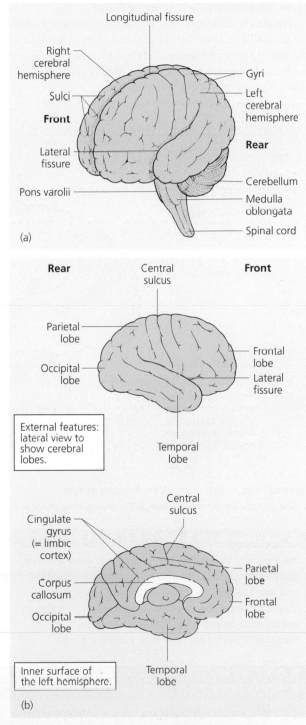

(a)

(b)

Figure 8.7 (a) External features of the brain. (b) The cerebral hemispheres.

Q. What is the corpus callosum?

A striking feature of the external appearance of the cerebrum is the occurrence of lobes, named after the bones of the skull that overlie them. There are four pairs of lobes (Figure 8.7(b)) – frontal, parietal, occipital and temporal – one member of each pair being found on each side of the brain. The frontal lobes are separated from the parietal lobes lying behind by a large involution called the central sulcus, while the temporal lobes are delineated on each side by an indentation called the lateral fissure.

Hindbrain structures that are visible externally include the cerebellum (a two-halved structure lying at the base of the brain; Figures 8.6 and 8.7(a)) and the pons varolii and medulla oblongata (distended areas of the part of the brain that lies at the top of the spinal cord).

Internally, sections through the brain reveal:

- white matter composed of myelinated nerve fibres that connect different parts of the brain;

- clusters of processing neurons (i.e. grey matter) called nuclei within the white matter . Note the distinction between brain nuclei and the nuclei of cells;

- fluid-filled spaces called ventricles (not to be confused with the ventricles of the heart). The fluid is called cerebrospinal fluid (CSF), which circulates around the brain and the spinal cord and helps to maintain a precise cellular environment (Figure 8.8).

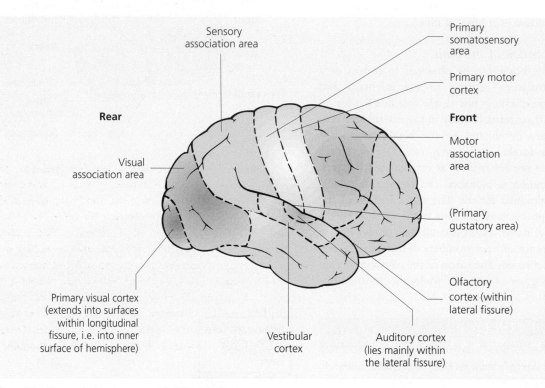

Figure 8.8   The cerebral cortex: general functional anatomy.
Q. How do these functional areas relate to the cerebral lobes shown in Figure 8.7 (a)?

pressure, due to excess cerebrovascular fluid, as in hydrocephalus and meningitis, or presence of a haematoma;

● toxin damage, e.g. the effects of ions of 'heavy metals' on brain development.

Some disorders in which (CNS) neurons degenerate are of unknown aetiology, although autoimmune responses or inherited causes have been implicated, e.g. in motor neuron disease and Alzheimer's disease.

Whereas peripheral damage may induce localized loss of function (see Box 8.1), loss of neurons in the central nervous system can cause disorders that are extensive and devastating. These include cognitive disorders (e.g. cerebral palsy, Alzheimer's disease, Creutzfeldt–Jakob disease), motor disorders (e.g. cerebral palsy, epilepsy, motor neuron disease, Creutzfeldt–Jakob disease), autonomic disorders (e.g. respiratory

dysrhythmias) and endocrine disorders (e.g. pituitary hyposecretion).

Correction may be aimed at removing the underlying cause, such as relieving raised intracranial pressure, or treating an infection. Drug treatments may be used to suppress any inflammation; tumours may be removed surgically, although additional damage may be incurred in the process. Generally, however, the correction of trauma is limited, and care is directed at alleviating symptoms, using therapies that reinforce remnant functions, and providing support.

In certain circumstances, non-progressive brain damage may be improved, but not reversed, by reinforcement of behavioural or social patterns (e.g. conductive therapy in children with cerebral palsy). This probably promotes the development of new neural synapses within the affected areas.

ANATOMY OF THE BRAIN

This section considers in more detail the neural organization of the central nervous system, and identifies some of the roles ascribed to parts of the brain. The major features discussed here are the forebrain, the midbrain, the hindbrain, the meningeal membranes, the fluid ventricles and cerebrospinal fluid, and the vasculature of the brain.

The forebrain

The forebrain consists of the most obvious external feature of the brain – the highly convoluted cerebrum – but also some deeper structures that together comprise the diencephalon (see Box 8.3).

The cerebrum

The cerebrum is divided into two hemispheres that are connected by a large bundle of myelinated axons called the corpus callosum (Figure 8.7(b)). This allows communication between the two hemispheres, and links geographically similar positions of the left and right hemispheres. Each hemisphere consists of outer areas that comprise the cerebral cortex, and deeper structures collectively referred to as cerebral nuclei, which may interact with each other, with the cerebral cortex, or with midbrain and hindbrain structures.

The hemispheres
The hemispheres have various functions, but some generalizations regarding perceptual functioning can be made (see Box 8.6).

The frontal lobes
The frontal lobes of the cortex are involved in the planning, execution and evaluation of actions, and their advanced development in humans (and dolphins and whales) is considered by evolutionary biologists to be an indicator of the acquisition of intelligence. The cortex includes an area called the motor association area (Figure 8.8), in which information concerning planned actions is collated and passed to the primary motor cortex area just forward of the central sulcus. This area determines most of the final efferent output to the muscles, including those of voluntary eye movements and speech (this latter especially involves the frontal lobe of the left hemisphere).

The parietal lobes
The parietal lobes are especially involved in sensory reception and perception. An area just behind the frontal lobe, and directly behind the motor cortex, called the primary somatosensory cortex (Figure 8.8) receives information from the somatosenses, i.e. the 'body' senses of touch, pressure, temperature and pain. Information from this area passes to various parts of the brain, including the sensory association area of the parietal lobes. This is a large area that extends into the occipital and temporal lobes (and so receives input from those lobes also), and is involved in the perception of a stimulus, the integration of various stimuli, and memory.

The occipital lobes
The occipital lobe consists mainly of the visual cortex (Figure 8.8), and so receives most of its input from the eyes. The primary visual cortex lies within the surfaces of the longitudinal fissure between the two hemispheres.

Curiously, the cortex of the right hemisphere receives most of its sensory information from the left side of the body, and the left hemisphere receives its information from the right side. Similarly, each hemisphere controls the contraction of muscles on the opposite side of the body. In this way, being left- or right-handed indicates that one hemisphere is dominant. People who are right-handed will have a dominant left hemisphere, while left-handed people will have a dominant right hemisphere. The left hemisphere seems to be more effective at analysing information presented to it in changing sequences, and is considered to be important in logic and mathematical analysis ('scientific' functions). The right hemisphere appears more effective in the analysis of shape, form and space ('artistic' functions), and studies have suggested that left-handedness gives a propensity to artistic abilities. This separation of functioning must be treated with caution, however, since both hemispheres will be involved in functions, and the effect is not powerful: there is no conclusive evidence that right-handed people are always better mathematicians.

Transmission of information between the hemispheres takes place via the corpus callosum that connects the two. Failure to transmit this information because of trauma in this area means that communication between the hemispheres will be affected. For example, the language centres on the left side of the brain might not communicate with the right side of the brain. Thus, a request for the individual to raise their left hand will not produce a response because muscle contraction on the left side of the body depends upon nerve activity from motor areas on the right side of the brain. Similarly, sensory stimuli applied to the left side of the body cannot be described, since sensory information from that side will pass to the right side of the brain but cannot be relayed to the language centres on the left side.

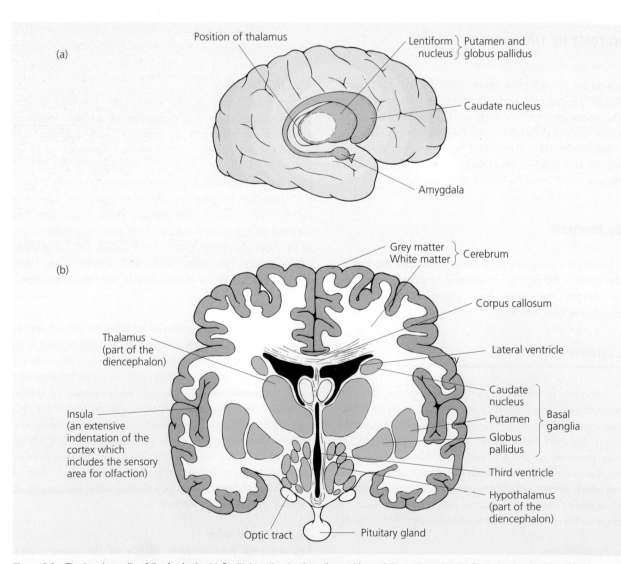

Figure 8.9 The basal ganglia of the forebrain. (a) Sagittal section to show the positions of the main nuclei. (b) Cross-section to show the main ganglia relative to other brain structures.

Q. What are the ventricles?

The temporal lobes

We have already mentioned the temporal lobe as consisting of part of the sensory association area. It also receives sensory information from the ears, and consists mainly of the auditory cortex (Figure 8.8).

Cerebral nuclei

Below the cerebral cortex there is substantial white matter, indicative of myelinated axons of nerve cells that convey information through the brain from one area to another. This subcortical region also contains nuclei of grey matter, which collectively comprise processing areas called the basal ganglia and limbic system. The basal ganglia are a collection of interconnected structures within both hemispheres (Figure 8.9) that are involved in the control of movement and so interact with the motor cortex. They

are described in more detail in Chapter 17 in relation to the control of muscle contraction and posture.

The limbic system, shown in Figure 8.10, is another collection of interconnected structures that surround the centre of the forebrain. Two of the most prominent of these structures are the hippocampus (named because of its passing resemblance to the shape of a sea horse) and the amygdala (= 'almond'). Some of the cerebral cortex also forms part of the limbic system, especially that along the lower edge ('limbus' = border) of the cerebral hemispheres, within the fissure between them. Much of the area is readily distinguishable from the rest of the cortex, and is called the cingulate gyrus (although it is frequently referred to simply as the limbic cortex) (See also Figure 8.7(b)). The limbic system has various functions, including roles in memory, behaviour and emotions.

The diencephalon

The diencephalon consists of cerebral nuclei deep within the cerebrum that separate it from the midbrain. They are distinguished from the cerebrum through embryological development See Figure 8.6. There are two major components: the thalamus and the hypothalamus (Figure 8.9(b)).

The thalamus is a large, two-lobed structure that acts as a relay centre for neural information (mainly from sensory receptors) on its way to the cerebral cortex. The thalamus itself is a heterogeneous structure. It can be divided into several functional component nuclei (Figure 8.11), from which axons pass to specific areas of cortex. For example, the lateral (i.e. at the sides) geniculate nuclei receive input

---

BOX 8.7 THE LIMBIC SYSTEM IN AROMATHERAPY

Evolutionary biologists consider the limbic system within the brain as being part of a 'primitive' brain that is found in all mammalian species and has been preserved during evolution. This would fit with its role in memory and behaviour, two faculties that are widespread in animals. In humans it has come to prominence in popular literature in recent years, especially with the increasing popularity of aromatherapy. Since activity in the olfactory nerve passes directly to limbic structures, smell can be highly evocative of memories of past events, and can also be mood enhancing.

Figure 8.10 The relative positions of major components of the limbic system.

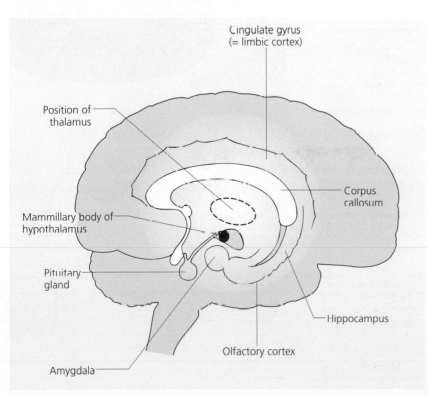

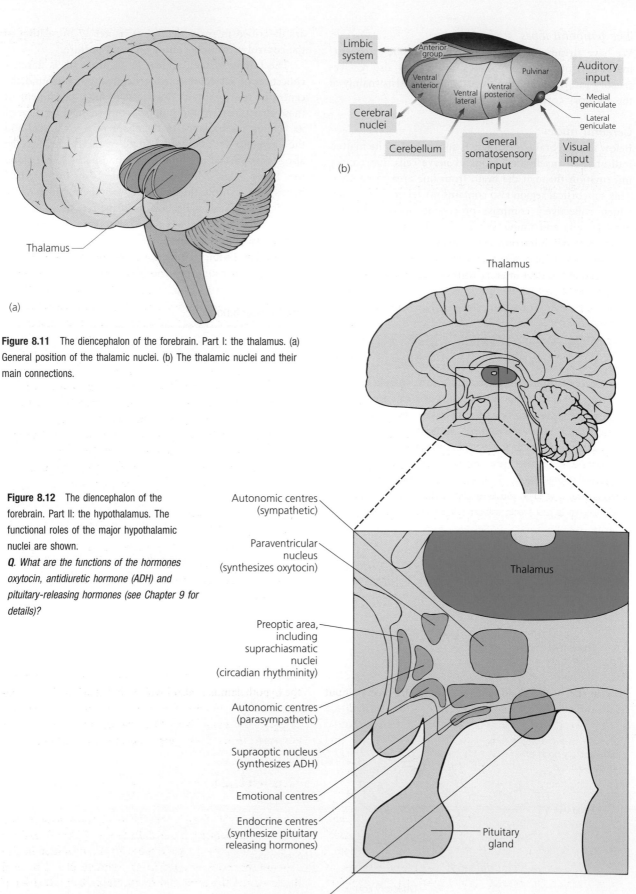

Limbic system

Anterior group

Ventral anterior

Cerebral nuclei

Ventral lateral

Ventral posterior

Pulvinar

Auditory input

Medial geniculate

Lateral geniculate

Cerebellum

General somatosensory input

Visual input

(b)

Thalamus

(a)

Figure 8.11 The diencephalon of the forebrain. Part I: the thalamus. (a) General position of the thalamic nuclei. (b) The thalamic nuclei and their main connections.

Thalamus

Figure 8.12 The diencephalon of the forebrain. Part II: the hypothalamus. The functional roles of the major hypothalamic nuclei are shown.

Q. What are the functions of the hormones oxytocin, antidiuretic hormone (ADH) and pituitary-releasing hormones (see Chapter 9 for details)?

Autonomic centres (sympathetic)

Paraventricular nucleus (synthesizes oxytocin)

Thalamus

Preoptic area, including suprachiasmatic nuclei (circadian rhythminity)

Autonomic centres (parasympathetic)

Supraoptic nucleus (synthesizes ADH)

Emotional centres

Endocrine centres (synthesize pituitary releasing hormones)

Pituitary gland

Mammillary body (olfaction relay centre)

BOX 8.8 NEURODEGENERATIVE DISORDERS

Some neurological disorders can be pinpointed to quite precise parts of brain anatomy. For example, Parkinson's disease is promoted by a decline in activity within neural pathways associated with a midbrain nucleus called the substantia nigra. In contrast, some disorders produce profound changes that are much more widespread. For example, Alzheimer's disease and Creutzfeldt–Jakob disease involve changes to intracellular and/or cell surface proteins, so the damage that arises is much less focused, although some of the consequences of the damage might relate to particular areas of the brain. Both diseases are progressive, disabling and ultimately fatal.

Alzheimer's disease

Alzheimer's disease (see Schweiger and Huey, 1999) still prompts debate as to whether it represents accelerated ageing or a specific disease state. This is because the extent to which ageing processes contribute to disorders of late adulthood is not always clear. Alzheimer's disease produces a loss of reasoning, abstraction, language and memory, and the failure of such cognitive functions through Alzheimer's disease and other causes is frequently referred to as 'dementia'. First described by Alois Alzheimer in 1907, the most obvious changes in brain anatomy are the formation of plaques and neurofibrillary tangles. The former are extracellular deposits of a protein called amyloid beta-protein, whilst the latter are dense tangles of proteinaceous fibres present within the cytoplasm of certain neurons. The plaques and tangles are not unique to the disease, however. Both occur to a lesser degree in the brains of elderly people, and an understanding of the aetiology of Alzheimer's disease could also give information as to how plaques develop in normal brains.

Much is now known about the genetics and molecular biology of Alzheimer's disease (Drouet et al., 2000), and plaque development is thought to result from a defective enzymatic processing of the precursor of amyloid beta-protein, a 'normal' protein found on cell membranes. In some people, there is a familial link with the disease involving genes on chromosome 21; people with Down's syndrome also exhibit a propensity to develop the condition. There is some evidence, therefore, that a propensity to the condition can be inherited.

The familial link is not especially strong, which suggests that Alzheimer's disease arises largely because the molecular changes that promote plaque formation are also influenced by environmental risk factors. This is a debatable area, but some studies have implicated smoking, alcohol and metal poisoning (e.g. aluminium) as risk factors.

Creutzfeldt–Jakob disease

Creutzfeldt–Jakob disease (CJD) (see Wallace, 1999) is a prion disease, i.e. it is caused by infection of the nervous system with a type of protein that seems to be capable of causing normal cell surface proteins to transform, and so become dysfunctional. Prions are resistant to the action of protease enzymes, and so can avoid digestion; they are normally taken up from a dietary source. With new-variant CJD (nv-CJD), the protein originates in cows, where it causes bovine spongiform encephalitis (BSE); it transfers to humans in food products that contain neural tissue from infected cows. The protein appears to make its way to the central nervous system, and possibly peripheral nerve cells. Within the brain, its resistance to proteases enables it to interact with cell surface proteins, possibly to cause them to change molecular shape. Very little is understood about prion diseases, but it has been suggested that some people have surface proteins that are more susceptible to change than those of other people, so perhaps there is a genetic susceptibility. The evidence is speculative at present, and in relation to nv-CJD is complicated by an incubation period that seemingly is of several years. The outcome is widespread degeneration of neural tissue, a process known as vacuolation, that produces sponge-like features.

---

from the eyes and relay it to the visual cortex, and the medial (i.e. at the middle) geniculate nuclei receive input from the cochlea of the ear and relay it to the auditory cortex. Not all thalamic nuclei receive sensory information directly, however. For example, the ventral (i.e. at the bottom) geniculate nuclei receive input from the cerebellum (part of the hindbrain) and relay it to the motor cortex in its role of mediating conscious movement.

The hypothalamus ('hypo-' = below) is a relatively small centre that lies at the base of the brain (Figures 8.9(b) and 8.12). It is a complex structure, containing several nuclei and tracts of axons. The nuclei modulate the autonomic nervous system and, via the pituitary gland, the release of several major hormones. The hypothalamus therefore provides an important link between the brain and the functioning of other physiological systems. Its role in this respect is described in the relevant chapters. In addition, the hypothalamus is also involved in behavioural organization, since it contains the centres of human 'drives', i.e. eating, drinking and sexual behaviours. The hypothalamus also contains the centre for temperature regulation.

The midbrain

The midbrain lies deep within the brain, and consists of two major component parts called the tectum (= 'roof') and the tegmentum (= 'covering') (Figure 8.13). The midbrain also contains the cerebral aqueduct, the centrally placed channel that connects the third and fourth fluid-filled ventricles of the brain and the periaqueductal grey matter which is involved in pain transmission (Chapter 21).

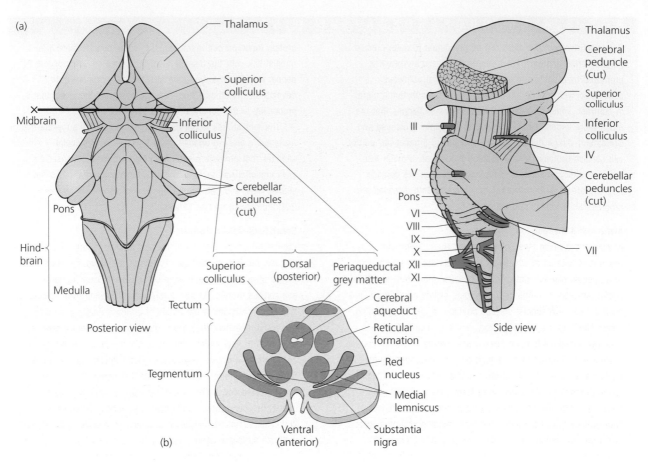

Figure 8.13 (a) Midbrain features and the brainstem. (b) Section through the midbrain at X—X in (a) to show the main nuclei.

Q. Which parts of the hindbrain are included as components of the brainstem?

Q. What is the cerebral aqueduct?

The tectum

The tectum forms the dorsal, or posterior, part of the midbrain. It consists of a number of nuclei, the most prominent ones being the pairs of superior (i.e. upper) and inferior (i.e. lower) colliculi, which appear as four bumps on the brainstem (Figure 8.13). The superior colliculi receive sensory input from the eyes, via the thalamus, and are involved in the control of eye movement. The inferior colliculi receive input from the ears.

The tegmentum

The tegmentum lies anterior to the tectum. It is a complex structure that contains many nuclei (Figure 8.13), including some of those involved in the control of movement:

● the *substantia nigra* (= 'black substance'; these neurons contain melanin) connects with certain basal ganglia of the forebrain. It is one of the centres for modulating impulses that will evoke muscle contraction. Parkinson's disease and Huntington's disease are both consequences of failure in some respect of these nuclei;

● the *red nucleus* projects to the spinal cord. It is part of the pathways that convey information out of the brain to the muscles. These pathways do not include those of the pyramids in the hindbrain (see below), so they are referred to as the extrapyramidal tracts (see chapter 17).

The tegmentum also contains part of the reticular (= 'net') formation, which is a diffuse area that extends into the hindbrain. It receives sensory information from the body, and relays it to the cerebral cortex via the thalamus. The reticular formation is more than just a simple relay station, however: it has been found to have a role in determining the sleep/wake cycle, and also in movement control. Some axons project from it to the spinal cord, i.e. efferent pathways carrying information away from the brain.

The hindbrain

The structures of the hindbrain visible as external features are the cerebellum, pons varolii and medulla oblongata (Figure 8.14(a)).

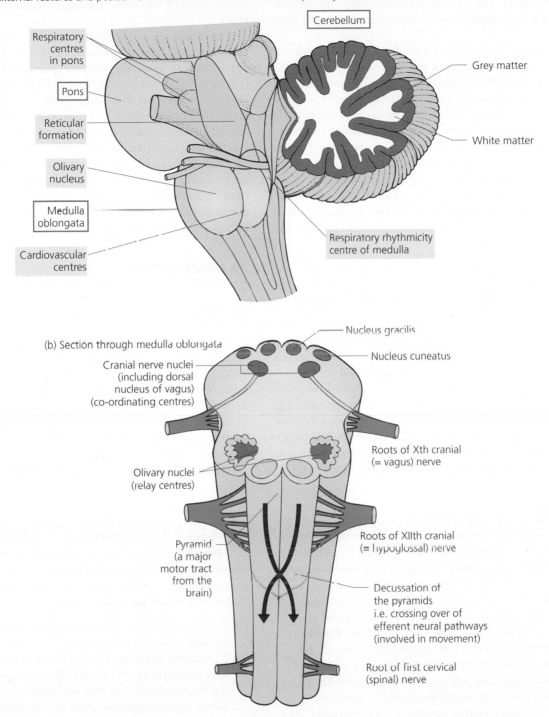

(a) External features and position of the cardiovascular centres and respiratory centres

Respiratory centres in pons

Cerebellum

Pons

Reticular formation

Olivary nucleus

Medulla oblongata

Cardiovascular centres

Grey matter

White matter

Respiratory rhythmicity centre of medulla

(b) Section through medulla oblongata

Nucleus gracilis

Cranial nerve nuclei (including dorsal nucleus of vagus) (co-ordinating centres)

Nucleus cuneatus

Olivary nuclei (relay centres)

Roots of Xth cranial (= vagus) nerve

Pyramid (a major motor tract from the brain)

Roots of XIIth cranial (= hypoglossal) nerve

Decussation of the pyramids i.e. crossing over of efferent neural pathways (involved in movement)

Root of first cervical (spinal) nerve

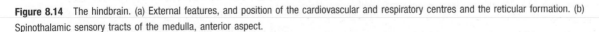

Figure 8.14 The hindbrain. (a) External features, and position of the cardiovascular and respiratory centres and the reticular formation. (b) Spinothalamic sensory tracts of the medulla, anterior aspect.

The cerebellum

The cerebellum (= 'little brain') is a large structure behind and below the rest of the brain. In general structure, it resembles the cerebrum: it has a cortex of grey matter that connects with a set of subcortical structures called the cerebellar nuclei. Three pairs of large tracts of nerve cells are associated with the cerebellum. The inferior cerebellar peduncles connect with the medulla oblongata of the hindbrain; the middle cerebellar peduncles connect with the pons varolii of the hindbrain; and the superior cerebellar peduncles communicate with the midbrain. The inferior and middle peduncles are primarily tracts of sensory nerve cells carrying information into the cerebellum, while the superior peduncle carries activity away from it.

The cerebellum receives input from the eyes, vestibular apparatus of the ears, and sensory receptors around the body. Information is then relayed to other areas involved in the control of movement, particularly the cerebral cortex. In addition, the cerebellum receives information from the cerebral cortex regarding the efferent output to muscles. The activities of the cerebellum provide a fine tuning of movement generated by neural activity from the cerebrum. The cerebellum, therefore, is important in the co-ordination of movement for standing and walking, the production of smooth movement, and the production of fine movements such as those involved in writing and playing sport.

The pons varolii

The pons is visible externally as a large bulge on the brainstem (Figure 8.14(a)). Some of its composite structures, such as the reticular formation, are continuous with those of the midbrain and medulla, and the tegmentum mentioned earlier forms the upper part of the pons. There are numerous nuclei of cells within the pons, e.g. those that comprise some of the respiratory centres. Many are the nuclei of various cranial nerves. Others are part of the pathways by which sensory information passes from the spinal cord to appropriate parts of the brain, or form part of the pathways by which efferent activity from motor areas of the brain converges before leaving the brain.

Converging sensory fibres entering the hindbrain from the spinal cord form the lemnisci (singular = lemniscus), which traverse both the medulla pons, and midbrain (Figure 8.14(b)) and pass to the thalamus and hence the cerebral cortex. Another large tract of fibres worth mentioning here are those that form the cerebellar peduncles. These carry sensory information arriving in the pons (via the spinal cord and cranial nerves) and pass it on to the cerebellum, and also relay information coming out of the cerebellum to the brainstem and cerebral cortex. These routes are therefore the means by which the cerebellum can modulate the output from the cerebral cortex and so help co-ordinate movement.

The medulla oblongata

The medulla is the section of hindbrain that links the brain with the spinal cord. Much of its anatomy involves tracts of the axons of nerve cells carrying information into and out of the brain. Large tracts, called the gracile and cuneate fasciculi (two of each), are noticeable on the posterior aspect of the medulla. These tracts carry sensory input into the brainstem from the spinal cord (Figure 8.14(b)). Two other large tracts, called the pyramids, pass through the anterior aspects of the medulla (from the pons and ultimately midbrain) that carry efferent activity to the muscles. It is in the medulla that the tract from the left side

---

BOX 8.9 THE BRAINSTEM AND 'BRAINSTEM DEATH'

The pons and medulla oblongata of the hindbrain, the midbrain, and parts of the thalamus of the forebrain are sometimes referred to as the brainstem. This is because the cerebellum of the hindbrain and the cerebrum of the forebrain appear to be attached to it, and activity passing into and out of these structures therefore arise or pass through brainstem structures. Brainstem structures act as a conduit for neural impulses passing into and out of the brain. This will apply to sensory/motor impulses from and to the rest of the body, but also includes impulses from the balance organs of the ear and also to and from muscles of the eye. The structures contain brain centres that are especially involved in the control of vital body functions, e.g. breathing and blood pressure.

The brainstem introduces important considerations in clinical practice. For example, the pons and medulla contain the reticular formation that is involved in arousal, and inhibited by general anaesthetics. The brainstem also contains the nuclei that are responsible for co-ordinating breathing, pulse rate, and blood vessel constriction/dilation, and also acts as a conduit for other features of the autonomic nervous system.

Accordingly, 'brainstem death' is considered to represent a condition that represents the death of the individual, and is an important factor in determining whether a person on life-support equipment is likely to recover. Tests include:

- an electroencephalogram (EEG) to monitor brain activity, especially in relation to sensory activity;
- the presence or absence of a pupil light response. The pupil of the eye is controlled by the nerve activity produced in response to the level of light stimulation of the retina (see Chapter 7). The nerve pathway involved includes brain centres within the hindbrain. Brainstem death will mean that the reflex does not occur;
- the presence or absence of a vestibulo-ocular reflex. Sudden movement of fluid within the vestibular apparatus of the inner ear (see Chapter 7) produces a reflex horizontal movement of the eye. The nerve pathway that stimulates this passes through the brainstem, so the reflex will be absent in brainstem death;
- the presence or absence of a corneal touch reflex. Blinking in response to contact with the cornea is a defence response that operates via a reflex passing through the brainstem. This reflex will be absent in brainstem death.

of the brain crosses over (called decussation) to the opposite side of the spinal cord (Figure 8.14(b)). In this way, one side of the brain mediates contraction of muscles on the opposite side of the body (remember that sensory information passing into the brain eventually passes to the hemisphere opposite to the side of the body from which it originated).

Internally, the medulla also contains nuclei that are associated with these tracts. For example, the gracile and cuneate fasciculi terminate at the gracile and cuneate nuclei, respectively, from which axons project toward the thalamus (Figure 8.14(b)). The presence of other nuclei within the medulla that are associated with cranial nerves also means that this part of the brain has a role in co-ordinating some of the activities of the autonomic nervous system. Thus, diffuse areas of neurons, and various nuclei, comprise the respiratory inspiratory and expiratory centres, and the cardiovascular accelerator and depressor areas (Figure 8.14(a)). Output from the respiratory centres, and hence the regulation of breathing rhythm, is normally controlled by input from an apneustic centre within the pons (see Chapter 14).

In addition to receiving afferent information from autonomic neurons, the areas of the medulla that are involved in promoting respiratory and cardiovascular responses also receive inputs from areas of the hypothalamus (which also receives input from the limbic system). These are responsible for the mediation of psychological influences on autonomic responses, e.g. in the stress response.

Two oval-shaped protrusions are also noticeable on the anterior surface of the medulla (Figure 8.14(b)). These are the olivary bodies, inside which are found the inferior olivary nuclei. These sac-like structures, together with accessory nuclei, act as relay centres for transmission of activity from various parts of the brain and spinal cord to the cerebellum.

The meningeal membranes

The brain and spinal cord are covered by three epithelial membranes, collectively called the meninges. The outer-most layer is called the dura mater; the innermost layer is called the pia mater; and the middle layer is called the arachnoid mater (Figure 8.15).

Dura mater

The dura mater is comprised mainly of the protein colla-gen. It forms a thick, tough protective/supportive layer. The layer has two components: an inner layer (sometimes confusingly referred to as the meningeal layer), which is continuous between the brain and spinal cord, and an outer layer, which is really the periosteum that coats the bones of the cranial cavity. Venous sinuses, which eventu-ally return blood flowing through the brain to the jugular veins, may be found between these two layers. The inner layer also provides a protective sheath around the cranial nerves and spinal nerves until they exit the skull and vertebrae, respectively, and forms inwardly folding membranes, or septa, that project into the major inden-tations of the brain and so help to support it. The most prominent of these septa is called the falx cerebri, which extends down into the longitudinal fissure between the two hemispheres.

Arachnoid mater

The arachnoid mater is a delicate membrane of loose connective tissue. A narrow space known as the subdural space separates it from the overlying dura mater. A much larger space called the subarachnoid space separates it from the underlying pia mater. The subarachnoid space contains the special tissue fluid called the cerebrospinal fluid (CSF; see below) that bathes the brain and spinal cord. The patency of the subarachnoid space is maintained by a meshwork of bridging strands called trabeculae between the arachnoid and pia maters. Enlargements of the subarachnoid space in certain parts of the brain, and at the base of the spinal cord, are used clinically to obtain samples of CSF.

In some places, the arachnoid mater penetrates the dura mater to project into the superior sagittal (blood) sinus. These projections are called arachnoid villi (= finger-like projections), and they provide the surface for the reabsorp-tion of CSF back into the blood.

BOX 8.10 SUBDURAL AND SUBARACHNOID HAEMATOMAS

Haemorrhage into the spaces between the meningeal membranes is often associated with head trauma (McNair, 1999). A subdural haemorrhage produces a clot (haematoma) within the subdural space between the dura mater and arachnoid mater. If acute, the haematoma may form within hours; if subacute, it may form in one or more weeks. The bleeding may also be chronic over weeks or even months. The mass of the haematoma compresses underlying brain tissue, commonly causing raised intracranial pressure.

In subarachnoid haemorrhage, the blood passes into the space between the arachnoid and pia maters. There is often an inflammatory reaction in these membranes, and the clot also impairs circulation of CSF and its reabsorption. Again, brain tissue is compressed and displaced by the blood mass. There is commonly a rapidly developing headache, visual and motor impairment, and loss of consciousness. Mortality rates are relatively high, and the possibility of re-bleeding and mortality major risks, especially in the first 24 h. For this reason, it is important to monitor for vital signs and general state of consciousness.

(a) Around the brain

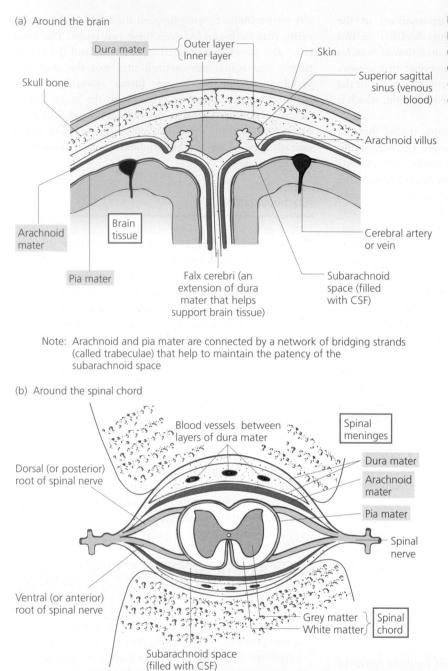

Figure 8.15 The meninges (a) around the brain and (b) around the spinal cord (exaggerated). Note how the dura mater extends along the spinal nerve roots.
***Q**. Where would a subarachnoid haemorrhage occur in (a)?*

Dura mater { Outer layer / Inner layer

Skull bone

Arachnoid mater

Pia mater

Brain tissue

Falx cerebri (an extension of dura mater that helps support brain tissue)

Skin

Superior sagittal sinus (venous blood)

Arachnoid villus

Cerebral artery or vein

Subarachnoid space (filled with CSF)

Note: Arachnoid and pia mater are connected by a network of bridging strands (called trabeculae) that help to maintain the patency of the subarachnoid space

(b) Around the spinal chord

Blood vessels between layers of dura mater

Dorsal (or posterior) root of spinal nerve

Ventral (or anterior) root of spinal nerve

Subarachnoid space (filled with CSF)

Spinal meninges

Dura mater
Arachnoid mater
Pia mater

Spinal nerve

Grey matter } Spinal chord
White matter }

BOX 8.11 MENINGITIS

This is an inflammation of the meningeal membranes induced by an infectious agent (Myers, 2000). Pain receptors are found in the meninges (but not in the brain tissue), and severe headache is experienced. Apart from localized effects of the inflammation on adjacent brain/spinal tissue, the meningeal vessels also become more permeable, leading to excess fluid secretion and raised intracranial pressure, which will have generalized cerebral effects; the condition is life threatening. Irritation of cranial and spinal nerves could explain associated symptoms, such as neck stiffness, tinnitus and head retraction.

Meningitis may be caused by infection with bacteria, viruses, fungi or parasites, or by the actions of toxins. Bacterial meningitis usually involves *Neisseria meningitidis* and is often referred to as meningococcal meningitis. Children and adolescents are particularly at risk. Other agents are *Streptococcus pneumoniae* and *Haemophilus influenzae*. The bacteria are common agents found within the nasopharynx, so the entry to the meninges remains unclear, although it is normally blood-borne. Viral meningitis normally produces milder symptoms.

Diagnosis usually entails the sampling of CSF. This is usually clear and colourless, but it becomes turbid if there is meningeal infection, because of the occurrence of large numbers of leucocytes. Differential white cell count is used to distinguish the occurrence of bacterial or viral meningitis.

Pia mater

The pia mater covers the actual surface of the brain and spinal cord, and forms a sheath around cranial nerves and spinal nerve roots as they traverse the subarachnoid space. The pia mater is comprised of loose connective tissue, and so resembles the arachnoid mater in structure, but it is additionally rich in blood vessels that supply the underlying neural tissue. The pia mater also lines the cerebral ventricles and forms the choroid plexus, the membrane that secretes the cerebrospinal fluid.

Cerebrospinal fluid (CSF)

As we explained earlier, the brain and spinal cord do not consist entirely of tissue: spaces filled with CSF are evident. The CSF provides the brain with:

● a protected environment;

● a hydraulic suspension of the brain matter;

● protection against mechanical damage to blood vessels and the membranous linings of the brain by preventing friction with the skull.

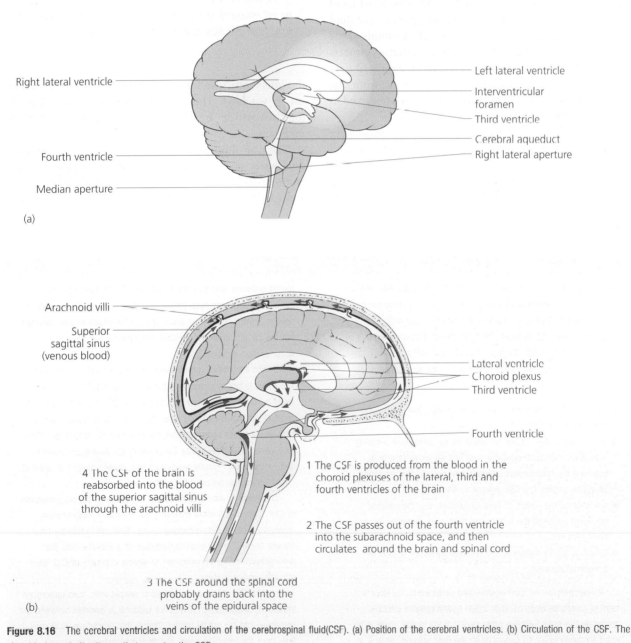

Figure 8.16 The cerebral ventricles and circulation of the cerebrospinal fluid (CSF). (a) Position of the cerebral ventricles. (b) Circulation of the CSF. The choroid plexus is the tissue that secretes the CSF.

Q. What is the role of the arachnoid villi?

The CSF provides the medium that bathes brain cells, and so is the medium with which the cell membranes interact. By their nature, neurons are particularly susceptible to changes in their intracellular/extracellular environment, and even the normal fluctuations of blood glucose concentration that arise through eating patterns would be disturbing for them (neurons do require glucose, but they operate most effectively if the extracellular concentration is held almost constant). To ensure an even tighter homeostatic control of extracellular environment, the central nervous system must, to a large extent, be physically isolated from the blood. The brain is, of course, dependent upon the circulation of blood for its nutrients, so the CSF must be produced from it; at the same time, it must be isolated from it. This is achieved be the fluid being secreted by cells lining the larger fluid spaces, i.e. the CSF is one of the transcellular fluids of the body (defined in Chaptr 6). Utilizing a secretory process means that the fluid composition can be regulated very closely, which helps to protect the neurons from the short-term, moment-to-moment fluctuations observed in the composition of blood plasma.

There are four main fluid spaces, or ventricles (Figure 8.16(a)). Three ventricles (two large lateral ventricles, and the third ventricle) lie deep within the forebrain, while the fourth is in the hindbrain. Most CSF is secreted into the lateral ventricles, which connect with the third ventricle via

BOX 8.12 THE BLOOD–BRAIN BARRIER AND DRUGS

The secretory epithelium that produces CSF forms a blood–brain barrier. Only lipid-soluble substances, or those with transport facilities within the epithelial cell membranes, can cross into the CSF. This barrier is clinically important, as drugs must be capable of crossing it if brain function is to be affected. For example, levodopa is a drug that is commonly prescribed for people with Parkinson's disease. This drug crosses the blood–brain barrier and enters the brain, where it is converted into dopamine, a neurotransmitter that is deficient in Parkinson's disease. Dopamine itself cannot be administered because it does not cross the barrier.

General anaesthetics and alcohol are lipid soluble and therefore are not influenced by the barrier. The rapid onset of action of these drugs is an indication of their rapid transit into the brain.

the interventricular foramina ('inter-' = between, 'foramina' = window). The third ventricle is connected to the fourth ventricle by the cerebral aqueduct within the midbrain.

The CSF flows from the ventricles into the subarachnoid space and then around the brain (Figure 8.16(b)). Some passes into the subarachnoid space of the spinal cord and so circulates around the cord neurons. Fluid flow is

BOX 8.13 EXCESS OR DEFICIENT CEREBROSPINAL FLUID

Normal ranges for CSF volume: child, 60–100 ml; adult, 100–160 ml.

The CSF is continuously being secreted from, and reabsorbed into, the blood plasma, so the volume present represents a homeostatic balance between the rate of secretion and rate of reabsorption (about 600 ml fluid is produced/reabsorbed each day in adults). Normally this is not problematic, but an increase in the volume present may be caused by:

- inflammatory conditions, such as meningitis, that disrupt the reabsorptive areas;
- brain trauma, e.g. stroke, in which tissue damage or bleeding disrupts the circulation of the fluid and so prevents it from reaching the reabsorptive areas. Consequently, the continued secretion causes the CSF volume to rise;
- blockage of the routes of fluid circulation, e.g. the cerebral aqueduct between the lateral and third fluid ventricles, by a brain tumour;
- failure in the formation of the cerebral aqueduct. This is a congenital disorder.

Raised intracranial fluid volume and pressure is therefore a form of (cerebral) oedema. It is called hydrocephalus (literally 'water on the brain'). Unlike other oedematous states, there is no room for brain tissue to expand with the fluid volume, since it is enclosed within the bony box of the skull. Consequently, tissue is

forced outward, and its impact with the skull disturbs neural functioning and may even cause neural loss if the compression is severe. Severe headaches and cognitive disturbances are common, but the compression can be fatal, especially if the fluid accumulation is rapid.

Benign intracranial hypertension (BIH) has a much slower onset. The cause is largely unknown, although previous history of head injury might be a factor. The slow accumulation of CSF produces a gradual onset of symptoms that may delay diagnosis. The outcome could be fatal. In congenital hydrocephalus, the presence of intracranial sutures for a period after birth makes the bones of the skull more movable, and the condition typically produces a high domed head. The onset of raised intracranial pressure is usually gradual.

Treatment is aimed at removing the cause of the accumulation of CSF. This might entail removing the source of inflammation, removing a blood clot, removing excess fluid until recovery from trauma occurs, or surgical implantation of a catheter into the subarachnoid space or ventricles to enable drainage of CSF back into the venous system.

Loss of CSF might be observed in people who have undergone intraspinal anaesthesia (in which a catheter is inserted between the vertebrae into the spinal cavity). During this procedure, fluid may leak from the insertion point. The fluid loss influences neural functioning; again, headaches are characteristic.

promoted by the action of cilia, although head and vertebral movements help. The fluid is eventually reabsorbed back into the blood plasma via projections of the middle meningeal membrane, the arachnoid mater. Clearly the rate of reabsorption must balance the rate of secretion if CSF volume is to be maintained. The means of regulation of the process is unclear.

Vasculature of the brain: the cerebral circulation

The brain is supplied with blood originating from the two common carotid arteries within the neck and from the two vertebral arteries (Figure 8.17(a)). Each common carotid artery divides into an internal and external branch. The external carotid arteries supply the pharynx, larynx and face with blood, but the internal carotids pass deeper and penetrate the base of the skull and so supply the brain. The vertebral arteries ascend the vertebral column, passing through the lateral or transverse foramina of the bones, and penetrate the skull via the foramen magnum, through which the spinal cord passes.

Upon entering the skull, each internal carotid artery divides to form an anterior and a middle cerebral artery, which supply blood to the anterior half to two-thirds of the brain. The vertebral arteries combine to form a single basilar artery. This runs along the anterior (ventral) aspect of the

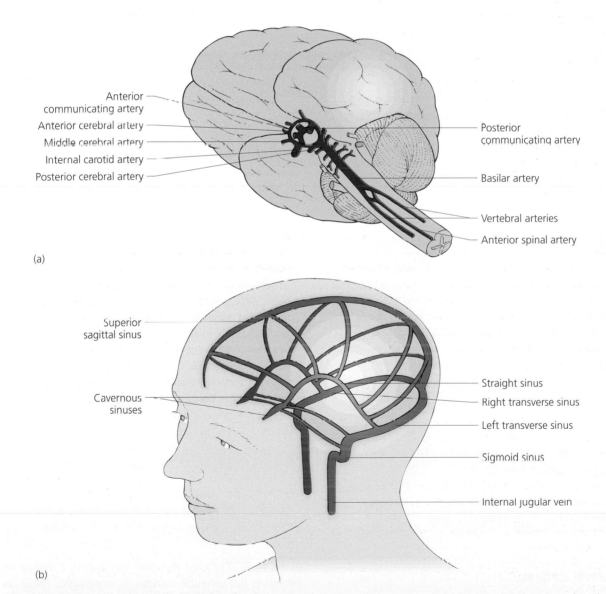

(a)

(b)

Figure 8.17 The cerebral vasculature. (a) Cerebral arteries. The anterior and posterior communicating arteries join the cerebral arteries to form the Circle of Willis. (b) Venous drainage.

Q. What is the advantage of having a Circle of Willis?

Q. To where do the jugular veins pass?

hindbrain and sends branches into the hindbrain and midbrain. It eventually divides to form a pair of posterior cerebral arteries that supply structures at the rear of the cerebrum.

Although the carotids and vertebral arteries would appear to be responsible for supplying blood to different parts of the brain, the internal carotids and the basilar artery are interconnected at the base of the brain. Communicating arteries branch from the sites of origin of the anterior cerebral and posterior cerebral arteries to form the circle of Willis, which encircles the stalk of the pituitary gland (Figure 8.17(a)). Blood can, therefore, pass from the carotid arteries to the posterior cerebral arteries, or from the basilar artery to the anterior and middle cerebral arteries. In view of its high metabolic activity, and the sensitivity of brain cells to disturbances

in their immediate environment, having four arteries supplying the brain, and having vessels that connect anterior and posterior vessels, are adaptations that help to prevent blood flow to the brain from being compromised.

Small veins drain the brain and empty into blood sinuses within the dura mater. The largest of these is called the superior sagittal sinus (Figure 8.17(b)), which lies within the fold of membrane called the falx cerebri. Most venous blood eventually drains into a pair of transverse sinuses, which run forward inside and along the base of the skull and empty into the internal jugular veins. Venous blood from other parts of the head and neck drain into the external jugular veins, which eventually fuse within the neck with the internal vessels to form the common jugular veins.

BOX 8.14 CEREBROVASCULAR ACCIDENT

A cerebrovascular accident (CVA, stroke) occurs when a portion of the brain is deprived of blood, and hence of oxygen and glucose. Cerebral thrombosis caused by clot formation at the site of an atherosclerotic plaque, cerebral embolism caused by drifting clots, fatty masses or air bubbles, and cerebral haemorrhages are all common causes of CVA, and may cause loss of neurons, or cause an increase in fluid pressure on underlying nerve cells.

Symptoms of CVA depend on which part of the brain is damaged, and therefore which cerebral artery is affected (see text):

- A CVA involving the anterior cerebral artery will particularly affect the motor and sensory cortex.
- A CVA involving the middle cerebral artery will have similar effects, but may also include speech and auditory defects.
- A CVA in the posterior cerebral artery will affect the visual cortex and the limbic system.
- Loss of blood supply via the basilar artery may partly be compensated for by blood passing through the circle of Willis. Nevertheless, damage to the cerebellum and brainstem can

be severe. Loss of brainstem functions will also affect autonomic control.

Initial symptoms of a stroke can be exaggerated by swelling of surrounding brain tissues and so neural function may improve with time as the swelling subsides. Care is directed particularly at facilitating neurological improvement (Petty, 2000).

Blockages to cerebral arteries can be temporary, in which case symptoms may be short lived. This is called a transient ischaemic episode (or attacks; TIA). A TIA can precede a more serious attack, though not necessarily. TIAs are most frequently observed in older people as a consequence of age-related changes to blood supply.

Anticoagulant therapy can help to reduce the likelihood of further clotting, and so prevent exacerbation of the problem. Surgical intervention to remove a haematoma may also be necessary to relieve raised intracranial pressure or to improve circulation. Preventive surgery, e.g. on aneurysms, is also possible in some cases. The reduction of risk factors, such as high blood pressure (hypertension), is an important part of health-promotion strategies.

ANATOMY OF THE SPINAL CORD

General features

The main functions of the spinal cord are to transmit motor activity from the brain to target tissues within the body, and to carry sensory activity from around the body

to the brain. The cord therefore increases in diameter on ascending the vertebral column as more nerve fibres are incorporated into it. The spinal cord is protected by the vertebral bones, passing through the spinal foramen of each bone, and is covered by the three meningeal layers noted earlier.

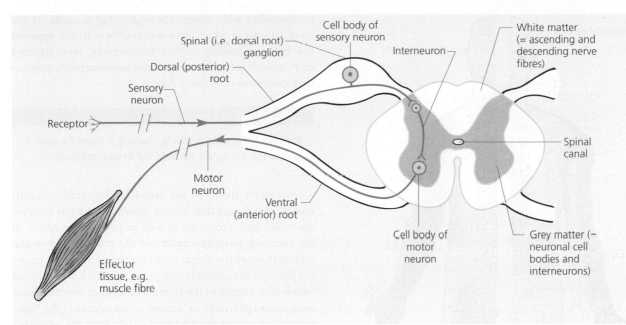

Figure 8.18 Spinal nerve roots and the general appearance of the cord.
Q. What do the terms 'ventral' and 'dorsal' mean?

In fact, the cord itself is not as long as the vertebral column. On reaching the level of the second lumbar vertebra, the cord divides into a mass of neural structures, which are the roots of various nerves that enter or exit the vertebral column below this point. The structure is reminiscent of a horse's tail, and so is called the cauda equina ('cauda' = tail, 'equina' = horse; see Figure 8.4).

Nerve roots leave the cord and cauda equina at intervals. At each vertebral joint there is a pair of posterior (or dorsal) and anterior (or ventral) nerve roots (Figure 8.18). The dorsal and ventral roots fuse after leaving the cord within spaces between the vertebrae (the vertebral foramen), thus forming the spinal nerves, of which there are 31 pairs:

- eight pairs arise from the cervical vertebrae;
- twelve pairs arise from the thoracic vertebrae;
- five pairs arise from the lumbar vertebrae;
- five pairs arise from the sacral vertebrae;
- one pair arises from the coccygeal vertebrae.

We noted earlier in this chapter that each spinal nerve consists of sensory (afferent) and motor (efferent) neurons. The sensory neurons form the dorsal nerve root, and the motor neurons form the ventral root, i.e. sensory information passing along the nerves to the cord enters the posterior aspect of the cord, and motor information passing from the cord into the nerves exits from the anterior aspect of the cord.

If you think back to the section on neuron structure, you may recall that sensory nerve cells are distinguished partly by the cell body that appears as an offshoot from the side of the cell. In fact, the cell bodies of afferent neurons are found in the same area of the dorsal root and produce the distension called a dorsal root ganglion (Figure 8.18). The cell bodies of motor neurons lie within the cord itself, so there is no comparable ganglionic structure in the ventral root.

The arrangement of paired spinal nerves suggests that each pair innervates a 'segment' of the body. To a large extent this is the case, and is particularly considered in relation to sensory nerves. Thus, epidural administration of an analgesic agent into the vicinity of the spinal cord could block pain transmission from a number of tissues, but they will be located in a similar part of the abdomen. The further away the nerve is from the spinal cord, the more dispersed the nerve endings tend to be, but even in the skin there are sensory areas that map to a particular spinal nerve; these areas are called dermatomes (Figure 8.19).

Structure of the spinal cord: white matter

The periphery of the spinal cord appears white in section (Figure 8.18) as a consequence of the presence of the fatty sheath, myelin, although unmyelinated fibres and glial cells will also be present. The white matter consists of neuronal fibres that descend or ascend the cord. It is highly organized, with the neurons forming 'columns' within the cord periphery called dorsal, lateral or ventral columns, according to the location. Within the columns, neurons passing to or from similar parts of the brain are arranged into distinct 'tracts' (Figure 8.20(a)). The dorsal columns are especially noticeable as an external feature of the cord and are comprised of the ascending neuronal tracts that

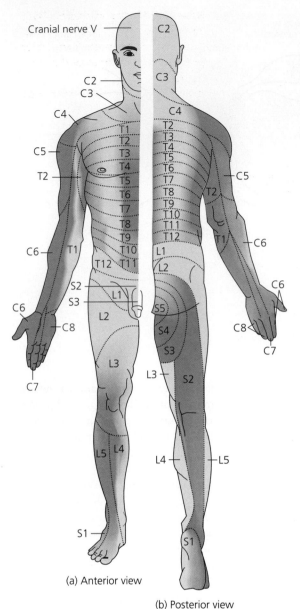

(a) Anterior view

(b) Posterior view

Figure 8.19 Distribution of dermatomes. The diagram provides a sensory map of the body surface. Each dermatome is an area of skin served by a pair of spinal nerves, or by cranial nerve V (trigeminal nerve). The letters and numbers refer to the origin of the nerve.
C = cervical, T = thoracic, L = lumbar, S = sacral
Q. Where would nerve activity stimulated by injury to the left little finger pass into the spinal cord?

transmit sensory information to the brain. The other columns consist of tracts of both ascending (sensory) and descending (motor) neurons.

Ascending (sensory) tracts

The dorsal columns consist of axons of sensory neurons that, on entering the cord, turn to ascend it. They terminate

by synapsing with nerve cells within the medulla of the hindbrain, from which neurons cross over to the opposite side before ascending further. Functionally, these neurons carry sensory information from mechanoreceptors, particularly cutaneous ones (see Chapter 7).

Ascending tracts of the lateral and ventral columns consist of neurons that convey information from temperature and pain receptors, as well as pressure receptors of the skin and proprioreceptors of the muscles and joints. Unlike those of the dorsal columns, the nerve axons entering the cord immediately synapse with others, the axons of which then ascend in the tracts. These other nerve cells are sometimes referred to as 'second-order neurons'; the 'first-order neurons' are the afferent neurons from the receptors. Some second-order neurons ascend on the same side as the afferent neuron enters the cord; others cross over to the opposite side before ascending the cord.

The destination in the brain of these tracts was considered in Chapter 7. Many eventually pass to the thalamus within the forebrain, from whence information passes out to other brain areas, especially the cerebral cortex. Accordingly, they are collectively referred to as spinothalamic tracts (perhaps preceded by anterior, lateral, etc.).

Descending (motor) tracts

There are various descending tracts within the lateral and ventral columns (Figure 8.20(a)). They are named according to where they originate within the brain, e.g. corticospinal tracts originate within the cerebral cortex. Each tract consists of motor neurons that eventually synapse with other efferent neurons, which pass to skeletal muscles or glandular tissue. Their names and functions are considered further in Chapter 16, where control of muscle function is described.

Structure of the spinal cord: grey matter

The central portion of the cord in section appears as an H-shaped (or butterfly-shaped) area (Figure 8.20(b)). This is the grey matter of the cord, which consists of neuronal cell bodies, axons and glial cells.

Sensory neurons entering the cord via the dorsal root of a spinal nerve pass into the grey matter. At this point, the grey matter is called the dorsal horn, since it is the 'arm' of the H-shape closest to the dorsal or posterior surface of the cord. The sensory neurons then either turn to enter the ascending white columns, or relay with small

(a) White matter

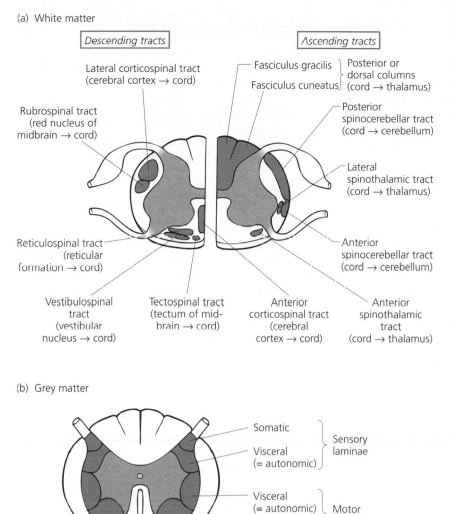

| Descending tracts | | Ascending tracts |

Lateral corticospinal tract (cerebral cortex → cord)

Rubrospinal tract (red nucleus of midbrain → cord)

Reticulospinal tract (reticular formation → cord)

Vestibulospinal tract (vestibular nucleus → cord)

Tectospinal tract (tectum of mid-brain → cord)

Anterior corticospinal tract (cerebral cortex → cord)

Fasciculus gracilis

Fasciculus cuneatus

Posterior or dorsal columns (cord → thalamus)

Posterior spinocerebellar tract (cord → cerebellum)

Lateral spinothalamic tract (cord → thalamus)

Anterior spinocerebellar tract (cord → cerebellum)

Anterior spinothalamic tract (cord → thalamus)

(b) Grey matter

Somatic

Visceral (= autonomic)

Sensory laminae

Visceral (= autonomic)

Somatic

Motor laminae

Note: Various laminae are present within each group, e.g. substantia gelatinosa within sensory groups

Figure 8.20 Structural organization of the white and grey matter of the spinal cord. (a) White matter; (b) grey matter. In (a) tracts on the left will also be found on the right, and vice versa.
Q. *What is it that makes white matter 'white'?*

interneurons (i.e. neurons between other neurons; sometimes called relay neurons), which may be confined entirely to the grey matter or may project to other parts of grey or white matter. These cells, therefore, provide communication channels in the cord. Other parts of the grey matter are comprised of the cell bodies of motor neurons, the axons of which project into the ventral root of a spinal nerve via the ventral or anterior horn (i.e. the 'arm' of the H-shape closest to the ventral surface of the cord). The cell bodies of these cells will receive information from descending neurons from the brain, or from interneurons within the grey matter.

Neurons of the lateral areas of the grey matter are particularly involved with the autonomic branch of the peripheral nervous system (see later).

The arrangement of cell bodies within the horns of grey matter conveys an image of layers of cell bodies and interneurons. Cells within the grey matter are said to have a laminar arrangement (rather than columnar, as in white matter). Laminae have been identified in which cell bodies/interneurons are found that are part of specific neural pathways, e.g. the laminae referred to as the substantia gelatinosa have a particular role in modulating the transmission of pain impulses (see chapter 21). In other words, there is once again a high degree of neural organization (Figure 8.20(b)). The types of cell present, and communication between them, reflect the three main functions of the grey matter:

● initial processing and/or relay of incoming sensory information;

● relay and/or final processing of outgoing motor activity;

● an integrative role modulating motor output in direct response to sensory input without involving the brain (i.e. reflex responses).

Spinal canal

The spinal canal lies at the centre of the cord and extends into the medulla of the hindbrain, where it communicates with the fourth ventricle, or fluid space, of the brain. The canal is filled with cerebrospinal fluid (CSF), which circulates down the cord and back to the brain by the action of the ciliated epithelium that lines the canal. As with CSF within the brain, the fluid provides a protected environment, a hydraulic support for the delicate tissue, and shock absorbance.

Vasculature of the spinal cord

The spinal cord has a complex arterial blood supply. Anterior and posterior spinal arteries descend the surface of the cord that are derived from the vertebral arteries and cerebellar arteries (branches of the basilar artery that supply the cerebellum of the hindbrain). Branches penetrate into the neural matter of the cord. In addition, this blood is joined by arterial blood supplied by small vessels that branch from intercostal, cervical and lumbar arteries, and penetrate the cord via spaces between the vertebrae.

NEURAL PHYSIOLOGY

There are generally three broad aspects to the basic functioning of the nervous system. First, if electrodes are placed close to a nerve, then electrical activity can be detected whenever neurons within it are active. Thus, the activity of neurons involves mechanisms that enable them to change their electrical properties in order to generate an impulse (a change in voltage), and to conduct the impulse to other areas.

Second, in conducting impulses neurons must have properties to ensure that they are conducted in the appropriate direction, and are transmitted from one cell to another. This latter process involves special junctions called synapses. Third, the passage of impulses to and from the brain, and within it, is by discrete pathways. The processing of information by the central nervous system is essentially one of an integration of these neural pathways, and involves various parts of the brain. Such integration is necessary for all the diverse properties associated with brain function, ranging from the somatic control of posture (see Chapter 17), to the autonomic regulation of blood pressure (see Chapter 12), to cognitive functions such as memory.

This section considers these three aspects in detail.

Membrane potentials: generating the nerve impulse

The resting membrane potential

The resting membrane potential is the voltage present across a cell membrane when it is at rest. It is present in most, if not all, cells but it has particular significance in nerve and muscle cells, and in some secretory cells.

The membrane potential arises because of the way in which electrolytes are distributed across the cell membrane. In Chapters 2 and 6, it was emphasized how the phospho-

lipid cell membrane has selective permeability properties. Although it is permeable to small, uncharged molecules, such as urea and carbon dioxide, the permeability to electrically charged substances such as ions is very low; this is important in the maintenance of a different ionic composition of intra- and extracellular fluids (see Chapter 6). Thus, sodium has the highest concentration in the extracellular fluids (about 10 times higher than inside cells), while potassium is about 30 times more concentrated within the cells. Likewise, the main anion outside cells is chloride (about 10 times more concentrated than in intracellular fluid), while proteins, amino acids, and phosphates are the main negatively charged electrolytes inside cells.

The net effect of this distribution of positive and negative electrolytes is complex, and relates to the permeability of the membrane to individual ions, and to its capacity to transport them actively. In practice, there is a 'leak', albeit slow, of positive charge from the cell, mainly as a consequence of the outward diffusion of potassium (K^+) ions. Although the long-term effects of this leak of charge is compensated for by the sodium/potassium exchange pump of the cell membrane, it is sufficient such that at any given time there is a residual positive charge on the external surface of the membrane. In other words, the membrane is *polarized*, and the situation is usually expressed as the inside of the membrane being negatively charged with respect to the outside (in relative terms, the loss of positive charge must mean that there is excess negative charge inside the cell).

The polarity of the cell membrane is therefore rather like that of a battery, and placement of microscopic electrodes across the cell membrane will detect a voltage. The value is minute, however, being of the order of 70 millivolts (usually written as -70 mV, i.e. negative inside with respect to outside the cell). The actual value varies slightly between cells depending upon the relative permeability of the cell membrane, especially to sodium and potassium ions.

The action potential

Nerve and muscle cells are 'excitable' because their cell membranes have the capacity to alter their ionic permeability in response to a stimulus. Their membranes contain specific ion channels, which are basically proteins through which ions may diffuse. In order to control this diffusion, however, molecular structures must provide 'gating' mechanisms. By regulating the opening or closing of these 'gates', the membrane can determine which ions are free to diffuse across it. Depending upon the ions that are free to move across the membrane, the voltage may move towards electrical neutrality (i.e. by making the inside of the cell less negative, a process called depolarization) or towards an even greater value (i.e. by making the inside of the cell more negative, a process called hyperpolarization).

Exercise

Nerve cells are stimulated physiologically by various means, e.g. receptor cells. Look back to Chapter 7 to identify the terms 'transduction' and 'generator potential'.

Nerve cells are stimulated by activity at either a sensory receptor or a synapse with another neuron (artificially, the same effect can be produced by application of an electric current, hence the devastating effects of electrocution). However it is produced, stimulation of the neuron causes the membrane to depolarize as sodium channels begin to open and sodium ions (i.e. positive charge) begin to diffuse into the cell, promoted by the concentration gradient and the net negative charge present within the resting cell. The value of the membrane potential will therefore begin to move towards electrical neutrality (Figure 8.21).

At a certain value, called the *membrane threshold,* the sodium channels open fully and sodium ions move rapidly into the cell (Figure 8.21). The movement is so rapid that the membrane potential actually assumes a positive value (about +30 mV, positive inside the cell with respect to outside) because of this influx of positive ions. The change in potential is referred to as an *action potential.* The generation of an action potential is, in some ways, a disturbance of cell membrane homeostasis. The action potential can be considered a positive feedback mechanism in which the slight potential change before threshold promotes further change, leading to the full response.

Once depolarized to this extent, the cell membrane cannot be restimulated; the membrane must be restored to or close to its original resting membrane potential if the neuron is to be capable of restimulation. *Repolarization* is achieved by the opening of potassium channels (Figure 8.21), which allow the diffusion of potassium ions (i.e. positive charge) out of the cell down their concentration and electrical gradients. The net loss of positive charge is

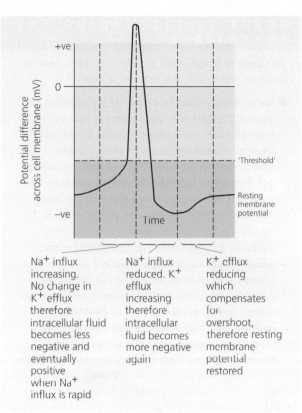

Figure 8.21 The action potential and changes in Na⁺ and K⁺ fluxes across the cell membrane. See text for explanation.

Q. How does the inside of the cell membrane become positively charged during an action potential?

transiently excessive, and the value of the membrane potential goes beyond its resting value (to about -90 mV, negative inside the cell with respect to outside). This hyperpolarization is advantageous, as it makes the membrane more difficult to stimulate (i.e. it is *refractory*) for a brief moment since a greater depolarization will be required to reach threshold. This means that once the nerve impulse has moved along a stage in the nerve fibre, retrograde stimulation is unlikely to occur and the impulse moves in just one direction.

The whole action potential from depolarization to full repolarization takes place in a millisecond or so. This extremely rapid response ensures that the impulse can be conducted rapidly, and that the membrane is quickly available for restimulation.

One further important feature to note concerning the action potential is that the response is *all or nothing*, since the membrane becomes fully permeable to sodium ions once the threshold potential has been attained. Graded responses are not possible, so the level of activity within a neural pathway is determined by how many action potentials are generated and conducted per second.

The ease at which the cell can be stimulated is a measure of its excitability, and depends upon how close the resting

BOX 8.15 DISTURBING THE GENERATION OF ACTION POTENTIALS

The capacity to generate action potentials is central to nerve cell functioning, and depends upon a number of factors:

● *The distribution of electrolytes across the cell membrane.* The influence of changes in ion concentrations in intra- and extracellular fluids was discussed in Chapter 6: the main ionic influences on neural function are the effects of altering potassium and calcium concentrations within the extracellular fluid. Such disturbances frequently arise as a consequence of disorders of fluid homeostasis induced by endocrine defects, renal failure or dietary deficiency. The effect of potassium changes is to alter the resting membrane potential, either depolarizing it toward threshold (in hyperkalaemia neurons become more excitable), or hyperpolarizing it away from threshold (in hypokalaemia, neurons become less excitable). Calcium ion disturbances influence the gating mechanisms, and therefore alter the threshold at which an action potential is generated. Thus, hypocalcaemia induces a lowering of the threshold (the membrane becomes more excitable) and hypercalcaemia raises it (the membrane becomes less excitable).

● *The presence of ion channels within the membrane.* Nerve cells will ordinarily possess such channels. In myelinated axons, however, the channels are concentrated at the nodes of Ranvier (Figure 8.22(b)). Should the insulative layer of myelin be lost, then current decrement from the membrane may be so extensive that subsequent nodes are not stimulated. This is one of the problems associated with multiple sclerosis.

● *The capacity to open and close the ion channels at appropriate times.* Provided that membrane potentials and the threshold potential are normal, then this should not be a problem. Some drugs, however, interfere with the gating mechanisms. This can be of clinical advantage, e.g. some anaesthetics have this effect.

● *Temperature.* Physiologically, body temperature will be controlled within tight limits. But in hypothermia, which is fairly common, particularly in elderly people, neural function is reduced throughout the body. This principle is often used in surgery, and in the 'freeze' sprays used to treat sport injuries.

---

membrane potential is to the threshold potential. Excitability is another example of homeostatic principle in action: the effects of altering parameters that influence either the membrane potential or the threshold potential enables a change in sensitivity when necessary. Thus, the presence of adrenaline during exercise, or in the stress response, seems to increase excitability (which improves reflex action), and the sinoatrial node of the heart undergoes faster cyclical depolarizations (that generate the heartbeat).

Conduction of nerve impulses.

Conduction along the nerve fibre

The generation of an action potential by a nerve cell is only one part of nerve cell function; the electrical activity must also be conducted to appropriate tissues. The basic process in propagating a nerve impulse is the destabilization of sodium channels in adjacent parts of cell membrane by the electric current generated by an action potential, thus causing an influx of positive charge and the shift in membrane potential towards threshold. When the resultant depolarization of adjacent cell membrane reaches the threshold potential, another action potential is generated (Figure 8.22(a)). In this way, an action potential is regenerated along successive parts of the membrane, i.e. along the axon, dendron or dendrite of the cell. We mentioned earlier how the nature of the action potential ensures unidirectional movement of the impulse.

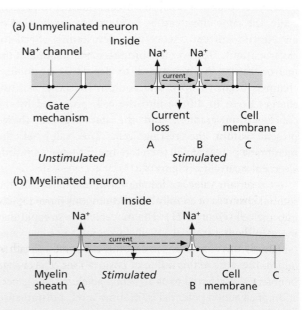

Figure 8.22 Sodium channels, membrane currents and conduction in (a) unmyelinated and (b) myelinated neurons. In each case, the sodium channels are fully open at A, so the membrane is fully permeable to Na⁺ and an action potential is generated. At B, the channels are beginning to open in response to the electrical current that was generated at A, so the membrane begins to approach threshold. At C, the channels are still closed but will subsequently respond to current produced at B. In this way, the impulse is said to propagate along the nerve cell. Note that the presence of myelin in (b) reduces loss of current out of the cell and so increases the distance between the sodium channels.

Table 8.3 Nerve fibre classification and properties

Class	Conduction velocity (m/s)	Myelination	Nerve fibre diameter (μm)
A			
Alpha (α)	50–120	Myelinated	8–20
Beta (β)	30–70	Myelinated	5–12
Gamma (γ)	10–50	Myelinated	2–8
Delta (δ)	3–30	Myelinated	1–5
C	0.5–2	Unmyelinated	< 1

C fibres normally comprise almost half the nerve fibres in a peripheral nerve, and all the post-ganglionic neurons of the autonomic system. An additional sensory nerve fibre classification is sometimes used, in which class I and II fibres correspond to Aα, Aβ and Aγ fibres, class III correspond to Aδ fibres, and class IV fibres correspond to C fibres.

The ease of conduction through a cell membrane of electric current generated by an action potential will be related to the electrical resistance of the membrane, and large diameter fibres have lower resistance than small-diameter ones. Large-diameter nerve fibres therefore conduct electric current more rapidly (and are also easier to stimulate). The rate at which a fibre conducts impulses is called its *conduction velocity*.

In general, only the smallest diameter axons are unmyelinated. The presence of myelin on axons of other neurons reduces current loss to the tissue fluids bathing the cell, and so increases the conduction velocity. Conduction velocities can be achieved that would otherwise require fibres of extremely large diameter if they were to be unmyelinated. Thus, myelinated nerve fibres conduct impulses at velocities of up to 120 m/s (more than 400 km/h!).

Myelin is secreted by certain neuroglial cells (called Schwann cells in the peripheral nervous system, and oligo-dendrocytes in the central nervous system; see earlier). The process of myelination results in the enveloping of the nerve axon by concentric layers of this insulative phospho-lipid. However, in spite of its insulative properties, the generated current still decrements as it leaks slowly through the myelin.

Clearly there must be gaps within the myelin sheath at which the cell membrane can be depolarized again to regenerate the current; these gaps are called the *nodes of Ranvier*. Current (i.e. impulses) can be envisaged as 'jumping' from node to node (note that ion channels will be concentrated only at the nodes; Figure 8.22(b)). This process is called *saltatory conduction*, and is in contrast to the continual conduction observed in unmyelinated neurons. There is still an influence of axon diameter, however, as this will determine the required distance between nodes, and therefore the number of times an action potential has to be generated along the axon.

The presence of myelinated and unmyelinated neurons, and neurons of different diameters, means that a range of conduction velocities can be observed within the nervous system. One of the main classifications of fibre type relates to conduction velocities and the presence or absence of myelin (Table 8.3).

Conduction between cells: the synapse

At some point within a neural pathway, the activity generated by action potentials in a nerve cell must be transmitted to another cell – either another neuron, a muscle cell, or a glandular cell. If there were physical contact between cells, then this would present little difficulty, and the impulse would be conducted as before. Such connections seem to be present in some parts of the brain, and between cells of cardiac muscle (which must also conduct electrical activity). Direct connections do not promote unidirectionality of the conduction of impulses, however, nor do they permit any kind of modulation, and most junctions between neurons, and between neurons and muscle or glandular cells, do not involve physical contact. These junctions are called *synapses*.

Figure 8.23 shows a diagrammatic synapse. It can be seen that a small, fluid-filled space exists between the neurons. This is called the *synaptic cleft* and, although microscopically small (of the order of 20 nm across), it represents a significant barrier to the direct conduction of the neural impulse. The neuron that is conducting an impulse terminates at the synapse as a distended bulb-like structure called a *synaptic end bulb* (sometimes called a *bouton*). When reference is made to synaptic function, this neuron is called the *presynaptic* neuron. The synaptic junction is made with either the next neuron in the pathway, which is referred to as a *post-synaptic* neuron, or with the (post-synaptic) membrane of a gland or muscle cell.

Microscopically, it can be seen that the terminal end bulb contains thousands of membrane-enclosed sacs, called *synaptic vesicles*. Each sac contains a small amount of a chemical synthesized in the cell body of the neuron and transported to the end bulb via the cytoplasm. When an action potential arrives at an end bulb of a presynaptic neuron, an influx of calcium ions from the bathing

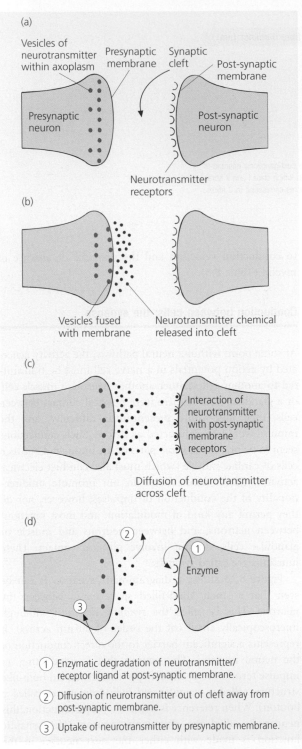

(a)

Vesicles of neurotransmitter within axoplasm

Presynaptic membrane

Synaptic cleft

Post-synaptic membrane

Presynaptic neuron

Post-synaptic neuron

Neurotransmitter receptors

(b)

Vesicles fused with membrane

Neurotransmitter chemical released into cleft

(c)

Interaction of neurotransmitter with post-synaptic membrane receptors

Diffusion of neurotransmitter across cleft

(d)

②

①

Enzyme

③

① Enzymatic degradation of neurotransmitter/ receptor ligand at post-synaptic membrane.

② Diffusion of neurotransmitter out of cleft away from post-synaptic membrane.

③ Uptake of neurotransmitter by presynaptic membrane.

Figure 8.23 The synapse and mode of activation. (a) Resting synapse. (b) Arrival of action potentials at the (presynaptic) membrane. (c) Activation of the post-synaptic membrane. (d) Restoration of the resting state.

Q. *What is the role of the neurotransmitter chemical?*

interstitial fluid occurs, which causes a few of the vesicles to move to the membrane (i.e. to the presynaptic membrane) and release their contents into the synaptic cleft (Figure 8.23). Molecules of the chemical then diffuse

across the cleft and interact with receptor molecules on the surface of the post-synaptic membrane. This interaction between chemical and receptor induces changes in the ionic permeability of the post-synaptic membrane, and hence in its membrane potential; collectively, these chemicals are therefore called *neurotransmitters*.

Having interacted with post-synaptic receptors, the neurotransmitter is removed by the actions of enzymes, which leaves the receptors free to interact with further chemicals should they be released from the presynaptic membrane. Excess neurotransmitter within the cleft either diffuses out of the synapse into the interstitial fluid, or is actively transported back into the presynaptic neuron.

The requirement of the presynaptic release of neurotransmitter also helps to ensure unidirectionality of neural pathways.

Excitatory and inhibitory synapses

The release of small amounts of a neurotransmitter from a single presynaptic end bulb does not produce an action potential in the post-synaptic neuron. It does cause slight change in the resting membrane potential, however, as sodium channels begin to open, and so brings the membrane potential close to that of threshold. This slight depolarization is called an *excitatory post-synaptic potential* (EPSP).

Although it does not trigger an action potential itself, the EPSP makes the membrane more easily stimulated, so should further neurotransmitter release occur, then the individual EPSPs that are generated may summate to reach threshold and trigger an action potential. This action potential will be propagated along the post-synaptic cell, as described earlier.

In practice, EPSPs last for only a few milliseconds, so summation will occur only if several adjacent end bulbs are activated more or less simultaneously (called spatial summation). Alternatively, the same synapse may be activated a few times in quick succession by the arrival of a train of impulses (called temporal summation). The whole process is highly complex, but it has a big advantage: nerve cells sporadically produce action potentials, perhaps because the local environment has been disturbed temporarily or because mechanical movement of the cell membrane activates it. These sporadic potentials will pass along the nerve axon but will not induce sufficient depolarization of the next cell within the pathway, so tissues, including the brain, do not receive what would otherwise be confusing messages.

Exercise

The concept of summating the minute changes in voltage means that sporadic occurrences are unlikely to cause the membrane to reach threshold, and hence the generation of an impulse. Refer to Figure 8.21, and review the ion changes and electrical variation that occur when a nerve cell is stimulated.

The picture presented so far is one of excitation: neurotransmitter excites the post-synaptic cell membrane and triggers another nerve impulse. The problem with this is that it means that pathways will always be excited when a nerve cell is stimulated. Flexibility to enable the nervous system to allow a pathway to be active or inactive is facilitated by the involvement of synapses that are inhibitory.

In inhibitory synapses, the release of small amounts of a neurotransmitter from a single synaptic end bulb causes a slight hyperpolarization of the post-synaptic membrane, rather than depolarization. This occurs because potassium channels and/or chloride channels open partly, and so promote either an efflux of positive charge out of the cell, or an influx of negative charge, respectively (remember that the gradient for potassium favours diffusion out of the cell, while that for chloride favours diffusion into it; both situations therefore increase the negativity of the inside of the cell with respect to the outside). The slight hyperpolarization produced is called an *inhibitory post-synaptic potential* (IPSP), and it can summate with other IPSPs to enhance the hyperpolarization. By causing the membrane potential to move further away from the threshold value, IPSPs make the membrane less responsive to excitatory potentials from other interacting nerve cells. Sufficient IPSPs make the membrane unresponsive under physiological conditions, i.e. 'switch off' the synapse.

Neurotransmitters that cause depolarization of the post-synaptic membrane, and therefore promote the forward continuation of the nerve impulse, are referred to as *excitatory neurotransmitters*. Those that induce hyperpolarization are called *inhibitory neurotransmitters*. Inhibitory synapses generally act in one of the following ways:

- Preventing the actions of the neurotransmitter from the end bulb of an excitatory neuron so that an action potential is not produced in the post-synaptic cell has a stabilizing effect on the post-synaptic membrane, and is therefore called *post-synaptic inhibition*. The means of membrane stabilization is much the same as described above, but note that only the actions – and not the release – of neurotransmitter are affected in this process (Figure 8.24(a)).

- Preventing depolarization of the end bulb of an excitatory presynaptic neuron, and thus effectively preventing the release of the excitatory neurotransmitter, is called *presynaptic inhibition*. This is the process described above. It seems to be the most common process (Figure 8.24(b)).

A variety of excitatory and inhibitory neurotransmitters have been identified (Table 8.4). Importantly, any presynaptic neuron can produce only one type of transmitter substance, hence the neuron will act only in an excitatory or an inhibitory fashion; it cannot do both. The neurotransmitter chemical produced also determines

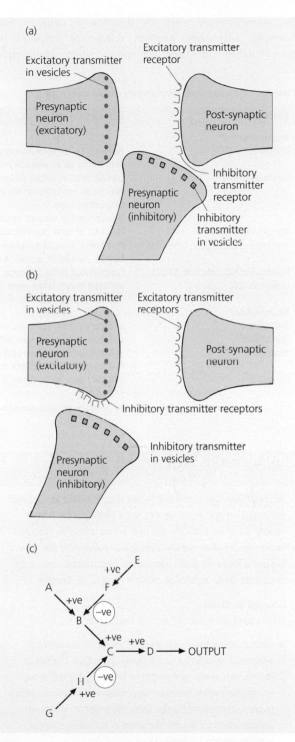

Figure 8.24 Inhibition of synapses, and its role in integrative responses. (a) Post-synaptic inhibition, in which the membrane is stabilized by the inhibitory neurotransmitter and so prevents generation of an action potential. (b) Presynaptic inhibition, in which the inhibitory neurotransmitter stabilizes the presynaptic neuron and prevents it from releasing its neurotransmitter. (c) Schematic integration. A – G are neurons. Note how activity from D will depend on the presence or absence of inhibitory influences from neurons F and H. In this way, output from D may be modulated according to the balance between the activation of neurons A, E and G.

Q. What is the role of inhibitory neurons?

the nomenclature used to describe a neuron. For example, adrenergic neurons release or respond to noradrenaline at their synapses, while cholinergic neurons produce acetylcholine. Similarly, drugs that mimic these chemicals are referred to as adrenergic or cholinergic drugs.

Table 8.4 Examples of neurotransmitters and neuropeptides

Substance	Homeostatic actions
Neurotransmitters	
Acetylcholine (ACh)	Released by some neuromuscular and neuroglandular synapses, and at neuronal synapses in the CNS
	Acts mainly as an excitatory neurotransmitter, but also has inhibitory functions
Serotonin (5-HT)	Concentrated in certain neurons in the brainstem
	Acts as an excitatory neurotransmitter
	May induce sleep
	Also involved in sensory perception, temperature regulation, and control of mood
Noradrenaline (NA)	Released at some neuromuscular and neuroglandular synapses
	Also found in neural synapses of the brainstem: mainly excitatory
	May be involved in arousal, dreaming, and regulation of mood
Gamma-aminobutyric acid (GABA)	Concentrated in the thalamus, hypothalamus, and occipital lobes of cerebrum; mainly inhibitory
Dopamine (DA)	Inhibitory in substantia nigra of midbrain
	Involved in emotional responses and subconscious movements of skeletal muscles
*Neuropeptides**	
Substance P	Excitatory in pain pathways within central nervous system (see Chapter 21)
Enkephalins	Inhibitory in pain pathways within the thalamus and spinal cord
Endorphins	Inhibitory (see Enkephalins) especially within the midbrain
	May have a role in memory and learning
Dynorphin	Inhibitory (see Enkephalins); 50 times more powerful than beta-endorphin

*Neuropeptides are neurotransmitters, but some are also neuromodulators that are produced elsewhere but will interact with the synapse where they are also found.

BOX 8.16 DETERIORATION IN CONDUCTION VELOCITY OF NEURONS

Reflex responses to stimuli will be depressed if conduction in those spinal neurons involved is reduced, but a slowing of conduction velocity within the brain will also have severe effects on integrated neural circuitry. Reductions in conduction velocity, or in the extreme a failure for action potentials to be conducted at all, arise because of either neuronal problems or synaptic dysfunction.

Neuronal problems

Some causes of reduced conduction velocity are:

● deterioration of the myelin sheath of axons, as in multiple sclerosis. This condition is still poorly understood. The rate of deterioration of myelin seems to be slowed by the use of anti-inflammatory drugs that slow the development of sclerotic (scar) tissue in demyelinated areas. Corrective treatment is not yet possible, and care is generally aimed at facilitating maximal possible function (Campion, 1997);

● hypothermia, which can reduce conduction velocity via its slowing effect on the generation of action potentials;

● a peripheral inflammatory demyelinating disease, such as the cause of Guillain–Barré syndrome. Motor dysfunction causes muscle weakness. Conversely, sensory activity may actually be enhanced in Guillain–Barré syndrome, presumably as a consequence of altered receptor sensitivity, with the patient experiencing heightened cutaneous sensation of pain, temperature and touch. This condition usually reverses, and care is directed at supporting the patient, with life support if necessary, until recovery occurs. Extensive rehabilitation is usually necessary (McMahon-Parkes and Cornock, 1997; Worsham, 2000).

Synaptic dysfunction

Synaptic function involves the synthesis and secretion of neurotransmitters, their interaction with receptors on the post-synaptic membrane, removal of excess transmitter chemical, and degradation of the chemical/receptor ligand so that the receptor is free to interact with more chemical when released. Errors can occur at all stages of the process. Myasthenia gravis is a condition in which muscle weakness occurs because of a defect at the neuromuscular synapse, probably because of a shortage of available post-synaptic receptors to the neurotransmitter acetylcholine, or because of an excess of acetylcholinesterase, the enzyme that removes acetylcholine from the post-synaptic receptors.

Parkinson's disease and Huntington's disease are disorders characterized, at least in early stages, by disorders of movement control. They are caused primarily by a deficiency in the neurotransmitters dopamine and gamma-aminobutyric acid (GABA), respectively, from certain neurons of the brain (see Chapter 17).

Correction of synaptic dysfunction is aimed at restoring the missing transmitter (see Box 8.17) or by prolonging the actions of the transmitter that is released, as in the administration of acetylcholinesterase inhibitors to myasthenia gravis patients.

Integrated functions

Synaptic integration

Neurons, especially those within the central nervous system, may synapse with more than one other neuron. Thus, a cell body of a brain cell may be influenced by synapses from several thousand others; some of these synapses will be excitatory, others inhibitory. Whether or not the post-synaptic membrane of the cell is stimulated depends on the balance between the summated excitatory and inhibitory synapses that are active at that particular time. Thus, a powerful input from inhibitory synapses might prevent the summation of EPSPs, and so prevent the depolarization of the post-synaptic membrane from attaining the threshold potential.

The importance of synaptic integration is that one neural pathway can be modulated by others. This is shown simplistically in Figure 8.24(c). In other words, the 'opening' and 'closing' of neural circuits forms the basis of neural processing in the central nervous system. Severe disorders can result if excitatory or inhibitory pathways are activated abnormally (Box 8.17).

Spinal reflexes as an example of integration

Reflexes are responses that do not involve extensive integration of activity by the brain for their initiation. The main advantage of having reflex neural pathways is that responses to sensory stimulation can occur much more rapidly than they would if processing by the brain was involved. The process is illustrated by the withdrawal reflex of a limb in response to pain (Figure 8.25).

Limb withdrawal requires contraction of the muscles that, when stimulated, move the limb away from the stimulus. For example, standing on a tack stimulates pain receptors at the puncture site, and the afferent activity passes to the spinal cord. Here, the afferent neuron

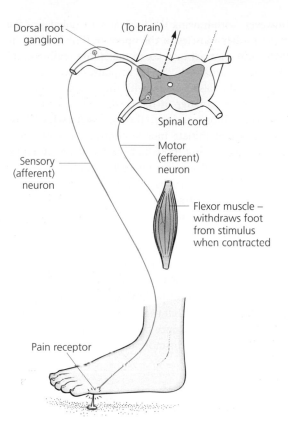

Figure 8.25 A simple monosynaptic reflex arc in response to a painful stimulus. Note that the brain is not involved, although neural information will be transmitted to the brain to keep it informed of the new limb positioning. The full response will be more complex, since other muscles will also be affected by the response (see also Figure 17.14).

synapses directly within the anterior horn of grey matter with the appropriate motor neuron that, when activated, causes the appropriate muscle to contract (Figure 8.25). This is a simple example of a *monosynaptic reflex arc*, i.e. the whole neural pathway has only one synapse, and thus only two neurons – one sensory and one motor – are involved. The neurotransmitter that is released in the synapse will be excitatory.

BOX 8.17 IMPORTANCE OF MAINTAINING A BALANCE BETWEEN INHIBITORY AND EXCITATORY NEUROTRANSMITTERS

Since the output from neurons within processing areas of the brain is determined by the net effects of excitatory and inhibitory inputs during the integration of nerve cell activities, a disturbance in one or other can have drastic effects on brain function. For example, the movement disorders of Parkinson's disease (see Chapter 17) result at least partially from the lack of the inhibitory transmitter dopamine, leading to excessive expression of excitatory pathways (producing the characteristic tremor). Correction is aimed at restoring the balance. Thus, levodopa (a precursor to dopamine) may be administered to people with Parkinson's

disease to replace the missing dopamine, or an anticholinergic drug may be used to reduce the activity of acetylcholine in the excitatory pathway.

Another example, which cannot at present be corrected in this way, is epilepsy. In this disorder, neural activity within the cerebral cortex seems to radiate out from a point to produce foci of intense activity (Moshé, 2000) that causes loss of consciousness and muscle contractions typical of fitting. Support, and help with prevention of episodes, are the main aims of care (Splevings, 2000).

However, withdrawing the limb acts to unbalance the body, and other muscles in the opposite limb and in the back will also contract or relax so that some semblance of balance is maintained. Such responses will involve interneurons that also synapse with the sensory neuron as it enters the grey matter of the cord. These in turn will synapse with motor neurons to these other muscles. Those interneurons that initiate muscle contraction will utilize excitatory synapses, but those that cause muscle relaxation will 'switch off' basal activity in the relevant motor neurons by utilizing inhibitory synapses. In this way, an integrated pattern of muscle contraction/relaxation is produced. The pattern may change quickly as other reflexes operate (called stretch reflexes); these are considered further in Chapter 17.

Note that the brain is not involved in the initial response, although information regarding the stimulus and the change in position of the limb will be transmitted to it. The role of the withdrawal reflex in homeostasis is evident in this example, since failure to withdraw the limb could potentially result in more damage to the tissues of the foot.

Examples of cerebral neural integration

The brain has an extensive role in the control of tissue and organ functions within the body, via the autonomic nervous system, the hypothalamic-pituitary gland axis, and the mediation of skeletal muscle contraction. These functions are dealt with later in Chapters 9 and 17, and this section will only concentrate on some of the brain's cognitive functions. The aim is to present, albeit simplistically, an overview of such functions, the intention being to emphasize the necessity of integrating the activity from various areas of the brain. Much of the physiology of cognitive function is still unknown, and in some instances insight has been gained only in recent years. What constitutes 'consciousness', however, remains an enigma: a physiological basis has not been ascertained. This is a complicated topic; readers interested in the subject are recommended to read the more 'popular' works of Susan Greenfield, especially Greenfield (2000).

Sleep

The electrical activity of the cortex undergoes four distinct phases during sleep, as shown in Table 8.5. The first two stages are characterized by irregular waveforms associated with shallow sleep or consciousness, but the 'deep' sleep of stage 3 is characterized by the occurrence of synchronized patterns of activity with a slow frequency, and so is called slow-wave sleep. The fourth stage is characterized by alternation between slow waves and patterns of activity reminiscent of stages 1 and 2. Such patterns produce changes in heart and breathing rates, and rapid eye movements are observed (stage 4 is called rapid eye movement (REM) sleep), while generally there is a pronounced muscular paralysis. Dreaming occurs in this stage, and it seems to relate to bursts of electrical activity passing from the pons of the brainstem to the visual cortex of the occipital lobe. Evidence suggests that sleep (especially stages 3 and 4) is a period during which information is sifted and its emotional impact assessed (Fox, 1999). Memory is updated accordingly.

Arousal is associated with increased activity in areas of the reticular formation within the upper pons and midbrain regions (Figure 8.14). The pathways utilize noradrenaline as an excitatory neurotransmitter, and the activity radiates to the thalamus, hypothalamus, cerebral cortex and other parts of the hindbrain (Figure 8.26). Sleep arises when activity from the reticular formation is inhibited.

BOX 8.18 NEURAL INTEGRATION AND SENSORIMOTOR DEVELOPMENT

It is thought that most neurons that the brain will have are present at birth. Thus, brain growth during childhood results from a proliferation of non-neuronal cells (the neuroglial cells) and the growth of processes from the neurons themselves. The latter establish communication links with neurons in the vicinity or at a distance. Much of the gross plan of the brain is established during fetal development, when axon growth is directed to appropriate areas by a 'scaffolding' of glial cells and by chemical attractants. Such connections are essential to the development of the circuitry of the brain, and it is their integrative functions that determine brain activities. Thyroid hormones are essential for this functional development of the brain in the fetus and early childhood, particularly in relation to cognitive functions.

Motor and sensory functions mature faster than cognitive functions, such as those of memory and reasoning. Early sensorimotor development is essential if the child is to be able to assume an upright posture, to walk, to acquire speech, and to gain voluntary control of urinary and anal sphincters. Autonomic efficiency will also increase, leading to better homeostatic regulation and improved physical performance. Fine motor skills therefore take time to become established.

The formation of synaptic connections between neurons is facilitated by reinforcement of their activities. Accordingly, physical activity, play and other primary and secondary socialization processes promote both sensorimotor and cognitive development. This increases the complexity of activities performed, which in turn facilitate further neural development. Readers are referred to Sheridan (1997) for an account of developmental changes.

Table 8.5 Electroencephalogram (EEG) patterns in (a) levels of consciousness and (b) stages of sleep

(a) Levels of consciousness

Wave	Frequency (cycles/s) of EEG waves	State of consciousness
Alpha (α)	8–23	Awake but quiet
Beta (β)	14–25	Awake but tense (note waves are asynchronous during normal increase in mental activity)
Theta (θ)	4–7	Emotional stress
Delta (δ)	< 3.5	Deep sleep, or anaesthesia (slow wave)

(b) Sleep stages

Sleep stage	Observed EEG
1	Low-voltage wave interrupted periodically by bursts of α-waves
2/3	Progressive decline to 2–3 cycles/s, i.e. δ-waves
4 (REM)	Bursts of desynchronized β-waves similar to those in wakefulness; lasts for 5–30 min, recurring approximately every 90 min

REM, rapid eye movement sleep, or paradoxical sleep.

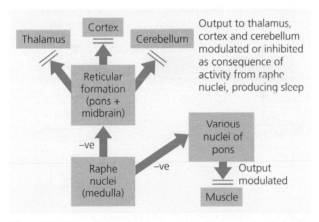

Figure 8.26 Interactions between structures of the brainstem during slow-wave sleep.

Q. *What would happen if the raphe nuclei were inhibited (i.e. 'switched off'')?*

Slow-wave sleep seems to involve an inhibitory action of nuclei within the medulla oblongata, particularly the raphe nuclei, via neurons that utilize the inhibitory transmitter serotonin. REM sleep, which includes a degree of cortical excitation, seems to involve noradrenergic neurons from the reticular formation, and also excitatory cholinergic neurons from various other nuclei within the pons. The latter are probably inhibited during slow-wave sleep, but the inhibition is modulated during REM sleep. The nuclei of the pons also seem to be responsible for the inhibition of spinal cord motor neurons (causing paralysis) during REM sleep (note that acetylcholine is excitatory, therefore the neurons must synapse with other inhibitory neurons for this effect to occur).

Sleep and wakening is an important biological rhythm that also appears to be associated with the suprachiasmatic nuclei of the hypothalamus (i.e. nuclei located above the chiasma, the 'cross-over' of optic nerve pathways; see Chapter 23). Neurons from this area pass to the brainstem and cortex and modulate the activities of the various brainstem nuclei. Although these nuclei can be said to induce sleep or wakefulness, it is less clear what regulates sleep. The presence of sleep-inducing substances released into the cerebrospinal fluid has been implicated, but their role remains debatable. What is clear is that the pattern of sleep changes through adulthood, and time spent in slow-wave sleep decreases (Van Cauter *et al.*, 2000).

Memory

Memory (see Markowitsch, 1998) is considered to consist of short- and long-term components. Short-term memory has a duration of several seconds or a few minutes at most, and has limited volume. Short-term memory can be converted into long-term memory by consolidation of the information.

Learning can be perceptual (visual), stimulus-response conditioning (an association between two stimuli), or relational (an association between two events). Perceptual learning utilizes the visual association area of the temporal lobe of the cortex, whilst conditional learning involves the amygdala nuclei of the limbic system, which seems to act as a mediator between sensory inputs and behavioural responses. The amygdala, however, has a complex circuitry and receives inputs from various parts of the brain, whilst neurons pass from it to the autonomic nuclei of the brainstem, and to the hypothalamus. Some areas of the cerebellum also appear to be involved in conditional learning.

Relational learning involves the hippocampus of the limbic system, which consolidates short-term memories. Various nuclei of the thalamus are also involved in the process, and also in the recall of information from long-term stores. Memory also involves the area of cerebral cortex called the limbic cortex.

Short-term memory seems to be associated with the persistent excitability of neurons within the cortex. Such changes seem to reverberate within neuronal circuits, the oscillation of activity remaining for perhaps several minutes before declining. Long-term memory is not associated with persistent neural activity, however. Experimental evidence suggests that the numbers of synaptic connections are increased, and that individual synapses are sensitized or primed so that they are more likely to be stimulated should similar sensory information arrive at a later date.

Acetylcholine is an important excitatory neurotransmitter of memory circuits within the hippocampus and the limbic cortex. Dopamine is also involved (probably as an inhibitory transmitter) in areas of the limbic cortex, whilst endogenous inhibitory or excitatory opiates are important in the amygdala. The complexity of memory is such, however, that various other neurotransmitters have also been implicated, which is evidence of complex, multiple neuronal circuits.

Speech and language

Areas of the left hemisphere dominate in the comprehension of language and the production of speech (Kent 2000). This seems to be most appropriate considering the general 'analytical' properties of that hemisphere. The right hemisphere includes cortical areas involved in the understanding of the meaning of words, and also applies emotional overtones to the voice.

Comprehension of speech begins within the auditory pathways, particularly in *Wernicke's area* of the auditory cortex in the superior aspect of the left temporal lobe (Figure 8.27). In contrast, speech is synthesized in a cortical area of the left frontal lobe, called *Broca's area*. Broca's area lies adjacent to the motor cortex responsible for producing movement of the tongue, lips and larynx in the

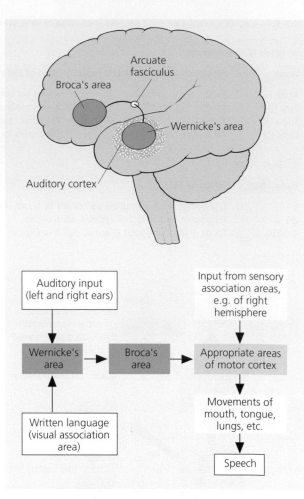

Figure 8.27 Speech areas of the left hemisphere.
Q. What might be the consequences of trauma to Broca's area?

enunciation of speech. It is thought that Wernicke's area in some way contains memories of the features of auditory sounds, turning them into words, whilst Broca's area contains memories of the motor output required to verbalize words. Neurons from Wernicke's area project to Broca's area via a tract of nerve fibres called the *arcuate fasciculus*.

The 'meaning' of words is stored within parts of the sensory association cortex, and the motivation to speak is supplied by areas of the motor cortex.

Emotional behaviours

'Behaviours' are diverse functions of the brain, but some generalizations can be made regarding the role of the limbic system. Thus, the amygdala nuclei convey a behavioural awareness and ensure that patterns of response are appropriate to an individual's situation. Different areas of the hippocampus are involved in different emotions, such as rage and passivity, and the limbic cortex appears to provide the association required between activity passing to and from various areas of cerebral cortex and the rest of the limbic system.

Aggressive behaviours especially involve medial (offensive behaviour) and dorsal (defensive behaviour) areas of the hypothalamus. Both project to the midbrain for expression. The amygdala is also involved, and neurons pass from here to the hypothalamus and midbrain. Interestingly, the amygdala responds to the presence of sex steroids, suggesting a role in sexual aggression.

Sexual behaviour involves various areas. The area of the basal forebrain lying anterior to the chiasma of the optic nerves determines copulatory behaviour and territorial aggression in males, and maternal behaviour in females. The ventromedial nuclei of the hypothalamus determine copulatory behaviour in females. Sexual behaviours are modulated by areas of the limbic cortex.

BOX 8.20 NEUROTRANSMITTERS AND MOOD STATES: DEPRESSION

Clinical depression is a mood disorder (or group of disorders) that seems to involve an imbalance of excitatory and inhibitory neurotransmission in certain parts of the brain (frontal lobe, limbic system, hypothalamus). Various neural pathways are involved, as evidenced by the range of drugs available:

● Serotonin (5-HT) agonists (e.g. fluoxetine or Prozac) stimulate the receptors to this excitatory neurotransmitter.

● Tricyclic antidepressants promote release of the excitatory neurotransmitter noradrenaline in adrenergic synapses.
● Monoamine oxidase inhibitors inhibit the breakdown of noradrenaline and therefore prolong its concentration in the synaptic cleft.
● Lithium enhances the release of serotonin (excitatory).

THE AUTONOMIC NERVOUS SYSTEM

The autonomic nervous system is the part of the nervous system that mediates the functioning of most organs of the body. It therefore has a dominant role in the homeostatic control of the internal environment. For this reason it is included here as a separate major subsection.

Anatomical organization of the autonomic nervous system

Exercise

Review the overview section at the beginning of this chapter on the general organization of the nervous system before commencing this section.

The autonomic nervous system is comprised of both central and peripheral elements. It is especially involved in the involuntary control of organs and tissues. Like other peripheral nerves, the nerves of this system are comprised of afferent (sensory) and efferent (motor) nerve cells. Earlier in this chapter we noted that the term 'motor' is used to convey an impression of promoting activity, especially in muscle cells. The term has to be used more broadly for the autonomic nerves because some will stimulate the target tissue when they are activated, but others will inhibit it. For example, autonomic nerves to the heart may increase heart rate, while others decrease it, and some nerves increase gut motility while others decrease it. In this way, tissue functioning can be enhanced or reduced by autonomic nerves according to the situation, which provides the level of flexibility that is required to maintain homeostasis.

An individual autonomic nerve, or nerve cell, will either increase or decrease the activity of tissue cells; it does not do both. If tissues are to be activated or deactivated according to circumstances, then different nerves/nerve cells must be present. Accordingly, the autonomic nervous system can be subdivided into the *sympathetic* and *parasympathetic* divisions (Figure 8.28), which usually act in a complementary way in various homeostatic control processes (Figure 8.29). There is no hard and fast rule as to which subdivision does what. In some instances, sympathetic nerves act to stimulate a tissue, and parasympathetic nerves inhibit it, while in other instances the reverse is true.

Parasympathetic division

The general layout of the nerves of the parasympathetic system is relatively straightforward. Basically it consists of the vagus nerve (cranial nerve X), neurons of various other cranial nerves, and nerves that originate from the sacral (lower back) region of the spinal cord (Figures 8.28 and 8.29). This is why this system is sometimes termed the *craniosacral* division.

As mentioned earlier, the vagus nerve passes from the brainstem, down through the thorax and abdomen, sending branches to various viscera as it goes along. The parasympathetic functions of the vagus and other cranial nerves are summarized in Table 8.1. The sacral nerves help to control lower abdominal functions such as micturition and defecation.

The layout of the parasympathetic division is actually slightly more complicated than this because the nerves

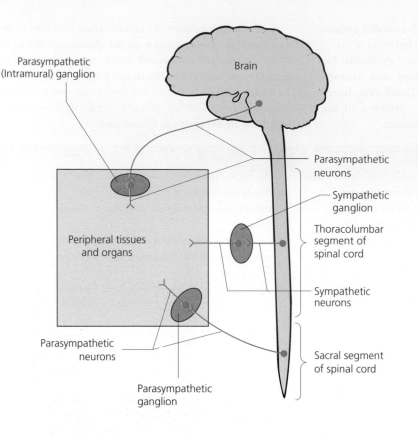

Figure 8.28 General organization of the autonomic nervous system.

Brain

Parasympathetic
(Intramural) ganglion

Parasympathetic
neurons

Sympathetic
ganglion

Thoracolumbar
segment of
spinal cord

Peripheral tissues
and organs

Sympathetic
neurons

Parasympathetic
neurons

Sacral segment
of spinal cord

Parasympathetic
ganglion

first synapse with shorter efferent nerves, which then interact with the target tissue. The aggregated cell bodies of these latter nerves form the intramural ganglia (Figure 8.28), which are usually found very close to (or even within) the tissues served by the nerves. The nerve cell axons leading from the cord to these ganglia are therefore usually referred to as preganglionic fibres, while the shorter ones from the ganglia to the target cells are post-ganglionic. These terms are used especially in pharmacology texts in relation to the actions of the neurotransmitters (see later).

Within the central nervous system, parasympathetic neurons synapse with cell neurons in various nuclei, which are also in communication with sensory areas of the cortex, the thalamus and hypothalamus, and other nuclei of the brainstem. The sacral nerves must also have projections along the spinal cord to and from the brain.

Sympathetic division

The anatomy of the sympathetic division can appear to be much more complex than that of the parasympathetic division (Figure 8.29). Sympathetic nerves leave the spinal cord (via the usual spinal nerve roots) at regular intervals between the sixth cervical and second lumbar vertebrae, hence the term 'cervicolumbar division' is sometimes used. The sympathetic nerves soon dissociate from the spinal nerves, however, and short nerves (containing preganglionic fibres) run to the sympathetic ganglia, which form

a chain alongside the vertebral column (Figures 8.29 and 8.30). The post-ganglionic neurons are generally much longer and extend from synapses within these ganglia to the target tissues. Modifications of this layout of sympathetic ganglia occur, however. For example, the *coeliac ganglion* lies some distance from the cord (Figure 8.29). This ganglion actually involves synapses from a number of sympathetic nerves from the cord, and is commonly called the solar plexus.

Within the central nervous system, the sympathetic division involves nerve cells that ascend or descend the spinal cord, and also includes various nuclei within the brain. As with the parasympathetic system, connections within the hypothalamus and brainstem are particularly important in sympathetic functions.

Summary of the physiology of the autonomic nervous system

The details of the functions of the sympathetic and parasympathetic divisions are outlined in Table 8.6, and the specific roles of autonomic nerves in regulating the functions of organs and organ systems are highlighted in the relevant chapters. The question as to which division is responsible for exciting a tissue is very much related to the situation under which they are activated. For example, exercise has a marked stimulatory effect on the sympathetic division (producing the 'fright/flight/fight' responses), and so is responsible for promoting responses

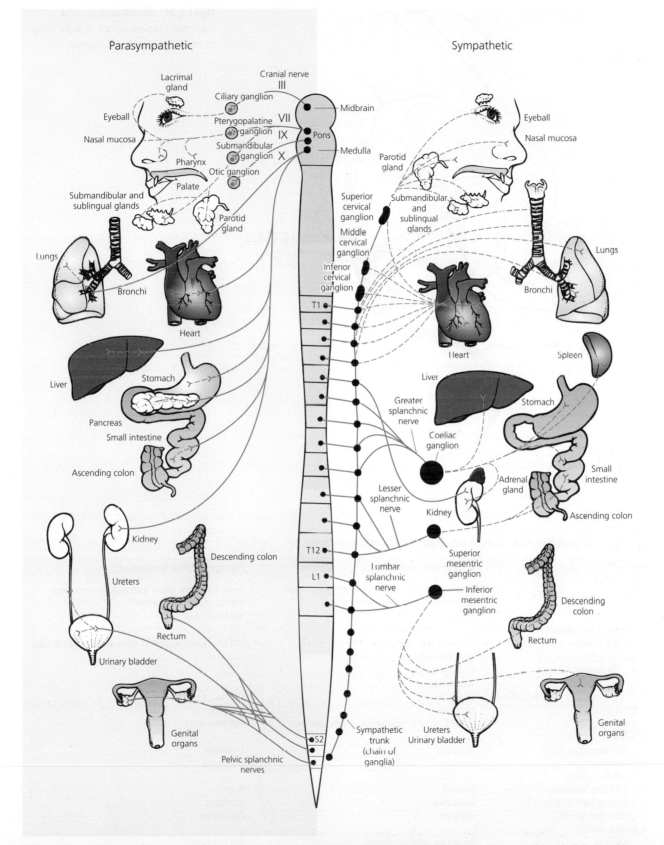

Figure 8.29 Innervation of the viscera by the autonomic nervous system. Although the parasympathetic division is shown only on the left side of the figure, and the sympathetic on the right, keep in mind that each division is found on both sides of the body. Solid lines = preganglionic neurons from the spinal cord to the peripheral ganglia; dotted lines = post-ganglionic neurons from the ganglia to the tissue cells.

Q. What is the advantage of having organs supplied with both parasympathetic and sympathetic nerves?

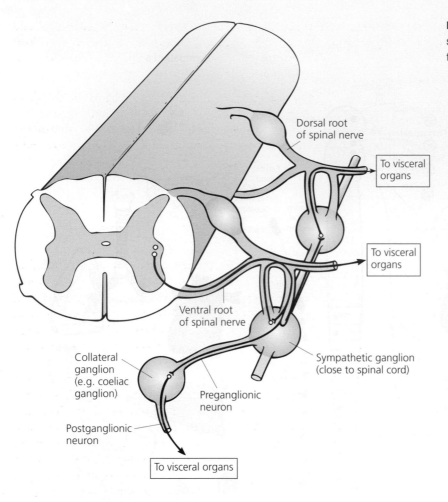

Figure 8.30 Efferent neurons of the sympathetic nervous system. Note the 'relay' function of the sympathetic ganglia.

Dorsal root of spinal nerve

To visceral organs

To visceral organs

Ventral root of spinal nerve

Sympathetic ganglion (close to spinal cord)

Collateral ganglion (e.g. coeliac ganglion)

Preganglionic neuron

Postganglionic neuron

To visceral organs

Table 8.6 Comparison of the sympathetic and parasympathetic nervous systems

Structure	Sympathetic innervation	Parasympathetic innervation
Eye	Dilates pupil; accommodation for distance vision	Constricts pupil; accommodation for near vision
Salivary glands	Concentrated secretion stimulated	Watery secretion stimulated
Sweat glands	Increased secretion	Not innervated
Cardiovascular system		
Blood vessels		Not innervated, except in penis and clitoris: dilation
To skin	Vasoconstriction	
To skeletal muscles	Vasodilation	
To digestive viscera	Vasoconstriction	
Heart, rate and force of contraction	Increases	Decreases rate
Blood pressure	Increases	Decreases*
Adrenal gland	Medulla secretes adrenaline + noradrenaline	Not innervated
Respiratory system		
Diameter of airways	Increases	Decreases
Respiratory rate	Increases	Decreases
Digestive system		
Sphincter muscles	Contract	Relax
General level of activity	Decreases	Increases
Secretory glands	Inhibited	Stimulated
Urinary system		
Kidneys	Decreases urine production	Not innervated
Bladder	Relaxes muscle of bladder, contracts internal sphincter	Contracts bladder muscle, relaxes internal sphincter
Male reproductive system	Increases glandular secretion; ejaculation	Erection through action on blood vessel

*Indirect effect as consequence of actions on heart rate.

that facilitate physical activity, e.g. cycling. Thus, changes in sympathetic nerve activity promote the following *excitatory* responses:

- Cardiac output is raised by increasing the heart rate and force of contraction.

- An initial vasodilation of muscles is induced to raise blood flow through them (although metabolic factors then become more important in this respect).

- Arterial blood pressure is maintained despite pronounced muscle vasodilation, by inducing vasoconstriction in various other tissues.

- Peripheral vision is enhanced by inducing dilation of the pupils.

- Excess heat produced by the raised metabolic rate is removed by stimulating sweat secretion.

- Glycogen stores in the liver and muscle are broken down to provide more glucose as fuel.

- Somatic nerve excitability is enhanced, thus speeding up reflexes and promoting more rapid movements.

In contrast, exercise is also facilitated through the actions of sympathetic nerves to *inhibit*:

- the motility and secretory activity of the gut (which is appropriate in view of the concurrent vasoconstriction in the gut);

- smooth muscle tone in the airways (bronchodilation then occurs, which facilitates lung ventilation).

The net effect of the responses of various systems is to maintain cellular homeostasis within the active muscles.

Exercise

Refer to the actions of adrenaline identified in Chapters 9 and 22, and compare these with the actions noted here of the sympathetic nervous system. Note the similarity. Why is this? You might refer to Table 8.6 for further help.

How quickly would the sympathetic nervous system change tissue functions? How long would adrenaline take to do likewise? Refer to the introduction in Chapter 9, which compares nervous and hormonal properties.

The parasympathetic division tends to be activated in response to emotional experiences. For example:

- contemplating the eating of food raises activity in the vagus nerve and induces gastric acid secretion and increases gut motility;

- relaxation therapy (which also reduces sympathetic activity) causes heart rate to decrease through stimulation of appropriate neurons within the vagus nerve;

- emotional shock promotes bronchoconstriction and may even inhibit the heart to the extent that blood pressure falls and fainting occurs, as a consequence of cerebral ischaemia;

- sexual stimulation induces vasodilation in the penis (male) or clitoris (female); these actions represent the main example of a direct effect of the parasympathetic nervous system on blood vessels (in contrast to sympathetic nerves, which have a pronounced effect on blood vessels within many tissues).

Neurotransmitters of the autonomic system

The principle of a single nerve cell being capable of producing only one particular transmitter is applicable also to the autonomic nervous system. The examples of autonomic actions described in the previous section indicate that the neurotransmitters can have either excitatory or inhibitory effects on tissues, depending upon the tissue.

The nerve endings of post-ganglionic neurons of the sympathetic nervous system release noradrenaline, which interacts with receptors on the membrane of cells within the target tissue (the hormone adrenaline, released when sympathetic nerves to the adrenal gland are stimulated, may also act on these receptors; Figure 8.31). Whether the response that ensues is stimulatory or inhibitory is determined by the type of receptor that is present. Receptor subtypes, classified as alpha and beta receptors, will be present in appropriate tissues (see Box 8.21). In addition, some sympathetic nerve cells release other transmitter chemicals that are related to noradrenaline, called dopamine and serotonin, which interact with their own receptors (of which there are further subtypes, e.g. dopamine receptors are referred to as D_1, D_2 or D_3 receptors). The interest in dopamine and serotonin is focused more on its actions as a central neurotransmitter, rather than its actions peripherally in the autonomic nervous system. Thus, D_1 and D_2 receptors are found in nerve terminals of the striatum, a collection of neural tissue that includes the cerebral nuclei called the caudate nucleus and the putamen. The terminals extend from the nucleus called the substantia nigra, and comprise what is referred to as the nigrostriatal pathway. The terminals secrete dopamine; disorders here, primarily of the D_1 receptor to the neurotransmitter, are implicated in Parkinson's disease. D_3 is of interest in relation to the actions of dopamine within the limbic system, especially in connection with schizophrenia, although this is a debatable area.

Post-ganglionic nerve cells within the parasympathetic division release acetylcholine. Receptor subtypes to this neurotransmitter, called muscarinic and nicotinic receptors, exist for this substance. Just to confuse matters,

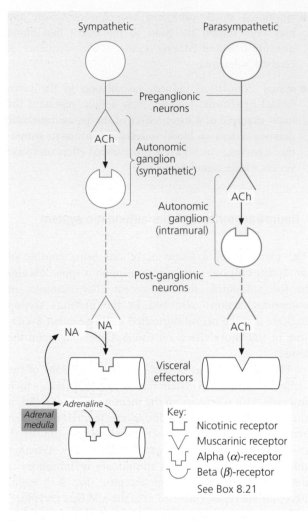

Figure 8.31 Neurotransmitters of the sympathetic and parasympathetic branches of the autonomic nervous system. NA, noradrenaline, ACh, acetylcholine.

Q. Which neurotransmitter is produced by the preganglionic neurons?

Q. Which neurotransmitters are produced by the post-ganglionic neurons?

acetylcholine is also the neurotransmitter released by preganglionic nerve cells within the sympathetic ganglia (Figure 8.31). Here, acetylcholine and drugs (e.g. nicotine) that act on nicotinic receptors for acetylcholine may provoke some sympathetic activities, such as a faster heartbeat.

BOX 8.21 AUTONOMIC NERVOUS SYSTEM: RECEPTORS AND DRUGS

Drugs acting on the autonomic nervous system are classed as adrenergic or cholinergic drugs according to the receptors that are activated or inhibited. Such receptors are those to the catecholamines (adrenaline, noradrenaline) and acetylcholine, respectively. Similar receptors are also found within the central nervous system, since both groups of chemicals also act as neurotransmitters there. Each category includes receptor subtypes according to subtle variations in the molecular structure of the receptor. Drugs have been developed that interact predominantly with one or other subtype, acting as agonists (i.e. activate the receptor) or as antagonists (i.e. no activation of the receptor, and receptor blockade against the intrinsic substance). They provide a means for therapeutic interventions on tissues and organs in which these subtypes are located.

Adrenergic receptors

Receptors for adrenaline and noradrenaline are classed as:

- α1, found especially in arterial muscle;
- α2, found mainly on platelets, post-synaptically on blood vessels, in the pancreas, and in brain synapses;
- β1, found on cardiac muscle cells;
- β2, found on smooth muscle in the bronchioles of lungs.

Other subtypes of both α and β receptors have been identified that are likely to result in the development of new pharmaceuticals.

Cholinergic receptors

These relate only to acetylcholine, but there are subtypes. Muscarinic receptors mediate most of the parasympathetic actions in peripheral organs. There are three main subtypes of muscarinic receptor, although no selective drugs are currently available:

- M1 receptors are found primarily in synapses in the central nervous system.
- M2 receptors are found on cardiac cells
- M3 receptors are found on gland cells, and smooth muscle cells of viscera.

Nicotinic receptors are another type of cholinergic receptor. There are two main subtypes:

- Ganglionic receptors are found in synapses in parasympathetic and sympathetic ganglia. Similar receptors are also found within the brain; it is these that promote the alertness associated with cigarette smoking.
- Muscle receptors are found in neuromuscular junctions with skeletal muscle.

Summary

1 Nerves, or more precisely nerve cells (neurons), provide the means of rapid communication necessary for the short-term regulation of many homeostatic processes.

2 The nervous system has two main anatomical divisions: the peripheral nervous system, which conducts neural activity to and from tissues, and the central nervous system, which analyses information before promoting a response.

3 The peripheral system is subdivided into the somatic system, which activates skeletal muscle in the regulation of body posture and movement, and the autonomic system, which is involved in the regulation of visceral functions. In general, we can exert considerable conscious control over the former, but the latter is under involuntary control.

4 Peripheral nerves enter/exit the spinal cord as spinal nerves between the vertebrae. Sensory neurons enter the dorsal (posterior) aspect of the cord, while effector (motor) neurons exit via the ventral (anterior) aspect.

5 The central nervous system consists of the brain and spinal cord.

6 The brain develops embryologically as three distinct components that increase in complexity during development; these are the forebrain, midbrain and hindbrain.

7 The forebrain consists of the cerebral hemispheres (with both cortical and subcortical processing areas) and deeper structures called the thalamus and hypothalamus. The cortex and subcortical areas have particular roles in cognitive processes, the control of movement, and the receipt and interpretation of sensory information. The hypothalamus is especially involved in the 'drives' of the body, stress responses, and co-ordinating circadian rhythms. The thalamus is predominantly a relay centre for information passing into and out of the forebrain.

8 The midbrain contains many brain nuclei and nerve tracts, and forms the area between the forebrain and the hindbrain. It provides aspects of movement control, but is also a route of information passage into and out of the brain.

9 The hindbrain consists of structures at the top of the spinal cord, but also includes the cerebellum, which have integrative functions particularly in relation to arousal, the control of movement, and the control of the autonomic system. Some of these structures (the pons varolii and medulla oblongata) form the brainstem with the midbrain.

10 The cerebrospinal fluid provides the environment that bathes cells of the brain and spinal cord. The fluid is secreted into fluid ventricles and circulates around the central nervous system. It is eventually reabsorbed into the venous blood across special areas of the meningeal membranes that surround the brain and cord.

11 The spinal cord has a precise organization, consisting of tracts of nerve cell fibres that ascend or descend the cord within the white matter, and layers of cells that integrate activity or act as relays within central grey areas. Integrative functions of the cord include the production of reflexes.

12 Nerve cell activity is generated by the movement of electrical charge across the cell membrane, as an action potential. The membrane can be stabilized (i.e. the action potential inhibited) by the antagonistic movement of other ions that prevent the action potential being generated. This forms the basis of neural integration, a switching mechanism within the nervous system, and takes place at junctions called synapses between nerve cells.

13 Synaptic function involves the release of neurotransmitters that modulate ionic movements across the membrane of the next cell in the pathway. Some chemicals are excitatory, others inhibitory. Within the central nervous system, the ionic environment surrounding the cells is controlled tightly (to enable membrane events to be regulated) by regulating the composition of the cerebrospinal fluid.

14 Many cognitive functions of the brain have now been attributed to various brain structures, and involve a variety of neurological features and neurotransmitters. The balance between excitatory and inhibitory pathways is essential for 'normal' functions.

15 The autonomic nervous system also operates via neurotransmitters. Numerous receptor subtypes to these chemicals have been identified that enable the system to exert complex control of visceral functioning. The system is subdivided into the sympathetic and parasympathetic branches, which, in general, exert opposing actions on tissues in response to visceral afferent input.

Review questions

1 Neurons are highly specialized to conduct messages throughout the body. By becoming so specialized, neurons have sacrificed the ability to divide. Thus nerves are unable to replace themselves once damaged. The greatest concentration of neurons is in the brain. Read about the following regions of the brain and make brief notes about them: (i) cerebrum (cerebral hemispheres); (ii) cerebellum; (iii) diencephalon (thalamus and hypothalamus); (iv) midbrain; (v) pons; (vi) medulla.

2 What are the meninges? Identify the three layers that comprise the meninges (drawing a diagram would be useful).

3 What is the composition and function of cerebrospinal fluid (CSF)? What happens if CSF becomes infected?

4 How does the cerebral circulation differ from the circulation in other parts of the body? What is a cerebrovascular accident?

5 Make brief notes on the anatomy of the spinal cord.

6 In order to understand how messages travel, we must first look at the resting membrane potential. How does the inside of a resting cell remain negatively charged in relation to the outside? If a cell dies, what will happen to the resting membrane potential?

7 How does a nerve impulse travel along a neuron? What is the role of the myelin sheath? At some stage, a neuron will connect with another cell. This could be another neuron, muscle tissue or a gland. There will be a gap between the two cells, which is called a synapse. How will the message cross this gap so it can continue to its destination? Defining these terms should help you: (i) presynaptic terminal; (ii) post-synaptic terminal; (iii) neurotransmitter; (iv) receptor.

8 The vast nervous system can be divided into the central nervous system (brain and spinal cord) and the peripheral nervous system (sensory and motor divisions). The motor division of the nervous system can be split into the somatic and autonomic divisions. What type of muscle tissue will nerves from the somatic division influence?

9 How does your body react if you are frightened, worried or excited? This is the sympathetic division of the autonomic nervous system reacting to stressor. It is called the 'fright/fight/flight' response, and happens in response to any stressor, whether physical (e.g. illness, pain) or psychosocial (fear, bereavement, financial hardship). Think about the effect on your blood pressure as your heart rate, breathing and digestion changes. These changes are not intended to promote homeostasis, but to mobilize you ready for action to deal with the stressor. Alternatively, they might be viewed as promoting homeostasis within muscles to be used in the response. Why might they be viewed in this way?

REFERENCES

Campion, K. (1997) Multiple sclerosis. *Professional Nurse* **13**(3): 169–72.

Drouet, B., Pincon-Raymond, M., Chambaz, J. and Pillot, T. (2000) Molecular basis of Alzheimer's disease. *Cellular and Molecular Life Sciences* **57**(5): 705–15.

Fox, M.R. (1999) The importance of sleep. *Nursing Standard* **13**(24): 44–7.

Greenfield, S. (2000) *The Private Life of the Brain*. London: Penguin.

Kent, R.D. (2000) Research on speech motor control and its disorders: a review and prospective. *Journal of Communication Disorders* **33**(5): 391–428.

Markowitsch, H.S. (1998) Cognitive neuroscience of memory. *Neurocase* **4**(6): 492–535.

McMahon-Parkes, K. and Cornock, M.A. (1997) Guillain Barre syndrome: biological basis, treatment and care. *Intensive and Critical care Nursing* **13**(1): 42–8.

McNair, M.D. (1999) Traumatic brain injury. *Nursing Clinics of North America* **34**(3): 637–59.

Moshé, S.L.(2000) Seizures early in life. *Neurology* **55**(5 Suppl 1): 15–20.

Myers, F. (2000) Meningitis: the fears, the facts. *RN* **63**(11): 52–8.

Petty, J. (2000) Stroke nursing: a national perspective. *Professional Nurse* **15**(12): 781–4.

Schweiger, J.L. and Huey, R.A. (1999) Alzheimer disease. *Nursing* **29**(6): 34–42.

Sheridan, M.D. (1997) *From Birth to Five Years: children's developmental progress*. London: Routledge.

Splevings, D. (2000) The nurse's role in achieving optimal epilepsy management. *Community Nurse* **6**(8): 34–5.

Van Cauter, E., Leproult, R. and Plat, L. (2000) Age related changes in slow wave sleep and REM sleep and relationship with growth hormone and cortisol levels in healthy men. *Journal of the American Medical Association* **284**(7): 861–8.

Wallace, M. (1999) Creutzfeldt–Jakob disease: assessment and management update. *Journal of Gerontological Nursing* **25**(10): 17–24, 52–3.

Worsham, T.L. (2000) Easing the course of Guillain Barre syndrome. *RN* **63**(3): 46–50.

FURTHER READING

Neurology is a large and complex subject area. This chapter can provide only an introduction to the clinical aspects of neurological problems. Interested readers may find the following useful:

Currie, D., Ritchie, E. and Stott, S. (2000) *The Management of Head Injuries*, 2nd edn. Oxford: Oxford University Press.

Neatherlin, J.S. (1999) Foundation for practice: neuro-assessment for neuroscience nurses. *Nursing Clinics of North America* **34**(3): 573–92.

O'Hanlon-Nichols, T. (1999) Neurologic assessment. *American Journal of Nursing* **99**(8): 44–50.

Temple, C.M. (1997) *Developmental Cognitive Neuropsychology*. Brighton, UK: Psychology Press.

Weiner, W.J. and Goetz, C.G. (1999) *Neurology for the Non-neurologist*. London: Lippincott Williams & Wilkins.

Chapter 9

The endocrine system

Introduction
Overview of the anatomy, physiology and chemistry of the hormonal system

Homeostatic functions of the hormones
Further reading

INTRODUCTION

Cells and tissues require an appropriate rate of delivery of specific nutrients if they are to function. This is achievable only by the regulation of the functions of other tissues and organs because of the 'division of labour' that is observed in the body. Physiological function therefore cannot be static, since systemic function must be responsive according to the needs of the individual at any given time. Although some tissues are able to exert limited intrinsic control on some of their activities, the overall regulation of tissues and the integration of organ functions are provided by the co-ordinating systems of the body: the nervous and hormonal systems.

Nerve cells and hormones provide a means of communication between different parts of the body. Whereas nerve cells provide an anatomical route by which 'messages' can be conducted directly between tissues, hormones are purely chemical messengers that are conveyed by the extracellular fluids from the site of their production to their target tissues. The principles of nervous function were described in Chapter 8, but it is worth considering here the advantages and disadvantages of the two co-ordinating systems in order to place hormones in the context of homeostatic regulation.

General comparison of neural and hormonal systems

Hormones are released from specific secretory cells in one part of the body, dispersed in extracellular fluid (usually blood plasma), and interact with target cells elsewhere. In contrast, nerve cells extend from one tissue to another, and provide a direct communication link. They also, however, depend upon the secretion of neurotransmitters into extracellular fluid (usually tissue fluid) at synapses, which must interact with receptors on target cells. The distances travelled by neurotransmitters are microscopic, and nerve cells have the advantage that they can convey 'messages' (i.e. impulses) very rapidly to the target cells. The disadvantages are that this direct link must be established with every target cell within a tissue; the link must be maintained, since neural damage may irreversibly prevent communication.

The rapidity at which neural impulses are conducted means that target cells can be induced to alter their activities within fractions of seconds. In contrast, the time taken to induce the release of hormones from stores within secretory cells (or to synthesize them first in some cases), and to conduct them to targets, means that responses are much slower, of the order of several minutes to 1–2 h, depending on the hormone. Hormones, therefore, are important in regulating medium- or long-term functions of tissues, such as controlling body fluid composition or growth. Hormone operation would clearly be unsuitable, for example, in the rapid change in cardiovascular function that is necessary to control blood pressure at the moment when we stand up.

Both systems can act concurrently in the regulation of an organ. For example, the rapidity of neural responses is

BOX 9.1 ANTAGONISTIC AND AGONISTIC DRUGS

The actions of hormones clearly depend upon an interaction with receptor chemicals on or in their target cells. Chemicals released at nerve endings are likewise dependent upon receptors. Drugs that influence hormone (and neurochemical) receptors are used widely in medicine. An *antagonistic* drug is one that will combine with the receptor chemical but not activate the resultant cell response. In doing so, it prevents the hormone gaining access to the receptor; these types of drugs are often referred to as 'blockers', e.g. a beta-blocker interferes with a (beta) receptor to

adrenaline. In contrast, *agonistic* drugs interact with, and activate, the receptor in the same way as the hormone would do, e.g. salbutamol mimics the actions of adrenaline on the airways, and so aids breathing in conditions such as asthma.

Antagonistic drugs, therefore, are useful when hormone activity must be reduced, and agonistic drugs are used when there is a hormone deficiency or when it would be useful to promote the hormone's actions in its absence.

---

advantageous in the moment-to-moment coordination of gut motility, but the slower response to hormones is more appropriate in the control of bowel secretions (although neural activity can also alter these).

Some nerve cells in the hypothalamus of the brain also synthesize hormones and therefore represent an overlap between the systems. It is partly through such secretions that the brain can alter body function.

Nervous activity modulates the release of certain hormones, and some hormones influence neural activity. The two systems, therefore, may not always act in isolation.

From a clinical viewpoint, the fact that both systems utilize the release of a chemical, and its interaction with target receptors, means that many drugs have similar modes of action, either as receptor antagonists or agonists (see Box 9.1), or as agents that interfere with chemical synthesis, storage or release.

The overlap in actions of nerves and hormones in determining biological functioning is illustrated by the stress response and by sexual behaviour. Part of the stress response

is referred to as the 'alarm' stage (see Chapter 23). In this stage, an individual's physiology is altered firstly by activation of the sympathetic nervous system, which produces an immediate response, and then by the hormone adrenaline, which provides a back-up to the neural actions. Both act to increase the output of blood from the heart, and to alter blood flow to the tissues, in preparation for physical activity. The response is very similar to that promoted by adrenaline alone (indeed, a similar chemical, noradrenaline, is produced at the endings of the sympathetic nerves), and sympathetic activation causes this hormone to be released; its actions support those of the nerves.

Sexual behaviour is complex. Basically, behaviour results from neurological functioning. Nerve cells within certain parts of the brain that are involved in such behaviours also act as target cells for the (gonadal) sex hormones, which modulate the functions of these cells, producing some of the features associated with female and male behaviours. Not all such behaviours can, of course, be attributed simply to hormone actions, but there is a hormonal influence.

OVERVIEW OF THE ANATOMY, PHYSIOLOGY AND CHEMISTRY OF THE HORMONAL SYSTEM

In order to have breadth of understanding as to how the hormonal system functions, it is necessary to consider:

- the nature of hormonal secretions;
- the chemistry of hormonal secretions;
- how secretory tissue is organized;
- how hormones induce a change in target cell activity;
- the general principles of how hormone release is regulated.

What is a hormone?

The term 'hormone' was coined almost 100 years ago. Translated, the term means 'I excite', which reflects the

role of hormones as chemical messengers that alter the activities of cells. The actual definition is much more involved, however. By definition, a hormone is *a substance produced by cells in one part of the body that is secreted into the blood in response to a specific stimulus and in amounts that vary with the strength of the stimulus, and has its actions in the body some distance from the site of secretion.*

This definition may be applied to the major hormones of the body, but various other chemical messengers are now recognized that do not fit it:

- *Autocrine secretions* are those that are released into the interstitial fluid but influence the activities of the cell that secreted them. An example is the way in which oestrogen hormones secreted by ovarian follicle cells during the menstrual cycle stimulate the same cells to secrete further oestrogen.

- *Paracrine secretions* are those that are released into interstitial fluid and influence the activities of other cells but again within the immediate vicinity. Delivery of the secretion to the target cells is by diffusion through the fluid; the secretion is not blood-borne. Prostaglandins (see later) are examples of paracrine secretions; these are synthesized by most, if not all, tissues and provide an intrinsic modulation of tissue functions.

- *Pheromones* are secretions that are released out of the body and change the behaviour of other organisms. There is considerable evidence for their presence in a variety of species, and it is thought that humans also produce pheromones as sexual attractants, probably via apocrine sweat.

The breadth of these secretions highlights the difficulty in defining precisely the term 'hormone'. This chapter uses the term in its broadest sense, as defined above, while recognizing that this still omits autocrine secretions.

Names of hormones

Hormones are often named after their actions or the processes involved in those actions. For example:

- *Testosterone:* secreted by and acts on the testes (the suffix '-sterone' indicates that this is a steroid hormone).

- *Oestrogen:* promotes oestrus (= female fertility; menstrual cycle).

- *Antidiuretic hormone:* prevents diuresis (the production of copious volumes of urine).

Some hormones are frequently referred to by a collective name. An example is the tropins, a term used to indicate that the hormone's action is to promote the release of another hormone. For example, gonadotropins are those hormones that act on the gonads to stimulate the release of testosterone (male) or oestrogens (female). You will become more familiar with the names of hormones as you read this and other chapters of the book.

Hormonal chemistry

Hormones are a diverse range of substances. Basically, they can be divided into four types: peptides, catecholamines, steroids and eicosanoids. Examples are given later, but some general features of their functional chemistry are noted here.

Peptides

Peptides are small molecules comprised of amino acids (Figure 9.1). They are soluble in water, but are only poorly soluble in lipid, so after synthesis they can be stored in vesicles within the secretory cells. Release can be almost immediate, and occurs by exocytosis of the vesicles following their fusion with the plasma membrane of the cell. The interaction of peptides with target cells requires the presence of specific receptors on the surface of those cells. Examples of peptide hormones include insulin, vasopressin and oxytocin.

Catecholamines

Catecholamine hormones are derivatives of the amino acid tyrosine, therefore they all share a similar chemical structure (Figure 9.2). They are only slightly soluble in lipid, so they can be stored in intracellular vesicles. They also require the presence of surface receptors on target cells for their actions. The similarity of their chemical structure may cause an overlap in those actions, although receptor subtypes are found in certain tissues that enable each hormone to have specific actions in those tissues. Adrenaline and noradrenaline are examples of catecholamines.

The hormone thyroxine (= tetra-iodothyronine) produced by the thyroid gland is also synthesized from tyrosine, and is stored within the thyroid gland. It also requires the presence of surface receptors on target cells. Although not strictly considered to be a catecholamine, its

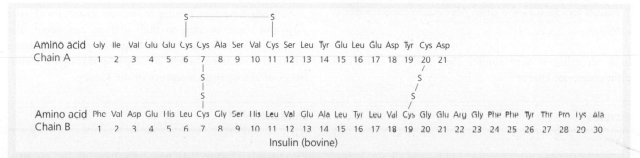

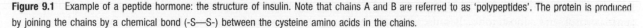

Figure 9.1 Example of a peptide hormone: the structure of insulin. Note that chains A and B are referred to as 'polypeptides'. The protein is produced by joining the chains by a chemical bond (-S—S-) between the cysteine amino acids in the chains.

(a) Precursor molecule

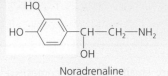

Tyrosine (an amino acid)

(b) Derivative hormones

   (i) Catecholamines

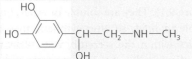

Noradrenaline

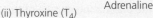

Adrenaline

   (ii) Thyroxine (T$_4$)

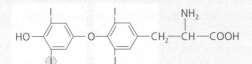

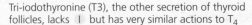

Tri-iodothyronine (T3), the other secretion of thyroid follicles, lacks I but has very similar actions to T$_4$

Figure 9.2 Structure of (a) tyrosine, (b) catecholamine hormones and (c) thyroxine (T4). Tyrosine is the precursor substance of catecholamines and thyroxine. Note the similarity in structure of adrenaline and noradrenaline; this helps to explain the overlap in their actions. Thyroxine is a derivative, but clearly contains some similar structural aspects. Note: I = iodine.

basic structure is very similar (but also has important differences; see later).

Steroids

Steroid hormones are modified lipids, and all are derivatives of cholesterol. Examples include testosterone, oestrogens, cortisol and aldosterone. Because they are highly

(a) Precursor molecule

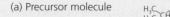

Cholesterol

(b) Derivative steroids

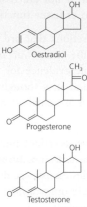

Oestradiol

Progesterone

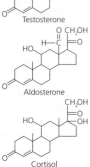

Testosterone

Aldosterone

Cortisol

Figure 9.3 Structure of (a) cholesterol and (b) some steroid hormones. Cholesterol is the precursor chemical. Note the similarity in structure of the steroids shown.

lipid soluble, they diffuse easily through cell membranes; therefore they cannot be stored, and must be synthesized as required. Steroid hormones pass into their target cells, where they interact with receptors within the cytoplasm. Their mode of action is quite different to that of other hormone groups, and necessitates the synthesis of proteins. All this means that responses that are dependent upon steroid release are relatively slow in onset, perhaps of the order of 1-2 h.

Steroids have very similar molecular structures (Figure 9.3), and some overlap in their actions can occur. For example, the influence of oestrogens on fluid balance during the menstrual cycle arises partly through a stimulation of aldosterone receptors in the kidney.

Eicosanoids

Eicosanoids (Figure 9.4) are derivatives of the essential unsaturated fatty acid arachidonic acid, which itself may be derived from essential dietary fatty acids, such as

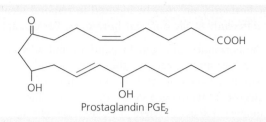

Figure 9.4 Simplified diagram of a prostaglandin molecule. This is a modified fatty acid. The 'arms' are chains of carbon atoms (see Chapter 5). The double-line segments in the 'arms' indicate that this is an unsaturated fatty acid.

linoleic acid and gamma-linolenic acid. They are, therefore, lipid soluble, and so must be synthesized as required. Eicosanoids act intracellularly in target cells.

Eicosanoids include the prostaglandins, thromboxanes and leukotrienes. The hormones are synthesised following the release of arachidonic acid from within the cell membrane, and their target cells are usually local to the site of synthesis. These hormones seem primarily to be intrinsic regulators of the tissue that produces them. Examples include prostaglandin E_2, prostaglandin F_{2alpha} and prostaglandin I_2 (also called prostacyclin).

Exercise

If you are unsure what an essential fatty acid is, re-read the section in Chapter 5.

Organization of secretory tissues: exocrine and endocrine glands

Cells that secrete chemicals are frequently collected into discrete areas of tissue that are collectively called glands. Some glands release their secretions onto the outer surface of the body (including into the lumen of the bowel, which strictly speaking is external[1]); these are called *exocrine glands*. Their secretions include mucus, saliva, digestive enzymes and sweat. Many exocrine glands, e.g. salivary glands, require ducts to transport their secretions. Not all exocrine glands are ducted, however; some cells that secrete digestive enzymes, and those that produce mucus, release their secretions directly. Hormones are not produced as exocrine secretions (although pheromones are

– which again highlights the difficulties of establishing a simple definition for hormones).

Those glands that secrete the major hormones of the body are referred to as *endocrine glands* (which is why the study of hormones is called 'endocrinology'). This process does not require the presence of ducts to transport the secretions, as they can be released directly into the extracellular fluid. Hence, these glands are sometimes referred to as ductless glands (this is a bad choice of term, since we noted above that some exocrine glands also do not have ducts).

In a few instances, a glandular tissue has both exocrine and endocrine functions. For example, the pancreas is an exocrine gland that releases digestive juices into the duodenum via the pancreatic duct, but also has 'islets' of endocrine tissue that secrete hormones such as insulin directly into the circulatory system. The pancreas, therefore, is a *mixed gland*. The gonads are also mixed glands.

Exercise

'Hormones are endocrine secretions.' Refer back to the earlier definition of a hormone and explain what this means.

Inducing a change in target cell activity: second messenger chemicals

Once a hormone has interacted with the target cell receptor, the responses of the target cell must involve an amplification of the signal until it is sufficient to produce an effective change in target cell activities. This is because the amount of hormone that is released is considerably diluted in extracellular fluid, and so interactions with target cell receptors are of a relatively low key, perhaps involving only one or two molecules. The amplification is provided by the generation of other messenger chemicals within the cytoplasm of the cell following the combination between the hormone molecule and cell receptor. In this way, the hormone is viewed as being the 'first messenger' and the chemicals produced within the target cell are 'second messengers'.

Second messengers to peptide, catecholamine and eicosanoid hormones

For these particular hormones, second messengers are produced when the hormone interacts with a receptor on the cell surface. There are a number of examples of second messengers, including cyclic adenosine monophosphate (cyclic AMP, cAMP), cyclic guanosine monophosphate (cyclic GMP, cGMP), calcium ions, and modified membrane lipids (in particular, inositol triphosphate), depending on the cell type. It is the deactivation of the

---

[1] Chapter 10 notes how the bowel is basically a tubular structure passing from the mouth to the anus. In spite of various modifications along the way, e.g. the stomach and intestines, the tube-like structure remains apparent. It is, in theory, possible to pass a thread from mouth to anus (we do not recommend that you try this!), so the lumen of the bowel can be considered to be continuous with the outer surface of the body. This is why secretions into the bowel are considered to be exocrine in nature.

second messenger process, and the enzymatic separation of the hormone molecule from its receptor result, that results in cessation of the target cell response to a hormone. The discovery of second messengers, and recent advances in understanding their actions, have opened up new avenues for pharmacological research. Some drugs that modulate their actions are available, e.g. phosphodiesterase inhibitors act on the enzyme phosphodiesterase to prevent the breakdown of cAMP and so prolong its actions; additional drugs and refinements can be expected in the future.

Second messengers promote the activation of a group of enzymes called protein kinases (note that 'kinase' has the same derivation as 'kinetic', i.e. these enzymes make certain proteins active) within the cell (Figure 9.5). These in turn activate further enzymes called phosphorylases ('phosphorylate' is a term used to indicate the chemical combination of a substance with a phosphate molecule) that then activate other proteins. The effect of having numerous stages of chemical activation is that a 'cascade' is produced. Thus, the second messenger/protein kinase system results in the activation of large numbers of enzymes. For example, just one molecule of the hormone glucagon, which promotes the breakdown of glycogen in liver cells, induces the generation of more than one million molecules of glucose. Hormones are therefore potent substances.

Having a second messenger system also provides other advantages. A single cell may act as a target for more than one hormone, and may be induced to respond identically or differently to the different hormones. For example:

- the hormones glucagon (a peptide) and adrenaline (a catecholamine) promote the same second messenger within a liver cell, and so both cause the release of glucose from glycogen stores. In this way, glucose can be mobilized under different circumstances: glucagon helps to prevent basal blood glucose concentration from decreasing too far, and adrenaline raises blood glucose concentration during times of physical activity (Figure 9.5(a));

- insulin promotes a second messenger that causes a liver cell to produce glycogen from glucose, but the same cell will also respond to glucagon by producing a different second messenger that results in the breakdown of glycogen into glucose. In this way, the same liver cell can respond to a situation when blood glucose concentration must be reduced (i.e. the insulin action), or when it has to be increased (i.e. the glucagon action), thus helping to maintain blood glucose homeostasis.

Second messengers for thyroid hormones and steroids

For thyroid hormones (thyroxine), the entire membrane receptor/hormone combination is internalized by the cell, and cell activation then results from a very different sequence of events from that observed during activation

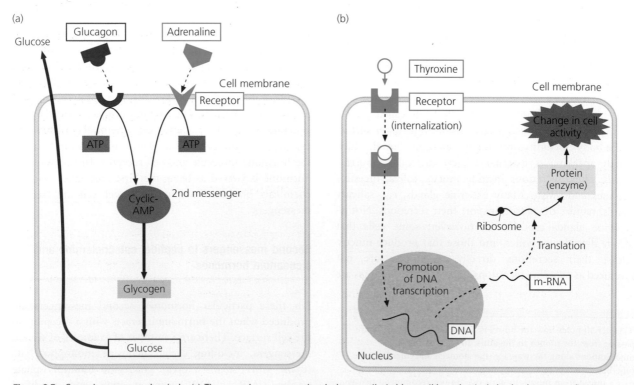

Figure 9.5 Second messenger chemicals. (a) The second messenger chemicals are activated by peptide and catecholamine hormones after their interaction with receptors in the cell membrane. (b) The interaction between steroids and thyroxine with their respective receptors triggers events directly within the cell.

by peptides and catecholamines. Thus, thyroxine triggers gene transcription and so will promote enzyme synthesis; it is these enzymes that then alter cell activity (Figure 9.5(b)). The principle of amplification and second messengers still applies, but this mode of action is generally slower than that of peptide hormones and catecholamines. It is perhaps of significance that thyroxine controls basal metabolic processes, so a rapid mode of action is not necessary.

The mode of cell activation by steroids is generally similar to that of thyroid hormones, except that steroids are lipid soluble and receptors to them are found within the cytoplasm of target cells, rather than on the cell membrane. Like thyroxine, steroids also promote gene transcription and enzyme synthesis. Similarly, steroid hormones are essentially concerned with processes (such as blood volume regulation and reproductive functions) that do not require an instant response.

Regulation of hormone release: general principles

Details of stimuli for the release of individual hormones, and the control of that release, are given in the next section. As an introduction, however, it is worth considering here general aspects of the stimulus required, and the regulation of secretion.

The stimulus

Many hormones have essential roles in the homeostatic regulation of physiological systems. The stimuli for their release therefore relate to a diverse range of parameters, such as the composition of body fluids, blood pressure, blood volume, body temperature, or nutrient content of digestive chyme. For example, the hormone vasopressin (antidiuretic hormone; ADH) plays a vital role in the maintenance of body water content. It is therefore appropriate that the release of this hormone is in direct response to the increased osmotic potential of body fluids

that occurs when we are dehydrated. As the osmotic potential is corrected, the stimulus declines and hormone release is reduced accordingly. The amount of vasopressin released, hence the extent of the kidney response is related directly to the magnitude of the change in osmotic potential.

In contrast to this role of a hormone in the maintenance of a constant environment, some hormones are released in order to induce change according to the needs of the body at that particular time. Thus, adrenaline has an important role in the heightening of cardiovascular responses during exercise; once the exercise has finished, the release of the hormone declines again. Adrenaline also induces metabolic change and will have widespread effects throughout the body. Under such circumstances, adrenaline is released through nerve activity to the adrenal gland from the brain.

Other hormones promote permanent change, e.g. sex hormones from the gonads control fertility in adulthood, but during puberty they are also responsible for instigating sexual maturity and the development of secondary sexual characteristics. This promotion of change requires a resetting of homeostatic parameter, much as responses to exercise did in the previous example, but this time the resets are permanent.

Principles of control

In the examples given of the actions of vasopressin during dehydration, and of adrenaline in exercise, removal of the stimulus directly reverses the change in hormone release. This is a simple negative feedback loop; it involves a 'short loop', since there is only one stage to the process (Figure 9.6(a)).

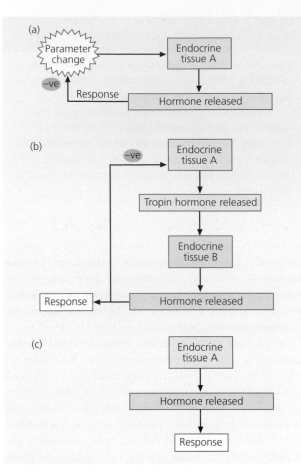

Figure 9.6 Feedback loops in the homeostatic control of the release and/or actions of hormones. (a) The feedback to hormone release operates as a 'short loop', and comes from the action of the hormone itself. (b) The feedback is 'long looped', and entails other hormones. (c) The loop is 'open', since there is apparently no feedback.

Q. Which of these feedback loops is likely to promote the most closely regulated control of hormone release?

The number of stages involved in the eventual secretion of some hormones, e.g. cortisol, utilizes a 'long-loop' feedback system. This is frequently observed when the initial stimulus for the release of a hormone must act through intermediary (i.e. tropin) hormones (Figure 9.6(b)). Negative feedback effects on the release of the intermediary hormone ensure that the final release of cortisol is regulated rigorously. Thus, the presence of cortisol in blood acts to 'switch off' the release of the intermediary, leading to a decline in cortisol release and hence the eventual 'switching on' of the release of the intermediary so that cortisol is secreted once again.

In contrast, there are occasions when certain hormones are released that do not appear to have a negative feedback mechanism to control their secretion. For example, growth hormone promotes a variety of metabolic actions, none of which could be envisaged as providing a stimulus to decrease its secretion. This is called an 'open-loop' system

Gland dysfunctioning is generally classed as causing either hyposecretion or hypersecretion. Specific examples are given later, but we will introduce the general principles here.

Hyposecretion

Inadequate secretion of hormone can have a number of causes:

● the gland cells may lack receptors to the activating stimulus, e.g. through the production of autoantibodies, as in the underactive thyroid disorder Hashimoto's disease. Ageing will also reduce hormonal secretion, partly because of receptor deficiencies as receptor production and maintenance decline as a consequence of the ageing process;

● hyposecretion might reflect an inability of glands to synthesize the hormone, as in insulin-dependent diabetes mellitus. Lack of synthesis usually results from genetic mutation, and may be inherited, congenital or acquired;

● a deficiency, usually dietary, of the precursor molecule may lead to inadequate synthesis, e.g. a lack of iodine in the diet may cause thyroxine deficiency. Overgrowth or hypertrophy of the gland as a consequence is an adaptive response to raise hormone secretion. Dietary deficiencies as causes of hormonal disorder are rare in Western societies.

Hyposecretion can sometimes be improved with drugs that stimulate synthesis and/or release of the hormone from the gland. Often, however, correction requires hormone replacement therapy. This term is frequently applied to the administration of oestrogens in post-menopausal women, but technically it can be used to mean any circumstance in which an individual is administered hormone therapy. The hormone is normally a synthetic form of the natural chemical.

Hypersecretion

Hypersecretion commonly results from a failure of the negative feedback mechanism that controls hormone release:

● The feedback failure usually results from a lack of receptors to the feedback signal to the gland cells, but what makes these receptors decline is unclear. Autoimmune responses are thought to be a frequent cause.

● Gland hypertrophy, and overactivity of its cells, is also seen when there is a tumour present, since tumour cells may 'escape' negative feedback processes. Alternatively, elevated plasma concentrations of a hormone might reflect non-glandular secretion of the hormone. Thus, the actual gland might continue to be regulated closely via a negative feedback, but tumours elsewhere, which do not have the appropriate receptors and are unresponsive to feedback control, could produce the hormone even when this is inappropriate. The secretion of a hormone by a site other than that of the gland is referred to as *ectopic*.

Principles of correction might involve using a drug to suppress hormone synthesis or to antagonize its actions. Availability of such drugs is limited at the present time. Surgery to reduce the gland is another option.

(Figure 9.6(c)), although it might just be the case that the feedback mechanism remains to be discovered.

Finally, there are a small number of instances when positive feedback operates. In positive feedback, the response to the hormone is to increase the stimulus, leading to yet greater hormone secretion. The cycle, therefore, is one of rapidly increasing hormone activity, rather than maintenance. An example is the effect of uterus tension during labour to stimulate the release of the hormone oxytocin, which then causes the development of further tension, and hence further hormone release.

Examples of feedback loops in the regulation of the secretory activities of individual endocrine glands are described in detail in the next section.

HOMEOSTATIC FUNCTIONS OF THE HORMONES

Hormones have essential roles in physiological homeostasis. Although hormonal actions are diverse, there is a degree of overlap, and examples have been given throughout this book in which interactions between secretions are important for the overall control of some parameters. For example, blood pressure regulation involves a number of vasoconstrictor hormones of different chemistries and origins. For clarity, however, this section will take a systematic approach, and describe the secretions of individual endocrine tissues, the locations of which are shown in Figure 9.7.

The hypothalamus and the pituitary gland

The hypothalamus lies at the base of the brain, and the pituitary gland is located just below it, attached to it by a 'stalk'. Together they form a functional unit often referred to as the 'hypothalamic-pituitary axis', since the hypothalamus mediates the secretion of hormones by the pituitary gland; however, it is convenient to consider the two separately.

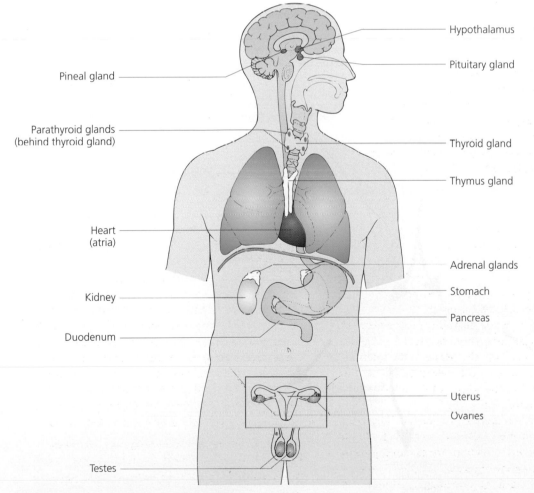

Figure 9.7 Location of the major endocrine glands.

The hypothalamus

The hypothalamus is a part of the forebrain (see Chapter 8). It has a diverse range of functions, including the control of 'drives' of human nature (feeding, drinking, sexual behaviour), the control of body temperature, and the establishment of a daily metabolic rhythm (circadian rhythm; see Chapter 23). It shares some functions with other parts of the brain, particularly with areas of the limbic system that are responsible for emotion, anxiety and aggression.

Being a part of the brain, the hypothalamus contains nerve cells. Some of these have a glandular role; cells that secrete the hormones are referred to as neuroendocrine cells, because they are both neurons and gland cells. The glandular cells of the hypothalamus will secrete their hormones when stimulated, but being neurological tissue, that secretion may also be influenced by higher brain centres. Thus, many of the psychological influences on physical function, such as stress and circadian rhythm changes, occur through the activities of the hypothalamus.

Most of the hormones produced by the hypothalamus are released into small blood vessels that form a direct link between the hypothalamus and pituitary (Figure 9.8). These hormones are conveyed to cells within the anterior lobe of the pituitary gland, which themselves produce further hormones, so the hypothalamic hormones involved are examples of tropins. They are referred to as either releasing or inhibiting hormones (or factors), according to their actions on the pituitary gland, and are usually named after the pituitary hormone that they influence (Table 9.1).

Other hypothalamic hormones are secreted directly from nerve endings within the posterior lobe of the pituitary. The hormone, having been synthesized in the cell body of the

> **Exercise**
>
> The blood vessels that pass from the hypothalamus to the anterior pituitary gland are examples of portal vessels, i.e. they carry blood directly from one capillary bed to another without passing through a vein or artery. Establishing this portal circulation from the hypothalamus is thought to determine the onset of puberty.
>
> The largest portal vessel in the body is the hepatic portal vein. Refer to Chapter 10 and identify why this is also a portal vessel. What does the blood within it carry?

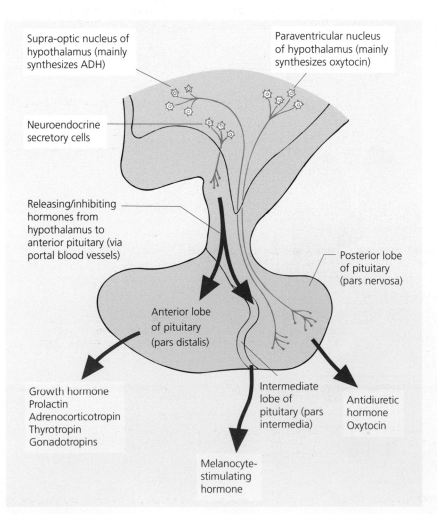

Figure 9.8 The hypothalamic-pituitary gland axis, and the main hormones secreted.

Supra-optic nucleus of hypothalamus (mainly synthesizes ADH)

Paraventricular nucleus of hypothalamus (mainly synthesizes oxytocin)

Neuroendocrine secretory cells

Releasing/inhibiting hormones from hypothalamus to anterior pituitary (via portal blood vessels)

Posterior lobe of pituitary (pars nervosa)

Anterior lobe of pituitary (pars distalis)

Growth hormone
Prolactin
Adrenocorticotropin
Thyrotropin
Gonadotropins

Intermediate lobe of pituitary (pars intermedia)

Antidiuretic hormone
Oxytocin

Melanocyte-stimulating hormone

Table 9.1 Summary of the secretions, actions and regulation of some of the major endocrine glands

Gland	Hormone	Target	Action	Homeostatic regulation
Hypothalamus	*Releasing hormones	Anterior pituitary	Release of various hormones (see text)	Negative feedback from target endocrine secretions Neural input to hypothalamus
	*Inhibitory hormones	Anterior pituitary	Inhibit release of various hormones (see text)	Unclear Neural input to hypothalamus
Anterior pituitary	Corticotropin (ACTH)	Adrenal cortex	Release of glucocorticoid hormones	Negative feedback from glucocorticoid Hypothalamic regulatory hormones
	Thyrotropin (TSH)	Thyroid follicles	Release of thyroxine	Negative feedback from thyroxine Hypothalamic regulatory hormones
	Gonadotropins, i.e. luteinizing hormone (LH), follicle stimulating hormone (FSH)	Gonads	Oestrogens and progestins (female), testosterone (male)	Negative feedback from gonadal hormones
	Growth hormone (GH, somatotrophin)	Various tissues	Metabolic (see text)	Unclear Hypothalamic regulatory hormones
	Prolactin	Breast (female) Unclear in male	Lactation (role in male unclear)	Unclear Hypothalamic regulatory hormones
	Melanocyte-stimulating hormone (MSH)	Melanocytes in skin	Promotes melanin synthesis	Unclear Hypothalamic regulatory hormones
Posterior pituitary	Vasopressin (antidiuretic hormone, ADH)	Kidney, arterioles	Water retention Vasoconstriction (blood pressure regulation)	Negative feedback from plasma osmotic pressure, and arterial blood pressure
	Oxytocin	Breast and uterus (unclear in male)	Lactation, labour Role in male unclear	Negative feedback from suckling Positive feedback from uterus during labour
Thyroid	Thyroxine (T3, T4)	Various tissues	Metabolic, especially role in basal metabolic rate	Thyrotropin from anterior pituitary gland
	Calcitonin	Bone	Promotes calcium deposition	Negative feedback from plasma calcium ion concentration
Parathyroid	Parathyroid hormone (PTH)	Bone, kidney	Promotes calcium resorption from bone Activates vitamin D in kidney (i.e. promotes calcium uptake from bowel)	Negative feedback from plasma calcium ion concentration
Adrenal cortex	Glucocorticoids, e.g. cortisol	Various tissues	Metabolic, permissive influence on other hormones	Corticotropin from anterior pituitary
	Mineralocorticoids, e.g. aldosterone	Kidney	Promote sodium reabsorption from renal tubule, promote potassium secretion (i.e. excretion)	Negative feedback from effects on blood volume (via changes in renin production), or plasma potassium concentration
	Gonadal steroids	Gonads	Influence on reproductive tract, but not regulatory	Unclear
Adrenal medulla	Catecholamines (adrenaline, noradrenaline)	Heart and circulation, also various other tissues (see text)	Promote cardiac function Promote vasoconstriction (BP regulation)	Sympathetic nervous system activity
Duodenum	Secretin and CCK-PZ	Digestive glands, gall bladder, pancreas, stomach	Promote secretion of pancreatic fluid and enzymes, bile secretion, regulate gastric emptying	Presence of food products in duodenum
Pancreas	Insulin	Liver, skeletal muscle	Promote glucose utilization	Negative feedback from blood glucose concentration
	Glucagon	Liver, skeletal muscle	Promote glucose mobilization from stores	Negative feedback from blood glucose concentration
	Somatostatin	Insulin- and glucagon-secreting cells of pancreas	Modulate release of insulin and glucagon	Presence of insulin or glucagon
Gonads: ovaries (female)	Oestrogens (e.g. oestriol), progestins (e.g. progesterone)	Reproductive tract, breast and secondary sexual characteristics	Regulation of menstrual cycle. Behavioural effects.	Gonadotropins (LH & FSH) from ant. pituitary.
Gonads: testes (male)	Androgens (eg testosterone)	Reproductive tract and secondary sexual characteristics	Regulation of spermatogenesis, and accessory glands of reproductive tract Behavioural effects	Gonadotropins (especially LH) from anterior pituitary

*Hypothalamic regulatory hormones include specific releasing and inhibitory hormones that act on the secretion of individual hormones from the anterior pituitary gland.

neuron located within the hypothalamus, is transported along the axon of the nerve cell to the terminals, where it is stored in vesicles ready for release. It is conventional, however, to consider these particular secretions as being pituitary rather than hypothalamic hormones.

The roles of hypothalamic secretions, and the control of their release, are considered below.

The pituitary gland

The pituitary gland (or hypophysis) is of mixed embryological origin: the anterior part is formed from an upgrowth of the oral cavity of the embryo, whilst the posterior part is a downgrowth from the overlying brain. This helps to explain how the anterior lobe is comprised of non-neural cells, while the posterior lobe is comprised of neural tissue.

The anterior lobe

The anterior lobe (or adenohypophysis) comprises some 75% of the pituitary by weight. It consists of two parts:

- the *pars distalis:* secretes most hormones of the anterior lobe;

- the *pars intermedia:* a small piece of glandular tissue that lies between the pars distalis and the posterior lobe of the pituitary gland (Figure 9.8). It is occasionally referred to as the intermediate lobe of the pituitary gland, but it is functionally linked to the pars distalis.

The hormones produced by the anterior lobe are identified, together with their main actions, in Table 15.1. All are peptides. Most are tropins that act on other endocrine tissues in the body, and therefore regulate the production of their secretions; for this reason, the anterior lobe has been called the 'master gland'.

Most of the secretory cells of the anterior lobe are subject to a long-loop negative feedback inhibition from the secretions of their target endocrine tissues (further details are given when the individual target glands are discussed). A schema was shown in Figure 9.6(b), and negative feedback was identified in Chapter 1 as the main means by which body functions, and hence homeostasis, can be regulated. The process places a high degree of control on the pituitary gland, and this need for precise control reflects the potency of its hormones.

Most hormones of the anterior lobe are released in response to the presence of hypothalamic releasing hormones. Some, namely growth hormone, melanocyte-stimulating hormone (MSH) and prolactin, are controlled primarily by hypothalamic inhibitory hormones, although the situation is complicated by the presence of releasing hormones. It is unclear why the control should be different to that of other anterior lobe secretions, but it may relate to their actions since they are not tropins and so have direct effects on non-glandular tissues: growth hormone has widespread metabolic effects (another name for growth hormone is somatotrophin; 'soma' = body, 'troph' = nutrition), MSH (which is the main secretion of the pars intermedia) promotes pigmentation of skin melanocytes, and prolactin promotes milk production during lactation.

The posterior lobe

We noted earlier that the posterior lobe (or neurohypophysis) is comprised of neural tissue. Thus, the lobe is sometimes referred to as the pars nervosa (= nervous part). The gland consists of axon terminals that contain vesicles of hormone produced by the cell bodies of the nerve cells within the hypothalamus. The posterior lobe secretes two hormones: vasopressin and oxytocin.

Vasopressin (antidiuretic hormone, ADH) is synthesized by cell bodies within a part of the hypothalamus

---

BOX 9.5 DYSFUNCTIONING OF THE ANTERIOR PITUITARY GLAND

Strictly speaking, such disorders include those arising from problems in the secretion of anterior lobe tropins, such as gonadotropin and thyrotropin, but these are considered in relation to the target glands (see Boxes 9.7 and 9.11). This box considers only disorders of growth hormone and prolactin, hormones that have direct effects.

Hyposecretion of growth hormone retards childhood growth, resulting in small stature but normal body proportions (a condition known as pituitary dwarfism). It is important that any growth deficiencies are identified during childhood, since the calcification of growth plates in the long bones at puberty will prevent further growth. Slowed growth is normally detected by regular attention to growth assessments. Synthetic growth hormone can be administered during childhood, if tests identify a deficiency, in order to improve growth rate. The hormone also has metabolic effects in the adult, and is released primarily during sleep.

Hyposecretion will therefore have metabolic consequences relating to slowed tissue maintenance.

Hypersecretion of growth hormone promotes excessive growth in children, leading to pituitary giantism. In adults, excessive secretion promotes growth of the skeleton, especially in the extremities, leading to exaggerated features (known as acromegaly), such as the frontal bone of the skull, mandibular bones, hands and feet . Hypersecretion may also occur from ectopic sites, such as tumours. Antagonistic drugs may be given, e.g. to counteract secretion from tumours, or alternatively destruction of part of the pituitary gland may be required. However, acromegalic changes are irreversible once they are established.

Hypersecretion of prolactin may be seen after birth when the hormone is released in increasing quantities to promote lactation. Drugs that promote the release from the hypothalamus of prolactin inhibitory hormone (PIH) may be used to reduce the hypersecretion.

called the supraoptic nucleus (i.e. they lie above the optic nerves close to where they cross over). Vasopressin is involved in the control of water balance via its retentive actions in the kidney (hence its alternative name), and the control of blood pressure via its vasoconstrictor actions. The hormone is released following the stimulation of osmoreceptors in the hypothalamus (responding to the effects of dehydration) or arterial baroreceptors (responding to hypotension). Correction of water balance or blood pressure removes the stimulus and provides the negative feedback that causes hormone secretion to decline.

Oxytocin is synthesized by cell bodies within the parts of the hypothalamus called the paraventricular nucleus (i.e. they lie alongside the cerebral ventricles). Oxytocin is involved in labour, and is released as a reflex response to increasing tension of the uterus wall. The hormone causes the uterus to contract, and a positive feedback operates that makes hormone secretion, and hence uterine tension, increase further. Delivery of the baby, and resultant loss of uterine tension, causes the hormone secretion to decline again. Oxytocin is also released during suckling, when it promotes the release of breast milk. Its release declines when the baby stops feeding, another negative feedback response. Some studies have suggested that oxytocin may also be involved in regulating fluid balance. Although debatable, such actions could help to explain its presence in males.

The thyroid gland

The thyroid gland has four lobes that straddle the lower end of the trachea. It secretes tri-iodothyronine (T3), tetra-iodothyronine (T4), and calcitonin.

T3 and T4

These are derived from the amino acid tyrosine (see Figure 9.2). Their names simply reflect the number of iodine atoms that are incorporated into each hormone molecule. They are released together and have similar actions, although T4 (commonly called thyroxine) is the main secretion.

The need for iodine to be incorporated into the molecules of thyroid hormones is one of the main reasons why iodine must be included in our diet. The iodide ion is actively taken up by the gland and initially incorporated into tyrosine molecules attached to a protein called thyroglobulin that is stored in extracellular spaces within the lobules of the gland (Figure 9.9). The gland therefore is able to concentrate iodine within it, and the uptake of administered radioisotopic iodine is a clinically useful means of monitoring thyroid function; it is also detectable following accidental exposure to emissions from nuclear explosion.

When required, T3 and T4 are generated quickly from thyroglobulin and released into the blood. Release is promoted by thyroid-stimulating hormone (TSH; increasingly known as thyrotropin) from the anterior pituitary gland, which in turn is released in response to TSH-releasing hormone from the hypothalamus (Figure 9.10). Both thyroxine and TSH have negative feedback actions on the hypothalamus and anterior pituitary cells, and there is, therefore, a tight control on thyroid hormone release. The need for this is clear when one considers that the main function of thyroxine is to determine basal metabolic rate.

Calcitonin

Calcitonin is secreted by pockets of cells located within the thyroid gland (Figure 9.9). Its main role is to promote the uptake of calcium ions by bone cells when plasma calcium concentration is elevated, thus returning blood calcium concentration to within its homeostatic range. As the concentration of calcium declines, the release of calcitonin is reduced. Calcitonin's activity forms only one part of the process by which plasma calcium concentration is regulated; its concentration reflects a balance between uptake from the intestine, incorporation or release from bone, and excretion in urine (Figure 9.11).

BOX 9.6 DYSFUNCTIONING OF THE POSTERIOR PITUITARY GLAND

Hyposecretion of vasopressin (or renal resistance to its actions) is known as *diabetes insipidus* (not to be confused with diabetes mellitus), and means that the kidneys are unable to conserve water efficiently. Copious volumes of dilute urine are produced because the urinary concentration mechanism is compromised (see Chapter 15), leading to persistent dehydration. Synthetic vasopressin is administered when the disorder is due to hyposecretion. Diabetes insipidus may be inherited or acquired, e.g. as a consequence of brain surgery in the area of the hypothalamus.

Hypersecretion of vasopressin is known as *syndrome of inappropriate ADH secretion* (SIADH). Water conservation is constantly promoted, even if the patient is well hydrated, and overhydration and body fluid dilution (called hypo-osmolality), and an expansion of body fluid volume (hypervolaemia), occur.

The main documented action of oxytocin is during birth. Hypersecretion of oxytocin is extremely rare, but its concentration in blood at stages of labour may be increased above that achieved by normal secretion by administration of synthetic hormone in order to progress labour.

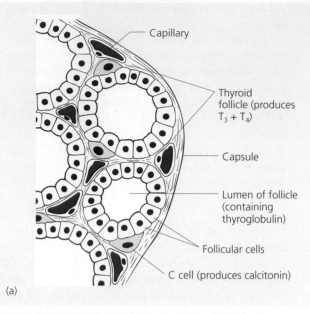

(a)

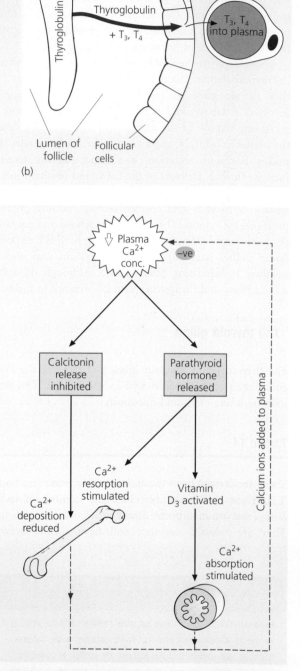

Figure 9.9 The thyroid gland. (a) Section through the gland, showing follicles, the glandular follicular cells, and the glandular C cells associated with the follicles. (b) Details of the synthesis of thyroxine (T3, T4) involving a complex protein called thyroglobulin within the lumen of a follicle. Note how the hormone is produced and stored within the follicle lumen, but is secreted from the follicular cells after removal of the thyroglobulin.

Q. Where does the iodine go? You might refer to Figure 9.2 for the answer.

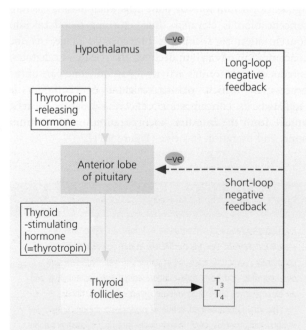

Figure 9.10 Feedback loops for the control of thyroxine release.

Q. How is the concentration in blood of thyrotropin (TSH) increased in people who produce insufficient thyroxine?

Figure 9.11 Hormonal regulation of calcium ion concentration in blood plasma. The responses to a decreased calcium concentration are shown. Note that the calcium concentration is largely a balance between calcium deposition in, or resorption from, bone, and uptake from the bowel. The latter must also compensate for losses in urine.

Q. How do the responses change if plasma calcium concentration is excessive?

Hyposecretion

Hypothyroidism arises when the secretion of thyroid hormones is deficient. Iodine deficiency was once a cause of this disorder, but supplemented diets and iodinated water have corrected this. A common cause is an autoimmune response when the gland becomes less sensitive to TSH (thyrotropin), a condition called Hashimoto's disease. Another cause is removal of thyroid tissue during excision of a tumour.

The lack of adequate hormone causes the basal metabolic rate to decline, leaving the individual feeling lethargic and apathetic. The person fatigues easily, and will usually have difficulties in keeping warm. Hair thinning is common, and the skin may become dry, scaly and thickened, a condition referred to as *myxoedema* (a non-pitting thickening of the skin that is distinct from the pitting oedema due to fluid retention). There will be a slowed pulse rate as a consequence of reduced metabolism.

Intervention is targeted at hormone replacement, using synthetic hormone preparations. Clearly, the dose taken must reflect the extent of hormone deficiency, so the individual's hormone status must be titrated. This usually entails an initial titration and periodic monitoring of the plasma concentration of TSH, since establishing a normal plasma concentration of thyroid hormones will promote a negative feedback action on the

pituitary gland, and so should reduce TSH secretion to normal values.

Hypersecretion

Hyperthyroidism is the name given to a syndrome of excessive secretion of thyroid hormones. A common cause is an autoimmune response that sensitises the gland to TSH (thyrotropin); this is called Grave's disease. The patient exhibits an elevated basal metabolic rate, readily observable as a raised pulse rate. The person will also feel very warm as a consequence of excessive heat generation. The individual may have insomnia and may even exhibit behavioural changes, appearing energetic, even compulsive. Structural changes can also occur to facial tissues (thyroid hormones also seem to influence certain proteins), producing a smooth texture to the skin. Protein deposition behind the eyes may also occur over time, causing the eyes to seemingly bulge forward, referred to as exophthalmos and produces visual disturbance.

Treatment is aimed at either surgically removing sections of the thyroid gland (thyroidectomy) to reduce the total secretion rate, using anti-thyroid drugs to prevent hormone synthesis, or using antagonistic drugs to block the actions of the hormones. Radioactive iodine may also be used to damage thyroid cells and reduce their secretory activity.

The parathyroid glands

The parathyroid glands are four small patches of tissue found on the posterior surface of the lobes of the thyroid gland. They secrete the peptide parathyroid hormone (PTH). PTH is released when the plasma calcium ion concentration is below its homeostatic range. It acts to stimulate osteoclast cells in bone to release calcium from bone mineral (Figure 9.11). It also promotes the activation of vitamin D within the kidneys. This vitamin is now recognized by many authorities to be a hormone (although it has retained its name), and increases calcium absorption from food contents in the bowel.

By stimulating directly the release of calcium from bone, and by enhancing indirectly the absorption of calcium from the gut, PTH rapidly corrects any deficiency in plasma calcium concentration. Release of the hormone becomes inhibited as the calcium concentration begins to rise above its homeostatic range.

The adrenal glands

As the name suggests, the adrenal glands lie adjacent to the kidneys; in fact they lie on top of them. Each gland can be subdivided into an outer layer, or cortex, and an inner

Hyposecretion

Since parathyroid hormone is responsible for raising plasma calcium concentration, its deficiency will promote a decrease in calcium (hypocalcaemia). Calcium ions influence the threshold for activation of excitable tissues, and hyposecretion of the hormone will therefore lead to increased neural excitability and even a pronounced muscle spasm called tetany. Tetany of the diaphragm muscle is life threatening. Synthetic hormone is available for hormone replacement treatment.

One cause of hyposecretion arises from the location of the gland cells in the thyroid gland. The removal of thyroid tissue to correct hyperthyroidism will more than likely entail the removal of some parathyroid tissue as well. Thus, correcting the thyroid

problem can potentially lead to deficient PTH secretion, and therefore lead to difficulties in maintaining normal calcium balance.

Hypersecretion

Excessive secretion of the hormone promotes demineralization of bone, since its actions are normally to regulate plasma calcium concentration through release of the ion from bone. A common cause of excess PTH is the ectopic production of PTH-like protein by tumours. In this case, the hypercalcaemia may be treated by elevating the blood calcitonin concentration by administering synthetic calcitonin. This in turn will increase uptake of calcium by bones. Hypercalcaemia makes excitable tissues less sensitive to stimulation.

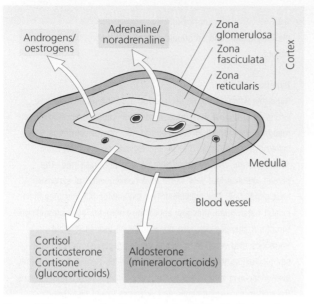

Figure 9.12 Cross-section through an adrenal gland to illustrate the cortical zones, the medulla, and the hormones secreted from them.

layer, or medulla. Cells in the cortex secrete steroid hormones, and cells in the medulla secrete catecholamine hormones (Figure 9.12).

The adrenal cortex

The cortex secretes a range of steroids that collectively are referred to as corticoids (= derived from the cortex). The steroids can be divided into:

● the *glucocorticoids:* have effects on glucose metabolism;

● the *mineralocorticoids:* have effects on the electrolyte composition of plasma;

● the *gonadocorticoids or sex steroids (androgens/oestrogens):* the amounts secreted are very small compared with the amounts produced by the gonads, but they do have some effects on secondary sexual characteristics.

Glucocorticoids

Glucocorticoids are produced by a layer of the cortex called the zona fasciculata (Figure 9.12). There are a number of glucocorticoids, with similar molecular structures and actions. The most important are *cortisol* and *corticosterone,* which have a variety of actions. In particular, they promote the breakdown of protein in skeletal muscle, the synthesis of glucose from the released amino acids, and the synthesis of glycogen from some of the synthesized glucose in the liver. The hormones also mobilize fatty acids from fats stored in adipose tissue, and inhibit the uptake of glucose by many tissues. The net effect is to:

● maintain glycogen stores in the liver that can be mobilized as and when required;

● increase plasma glucose concentration. and so raise the availability of glucose for metabolism by various tissues;

● increase free fatty acid concentrations in blood plasma, and so raise their availability for metabolism by tissues.

Glucocorticoids also exert 'permissive' effects that enhance the actions of other hormones, e.g. adrenaline. Other effects are to stimulate red blood cell production, and to reduce inflammation.

Clearly, the glucocorticoids have wide-ranging effects on the body. The actions detailed above would be particularly useful during times of physical activity, and following trauma, when there may be wound healing and a need to re-establish a 'normal' state of homeostasis generally. It is perhaps not surprising that they are released when the body is under stress, including that produced by surgical trauma. They have been called the 'hormones of stress', and our capacity to cope with demands is markedly reduced in their absence (see Chapter 22).

The release of glucocorticoids is stimulated by adrenocorticotropic hormone (ACTH; often called corticotropin) from the anterior pituitary gland (Figure 9.13). This in turn is released in response to the secretion of corticotropin-releasing hormone from the hypothalamus. The glucocorticoids normally exert inhibition (negative feedback) on the release of both hormones, and therefore provide a high degree of control of their own secretion. The secretion rate can be modulated, however, by neurological inputs to the hypothalamus; this is how perceptions of stress can increase secretion.

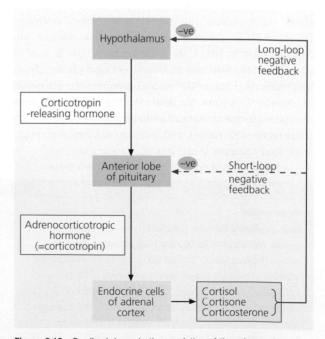

Figure 9.13 Feedback loops in the regulation of the release of glucocorticoid hormones (e.g. cortisol). Compare with that for thyroxine in Figure 9.10.

Q. What would happen to this control in a person with a corticotropin-producing tumour in the pituitary gland?

Mineralocorticoids

Mineralocorticoids are steroids that are secreted by cells of the zona glomerularis of the adrenal cortex (Figure 9.12). The main mineralocorticoid is aldosterone, the release of which is stimulated by sodium deficiency or by an increased plasma potassium concentration. It has an important role in the maintenance of sodium (and hence water) and potassium balance (see Chapter 15). Its actions are:

● in the kidney, to stimulate sodium uptake in exchange for potassium or hydrogen ions, thus conserving sodium but increasing the urinary excretion of potassium/ hydrogen ions (these are the main actions of the hormone);

● in sweat and salivary glands, to promote sodium reabsorption from sweat and saliva, thus diluting the sweat and conserving sodium ions;

● in the gut, to stimulate sodium absorption, thus adding sodium to body fluids.

Sodium deficiency results in a reduced extracellular fluid volume (see Chapter 6); aldosterone release in these circumstances is mediated by increased generation of the hormone angiotensin (Figure 9.14). This peptide hormone is produced from a precursor (a protein called angiotensinogen) found in plasma, although final activation is produced by the actions of angiotensin-converting enzyme (ACE) as blood passes through the lungs. The initial conversion of angiotensinogen is induced by the

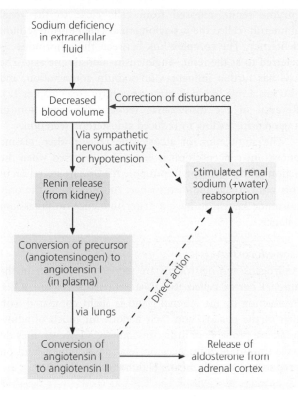

Figure 9.14 The renin-angiotensin-aldosterone axis, and its role in the regulation of sodium balance. Note that aldosterone is only one of the hormones that influences sodium regulation (see Chapter 15). Angiotensin is also involved in the regulation of arterial blood pressure (see Chapter 12).
Q. How would an angiotensin-converting enzyme (ACE) inhibitor drug alter this response?

Hyposecretion of glucocorticoids and mineralocorticoids

Deficiency of cortisol secretion produces Cushing's syndrome, in which decreased blood glucose concentration of cortisol leads to lethargy and muscle weakness. Blood pressure may also be low, since the permissive effect of cortisol on the heart is reduced. Intervention is by hormone replacement through administration of synthetic steroid.

Hyposecretion of aldosterone can adversely affect sodium balance, although compensatory mechanisms will often ensure that balance is reasonably maintained. However, aldosterone is the body's only potassium-regulating hormone, so plasma potassium concentration will be elevated (hyperkalaemia), leading to disorders of nerve and muscle functions. Intervention is by administration of synthetic steroid.

Hypersecretion of glucocorticoids and mineralocorticoids

Excess cortisol (called Addison's disease) mobilizes fatty acids, causing a redistribution of fat stores, and may produce a 'moon face' or 'buffalo hump'. Excessive oedema is observed, including that of the abdomen called ascites, partly because of the overlap in actions with the mineralocorticoid aldosterone (see below). Striations may be observable on the abdomen if distension is extreme. The person becomes prone to bruising, and wound

healing is usually poor (glucocorticoids suppress leucocytes; this action is exploited in the treatment of inflammation and some types of leukaemia).

Excess aldosterone causes aldosteronism. Primary aldosteronism is excessive secretion of the hormone due to a disorder of the gland itself; secondary aldosteronism is excessive secretion due to another disorder, such as renal failure (via increased generation of angiotensin). The problem is characterized by low plasma potassium concentration (hypokalaemia), leading to disorders of nerve and muscle functions. Sodium retention will also be observed. Aldosterone antagonists may be used to block the actions of the hormone on the kidneys.

Gonadocorticoids

Sex steroids from the cortex are secreted at a very low rate compared with from the gonads. They are not considered to be significant in sexually mature adults, but they can be problematic when gonadal function is deficient, e.g. cortical oestrogens may promote breast development in boys, while androgens may cause voice deepening, hair loss, changes in skin texture, and facial hair in postmenopausal women. Under these circumstances, the psychological effects can be profound.

enzyme renin, released from cells close to the renal glomeruli (called the juxtaglomerular cells) during sodium deficiency. The complex link between these hormones is referred to as the renin–angiotensin–aldosterone axis. The axis has further influences on sodium conservation, and also has a role in blood pressure control (see Chapter 12). Reversal of the disturbance reduces the activation of angiotensin, leading to reduced aldosterone secretion.

The stimulation of aldosterone release when plasma potassium concentration is elevated is reversed when the action of the hormone to promote the urinary excretion of this ion corrects the disturbance. Aldosterone is the only hormone known to have a major influence on potassium balance.

Gonadocorticoids

Androgens and oestrogens are secreted by a layer of the adrenal cortex called the zona reticularis (Figure 9.12). Production by the adrenal gland is slight compared with that of the gonads, and their actions for much of adulthood are probably of little consequence. However, they do have important influences on fetal development, and on prepubertal growth during childhood (see Box 9.9).

The adrenal medulla

The adrenal medulla secretes the catecholamine hormones adrenaline and noradrenaline; adrenaline is the main secretion. These hormones are synthesized and released by cells that develop from neurons in the embryo, and are modified cells of the sympathetic nervous system.

The hormones are released when sympathetic nerves to the adrenal glands are activated. Their actions support the activities of this branch of the autonomic nervous system. Particular effects are to promote responses that facilitate physical activity (the fright/fight/flight responses):

- cardiac function is increased, with greater force of contraction and increased pulse rate;
- selective vasoconstriction and vasodilation are induced, which helps to raise blood pressure and redistribute blood to active tissues;
- sweat production is increased, which helps to dissipate excess heat from increased metabolism;
- bronchodilation is induced, which lowers airway resistance and facilitates alveolar ventilation;
- motility is decreased, reducing the demands on bowel muscle cells and diverting blood from the bowel to active tissues;
- metabolic fuels (glucose and fatty acids) are mobilized to meet the needs of increased metabolic activity.

Sympathetic nerve stimulation is usually transient, and its activity declines once the demand for activity has passed. Hormone release will normally be reduced as a consequence.

The gonads

The testes and ovaries produce steroid (mainly) and peptide hormones. The gonadal steroids produced by males are collectively called androgens, the main one being *testosterone*. Testosterone is essential for determining the production of spermatozoa (= spermatogenesis), and is responsible for promoting their capacitation (i.e. bringing to functional capacity).

The gonadal steroids produced by females are of two types: *oestrogens*, the main ones being *oestriol*, *oestradiol* and *oestrone*, and *progestins*, the main one being *proges-*

BOX 9.10 DYSFUNCTIONING OF THE ADRENAL MEDULLA

Hypersecretion

Sympathetic nerve activity and catecholamine secretion may be sustained in severe distress as a consequence of the limbic-hypothalamic modulation of autonomic nuclei in the brainstem (see Chapter 22). Such stress-related responses may have long-term costs to the individual, e.g. hypertension may develop arising from the cardiac and vascular actions. Other problems relate to disturbances of gastrointestinal functions, although these are not always easy to separate from those caused by dietary and behavioural responses to prolonged stress.

Intervention is targeted at antagonizing catecholamine receptors, e.g. using beta-blockers to reduce heart rate, or using alpha-receptor antagonists to induce vasodilation. (See chapter 8 for explanation of beta- and alpha-receptors.)

Hyposecretion

This is unlikely to have a major consequence, since sympathetic nerve activity will normally compensate. One functional disorder of note, however, is that of circulatory shock, in which nerve activity and hormone release are ineffective, due to either cardiac dysfunction or profound vasodilation as a consequence of hypoxia or toxins. Although this is not actually due to hyposecretion of the hormone, it serves to illustrate the need for appropriate activity when required. Adrenaline itself may be administered, but drugs that stimulate catecholamine receptors may also be used, e.g. beta-receptor agonists to raise heart rate, or alpha-receptor agonists to induce vasoconstriction. However, the fact that sympathetic activity and hormone secretion will actually be occurring in this state means that such intervention may have limited success.

BOX 9.11 EXCESSIVE CHANGES IN GONADAL STEROID SECRETION

Hyposecretion

Deficiency of these hormones causes a failure of puberty in adolescents, or loss of fertility in adults (referred to as hypogonadism, because the gonads are underactive). In adult men, lack of testosterone produces castration syndrome, in which there is a heightening of voice tone, changes to skin and facial characteristics, a loss of libido, and a 'feminizing' of behaviour as a consequence of reduced secondary sexual characteristics. Adult women deficient in oetrogens may experience loss of libido, and changes to the cervix and breasts. Menstrual cycle will be irregular, or may even stop.

Hyposecretion may be due to a disorder of the production of gonadal hormones, or it may reflect inadequate gonadotropin release from the anterior pituitary. In the former case, administration of sex steroid may improve the situation, whilst in the latter, synthetic gonadotropins may be administered to trigger sex steroid release from the gonads. Giving gonadotropin-releasing hormone to stimulate the pituitary to release gonadotropin has also been used.

Menopause

The declining secretion of oestrogens during the menopause has effects in addition to causing atrophy of the reproductive system, including vasomotor changes ('flushes' and sweats) associated with altered autonomic nervous system activities. Psychological effects may also be apparent, although these do not appear to result directly from the loss of the steroids. The withdrawal of ovarian steroids may facilitate expression of the actions of testosterone, which is produced in small quantities throughout life by the adrenal cortex of both sexes. This androgen can cause the growth and coarsening of facial hair, and a deepening of the voice in post-menopausal women.

In the long term, the most serious consequences for physical health are reductions in the ratio of high- to low-density lipoproteins in blood plasma, which begins to favour the deposition of cholesterol in blood vessels (possibly resulting in heart disease and strokes), and the loss of bone matrix and mineral, leading to osteoporosis. Although such changes will be initiated in the perimenopausal period, their progress is gradual, and effects are most likely to be observed many years later. Studies indicate that hormone replacement therapy during the perimenopausal and post-menopausal years prevents, or at least reduces, these changes, although concern regarding the possibility of oestrogen-induced tumours makes the therapy debatable.

The menopause appears to have no comparable process in males, but this is a debatable area, especially from the psychological perspective. Biologically, although testosterone secretion declines with age, its metabolism also declines, so plasma concentrations decline only slowly if at all. Sperm production continues well into late adulthood, although the numbers of sperm and their viability may be decreased slightly. Men whose testosterone secretion significantly diminishes may exhibit castration syndrome, a term that reflects the voice heightening and facial changes (a 'softening') that are characteristic of losing the secretion of this hormone through trauma.

Hypersecretion

In men, excess testosterone is thought to promote aggressive behaviours. In women, excess oestrogens and progesterone may cause irregular menstrual cycles with particularly heavy blood loss. Behavioural changes may also be observed. The long-term health risks are the potential for cardiac damage, and development of cancerous tumours of the breast and cervix. Long-acting drugs that suppress the release of luteinizing hormone have been found to be useful to treat endometriosis (growth of endometrial tissue outside the uterus) by suppressing development of the corpus luteum and so preventing progesterone release.

---

terone. Oestrogens and progesterone determine and regulate the menstrual cycle and breast development.

The gonads also produce the peptide *inhibin*, which, although poorly understood, seems to modulate steroid production and gametogenesis.

The roles of these hormones are explained in detail in Chapter 18, but it is worth noting here that the control of their release is via gonadotropins from the anterior pituitary, follicle-stimulating hormone (FSH) and luteinizing hormone (LH). These peptide hormones are named after their effects in the female, but are they are chemically identical in both sexes. They are released in response to the presence of gonadotropin-releasing hormones (GnRH) produced by the hypothalamus. Regulation is exerted by negative feedback effects of the gonadal steroids on both the hypothalamus and pituitary (see Chapter 18).

The gut and pancreas

The gut

The bowel produces a wide variety of hormones that mediate digestive functions (see Chapter 10). These are peptides, the main ones being:

- *gastrin*, produced by cells lining part of the stomach;
- *secretin*, produced by cells lining the duodenum;
- *cholecystokinin pancreozymin* (CCK PZ), produced by cells lining the duodenum.

Gastrin

Gastrin release is stimulated by the presence of food in the stomach. It has a role in gastric acid secretion. Gastrin also stimulates gastric motility, and the muscular contractions mix the chyme and empty the gastric contents into the duodenum. Its release is inhibited, however, if the acidity of the chyme becomes intense, since this acts as the negative feedback signal on the hormone-secreting cells.

Secretin

Secretin was the first hormone to be identified (the term 'hormone' was coined after its discovery). It is secreted by mucosal cells lining the duodenum in response to the presence of acidic chyme, i.e. when chyme has entered the duodenum from the stomach. The hormone acts to neutralize and then alkalinize the chyme by stimulating the secretion of a bicarbonate-rich fluid from the pancreas. As the acidity falls, the release of secretin declines.

Cholecystokinin-pancreozymin

This hormone's name is a clumsy combination of what was once thought to be two distinctive hormones – cholecystokinin (CCK) and pancreozymin (PZ) – that were discovered independently. The two names relate to the dual actions of the hormone. CCK-PZ is released from mucosal cells lining the duodenum in response to the presence of chyme. The stimuli seem to be the major foodstuffs of the chyme, i.e. carbohydrates, fats and semi-digested proteins. The hormone then promotes the secretion of digestive enzymes by the pancreas (hence the 'pancreozymin' component of the name). It also has other actions in relation to fat digestion: it promotes the release of bile from the gall bladder, and so facilitates emulsification of fats, and it reduces gastric emptying, and so increases the time that chyme remains in the duodenum ('cholecystic gland' is an old term for the gall bladder, hence the 'cholecystokinin' component of the name).

Other gut hormones

The gut also produces a host of putative hormones, i.e. substances that seem to have an effect on the organs but have yet to be researched to the extent required for their recognition as hormones. One such substance is a peptide called motilin, which some authorities do consider to have hormone status. Motilin is secreted by cells lining the ileum. It appears to have a role in co-ordinating the pattern of motility (i.e. contractions) of the ileum as it changes from that observed between meals to a pattern associated with standing waves and peristalsis when chyme is present.

Another example is gastric insulinotropic peptide (GIP), released in response to the presence of monosaccharides in the digestive chyme. Its name reflects the main documented action to act as a tropin and stimulate the release of insulin. This is seen as being anticipatory of a glucose load entering the circulatory system (see below). Its alternative name, gastric inhibitory peptide (also GIP), reflects its other action to reduce gastric emptying.

The pancreas

The endocrine tissue of the pancreas is found as discrete clusters of cells, called the islets of Langerhans. These gland cells produce peptide hormones (Table 9.2):

- *insulin*, produced by the B-cells (beta-cells) of the islets;

- *glucagon*, produced by the A-cells (alpha-cells) of the islets;

- *somatostatin*, produced by the D-cells (delta-cells) of the islets.

Insulin

Insulin release is promoted when blood glucose concentration is elevated beyond its homeostatic range. Insulin acts to stimulate the uptake and utilization of glucose by the liver and skeletal muscle cells. Energy is released by cellular respiration, and glycogen synthesis is promoted to replenish carbohydrate stores. The conversion of glucose into certain amino acids and glycerol promotes further storage of metabolic fuel. Insulin release decreases again as plasma glucose concentration declines. Insulin is the only known hormone that reduces blood glucose concentration.

Glucagon

In contrast, glucagon release is stimulated by a decrease in the glucose concentration of plasma below its homeostatic range. Its actions are the opposite of those of insulin, promoting the mobilization of glucose via the breakdown of glycogen and via the synthesis of glucose from glycerol and amino acids. Glucagon release declines as the plasma glucose concentration increases.

Somatostatin

Somatostatin release is stimulated by both glucagon and insulin. It seems to act as a paracrine secretion, and modulates the release of the other two hormones, thus preventing excessive secretion. Control of the release of glucagon and insulin is also provided by their actions to promote the other's release (their antagonistic actions will help to prevent excess responses to either).

Table 9.2 Factors influencing the release of insulin and glucagon

Excitatory influences	Homeostatic relevance	Inhibitory influences	Homeostatic relevance
Insulin			
Direct influence of elevated blood glucose concentration	Increased glucose utilization after food intake Promotes glycogenesis	Blood glucose deficit	Reduction of glycogenesis, leaving more glucose available for cellular respiration
Increased parasympathetic nervous activity from hypothalamus to pancreatic B-cells (in response to elevated blood glucose)	Increased glucose utilization after food intake Promotes glycogenesis	Increased sympathetic nervous activity from hypothalamus to pancreatic B-cells (in response to stress or exercise)	Reduction of glycogenesis, leaving more glucose available for cellular respiration
Duodenal hormones (e.g. CCK-PZ) in response to glucose present in digestive chyme	Feed-forward release of insulin in preparation for glucose load from gut	Somatostatin (released by direct stimulation of pancreatic D-cells by insulin)	Fine control of insulin release in presence of stimulatory factors
Glucagon			
Direct influence of blood glucose deficit	Promotion of glycogenolysis and gluconeogenesis to provide glucose for cellular respiration	Direct influence of elevated blood glucose concentration	Decreased glycogenolysis/ gluconeogenesis Increased glucose utilization (via promotion of insulin release)
Increased parasympathetic nervous activity from hypothalamus to pancreatic A-cells (in response to blood glucose deficit)	Promotion of glycogenolysis and gluconeogenesis to provide glucose for cellular respiration	Somatostatin (released by direct stimulus of pancreatic D-cells by glucagon	Fine control of glucagon release in presence of stimulatory influences

BOX 9.12 DYSFUNCTIONING OF THE PANCREATIC ISLETS

Hyposecretion

Diabetes mellitus is observed when there is a deficiency of the hormone insulin (see also Box 4.11). The effects are to increase blood glucose concentration (hyperglycaemia), leading to excretion of glucose in the urine (glycosuria) and dehydration. Urinary tract infections may also be observed. Medium-to long-term hyperglycaemia has the potential to damage the eye (retinopathy), the nervous system (neuropathy) and the renal system (renopathy) as a consequence of the direct effects of glucose on tissues and the shift towards fat metabolism that is also observed in this condition. Unstable regulation of blood glucose concentration can also result in episodes of hypoglycaemia, which has behaviour-inducing consequences (frequently aggression), and may induce poor co-ordination, confusion and even coma as a consequence of poor delivery of glucose to brain cells.

The condition is subdivided into the form in which the individual is incapable of producing the hormone (insulin-dependent diabetes mellitus, IDDM), and the form in which the individual exhibits poor release of the hormone and/or poor tissue responses to it (non-insulin-dependent diabetes mellitus, NIDDM). The former typically occurs in children or adolescents, and the latter during adulthood. (IDDM is sometimes still referred to by the earlier names, Type 1, early onset or juvenile diabetes. NIDDM may be referred to as Type 2 or late onset diabetes).

Care for IDDM patients revolves around a need to take insulin as a hormone replacement, and to pay particular attention to dietary habits and foods eaten, especially in relation to the timing of insulin administration. The intention is to provide extrinsic control of blood glucose concentration, preventing excessive hyperglycaemia or hypoglycaemia.

Care for NIDDM patients has similar objectives, and will also involve dietary advice. However, this form of diabetes may also be treated pharmacologically, depending upon the actual problem. For example, a drug may be used to stimulate the pancreas to release its insulin, or a metabolic stimulant drug may be used to promote metabolism of glucose.

The thymus

The thymus is a lymphoid gland found in the neck. It has an important role in the differentiation of T-lymphocytes in immune responses. Differentiation is not understood completely, but it is promoted by peptide hormones released within the thymus called *thymin*, *thymosin* and *thymopoietin*. They appear to have similar actions, but the mechanism of their control is unknown.

The thymus gland involutes and begins to atrophy early in adulthood, by which time the secondary lymphoid tissues will have a full complement of the T-cells necessary for immunity. This suggests that the hormones perform most of their roles relatively early in life.

The pineal gland

The pineal gland is an outgrowth of neural tissue situated in the roof of the third cerebral ventricle, deep within the brain. Its main secretion is the peptide *melatonin*. Documented actions of this hormone include the induction of sleep, but it has also been shown to prevent ovulation via an inhibition of the release of gonadotropin-releasing hormone from the hypothalamus (therefore overproduction of melatonin can delay puberty). Links with the human menstrual cycle have not been established, however. There is some evidence that melatonin influences the secretion of other pituitary hormones, and the rich innervation of the pineal gland by sympathetic neurons would seem to suggest further roles.

One documented role is that of a mediator of circadian rhythms (see Chapter 23). The gland receives impulses from the eyes, and is postulated to be involved in the light/dark synchronization of the rhythmicity observed for some physiological parameters, presumably via its neural links with the hypothalamus and thence the pituitary gland. The role of the hormone in regulating sleep is entirely in keeping with this further role in determining biological rhythms. The gland calcifies during adulthood, and its activities are thought to become less efficient, thus making circadian rhythms less effective in elderly people.

The gland is also of interest for historical reasons. Its central position in the brain and its unclear functions led to it for many years being postulated to be the 'spiritual' centre of the brain, conveying conscience as a human faculty. There is no evidence for this, although it could also be argued that 'conscience' is an indeterminate faculty.

The placenta

This gland is obviously only functional in pregnant women. The placenta is often considered in its role in providing nutrients and oxygen to the developing fetus, but it also has important endocrine functions. The placenta produces large amounts of oestrogens throughout the pregnancy, which help the mother to maintain her pregnancy, promote changes in the mother's physiology that will support fetal development, facilitate breast development, and help to prepare the reproductive tract for the birth process. Oestrogen production by the fetal adrenal gland is also an important source of the hormones.

(Human) chorionic gonadotropin (hCG) is a hormone produced by the early placenta that helps to maintain oestrogen and progesterone production by the corpus luteum within the mother's ovary until the placenta is sufficiently developed in this respect. The hormone continues to be produced by the placenta for the duration of the pregnancy, albeit at a lower rate than in the first few weeks, but its role in the pregnancy is unclear. The term 'chorionic' indicates that the source of the hormone is from embryonic cells within the placenta

---

BOX 9.13 HORMONAL CONTROL OF BREAST DEVELOPMENT IN PREGNANCY, AND LACTATION

Breast development and lactation provide illustrations of altered set points in homeostasis, induced by hormone release that is linked to the need for the development of specific tissues and functions.

Breast development

In this case, we see the roles of increased production of gonadal steroids (although these are released mostly from the placenta), and their interaction with placental lactogen. Progesterone from the placenta promotes the growth of breast alveoli, i.e. the glandular tissue that secretes milk. Oestrogens from the placenta stimulate growth of lactiferous ducts that will conduct milk to the nipple. Placental lactogen has a permissive role, i.e. the actions of oestrogen and progesterone on the breast will be effective only in the presence of this hormone. Placental lactogen also inhibits the release of prolactin from the pituitary gland. This hormone has a central role in lactation (see below), and its inhibition during pregnancy prevents milk secretion from the developing alveoli.

Lactation

Lactation is the process of milk secretion. It is clearly most effective if milk is secreted according to need, i.e. when a baby is suckling. Suckling promotes a number of hormonal responses:

- Prolactin release from the pituitary gland is stimulated via neural input to the hypothalamus (remember that the release of hormones from the anterior pituitary gland involves releasing or inhibitory hormones from the hypothalamus). Prolactin causes secretion of milk by the alveoli of the breast.
- Neural inputs to the hypothalamus also promote the release of oxytocin from the pituitary gland. This hormone contracts the lactiferous ducts and so enables milk to be conveyed to the surface. Oxytocin release stimulated by suckling may also help to contract down the uterus after birth (remember that oxytocin is a vital hormone in labour).
- Neural inputs to the hypothalamus also cause the pituitary to release less gonadotropin, which then reduces oestrogen release from the ovarian follicles. This may be a mechanism to reduce the likelihood of another pregnancy while the infant is dependent upon the mother – but it is not unfailingly effective.

(the chorion is one of the extra-embryonic membranes; see Chapter 20).

Placental lactogen (also called chorionic somatomammotrophin) is involved in breast development during pregnancy (see Box 9.13). It is also a metabolic hormone, and alters maternal glucose and fat metabolism. Its release increases during pregnancy, and it is used clinically as an index of placental function. Again, the term 'chorionic' is of note – the hormone derives from embryonic cells within the placenta.

Relaxin is a hormone that relaxes the symphysis pubis joint in the mother's pelvis, and promotes dilation of the cervix during birth.

These secretions emphasize how maternal physiology is influenced by the placenta, the cells of which are derived partially from the fetus. Who is controlling whom? It may be the mother who is supporting the fetus, but fetal secretions are instrumental in ensuring that this occurs. In endocrine terms, the placenta is often referred to as a fetoplacental unit, a name that recognizes that the fetus makes a contribution to the hormonal secretion.

Other hormones

Various other hormonal secretions have been identified, secreted by cells that do not form identifiable glands. Their numbers continue to grow. In addition to those substances now accepted as hormones, a host of others are putative ones. A comprehensive list of all these secretions is not possible, but some of those recognized as hormones are discussed here.

Atrial natriuretic factor is a peptide hormone that originates from cells lining the atria of the heart (particularly the right atrium). The hormone is named because of its actions to increase urinary sodium excretion (natriuresis), but it also has an important role in promoting dilation of veins. It is released when an increase in blood volume stretches the atrial wall. Although this could occur transiently, e.g. when venous return is increased during exercise, the main role of the hormone is probably in the longer-term regulation of blood volume. Its dilatory actions on veins help the circulatory system to accommodate any increase in volume (and therefore avoid arterial hypertension), while the renal actions help to reduce blood volume (by excreting sodium chloride and water).

Prostaglandins are local eicosanoid hormones; they were named after they were first identified as secretions in seminal fluid from prostate glands. They are produced by most, if not all, body tissues, and probably only influence cells in the vicinity of their secretion, i.e. they are paracrine secretions. There are various kinds of prostaglandin, E_2, F_{2alpha} and PGI_2 being the main ones, and their roles vary with the tissue. For example, prostaglandins help to maintain blood flow to tissues such as the stomach; they

influence transport mechanisms in the kidney; they contract the cervix after coitus, and the uterus during birth; and they produce pain and inflammation when tissues are damaged (see Chapter 21). They act either directly or by modulating the actions of other hormones. *Thromboxanes* are another group of eicosanoids that also act locally, e.g. they are part of the clotting factor secretion produced by blood platelets. *Leukotrienes* are also eicosanoids. One documented action of these is in promoting contraction of bronchial smooth muscle during asthma.

Erythropoietin is a peptide hormone produced by conversion of a precursor (erythropoietinogen) in plasma by the enzyme erythrogenin, which is released from the kidney when blood perfusing the organ is deficient in oxygen. The hormone promotes production of red blood cells (a process called erythropoiesis) by bone marrow (see Chapter 11).

Endothelium-derived relaxing factor (EDRF) is a substance produced by capillary endothelial cells. It has an important role in the intrinsic regulation of vascular resistance in tissues. Its actions are to stimulate the production of nitrous oxide by the cells, which in turn causes vasodilation.

It may seem odd to include *vitamin D* in a chapter on hormones, but many authorities now recognize it to be a hormone. Vitamin D_3, also called cholecalciferol, is obtained either from the diet or from the conversion of a steroid precursor in the skin through the actions of sunlight. However, this must then be converted to an intermediary in the liver, and then into the active form (1,25-dihydroxycalciferol) in the kidneys. In this form, it promotes the uptake of calcium from the intestine. It is the intrinsic production in the skin of a precursor and the conversion to the active form that is observed when calcium concentrations are beginning to decrease, that have promoted the view that it is a hormone.

Leptin is a peptide secreted by adipose tissue when adipose cells increase their fat content. It crosses the blood–brain barrier, and acts on centres within the hypothalamus to promote satiety, and to cause a decrease in food intake. Leptins were only discovered during the 1990s, but they have attracted a tremendous amount of interest, not least because they are considered to be one of the regulators of body weight (see Box 4.12).

A host of peptide growth factors have also been identified, e.g. *epidermal growth factor* has a role in regulating cell division by mitosis (not necessarily confined to the epidermis). *Neurogenic (or nerve growth) factor* has a role in nerve axon growth in the embryo/fetus and infant, and also if there is nerve damage. These peptides probably have localized actions, and so are paracrine or autocrine secretions. Although the actions of these and other 'tissue' hormones have been documented, the control of their secretions is generally poorly understood.

Summary

1 Hormones are chemical messengers that provide a means of communication between tissues in different parts of the body, and therefore are part of the co-ordinating mechanisms of the body.

2 The process of hormone synthesis/release, transportation in extracellular fluid, and interaction with target cells means that responses are slower than those of nerve stimulation, so hormones are generally not involved in responses that must occur rapidly, i.e. within seconds.

3 Hormones are secreted by glands, although not all glandular secretions can be considered to be hormones. Hormone-secreting glands are generally referred to as endocrine glands.

4 Hormones are either peptides, catecholamines (modified amino acids), steroids (modified lipids) or prostaglandins (modified fatty acids). Their diverse actions help to regulate the range of physiological parameters vital for health.

5 Hormones are able to produce a large response by target cells because the cell activation is amplified through the cascade effect of second messenger activation (hormones are the first messenger chemicals).

6 Many hormones are tropins, i.e. they promote the release of further hormones from target gland tissue. Others are released in response to non-hormonal stimuli, and promote a change in those parameters.

7 Hormone release is usually controlled by negative feedback mechanisms. Some glands utilize short-loop control, others long-loop.

8 This chapter identifies over 40 important hormones and the glands that produce them. The stimuli that release them are largely identified, as are the feedback processes (where applicable) that control their secretion.

9 Disorders of hormone function arise from a failure to control hormonal secretion, or from a lack of response of target tissues to the hormone after it is released. Clinical intervention is directed at correcting the secretory defect, replacing the hormone (if it is deficient in blood), preventing/promoting hormone action with appropriate antagonistic/agonistic drugs, or stimulating tissue function by other pharmacological means.

Review questions

1 What are hormones?

2 How do hormones reach their target sites?

3 How do hormones recognize target cells?

4 Which type of hormone is lipid soluble?

5 Name three ways in which endocrine organs can be stimulated to release hormones

6 Insulin is a hormone that lowers blood glucose levels. How is this achieved? What is glycosuria, and when does it occur?

7 Name five endocrine organs, and state the hormone(s) that each produces. Identify the functions of these hormones, and list the signs and symptoms associated with increased or decreased levels (hyposecretion and hypersecretion).

FURTHER READING

Most generic texts on human functioning will include discussion of hormones. Alternatively, a specialist text might be consulted that extends the discussion, e.g.

Gard, P.R. (1998) *Human Endocrinology*. London: Taylor & Francis.

Section Four

Effectors of homeostasis

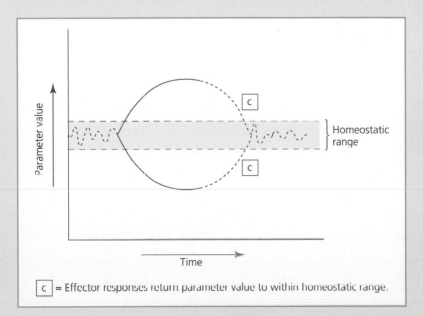

c = Effector responses return parameter value to within homeostatic range.

Chapter 10

The digestive system

INTRODUCTION: RELATION OF THE DIGESTIVE SYSTEM TO CELLULAR HOMEOSTASIS

The digestive system aids the correct functioning of cell by ensuring that the body is provided with the 'normal' requirements of molecules necessary to maintain cellular metabolism at a rate compatible with life. The importance of a balanced diet was discussed in Chapter 5, which emphasized that the food humans consume consists of a diversity of molecular compounds. The bulk of the diet is provided by three main classes of food: carbohydrates, lipids and proteins (and also nucleic acids). These are usually consumed as large, insoluble molecular complexes, and must be reduced in size and made soluble before they can be absorbed into blood, transported to their site of action, and utilized in cellular metabolism, for growth, repair of component parts, production of energy, etc.

The breaking down and increase in solubility of ingested molecules is called digestion. In addition to the three main classes of food, dietary constituents must also include water, vitamins and minerals. These molecules are already soluble, and are small enough to be absorbed into blood, hence their digestion is unnecessary.

This chapter is concerned with how food intake is regulated, the process of digestion, and the liver's role in determining the fate of the majority of these end products of digestion.

REGULATION OF FOOD INTAKE

Many areas of the brain have been identified as having a role in feeding and satiety. However, the most important area is the hypothalamus, which has two centres involved in the regulation of food intake: the hunger (feeding) centre, and the satiety (cessation of feeding) centre.

The hunger centre is constantly active, unless it is inhibited by input from the satiety centre. There are many theories as to the regulatory factors associated with food intake:

● The *glucostat theory* suggests that low levels of plasma glucose initiate feeding, by stimulating the hunger centre activity and depressing the inhibitory action of the satiety centre. Conversely, a high plasma glucose concentration results in inhibition of hunger centre activity and thus stops feeding.

● The *amino acid theory* is based on the same reasoning, but with reference to plasma levels of amino acids instead of glucose. Amino acid responses appear to be less effective than glucose responses. Lipids have also been indicated as important factors.

- The *fat cell theory* states that leptins released by fat cells signal the synthesis of triglycerides, thus the rate of feeding decreases as the volume of adipose tissue increases.

- The *signalling chemicals theory* states that chemicals in the blood act on the hypothalamus to decrease appetite and increase energy expenditure; such chemicals include several hormones (e.g. noradrenaline, cholecystokinin, glucagon). Conversely, other signalling chemicals in the blood act on the hypothalamus to increase appetite and decrease energy expenditure (e.g. the hormones adrenaline, growth hormone releasing factor, glucocorticoids, insulin, somatostatin and progesterone).

- *Psychological factors* are also an important consideration, since they can override the usual intake mechanisms; this occurs in obesity, anorexia nervosa and bulimia.

- The *body temperature theory* attempts to explain why it is that we tend to eat more in winter, linking this with the colder environmental temperatures that result in a lowering of the body temperature and a stimulation of the hunger centre. The reverse reasoning is given to explain why we tend to eat less in hot summer months. This theory may partly explain why we tend to gain a little weight in the winter months, but many other contributory factors are also important.

- The *gastrointestinal stretch receptor theory* has received most recognition in controlling food intake and the cessation of intake (Figure 10.1). This suggests that distension of the stomach and duodenum by the presence of food stimulate stretch receptors in these organs above their 'normal' or baseline firing range. These receptors send sensory impulses to the hypothalamic satiety centre,

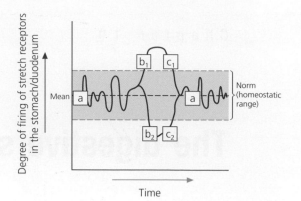

Figure 10.1 The regulation of food intake. (a) 'Normal' level of firing of stretch receptors. Stimulus is not enough to stimulate satiety centre and the degree of hunger centre output is not sufficient to seek food. (b_1) Increased rate of firing of stretch receptors above their baseline level, resulting in sensory input to the satiety centre. This centre inhibits the hunger centre's output, and so causes the cessation of food intake. (b_2) Decreased rate of firing of stretch receptors below their baseline level, resulting in a decrease in sensory fibre input to the satiety centre (i.e. insufficient to stimulate it), thus stimulating the hunger centre activity, causing the individual to seek food. (c) Restoration of 'normal' stretch receptor activity by appropriate changes in satiety (c_1) and hunger (c_2) centre activity.

Q. List the theories that attempt to explain the control of food intake.

which in turn inhibits hunger centre activity, bringing about cessation of food intake. Conversely, if the degree of stretching falls below the baseline-firing rate, then the sensory information is not sufficient to stimulate the satiety centre output. Thus, the inhibition to the hunger centre is removed, with the result that feeding is promoted.

See the case study of an adolescent girl with anorexia nervosa in Section 6.

OVERVIEW OF THE ANATOMY AND PHYSIOLOGY OF THE DIGESTIVE SYSTEM

The anatomy and physiology of the digestive system evolved in humans to convert consumed food into a form that could be used by the cells. The conversion can be divided into five principal physiological processes:

1 *Ingestion (eating):* the process of taking food into the mouth.

2 *Digestion:* the physical and chemical breakdown of food; both processes are necessary to render food into a state for the third process of absorption.

3 *Absorption:* the passage of the end products of digestion from the digestive tract into the transporting (cardio-

vascular and lymphatic) systems, which distribute these metabolites to the cells that require them.

4 *Assimilation:* the liver's homeostatic involvement in maintaining blood composition optimal for cellular metabolism.

5 *Defecation (egestion):* the elimination of indigestible substances, such as fibre, certain excretory products (e.g. bile salts and bile pigments), and unabsorbed substances (e.g. some water and electrolytes) from the body.

The digestive system, as shown in Figure 10.2, is adapted to perform these functions. Thus, regional

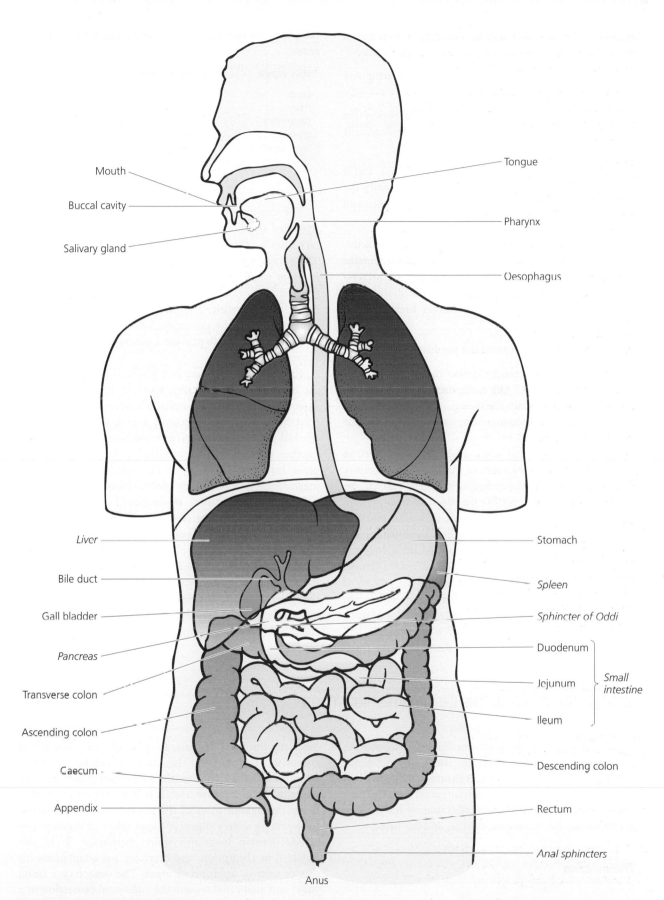

Mouth

Buccal cavity

Salivary gland

Tongue

Pharynx

Oesophagus

Liver

Bile duct

Gall bladder

Pancreas

Transverse colon

Ascending colon

Caecum

Appendix

Stomach

Spleen

Sphincter of Oddi

Duodenum ⎤
⎥
Jejunum ⎥ Small
⎥ intestine
Ileum ⎦

Descending colon

Rectum

Anal sphincters

Anus

Figure 10.2 The human alimentary canal.

Q. Describe the general histological features associated with the wall of the alimentary canal.

anatomical differentiation can be identified that facilitates the performance of specialized functions. In particular:

- the structure of the mouth is suited to the chewing and moisturizing of food, and swallowing;

- the stomach provides a large, distensible region for holding food, 'sterilizing' food, and the commencement of protein digestion;

- the small intestine continues the digestive process, and is supported by the release of bile and enzymes from the pancreas. Distal parts of the small intestine are concerned particularly with the absorption of food products;

- the large intestine also exhibits limited absorptive activities. Its main role is to consolidate undigested remains into semi-solid faecal masses. A number of bacteria present within the large intestine also contribute to the digestive process by promoting further breakdown of undigested material;

- the liver assimilates many of the products.

The organs of the digestive system can be divided into two groups (Table 10.1): the main organs of the alimentary or gastrointestinal tract, e.g. the stomach and intestines, and the accessory digestive organs, e.g. the pancreas and liver.

The alimentary tract is a continuous tube about 10 m long extending from the mouth to the anus. The accessory organs associated with the digestive system (except the tongue) are positioned outside the digestive tract and are involved in the production and release of various digestive secretions. The glandular part of the lining epithelium also produces secretions, which are transported along channels called ducts to their sites of action. Most secretions (except for bile) contain enzymes, which accelerate the process of chemical digestion. For the process to operate efficiently, however, physical churning and softening of foodstuffs must also occur. The processes of both physical and chemical digestion can be identified throughout the tract.

Table 10.1 The main organs and accessory organs of the digestive system

Main organs	Accessory organs
Mouth	Lips, teeth, tongue, salivary glands, palate
Pharynx	
Oesophagus	
Stomach	
Small intestine	Pancreas, gall bladder, liver
Large intestine	

The major regions of the gastrointestinal tract are separated from one another by circular rings of involuntary muscle called sphincters, or by a valve-like structure. The pyloric sphincter, for example, separates the stomach from the small intestine, and the ileo-caecal valve separates the terminal region of the small intestine from the first part of the large intestine. The functional significance of these structures is to aid movement of food in one direction along the tract, and to provide a means of control over that movement.

Exposure to pathogens is a potential problem, because the openings of the digestive tract are in contact with the external environment. Lymphatic 'patches' throughout the tract help to remove infectious agents. Furthermore, the marked pH changes observed throughout the tract provide another external defence mechanism to potential pathogenic invaders. However, if the invaders survive these mechanisms and gain entry into the blood, then our internal defence mechanisms are activated in an attempt to destroy these organisms (see Chapter 13).

The remainder of this chapter discusses the individual regions, their associated physical and chemical digestive processes, and the regional homeostatic imbalances and developmental issues regarding this organ system. First, though, it is important that you become familiar with the types of cells and membranes found in the alimentary canal; reference to Chapter 2 may be useful while you are reading this section.

GENERAL HISTOLOGY OF THE GASTROINTESTINAL TRACT

The basic structure of the gastrointestinal tract follows the same pattern from mouth to anus, with some functional adaptations throughout. Figure 10.3 illustrates the generalized histological appearance of the gastrointestinal tact. The tract has four principal layers or coats called tunicae: the mucosa, the submucosa, the muscularis externa, and the serosa.

The mucosa

The mucosa is a mucous membrane that forms the innermost lining of the tract. The function of mucous is to lubricate the food to ease its passage. The membrane comprises two layers. The inner glandular epithelial membrane is the layer exposed to the lumen and thus the contents of the digestive tract. It is glandular simple epithelium (throughout most of the tract), hence it is adapted for secreting watery digestive juices. Most of the digestive glands develop from this inner membrane. It is also involved in absorption, and therefore has adaptations for this process in appropriate areas. The oesophagus (food tube) and anal canal require the additional protection of a stratified (layered) epithelium, as they are exposed to much wear and tear.

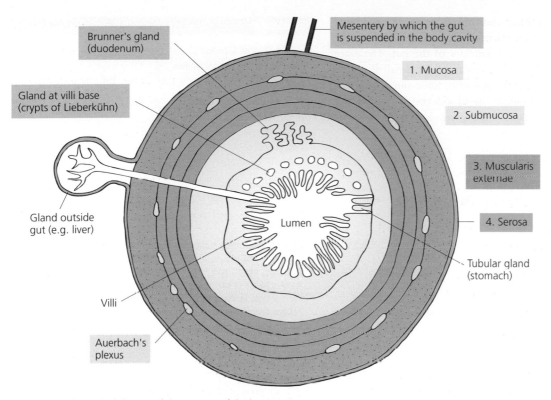

Figure 10.3 Generalized diagram of the structure of the human gut.

Q. Using boxes 10.1 and 10.2, identify a gastrointestinal investigation associated with each main region of the gastrointestinal tract.

The outer membrane, or lamina propria, is a loose connective tissue that supports the glandular epithelium. It accommodates digestive glands, and blood and lymph vessels, providing nutritive and defence functions to the glandular epithelial layer. The propria is attached to a layer of smooth muscle called the muscularis mucosa. This muscle's fibres are subjected to a sustained tonic state of contraction, and are responsible for the folded appearance of the digestive and absorptive surfaces.

The submucosa

The submucosa contains blood vessels and nerves (the nerve cells form a meshwork called the Meissner's plexus). The layer also contains a large amount of collagen and elastic fibres. It functions to control the tract's secretory

activities, and to bind the mucosa to the third coat, the muscularis externa.

The muscularis externa

In most regions, the muscularis externa consists of an outer sheet of longitudinally arranged involuntary (smooth) muscle fibres and an inner sheet of circularly arranged muscle fibres. A meshwork of nerves, called Auerbach's or myenteric plexus, lies between these sheets of muscle fibres, and is responsible for co-ordinating their activity. Contraction of these fibres generates the specialized movements of the gastrointestinal tract that move food along the tract, aid the mixing of its contents, and therefore facilitate the digestive process.

The serosa

The serosa is part of a serous membrane called the peritoneum. The serosa of the gut is known as the visceral peritoneum, as it is attached to the surface of the digestive organs. Its counterpart, the parietal peritoneum (not a part of the gut serosa), lines the wall of the abdominal cavity. The fluid-filled space between these serous membranes, called the peritoneal cavity, provides a protective cushioning of the gut during digestion and upon changes in intra-abdominal pressure associated with breathing movements. An extension of the peritoneum forms the mesenteries of the gut. These are outward folds of the serous coat of the small intestine that bind this organ to the posterior abdominal wall. The mesenteries accommodate the blood vessels, lymphatics and neurons that supply this region.

The regional adaptations of the membranes in the gut are summarized in Table 10.2.

Table 10.2 Regional histological features of the alimentary canal

Oesophagus

Folded mucosa
Stratified squamous epithelia
Thick muscularis mucosa
Some glands are present
Absence of serosa
Thickest muscularis externa; upper third is voluntary, the mid-third is a mixture of voluntary and involuntary, and the latter third is involuntary
Papillae project into the epithelium

Stomach

Large mucosal folds – rugae
Thick muscular wall
Numerous gastric pits
An abundance of exocrine glands in the lamina propria
Parietal cells in the fundus
Oblique layer in the muscularis externae
No villi or goblet cells

Small intestine

Duodenum
    An abundance of villi compared with jejunum and ileum; villi are short and leaf-shaped
    Two types of epithelial cells
    Goblet cells
    Intestinal folds – plicae
    Brunner's glands
    Crypts of lieberkühn

Jejunum
    As for duodenum except taller plicae, and villi are tongue-shaped

Ileum
    As for duodenum except fewer or no plicae, and finger-shaped villi
    Aggregates of lymph nodules – Peyer's patches

Large intestine

Appendix
    Lymphatic tissue, with lymphocytes between the crypts
    Narrow lumen

Colon
    No villi
    Long tubular glands
    Few goblet cells
    Thin muscularis externa consisting of three muscular bands – taeniae (giving this region a pouched appearance)
    Large lumen
    Peyer patches project into submucosa

Rectum
    As for colon, except no taeniae, and thick muscularis externae
    Stratified epthelium near the retroanal junction
    Longest glands

BOX 10.2 EMBRYOLOGICAL FORMATION OF THE GUT

The embryo cells flatten during the fourth week of development, and become folded to form an enclosed tube. The lumen of the tube lined with epithelium will form the gut. The epithelium is derived from embryonic endoderm, with the exception of the epithelia lining the anal canal and parts of the mouth cavity, which is of ectoderm origin. The wall layers beyond the endoderm lining are formed from embryonic mesoderm. Suckling movements are apparent from the twenty-fourth week of gestation, and the fetus takes in a substantial amount of amniotic fluid during the gestational period.

The digestive glands along the wall of the digestive tube are formed from endoderm. The primitive gut is divided into foregut, mid-gut and hindgut. The foregut comprises the pharynx, oesophagus, stomach, duodenum and, as far as where the bile and pancreatic ducts drain into the gut, the pancreas and liver. The mid-gut develops and continues from the duodenum to the jejunum, ileum, caecum and appendix, and up to the transverse colon. The mid-gut herniates into the umbilical cord during the fifth week of gestation. The hindgut develops into the remainder of the colon, the rectum and the proximal anal canal. The gut fills with meconium, which contains digestive secretions.

Developmental abnormalities can occur during the gestation period, e.g. regions of the digestive tube may become stenosed, as in pyloric stenosis (see Box 10.10).

PHYSIOLOGY OF THE DIGESTIVE SYSTEM

Digestion is the sum total of all the processes involved in breaking down consumable food from large, complex, insoluble molecules to simple, soluble molecules, so that these substances can be absorbed readily into the blood for carriage to cells that utilize them. There are two processes involved in this breakdown:

1 *Physical digestion* involves a variety of structural components of the digestive tract, which mechanically reduce the size of the ingested food particle (Figure 10.4(a)). The function of physical digestion is to increase the surface area of the food particles to aid chemical digestion.

2 *Chemical digestion* involves the breakdown of chemical bonds within molecules too large to be absorbed directly into the blood. Enzymes accelerate (catalyse) this breakdown by promoting hydrolysis of the molecules. Hydrolysis is the chemical breakdown using water, whereby a hydrogen group from the water molecule is added to one of the products of this breakdown, and a hydroxyl group is added to the other (Figure 10.4(b)). Figure 10.4(b) shows that heat is also given off as a result of this process, so the actions of digestive enzymes also contribute to the thermoregulation of cells and extracellular fluid.

Physical and chemical digestion occur simultaneously. For convenience, however, the processes will be described individually for each anatomical region of the gut. Pancreatic and liver functions will also be separately described, but it should be remembered that integration of regional functions determines the final outcome of the digestive/assimilative processes.

A person's nutritional status can be compared with scientific tables of 'ideal' weight for height and build, or can be explored more specifically. The boxed text in this chapter is concerned mainly with the common regional problems associated with the alimentary canal, starting at the mouth and terminating at the anus.

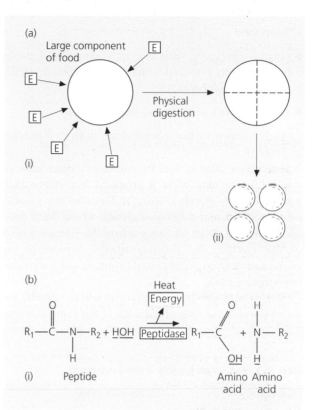

Figure 10.4 (a) Physical digestion — an aid to chemical digestion. (i) Before physical digestion, the enzymatic action is limited to the area surrounding the food component. (ii) After physical digestion, a greater surface area is available for enzymatic action. Note that physical and chemical digestions occur simultaneously. Physical digestion merely makes chemical digestion more efficient by increasing the available surface area for enzymatic attack. (b) Hydrolysis of peptides. During hydrolysis (accelerated by enzymatic action), a water molecule (as hydrogen, H and hydroxyl, OH) is added to the two breakdown products (i.e. amino acids), breaking the chemical bond (called a peptide bond) that is holding the products together.

E, enzyme.

Q. Differentiate between the processes of chemical and physical digestion.

The mouth, pharynx and oesophagus

The mouth

The mouth (oral or buccal) cavity is the opening of the alimentary canal, which aids ingestion. This is the only region that is surrounded by bony skeletal structures, i.e. the upper and lower jaws (the maxilla and mandible, respectively). The muscles associated with these bones are responsible for controlling the overall size of the mouth. The muscular lips or labia guard the opening. The hard

and soft palates, the latter tapering backwards, form the roof of the buccal cavity, terminating in a projection called the uvula. The cheeks form the sides of the mouth, and the tongue forms the floor. The jaws support the cavity and contain the sockets that accommodate the teeth. The mouth is lined with a mucous stratified epithelial membrane, reflecting the wear and tear associated with this area.

Salivation

Water makes up 90–95% of saliva; the remaining 5–10% comprises dissolved solutes, including:

- ions, such as bicarbonate (HCO_3^-), chloride (Cl^-), phosphate (PO_4^{2-}), sodium (Na^+) and potassium (K^+);

- the enzyme salivary amylase;

- lysozymes;

- organic substances, such as urea, albumins and globulins (especially gammaglobulins or antibodies, in particular immunoglobulin A);

- mucin, derived from mucus-secreting cells.

Each component has a homeostatic role, as illustrated in Table 10.3.

The pH of saliva is 7–8. Its production varies between 1 and 1.5 l per day. Most is produced from three main pairs of salivary glands (Figure 10.5), called the parotid, submandibular and sublingual glands, whose ducts open into the buccal cavity on either side of the internal surface of the mouth. The parasympathetic division of the autonomic nervous system largely controls saliva secretion from these glands.

The parotid glands are the largest salivary glands, but are responsible for only about 25% of the daily secretion. Their cells are specialized for contributing to the watery and enzyme-rich component of saliva. They are positioned just below and in front of the ears, and their ducts (called Stenson's ducts) open at a point opposite the second upper molar teeth. The glossopharyngeal (IXth cranial) nerve

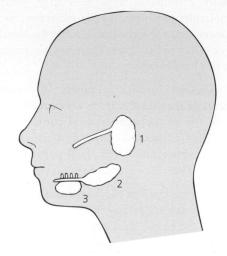

Figure 10.5 Human salivary glands. 1, parotid glands (Stenson's duct); 2, submandibular glands (Wharton's duct); 3, sublingual glands.
Q. Identify the major salivary glands and the main constituents of saliva.

Table 10.3 Homeostatic functions of saliva components

Saliva components	Homeostatic roles
Water	Dissolves food for the appreciation of taste Vital for digestion (hydrolysis) and to provide the necessary aqueous medium for the enzyme's maximum breakdown efficiency
Bicarbonates and phosphates	Buffering action keeps the pH within its homeostatic range (6.35–6.85), essential for enzymatic action; pH changes to slightly alkaline during chewing, which is important for maximizing the effects of salivary amylase, and for destroying the enzyme of acid-liking bacteria
Amylase	Initiates carbohydrate digestion
Lysozymes and antibodies	Destroy bacteria, hence prevent infection
Mucin	Forms soluble mucus in the presence of water, which has a lubricating and moisturizing action
Urea	Excretory products of amino acid metabolism
Chloride	Being a cofactor, it aids salivary amylase

B O X 1 0 . 3 M U M P S

The mumps virus (myxovirus) typically attacks the parotid glands. The condition, mumps (or parotitis), is an enlargement and inflammation of the parotid glands. Swelling occurs on one or both sides of the face. Inflammation of these glands cause electrolytes to become concentrated, and may result in salivary stone formation, causing blockage of the glandular ducts, leading to a swelling of the affected gland. Other accompanying symptoms are moderate fever, general discomfort (malaise), and extreme pain in the throat, especially when swallowing.

In about one-third of males infected after puberty, the testes also become inflamed. Usually only one testis is affected, so sterility rarely occurs. The incidence of mumps has declined following the availability of a vaccine since 1967.

Tumours of the nerve or the blood vessel supplying the glands (particularly the parotid glands) also give rise to painful swelling.

supplies the parotids. This saliva is rich in both enzymes and antibodies (IgA).

The submandibular glands are positioned under the base of the tongue in the posterior aspects of the mouth. Their ducts (called Wharton's ducts) extend centrally along the floor of the mouth, opening behind the lower central incisors. They are responsible for approximately 70% of the daily production of saliva. Their cells are specialized to function in a similar way to the parotid cells, but they also secrete mucous and so produce a more viscous secretion.

The sublingual glands are the smallest of the paired glands, and are responsible for about 5% of the daily production of saliva. Their cells are mainly mucous-secreting cells, and are responsible for producing a very viscous secretion, with little enzyme present. These glands are positioned under the tongue, and have several Rivinus's ducts, which open onto the floor of the mouth.

The submandibular and sublingual glands are responsible for the spray of saliva that sometimes flows out when one yawns. Both of these pairs of glands are supplied by the facial (VIIth cranial) nerve.

Other salivary glands are also present over the palate and tongue, and upon the inner side of the lips. They respond to mechanical stimulation from the presence of food in the mouth, rather than neural activity to the gland.

Control of salivation

Saliva production by the paired glands is controlled mainly via parasympathetic neurons originating in the brainstem. There is always a constant flow of saliva in moderate amounts, because it has homeostatic functions as well as a role in digestion (Table 10.3).

An increase in the basal level of saliva secretion (and stomach secretions) occurs with the sight, smell and touch of food, together with the sound of food preparation, or the anticipation of food intake. This is known as a Pavlovian nervous conditioning response, after the Russian

psychologist who first described the principle. The stimuli increase salivary flow as a result of conditioned reflexes set up from our association areas and memory regions of the brain (see Chapter 8). Such responses are important, as they allow the mouth to lubricate food and commence chemical breakdown as soon as it enters. The presence of ingested food stimulates an even greater salivary flow, by stimulating taste buds on the tongue and other regions in the mouth. Any object rolled on the tongue has the same effect. Once the food is swallowed, a large flow continues that cleanses the mouth, 'washing' the teeth and diluting food residues.

The tongue

The tongue is an accessory organ of the digestive system. The tongue's extrinsic muscles are important in moving it from side to side and in and out; its intrinsic muscles are responsible for changing its shape. The superior surface and the sides of the tongue contain projections called

---

BOX 10.4 THE EFFECTS OF DEHYDRATION AND STRESS ON SALIVA SECRETION

Saliva glands cease to secrete a watery saliva in states of dehydration, as part of the homeostatic conservation of body water. As a result, the mouth becomes dry and may become coated with a thick viscous saliva secretion; this stimulates the sensation of thirst. Liquid intake restores body fluid volumes to within their homeostatic ranges. The nurse should frequently and repeatedly cleanse the mouth of a patient who is dehydrated, so as to remove this viscous secretion and the sensation of thirst.

The tongue may also appear temporarily dry when an individual is anxious, nervous or frightened, as sympathetic nervous system activity inhibits the flow of watery saliva and stimulates a viscous secretion.

BOX 10.5 NORMAL AND ABNORMAL APPEARANCES OF THE TONGUE

The visual appearance of the tongue is of concern to many people, but the following appearances are only cosmetically displeasing, as they are considered quite 'normal':

● Furring, common in mouth breathers.
● Fissuring, common in elderly people. This may be an indication of the wear and tear associated with the ageing process.
● Sublingual vein varicosities.

There are, however, many deviations from the tongue's normal, moist, pink appearance, which are indicative of deficiency diseases, such as the pallor associated with anaemia, the smooth, red appearance of a patient with pernicious anaemia, and the 'dry' tongue seen in dehydration. Tongue movements, particularly during swallowing, will be affected adversely as a consequence of certain

neural lesions involving areas of the brain, especially the brainstem, which regulates the movements, and the cranial nerves, which supply the tongue.

Superficial inflammation of the tongue, called glossitis ('glossa' = tongue), may be associated with people with inflammation of the mouth, generally referred to as stomatitis ('stoma' = mouth). Glossitis may arise in people who experience dental caries, gum infection, gastric disorders, or mucous membrane infections, and in people who smoke and drink alcohol excessively. Treatment varies with each case, and an important part of treatment is allaying the person's fear of cancer.

Q. Differentiate between the actions of parasympathetic and sympathetic innervation on saliva flow and saliva water content.

papillae. The papillae are associated with the sensation of taste, as they contain the taste buds; the details of taste are discussed in Chapter 7.

Tongue movements alter the shape and volume of the mouth cavity, and are also vital in forming speech.

Physical digestion in the mouth

Physical digestion reduces the size of the food particles to aid the chemical processes involved in digestion. It involves the action of the jaw muscles, the teeth and the tongue. The size of the mouth opening, together with the biting action of the teeth, are responsible for determining the size of the food particle ingested. Powerful jaw muscles voluntarily control mouth opening, and the size of this opening is restricted by the perimeter of the muscular lips and the joint between the mandible and the cranium. The teeth are considered in detail in Box 10.6 and Figure 10. 6. The incisors, or biting teeth, mainly control the size of the particle we take in. The canines are used to a limited extent for tearing and shearing fleshy meat from its bone, although as man's diet and social eating habits have changed, these teeth have become less important in ingestion and have become much less prominent in modern man.

Once the food particles are inside the mouth, the premolars and molars crush and grind them, reducing their size. This is controlled by the jaw muscles, and the mechanical process is termed 'mastication' (chewing). Also important in this chewing process is the involuntary movement of the tongue, which moves food particles around the oral cavity; in doing so, the tongue produces friction between the particles and structures that they rub against, and the particle are fragmented as a result. Simultaneous with this physical breakdown is the mixing and lubrication of food with saliva. Saliva contains the enzyme amylase, which initiates the chemical breakdown of carbohydrate within the food.

Chemical digestion in the mouth

The chemical breakdown of large, insoluble molecules begins in the mouth. Salivary amylase ('amyl-' = starch), previously known as ptyalin, initiates the breakdown of the carbohydrate starch by breaking the bonds between the monosaccharide subunits from which starch is constructed (Figure 10.7(a)).

Most dietary carbohydrates are in the form of polysaccharides (see Chapter 5). In theory, amylase is capable of converting starch into the disaccharide maltose, which

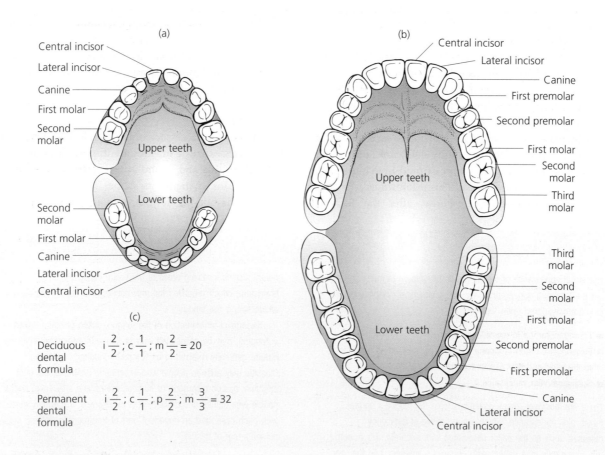

Figure 10.6 Dentitions and dental formulae. (a) Deciduous dentition. (b) Permanent dentition. (c) Dental formulae include the number of teeth associated with one-half of either the lower or upper jaw.

Q. How are the various types of teeth adapted to provide specialized functions?

BOX 10.6 TEETH AND THE ORAL CAVITY

The development of teeth, essential for biting and chewing solid food, begins during fetal life, but teeth do not begin to erupt until about 6 months after birth. These are the deciduous (milk) teeth; on average, one tooth erupts each month until all 20 are present (Figure 10.6(a) and (c)). The incisors erupt first; these are chisel shaped for biting. The cuspid or canine teeth erupt next; these are used to tear and shred food. The molars are the last to erupt; they are used to crunch and grind food.

Deciduous teeth are shed from about 6–7 years of age, and are replaced with permanent teeth that are normally in place by about 12 years of age, although a further four 'wisdom teeth' may erupt during teenage or early adulthood years. The wisdom teeth may be a source of pressure and pain, as the relative size of the jaw recedes with age. If this is the case, these teeth may be removed surgically.

Excluding the wisdom teeth, there are 28 permanent teeth, comprised of four incisors, two canines, four premolars and four molars in each jaw (Figure 10.6(b) and (c)). Since there are only 20 deciduous teeth, some permanent teeth do not have deciduous predecessors. Permanent teeth have extensive roots, but they have the same basic structure as the deciduous teeth.

The ageing process is associated with the following changes:

● Tooth enamel and dentine wear down, so cavities are more likely.
● Teeth are lost as a result of periodontal disease and roots that break easily.
● Taste and smell diminishes.
● Saliva secretion decreases.

The overall result of these changes is that eating becomes less pleasurable, appetite is reduced, and food is not chewed or lubricated sufficiently, so swallowing becomes difficult for the older person.

A general problem associated with teeth is the accumulation of plaque, which may lead to inflammation of the gums (gingivitis), dental decay and caries formation, leading to loss of teeth. Prevention is necessary, and involves avoiding foods that have a greater tendency for plaque formation, and adequate oral hygiene.

During pregnancy, the gums have a tendency to swell and become spongy. As a consequence, bleeding may occur. This has implications on the dental health of a woman, and for this reason dental care is provided during pregnancy until 1 year after birth. A dental hygienist may also offer advice, e.g. using a soft toothbrush to reduce the aggravation of the gums.

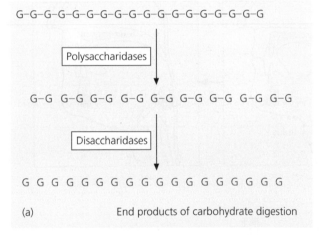

(a) End products of carbohydrate digestion

(b) End products of lipid digestion

(c) End product of protein digestion

Figure 10.7 Digestive enzymes. Endopeptidases break down the bonds between amino acids other than the terminal bonds. Carboxyexopeptidases are involved in breaking the terminal peptide bond associated with the amino acid in which its carboxyl acid group is exposed. Aminoexopeptidases are involved in breaking the terminal peptide bond associated with the amino acid in which its amine group is exposed. (a) The mode of action of carbohydrases. (b) The mode of action of lipases on a triglyceride (most dietary fats are in the triglyceride form). (c) The mode of action of proteases. (i) and (ii) are polypeptide chains (protein molecules consist of two or more polypeptide chains).

AA, amino acid; COOH)AA, carboxylic acid terminal amino acid; FA, fatty acid; FFA, free fatty acid; G, monosaccharide (e.g. glucose); (NH$_2$)AA, amino terminal amino acid.

Q. Reflect on your understanding of how enzymes are named.

consists of two glucose molecules joined together. However, this takes time. In practice, the food is in the presence of amylase for only 15–30 min: food is usually in the stomach within 4–6 s of eating it; it remains for a while in areas of the stomach in which gastric acid is not present, thus amylase continues to work. Eventually the food is passed to acidic areas of the stomach, where the acidity denatures and inactivates the amylase, so at this stage carbohydrate digestion ceases. Thus, the carbohydrate components of the food at this point are starch molecules that have not been in contact with amylase, dextrins (intermediate breakdown products between starch and the disaccharide maltose), and to a small extent maltose itself. No other foods are chemically broken down in the mouth, or on the food's journey to the stomach. As a result of the physical and chemical processes, the food leaving the mouth is reduced to a soft, flexible ball (called a bolus; plural = boli) that is swallowed easily.

Exercise

Reflect on your understanding of the physical and chemical digestive functions of the mouth.

The pharynx and oesophagus

The pharynx, or throat, is a cone-shaped cavity approximately 12 cm long. It is subdivided into:

- *the nasopharynx*: the area behind the nasal passageways concerned with the flow of air through the respiratory pathways;

- *the common pharynx or oropharynx*: contains the tonsils on its lateral walls. The mouth is anterior to this region;

- *the laryngeal pharynx*: the area around the larynx that bifurcates into the larynx (voice box) and oesophagus.

The oesophagus is a collapsible muscular tube approximately 25 cm long running from the pharynx to the stomach, anterior to the thoracic vertebrae, but behind the trachea. The oesophagus penetrates the diaphragm before entering the stomach via the oesophageal hiatus, more commonly called the cardiac sphincter.

The pharynx and the oesophagus are lined with a stratified mucosal membrane (see Chapter 2), as these regions are associated with a great deal of wear and tear during the passage of food.

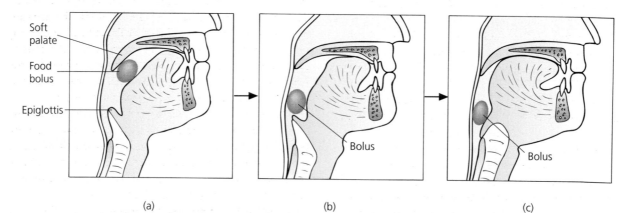

(a) (b) (c)

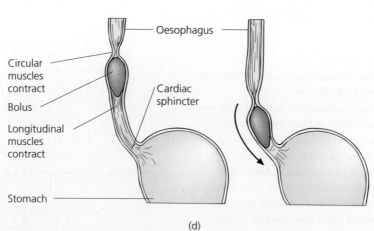

(d)

Figure 10.8 Deglutition. (a) Voluntary stage (the tongue rises against the palate); (b) and (c) involuntary pharyngeal stage (nasal and laryngeal passages sealed off); (d) oesophageal stage (peristaltic motion and entry to the stomach).

Q. Describe the mechanisms involved in the swallowing reflex.

The swallowing process

The swallowing of food, called deglutition, is aided by the moist consistency of the bolus of food resulting from the presence of saliva and mucous secreted from the lining of the mouth and oesophagus. In addition, the absence of cartilage from the posterior surface of the trachea helps to reduce friction as the food passes down the oesophagus. This is because the anterior surface of the upper section of the oesophagus lies against the posterior surface of the trachea; the presence of cartilage would make swallowing extremely uncomfortable.

The swallowing process involves a triad of responses (Figure 10.8):

1 *The voluntary stage.* The tongue voluntarily moves the bolus of food to the back of the mouth, and then into the oropharynx. This involves the tongue rising and pushing itself against the soft palate (Figure 10.8(a)).

2 *The involuntary pharyngeal stage.* This begins with the bolus stimulating receptors in the oropharyngeal region, resulting in an involuntary swallowing reflex. Sensory impulses ascend to the deglutition (swallowing) centre of the medulla and lower pons of the brainstem. Parasympathetic motor output causes the soft palate, and its extension the uvula, to move upwards, thus sealing off the nasal passageways and preventing food from entering the nasal cavity (Figure 10.8(b)). Parasympathetic motor impulses also cause the larynx to move upwards, sealing off the opening of the larynx, called the glottis, with the epiglottis (Figure 10.8(c)), and widening the space between the laryngeal pharynx and oesophagus. This aids the passage of the bolus. Once food has moved into the oesophagus, breathing is resumed with the opening of the respiratory pathway. Occasionally, when we drink liquids very quickly the sealing of the nasal passageways is too slow and the drink passes into them. Alternatively, food particles may be swallowed so fast that the sealing of the glottis is incomplete and food becomes lodged at the top of the larynx, stimulating the coughing reflex and expelling the irritant particles from the larynx.

3 *The oesophageal stage.* Once the bolus has entered the oesophagus, muscular movements (peristalsis) are responsible for its transport to the stomach. Although the main function of peristalsis is to propel the food along the tube, it is inevitable that there will be friction between food boli and the oesophageal surfaces as they 'rub' against each other. This aids physical digestion to a limited extent. Peristaltic movement of food occurs throughout the gastrointestinal tract, from the oesophagus to the final elimination via the anal canal.

The medulla of the brainstem controls the events in the first part of the oesophagus via parasympathetic motor impulses, and may influence gut movements in other sections of the tract. A myenteric plexus ('mysenteric' = within muscle, 'plexus' = collection of nerve cells) is capable of generating peristaltic movements in the absence of extrinsic stimulation, however. Figure 10.8(d) illustrates the peristaltic process. Circular muscle fibres contract immediately behind the bolus, which constricts the oesophagus in this region and forces the bolus downwards. Longitudinal fibres immediately in front of the bolus simultaneously contract, thus shortening and expanding the diameter of the section, and allowing the forward propulsion of the bolus. The co-ordinated action of these muscular movements provides the appearance of a continuous wave of contraction. Swallowing also promotes the relaxation of the normally contracted cardiac sphincter, and allows passage of the bolus into the stomach.

The duration of swallowing depends upon the consistency of the food (fluid-like foods travel quicker) and the body's position (an upright body position facilitates a more rapid descent). Taking these extremes into consideration, the time for the passage of boli from entering and leaving the oesophagus ranges from 1 to 8 s.

Table 10.4 summarizes the regulation of alimentary canal activities.

Table 10.4 Regulation of the alimentary canal's activities

Region	Functional activity	Regulator of function
Mouth	Opening via jaw muscular movement	Mainly by the trigeminal nerve, but also the facial nerve
	Taste	Glossopharyngeal nerve – sensory to posterior third of tongue – and facial nerve – sensory to anterior two-thirds of the tongue
	Mastication	Trigeminal nerve
	Tongue movements	Facial nerve
	Salivary flow	Facial nerve (submandibular and sublingual glands), glossopharyngeal nerve (parotid glands)
Swallowing reflex	Upward movement of soft palate	Facial nerve
	Movement of the epiglottis over the larynx	Vagus nerve
	Oesophageal peristalsis	Facial nerve and mesenteric/Auerbach's plexus
Stomach	Entry via relaxation of the cardiac spincter	Innervated by vagus nerve
	Churning	Innervated by vagus nerve
	Gastric juice secretion	Innervated by vagus nerve; actions of gastrin (gastric and duodenal)
	Exit via the relaxation of the pyloric sphincter	Innervated by vagus nerve
Small intestine	Peristalsic segmentation	Vagus nerve
	Pancreatic juice secretion	CCK-PZ and secretin
	Bile secretion from the gall bladder	CCK-PZ
	Succus entericus secretion	Vagus nerve
Large intestine	Entry from the small intestine through the ileocaecal valve	Gastrocolic reflex controlled by vagus nerve
	Peristalsis	Vagus and pelvic nerves
	Exit via:	
	1 Relaxtion (opening) of the internal sphincter	Pelvic nerve
	2 Relaxation (opening) of the external sphincter	Controlled voluntarily

Q. Discuss the importance of pH variation in the alimentary canal.

CCK-PZ, cholecystokinin-pancreozymin.

The stomach

The stomach is a J-shaped muscular organ, located immediately below the diaphragm on the left side of the abdominal cavity. Its size and shape varies according to content (the stomach's folds, or rugae, disappear when the stomach is distended), and according to which part of the respiratory cycle the person is in. Upon inspiration, the diaphragm is pulled down, which displaces the stomach downwards slightly. With expiration, the stomach extends upwards. The opening from the oesophagus, and the exit into the first region of the small intestine, are guarded by the cardiac and pyloric sphincter muscles, respectively. These are normally contracted, thus preventing passage of stomach contents. The stomach is held in position by the mesenteries of the peritoneum.

Figure 10.9 (a) illustrates the four main regions of the stomach:

- The cardiac region surrounds the cardiac sphincter muscle.

- The fundic region is the elevated rounded part around and to the left of the cardiac portion.

- The body region occupies most of the stomach; it lies between the fundic and pyloric parts.

- The pyloric region is the most inferior part of the stomach, lying superior to the pyloric sphincter.

BOX 10.8 HIATUS HERNIA, PREGNANCY AND HEARTBURN

Hiatus hernia occurs when part of the person's stomach herniates, or distends, through the oesophageal gap (hiatus) in the diaphragm. It may be congenital or may result from an acquired weakness. Often there are no symptoms, but pain and 'heartburn' from the reflux of gastric acid can occur. Correction involves external manipulation of the herniated region back into the abdomen. If this is unsuccessful, then a simple and effective operation can remove the problem.

Heartburn is also a common disorder of pregnancy. Increased levels of the hormone progesterone during pregnancy relax the cardiac sphincter. This slows digestion of food, which may make the woman feel nauseous after meals. Therefore, pregnant women are encouraged to eat smaller meal portions, e.g. five small meals a day instead of the usual three (Blamey, 1998).

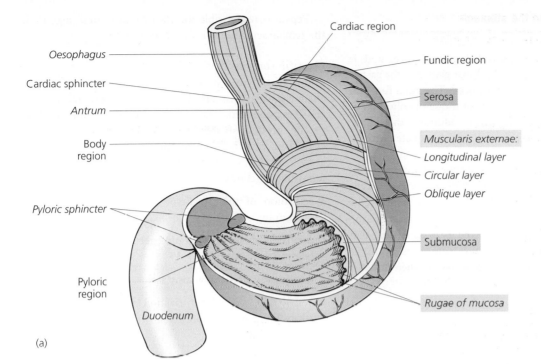

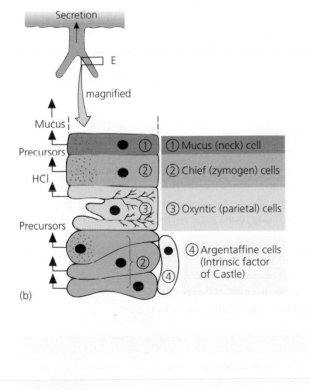

Figure 10.9 (a) The stomach. (b) The gastric (tubular) gland.
Q. Describe the sphincter functions of the stomach when (i) food is approaching the stomach, (ii) food is being digested within the stomach, and (iii) food has been digested by the stomach.

Entry of food

The cardiac sphincter relaxes and opens when food is present in the lower oesophagus, allowing entry of boli into the stomach. Simultaneously, the pyloric sphincter, which guards the exit from the stomach, contracts so that food cannot pass immediately into the small intestine without first undergoing gastric digestion.

Physical digestion in the stomach

The stomach 'churns' food using a mechanism peculiar to this organ. A three-dimensional muscular movement is brought about by the presence of an additional oblique muscular layer (Figure 10.9(a)). This movement increases the efficiency of physically breaking down food boli that have entered this region, and mixes food with the stomach's chemicals, or gastric juice, thus facilitating chemical digestion.

There is regional variation in the peristalsis movements of the stomach. The fundic region exhibits only a few peristaltic waves, as this is the 'storage' area of the stomach; food is not mixed with gastric secretions, so salivary amylase continues to work here. The waves of contraction beginning in the body of the stomach become more vigorous in the inferior regions, becoming very forceful in the pylorus region. These latter waves of contraction allow liquidized foods a more rapid exit from the stomach should the pyloric sphincter relax. Contraction of the sphincter, however, normally seals off the exit from the stomach, resulting in the temporary backward movement of the food within the pylorus, producing a more efficient mixing of the gastric contents.

Chemical digestion in the stomach

The stomach's secretion is called gastric juice, and is produced from the compound tubular glands of the gastric pits. About 2–3 l per day are produced. The main function of the secretion is the conversion of the semi-solid boli of food into a semi-liquid chyme. In addition, the gastric juice contains a protease enzyme, which initiates protein breakdown.

Each gastric gland possesses four types of secretory cells (Figure 10.9(b)) – mucous cells, chief cells, oxyntic cells and argentaffine cells – which secrete separate components of the gastric juice. A fifth type of cell is also present in the gastric mucosa; these are specialized endocrine cells that secrete the hormone gastrin, which stimulates a greater flow of gastric juice. Gastrin is released when food is present in the stomach.

Mucous cells

Normally, the gastric cells are protected by mucous and by intact gastric cell membranes with low permeability to hydrogen irons and tight junctions between the cells. Mucous (or neck) cells are located mainly in the neck of the gland, and secrete the mucous part of the juice. Mucous adheres to the gastric mucosal surface. It prevents autodigestion of the stomach wall by the hydrochloric acid and proteolytic enzymes present in gastric juice. The mucous layer normally is about 1 mm thick.

Chief cells

Chief (or zymogen) cells produce two enzyme precursors (inactive enzymes), pepsinogen and prorennin. These are activated by the acidic gastric juice to pepsin and rennin, respectively. Both enzymes accelerate protein digestion. Pepsin converts proteins into polypeptides (long chains of amino acids); it is an endopeptidase enzyme, so it breaks the peptide bonds in places other than at the terminal peptide positions (Figure 10.7(c)). Rennin converts the soluble protein of milk into an insoluble form, in order to retain it in the stomach for longer periods so pepsin can have its proteolytic effects.

Pepsin is responsible for 10–15% of protein digestion; the remainder occurs in the small intestine.

Oxyntic (or parietal) cells

The oxyntic (or parietal) cells contain intracellular channels, called canaliculi, in which hydrochloric acid (HCl) is produced. The initial chemical reactions leading to the production of hydrochloric acid occur in the cytoplasm, but the final reactions occur in the channels away from the cytoplasm. The acid in gastric juice has the following functions:

- activation of the precursor enzymes pepsinogen and prorennin;
- provision of the optimal pH (pH 2–3) for the action of pepsin (and rennin);
- inactivation of salivary amylase;
- destruction (i.e. denaturization) of the enzymes of alkali-liking bacteria present in ingested food (i.e. HCl is bactericidal);
- dissolves splinters of bone that may have been swallowed.

Argentaffine cells

Argentaffine cells are small and fairly uncommon, and are responsible for producing intrinsic factor of Castle. This chemical is essential for the carriage of vitamin B_{12} through the stomach, and for its absorption by the small intestine. People without this factor exhibit the homeostatic imbalance of pernicious anaemia (see Chapter 11).

Exit of food

The pyloric sphincter is usually partially open when food is present in the stomach, thus allowing liquid material to pass through very quickly. However, the end product of stomach digestion called chyme is semi-liquid and requires

Exercise

Reflect on your understanding of the chemical and physical digestive processes of the stomach.

BOX 10.9 LACTATING INFANTS

The digestive system of neonates cannot synthesize the full range of digestive enzymes necessary for a mixed diet, and gastric secretion is inadequate. The infant is therefore dependent upon milk feeds, and the tongue of babies is in a forward position to facilitate suckling. The relative position of the tongue changes gradually, and digestive enzyme secretion increases in capacity and variety, so the baby becomes able to cope with semi-solid foods.

The reliance of the infant on milk feeds necessitates the production of the gastric enzyme rennin. This coagulates milk protein, and so slows its advance through the stomach, giving

more time for its digestion. Rennin is not to be confused with the renal enzyme renin, which generates the hormone angiotensin from its blood precursor angiotensinogen (see Chapter 12).

Gastric lipase is another enzyme that is secreted into the gastric juice of infants. This breaks down butterfat molecules in milk. It requires a pH of 5–6 for its actions, however, and so has a limited role in the adult stomach where pH values are generally lower. Adults rely on lipases secreted into the small intestine to digest lipids.

Tooth development begins during fetal life (see Box 10.6).

BOX 10.10 PYLORIC STENOSIS AND PYLOROSPASM

Pyloric stenosis

This is a major disorder of gastric emptying. The pyloric sphincter grows or hypertrophies, causing a narrowing of the lumen of the stomach's exit, and dilation of the stomach. An extra peristaltic effort is therefore needed to force the gastric contents through the narrowed pyloric sphincter, thus the muscle layers of the stomach may also become hypertrophied.

The condition is more common in small babies. It usually appears by the third week of extra-uterine life. Pyloric stenosis is five times more common in males (5 in 1000 births) than in females. The condition is also more common in children with Down's syndrome (Huether and McCance, 1996). Pyloric stenosis is inherited as a multifactorial trait; an increase in gastrin secretion by the mother in the last trimester of pregnancy also increases the likelihood of pyloric stenosis in the infant.

The hallmark symptom of pyloric stenosis is projectile vomiting – the spraying of liquid vomit some distance from the infant. The vomiting may lead to malnutrition, dehydration and electrolyte imbalances. Standard treatment for hypertrophied pyloric stenosis in those cases that do not resolve themselves is a pyloromyotomy, in which the muscles of the pyloric sphincters are separated. As part of the care and discharge planning, the patient should be given dietary advice regarding the necessity to take small, frequent meals. See the case study of a child with hypertrophied pyloric stenosis in Section 6.

Pylorospasm

In this condition, the muscle fibres of the pyloric sphincter fail to relax normally, so food does not pass easily from the stomach to the duodenum. The stomach becomes overfull, and the infant vomits often to relieve the pressure build-up. Antispasmodic drugs are given to relax the pylorospasm, and the infant is re-fed after vomiting.

---

the sphincter to be completely open to allow the passage of large quantities per unit time.

Regulation of gastric functions

The secretion of gastric juice is usually related to the presence, or anticipation, of food. Three phases are responsible for controlling the secretion of gastric juice:

- *The cephalic stage:* this involves parasympathetic nerve stimulation of the stomach via the vagus nerve. It is a conditioned association reflex that occurs when we smell, see or taste food, i.e. it is preparatory for the arrival of food. It is responsible for inducing contractions of

---

BOX 10.11 GASTRITIS AND PEPTIC ULCERS

Gastritis

This is inflammation of the stomach mucosa, often caused by prolonged exposure to certain substances (e.g. aspirin and other nonsteroidal anti-inflammatory drugs, alcohol), that disturbs the cell arrangement of gastric mucosa, and increases the permeability of the cell membranes to hydrogen ions. This lowers the cellular pH, and so decreases optimal enzyme functioning. The subsequent cell damage may result in gastric inflammation (gastritis) and bleeding, hypoxia, and eventually necrotic areas of gastric mucosa, and can lead to the formation of an ulcer. Patients with arthritis who are prescribed long-term aspirin as an analgesic are often given enteric-coated aspirin; the enteric coat prevents the absorption of aspirin from the stomach.

Treatment for chronic gastritis is a soft bland diet, and avoidance of irritant foods, smoking and alcohol. Patients are encouraged to minimize anxiety-causing situations that initiate gastric secretion when the stomach is 'empty'.

Diagnosis can be made by gastroscopy. *Helicobacter pylori* (H. pylori) bacteria are often present on biopsy.

Peptic ulcers

Peptic ulcers are breaks in the protective mucosal lining caused by gastric secretions. They may be gastric, duodenal or (occasionally) oesophageal in origin. The presence of ulcers is a sign of a homeostatic imbalance associated with either excessive secretion of gastric juice, reduced resistance of the gastric mucosa to the secretion, or the presence of a short stomach. The most common

cause is infection of the affected region with *H. pylori*. Other contributory causal factors are:

- hereditary tendency;
- use of steroids, as these decrease mucosal resistance;
- habitual use of nonsteroidal anti-inflammatory drugs (NSAIDs), alcohol and heavy smoking;
- a 'stress' or 'type A' personality (although this is controversial nowadays);
- chronic diseases, such as emphysema, rheumatoid arthritis or cirrhosis.

Although both gastric and duodenal ulcers are classified as peptic ulcers, they have different symptoms. For example, the boring/burning pain of gastric ulcer comes soon after eating and is not relieved by eating more food, whereas duodenal ulcer pain comes approximately 2 h after a meal, when chyme exits the stomach, and is relieved temporarily by further eating because this stops gastric emptying for a while.

Diagnosis can be made by gastroscopy. *H. pylori* bacteria are often present on biopsy.

Principles of correction are based upon the patient eating an easily digestible meal, using antacid preparations to neutralize the gastric acids, or using other drugs to diminish gastric secretions and/or motility. For gastric ulcers, mucous secretion can be increased by the administration of carbenoxolone (a liquorice derivative).

stomach muscle, which bring about churning, and an increased rate of gastric juice secretion.

● *The gastric phase:* the presence of food in the pyloric region of the stomach results in the release of the hormone gastrin, which aids gastric motility (muscular movement) and stimulates the increased secretion of gastric juice.

● *The intestinal phase:* once food comes into contact with the mucosa of the first region of the small intestine, called the duodenum, a variety of hormones (e.g. cholecystokinin-pancreozymin (CCK-PZ), gastric inhibitory peptide (GIP) and secretin) is released. Most of these hormones inhibit gastric motility and gastric secretion, and so delay gastric emptying. This allows more time for digestion (particularly of lipids) in the duodenum. In addition, these hormones help prevent homeostatic imbalances, such as gastric ulcers, occurring in the stomach as a result of excessive gastric acid secretion in the absence of food. Conversely, duodenal gastrin may also be released when the chyme is rich in proteins and polypeptides. This is identical to the stomach's gastrin, and promotes protein digestion of food remaining in the stomach.

The small intestine, pancreas and gall bladder

The small intestine

The small intestine extends from the pyloric sphincter to the ileo-caecal valve located at the junction with the large intestine. It is about 6.5 m, with a diameter of 2.5 cm. The small intestine is a coiled structure occupying a large part of the abdominal cavity. It is suspended by the mesenteries, which carry the nerves, and blood and lymphatic vessels that support this area. The small intestine is the main area of digestion and absorption, and is divided anatomically into three distinct regions (Figure 10.2):

● The *duodenum* is the shortest section of the small intestine, extending from the pyloric sphincter for

BOX 10.12 NAUSEA AND VOMITING

Nausea

Nausea is an unpleasant sensation that may occur as a result of an emotional disturbance, indigestion, gastritis, or unpleasant sights and smells. Nausea may be accompanied by autonomic nervous stimulation, resulting in one or more of pallor, sweating, and a sudden secretion of saliva into the mouth.

Vomiting

Vomiting (emesis) is forceful expulsion (regurgitation or antiperistalsis) of the contents of the gastrointestinal tract, usually preceded by nausea and excessive salivation. It is a reflex resulting in:

1 Closure of the larynx via the epiglottis, sealing the glottis.
2 Closure of the nasal passageways in order to prevent the entrance of the vomitus.
3 Forceful contraction of the diaphragm and abdominal wall muscles.
4 Closure of the pyloric sphincter, which increases the stomach pressure, causing gastric regurgitation.

The responses are determined by neural output from the vomiting centre of the medulla of the brainstem. The centre sends motor impulses to the above areas to initiate the act, in response to sensory impulses from one (or more) of the following:

● gastrointestinal irritation by chemicals, micro-organisms, or handling of the viscera during surgery, thus acting crudely as a 'protective' response to remove the initiating stressor;
● cerebral tumour or raised intracranial pressure;
● higher cerebral centres in response to intense fear, anxiety, unpleasant smells, etc.;

● impulses from the vestibular apparatus (balance organ of the ear), e.g. in seasickness;
● some drugs, e.g. morphine, digitalis and emetics (e.g. ipecacuanha); thus the principle of pharmacological correction is the use of anti-emetic drugs;
● general anaesthetics.

Examination of the products of the vomit (called vomitus) is indicative of the associated aetiological factor. For example, the presence of blood may indicate gastric (peptic) ulceration, whereas the presence of undigested food could indicate an obstruction to the pyloric sphincter.

The consequences of vomiting, particularly if chronic, are reduction of nutrient uptake, and a change in body fluid composition. There is a loss of fluid and electrolytes. The loss of gastric acid can result in metabolic alkalosis, although chronic vomiting may induce a metabolic acidosis because the body utilizes body fats as an energy source to compensate for reduced carbohydrate intake.

Weight loss and nutritional disturbances occur if vomiting is prolonged. In addition, inhalation of vomit can lead to aspiration pneumonia, and ultimately death. To prevent any potential vomitus from being inhaled, the unconscious patient must be placed in a semi-prone position to encourage vomitus to be 'drained out' via gravity.

The principles of correction of nausea and vomiting vary according to the aetiology, e.g. the avoidance of gastric irritants such as alcohol. The secondary consequences may also require correction, including fluid replacement and/or buffer therapy (see Chapter 6).

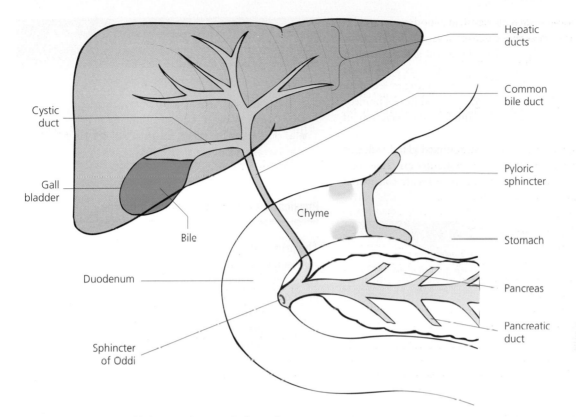

Figure 10.10   The relationship between the stomach, liver and pancreas.

Q. What is the hallmark symptom of infantile pyloric stenosis?

Q. Describe the mechanisms involved in the gastrocolic reflex.

about 25 cm. It forms a loop inferior to the stomach, and encloses the body of the pancreas. The united ducts from the gall bladder and the pancreas empty into the duodenum via the circular ring of involuntary muscle called the sphincter of Oddi (Figure 10.10).

● The *jejunum* is about 2.7 m long. It extends from the duodenum to the final part of the small intestine, or the ileum. The duodenum and jejunum are both concerned mainly with digestion.

● The *ileum* is about 3.6 m long. It connects the small intestine with the large intestine, or caecum, via the ileocaecal valve. It is the main area of absorption.

The mucosal epithelium of the small intestine has circular folds, or plicae. Projecting from these plicae are finger-like projections called villi. The villi bear further projections called microvilli. These folds and projections increase the surface area available for digestion of the chyme and for the process of absorption. At the base of the villi are intestinal glands called crypts of Lieberkuhn. These are responsible for secreting the intestinal juice. Brunner's glands in the duodenal submucosa produce an alkaline mucus, which, together with pancreatic and bile salts, neutralize the acidic chyme as it enters the duodenum from the stomach. The pH actually becomes slightly alkaline, which is conducive

to the activation of pancreatic precursor enzymes and the optimal functioning of enzymes within the intestines. Mucous partially protects the intestinal wall from autodigestion by the multiple enzymes (particularly the proteases) secreted into the intestine.

The pancreas

The pancreas is a soft, tapering gland. Its head lies within the loop of duodenum, and the whole structure positions itself inferior and horizontal to the stomach (Figure 10.10). The pancreas is about 12–15 cm long and 2.5 cm thick. It contains both exocrine and endocrine secretory cells. Exocrine (or acini) cells have a role in digestion. They are responsible for secreting precursor and active digestive enzymes into the duodenum via the pancreatic duct. Other acini cells produce the bicarbonate-rich, alkaline fluid into which the enzymes are secreted before being released into the duodenum.

Endocrine cells (islets of Langerhans) include:

● *alpha cells*, which produce the hormone glucagon;

● *beta cells*, which produce the hormone insulin;

● *delta cells*, which produce the hormone somatostatin.

These hormones are important in blood sugar regulation. Insulin lowers blood glucose (it is a hypoglycaemic agent), whereas glucagon raises the blood glucose level (it is a hyperglycaemic agent). Somatostatin has a paracrine (or dual) role, and inhibits insulin and glucagon secretion when the blood glucose concentration is within its homeostatic range. Somatostatin also inhibits the secretion of pancreatic enzymes.

The pancreas is referred to as a 'mixed gland', since it has both endocrine and exocrine tissue. Its exocrine roles are described below, and its endocrine roles are considered in more detail in Chapter 9.

Exercise

Refer back to Chapter 9 and distinguish between the terms 'exocrine' and 'endocrine' in relation to the function of the pancreas.

The gall bladder

This pear-shaped organ is about 7–9 cm long. It is attached to the undersurface of the liver. Its function is to store and concentrate bile, and to secrete it into the bile ducts, which unite with the pancreatic duct and enter the duodenum via the sphincter of Oddi (Figure 10.10). Bile is synthesized within the liver.

BOX 10.14 AGEING AND THE ASSOCIATED GLANDS OF DIGESTION

The following are associated with the ageing process:

● fibrosis, fatty acid deposits, and pancreatic atrophy;
● decrease in secretions of digestive enzymes;
● no changes occur to the gall bladder or bile duct, but there is an increased prevalence of gallstones.

Physical digestion in the small intestine

The principal movement within the small intestine is called segmentation (Figure 10.11). This mechanism involves a series of isolated contractions in alternating localized positions. The contractions of circular muscle fibres constrict the tube, segmenting the food chyme into smaller masses. Next, the muscle fibres within the individual segments contract, with the result that further smaller masses are produced. As the muscle fibres relax, the larger segments are reformed. The overall results are that food particles are broken mechanically into smaller particles, and there is a thorough mixing of the food with digestive juices.

Segmentation stops periodically, and a wave of peristalsis then moves the food further along the intestine. This

BOX 10.13 PANCREATITIS

Pancreatitis (inflammation of the pancreas) is relatively rare and potentially serious; it can carry a 10–15% mortality rate (McArdle, 2000). Pancreatitis may be acute or chronic. In acute pancreatitis, the more severe condition, which may be associated with heavy alcohol intake or biliary tract obstruction, the pancreatic cells release trypsin instead of its precursor trypsinogen; the trypsin begins to digest the pancreatic cells. Patients with chronic pancreatitis are 16 times more likely to develop pancreatic cancer than other people (Chowdhury and Rayford, 2000).

The patient will often present with abdominal pain, and investigations are often made on abdominal ultrasound and blood

amylase analysis. A raised amylase (over 1000 IU/l in the last 48 h) is indicative of pancreatitis.

Patients usually respond to treatment, but recurrent attacks often occur. Treatment involves narcotics (e.g. demerol) to relieve the pain; oral foods are withheld, and gastric suction is instituted to 'rest' the gland. Parenteral fluids are given to restore blood volume. Cimetidine may be administered to prevent stimulus of the pancreas. Surgical drainage may be necessary.

Common laboratory tests of pancreatic function are summarized in Table 10.5.

Table 10.5 Common laboratory tests of pancreatic function

Test	Normal range	Clinical significance
Serum amylase	60–180 Somogyi units/ml	↑ levels with pancreatic inflammation
Serum	1.5 Somogyi units/ml	↑ levels with pancreatic inflammation (may be elevated with other conditions; differentiates with amylase isoenzyme study)
Urine amylase	35–260 Somogyi units/h	↑ levels with pancreatic inflammation
Stool fat	2.5 g/25 h	Measures fatty acids; decreased pancreatic lipase increases stool fat

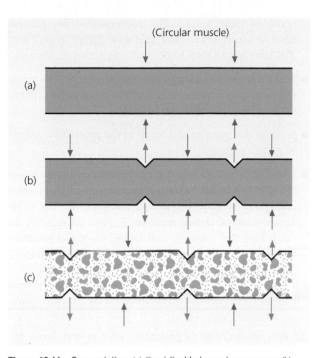

(Circular muscle)

(a)

(b)

(c)

Figure 10.11 Segmentation. (a) Semi-liquid chyme in one mass; (b) chyme segmented via isolated contraction of circular muscle fibres; (c) chyme segmented further as other areas contract. Note that relaxation is an inevitable consequence of contraction.

Q. How does segmentation differ from peristalsis?

movement also contributes to the physical breakdown of food, as friction occurs between the food and the intestinal wall. Peristaltic movement is weaker in this region than in the oesophagus and stomach, so food is retained in the small intestine for longer, reflecting the time required for digestion to be completed.

Bile

Bile is a yellow-green alkaline (pH 7.6–8.6) fluid. About 80–100 ml of bile are produced by the liver daily. It is transported to the gall bladder by the hepatic and cystic ducts (Figure 10.10). Bile is stored and concentrated in this organ until it is required in the small intestine. Bile is mainly a watery secretion; other components include bile salts, bile pigments, cholesterol, lecithin, mucus and several ions. It has two principal functions: physical digestion and excretion.

Physical digestion by bile

Bile is frequently not recognized as being involved in physical digestion because it is a chemical secretion. Bile salts (sodium taurocholate and sodium glycocholate) and lecithin, however, are responsible for emulsification, i.e. the reduction of large globules of fat (lipids exist as globules, in a watery intestinal chyme solution) into small droplets. This process falls more under the broad heading of physical breakdown since no enzymes are involved. The increased surface area produced by emulsification aids the actions of digestive enzymes (lipases) to speed up the chemical breakdown of lipids. The emulsification process is rather like pouring cooking oil into water. As the large globule of oil enters the water, it disperses into smaller fat droplets, increasing the total surface area. Bile also prevents the droplets coalescing into larger ones.

After bile salts have performed their digestive function, they are involved in another homeostatic function by aiding the absorption of long-chain fatty acids (see later). Most of the salts are reabsorbed in the process and recycled by the liver into bile. Bile salts also contribute to the alkaline medium within the intestine, which buffers the acidic chyme and produces a pH at which intestinal enzymes operate with maximum efficiency.

BOX 10.15 GALLSTONES (CHOLELITHIASIS)

The production of stone-like concretions of the gall bladder in a person is a result of either:

- inadequate bile salts or lecithin in the bile, which results in multiple-faceted stones, composed of calcium and bile pigments;
- excessive cholesterol, resulting in its precipitation out of solution and crystallization. These cholesterol crystals coalesce; they are responsible for 85% of all gallstones.

Gallstones often go undetected in the body, but as they increase in size, they may be responsible for minimal, intermittent or complete obstruction to the flow of bile from the gall bladder into the duct system (Agrawal and Jonnalagadda, 2000).

The more common situation is partial obstruction to the outlet from the gall bladder, resulting in a heartburn pain or discomfort (called biliary colic) after eating, when digestive enzymes, notably CCK-PZ, are released and contract the gallbladder. The inflammation produced is called cholecystitis, after the old name of the gall bladder, the cholecystic gland. If the stone becomes mobile and lodges itself, there is intense pain and fever, with the yellow coloration of the skin characteristic of obstructive jaundice appearing in due course. Complete obstruction of the flow may even be fatal. Bile pigment accumulation in the blood may cause intense itching of the affected area. Frequent bathing and the use of a soothing lotion, such as calamine, is sometimes helpful to the patient.

Investigations performed to detect gallstones may include X-ray, intravenous cholangiogram, endoscopic retrograde cholangiopancreatography (ERCP), or laparotomy (see Box 10.16).

Correction involves administering gallstone-dissolving drugs, e.g. chenodeoxycholic acid, or fragmentation of stones using high-frequency sound waves (called lithotripsy). Surgical removal of the gallstones may be necessary if non-invasive treatments are ineffective; often, a cholecystectomy will be performed to remove the gallbladder and the stone inside.

Excretory function of bile

The bile pigments, bilirubin ('rub-' = red) and biliverdin ('verd-' = green), are produced by the liver from the breakdown of haemoglobin released when old erythrocytes are destroyed. The liver removes the iron and protein (globin) part of haemoglobin; these are then homeostatically recycled (see later). The remaining parts of haemoglobin comprise the bile pigments, the principal one being bilirubin. When the bile is secreted into the intestine, this pigment is converted into urobilinogen and stercobilin. The former is absorbed into blood and then transported to the kidneys where it is converted into urochrome, which is responsible for the yellow colour of urine. Stercobilin remains in the intestine, where it is responsible for colouring the faeces. These components of faeces and urine are genuine excretory products, as they have been involved in cellular metabolism (which differentiates them from the indigestible material present in faeces).

Exercise

Describe how bile contributes to physical digestion within the small intestine

Chemical digestion in the small intestine

Chyme entering the small intestine consists of a mixture of nutrients (Table 10.6). These include:

- *carbohydrates:* various polysaccharides arising from partially digested starches. Some disaccharides, such as maltose, may be present, reflecting some success on the part of salivary amylase activity. In addition, depending upon the food that was consumed, other disaccharides may be present, such as lactose (milk sugar) and sucrose (cane or table sugar). The monosaccharides glucose, fructose (fruit sugar) and galactose (grape sugar) may also have been taken in;

- *fats:* these are not chemically digested up to this point; they enter the small intestine in their consumed chemical form, i.e. mainly triglycerides;

- *polypeptides:* present as a result of the proteolytic actions of gastric pepsin;

- *vitamins, minerals and water:* together with monosaccharides, these are not digested because they are small enough to be absorbed across the gut wall. The other components of chyme must be digested chemically; the small intestine initiates and completes these processes via secretions of the pancreas and the intestinal mucosa.

Digestive secretions of the pancreas

About 1200–1500 ml of pancreatic juice are produced and secreted daily. Water is the main constituent of this clear, colourless secretion. Other constituents include pancreatic salts, 'protein'-digesting enzymes, carbohydrate-digesting enzyme, fat-digesting enzyme, and nucleic-acid-digesting enzymes. *Pancreatic salts*, the most common of which is sodium bicarbonate, contribute to the alkalinity (pH 7.1–8.2) of pancreatic juice. We have already described the neutralizing effects of the juice, bile salts and intestinal secretions on gastric acid as it enters the duodenum.

Pancreatic juice contains two *endopeptidases*, 'protein'-digesting or, more accurately, polypeptide-digesting, enzymes. (i.e. enzymes that act on peptide bonds within the protein molecule), called trypsin and chymotrypsin. Figure 10.12 illustrates how both are secreted into the duodenum as the precursors trypsinogen and chymotrypsinogen,

Table 10.6 Actions of the enzymes of the human alimentary tract

Enzyme	Site of secretion	Site of action	Substrate acted upon	Products of action
Salivary amylase	Mouth	Mouth	Starch	Disaccharides (few), dextrins (mainly)
Pepsinogen→pepsin	Stomach	Stomach	Proteins	Polypeptides
Pancreatic amylase	Pancreas	Small intestine	Starch	Disaccharides (maltase)
Enterokinase	Small intestine	Small intestine	Trypsinogen	Trypsin
Trypsinogen→trypsin	Pancreas	Small intestine	Polypeptides/chymotrypsinogen	Peptides/chymotrypsin
Chymotrypsinogen→chymotrypsin	Pancreas	Small intestine	Polypeptides	Peptides
Carboxypeptidases	Pancreas	Small intestine	Peptides	Smaller peptides (oligopeptides)
Aminopeptidases	Pancreas	Small intestine	Peptides	Smaller peptides (oligopeptides)
Lipase	Pancreas	Small intestine	Triglycerides	Diglycerides, monoglycerides, fatty acids, glycerol
Nucleases	Pancreas	Small intestine	Nucleic acids	Nucleotides
Disaccharidases (maltase, sucrase, lactase)	Small intestine	Small intestine	Disaccharides (maltose, sucrose, lactose)	Monosaccharides (glucose, fructose, galactose)
Peptidases	Small intestine	Small intestine	Oligopeptides	Amino acids
Nucleotidases	Small intestine	Small intestine	Nucleotides	Nucleosides, phosphoric acid
Nucleosidases	Small intestine	Small intestine	Nucleosides	Sugars, purines, pyrimidines

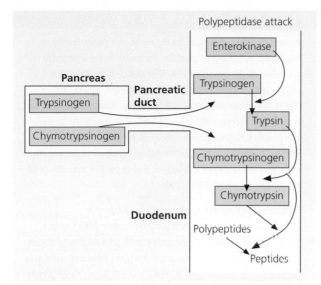

Figure 10.12 Action of trypsin/chymotrypsin (endopeptidases).
Q. Which hormones stimulate the release of pancreatic juice?

respectively. These are activated rapidly within the duodenum. An enzyme called enterokinase secreted from the duodenal mucosa activates trypsinogen. Once trypsin is produced, this activates further conversion of trypsinogen into trypsin (an example of a positive feedback response), and converts chymotrypsinogen into its active form, chymotrypsin. Being endopeptidases, they break down large polypeptide fragments into smaller and smaller subunits called peptides (Figure 10.7(c)).

A further role of trypsin is the activation of another pancreatic precursor, procarboxypolypeptidase. Once activated, this operates as an exopeptidase (an enzyme that acts on peptide bonds at the end of a protein/polypeptide molecule), breaking down the terminal peptide bond and exposing the carboxylic acid part of the amino acid molecule (Figure 10.7(c)). Exopeptidases remove terminal amino acids one at a time from the ends of the chain, until a dipeptide (two amino acids connected by a peptide bond) is formed.

Carbohydrate-digesting enzyme, or pancreatic amylase, breaks down remaining polysaccharides into the disaccharide sugar maltose (Table 10.6).

Fat-digesting enzyme, or pancreatic lipase, together with intestinal lipase, detaches fatty acids from glycerol one at a time (remember that a triglyceride molecule consists of three fatty acids attached to a glycerol molecule; see Chapter 5). A mixture of triglycerides, diglycerides, monoglycerides, glycerol and free fatty acids may therefore be found in the duodenum (Figure 10.7(b)). Lipases continue their breakdown actions until all the fatty acids are removed from the ingested lipids.

Nucleic-acid-digesting enzymes, or nucleases, include ribonucleases, which act on RNA, deoxyribonucleases, which act on DNA, and nucleosidases and nucleotidases, which act on DNA fragments (Table 10.6). These enzymes are essential, since all foods consumed are of cellular origin

and will usually contain nuclear components. Thus, we must break down the components present, rendering them into a form that can be utilized within our own cells for the synthesis of our own nucleic acids during cell division.

Digestive secretions of the intestinal mucosa

Intestinal juice, called succus entericus, is a clear, yellow, alkaline (pH 7.6) fluid produced at a rate of 2–3 l per day from Brunner's glands in the duodenum and from the crypts of Lieberkuhn in the ileum. The juice is mostly of a watery constitution, but it also includes a variety of digestive enzymes (Table 10.6). These enzymes are concerned with the final chemical breakdown of ingested foods. They include:

● *'protein'-digesting enzymes, more correctly termed peptidases:* a variety of dipeptidases are present in intestinal juice. These enzymes are responsible for breaking down dipeptides into individual amino acids. At this point, protein digestion is complete, and the end products of protein digestion, amino acids, can now be absorbed into the circulation;

● *carbohydrate-digesting enzymes, or disaccharidases:* this group includes three enzymes that are responsible for digesting disaccharides (molecules of two simple sugar units) into their constituent monosaccharides. The enzymes are named after the disaccharide that they break down, i.e. maltase converts the disaccharide maltose into its two constituent glucose molecules, lactase breaks down lactose into glucose and galactose, and sucrase converts sucrose into glucose and fructose. Carbohydrate digestion is now complete, and monosaccharides can be absorbed into blood;

● *fat-digesting enzymes, or lipases:* these operate in the same way as pancreatic lipases, i.e. they remove fatty acids from glycerol. The breakdown products of fats are now absorbed into the blood and lymphatic circulation;

● *intestinal nucleases:* these share the breakdown functions with pancreatic nucleases; they break down nucleic acids within the food chyme.

Exercise

List the enzymes associated with the pancreas. Identify their substrates and the breakdown products.

Regulation of the functions of the small intestine

The control of intestinal motility and secretions is mainly hormonal. However, parasympathetic neurons (via vagus, splanchnic and pelvic nerves) also play a part. The presence of food, and the resultant mechanical stimulation

BOX 10.16 UPPER GASTROINTESTINAL ENDOSCOPY

The development of endoscopes has aided the internal examination of body cavities. Endoscopy is a general term used to describe this visual inspection.

Upper gastrointestinal endoscopy

This investigation, also called oesophagogastroduodenoscopy (OGD), allows visualization of the oesophagus, stomach and proximal duodenum via a flexible scope with a light at the tip. The operator guides the end of the scope through the mouth, and passes it into the oesophagus as the patient swallows. The passage of the scope is monitored either using a television screen connected to the probe (video gastroscopy), or by the operator looking directly through the scope. The tip can be bent in several directions. Channels are used for suction and irrigation, and to take biopsies if necessary. The scope can also dilate constrictions, remove unwanted objects, and arrest bleeding in some vessels.

The patient should be consented for this procedure. The patient lies on their left side. Often, an intravenous sedative is given before the tube is introduced. A mouth guard stops the patient biting on the tube, and protects the teeth. The patient must have an empty stomach for effective visualization.

Understandably, OGD can present risks. The most common danger is an adverse reaction to the sedative administered (Cotton and Williams, 1996), which may result in respiratory depression. In addition, perforation and haemorrhage are possible. If a local anaesthetic is used in the throat to aid tolerance of the scope, eating and drinking will not be possible until this has worn off. The patient must also be comfortable undergoing the procedure, so

explanation and reassurance by the nurse and doctor is vital to keep them as relaxed as possible. The nurse in the endoscopy unit is involved in the important task of cleaning, disinfecting and storing used scopes, to ensure optimal infection control, and assists the doctor performing the procedure. Another nurse will be in charge of checking the patient's vital signs during the procedure and providing reassurance. Recovery of the patient after OGD involves monitoring vital signs, providing advice on managing any symptoms or the patient's condition, and explaining side effects of the sedatives used (D'Silva, 1998).

Endoscopic retrograde cholangiopancreatography

Endoscopic retrograde cholangiopancreatography (ERCP) uses a side-viewing endoscope so the sphincter of Oddi (Figure 10.2) can be viewed. ERCP is performed under X-ray, as radio-opaque dye is introduced into the bile duct to locate any blockages. Small stones can often be removed via this method. A wire can be introduced down the scope, which is inserted past the stone, then a basket or balloon on the end of the wire can be opened, and the wire withdrawn. This procedure can drag the stone into the duodenum, where it can be passed normally. If the bile duct has become blocked, a sphincterotomy can be performed, in which the end of the duct is cut and enlarged. Stents can also be inserted into the bile or pancreatic duct to allow free drainage of contents, correcting any narrowing.

ERCP carries more risk than OGD. In addition to the risks of OGD, there is a potential for this procedure to cause pancreatitis or infection of the bile duct. However, ERCP can eliminate the need for surgical removal of gallstones.

Exercise

Identify the nursing observations that are performed to ensure respiratory depression is detected early.

of the intestinal walls by food, causes a release of a variety of hormones, the main ones of which are:

- *secretin*: released in response to the presence of an acidic chyme in the duodenum; causes the release of an alkali-rich pancreatic juice in order to buffer this acidity;

- *cholecystokinin-pancreozymin (CCK-PZ):* stimulates the release of bile from the gall bladder and an enzyme-rich pancreatic juice. The stimulus for its release is a nutrient-rich chyme in the duodenum, in particular the presence of fats (note the role of bile in fat digestion);

- *motilin*: responsible for stimulating a more forceful contraction of the intestinal muscles. It is thought to have a role in promoting a greater movement of food along the tract, particularly in the small intestine.

The secretion of intestinal 'juice' is thought to result from the mechanical contact of food with the intestinal mucosa. It is uncertain whether the mechanism of release is controlled hormonally or neurally. The intestine is a rich source of putative hormones, i.e. substances with demonstrable action but that have yet to be accepted as genuine chemical messengers.

Absorption

Absorption is the process whereby the end products of digestion and the ingested 'soluble' nutrients, which do not need to be broken down, are transported from the lumen of the alimentary tract into the body's transporting systems. Most nutrients are absorbed directly into blood, although long-chain fatty acids are absorbed into the lymphatic circulation. The ileum accounts for 90% of absorption, and is anatomically adapted for this process (Figure 10.13). Adaptations include:

- a large surface area. The ileum is very long (approximately 6.5 m), and the surface area of its lining is increased by many circular folds (plicae) and the finger-like projections, villi and microvilli;

- a very thin absorptive epithelium. The mucosal membrane is a simple columnar epithelium. This is constantly being damaged and worn away, so cells must be mitotically active (especially at the bases of the villi) in order to replace the cell loss;

- an extensive blood and lymphatic supply to the villi;

- a small extracellular space between the absorptive cell and the blood capillaries and lymphatic vessels;

- the walls of the blood and lymphatic vessels consist of a squamous (i.e. thin) endothelium.

The mouth, stomach and large intestine absorb the remaining 10% of the end products of digestion.

BOX 10.17 ABSORPTION OF GLYCERYL TRINITRATE

Oral absorption is clinically useful. For example, the drug glyceryl trinitrate (GTN), used to treat angina, is absorbed sublingually (under the tongue), providing quick entry to the blood. The result is a rapid dilation of coronary blood vessels, leading to an improved delivery of arterial oxygen to the cardiac muscle, and so removing the ischaemic pain of angina.

Substances absorbed by the stomach include glucose, salts, a little water, and vitamin B_{12}. Alcohol is absorbed mainly in the small intestine (80%); the stomach absorbs the remainder, hence its rapid effects. A large intake of protein decreases the rate of alcohol absorption from the stomach. Absorption by the large intestine, particularly the colon, is mainly that of water, although most of this is absorbed by the ileum.

Nutrient absorption in the ileum

Absorption of materials occurs specifically through the epithelial membranes of villi. The process depends upon mechanisms involving facilitated and passive diffusion, osmosis, active transport, and pinocytosis. These mechanisms were discussed in Chapter 2, and you are advised to re-familiarize yourself with these processes. Figure 10.14 summarizes the main processes involved in absorption.

There are two stages to the absorption process. First, the nutrient components must enter the luminal side (i.e. the apical membrane) of the epithelial cell, which involves a variety of different mechanisms, described below. Second, the materials must leave via the lamina propria (i.e. basolateral membrane) surface of the mucosal epithelial cell into the blood capillaries and central lymphatics, or lacteals. This relies mainly on passive diffusion.

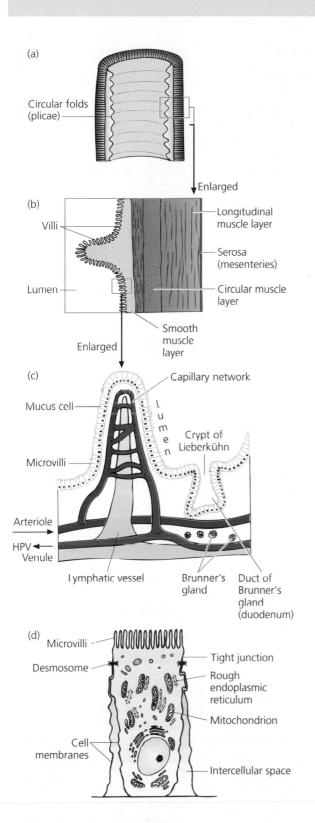

Figure 10.13 Villi. (a) Longitudinal section of duodenum showing circular folds; (b) vertical section through one circular fold; (c) vertical section through one villus; (d) enlarged intestinal cell.

HPV, hepatic portal vein.

Q. List the enzymes associated with pancreatic and intestinal juices, and identify their substrates and the breakdown products from these.

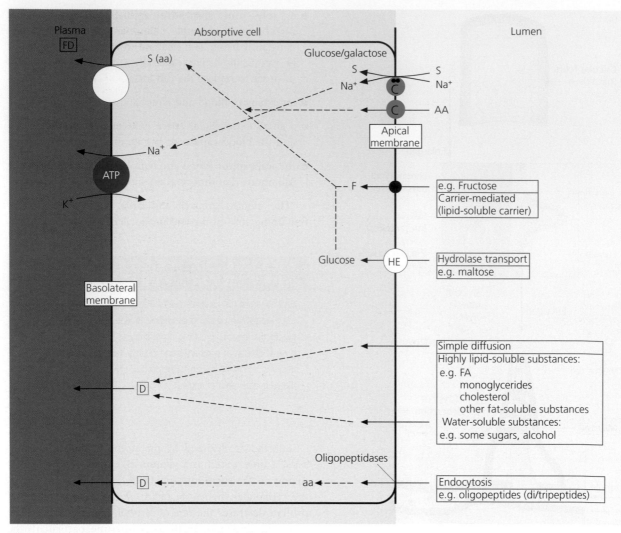

Figure 10.14 The transport mechanism of absorption in the ileum.

AA, amino acid; C, carrier; D, diffusion; FA, fatty acid; FD, facilitated diffusion; HE, hydrolysing enzyme; S, sugar.

Q. How does passive diffusion differ from facilitated diffusion?

Monosaccharide absorption

Fructose is transported into the epithelial cell by carrier-mediated facilitated diffusion. Glucose and galactose are transported in a similar way, but they are co-transported with sodium. Glucose and sodium share the same carrier protein, which contains two specific receptor sites (one for glucose, the other for sodium), both of which must be occupied before transport can take place. Monosaccharide absorption is completed by the terminal part of the ileum.

Amino acid absorption

This occurs mainly in the duodenum and jejunum. Facilitated diffusion co-transporting with sodium is the mechanism involved. Occasionally, dipeptides and tripeptides are absorbed into epithelial cells by pinocytosis, and the final stages of digestion occur within those cells.

Fatty acid absorption

There are two mechanisms for the absorption of fatty acids, depending on the length of the fatty acid chain. Short-chain fatty acids (i.e. those with fewer than 10–12 carbon atoms) pass into the epithelial cell and then into the circulation by simple diffusion because of their high lipid solubility. This accounts for approximately 20% of fat transported. Most dietary fats, however, contain long-chain fatty acids (those with more than 12 carbons atoms); these must combine with fat-soluble vitamins (A, D, E and K), glycerol, monoglycerides and bile salts to form a micelle-like structure, which is pinocytosed into the epithelial cell (Figure 10.15). Once inside the cell, the micelle breaks down into its component parts. The bile salts and fat-soluble vitamins diffuse into the blood; the free fatty acids are combined with glycerol and

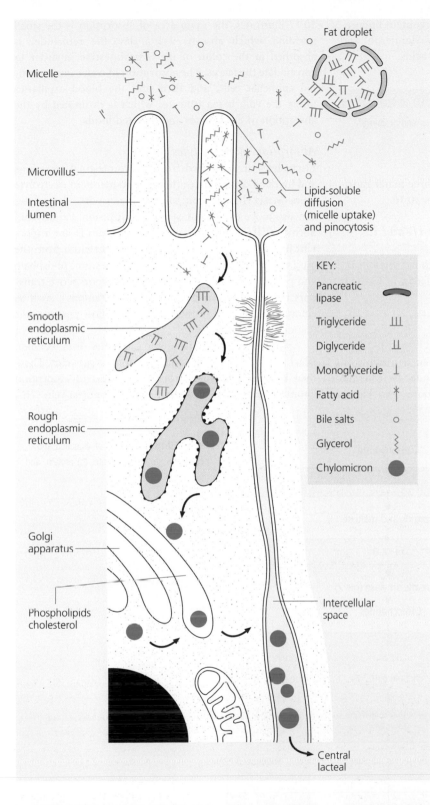

Micelle

Microvillus

Intestinal lumen

Fat droplet

Lipid-soluble diffusion (micelle uptake) and pinocytosis

Smooth endoplasmic reticulum

Rough endoplasmic reticulum

Golgi apparatus

Phospholipids cholesterol

Intercellular space

Central lacteal

KEY:

Pancreatic lipase	⌒
Triglyceride	⊥⊥⊥
Diglyceride	⊥⊥
Monoglyceride	⊥
Fatty acid	⋇
Bile salts	○
Glycerol	⌇
Chylomicron	●

Figure 10.15 Transport of lipids from intestinal lumen through absorptive cells and into the interstitial space. Products of triglyceride digestion — monoglycerides, fatty acids and glycerol — form micelles with the bile salts in solution. They enter the absorptive cell by pinocytosis across the microvillous membrane. Within the cell, the products accumulate in the smooth endoplasmic reticulum, from which they are passed to the rough endoplasmic reticulum. There, they are resynthesized into triglycerides and, together with a smaller amount of phospholipids and cholesterol, are stored in the Golgi apparatus as chylomicrons , droplets about 150 nm in diameter. These then leave the basolateral portions of the cell by exocytosis.

Q. *Identify the path of flow of long-chain fatty acids through the cardiovascular system from their entrance in the neck region to the liver.*

monoglycerides to form triglycerides. Thus, the initial digestion of dietary fats is simply to facilitate the formation of this micelle so that fats, fat-soluble vitamins, and bile salts can collectively pass over the apical membrane of the epithelial cell.

Within the epithelial cell, the triglycerides become coated with a lipoprotein coat to form water-soluble struc-

tures called chylomicrons. These diffuse into the lymphatic minor drainage vessels or lacteals of a villus, and are transported via the lymphatic system into the thoracic lymphatic duct, which drains into the circulation at the junction of the left subclavian and left jugular veins in the neck (see Figure 13.3). Finally, they arrive at the liver through the hepatic artery.

Cells that metabolize these substances contain lipoproteases, to break down the coat of the chylomicron, and triglyceridases, to release individual fatty acids.

The digestion and absorption of the three major nutrients of the diet are summarized in Figure 10.16.

Absorption of water-soluble vitamins (B and C complexes)
These are absorbed by diffusion, although for vitamin B_{12} conjugation with the stomach's intrinsic factor of Castle is necessary.

Water absorption
About 10 l of water a day are absorbed. Of this, 1–2 l are from ingested (i.e. liquid and solid) sources (depending on thirst and social habits), and the remainder is from the accumulation of gastrointestinal secretions. As Figure 10.17 illustrates, the main area of absorption is the small intestine, which absorbs 9 l a day; the remainder is absorbed in the colon of the large intestine in order to consolidate the faeces. The absorption of water into intestinal epithelial cells, and then into the blood capillaries lining the villi, is via osmosis, which is promoted by the absorption of electrolytes and digested foods.

Absorption of electrolytes
Electrolytes are absorbed from gastrointestinal secretions and ingested components; they help to maintain electrolyte homeostasis. In addition to active transport, electrolytes can also move in and out of cells by diffusion. Parathyroid hormone (PTH) and, in particular, vitamin D are important in regulating the active transport of calcium from the gut (see Chapters 9 and 15). Iron, magnesium, phosphate and potassium absorption is dependent upon active transport methods. Negatively charged ions (anions), such as chloride, iodide and nitrates, passively follow positive ions (cations), such as sodium.

Absorbed products pass via capillaries into venules, which drain from the intestinal wall into larger veins. These then link up with veins from other areas of absorption (stomach and colon) to form the hepatic portal vein. This

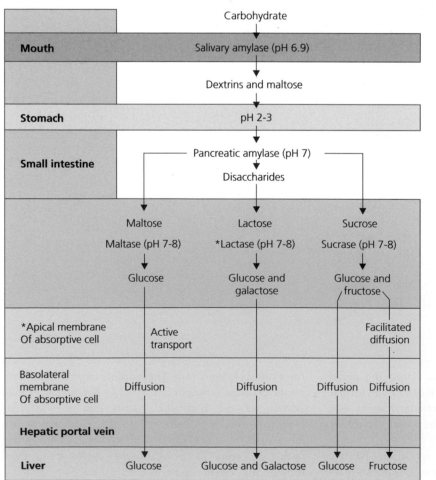

Figure 10.16 Summary of digestion and absorption. (a) Carbohydrate, (b) protein, and (c) fat.

(a)

Figure 10.16 *Continued*

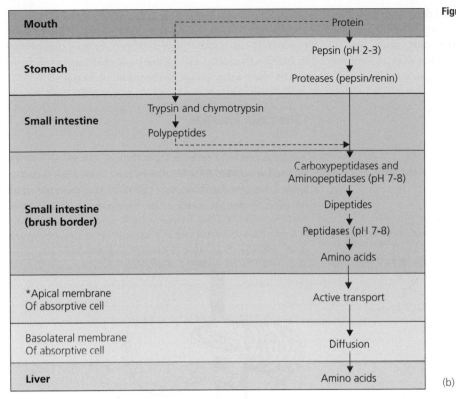

(b)

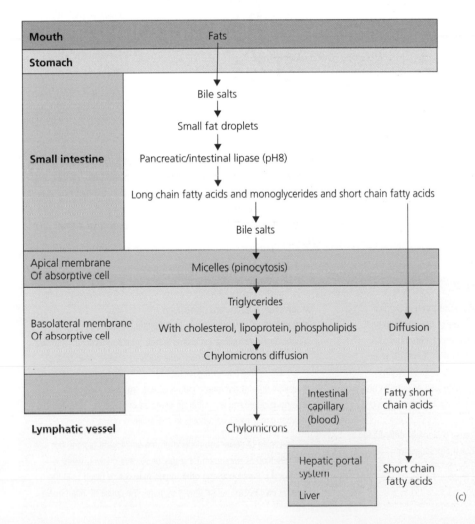

(c)

large vessel carries the end products of digestion directly to the liver (Figure 10.18). All the absorbed components take this route, except for long-chain fatty acids, which pass to the liver via the hepatic artery after being drained into the lymphatic system, as discussed earlier. The liver assimilates the products, and has a role in the homeostatic control of the blood concentrations of some components. Some products of digestion or liver synthesis are then transported in blood to specific cells of the body that require them to sustain their intracellular homeostatic processes.

The large intestine

The large intestine extends from the ileo-caecal valve to the external sphincter muscle of the anus. It is about 1.5–2 m long. It has a wider diameter (about 6.5 cm) than the small intestine, hence its name. The longitudinal muscle layer

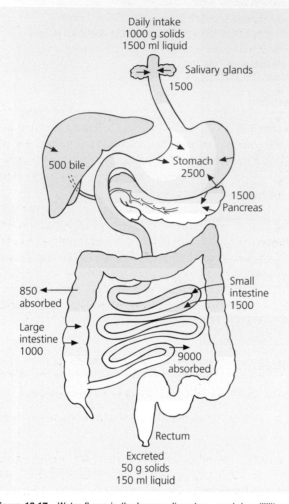

Figure 10.17 Water fluxes in the human alimentary canal, in millilitres. Figures vary with the condition and size of the subject.
Q. How much water is absorbed each day?

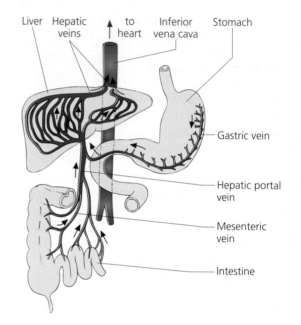

Figure 10.18 The hepatic portal system. Blood is carried directly from the stomach and intestines to the liver via the mesenteric, gastric and hepatic portal veins. Hepatic veins then convey it to the heart by way of the inferior vena cava.
Q. What differentiates the portal vessels in the body from arteries and veins?

BOX 10.18 SURGICAL LESIONS AND GASTROENTERITIS

Disorders of the small intestine commonly arise through surgical lesions, or as a consequence of inflammation of the stomach and the intestines (a condition called gastroenteritis). There is no appreciable difference in digestive and absorptive functions when quite a large amount (up to 50%) of the intestine is surgically removed. However, if less than 25%, digestion and absorption are so reduced that the patient can only survive via parenteral feeding, i.e. infusion of nutrients into a large vein.

Diarrhoea, vomiting, high temperature, and signs of dehydration characterize gastroenteritis. There are four main causes of gastroenteritis:

- infection, e.g. cholera, dysentery;
- metabolic and/or absorptive homeostatic imbalances, e.g. indigestion following excessive starch intake, diarrhoea following too much protein, and conditions such as coeliac disease that exhibit an inability to digest fat;
- emotional and nervous conditions, e.g. 'nervous diarrhoea';
- various other causes, such as allergies or tumours, although the latter occur most commonly in the colon.

Principles of correction depend on the aetiological factors, but generally food is withdrawn for a day or so, and drinking water is encouraged. Antibiotics and other drugs may not be given until the cause is established, since they may mask the cause of inflammation.

forms three bands, called taeniae, which are maintained in a tonic state of contraction, giving this part of the intestine a 'pouched' appearance. Structurally, the large intestine has four main areas: the caecum, colon, rectum and anal canal.

The caecum is the first pouch. Inferiorly, it leads to a blind-ended tube of lymphatic tissue called the appendix.

The colon consists initially of the ascending colon, which is superior to the caecum on the right abdominal side. The ascending colon passes vertically to the transverse colon, which lies just under the inferior surface of the liver (as the hepatic flexure). This extends across the abdominal cavity until it becomes the descending colon on the left side of the abdomen. After descending, the colon becomes the sigmoid colon, which projects to become the third principal part, the rectum.

The rectum is about 16–20 cm long, and lies anterior to the sacrum and coccyx bones. Its terminal 2–3 cm become the fourth principal part of the large intestine, the anal canal.

The anal canal is richly supplied with arteries and veins. Its opening to the exterior is called the anus, which is regulated by two sphincter muscles. The internal sphincter muscle is controlled involuntarily, whereas the external sphincter is under voluntary control.

Homeostatic functions of the large intestine

Homeostatic functions of the large intestine include:

- storage of indigestible food until it is eliminated from the body;

- secretion of mucus, which ensures lubrication of the faeces and eases the elimination process. Mucus also contributes to the alkaline pH of this region, because it contains HCO_3^- ions.

- absorption of most of the remaining water, electrolytes, and some vitamins. The amount of water absorbed depends upon the length of time that the residue of food remains in the colon. Of this residue, 70% is eliminated within 72 h of ingestion; the remainder may stay in the colon for a week or longer. The longer it stays there, the more water will be absorbed.

   Symbiotic bacteria within the colon produce vitamin K and some of the vitamin B complexes (B_1, B_2 and folic acid). The small amounts of vitamin synthesized are not nutritionally significant, unless the individual has a diet that is deficient in these vital nutrients, in which case this may be regarded as a crude homeostatic mechanism for the maintenance of these vitamins in blood. The small amount of vitamin B_{12} produced in this region is also insignificant, as the vitamin is absorbed only in the small intestine, thus any produced or remaining in the colon is eliminated.

   Bacteria also ferment any remaining carbohydrates, releasing gases (carbon dioxide, hydrogen and methane), which contribute to flatulence. The amount of flatulence varies according to the amount and type of food consumed, e.g. baked beans and onions increase the rate of fermentation, and so lead to increased flatulence. Bacteria also break down any remaining proteins and fatty acids in the gut, and convert bilirubin into urobilinogen and

---

BOX 10.22 DIARRHOEA AND CONSTIPATION

Diarrhoea

Diarrhoea usually occurs when the intestinal movements are too rapid for adequate absorption of water, resulting in a large amount of water being eliminated. Other causes are disorders of nutrient absorption, e.g. the effects of cholera toxin on electrolyte transport. Severe diarrhoea results in a large loss of water and electrolytes (particularly sodium and potassium bicarbonate), resulting in dehydration and electrolyte imbalance. Chronic diarrhoea produces hypokalaemia (low blood potassium), and the loss of alkaline digestive juices of the intestine may cause metabolic acidosis. The causes of diarrhoea are summarized in Table 10.7.

   Principles of correction depend upon the cause. However, routine treatment of simple cases is usually based on kaolin or chalk mixtures, which absorb toxins and allay intestinal irritation. Antibiotic therapy may also be used. Since there is fluid loss, sweetened drinks with a little salt are useful in restoring water and electrolyte balance. Severe diarrhoea may require intravenous infusion of a suitable solution (see Chapter 6).

Constipation

Constipation refers to a failure or difficulty with the passage of hard stools. It is the opposite of diarrhoea, in that the faeces are hard due to the absorption of most of the water, usually as a consequence of food residues remaining in the colon for long periods of time, e.g. when there is little fibre in the diet. Faeces become difficult and often painful to eliminate. Abdominal distension may become evident because of food retention. In addition, halitosis, a furred tongue, headache, irritability and flatulence may also occur. The passage of hard stools may also result in the development of haemorrhoids (see Box 10.21). The causes of constipation are summarized in Table 10.7.

   Although constipation is a common problem of ageing (Camilleri *et al.*, 2000), everyone at some time in their lives experiences constipation, and one should not be overly concerned about this. However, if the condition becomes a chronic problem, then this is usually indicative of underlying pathology, e.g. bowel obstruction or poor bowel motility as a consequence of chronic hypokalaemia (as occurs with certain diuretic drug therapies), chronic hypercalcaemia (as occurs with PTH-secreting tumours), or use of analgesics such as morphine.

The principles of correction of constipation involve the use of mild laxatives that induce defecation, and treatment of the underlying pathology.

   The management of constipation is a common routine hospital function. The patient should be encouraged to adopt a comfortable squatting position; this is much more efficient for the process of defecation where possible, because sitting on a bed pan is uncomfortable and therefore does not aid defecation. The following preparations are commonly used in the hospital environment:

- oral or rectal lubricants, e.g. orally administered liquid paraffin, or rectally administered glycine suppositories, serve to soften the faeces. Frequent use should be avoided, since the lubricants may interfere with the absorption of fat-soluble vitamins (A, D, E and K);
- bowel stimulants (aperients), e.g. senna derivatives, bisacodyl and cascara, irritate the mucosa of the colon, and thus aid defecation;
- osmotic aperients, e.g. orally administered magnesium sulphate (= milk of magnesia), or phosphate and lactulose administered as enemas, draw water into the lumen of the gut and the surrounding blood capillaries, causing a large watery stool;
- bulking agents, e.g. methylcellulose derivatives (e.g. dietary fibre, Normacol®, Celevac®), reduce the mouth-to-anus transit time by attracting water to the gut contents, thus, providing a bulky, relatively soft stool;
- manual evacuation of faeces: if the above methods fail to manage constipation, then manual removal may be performed in extreme circumstances. The patient will need an analgesic or sedative before this potentially painful and embarrassing procedure.

Constipation during pregnancy

Constipation is considered a minor disorder of pregnancy. It usually occurs as a result of the effects of progesterone on the smooth muscle of the gut. This reduces the peristaltic action and, together with increased water reabsorption of the colon, increases the risk of constipation. Pregnant women are encouraged to keep to a diet rich in fruit and vegetables, and to increase their fluid intake. In addition, bran foods are also recommended.

Table 10.7 Causes of diarrhoea and constipation

Diarrhoea	Constipation
Foods rich in spices, fruits such as gooseberries and prunes, high alcohol intake	Deficiency in dietary fibre
Distress	Depression and dementia
Drugs, e.g. antibiotics, iron preparations, laxatives	Drugs such as narcotic opiates (codeine, morphine, etc.), some antihypertensives (e.g. methyldopa), anticholinergics, and aluminium antacids
Neoplasms: malignant growths may result in a change in bowel habit, such as alternating periods of diarrhoea and constipation	Neoplasms: change in bowel habits brought about by intestinal growths can lead to alternating bouts of diarrhoea and constipation
Inflammation conditions of the gut, e.g. ulcerative colitis, irritable bowel syndrome, Chrohn's disease (this increases peristaltic motions)	Inactivity
Malabsorption syndrome	Weak pelvic floor musculature
Pathogenic infective organisms, such as *Salmonella*, usually as a result of ingestion of contaminated foods; other symptoms include abdominal pain and nausea	Dehydration
Diverticulosis	Haemorrhoids
Thyroidtoxicosis	Hyperthyroidism

BOX 10.23 PERITONITIS

Sluggish colonic movement is conducive to bacterial growth. These bacteria are potentially pathogenic if released into other areas of the body, e.g. if released into the abdominal cavity via intestinal perforation, or rupture of abdominal organs such as the appendix, they may cause life-threatening acute inflammation of the peritoneum (called peritonitis). Long-term antibiotic therapy results in a loss of these symbiotic bacteria, and encourages the colonization of this area with other potentially pathogenic antibiotic-resistant bacteria. A less serious form of peritonitis can result from the rubbing together of inflamed peritoneal membranes.

BOX 10.24 LOWER GASTROINTESTINAL ENDOSCOPY AND NURSING ASSESSMENT OF THE BOWELS

Lower gastrointestinal endoscopy includes colonoscopy and flexible sigmoidoscopy. This technique has replaced diagnostic laparotomy (Cotton and Williams 1996). Colonoscopy allows the trained operator to view the whole of the large intestine. A flexible colonoscope, similar in design to the endoscope, can reach approximately 175 cm, while a flexible sigmoidoscope can view up to 60 cm of the bowel. This is useful in detecting abnormalities that occur mainly in the descending colon, rectum and anal canal (79% of cancers in the large intestine affect these regions (Davies *et al.*, 1998)). These instruments are inserted into the anus, and pushed carefully along the bowel, guided by images projected onto a television screen. Similarly to OGD, treatment such as the removal of polyps can be carried out, and biopsies can be taken.

To view the colon effectively, the bowel must be cleared. This will possibly commence the day before the examination, or an enema may be administered before the investigation. The method used often depends on the choice of the doctor performing the procedure.

The anal canal and rectum can also be viewed by rigid sigmoidoscopy, which, as its name suggests, is a rigid tube illuminated at one end. Carbon dioxide gas can be passed into the lower descending colon to view the mucosa. Proctoscopy can also examine the anorectal region.

The processes of colonoscopy and flexible sigmoidoscopy carry risks. Perforation can occur, especially in a bowel wall that has already been weakened by inflammation or disease. The necessity of carrying out the investigation should therefore be considered carefully.

The preparation for, and course of, these investigations can obviously be distressing and very embarrassing for the patient. Therefore, explanation of the need for the procedure and what it involves can put the patient more at ease. Reassurance should be given throughout the procedure, even if the patient is sleepy.

Nursing assessment of the patient's bowel habits

Although bowel problems may not be central to the patient's need for care, they can aggravate the primary problem if allowed to develop. It is therefore important to assess the patient's bowel function, including the state of hydration, the smell of the patient's breath, the condition of the patient's tongue, food and fluid intake, and activity levels. The nursing assessment includes:

- frequency of bowel actions;
- quantity of stool and variation from the norm, e.g. stool volume will be increased in patients taking large amounts of fibre;
- consistency of stool passed, e.g. patients with high-fibre diets will produce soft, large stools, which should float in the lavatory;
- stool containing mucus (may signify an inflammatory condition in the gut);
- stool containing undigested food (occurs in conditions of intestinal hurry);
- colour of stool (a very bright red blood content may indicate damage to the rectal blood vessels, tarry stools may indicate bleeding from the gastric or upper-intestinal regions, and pale stools may be the result of obstructive jaundice);
- odour of stool (a change may occur with malabsorption states);
- pain on passing stools (may indicate the presence of haemorrhoids, anal fissure or constipation).

stercobilirubin, which are responsible for the characteristic colours of the urine and faeces, respectively.

The caecum and ascending colon continue to absorb water, and the semi-liquid chyme is converted to semi-solid faeces. Components of the faeces include:

- water;
- inorganic salts;
- bacteria and components of bacterial decomposition;
- alimentary canal cells that have sloughed off;
- indigestible remains (cellulose and vegetable fibres, known as roughage or fibre);
- small amounts of the end products of digestion that have not yet been absorbed;
- excretory products (bile salts, bile pigments and mucus).

Rectal distension as a consequence of the accumulation of faecal matter stimulates rectal wall receptors, which send sensory neuronal input to the sacral region of the spinal cord. This results in parasympathetic motor output to the rectum and anal canal, thus completing the reflex arc. Simultaneously, impulses pass via the spinal cord to the cerebral cortex, so that we can voluntarily inhibit defecation if necessary, especially through the control of the external sphincters.

Defecation results from longitudinal muscle contraction, which causes a reduction in the length of the rectum, thus increasing the pressure within it. This increased pressure, together with voluntary contractions of diaphragmatic and abdominal muscles, forces the internal sphincter open; the faeces are expelled through the anus via the voluntarily relaxed external anal sphincter muscle (which is usually in a state of tonic contraction). The degree of rectal muscle contraction and straining required depends on the consistency of the faeces.

The gastrocolonic reflex is an important stimulus for defecation. This autonomic neural reflex occurs two to three times daily, usually following meals, and increases peristaltic wave activity to move food along the colon. This is more noticeable after breakfast, because it is eaten when the stomach is empty. The gastrocolonic reflex results in an increased contraction of the terminal ileum, relaxing the ileo-caecal valve and stimulating colonic peristalsis. This reflex, therefore, allows filling of the colon; consequently, a mass movement of food residue occurs. The person becomes aware of this only when the faeces enter the rectum.

Exercise

Describe the mechanism involved in defecation.

BOX 10.25 INFLAMMATORY BOWEL DISEASE AND FAECAL INCONTINENCE

Inflammatory bowel disease

This term encompasses the two inflammatory conditions ulcerative colitis and Crohn's disease, which are believed to be different versions of the same autoimmune disease (O'Keefe, 2000). These conditions are characterized by spells of inflammation. In ulcerative colitis, the mucosa and submucosa of the large intestine are affected. In Crohn's disease, all layers of the tissue structure are affected, and inflamed segments can occur anywhere in the gastrointestinal tract. The inflammatory events caused by exacerbations of Crohn's disease can lead to fistula formation and narrowing, while the risk of colorectal cancer is increased by ulcerative colitis. Both conditions cause weight loss, diarrhoea, the passage of blood, and pain; the absorption of nutrients is impeded.

Detection of inflammatory bowel disease is performed by examination of diarrhoea, endoscopic examination, and ultrasound to detect any abscesses.

Principles of correction depend on the severity of the symptoms. It is often treated with sulfasalazine (a combination of sulfa drugs and aspirin). Steroids are also given to suppress the inflammatory response and alleviate the cramping pain. Broad-spectrum antibiotics are prescribed if bacterial infection is suspected. If the condition becomes chronic and severe, then the patient is admitted to hospital and IV fluids administered.

If there is persistent severe disease, or the risk of carcinoma is high, surgical intervention may be required, such as removal of part or all of the colon (called colectomy), or externalization of the ileum (called ileostomy), which bypasses the colon.

Faecal incontinence

Defecation is a reflex response to rectal distension. Faecal incontinence is an inappropriate emptying of the bowel, and may result from any of the following:

- severe fluid diarrhoea, because the sphincters are adapted to retain semi-solids or solid material and are inefficient at retaining fluids;
- fluid leakage around an impacted mass of hard faeces;
- profuse fluid discharge from some kinds of rectal growth.

Faecal incontinence is more common in older people. These people also have a greater risk of cerebrovascular accidents (strokes), following the sharp rise in blood pressure associated with exertion during elimination, especially during constipation. Older people also commonly exhibit deterioration of cerebral and spinal cord functions, which may result in defecation as soon as rectal distension occurs (Norton and Chelvanayagam, 2000).

Principles of correction vary. Rehabilitation through education removes the problem for some people. For others, the problem is incurable, in which case management may involve the use of incontinence pads and rubber sheeting.

The liver

The liver is the largest gland in the body. The bulk of the liver occupies the right upper quadrant, or hypochondrium, of the abdominal cavity under cover of the lower ribs, which function to protect it (see Figure 1.4). On the left side of the abdomen, the liver lies superior to the upper part of the stomach, the presence of which explains why the bulk of the liver is on the right. Above the liver is the diaphragm, anterior to it is the anterior abdominal wall, and below it are the stomach, gall bladder, bile ducts, duodenum, right colonic flexure of the colon, the right kidney, and adrenal glands (Figure 10.2).

The liver is soft, and is extremely red due to its rich blood supply (approximately one-fifth of its weight is blood). Lacerations of the liver are dangerous, as the individual bleeds profusely and such injuries are difficult to repair.

Anatomy of the liver

The liver is covered almost entirely by peritoneum. It has two main lobes – a large right lobe and a smaller left lobe – separated from by ligaments. The right lobe is associated with two further lobes called the inferior quadrate and posterior caudate lobes. The hepatic portal vein from the gastrointestinal tract enters the liver on its lower surface, and subdivides into smaller and smaller vessels, which finally enter a connecting (or anastomosing) system of smaller blood spaces called sinusoids.

The lobes of the liver are composed of microscopic structural and functional units known as the liver lobules (Figure 10.19(a)). A hexagonal capsule of connective tissue, called Glisson's capsule, surrounds each lobule. Internally, each lobule consists of chains or cords of cells referred to as hepatocytes. The cords are arranged radially around a central vein. Between the cords are the blood and bile sinusoids, which are equivalent to the circulatory capillaries of other tissues; they allow an exchange of substances between hepatocytes, blood and bile channels.

The blood sinusoids carry hepatic arterial (from an interlobular arteriole) and hepatic portal (from interlobular veins) blood from the edge of each corner of the hexagonal capsule to the central intralobular vein.

Of the hepatic circulation, 80% of the blood is from the portal vein and 20% is from the hepatic artery, so these sinusoids contain a mixture of nutrient-rich (portal) venous blood and oxygen-rich arterial blood. Oxygen, nutrients and some poisons, such as alcohol, are extracted by the hepatocytes for assimilation or detoxification (see below). Also present within the sinusoids are reticuloendothelial (Kupffer) cells, which destroy bacteria and old erythrocytes and leucocytes. Sinusoidal blood drains into the intralobular (central) vein, which is a tributary of the hepatic vein that drains blood from the liver into the inferior vena cava and thence to the heart.

Bile channels are concerned with the transport of bile produced from the hepatocytes lining them. Flow of bile is in the opposite direction to that of blood, and so flows towards one of the small bile channels (bile canaliculi) at the corners of the hexagonal capsule (Figure 10.19(b)).

The corners of each liver lobule thus contain branches of the hepatic artery, the hepatic portal vein, and a bile canaliculus. This collection of vessels is sometimes referred to as a hepatic triad (Figure 10.19(a)). Bile canaliculi drain into the right and left hepatic ducts, which then form the common hepatic duct. This transports the bile into the gall bladder via the cystic duct (Figure 10.19(c)). Bile is stored and concentrated in this bladder until the duodenum requires it. We discussed bile production and the regulation of its release earlier in this chapter.

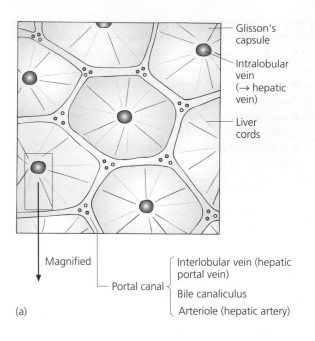

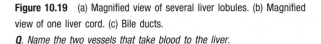

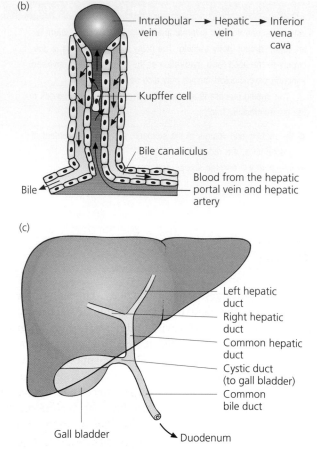

Figure 10.19 (a) Magnified view of several liver lobules. (b) Magnified view of one liver cord. (c) Bile ducts.

Q. Name the two vessels that take blood to the liver.

Homeostatic roles of the liver

The liver is an extremely important homeostatic organ. It is vital in the intermediate metabolism of many end products of digestion, and it has a homeostatic role as an assimilatory organ. It also has an exocrine role in the secretion of bile, which is conveyed to the gall bladder.

Assimilation

The liver is part of the reticuloendothelial system, which is involved in breaking down worn-out erythrocytes (see Chapter 11) and removing the useful components of haemoglobin. For example, iron is extracted and used to maintain its homeostatic range within blood, in order to support the metabolic reactions that require it, such as the production of 'new' erythrocytes to replace the loss of 'old' ones. The globin part of the haemoglobin molecule is converted into its constituent amino acids, which are added to the essential and non-essential amino acid pools within the blood to help maintain their individual homeostatic values. If some of the non-essential amino acids are already within their homeostatic range, they can be converted (or transaminated) into other non-essential amino acids if necessary (Figure 10.20(a)). Conversely, if these amino acids are already within their homeostatic

range, the excess may be broken down (or deaminated) into urea by the ornithine cycle of reactions and into glucose-like compounds, which are use to produce energy via glycolysis and the Krebs cycle (see Chapter 4). Figure 10.20(b) summarizes the metabolic pathway for amino acids.

Excess glucose molecules are taken from blood sinusoids into the hepatocytes to maintain blood glucose concentrations homeostatically (Figure 10.21(a)). As a consequence, the intracellular glucose within the hepatocytes may rise above its homeostatic range; this excess must be removed. Some of the excess is used in cellular respiration to sustain normal metabolic processes; the remainder is converted into the storage component glycogen by a process called glycogenesis. If there is still an intracellular excess of glucose when the cell stores of glycogen are full, it is converted into glycerol and hence fat by a process called lipogenesis. Note that these mechanisms are reversible, so when blood glucose concentrations are low, the glucose stores (first glycogen, then fats) are converted back to glucose to raise the blood glucose level to within its homeostatic parameters. The metabolic pathways for glucose and fatty acids are summarized in Figure 10.21 (b) and (c).

The fat-soluble vitamins (A, D, E and K), and the minerals iron (Fe) and copper (Cu), are stored by hepatocytes

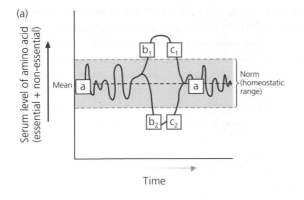

(a)

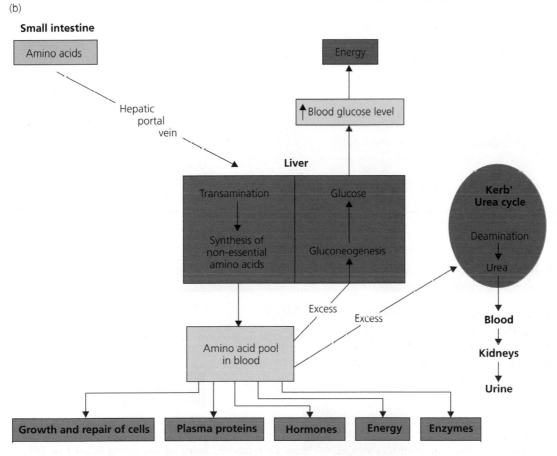

Figure 10.20 (a) The liver's utilization of the end products of globin breakdown. (a) Homeostatic pool of serum amino acids. (b₁) Amino acids above their homeostatic range as a result of post-absorption of a protein-rich meal and/or excessive haemolysis (breakdown) of erythrocytes. (b₂) Amino acids below their homeostatic range due to insufficient dietary protein. (c₁) Restoration of serum non-essential amino acids levels by deamination of the excess into urea (ornithine cycle) and energy (glycolysis and Krebs cycle). (c₂) Increased non-essential amino acids by transaminating excess of some amino acids into those below their homeostatic range and/or proteolytic breakdown and/or increased dietary intake, increased essential amino acids via increased dietary intake.

(b) Summary of the metabolic pathway for amino acids.

Q. When does transamination occur?

when the absorption of a meal produces blood levels in excess of their individual homeostatic ranges. Excess water-soluble vitamins (C and B complexes), water and other minerals pass through the sinusoids, except for that taken into hepatocytes for their metabolic needs, as the liver cannot store them, transfer them into other substances, or destroy them. The body's excretory organs then remove these excesses in order to maintain their individual homeostatic levels (Figure 10.22).

Excess fatty acids and glycerol are converted into glucose only if hypoglycaemia is present and there are inadequate glycogen stores. Otherwise, these substances pass through the liver to the storage regions of the body, i.e. the adipose tissues under the skin and surrounding organs such as the heart and kidneys.

Secretory functions

The liver secretes bile salts, which are important in emulsification (described earlier) and the absorption of fats, phospholipids and lipoproteins. The anticoagulant heparin, and the plasma proteins, are also produced and secreted by the liver.

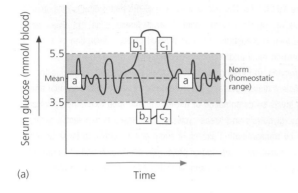

(a)

Figure 10.21 (a) The liver's role in blood glucose regulation. (a) Normal blood glucose level. (b_1) Elevation post-absorption of a meal. (b_2) Decreased glucose levels due to greater cellular uptake for increased metabolism. (c_1) Glucose in excess of its homeostatic range taken into hepatocytes and skeletal muscle cells mediated by effects of insulin. Consequently, intracellular levels rise; this excess is used in cellular respiration and in promoting a glucose store in the form of glycogen (glycogenesis). If glycogen stores are full, then the excess glucose is converted into fat (lipogenesis) within fat stores throughout the body. (c_2) Depressed glucose levels in the blood are corrected by measures such as glycogenolysis (i.e. glycogen is converted to glucose). If levels remain low, lipolysis (fat breakdown) and proteolysis (protein breakdown) occur. The latter occurs only in severe starvation states. (c_2) Events mediated by glucagon, somatomedin, adrenaline, noradrenaline, thyroxine and the sympathetic nervous system act to increase glucose availability.

Q. Explain the paracrine role of somatostatin (refer to Chapter for help).
(b) Summary of the metabolic pathway for monosaccharides (glucose, galactose and fructose).

(b)

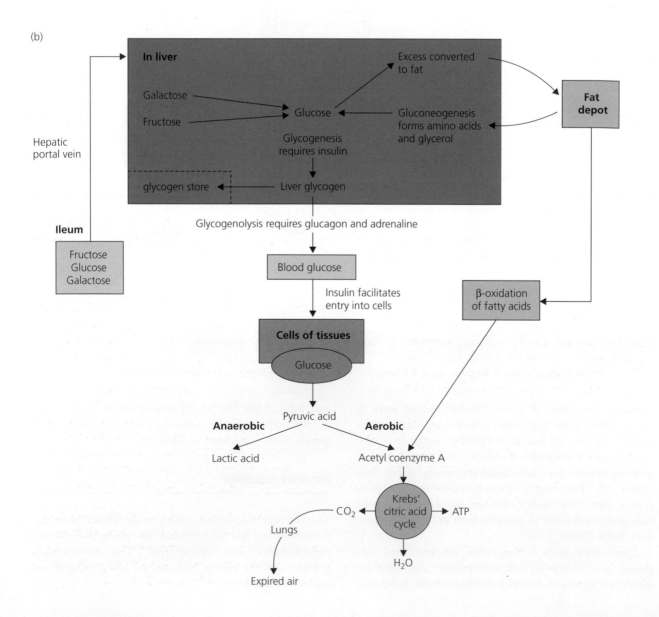

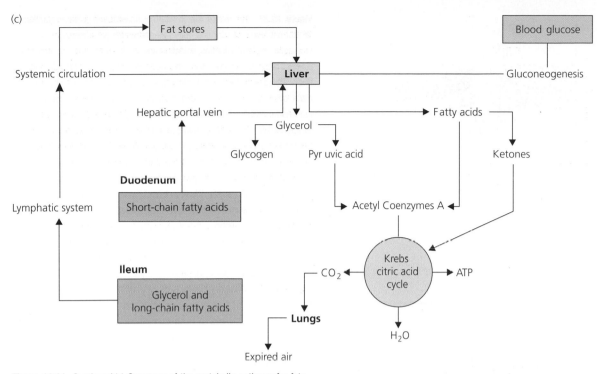

Figure 10.21 *Continued* (c) Summary of the metabolic pathway for fats.
Q. What general name is given to enzymes involved in lipid digestion?

Detoxification/deactivation functions

The liver contains detoxifying enzymes, which are responsible for transforming poisons such as alcohol into harmless substances. Similarly, ammonia produced when excess amino acids are deaminated to provide energy is converted into urea. Moderate amounts of urea are harmless to the body, and the kidneys and the sweat glands easily excrete the excess. The liver also deactivates various hormones, thus reducing their blood concentrations and hence their physiological activities.

Storage functions

In addition to the storage of the various nutrients, the liver also stores some poisons (e.g. DDT) that cannot be broken down and excreted.

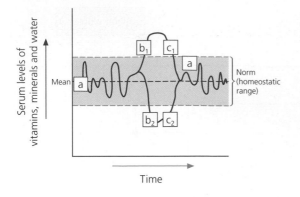

Serum levels of vitamins, minerals and water

Mean

Time

Figure 10.22 The liver's role in vitamin, mineral and water regulation. (a) Normal levels of vitamins, minerals and water pre-absorption. (b_1) Increased levels of vitamins, minerals and water above their homeostatic ranges following dietary intake. (b_2) Decreased levels of vitamins, minerals and water below their homeostatic ranges as these nutrients are used in metabolism. (c_1) Excess fat-soluble vitamins (A, D, E and K) and minerals (iron and copper) are stored in hepatocytes. Excess water-soluble vitamins (C and B complexes), other minerals and water pass through the liver to the excretory organs in order to restore their homeostatic ranges. (c_2) Corrective measures to restore these nutrients to within their serum homeostatic ranges, i.e. the liver releases its stores of fat-soluble vitamins, iron and copper. Water-soluble vitamins, other minerals and water must be consumed to restore their homeostatic ranges.
Q. *Describe the secretory, storage and detoxification assimilative roles of the liver.*

Other functions

Because liver cells have hundreds of enzymes, the organ is responsible for at least as many important homeostatic functions, some of which remain to be identified. For example, the liver, together with the kidneys, is involved in the activation of vitamin D, and it contributes indirectly to the regulation of blood pressure by synthesizing angiotensinogen, the precursor of the hormone angiotensin. The liver's role in cholesterol metabolism is discussed in Chapter 10.

As a result of the liver being involved in a large number of metabolic reactions, it is inevitable that many of these give off heat. Thus, the liver is an important contributor to thermoregulation.

BOX 10.28 DEVELOPMENT OF THE LIVER

The liver is responsible for approximately 55% of the total body weight at birth, and is largely responsible for the protuberant abdomen of infancy. As growth rate slows during childhood, there is a corresponding decline in metabolism and, as a result, the liver becomes proportionally smaller; in the adult, the liver represents approximately 2.5% of the body weight. As a result of the ageing process, the size and weight of the liver decrease, and blood flow to the liver decreases, decreasing the efficiency of drug metabolism.

BOX 10.29 HEPATITIS

Hepatitis is an inflammation of the liver that may arise as a result of poisoning from various drugs or, more commonly, from one of five types of viral infection. Hepatitis A virus (HAV) (previously known as infectious hepatitis) tends to occur as local outbreaks, and is transmitted by the faecal-oral route, i.e. faecal contamination of food. An attack usually starts with the appearance of jaundice and bile-coloured urine, following signs of toxaemia, loss of appetite and fever. It does not cause lasting liver damage, and most patients recover in 4–6 weeks.

Hepatitis B virus (HBV) (formerly known as serum hepatitis) may be transmitted through contaminated syringes and transfusion equipment, or via other body secretions, such as tears, saliva or semen. The virus may produce chronic liver inflammation, which can persist throughout the person's lifetime. HBV is a hazard that must be considered during blood transfusion, renal dialysis, and transplant surgery. Infected patients are also at increased risk of cirrhosis. Even when recovery is complete, patients can remain carriers of the virus.

Hepatitis C virus (HCV) is similar to HBV, and is often transmitted through blood transfusion. Hepatitis D virus (HDV) and hepatitis E virus (HEV) have also been identified.

These infections can all cause acute hepatitis; HBV and HCV can also cause chronic hepatitis.

There is no specific treatment for acute viral hepatitis. In most patients the disease is self-limiting with full recovery. A low-fat, high-carbohydrate diet is beneficial if bile flow is obstructed. Physical activity may be restricted. Interferon alfa can be useful in the treatment of chronic hepatitis B and hepatitis C, and thymosin may be a promising new treatment for hepatitis B.

To prevent transmission of hepatitis A, washing the hands and using gloves for disposing bedpans and faecal matter are imperative. The administration of immunoglobulins before exposure or early in the incubation period can prevent hepatitis A and hepatitis B. Vaccines are available to protect against hepatitis A and hepatitis B infections. Prophylaxis is recommended for healthcare workers and others who are at risk of contact with infected body fluids, particularly children (Jefferson *et al.*, 2001).

The common laboratory tests of liver function are summarized in Table 10.8.

Identify a homeostatic failure associated with each region of the gut. Suggest the principles of correction associated with the failures you have named.

Table 10.8 Common laboratory tests for liver function

Test	Homeostatic range	Clinical significance
Serum enzymes		
Alkaline phosphatase	13–39 U/ml	↑ with biliary obstruction and cholestastic hepatitis
Aspartate amino transferase	5–40 U/ml	↑ with hepatocellular injury
Lactate dehydrogenase (LDH)	200–500 U/ml	↑ isoenzyme LDH_5 with hypoxic and primary liver injury
Bilirubin metabolism		
Serum bilirubin		
Indirect (unconjugated)	< 0.8 mg/dl	↑ with haemolysis
Direct (conjugated)	< 0.2–0.4 mg/dl	↑ with hepatocellular injury or obstruction
Total	< 1.0 mg/dl	↑ with biliary obstruction
Urine bilirubin	0	↓ with biliary obstruction
Urine urobilinogen	0–4 mg/24 h	↑ with haemolysis
Serum proteins		
Albumin	3.5–5.5 g/dl	↓ with hepatocellular injury
Globulin	2.5–3.5 g/dl	↑ with hepatitis
Total	6–7 g/dl	
Transferrin	250–300 µg/dl	Liver damage with ↓ values, iron deficiency with ↓ values
Blood clotting functions		
Prothrombin time	11.5–14 s	↑ with chronic liver disease (e.g. cirrhosis) or vitamin K deficiency
Partial thromboplastin time	25–40 s	↑ with sever liver disease or heparin therapy

BOX 10.30 COMMON CANCERS OF THE GASTROINTESTINAL TRACT

Oesophageal carcinoma

A tumour in the oesophagus is linked with smoking, high alcohol intake, and a history of oesophageal trauma or gastro-oesophageal reflux (Miller *et al.*, 1994). The patient tends to present late with dysphagia (difficulty in swallowing). The majority of tumours appears in the lower two-thirds of the oesophagus, and can be detected by gastroscopy, computerized axial tomography (CAT or CT) scan and ultrasound.

Carcinoma of the stomach

Most tumours are located at the pyloric region, and have a poor overall prognosis. Patients often present late with anorexia and pain. Diagnosis can be made from biopsy during gastroscopy.

Carcinoma of the liver

Secondary tumours occur most frequently in the liver (Miller *et al.*, 1994), although primary lesions also occur, usually in the right lobe, which can infiltrate the portal vein, causing portal hypertension. Secondary deposits can occur anywhere in the liver. Spread is possible into nearby lymph nodes or pleura. As the liver enlarges, its capsule stretches, causing pain.

Blood tests and biopsy can detect the carcinoma. Ultrasound or CT scan can indicate the extent of the lesion.

Cancer of the pancreas

Cancer of the pancreas is the fourth and sixth most common cancer experienced in men and women, respectively (Miller *et al.*, 1994). It is often found in the head region of the organ. Frequently, the patient experiences jaundice and weight loss. An obstruction of the bile duct may be cleared by ERCP, but this condition carries a poor prognosis for the patient, as spread is common.

Colorectal cancer

This type of malignancy is very common today, and is linked to a low-fibre diet. A higher risk of colonic cancer is evident in ulcerative colitis. As in carcinoma of the stomach, patients often present late, as symptoms are often vague and unthreatening, such as a change in bowel habit. Endoscopy can be employed to detect a mass, and ultrasound or CT scanning can search for any spread to surrounding tissues. The system of Dukes staging is often used to class the severity of the carcinoma once it has been detected (Table 10.9).

Table 10.9 Dukes staging of colorectal cancer

Dukes stage	Severity of the cancer
A	Only mucosa and submucosa effected
B	Muscle wall involved, but no lymph node Involvement
C	Lymph nodes have been infiltrated
D	Metastases present, or severe spread – cure impossible

Summary

1 Providing that a balanced diet is ingested, the digestive system ensures that cells receive the nutrients (metabolites) necessary for their correct functioning (metabolism).

2 Digestion is the breakdown of food. It involves physical processes (provided mainly by specialized gut movements), and chemical processes (i.e. hydrolysis). Chemical digestion is accelerated by specific enzymatic actions.

3 Hydrolysis converts large, insoluble molecules into small, soluble molecules, which can be absorbed into the blood.

4 The digestive system consists of an alimentary canal and several accessory organs.

5 Various regions of the canal are adapted to perform specialized functions:

   (a) The mouth is adapted to receive food, initiate digestive processes, and perform a limited amount of absorption. It also serves as the organ of speech.

   (b) The salivary glands secrete saliva, which moistens food, helps bind food particles together, initiates carbohydrate digestion, makes taste possible, and helps cleanse the mouth, gums and teeth.

   (c) The pharynx and oesophagus act as passageways for boli of food.

   (d) The stomach receives boli of food, mixes them with gastric juice, initiates protein digestion, performs limited absorption duties, and passes chyme into the small intestine.

   (e) The small intestine receives secretions from the pancreas and the gall bladder, completes digestion of food, absorbs most of the end products of digestion, and transports the indigestible remains to the large intestine.

   (f) The large intestine absorbs water and electrolytes, and stores and expels the faeces.

   (g) The pancreas is a mixed gland, having both endocrine and exocrine tissue. Its exocrine secretion, pancreatic juice, contains many enzymes that, together with intestinal juice and bile components, complete the digestive process.

   (h) The gall bladder receives bile from the liver, and stores and concentrates it until it is required by the small intestine. Bile is involved in emulsification.

   (i) The liver assimilates most of the absorbed nutrients in order to prevent nutrients becoming in excess of their homeostatic ranges within blood, and to synthesize other vital biochemicals.

6 Food is moved through the alimentary canal principally by peristalsis.

7 Homeostatic imbalances can result from:

   (a) malnutrition (i.e. insufficient intake of nutrients, or from an overindulgence of nutrients);

   (b) disturbances in the ability to chew or swallow food. In the mouth, such disturbances can result from poor functioning of the mucous membranes, teeth, gums, tongue or salivary glands;

   (c) problems affecting pharyngeal or oesophageal function, including tonsillitis, hiatus hernia and oesophageal diverticulosis;

   (d) disorders of the stomach, the symptoms of which are often exacerbated by the high acidity of gastric juice. Disorders may arise because of localized inflammation (e.g. gastritis), and ulceration of the gastric mucosa is a relatively common disorder. Nausea and vomiting are frequently associated with stomach disorders;

   (e) disorders of the small intestine, which commonly relate to disturbances in enzyme or mucous secretion, or in absorption. Since many digestive enzymes originate from the pancreas, pancreatic infections (pancreatitis) or blockage of ducts (as in cystic fibrosis) will disturb the digestive process. More commonly, however, disorders arise through surgical lesions or as a consequence of gastroenteritis;

   (f) disorders of the large intestine, which are relatively common, and include inflammation, which may be localized as in appendicitis, ulcerative colitis and diverticulitis. Rectal function disturbance as a result of blood vessel congestion (haemorrhoids) is also relatively common;

   (g) disorders of the liver influence, which may compromise the utilization of the products of digestion and the production of bile.

Review questions

Constipation and diarrhoea are common problems encountered in all branches of nursing. There are many reasons why an individual may become constipated or have diarrhoea.

Constipation

1 Define constipation.

2 Do all individuals open their bowels once per day? If not, does this mean they are constipated?

3 Investigate the possible causes of constipation. Explain how these would cause constipation.

4 What are the signs and symptoms of constipation?

5 What other problems are associated with constipation?

6 Consider your role in the care of a person who presents with symptoms of constipation. What factors would be important to include in your assessment?

7 How could you help to promote defecation? Note that purgatives should not be the first choice.

8 What are purgatives/laxatives? Identify the different types of purgatives used.

Diarrhoea

9 What is diarrhoea?

10 Identify the causes of diarrhoea.

11 What are the signs and symptoms of diarrhoea?

12 What factors would be important to include in your client assessment?

13 How would you care for a client with diarrhoea?

REFERENCES

Agrawal, S. and Jonnalagadda, S. (2000) Gallstones, from gallbladder to gut: management options for diverse complications. *Postgraduate Medicine* **108**(30):143–6, 149–53.

Blamey, S. (1998) Classifying hiatus hernia: does it make a difference to management? *Australian Family Physician* **27**(6): 481–5.

Camilleri M., Lee, J.S., Viramontes, B., Bharucha, A.E. and Tangalos, E.G. (2000) Progress in geriatrics. Insights into the pathophysiology and mechanisms of constipation, irritable bowel syndrome, and diverticulosis in older people. *Journal of the American Geriatrics Society* **48**(9): 1142–50.

Chowdhury, P. and Rayford, P.L. (2000) Smoking and pancreatic disorders. *European Journal of Gastroenterology and Hepatology* **12**(8): 869–77.

Cotton, P. and Williams, C. (1996) *Practical Gastrointestinal Endoscopy*, 4th edn. Oxford: Blackwell Science.

Davies, P., Button, C. and Foster, M. (1998) Rectal bleeding. *Nursing Times* **16**: 46–9.

D'Silva, J. (1998) Upper gastrointestinal endoscopy: gastroscopy. *Nursing Standard* **12**: 45, 49–54.

Fass, R., Pulliam, G., Johnson, C., Garewal, H.S. and Sampliner, R.E. (2000) Symptom severity and oesophageal chemosensitivity to acid in older and young patients with gastro-oesophageal reflux. *Age and Ageing* **29**(2): 125–30.

Huether, S.E. and McCance, K.L. (1996) *Understanding Pathophysiology*. London: Mosby.

Jefferson, T., Demicheli, V., Deeks, J., MacMillan, A., Sassi, F. and Pratt, M. (2001) Vaccines for preventing hepatitis B in health-care workers. The Cochrane Library, Issue 1. Oxford: Update Software.

McArdle, J. (2000) The biological and nursing implications of pancreatitis. *Nursing Standard* **14**: 48, 46-51.

Miller, R., Howie, E. and Murchie, M. (1994) The gastrointestinal system, liver and biliary tract. In: Alexander, M.F., Fawcett, J.N. and Runciman, P. *Nursing Practice Hospital and Home: the adult*. Edinburgh: Churchill Livingstone.

Norton, C. and Chelvanayagam, S. (2000) A nursing assessment tool for adults with fecal incontinence. *Journal of Wocn* **27**(5): 279–91.

O'Keefe, T. (2000) Irritable bowel syndrome (IBS): holistic treatment approach. *Positive Health* (59): 35–7.

FURTHER READING

Bartlett, D. and Davidhizar, R. (1999) What the nurse manager can do to avoid an ulcer. *Seminars for Nurse Managers* **7**(2): 67–70.

Bazaldua, O.V. and Schneider, F.D. (1999) Evaluation and management of dyspepsia. *American Family Physician* **60**(6): 1773–84, 1787–8.

Cooley, C., Adeodu, S., Aldred, H., Beesley, S., Leung, A. and Thacker, L. (2000) Literature review. Paediatric palliative care: a lack of research-based evidence. *International Journal of Palliative Nursing* **6**(7): 346–51.

Lundell, L., Miettinen, P., Myrvold, H.E., Pederson, S.A., Thor, K., Lamm, M., *et al.* (2000) Long-term management of gastro-oesophageal reflux disease with omeprazole or open antireflux surgery: results of a prospective, randomized clinical trial. *European Journal of Gastroenterology and Hepatology* **12**(8): 879–87.

Chapter 11

The cardiovascular system 1: blood

INTRODUCTION

The circulating blood acts as an intermediary between the external environment (outside the body) and the internal environment (tissue fluid and cells). Figure 11.1 illustrates the constant interchange between the external environment and body fluids for the maintenance of extracellular and intracellular homeostasis. The importance of blood as an intermediary tissue cannot be overemphasized: any area of the body deprived of the contents of circulating blood will be subjected to functional impairment, resulting in tissue death within a matter of minutes if the circulation is not restored. A number of homeostatic functions can therefore be ascribed to blood and the circulatory system in relation to the composition of the internal environment, but also in relation to defence of tissues.

Respiratory gases

The blood transports oxygen from the lungs to cells for the process of cellular respiration (i.e. the energy-producing process involving the breakdown of food). Carbon dioxide is a product of cellular respiration, and the excess (i.e. level above its homeostatic range) must be removed from the cells to prevent imbalance. Carbon dioxide diffuses into blood, which then transports it to the lungs for excretion. This removal from the blood is necessary to prevent homeostatic imbalances also occurring in this body fluid (see Chapters 6 and 14).

Metabolic wastes

Metabolic wastes are generally considered to be substances that cannot be metabolized by cells. They also include useful substances in excess of their homeostatic ranges that cannot be stored, destroyed, or transferred into other metabolites. The blood transports these substances from the tissues to the excretory organs for removal from the body, in order to prevent consequential build-up to toxic levels (see Chapter 15).

Nutrients

The end products of digestion are transported to the liver for processing or assimilation (see Chapter 10). Nutrients from storage areas, e.g. fats from adipose tissue and proteins from muscle tissue, are transported to cells requiring them for their own metabolic processes. Fats and proteins can be used to produce energy in cells when the body has depleted its carbohydrate reserves, and may also be assimilated into other cellular processes.

Regulatory materials

Enzymes and hormones are taken from their sites of production to their target cells (see Chapter 9).

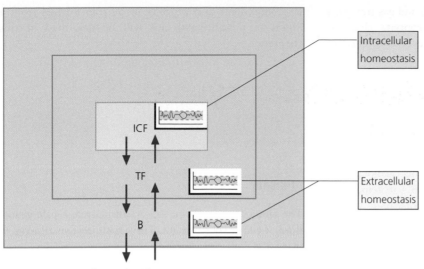

Figure 11.1 The interchange between external and internal environments in order to maintain homeostasis. Component intake must match component output in order to achieve extracellular and thus intracellular homeostasis.

B, blood; ICF, intracellular fluid; TF, tissue fluid.

Q. Suggest why the composition of blood is important for intracellular homeostasis.

pH and electrolyte composition

Buffer chemicals in blood and intracellular fluid contribute to the homeostatic regulation of body fluid pH (acid/base) balance and, to some extent, the electrolyte composition of the body fluids. Acid/base regulation is essential for the optimum functioning of enzymes, and hence metabolism, within these fluid compartments (see Chapter 6). Blood pH is slightly alkaline (mean 7.4), while the pH of cells is slightly acidic (mean 6.8).

Exercise

Refer to previous chapters to reflect on your understanding of the following: the liver's role in assimilation (Chapter 10), enzymes as the 'key chemicals of life'(Chapters 1 and 4), and the role of genes in the process of protein (enzyme) synthesis (Chapter 2).

Thermoregulation

Cells must release heat generated by metabolism in order to prevent intracellular imbalances, since optimal enzyme action occurs within a narrow temperature range. The removal of heat from cells by blood may cause blood temperature to rise above its homeostatic range. This occurs when cellular metabolism is high, as in strenuous exercise, fever and illness, and times of distress. The excess heat is distributed to the skin surface, where it is dissipated. Alternatively, heat may be redistributed to areas of the body that require warming, when their regional temperatures have fallen below their homeostatic ranges. Normally the temperature of blood is about 38°C; the normal body temperature varies between different sites in the body (see Chapter 16).

Haemostasis

Blood clotting helps preserve body fluid homeostasis by restricting fluid loss through damaged vessels or injury sites, a process called haemostasis. This helps prevent excessive loss of extracellular fluids, which could seriously affect blood pressure and cardiovascular function.

Cellular defence mechanisms

White blood cells and antibodies in the blood are instrumental in defending the body against potential disease-causing microbes (pathogens) and their poisonous chemical secretions (toxins). These processes are described in more detail in Chapter 13. The blood also transports toxic substances to the liver and kidneys, where they are detoxified and excreted.

Blood is in constant interaction with tissues, hence its functions will clearly overlap with those of various tissues and organs (see Box 11.1). Many of these roles, such as

BOX 11.1 ELECTROLYTE DISTURBANCES

Blood electrolyte disturbances in individuals are a reflection of intracellular imbalances (see Table 1.3 for normal values). For example, hyponatraemia (sodium deficiency in the blood) can be a result of severe diarrhoea and vomiting (often abbreviated as D&V). It causes a reduction in extracellular fluid volume, resulting in hypotension (low blood pressure), weakness, dizziness, mental confusion and fainting due to the diminished transport of metabolites to the cells. Details of electrolyte disturbances can be found in Chapters 6 and 15.

pH regulation, temperature regulation, and gas transport are described elsewhere in the appropriate chapters. Blood is a tissue in its own right, however, and its cellu- lar components and capacity to be transformed from a liquid to a semi-solid clot will be described in this chapter.

OVERVIEW OF THE COMPOSITION OF BLOOD

The volume of blood circulating in the cardiovascular system averages 5–6 l in males and 4–5 l in females. It accounts for approximately 8% of the total body weight. Blood appears to be a uniform (homogeneous), dark red, viscous liquid that, if left to stand for a few minutes, normally clots or solidifies. Microscopic investigation reveals, however, that blood is a mixture of cell types, suspended in a fluid compartment called plasma. Plasma and red blood cells account for about 55% and 44% of a blood sample, respectively. The remaining 1% consists of white blood cells and platelets (Figure 11.2).

Plasma

The blood contains some 2.5–3 l of plasma, a pale yellow fluid of which 90% is water. The remaining constituents of plasma include:

- plasma proteins (albumins, globulins, fibrinogen);

- regulatory chemicals (enzymes, hormones);

- various other organic chemicals, including nutrients (e.g. glucose, amino acids, fatty acids, glycerol), choles-

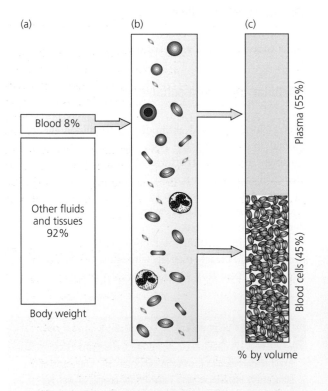

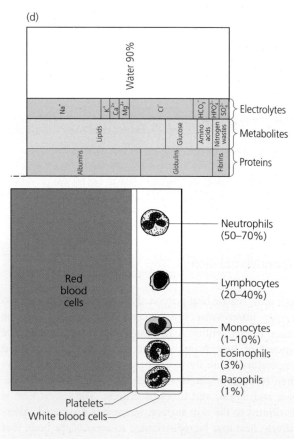

Figure 11.2 The homeostatic composition of body fluids and blood. (a) Body fluids. (b) Whole blood. (c) Centrifuged blood. (d) Separate components of blood.

Q. Name the cellular elements and non-cellular components of blood.

terol, and waste products of metabolism (e.g. urea, creatinine);

● inorganic substances (electrolytes).

These components give plasma a greater density and viscosity than water. The dissolved proteins make this fluid sticky, cohesive and resistant to flow.

Exercise

Define the following terms: (i) organic; (ii) inorganic; (iii) density; (iv) viscosity.

Blood cells

The cellular components of blood are:

● *red blood cells (erythrocytes; 'erythro-' = red):* transport respiratory gases to and from cells, and define the person's blood group;

● *white blood cells (leucocytes; 'leuco-' = white):* important components of the body's immune system, concerned with defending the body against pathogens and their toxin secretions;

● *platelets (thrombocytes):* of fundamental importance in blood clotting. Their homeostatic role is in haemostasis, i.e. they prevent blood loss, and thus help maintain body fluid balance following injury to a blood vessel.

Blood production

Blood production (haemopoiesis) occurs in three stages, according to the individual's period of growth and development. These are referred to as the mesoblastic, hepatosplenic and myeloid stages.

The mesoblastic stage

The first blood cells to be produced in the unborn child originate from the embryonic mesodermal cells that migrate to the yolk sac, where they form 'blood islands' (see Figure 20.4). These become hollow tubes that secrete a plasma-like fluid from their walls. Proliferation of cells lining these tubes forms the early cells of the circulation. These nucleated cells (called megaloblasts of Ehrlich) contain the pigment haemoglobin; their sole purpose is to transport oxygen to the developing embryonic tissue cells. Blood production from these cells is sufficient for the first few weeks of embryonic life, but is inadequate to support further development.

Exercise

Use appendix C to look up the meaning of the prefix 'mes-' and the root '-derm'. Using a medical/nursing dictionary, differentiate between the embryo and fetal stages of development. Note that a 'blast' is an embryonic cell that has not undergone final differentiation.

The hepatosplenic stage

This stage of blood production begins at about the sixth week of gestation; it is mainly responsible for the relatively large size of the liver between the seventh and ninth weeks of gestation. It is necessary because the fetus is growing at a fast rate, and its tissues require a correspondingly greater blood supply to sustain this activity. The liver ('hepato-') and spleen ('-splenic') become the main contributors of this enhanced blood production, although the thymus is also involved. The liver becomes the major haemopoietic site between weeks 13 and 17 of gestation, and continues to produce blood until the later stages of pregnancy.

BOX 11.2 TAKING A BLOOD SAMPLE

Taking blood samples for laboratory analysis is called venepuncture. This is a straightforward procedure that involves withdrawing a specimen of blood from a vein using a hypodermic needle and a syringe. Blood is usually taken from the median cubital vein, which is anatomically anterior to the elbow (see Figure 12.19(b)) A tourniquet is wrapped around the arm above the venepuncture site to cause the build-up of blood in the vein. If the patient repeatedly makes a fist, the visibility of the vein increases, enhancing the success rate of the procedure.

A specimen of blood may be taken from a finger stick, e.g. in people with diabetes mellitus who need to check their blood sugar levels during the day. The heel stick specimen (analysed by the Guthrie test) is used to check for neonatal abnormalities such as phenylketonuria, galactosaemia and hypothyroidism. Due to the interdependence of body parts (see Chapter 1), if any part of the body is functionally abnormal, this is almost always reflected in the composition of blood.

Healthcare workers need to exercise care to avoid infection with pathogens, such as HIV and hepatitis B virus, when handling blood, other body fluids, and potentially contaminated items such as needles, syringes, intravenous equipment and linen. The UK Department of Health (1996) suggests the following precautions when handling such products:

● Wear protective gloves, plastic aprons, masks and, where appropriate, gowns and eye goggles.
● Dispose of used items such as 'sharps', i.e. anything capable of inflicting cuts, scratches or punctures.

The myeloid stage

The term 'myeloid' refers to the activities of immature blood cells (called precursor cells) in bone marrow. The bone marrow becomes active in blood cell production from the fifth month onwards, establishing itself as the major haemopoietic organ of the fetus at about 7 months. Production from this site continues throughout life. At birth, all the marrow is active in blood production; it is called red active marrow, because although it produces all blood cells, the extensive number of erythrocytes colours it red. As the infant grows, the active red marrow of the long bones is replaced by yellow inactive (or fatty, lymphoidal) marrow. The tibia and radius bones of the limbs are the first bones to lose this haemopoietic ability, followed by the femur, and then the humerus. In the young adult, the active marrow is found in the flat bones, such as the cranium, ribs, sternum and pelvis, and in the vertebrae. The liver, spleen and the yellow inactive marrow, are, however, capable of reverting back to their erythrocyte production function when erythrocyte numbers are deficient in severe anaemias, and so act as homeostatic regulators.

The marrow's haemopoietic functions can be divided into erythropoiesis (red cell production), leucopoiesis (white cell production) and thrombopoiesis (platelet production). These processes will be discussed later.

BOX 11.3 HAEMOPOIESIS

All blood cells originate from a common stem cell called the haematocytoblast (Figure 11.3). These stem cells are a result of cell specialization, since they are differentiated from other cells within the body once the particular genes for blood cell development are expressed. Once this initial specialization has taken place, producing the common stem cell, the cells divide mitotically and specialize further into red blood cells, white blood cells or platelets. This differentiation of the stem cell into blood cells is again by specific gene expression. Furthermore, once a cell has become specialized, it cannot be transformed into another cell (blood cell or otherwise).

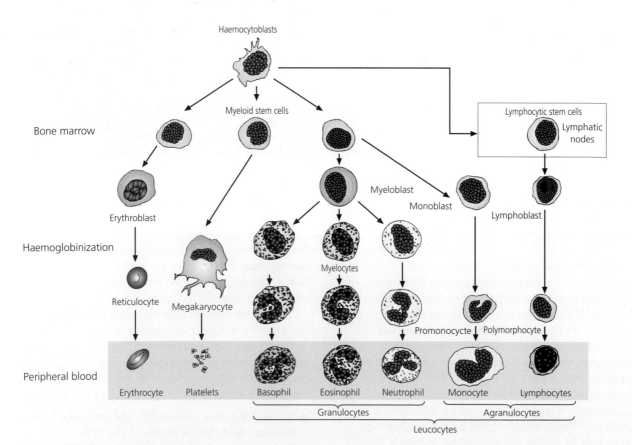

Figure 11.3 Haemopoiesis. The origin and differentiation of blood cells.

Q. Distinguish between neutrophils and eosinophils, and erythropoiesis and leucopoiesis.

Q. What do the granules represent in granulocytes?

BOX 11.4 HAEMATOLOGY

The study of blood is called haematology. It involves estimating:

- the number of cells and values of non-cellular blood components, and comparing these with the homeostatic ranges expected;
- the shape (morphology) and size of the cellular components, using a stained blood film.

Full complete blood count

A full complete blood count (FCBC) screens for anaemia, various infections, and blood-clotting disorders; it is also very important in pregnancy, especially with pre-eclampsia and HELLP syndrome. It includes counts of the red blood cells (RBCs), white blood cells (WBCs) and platelets, a differential white cell count, and an estimate of the haematocrit and haemoglobin values (see Boxes 11.12 and 11.13). Figure 11.4 shows a laboratory slip used in clinical blood analysis.

Bone marrow biopsy

This clinical test may confirm a diagnosis suggested by clinical examination and blood investigations. It provides information about the homeostatic status of haemopoiesis, the number of the respective cellular components, and the presence of abnormal cells, as found in metastatic cancers and Hodgkin's disease.

The biopsy procedure involves puncturing the bone with a needle, then taking (i.e. aspirating) a specimen of the bone marrow with a syringe. The iliac crest and sternum are common sites of biopsy in adults, and the tibia is a common site in children, since these areas have relatively thin layers of bone above the marrow. Alternatively, small sections of bone may be removed using a bone-biopsy terrapine needle. The procedure is unpleasant for the patient because of the pressure that needs to be applied to penetrate the bone. Local anaesthetic is used to ensure no pain is perceived; a general anaesthetic may be used in children.

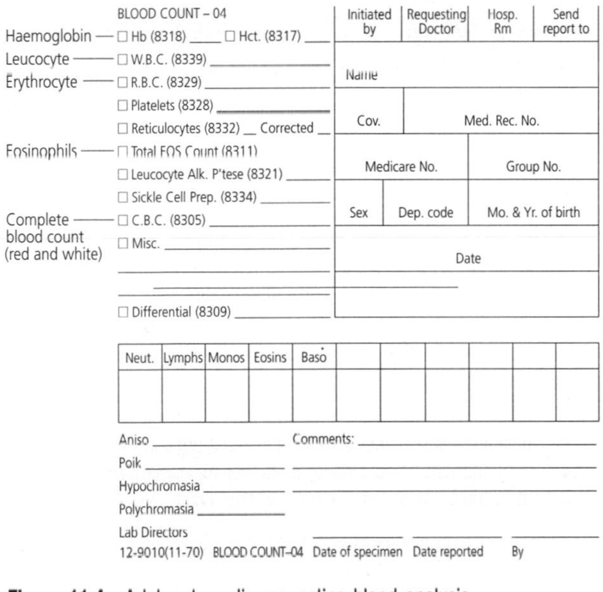

BLOOD COUNT – 04

Haemoglobin — ☐ Hb (8318) ____ ☐ Hct. (8317) ____
Leucocyte — ☐ W.B.C. (8339) ____
Erythrocyte — ☐ R.B.C. (8329) ____
☐ Platelets (8328) ____
☐ Reticulocytes (8332) ____ Corrected ____
Eosinophils — ☐ Total EOS Count (8311)
☐ Leucocyte Alk. P'tese (8321) ____
☐ Sickle Cell Prep. (8334) ____
Complete blood count (red and white) — ☐ C.B.C. (8305) ____
☐ Misc. ____
☐ Differential (8309) ____

Initiated by	Requesting Doctor	Hosp. Rm	Send report to
Name			
Cov.	Med. Rec. No.		
Medicare No.	Group No.		
Sex	Dep. code	Mo. & Yr. of birth	
Date			

Neut.	Lymphs	Monos	Eosins	Baso						

Aniso ____ Comments: ____
Poik ____
Hypochromasia ____
Polychromasia ____
Lab Directors
12-9010(11-70) BLOOD COUNT-04 Date of specimen Date reported By

Figure 11.4 A laboratory slip requesting blood analysis.

Q. *Distinguish between whole blood, serum and plasma.*

Q. *What is the blood volume of a healthy adult female?*

BOX 11.5 CHANGES TO BLOOD COMPOSITION DURING PREGNANCY

During pregnancy, there is a maximum rise in plasma volume and red blood cell volume of 50% and 20%, respectively; this is called haemodilution. Plasma volume begins to increase in the first trimester (trimester = period of three months), then increases rapidly during the second trimester, with a further slight increase in the third trimester. Red cell volume begins to increase in the second trimester, with the greatest increase in the third trimester

Due to the different pace of the changes in plasma and red cell volumes, the haemoglobin and packed cell volumes reduce progressively until approximately 30 weeks gestation. After 30 weeks gestation, there is a reversal as the increase in red cell volume outweighs the plasma volume.

COMPOSITION AND PHYSIOLOGY OF THE BLOOD

Plasma

Plasma forms approximately half of the total blood volume, and one-fifth of the total volume of extracellular fluid (male value, 52–83 ml/kg; female value, 50–75 ml/kg). Plasma and tissue fluids are very similar in composition, apart from the total amount of protein present. This is not surprising, as the membrane of a blood capillary (i.e. tiny blood vessel) separates these two fluids and is permeable to most substances. Tissue fluid is derived from plasma at the arterial side of the capillary, and returns to the plasma at the venous side (see Figure 12.32). However, despite this interchange of plasma and tissue fluid, there remain some differences in their composition.

One of the most noticeable differences is in the concentration of the respiratory gases. Plasma has a higher concentration of oxygen, while tissue fluid has a higher concentration of carbon dioxide. As a result, oxygen diffuses from blood into tissue fluid, and carbon dioxide diffuses into the plasma. Diffusion, as discussed in Chapter 2, could be expected to result in a uniform distribution of the gases, but this is not the case, because cells are constantly removing and using oxygen from tissue fluid, and supplying carbon dioxide to it, in order to maintain cell homeostasis. Thus, diffusion is a working concept to explain the movement of molecules down their concentration gradients. Another notable difference between plasma and tissue fluid is the large presence of dissolved proteins in the plasma (70 g/l compared with 20 g/l in tissue fluid). Plasma proteins are macromolecules that are too large to pass through pores in the capillary membranes, and thus generally in health do not pass into tissue fluid. Intracellular fluid has a different composition to plasma and tissue fluid because of the selectively permeable properties of cell membranes (see Chapters 2 and 6).

Plasma proteins

Plasma contains three principal types of proteins: albumins, globulins and fibrinogen. The latter is a protein involved in blood clotting. The plasma also contains other proteins associated with clotting, e.g. a globulin called prothrombin. Most plasma proteins are produced in the liver.

Albumins

Approximately 70% of the solutes found in plasma are proteins. Albumins comprise about 55–60% of this protein component, and thus are important determinants of the viscosity of blood, i.e. the plasma proteins slow down the flow rate of blood. Albumins osmotically draw water (and its dissolved components) from the tissue fluid back into the venous side of the blood capillary, and so facilitate the capillary exchange process. This helps to maintain the blood

Table 11.1 Chemical composition, description and homeostatic functions of plasma components

Component	Description	Homeostatic function
Water	Liquid portion of blood; constitutes approximately 90% of the plasma Water is derived from absorption from the digestive tract and from cellular respiration	Transports organic and inorganic molecules, blood cells, and heat

Solutes
  Proteins
  Albumins
	Constitutes approximately 7% of the plasma
	Produced by the liver
		Provides blood with viscosity, a factor related to the homeostatic regulation of blood pressure
		Exerts considerable osmotic pressure to maintain water balance between blood and tissues hence, homeostatically regulates blood volume and thus blood pressure
		Binding functions
		Transports lipids

Globulins	Group to which antibodies belong	Gammaglobulins (antibodies) attack pathogenic organisms Include an important blood-clotting precursor molecule (prothrombin) Important in transport of ions, hormones and lipids
Fibrinogen	Produced by the liver	Homeostatic role in blood-clotting, when it is converted into insoluble fibrin
Non-protein nitrogen-containing substances	Include urea, uric acid, creatinine, and ammonium salts	Byproducts of protein metabolism; these are excreted to prevent toxic build-up
Food substances	Products of digestion passed into blood for distribution to all body cells; products include amino acids (from proteins), glucose (from carbohydrates), fatty acids and glycerol (from fats), and vitamins	Used for energy production, growth, and repair and maintenance of cells
Regulatory substances	Enzymes and hormones	Enzymes catalyse chemical reactions to a rate compatible with life
Respiratory gases	Oxygen and carbon dioxide; these gases are also associated with haemoglobin or red blood cells	Hormones regulate metabolism Oxygen has a homeostatic role in cellular respiration (Krebs cycle) Carbon dioxide is important in the regulation of pH of body fluids
Electrolytes	Inorganic salts of plasma Cations include Na^+, K^+, Ca^{2+} Anions include Cl^-, HCO_3^-	Help to maintain osmotic pressure, normal pH, and physiological balance between tissues and blood

Q. Describe the origin and functions of plasma proteins.

volume and hence blood pressure. Other plasma proteins, being macromolecules, also contribute to the viscosity and osmotic potential of blood. Albumins also have important transport functions, e.g. they bind to calcium and bilirubin, thus maintaining the homeostatic concentration of these 'free' chemicals in body fluids (both are physiologically active only when unbound). Albumins also bind to certain drugs, e.g. aspirin. Although largely retained in plasma, a small amount of albumin is found in the tissue fluid, where it has similar properties to that in plasma.

Globulins

Globulins comprise about 33–38% of the plasma proteins. They are much larger molecules than albumins. Globulins are subdivided into the following fractions:

- *Gamma globulins.* Consist mainly of most of the known antibodies, and so are produced in the circulation and the lymphatic systems in response to an 'antigenic insult' (see Chapter 13). They are concerned with protecting the body from pathogens and their toxins, hence their alternative name, 'immunoglobulins'. Globulins are used as a basis for therapeutic administrations, e.g. anti-tetanus injections consist of an antibody-rich gamma globulin fraction of horse serum.

- *Alpha globulins.* These have several transport functions. They bind to smaller proteins, and certain electrolytes, and so prevent these substances from passing out in the urine.

- *Beta globulins.* These also have several transport functions. Some contain specific metal-combining groups, e.g. transferrin is a protein that transports iron, and some carry fat-soluble vitamins. Others contribute to the blood clotting process.

Fibrinogen and prothrombin

Fibrinogen and prothrombin (a beta globulin) act as precursors of the active clotting proteins, fibrin and thrombin, respectively (see Wound healing section later)

General roles of plasma proteins

In addition to the specific functions mentioned above, plasma proteins have some more generalized roles. In the 'normal', slightly alkaline plasma, proteins carry a negative charge. As ions, they are capable of 'mopping up' positively charged hydrogen ions when these are in excess of their homeostatic range, e.g. as occurs when the metabolic rate is increased. This important buffering action contributes to the homeostatic maintenance of blood pH, which is essential for optimum enzymatic activity.

Plasma proteins also act as a protein reservoir, i.e. they can be used in times of chronic dietary protein deficiency. This may lead to protein depletion in the plasma (hypoproteinaemia), however, which has consequences for fluid distribution.

Table 11.1 summarizes the homeostatic functions of plasma constituents.

BOX 11.6 SERUM ANALYSIS

Plasma is frequently the subject of clinical biochemical analysis as an indication of a person's state of health (Figure 11.5). Table 1.3 shows the homeostatic ranges of various organic and inorganic components within plasma. Deviations from these values are indicative of an individual's fluctuating physiological condition, or may be a sign of underlying pathology. Thus, such levels are used as aids to diagnose specific disorders. Analysis of plasma components could be potentially difficult, as samples coagulate (clot) within a matter of minutes after taking them. Thus, plasma analysis also involves adding an anticoagulant removing the clotting proteins (fibrinogen and prothrombin). The remaining plasma like fluid is called serum.

Homeostatic failures of the plasma proteins

Albumin deficiency (hypoalbuminaemia) occurs when there is damage to the glomerular capillaries of the kidneys (see Figure 15.5), which results in albumin being filtered and passing out in the urine. Albumin synthesis by the liver is such that its deficiency results only when there are large amounts of albumin lost from the body, or when inadequate dietary amino acids prevent its synthesis. This condition, together with other hypoproteinaemias, causes a decrease in the plasma osmotic pressure, resulting in an accumulation of the tissue fluid called oedema (see Figure 12.32). There are other causes of oedema, e.g. healthcare professionals and carers will often see gravitational oedema of the lower limbs in static elderly patients. Liver diseases, protein malnutrition, inflammation and allergic reactions cause such deficiencies in plasma proteins.

Gamma globulin excess (hypergammaglobulinaemia) is indicative of chronic infection states, collagen diseases, and parasitic infections, and reflects the increased antibody production in these conditions. Gamma globulin deficiency (agammaglobulinaemia) may occur as a congenital disease (congenital = present at birth) and in patients who are subjected to recurrent infection, and so reflects a failure or decline in antibody response to infection.

Fibrinogen excess (hyperfibrinogenaemia) occurs in pathological acute infections, and in pregnancy. Increased fibrinogen levels result in a faster erythrocyte sedimentation rate (ESR; see Box 11.12). Fibrinogen and prothrombin deficiencies (hypofibrinogenaemia and hypoprothrombinaemia, respectively) cause longer bleeding and clotting times. Hypofibrinogenaemia occurs in liver diseases, such as cirrhosis, and can also cause problems in pregnancy.

Clinical correction of such disorders involves plasma transfusions. An immune response in the recipient is avoided by infusing 'conditioned' plasma (i.e. plasma minus the antibodies it may contain). Table 11.2 summarizes the clinical use of infused plasma components in re-establishing a patient's plasma homeostatic balance.

Figure 11.5 Clinical analysis of plasma components using homeostatic principles. (a) Homeostatic dynamism. Value fluctuating within the component's homeostatic range (see Table 8.2). The fluctuation is a result of the component entering and leaving the plasma. For example, some plasma components such as nutrients leave blood at the arterial side of the capillary bed, whilst others, such as metabolic wastes, enter the blood at the arterial side of the capillary bed. Consequently the component's level fluctuates.

(b_1) Plasma component in excess of its homeostatic range. The excess could be indicative of a clinical condition, e.g. the presence of the cardiac-specific enzyme creatinine phosphokinase above serum baseline level, which occurs after a myocardial infarction (heart attack). Alternatively, the excess may be indicative of a 'normal' temporary change in the plasma level of the component, e.g. elevated glucose concentration after absorption of a carbohydrate-rich meal. (b_2) A decrease in the component level below its homeostatic range. This could be indicative of a clinical condition, e.g. low levels of plasma proteins might be indicative of liver damage (as occurs in tissue fibrosis due to cirrhosis), since the hepatocytes produce plasma proteins, and fibrosis impairs this synthesis. Alternatively, the low levels

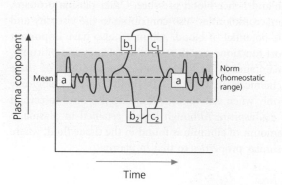

could be a 'normal' temporary change, e.g. hypoglycaemia, which occurs 1 h after absorption of a carbohydrate-rich meal due to the long-duration effects of the hypoglycaemic agent insulin.

(c) Clinical intervention, or the body's normal negative homeostatic feedback mechanisms, which correct the temporary pathological (see Table 11.2) and normal physiological homeostatic imbalances, respectively.

Q. List seven functions of the circulating blood.

Table 11.2 Plasma components for clinical use in redressing plasma component homeostasis

Plasma component	Clinical homeostatic correction
Plasma protein fraction	Plasma replacement Blood volume expansion
Human albumin	Albumin replacement in hypoalbuminaemia, e.g. in nephrosis
Fresh frozen plasma	Clotting factor deficiencies, e.g. in liver disease.
Cryoprecipitate (factor VIII, fibrinogen)	Classical haemophilia (haemophilia A) Von Willebrand's disease Fibrinogen deficiency
Factor VIII concentrate and freeze-dried factor VIII	Classical haemophilia A
Factor IX concentrate	Christmas disease (haemophilia B)
Human immunoglobulin (Ig)	Hypogammaglobulinaemia, e.g. to produce passive immunity to viral diseases such as rubella (German measles)
Human-specific globulin (specific antibodies) Apply principles shown in Figure 11.5.	To produce passive immunity to rare, life-threatening disease, e.g. tetanus.

Cellular components of blood

The cellular components of blood make up about 45% of whole blood (Figure 11.2(c)). The three principal cell types are classified as follows:

- *erythrocytes*;
- *leucocytes:* divided into two main groups, granulocytes (subdivided into neutrophils, eosinophils and basophils) and agranulocytes (subdivided into lymphocytes and monocytes). Granulocytes have granules (i.e. potent enzymes) within their cytoplasm; agranulocytes do not;

- *thrombocytes (platelets):* have an essential role in promoting blood clotting, hence the name ('thrombus' = clot).

Table 11.3 summarizes the homeostatic functions of blood cells.

Erythrocytes

Structure

Microscopically, red cells appear as biconcave discs. Each cell has a doughnut shape, having a thick outer margin and a very thin middle region. Erythrocytes are approximately

Table 11.3 Various types of blood cells. A differential white cell count is taken by examining a stained blood smear; the values in this table represent the numbers of each type encountered in a sample of 100 leucocytes. Reproduced from Craigwyle, M.B.L. (1975) *A Colour Atlas of Histology.* London: Wolfe Medical Publications.

Leucocytes	Blood cell	Diameter (μm)	Number/mm³ (homeostatic range)	Differential white cell count (%)	Homeostatic function
	Erythocytes	7.0–7.7	4.2–6.2 million		Transportation of respiratory gases (particularly oxygen)
Granulocytes	Neutrophils	9–14	3000–6750	60–65	Phagocytic – engulf pathogens or debris in tissues
	Eosinophils	10–14	100–360	2–4	Phagocytic – engulf items in tissues that are labelled with antigens (combat allergies)
	Basophils	8–10	25–90	0.5–1.0	Enter damaged tissue release histamine (combat allergies)
Agranulocytes	Lymphocytes	6–12	1 000–2700	20–35	Cells of the lymphatic system provide defence against specific pathogens or toxins
	Monocytes	10–15	150–170	3–8	Mobile and fixed macrophages, engulf pathogens or debris
	Thrombocytes	2–4	150 000–400 000		Blood clotting

Q. Give a function for each of the following: (i) basophils, (ii) fixed macrophages, and (iii) megakaryocytes.

7.2 μm in diameter and are 2.2 μm thick; the central portion narrows to 0.8 μm (Figure 11.6). The biconcavity provides a large surface area with respect to volume (compared with a spherical shaped cell), thus maximizing the available membrane surface for the exchange of respiratory gases. This structural adaptation also gives these cells greater flexibility, enabling them to pass through capillaries that are even narrower than the diameter of the erythrocyte. The membrane, as with all cellular membranes, contains surface chemical markers called antigens. Some of the blood cell antigens, namely A, B and D (rhesus) types, together with specific plasma antibodies, determine an individual's ABO and Rhesus blood group (described later).

The cytoplasm of the erythrocyte consists mainly of the red pigment haemoglobin. This pigment accounts for approximately 95% of the intracellular protein, and is responsible for approximately one-third of the cell's mass. Its main functions are the transportation of respiratory gases (primarily oxygen) and the regulation of blood pH

(when haemoglobin is not transporting respiratory gases, it has a buffering action).

Table 11.4 illustrates the clinical importance of homeostatic values concerning the erythrocyte.

Table 11.4 Clinical importance of the homeostatic ranges concerning erythrocytes

Measure	Homeostatic range
Erythrocytic count	
Infant (6y)	4–5.2 million/mm³
Adult male	4.5–6.5 million/mm³
Adult female	4.5–5 million/mm³
Packed cell volume (PCV) (haematocrit)	
Infant (6y)	0.40 (40%)
Adult male	0.47 (47%)
Adult female	0.42 (42%)
Haemoglobin (Hb)	
Infant (6y)	14–20 g/ml
Adult male	13 18 g/ml
Adult female	11.5–16.6 g/ml

Q. Why is circulating blood not white?

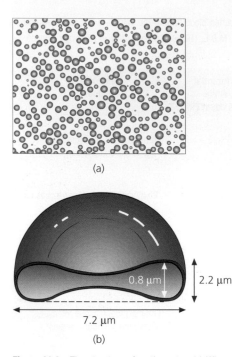

(a)

(b)

Figure 11.6 The structure of erythrocytes. (a) When viewed in a standard blood smear, erythrocytes appear as two-dimensional doughnut-shaped objects. (b) In cross-section, erythrocytes appear as three-dimensional. The biconcavity produces a greater surface area for the process of gaseous exchange. The dashed line represents the smaller surface area of a spherical cell.

Q. Under what physiological conditions is erythropoietin released?

Production of erythrocytes

The number of red blood cells remains similar throughout life. Erythrocytes have a lifespan of 100–120 days. Their production must therefore match their loss in order to homeostatically control the number of red cells present. Approximately 1% of circulating red cells are replaced daily; this may seem a small proportion, but it actually means that three million erythrocytes enter the circulation every second!

Figure 11.3 simplifies the processes involved in erythropoiesis. The main characteristic changes for the development of a mature erythrocyte take about 1 week. During this time, the cell gradually becomes smaller and smaller. The nucleus 'ripens', with the loss of the nucleoli and the condensation of nuclear material. The cytoplasm 'ripens' due to the process of haemoglobinization. Some of the organelles and inclusions (e.g. nucleus, mitochondria and ribosomes) are removed to increase the available space for haemoglobin. Mature erythrocytes therefore cannot divide or produce proteins, and they are dependent upon anaerobic respiration for their ATP source. This form of respiration (see Chapter 14) produces much less energy from glucose breakdown. Perhaps red cells come to the end of their lives when their ATP and enzyme levels fall below the requirements necessary to maintain their homeostatic

roles, and consequently metabolism is reduced so much that it becomes incompatible for the continued existence of the cell.

There are many factors that regulate the maturation process. These can be divided broadly into those that stimulate erythropoiesis (e.g. hypoxia and hypersecretion of the metabolic hormones – thyroid-stimulating hormone, thyroxine, adrenocorticotropic hormone, growth hormone and androgens), and those that inhibit erythropoiesis (e.g. an oxygen-carrying capacity of the blood above or within its homeostatic range, and an undersecretion of the hormones mentioned above).

The process of erythropoiesis is controlled by the release of a factor called erythrogenin from the kidney tissue in response to hypoxia. This factor converts a precursor protein in plasma, erythropoietinogen, into erythropoietin, which activates the erythropoietic tissues to increase red cell production and release them into the circulation (Figure 11.7). At sea level, the atmospheric oxygen conditions are sufficient to meet the metabolic demands of humans. When erythrocyte production exceeds the homeostatic range (e.g. values greater than 6.5 million/mm^3 for men and 5 million/mm^3 for women; see Table 11.4), production is inhibited because the secretion of erythrogenin is prevented. This is an example of a negative feedback mechanism. As time passes, the numbers of erythrocytes return to their normal homeostatic levels, because cells are still being destroyed at their normal rate of breakdown. At this point (within the homeostatic range), production must begin again at a rate that matches that of destruction, in order to maintain the 'normal' levels. The levels of erythropoietin then rise, due to erythrogenin secretion and its activation of erythropoietinogen. Erythropoietin release is, therefore, controlled tightly within its 'normal' parameters. A change outside these parameters occurs, for example, when erythrocyte destruction becomes greater than production, resulting in low levels of erythrocytes, as is observed in haemolytic diseases.

Table 11.5 summarizes the dietary components essential for erythropoiesis to occur.

BOX 11.7 BLOOD DOPING

Some athletes have used blood doping and the administration of erythropoietin in an attempt to improve their performance, particularly during endurance events (Browne *et al.*, 1999). This involves removing blood cells from the body, storing them for 4–5 weeks, then reintroducing them into the body a couple of days before the athletic event to increase the oxygen-carrying capacity of blood. Blood doping is banned by the International Olympics Committee because of the extra workload it enforces on the heart due to the increased viscosity of blood resulting from the addition of extra erythrocytes.

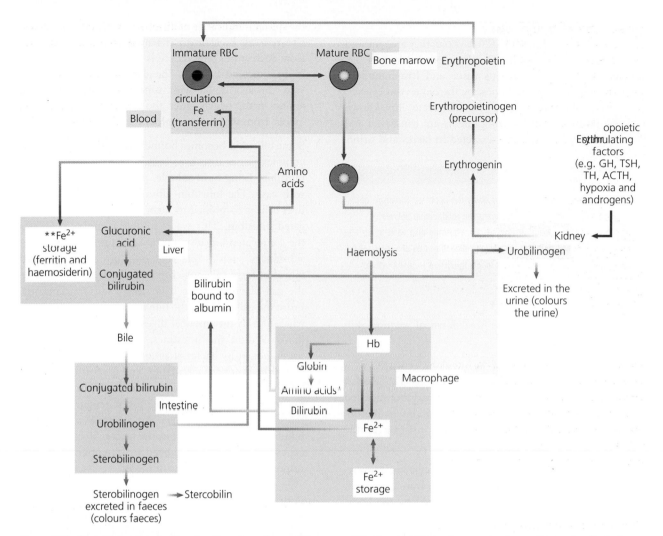

Figure 11.7 Production and destruction of erythrocytes: a homeostatic process. This diagram indicates the normal pathways for recycling the amino acids and iron content of old or damaged erythrocytes, and the pathway associated with red cell production.

ACTH, adrenocorticotropic hormone; GH, growth hormone; PN, pyrrol nuclei; RBC, red blood cell; TSH, thyroid-stimulating hormone.

*Transamination (deamination if the amino acid pool is above the homeostatic range). **Occurs if circulatory iron is in excess of its homeostatic range.

Q. Describe the process of red blood cell breakdown.

Table 11.5 Dietary components necessary for erythropoiesis

Dietary component	Homeostatic important in erythropoiesis
Protein	Synthesis of globin part of haemoglobin Synthesis of other cellular proteins, including conjugated molecules, e.g. lipoproteins, glycoproteins
Iron	Contained in the haem part of haemoglobin
Vitamin B_{12} and folic acid	Synthesis of DNA
Vitamin C	Facilitates the absorption of iron by reducing ferric iron to ferrous iron Important in normal folic acid metabolism
Vitamin B_6, riboflavin, and vitamin E	Important for normal erythropoiesis, since deficiency of these substances has been associated with anaemia
Copper and cobalt	Copper is essential for haemoglobin synthesis Cobalt is important in vitamin B_{12} synthesis in other organisms Therefore, these trace elements may have a role in human erythropoiesis

Destruction of erythrocytes

When red cells are about 100–120 days old, they are removed from the circulation by the reticuloendothelial system (i.e. the spleen, liver, subcutaneous tissue and lymph nodes), where phagocytes ingest and destroy the old erythrocytes.

Haemoglobin undergoes an elaborate breakdown process. Its most valuable components are conserved and re-utilized. The remainder is excreted in faeces and urine.

Exercise

Before continuing, we suggest you study the sections 'Structure of haemoglobin' and 'Factors influencing the relationship between oxygen and haemoglobin' in Chapter 14. You may also wish to re-familiarize yourself with the intracellular digestion role of lysosomes, since this organelle is vitally important in phagocytosis of red cells.

The stages involved in the breakdown of haemoglobin (Figure 11.7) are as follows:

1   The haem component of haemoglobin consists of a porphyrin ring compound, with a ferrous (Fe^{2+}) ion at the centre of each ring (see Figure 14.8). Once ingested by macrophages, this ring is opened by oxidation, forming a straight-chain molecule consisting of the components of haem, and globin, called choleglobin.

2   Iron and globin are removed from choleglobin, converting it into bilirubin (red bile pigment). Iron and globin are useful substances, and are re-utilized by the body. Some of the iron is used for the re-synthesis of haemoglobin and other iron-containing compounds. However, if the iron released from the haemoglobin causes its availability to go above the homeostatic range, the excess is transferred into iron storage compounds called ferritin and haemosiderin. Thus, an increased haemosiderin concentration (above its normal range) in the liver and

the spleen is indicative of diseases in which there is excessive red cell breakdown (haemolysis). Iron is released from such stores when there is insufficient in the blood to meet metabolic needs. The globin molecule is hydrolysed (broken down with water) into its constituent amino acids, which enter the amino acid body fluid 'pools' from which haemoglobin is re-synthesised.

3   Some bilirubin becomes bound tightly to albumin. This complex passes into liver cells. Other free or unbound bilirubin, being lipid soluble, passes into the liver cells with ease. The bilirubin–albumin complex within the liver cells is combined to form a complex called conjugated bilirubin. This water-soluble complex facilitates the conjugated bilirubin excretion. Together with other substances, such as bile salts, bilirubin and conjugated bilirubin form bile, which is secreted from the liver to the gall bladder, where it is stored and concentrated. From the gall bladder, the bile is passed to the intestine, where it aids the physical digestion (emulsification) of lipids. Within the intestines, bilirubin is reduced to urobilinogen by bacterial action. Some urobilinogen is reabsorbed into the circulation and is re-utilized by the liver, although some is excreted in the urine, contributing to its colour. The urobilinogen remaining in the intestines is converted via gut bacteria into stercobilinogen, and is excreted in the faeces. Stercobilinogen exposed to the air is oxidized to stercobilin, which is responsible for the colour of faeces.

Anaemia

Anaemia is a sign of a disease, rather a disease in itself. It is defined as a low oxygen-carrying capacity of blood, and occurs when the number of erythrocytes, or the amount of haemoglobin, is below its homeostatic range. Erythrocytes and haemoglobin and are at first reduced equally, but as the bone marrow replaces lost erythrocytes, blood investigations may reveal an adequate number of red cells with

BOX 11.8 ABNORMAL RED CELLS

It is still a mystery as to how tissues recognize aged red cells, but we do know that the spleen is involved. An enlarged spleen (referred to as splenomegaly) is observed in conditions associated with abnormal red cells, e.g. sickle cell anaemia (see the case study of a child with sickle cell disease in Section 6).

BOX 11.9 IRON LOSS

Normally, very little iron is lost from the body, although significant amounts may be lost in women who frequently experience heavy menstrual flow. Modern diets in the UK are generally sufficient to replace the iron that is lost, although iron-deficiency anaemia is not unusual in people whose diets lack iron.

BOX 11.10 JAUNDICE

The conjugation of bilirubin by liver cells is used diagnostically in determining whether jaundice, a retention of bilirubin in the body, is due to a liver problem or something else. In this way, the ratio of conjugated to free bilirubin in bile is an important assessment. Jaundice is explained in detail in Chapter 10.

BOX 11.11 NEONATAL EXCRETION OF CONJUGATED BILIRUBIN

In the gut of the neonate, bacterial cultures take time to establish. Consequently, the conjugated bilirubin is not converted, but is excreted intact, hence the different faecal colour observed in neonates.

BOX 11.12 HOMEOSTATIC FAILURES AFFECTING THE ERYTHROCYTE POPULATION

Reticulocyte count

Erythrocyte imbalances are due to a mismatch between erythrocyte production and destruction. In order to investigate such imbalances, a reticulocyte count is taken. Reticulocytes are immature erythrocytes that account for 0.5–1.5% of the erythrocyte population in a normal blood sample. Reticulocyte counts of less than 0.5% indicate that blood production cannot match the loss; this occurs in patients with pernicious anaemia and iron-deficiency anaemia, and during radiation therapy. Low reticulocyte counts may also be due to a deficiency of erythrogenin and/or erythropoietinogen and/or erythropoietin. If the count is above 1.5%, production is greater than destruction. This occurs in response to a number of conditions, including haemolytic anaemia, leukaemia and carcinoma. High reticulocyte counts, however, may also indicate a good red bone marrow response to previous blood loss, or to iron therapy in someone who has been iron deficient (Figure 11.8).

Erythrocyte sedimentation rate

The erythrocyte sedimentation rate (ESR) is the rate at which red blood cells in a vertical tube containing an anticoagulant fall under gravity out of suspension, and then settle on the bottom of the tube. This tendency to sediment is dependent on the relative concentration of the plasma components and plasma viscosity. The ESR is determined by measuring the length of the column of clear plasma above the red blood cells after 1 h. The homeostatic range for men is 1–5 mm/h, and for women 5–15 mm/h.

The ESR is raised in inflammatory diseases, some forms of cancers, and pregnancy. An ESR of 12 mm/h is usually indicative of disease. Values in excess of 100 mm/h are found in chronic infections, such as tuberculosis. It is still unclear why such a condition should alter the ESR.

Haematocrit

Measuring the packed cell volume (or haematocrit) as a percentage of whole blood is another routine clinical test. A haematocrit value of 40 means that 40% of the total volume blood is composed of red blood cells. The normal range of the haematocrit in adult males is 40–54% (mean 47%), and in adult females 38–46% (mean 42%). Thus, red cells account for nearly half the volume of whole blood. Higher numbers of erythrocytes exist in men, (i.e. 5.4 million/mm^3) than in women (4.8 million/mm^3) due to the need to transport more oxygen to support the male's greater metabolic rate, which accounts for the gender differences in haematocrit. When assessing the haematocrit, the patient's state of hydration must always be taken into consideration.

Figure 11.8 The homeostatic and clinical control of the number of erythrocytes, using a reticulocyte count as an indicator of the red cell number. The reticulocyte count is the percentage of reticulocytes within the total number of erythrocytes. (a) Normal homeostatic levels of reticulocytes, 'hunting' about the mean. This indicates that the erythrocyte homeostatic range is being achieved, i.e. red cell production rate matches destruction rate.
(b$_1$) Reticulocyte count is beyond the homeostatic range (i.e. (1.5% of mature erythrocytes), indicating production is greater than destruction of red cells, resulting in polycythaemia. The excessive production can be considered a normal physiological reaction in response to altitude hypoxia, which results in hypersecretion of the hormone erythropoietin. Alternatively, polycythaemia may be indicative of a pathological homeostatic imbalance, as experienced with cancers of erythropoietic sites and/or kidney cells, resulting in hypersecretion of erythrogenin. (b$_2$) Reticulocyte count is below the homeostatic range (0.5%), indicating production is less than destruction. The low levels may be indicative of pathological homeostatic imbalances, such as anaemias (Table 8.9), liver

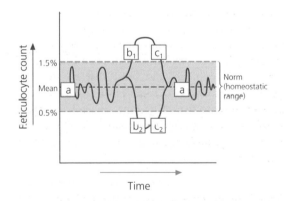

or kidney diseases that cause hyposecretion of erythrogenin, resulting in less erythropoietin reaching the erythropoietic sites, or conditions that cause a hyposecretion of the hormone precursor erythropoietinogen. (c$_1$) Clinical correction of pathological polycythaemia involves 'bleeding' therapy. (c$_2$) Clinical correction of red cell deficiency involves red cell infusions.

BOX 11.13 HAEMATOCRIT VALUES AND ANAEMIA

The higher red cell count and haematocrit value in males is associated with the presence of testosterone. This hormone stimulates synthesis of erythropoietin by the bone marrow and kidney. Lower values in females during their reproductive years may be due to excessive loss of blood during the menstrual flow. A haematocrit value of 15% is extremely low, and a value of 65% is extremely high; such values reflect the homeostatic imbalances of severe anaemia and polycythaemia, respectively

Iron deficiency is commonly seen in communities when babies are weaned late and given a diet deficient in iron. Nurses should be alert to the vulnerable groups, so they can give culturally sensitive nutritional information.

BOX 11.14 HAEMOGLOBIN DEFICIENCY AND ANAEMIA

Haemoglobin values of below 13.5 g/dl in adult males, 11.5 g /dl in adult females, and 11 g/dl from 3 months to puberty indicate anaemia. A value of 15 g/dl is the lower normal limit at birth. The newborn has a relatively high amount of haemoglobin, including the form required for intrauterine life, referred to as fetal haemoglobin (Hb-F; see Chapter 14).

The severity of symptoms will depend upon the level of haemoglobin and the length of time over which the problem has developed. For example, adults with chronic anaemia do not normally experience health problems until the haemoglobin values are below 8 g/dl, an older person in whom blood supply and respiratory efficiency are compromised may have symptoms with values of 11 g/dl.

Table 11.6 Classification of anaemia

Increased blood loss	
Haemorrhage	Acute, e.g. road traffic accident
	Chronic, e.g. menstruation, peptic ulcer
Haemolysis	Intracellular cause, e.g. abnormal haemoglobin variant such as sickle cell anaemia, thalassaemia
	Extracellular cause, e.g. bacteria, drugs, severe infection
Decreased blood production	
Nutritional deficiency, poor absorption of nutrients	Lack of iron results in small red blood cells (microcytic anaemia) with reduced haemoglobin
	Lack of vitamin B_{12} results in macrocytic or megaloblastic anaemia (so-called because of abnormal red blood cells precursors); vitamin B_{12} can also be deficient due to a lack of the stomach's intrinsic factor of Castle, which aids its absorption, thus occurs when the stomach lining atrophies after a gastrectomy (pernicious anaemia)
	Folate may not match the demand, e.g. in pregnancy
Bone marrow failure (aplastic anaemia)	Primary, e.g. congenital
	Secondary, e.g. acquired (e.g. ionizing radiation), cytotoxic drugs (e.g. bulsulfan), bone cancer

abnormally low levels of pigment present, i.e. each cell is deficient in haemoglobin.

Anaemia is classified according to its causal factors, and is divided broadly into conditions that are a consequence of an increased blood loss and those that are due to a decreased blood production (Table 11.6).

In general, irrespective of its type, anaemia affects all organ systems. It is characterized particularly by signs and symptoms of oxygen shortage at peripheral tissues, including:

- pallor of the skin, especially noticeable on the lips and eyelids, where the outer layer of the skin is relatively thin;

- a feeling of tiredness and listlessness;

- a full, soft pulse, with pulse and respiratory rates increasing unduly on slight exertion;

- a tendency for the ankles to swell, due to peripheral oedema;

- an appearance of central nervous system symptoms (only in severe anaemia), such as tinnitus (ringing in the ears), headaches, spots before the eyes, fainting and giddiness.

Minor signs aid differential diagnosis. For example, haemolytic anaemias often show the classical jaundice appearance due to the deposition of bile pigments in skin (bilirubin is excessive because of the haemoglobin and release of haemoglobin). However, standard laboratory tests based on the number, size and morphology of erythrocytes, and cellular haemoglobin contents, are required for accurate diagnosis. It is important that the underlying cause is identified, as this forms the basis of correction. For example, iron-deficiency anaemia is treated with digestible iron salts (such as ferrous sulphate tablets), whilst simultaneously ensuring that the patient eats an appropriate diet. Severe anaemias may require blood transfusions, although this has the associated risk of fluid

BOX 11.15 ANAEMIA AND HAEMOPOIETIC GROWTH FACTOR

Haemopoietic growth factor (HGF) is a chemical similar to erythropoietin that promotes blood cell synthesis in bone marrow. It is made available through recombinant DNA technology. HGF has tremendous potential for treating patients who have diminished ability to produce blood cells. Recombinant or genetically

engineered erythropoietin (epoietin) is extremely effective in alleviating the extreme tiredness and breathlessness in people with chronic kidney disease. The use of epoietin potentially also has benefits for anaemic patients with associated chronic inflammatory diseases, such as arthritis.

overload, unless the anaemia is caused by acute haemor-rhage, as occurs in traumatic accidents or major surgery.

Concentrated (packed) red cells are preferable to whole blood transfusions, in order to restore the oxygen-carrying capacity of blood without greatly disturbing the blood volume. Washed red cells may be administered to remove antigenic substances (e.g. plasma proteins) attached to the erythrocytes. Frozen preparations may also be used, because freezing lowers the leucocyte and thrombocyte content and eliminates pathogenic organisms.

Polycythaemia

Blood with an increase of 2–3 million red cells/mm^3 above the normal homeostatic range is considered to be polycythaemic ('poly-' = many, 'cyte' = cell, '- aemia' = of blood). The presence of excessive cells increases the blood viscosity, and therefore slows the flow rate of blood. This increases the risk of intrinsic blood clotting (described later) and its potential consequences, such as ischaemic attacks and thrombotic infarctions. Polycythaemia occurs in dehydrated patients, as all body fluids are concentrated, with the result that erythrocytes become relatively more numerous in any measured quantity of blood, or in situa-tions of chronic oxygen shortage.

There are various pathological conditions of the heart, circulation, lungs and bone marrow that cause the body to manufacture extra erythrocytes. In order to carry sufficient quantities of oxygen to support metabolic demands, sometimes twice the normal amount of red cells are produced. An increase in erythrocytes also occurs during prolonged hypoxia (deficiency of oxygen in the tissues) when living at high altitudes. This is referred to as physiological polycythaemia, and it occurs as a homeostatic adaptation, whereby it becomes 'normal' and necessary to have a large number of red cells as a compensatory mechanism for the low levels of atmospheric oxygen. Polycythaemia therefore is not always a sign of pathology, but may be a consequence of the homeostatic set points being reset. Mountaineers and people living above 10 000–12 000 feet may have haemat-ocrit values as high as 65%.

Leucocytes

Structure

Leucocytes are nucleated and do not contain haemoglobin, so they appear 'white' in contrast to red blood cells. Leuco-cytes fall into two main groups: granulocytes (neutrophils,

BOX 11.16 BLEEDING POLYCYTHAEMIC PATIENTS

The causes of polycythaemia are largely unknown, but various hormones are known to affect the rate of erythropoiesis. Polycythaemia, therefore, may be a clinical sign of certain endocrine disorders, e.g. the hypersecretion of cortisol in Cushing's syndrome.

True polycythaemia is one of the very few diseases for which bleeding is still employed as a principle of correction of a homeostatic imbalance. Modern methods include the insertion of a wide-bore needle into a vein; this has superseded the traditional methods of vein cutting, or applying blood-sucking leeches.

eosinophils and basophils) and agranulocytes (lymphocytes and monocytes). The cytoplasm of granulocytes contains granules; that of agranulocytes does not. Granulocytes are classified according to their reactions to staining techniques and to their size. All granulocytes have a lobed nucleus, whereas agranulocytes possess spherical (lymphocytes) or kidney-shaped (monocytes) nuclei.

White cells are far less numerous than red cells and platelets, with an average of 5000–9000/mm^3. The range represents a large variation in the number of leucocytes within individuals. The numbers vary even on an hour-to-hour basis, according to various accompanying physiolog-ical and psychological factors, such as exercise and emotions. A greater fluctuation arises in response to underlying pathology.

Homeostatic functions of leucocytes

White cells are components of the immune system. As they circulate in blood vessels, they are 'looking' for signs of pathogenic invasion in adjacent tissues. Leuco-cytes are attracted chemically (a process called chemo-taxis) to the site of inflammation by, for example, the toxic secretions of pathogens and components of the inflammatory and immune responses. This chemotaxic response attracts the white cells to the invaders, damaged tissues and other white blood cells. The movement of the leucocytes across capillary membranes is called diapedesis. In this way, most white cells are located in the peripheral tissues, since there is no human tissue that is not susceptible to pathogenic invasion; the mucous membranes and the skin are under constant threat, whereas deeper body tissues are less threatened. Thus, white cells present in blood represent only a small fraction of the total population of leuco-cytes. The generalized homeostatic function of white cells is to protect the body by combating microbes and non-self substances (collectively called antigens) using two processes, phagocytosis (see Figure 13.9) and antibody production (see Chapter 13). The entire collec-tion of leucocytes has the sole purpose of defending the body against pathogenic invasion, including the removal of toxins, waste products of microbial metabolism, and abnormal or damaged cells.

The homeostatic ranges and a summary of the homeostatic functions of leucocytes are shown in Table 11.3

Classification

The granular components within granulocytes contain potent enzymes and chemicals that kill bacteria. Neutrophils account for the largest proportion (about 60–65%) of the circulating leucocyte population. They are so-called because they are difficult to stain with either acid or basic dyes, but neutral dyes stain their granules purple (see Table 11.3). Neutrophils have a distinctive lobed nucleus, hence the alternative name polymorphonucleocytes ('polymorph-' = many forms). Neutrophils are 9–14 µm in diameter. Neutrophils are very mobile, and they are the first cell type to arrive at a site of injury; they are also the most active phagocytes in response to tissue destruction by bacteria. Large numbers of neutrophils are destroyed in any bacterial infection. These, together with dead bacterial cells and their contents, form the pus that occurs at the injured site. Some bacterial toxins are fever-producing substances (called pyrogens). It is thought that they activate neutrophils to produce further pyrogens that cross the blood–brain barrier and affect the temperature-regulating centre within the hypothalamus of the brain.

Eosinophils represent about 2–4% of the circulating white cells. They are generally only slightly larger than neutrophils. Eosinophils have bilobed nuclei, and easily take up acid dyes like eosin, hence the name (see Table 11.3). Eosinophils are mobile and phagocytic, but not as phagocytic as neutrophils and monocytes. Eosinophils phagocytose bacteria more readily if the bacteria are coated with antibodies (see Figure 13.14 (b) and (c)). These white cells also combat irritants that cause allergies, thus their numbers gradually increase in allergic reactions and parasitic infections. Their granules contain lysosomal enzymes and, by their involvement with antibody- (i.e. immunoglobulin E, IgE) mediated immune responses, they function to neutralize and limit the effects of inflammatory substances, such as histamine and bradykinin, produced by damaged tissue. Eosinophils especially collect at the site of allergic reactions, e.g. in the respiratory mucous membranes in hay fever and asthma. Eosinophils and neutrophils are often collectively called microphages to avoid confusion with the larger phagocytes (macrophages) found in the blood and peripheral tissues.

Basophils account for about 0.5–1% of circulating white blood cells. Their granules stain easily with basic dyes, hence the name (see Table 11.3). Basophils are important in allergic reactions. They become mast cells in inflamed tissues, and secrete their granular contents (heparin, serotonin and histamine), which exaggerate the inflammation response at this site. Other chemicals released by activated basophils attract eosinophils and further basophils to the affected area. Basophils bind to their surface specific IgE antibodies, which are released in response to allergic irritants. Secretion and breakdown of basophil granules occur upon subsequent exposure to the antigen, for which the bound IgE is specific (see Figure 13.23). Basophils release histamine, and are also involved in hypersensitive reactions to allergens (i.e. antigens that cause allergies). Histamine is a vasodilator; large quantities may cause a decrease in blood pressure, with a resultant increase in the heart rate. Itching and pain are also associated with hypersecretion of histamine.

Exercise

Reflect on the physiological principals underpinning the use of antihistamine cream and tablets (see Chapter 2).

Lymphocytes account for 20–35% of the leucocyte population. Most are found outside the blood within the lymphatic system, although they may appear in blood, especially when there is an infection. Morphologically, they are divided into large (10–12 µm) and small (8–10 µm) lymphocytes. The smaller cells are approximately the same size as red cells, and their nucleus occupies most of the cytoplasm (see Table 11.3). Functionally, lymphocytes are subdivided into T- and B-lymphocytes. These cells also have a number of subdivisions, which are discussed in Chapter 13. To summarize, T-lymphocytes attack the microbes directly in the cellular immune response, and B-lymphocytes differentiate into large 'plasma' cells characterized by the production of vast quantities of rough endoplasmic reticulum. These cells produce and secrete the antibodies (gamma globulins) that attach to antigenic material. There is a high degree of specificity with regard to antibody–antigen binding. Once formed, the covered or bound antigen (e.g. microbe or bacterial toxin) cannot come into contact with any other chemical in the body; as a result, the antigen is rendered harmless to body tissues. Antigen–antibody binding therefore helps combat infection, and gives the body immunity to some diseases.

Monocytes account for 3–8% of circulating leucocytes. These cells are easily recognizable under the microscope because of their large size (they are approximately 10–15 µm in diameter, nearly twice the size of a red cell) and distinctive kidney-shaped nuclei. These characteristics are illustrated in Table 11.3. There are a number of different categories of monocytes:

- Free monocytes ('mobile' macrophages) are found outside the blood. They are extremely mobile, and so have an abundance of mitochondria. They arrive at the site of injury very quickly, and are phagocytic.

Macrophages release chemicals that attract other macrophages, phagocytes and fibroblasts to the inflamed area. Fibroblasts secrete a fibrous material that 'walls off' the injured area. Macrophages (and granulocytes) respond to a diverse range of stimuli, unlike lymphocytes, which respond to specific antigens (microbes and their antigens). Monocytes entering the infected tissues are called 'wandering' or 'scavenger' macrophages, as they clean up the debris following injury.

- Immobile (fixed) monocytes are found in most connective tissues. They are slower to respond, and take longer to reach the site of invasion. Despite this, they destroy more microbes, due to the vast quantities that enter the site of infection.

The monocytes that migrate into reticulendothelial tissues (bone marrow, spleen, liver and lymph nodes) develop into larger specialized cells, e.g. the liver's Kupffer cells. These survive for long periods of time, and are important in the destruction of aged erythrocytes.

Production and destruction of leucocytes

Leucopoiesis is the general term used for the production of all white cells. The process is subdivided, and other terms are employed to describe specific leucocyte production and maturation. These include granulopoiesis (synthesis of granulocytes), lymphopoiesis (synthesis of lymphocytes), and monopoiesis (synthesis of monocytes). The developmental processes associated with leucopoiesis are summarized in Figure 11.3.

Granulopoiesis occurs in the red active bone marrow. The condensation and lobulation of the nucleus, the loss of some organelles such as the mitochondria, and the formation of cytoplasmic granules characterize the development processes. Although the homeostatic regulation of granulopoiesis has yet to be identified, it is known that the maturation process takes about 14 days. Approximately 50% of these newly formed mature cells adhere closely to the endothelial lining of blood vessels, and are referred to as marginating cells. The remaining granulocytes circulate in the blood. Within a matter of hours, however, some of these circulating cells enter the tissues requiring their services; these never return to blood.

Some agranulocytes, i.e. lymphocytes and monocytes, are produced in the red bone marrow, but other areas, however, are also involved. For example, before birth, and for a few months after birth, some lymphocytes (T-cells) are produced in the thymus gland. Subsequently most lymphocytes (T- and B-cells) and monocytes are formed within the lymph nodes and other lymphatic tissue, such as the spleen, adenoids, tonsils and appendix (see Figure 13.4).

The lifespan of a leucocyte is the shortest of all the cellular components of blood. Whilst red cells live for 100–120 days and platelets for 5–9 days, in a healthy body white cells will survive for only 4–5 days. Neutrophils have an even shorter lifespan – 12 h or less – when they are actively phagocytosing bacteria, as the bacterial antigens interfere with metabolism and accelerate cell death.

Homeostatic failures affecting the leucocyte population

Leucocytosis and leucopenia are general terms used to indicate leucocyte levels above and below, respectively, the homeostatic range. The suffixes '-osis' and '-penia' are used to indicate a specific leucocytic excess or deficiency, respectively, e.g. granulocytosis or granulocytopenia.

BOX 11.17 DIFFERENTIAL WHITE BLOOD COUNT

A differential white cell count is taken by examining a stained blood smear. The values obtained represent the number of each type of leucocyte encountered in a sample of 100 white cells. It confirms which specific white cell imbalance is present, and it is therefore a diagnostic aid for certain clinical conditions:

- Neutrophil leucocytosis occurs in acute bacterial infection (e.g. appendicitis, pneumonia), and inflammatory reactions associated with tissue cell death (e.g. cerebrovascular accident (stroke), myocardial infarction (heart attack)).
- Lymphocytosis occurs in chronic infection, such as measles, mumps, or hepatitis.
- Eosinophilia occurs in allergic reactions and in parasitic invasion of the body.

Figure 11.9 illustrates the homeostatic and clinical control of the leucocyte population.

Table 11.7 shows the classification of homeostatic imbalances associated with blood cells. Slight temporary increases in leucocytes occur during digestion, and an increase of longer duration exists in pregnancy. The latter requires the homeostatic set points to be changed to accommodate the altered metabolic requirements. In most situations, however, leucocytosis implies a normal protective reaction to a variety of potential pathological conditions, especially in response to inflammation or infection. In any infection, leucocytosis representing an increase from 9000 to 15 000/mm^3 is a good sign, indicating that white cells are responding to the challenge. Conversely, no increase, or an inadequate increase, in leucocytes is an unfavourable sign. Once the infection subsides, the number of leucocytes returns to the normal homeostatic parameters.

Figure 11.9 The homeostatic and clinical control of the number of leucocytes. (a) Homeostatic levels of the number of leucocytes, i.e. production rate = destruction rate.

(b_1) Leucocytosis: white cells in excess of their homeostatic range (i.e. (11 000/(l). The excess can be a result of the homeostatic set points being changed in response to altered states of health, e.g. pregnancy, in which case, the excess can be considered a normal adaptation to changing metabolic demands. Alternatively, the excess may be an indication of a protective response to infection and/or an underlying pathology. A differential white cell count indicates which leucocytic imbalance is present. The differential white cell count is an important diagnostic aid (see Tables 11.8 and 11.9). (b_2) Leucopenia: white cells below the homeostatic range (i.e. (4000/(l). Leucopenia can be a lack of all white cells, or a result of inadequate levels of specific white cells (see Table 11.7).

(c_1) Clinical correction of leucocytosis includes chemotherapy and radiotherapy. Bone marrow transplantation may be required for those patients experiencing very high-dose chemotherapy, as this destroys all residual leucocytes. (c_2) Clinical correction of agranulocytosis includes

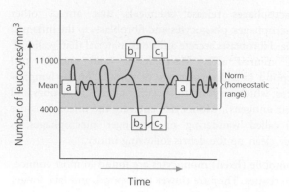

removal of the aetiological factor (e.g. rapid withdrawal of offending drugs, such as sulphonamides and antihistamine), and injections of hydrocortisone or adrenocorticotropic hormone (ACTH). Granulocyte transfusions are still at the experimental stage, and are used when antibiotic therapy is ineffective in controlling severe infections in patients with bone marrow neutropenia.

Table 11.7 Classification of homeostatic imbalances of blood cells

Blood cells	Excess (may indicate)	Deficiency (may indicate)
Leucocytes		
General	Leucocytosis	Leucopenia
Granulocytes	Neutrophilia (bacterial infection, burns, stress, inflammation, myocardial infarction)	Neutropenia (radiation exposure, drug toxicity, cytotoxic drug therapy, vitamin B_{12} deficiency, systemic lupus erythematosus (SLE))
	Basophilia (allergic reaction, leukaemia, cancer, hypothyroidism)	Basopenia (pregnancy, ovulation, stress, hyperthyroidism) Eosinopenia (drug toxicity, stress)
	Eosinophilia (allergic reaction, parasitic infection, autoimmune disease)	
Non-granulocytes	Lymphocytosis (some leukaemias and viral infections, particularly Epstein–Barr virus and agents of glandular fever) Monocytosis (viral or fungal infection, tuberculosis, some leukaemias, other chronic diseases)	Lymphopenia (prolonged illness, malignant disease, e.g. Hodgkin's disease, immunosuppression cytotoxic therapy, treatment with cortisol) Monopenia (bone marrow depression, treatment with cortisol)
Thrombocytes	Thrombocytosis	Thrombocytopenia
Erythrocytes	Polycythaemia	Anaemia (see Table 11.6)

Q. Differentiate between a physiological and a pathological polycythaemia.
Q. Give two conditions that are associated with examples of thrombocytosis and thrombocytopenia.

BOX 11.18 LEUKAEMIA

Leukaemia is a group of diseases characterized by gross excessive activity of the leucopoietic organs (bone marrow, spleen, lymph glands). Leukaemia is frequently called 'cancer of the blood', because of the vast quantities of circulating leucocytes. These proliferating white blood cells crowd out other cells produced in the marrow, so symptoms usually include a deficiency in red blood cells and platelets, i.e. anaemia and thrombocytopenia, respectively. The causes of leukaemia are largely unknown, although a few have been identified. For example, some people have a genetic predisposition that is triggered by environmental factors, such as radiation or viruses. Leukaemias are classified according to the cell type involved (Table 11.8) and according to the rate of development, i.e. acute and chronic leukaemias.

The most common cause of death from leukaemia is internal haemorrhaging, especially within the brain. Another frequent cause of death is uncontrolled infection owing to the lack of mature, or normal, leucocytes. In this case, leucocyte production is so fast that the cells do not mature and are dysfunctional. Treatment is aimed at correcting this abnormal accumulation of white cells using radiotherapy and anti-leukaemic (cytotoxic) drugs. Partial or complete remission may be induced, lasting perhaps for as long as 15 years. Table 11.9 compares the typical results of a differential white cell count of a normal person and a patient with leukaemia. See also the case study of a boy with lymphoblastic leukaemia in Section 6.

Table 11.8 Types of leukaemia and the cells involved

Type	Cells involved
Myeloid (myelocytic, myeloblastic)	Granulocytes
Lymphocytic (lymphoblastic)	Lymphocytes
Monocytic	Monocytes

Table 11.9 Typical results for a differential leucocyte count (values are percentage of total leucocyte population) in blood from a normal person and blood from a patient with leukaemia

Leucocytes	Normal person	Leukaemia patient
Neutrophils	65	3
Monocytes	8	1
Lymphocytes	24	96
Eosinophils	2	–
Basophils	1	–

BOX 11.19 GRANULOCYTE COLONY-STIMULATING FACTORS AND BONE MARROW TRANSPLANT

Granulocyte colony-stimulating factors (GCSFs) are administered to cancer patients who are taking nonspecific cytotoxic drugs. These cytotoxic drugs kill off cancer cells surrounding bone marrow cells, which are also often damaged in the process. The GCSFs help to promote replacement of these marrow cells.

GCSFs and the recombinant epoietin are also given to patients who have received bone marrow transplants to improve the outcome of the procedure.

Bone marrow transplants are an exciting addition to the therapeutic possibilities for haematological disease. Transplant may be used to treat patients with aplastic anaemias, haemolytic anaemias, sickle cell disease, acute leukaemia, Hodgkin's and non-Hodgkin's disease, thalassaemia, infrequent congenital immune deficiency and haemopietic disorders, and breast, ovarian and testicular cancers (Johns, 1998). The transplant involves the intravenous transfer of red bone marrow stem cells from the healthy donor to the recipient. The aim is to provide a normal haemopoietic function. The transplanted cells travel immediately to the marrow spaces that have been emptied by disease (e.g. aplastic anaemia); in patients with cancer, the defective red bone marrow first must be destroyed by high doses of chemotherapy and whole-body radiation. Although a transplant is the best chance of a cure for such patients, it has potential risks. The donor cells proliferate in the marrow, releasing functional cells into the peripheral circulation. Complete marrow recovery may take 6–8 weeks.

The major barrier to the success of bone marrow transplant is the antigenic differences between donor and recipient. Identical twins are ideal donors for each other as they have identical human leucocyte antigen (HLA), therefore bone marrow transplants between identical twins are nearly always successful. More commonly, the donor is an HLA-identical brother, sister or parent; these transplants are often successful. If the patient and donor are not HLA-identical, immunosuppression is necessary.

Smith (1998) explores the psychosocial implications of bone marrow transplants.

BOX 11.20 LEUCOPENIA

A marked reduction of white blood cells – leucopenia – is usually known as a neutropenia, since the most significant reduction is usually the neutrophil population. Neutropenia is usually a consequence of bone marrow depression, often as a result of the toxic side effects of drugs, e.g. chlorpromazine or the sulphonamides, in people with high sensitivity. It may also arise as a consequence of a radiotherapy and anti-cancer drug therapy. It is also associated with overwhelming infections, such as malaria, typhoid fever and hyposplenis (a condition in which the spleen destroys neutrophils at an accelerated rate).

Management of leucopenia is by the withdrawal of any possible offending drugs; if the granulocyte count is very low, the patient is protected form obvious sources of infection. The aim of treatment is to abolish the factor responsible for the bone marrow depression. Spontaneous restoration of marrow function often occurs in 2–3 weeks.

Thrombocytes

Structure

Thrombocytes (platelets) are more numerous than leucocytes, but less numerous than erythrocytes; there are approximately $250\,000/mm^3$. Thrombocytes are the smallest cellular components of blood, being only 2–4 μm in diameter. They do not have a nucleus; microscopically, they appear as a disc-shaped structure with a colourless cytoplasm. Their membranes are the sites of many enzymatic reactions, and contain specific receptors for collagen and the hormones serotonin and adrenaline. It is these receptors that enable platelets to respond to tissue damage and trauma. Microfilaments in the cytoplasm are composed of a contractile protein called platelet actomyosin. These filaments function in the haemostatic process of clot retraction (see later). Thrombocytes possess numerous cytoplasmic granules that contain enzymes (or factors) that are released when platelets aggregate together and/or are lysed. These enzymes are important in the homeostatic function of blood coagulation.

Production and destruction of thrombocytes

Thrombocytes are formed in the red marrow, lungs and, to some extent, the spleen and liver, by the fragmentation (platelet budding) of very large cells called megakaryocytes (Figure 11.10). The rate of platelet production (thrombopoiesis) is regulated tightly between the two interchangeable platelet 'pools' of the circulation and spleen. The feedback mechanism for thrombopoiesis and this interchange has yet to be identified. It must be stimulated, however, by a low platelet count (thrombocytopenia). A platelet's lifespan is about 5–9 days, after which it is destroyed by specialized macrophages of the liver and spleen.

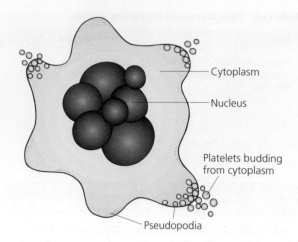

Figure 11.10   A megakaryocyte, showing platelet budding.
Q. *Where do megakaryocytes originate?*

WOUND HEALING

Wound healing is a remarkable process. Without it, surgery would be impossible; furthermore, the more surgery advances, the greater becomes the problem of wound healing. For patients with systemic ischaemia, infection, pre-existing medical conditions such as jaundice and diabetes mellitus, or malnutrition, and in patients taking anti-inflammatory and steroidal drugs, the problems are numerous, but the requirements are the same, i.e. a safely healed wound after surgery.

Wound assessment has traditionally been the responsibility of nursing staff, and has tended to be subjective, often relying on anecdotal evidence that frequently fails to report accurate information (Flanagan, 1997). It is our view that accurate wound assessment and management are dependent on an understanding of the biochemistry of healing, the factors that delay the process, and the optimal conditions required at the wound surface to maximize healing.

A wound may be defined as 'an interruption to the continuity of the external surface of the body, which may be due to accidental injury, planned surgery, thermal injury, pressure, or disease process such as leg ulceration or carcinoma' (Norfolk Health, 1996). Clancy and McVicar (1997) define wound healing as 'the physiological process by which the body replaces and restores the function of damaged tissue'.

Skin is predominantly affected. Other tissue (e.g. muscle) may be torn, bones fractured, and blood flow disrupted during a major surgical procedure such as open-heart surgery. This section considers only the healing of skin wounds. Bone healing is discussed in Chapter 3.

The extent of tissue injury or tissue death (necrosis) depends largely on the intensity and duration of the exposure to the injurious agent, as well as the type of tissue involved (Clancy and McVicar 1996a). Thus the homeostatic responses of tissue repair, regeneration and replacement are necessary following tissue injury or tissue death to maintain the numbers of cells within their homeostatic limits, and so as not to compromise cell, tissue and organ system functional integrity. Tissues can be divided into three categories according to their repair, regeneration and restoration capabilities (Figure 11.11).

Chapter 1 discussed the importance of the interdependency of organ systems in maintaining intracellular homeostasis. This interdependence is vital in producing the optimal physicobiochemical conditions required at the wound surface to maximize the healing process. For example:

● efficient digestive functioning provides essential intracellular nutrients (metabolites and products of metabolism) for repair, regeneration and restoration of tissue integrity following injury (Table 11.10; Figure 11.12);

● efficient circulatory functioning is necessary to transport leucocytes (to protect the integrity of undamaged cells), nutrients, oxygen and biochemicals important to the wound-healing process to the site of tissue damage;

● the lymphatics prevent the accumulation of tissue fluid via their drainage facilities, and so minimize the discomfort (oedema and associated pain) that can accompany

Figure 11.11 Repair, regeneration and restoration of a tissue's structural and functional integrity following injury. (a) Structural and functional integrity of body tissues intact. (b) Compromised structural and functional integrity of the body's tissues due to tissue loss. (c) Speedy and complete repair and regeneration with complete restoration of the functional integrity of body tissues. Labile tissues, such as the skin, undergo mitosis throughout life, and therefore have excellent repair capabilities. (d_1–d_2) Complete or partial repair and regeneration, with only partial restoration of the functional integrity of body tissues following injury. Stable tissues, such as the liver, normally exhibit little mitotic activity during adult life but are capable of increasing the rate of cell division if they are damaged. Although such tissues may heal, their complex

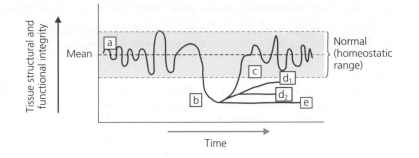

architecture may not regenerate, and they may not necessarily be restored to full function. (e) Minor repair and regeneration, with loss of functional integrity of tissue following injury, resulting in scarring of the damaged area. Permanent tissues, such as the brain, spinal cord and skeletal muscle, exhibit little mitotic activity during adult life. They are so complex that little repair, other than scarring, can be achieved following injury.

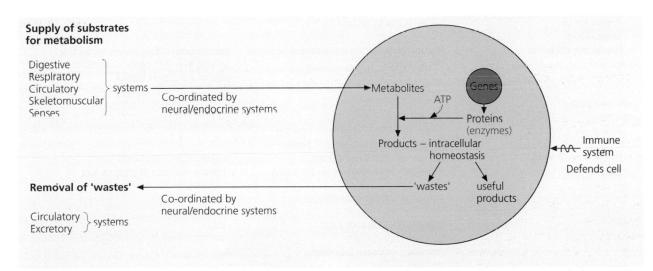

Key:
Intracellular metabolites include: Micronutrients (see Table 11.10)
Intracellular products include: Macronutrients (see Table 11.10) and products of metabolism which are important in the healing process. These include: Serotonin (released from basophils), histamine (released from basophils, platelets and cells that have been damaged), prostoglandins and kinins (released from cells that have been damaged), clotting factors (released from cells that have been damaged and platelets), antibodies (released from B-lymphocytes), collagen and elastin (released from fibrocytes), macrophage attracting substances such as compliment (released from liver cells), prothrombin and fibrinogen (released from liver cells) and cytotoxic substances (released from T-lymphocytes), mitotic growth factors (released from cells which have no contact inhibition).

Figure 11.12 The interdependency of organ systems in providing intracellular metabolites and products necessary for wound healing.

inflammation as a result of fluid compression on surrounding soft tissues;

- the excretory organs remove cellular/chemical debris from the damaged site. This decreases the likelihood of septicaemia (the presence of a large number of bacteria and their toxins) and toxaemia (poisoning of the blood by absorption of bacterial toxins), particularly during injury accompanied by an infection;

- the co-ordinators (neural/hormonal mediators) of body functions direct the systemic interactions listed above

involved in providing the optimal physicobiochemical conditions for the wound-healing process.

Therefore, it should not come as any surprise that an inefficiency of one component part of the body leads to functional disturbances of other parts. For example, if cardiovascular function is compromised (e.g. progressive atherosclerosis), as occurs in older people and in people with diabetes mellitus, wound healing is delayed due to inadequate cardiovascular homeostatic responses to tissue damage.

Table 11.10 Role of nutrients in the process of wound healing. Note that nutrients are intracellular metabolites and/or products of metabolism

Intracellular metabolites/products vital for wound-healing process		Role of nutrients in providing intracellular products vital for wound healing	Nutrient deficiency: the effect on wound healing
Macronutrients			
Proteins			
General role of proteins		Metabolism of cell membranes Enzymes synthesis	Prolonged inflammation Impairs fibroplasia
Specific role of some amino acids	Cysteine	Important role in collagen synthesis	Delays collagen synthesis Delays angiogenesis Delays wound remodelling
	Argenine	Enhanced collagen synthesis Enhances immune response	Weaker wounds
Lipids			
General roles of lipids		Concentrated energy source Metabolism of cell membranes	
Specific role of some fatty acids	Linoleic acid	Maintains integrity and function of cellular unit membranes Prostaglandin precursor	Rare
Carbohydrates			
General role of carbohydrates		Energy source for all cells	
Specific role of glucose		Primary energy fuel for metabolism of leucocytes and fibroblasts	Gluconeogenesis from protein metabolism resulting in protein energy malnutrition in patients with severe injuries
Micronutrients			
Vitamins			
General role of vitamins		Cofactors, therefore important for general metabolism and maintenance of health	
Specific roles of some vitamins	Vitamin C	Cofactor for several amino acids Antioxidant factor enhances wound healing	Wounds healing inefficiently Increases likelihood of pressure sore development
	Vitamin B complex	Involved in collagen cross-linkages	Rare
	Vitamin A	Epithelial proliferation/migration *Collagen cross-linkages	Rare
	Vitamin E	Antioxidant may work with Vitamin C	Rare
Minerals			
General role of minerals		Cofactors, therefore important for general	
Specific roles of minerals		metabolism and maintenance of health	
Iron		*Cofactor important in collagen synthesis	Anaemia, therefore delays the wound-healing process Decreased collagen synthesis/cell proliferation
Zinc		*Cofactor important in collagen synthesis, protein synthesis	Decreased wound-healing processes
Copper		*Cofactor important in collagen cross linkages	
Calcium		*Remodelling of collagen	
Magnesium		*Synthesis of collagen	

*Important in remodelling of collagen; deficiencies lead to decreased collagen cross-linkages, therefore reducing strength of scar tissue.

Local and general responses to injury

The homeostatic responses to injury are divided into two types of response:

- *local responses:* responses in the injured tissues (the focus of this chapter);

- *general responses:* responses elicited in the rest of the body by the local response. These responses can be referred to as 'shock'. Many forms of shock exist, each of which describes the pattern of responses to a particular injury or 'antigenic insult', e.g. cardiogenic shock is a response to heart failure, haemorrhagic shock is a response to haemorrhage, traumatic shock is a response to trauma, and septic or endotoxic shock is a response to infection (Clancy and McVicar, 1996b).

Wound healing does not, of course, apply only to the skin, although the skin is more susceptible to damage than

BOX 11.21 CLASSIFICATION OF WOUNDS

Wounds are conventionally classified as either superficial (non-bleeding) or deep (bleeding). Damage to the epidermis will not result in bleeding, since this layer does not contain blood vessels. Its main function is to form a protective covering from the external environment. Wound healing of this tissue involves the replacement of cells known as the germinating layer, since the layers above it are derived from the mitotic activity of this layer (Figure 11.13(a)).

Damage to the deeper dermal layer results in a bleeding wound, since blood vessels are present in this layer of the skin (Figure 11.13(b)). This type of injury involves a more complicated type of wound healing. The initial homeostatic responses are involved in repairing and regenerating damaged blood vessels, thus restoring transport of the vital factors essential for the wound-healing process of the tissue above it, i.e. the epidermal cells. Of course, if blood vessels are damaged directly, blood will also be lost at the site of the injury, either escaping to the outside or being retained in the tissue as a bruise (haematoma). Wound healing of connective soft tissues is similar. It involves the formation of new

epithelium and contraction of healthy granulation tissue beneath to form a fibrous scar.

There are two basic types of wound healing: primary and secondary intentions. Healing by primary intention (or closure) is the most common type of healing following surgery. It occurs when the tissue edges are maintained in apposition. The lower layers are stitched with a dissolvable suture, and the skin is either sutured or clipped together (Figure 11.14(a)). This should be achieved in all incised surgical wounds and primarily sutured fresh traumatic lacerations. The wound heals quickly with minimal scarring (Collier, 1996).

In secondary intention healing, the wound edges are distant from each other. The defect fills via granulation tissue from the lowest part of the wound upwards, with the epithelial layer being the last to grow (Figure 11.14b). This type of wound closure is sometimes achieved in full-thickness burns, chronic leg ulceration, after surgical excision of necrotic tissue, and when the wound is infected.

A wound may also be categorized as clean, bacterially contaminated, or infected.

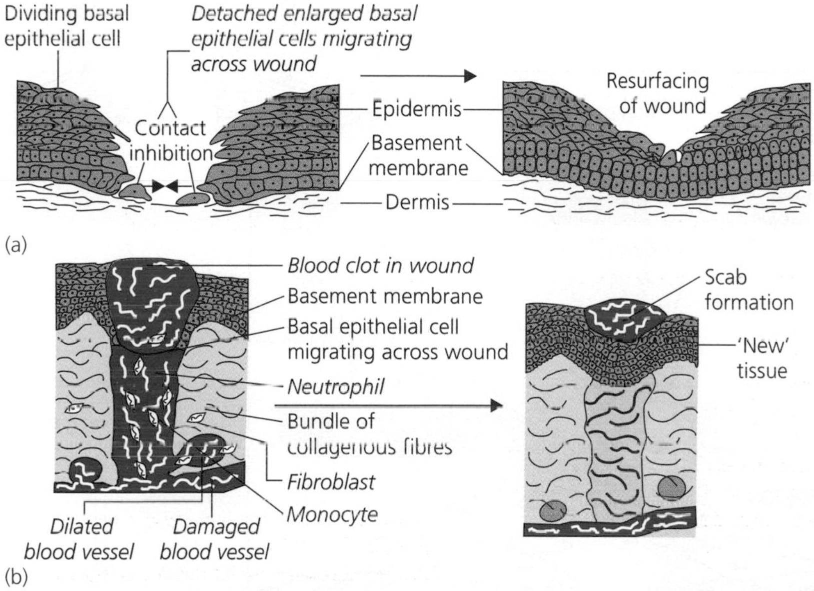

Dividing basal epithelial cell

Detached enlarged basal epithelial cells migrating across wound

Contact inhibition

Epidermis

Basement membrane

Dermis

Resurfacing of wound

(a)

Blood clot in wound

Basement membrane

Basal epithelial cell migrating across wound

Neutrophil

Bundle of collagenous fibres

Fibroblast

Monocyte

Scab formation

'New' tissue

Dilated blood vessel   *Damaged blood vessel*

(b)

Figure 11.13 (a) Epidermal wound healing following superficial injury, e.g. a mild abrasion of the skin. Basal (germinating) cells divide and migrate across a superficial wound. (b) Epidermal wound healing following injury to deep layers of the skin, e.g. a surgical incision. This involves generation of a new blood supply (angiogenesis) before the division and migration of basal (germinating) cells across the surface of the wound.

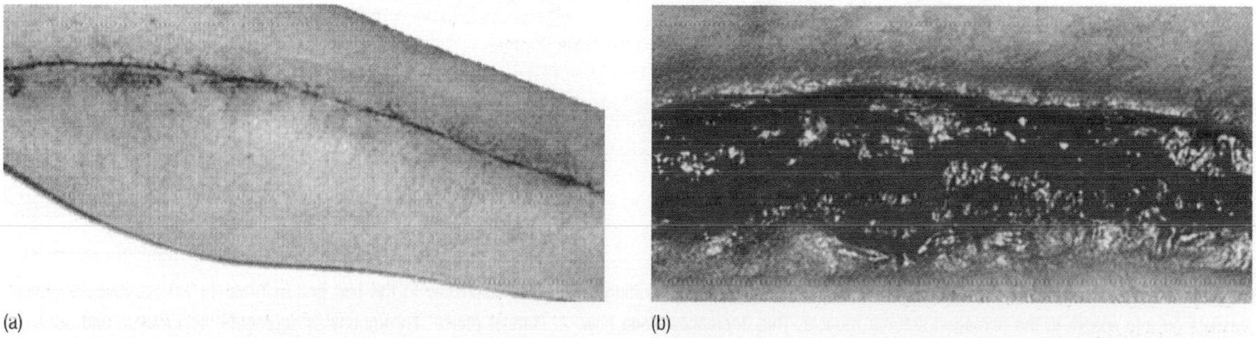

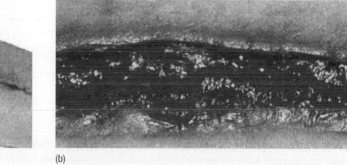

(a)   (b)

Figure 11.14 (a) Wound healing by primary intention or closure, e.g. as occurs with surgical incision. The wound is closed to eliminate the dead space, and is held together by sutures or clips. There is minimal granulation and a low risk of scarring. If scarring is present, it fades with time and disappears when wound healing is matured. Primary closure is not appropriate for infected or long-standing wounds. (b) Wound healing by secondary intention or closure, e.g. as occurs with leg ulceration when there is a lot of tissue lost or when there is a risk of infection. The wound is left open to heal by granulation. Cosmetically, the results are comparable to primary intention wound healing.

other underlying tissues. However, the healing process following injury to the skin is a good illustration of the basic processes of healing.

Exercise

Before continuing, read about the structure and associated functions of the skin in Chapter 16.

The wound-healing process

The healing process occurs as a set of homeostatic responses brought about by trauma. The process can be divided conveniently into four main stages: the vascular, inflammation, proliferation and maturation stages. Substages or phases exist within the main stages, e.g. the

platelet and blood coagulation phases of the vascular stage. There is, however, considerable overlap between the stages/phases, and in the time required by an individual to progress to the next stage/phase of healing.

The vascular stage

The vascular stage comprises five principal phases: the vascular, platelet, coagulation, clot retraction, and clot destruction phases. The process is summarized in Figure 11.15.

The vascular phase
Seconds after damage to blood vessels, the muscular wall (the tunica media; see Figure 12.12(a)) contracts, a process called vasoconstriction ('vaso-', = vessel). This muscle spasm decreases blood flow and therefore minimizes blood loss for up to 30 min, thus aiding other homeostatic

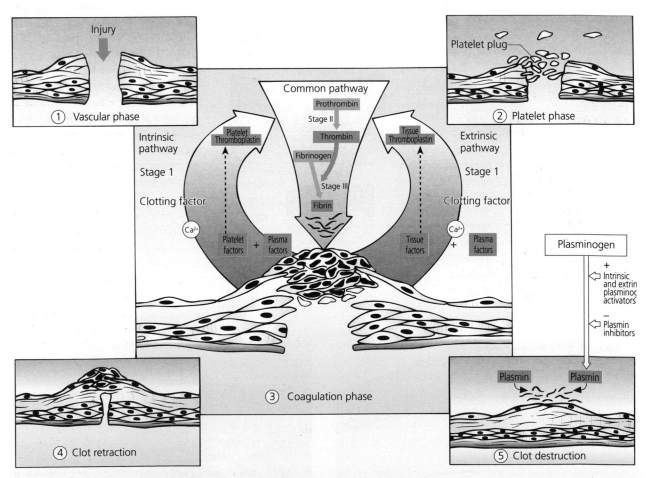

Figure 11.15 The clotting mechanism. (Details of plasma and platelet clotting factors are discussed in the text and in Table 11.11). 1. Vascular phase. Vessels go into spasm in the damaged smooth muscle. This decreases blood flow. 2. Platelet phase. Thrombocytes aggregate, accumulate and adhere to the damaged vessels, forming the platelet plug. 3. Coagulation phase. Activation of clotting and clot formation. 4. Clot retraction. Involves the contraction of the blood clot. 5. Clot destruction. Enzymatic (plasmin) destruction of the clot.

Q. Why does whole blood fail to clot when calcium ions are removed?

Q. What are the outcomes of the first, second and third stages of clotting?

+, stimulatory; —, inhibitory.

responses within the haemostatic response (responses associated with arresting bleeding). In addition to the vascular stage of haemostasis, the platelet and blood coagulation phases also act to prevent blood loss. These mechanisms are adequate as homeostatic controls in preventing blood loss if the damage is to small blood vessels. If larger blood vessels are involved (resulting in mass haemorrhage), these mechanisms are inadequate.

The platelet phase

The platelets (thrombocytes) that come into contact with the damaged vessel enlarge. They become irregular in shape, and extremely sticky, adhering to the collagen fibres of the vessel wall. These thrombocytes secrete substances (e.g. thromboxane A2, TXA2) that activate more platelets, causing them to stick to the original platelets. The aggregation and attachment of platelets forms a platelet plug almost immediately after the damage. The plug becomes strengthened by fibrin threads formed during the coagulation process, and is extremely effective in preventing blood loss from small vessels.

The blood coagulation phase

Coagulation is a complicated metabolic pathway involving many interdependent enzyme-controlled reactions. Collectively, these reactions are called the clotting cascade. This cascade is a multiplicative process. Proenzymes (inactive enzymes) interact; the conversion of one proenzyme creates an enzyme that activates a second proenzyme, which activates a third proenzyme, and so on, in a chain reaction. Many clotting factors are involved (Table 11.11), including plasma factors (numbered I–XIII) and platelet factors (labelled Pf1–4). The cascade occurs rapidly once stimulated; when blood is taken in a blood test, or when a vessel is damaged, blood is converted quickly from its usual liquefied state into a gel-like clot. The process is initiated within 30 s of damage, and completed after several minutes. The coagulation phase can be summarized as a sequence of three stages:

1 *Stage I:* formation and release of a collection of enzymes collectively called thromboplastin or thrombokinase.

2 *Stage II:* thromboplastin converts plasma prothrombin into thrombin.

3 *Stage III:* thrombin converts the soluble plasma protein fibrinogen into insoluble fibrin, then forms the threads of the clot.

The initiating enzyme (thromboplastin) is released from damaged tissue cells, triggering the extrinsic coagulation pathway, and/or by the lysis of platelets, which triggers the intrinsic coagulation pathway. The extrinsic pathway is initiated by the release of a tissue factor (an enzyme) from damaged peripheral cells and/or damaged capillary endothelial cells. This enzyme, together with certain plasma factors (IV, V, VII and X), forms extrinsic or tissue thromboplastin, which is equivalent to stage I of the clotting cascade (Figure 11.15). The second stage utilizes extrinsic thromboplastin to convert prothrombin into thrombin. The second stage is then promoted, with the conversion of fibrinogen into fibrin by the action of thrombin and plasma factors IV and XIII. Most steps in the extrinsic mechanism also require the presence of calcium ions.

The intrinsic pathway is normally activated when there is damage to the internal lining of the blood vessels. It is also activated by the presence of a rough surface, such as fatty plaques or calcium deposits attached to the internal lining of the blood vessel (see Figure 12.13). This stimulus removes the normal repulsion activities between platelets and endothelial cells lining the blood vessels, with the result that platelets adhere to the rough surface. The aggregation and clumping of platelets bring about their lysis, releasing platelet coagulation factors (Pf1–4) into the plasma. The clumping reaction is sometimes all that is necessary to plug a lightly damaged area.

Stage I of the intrinsic pathway involves four platelet factors (Pf1-4) and seven plasma factors (IV, V, VIII, IX, X, XI and XII) to form intrinsic thromboplastin. The second stage involves the conversion of prothrombin into thrombin by thromboplastin. The third stage is the same for both intrinsic and extrinsic pathways. The difference in the second stages is that intrinsic thromboplastin and extrinsic thromboplastin initiate the prothrombin conversion from their respective pathways. All stages of the intrinsic pathway require the presence of calcium ions.

Thrombin is a key chemical because of its involvement in the third stage. It stimulates more platelets to adhere to one another, resulting in a further lysis of

Table 11.11   The homeostatic importance of coagulation factors

Coagulation factors	Homeostatic importance
Plasma coagulation factors	
I Fibrinogen	Important factor in stage III of clotting, in which it is converted to fibrin
II Prothrombin	Important in stage II of clotting, in which it is converted into thrombin
III Thromboplastin (thrombokinase)	In extrinsic pathway, referred to as extrinsic thromboplastin; formed from tissue thromboplastin In intrinsic pathway, referred to as intrinsic thromboplastin; formed from platelet disintegration Formation of thromboplastin signifies the end of stage I
IV Calcium ions	Involved in all three stages of clotting Removal of calcium or its binding in the plasma prevents coagulation
V Proaccelerin or labile factor	Required for stages I and II of both extrinsic and intrinsic pathways
VI No longer used in coagulation theory	
VII Serum prothrombin accelerator or stable factor	Required in stage I extrinsic pathway
V III Antihaemophilic factor	Required for stage I of intrinsic pathway Deficiency causes classical haemophilia A
IX Christmas factor or plasma thromboplastin component	Required for stage I of intrinsic pathway Deficiency causes haemophilia B
X Stuart factor or Stuart–Prower factor	Required for stages I and II of extrinsic and intrinsic pathways Deficiency results in nose bleeds, bleeding into joints, or bleeding into soft tissues
XI Plasma thromboplastin antecedent	Required for stage I of intrinsic pathway Deficiency causes haemophilia C
XII Hageman factor	Required for stage I of intrinsic pathway
XIII Fibrin stabilizing factor	Required for stage III of clotting
NB. Vitamine K is required for the synthesis of Factors II, VII, IX ad X. Vitamine K deficiency often leads to uncontrolled bleeding	
Platelet coagulation factors	
Platelet factor 1 – Pf1	Essentially the same as plasma coagulation factor V
Platelet factor 2 – Pf2	Accelerates formation of thrombin in stage 1 intrinsic pathway and the conversion of fibrinogen to fibrin
Platelet factor 3 – Pf3	Required for stage I of intrinsic pathway
Platelet factor 4 – Pf4	Binds heparin, an anticoagulant during clotting

platelets, and thus the consequential release of further platelet factors. The more thrombin that is released, the more platelet factors are released, resulting in more thrombin production, hence a greater clot formation. This cyclical process is therefore a positive feedback mechanism. It ensures continual platelet lysis until the clot is formed, so the healing process can proceed appropriately. For example, bleeding activates both extrinsic and intrinsic pathways to maximize clot formation and arrest bleeding.

The clot retraction phase

Once the fibrin meshwork has been formed, the platelets and erythrocytes stick to its strands. The platelets contract, with the result that the entire clot retracts, bringing the torn edges closer together, and stabilizing and consolidating the injury. Microfilaments can be observed in platelet cytoplasm composed of a contractile protein called actomyosin. The clot plugs the damaged vessel to prevent further blood loss, and the retraction makes it easier for

fibroblasts, smooth muscle cells, and endothelial cells to perform their homeostatic repair functions.

The clot destruction phase

Once the area is repaired, the clot is dissolved via the process of fibrinolysis, which involves tissue factors (intrinsic and extrinsic) that activate the precursor plasminogen into the clot-dissolving enzyme plasmin.

Exercise

List the three stages of the clotting reaction. Describe the role of extrinsic and intrinsic thromboplastin.

The inflammation stage

This is the part of the nonspecific response to infection. When a tissue is damaged via mechanical, thermal or chemi-

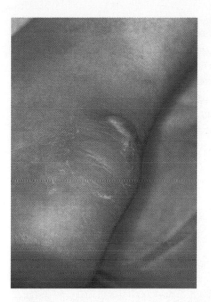

Figure 11.16 Wound showing the classical signs of inflammation. *Q. List the classical signs of inflammation.*

cal causes, or in response to a hypersensitive reaction or a pathogenic invasion, the body reacts in the same way. The tissue soon shows the four classic signs of inflammation (see Figure 11.16), which provide a reassurance that normal homeostatic responses have been activated following injury (DeCruz, 1998). These signs are redness, an increase in tissue temperature, swelling, pain and discomfort. These signs may be followed by an additional loss of function. The first three responses are characteristic to changes in the microcirculation in the injured tissue. The redness (erythema) is due to vasodilation of the arterioles (smallest arteries); heat is due to increased blood flow; and swelling (oedema) is due to an increase in the extravascular fluid content of the injured tissues. This post-traumatic oedema is promoted by an increase in microvascular permeability; the consequential loss of blood components is called exudation.

The permeability changes are in response to the secretion from the site of injury of cellular products of metabolism (Figure 11.12), such as:

- histamine, released from mast cells (basophils), platelets and damaged cells at the site of injury;

- serotonin and heparin, released from mast cells;

- kinins and prostaglandins, released from injured cells.

The role of the exudate is to promote the entrance of proteins and phagocytic white cells into the wound from the plasma. Generally, the proteins in the tissue fluid create a colloidal osmotic pressure, promoting fluid leakage from plasma, resulting in the accumulation of tissue fluid (McVicar and Clancy, 1997). The increased blood flow to the area, and the accumulation of fluid in the soft tissues, eventually exerts pressure on sensory nerve endings, making the wound feel uncomfortable and/or painful (Flanagan, 1996). Pain is also a result of the presence of kinins and prostaglandins, which stimulate pain receptors (see Figure 21.1). Specifically, proteins such as prothrombin and fibrinogen stimulate the clotting process – an adaptive homeostatic reflex to create a physical protective barrier between the external and internal environments of the body.

The next part of the process of inflammation involves the removal of debris and microorganisms (DeCruz, 1998). Phagocytes, such as neutrophils and macrophages, dispose of damaged tissue cells, foreign material and microorganisms via phagocytosis (see Figure 13.9). This process is facilitated by the presence in the exudate of other white cells (T- and B-lymphocytes) and various proteinaceous components, collectively called complement. Complement facilitates the phagocytic and lymphocytic responses to either prevent or fight infection (see Figure 13.14).

> **Exercise**
>
> Refer to Chapter 13 for the details associated with the phagocytic response, the lymphocytic responses, and the role of complement.

To summarize, neutrophils are attracted into the wound first, usually within a few hours of injury; they are followed by macrophages. The activity of lymphocytes essentially cleanses the wound bed. Macrophages secrete growth factors, prostaglandins and complement factors, which aid antibody–antigen complexing. Since these chemicals promote healing, macrophages are usually present during all stages of wound healing. In clean wounds, the inflammatory phase lasts approximately 36 h; in necrotic or infected wounds, the process is prolonged (Flanagan, 1996).

The biochemical constitution of the exudate reflects the intensity and duration of the injurious agent. For example:

BOX 11.23 INFLAMMATION

The process of inflammation is considered beneficial since it involves the homeostatic responses that restore tissue homeostatic integrity by neutralizing and destroying antigens locally at the site of injury. The process is referred to as a biological emergency response, since there is a latent stage of approximately 12 h before any obvious healing begins (Silver, 1994). Therefore, during the inflammatory process the patient may feel generally ill. Signs and symptoms may include fever, loss of appetite, and tiredness. The process of wound healing may also instigate harmful effects, such as:

- oedema in vital organs, such as the lungs, heart and brain. Cerebral oedema is a common cause of raised intracranial pressures in head injury;
- autolysis (self-destruction) of local body tissues, due to the release of lysozymes from the large numbers of phagocytes presents in the exudate;
- complications caused by the lodging of antigen–antibody complexes.

- serous exudate has a low protein content, indicating that there is superficial and minimal damage, as occurs with blistering of the skin;

- fibrinous exudate indicates damage of a more intense nature, since this type of wound requires the development of a protective fibrin clot. The material must be removed if a scar is not to form;

- haemorrhagic exudate has the same biochemical constitution as a fibrous exudate, with the additional presence of erythrocytes, indicating that the injury has damaged blood vessels;

- purulent exudates are wounds that contain pus (a mixture of living and dead body cells, dead microbes, cell debris such as proteinaceous fibres, and bacteria toxins). Such an exudate is detrimental to the healing process.

Exercise

Refer to Chapter 13, in particular Figure 13.14, to review the antigen–antibody complexing process.

The proliferation stage

Following the vascular and inflammatory stages, replacement, repair and regeneration of injured cells must occur. This stage is referred to as proliferation, during which the wound is filled with new connective tissue. The three processes involved are granulation, contraction and epithelialization.

Granulation

The filling of the deep wound with tissue during proliferation is usually referred to as granulation (Figure 11.13(b)). Initially, this process involves the creation of new capillaries (a process called angiogenesis) in the wound bed to support the mitotic activity that provides replacement cells. Angiogenesis is stimulated by the tissue hypoxia that is caused by the disruption of blood flow at the time of injury (Flanagan, 1997). Capillary 'buds' develop from the periphery of the wound and grow into the site at about 0.5 mm/day (Collier, 1996). Macrophage activity (arising from the process of inflammation) stimulates the production and multiplication of fibroblasts. These cells migrate along the fibrin threads (produced in the vascular phase), lay down a ground substance, and begin the secretion of collagen. This substance will ultimately form the scar of the wound.

The characteristics of healthy and unhealthy granulation tissue are summarized in Figure 11.17.

Wound contraction

Following the deposition of connective tissue, the fibroblasts that have congregated at the wound margins develop

BOX 11.24 ANGIOGENESIS

The importance of an adequate blood supply in granulation is illustrated by the slow rate of healing induced by circulatory deficiencies in conditions such as diabetes mellitus. Granulation is also slowed in elderly people, partly because of reduced cardiovascular efficiency, but also because rates of cell division and cell metabolism decline with age.

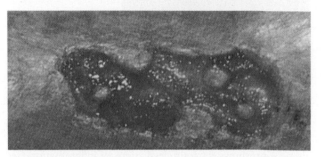
(a)

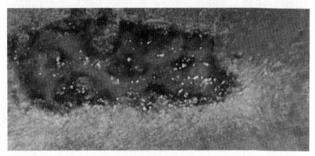
(b)

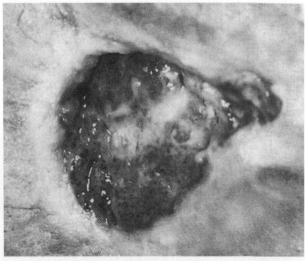
(c)

Figure 11.17   (a) Wound showing signs of healthy granulation. Note that the wound has a bright red, moist, shiny appearance. (b) Wound showing signs of unhealthy granulation. Note that the wound has a dark red colour (in parts), and a dehydrated and dull appearance. Wound showing the process of epithelialization. Note the pinkish-white skin around the edges of the wound.

contractile proteins and use their properties to pull the edges of the wound together, thus reducing the size of the wound (see The clot retraction phase above).

Wound epithelialization

The proliferating, migrating new epithelial cells from the wound edge, and, in skin, remnants of hair follicles, sweat and sebaceous glands (see Figure 16.1), move across the surface of the wound until the wound is closed. It is not understood completely why cells should begin to migrate, but it is thought that the loss of contact between neighbouring cells causes the movement, i.e. 'contact inhibition' is removed (Figure 11.13(a)). This concept has been refined in recent years, and it is clear that cells adjoining each other communicate and modulate each others' behaviour. Movement stops when others surround the cell, although these cells however must be of the same 'type' (e.g. cancer cells appear to lose contact inhibition). Once the migrated cells have formed a new germinating layer, they will divide, and new epidermal strata will be formed. Newly formed epithelial cells have a translucent appearance; they are usually whitish-pink (Flanagan, 1996; Figure 11.17(c)) and are 'raised' to some degree in relation to the surrounding tissue (Collier, 1996). The signs of inflammation should subside, thus the amount of wound exudate decreases and becomes more manageable.

Complete healing is possible only once the epithelial cells have completely bridged the surface of the wound. Any scab over the wound will slough away, and the new epidermis will become toughened by the production of the protein keratin. The whole process normally takes place over 24–48 h after injury, although epithelialization may continue for up to a year or more in injuries sustaining substantial tissue loss.

The maturation stage

Once the granulation, wound contraction and epithelialization phases are completed, the final stage of wound healing – maturation occurs. This stage can take from 24 h to 2 years to complete, depending upon the severity of the wound and tissue involved. In the maturation phase, the fibrocytes begin to disappear. Collagen fibres form a mesh, strengthening the tissue, and become indifferent to the surrounding area in both colour and texture (DeCruz, 1998). The original clot is removed by the action of plasmin (Figure 11.15; see also The clot destruction phase above).

As the scar tissue matures, its blood supply decreases, and the tissue contracts, causing the scar to become flatter, paler and smoother. Mature scar tissues contain no hairs, or sebaceous or sweat glands.

In summary, wound healing following injury is a dynamic process involving the precise co-ordination of a number of homeostatic responses at a cellular and biochemical level. These responses are, only as a matter of convenience, divided into a number of stages and phases of wound healing.

See the case study of a man with a surgical wound in Section 6.

BOX 11.25 HOMEOSTATIC FAILURES OF THE CLOTTING MECHANISM

Read this box in conjunction with Figure 11.18, which summarizes the homeostatic and clinical control of blood clotting.

Thrombocyte imbalances

Thrombocytosis is an abnormally high platelet count. This is a common sign of many diseases, including certain leukaemias, such as myeloid leukaemia, and is observed immediately after a splenectomy ('-ectomy' = removal).

Thrombocytopoenia is a deficiency of platelets. This may be due to either a decrease in platelet production or an increased rate of destruction. The latter may be a result of thrombocytes being crowded out of the bone marrow in some bone diseases, such as certain leukaemias, pernicious anaemia or malignant tumours. X-irradiation, radioactive isotopes, cytotoxic drugs and other drugs, such as sulphonamides and phenylbutazone, may also reduce the thrombocyte concentration. Thrombocytopenia is evident in patients with various types of purpura, a condition characterized by small multiple haemorrhagic spots (petechiae) or large, blotchy areas on the skin and mucous membranes. Purpura is also a complication of other blood diseases, such as leukaemias and severe anaemias, and may also result from antibiotic and corticosteroid therapies.

Clotting factor imbalances

The cascade of enzymatic conversions during clotting means that a disorder that affects any individual clotting factor disrupts the whole clotting mechanism. Many clinical conditions can therefore result in clotting abnormalities, particularly those that disrupt calcium and vitamin K metabolism. Calcium ions are important in most of the cascade reactions, so calcium imbalance has a direct effect on coagulation. Vitamin K is required for the synthesis of five clotting factors (including prothrombin), and its deficiency results in a breakdown of the common pathway. Deficiency can be due to insufficient dietary intake, malabsorption problems, or incorrect utilization. Dietary deficiencies are uncommon, as gut bacteria usually supply the individual with sufficient levels of this vitamin. Deficiencies can occur, however, if these bacteria are interfered with, e.g. after sterilizing treatments of the bowel. Malabsorption of vitamin K is the most common cause of depressed circulating levels. The vitamin requires bile salts for its absorption, thus low

Figure 11.18 The homeostatic and clinical controls of blood clotting. (a) Normal ability to coagulate blood, i.e. thrombocyte and clotting factors are within their homeostatic ranges. (b_1) An increased ability to clot the blood. This may be due to other homeostatic imbalances, e.g. hyperlipidaemia or hypercalcaemia, responsible for an increased tendency for atherosclerotic plaque and calcium deposit formation, respectively. Both precipitate blood clotting. Alternatively, the increased clotting ability may be a result of a normal physiological homeostatic mechanism (haemostasis) that goes into operation when a blood vessel is damaged. (b_2) Decreased ability to produce blood clots. This may be due to a homeostatic imbalance of the factors involved in blood clotting, e.g. hypocalcaemia, hypoprothrombinaemia, hypofibrinogenaemia, or inadequate levels of vitamin K or factor VIII (haemophilia, etc.). (c_1) Clinical correction involves fibrolytic enzyme (streptokinase or urokinase) therapy. (c_2) Clinical correction of prolonged bouts of bleeding involves

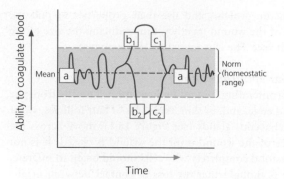

the administration of the deficient aetiological factors, e.g. factor VIII therapy in classical haemophilia A.

Q. How could an enzyme, such as streptokinase, assist in preventing unwanted clotting and removing clots already formed?

BOX 11.25 CONTINUED

circulating levels can occur in liver diseases, in prolonged biliary tract obstruction, and in any other disease that impairs fat absorption (e.g. coeliac disease). Pancreatic disease and chronic diarrhoea may also be responsible for Vitamin K deficiency. Conversely, levels in excess of the homeostatic range of vitamin K or calcium may result in inappropriate clot formation (thrombosis).

Increased fragility of capillary walls

Increased fragility of capillary walls results in bleeding, appearing as bruising under the skin, even when there is minimal damage. The main causal factors are thrombocytopenia and autoimmune diseases, and the use of some drugs, e.g. penicillin and aspirin.

Plaques

Hyperactivity of the clotting mechanism may result from a roughened or irregular surface within the cardiovascular system, causing platelet aggregation and/or lysis. In aggregation, platelets stick to the roughened inner (endothelial) coat of intact vessels. This adhesion may be due to the presence of endothelial fatty streaks (precursors of atherosclerotic plaques), or calcium deposits. Both situations are essentially consequences of the ageing process, are the result of a modern lifestyle, and may result in intravascular thrombosis.

Thrombosis

A clot is called a thrombus when it forms within an intact vessel. Once formed, the clot progressively enlarges, obliterating more and more of the lumen. This may progress until the clot severely impairs blood flow to the tissue's cells. If the oxygen supply is not restored, cells surrounding the area of the clot die (necrosis). This is referred to as an infarction. Alternatively, a part of the clot may break off (dislodged thrombi are called emboli) and become lodged in small blood vessels, producing ischaemic changes and infarction at those sites. The lungs are common embolic sites, where the emboli will produce a pulmonary infarction. Emboli are also being as a result of platelet lysis.

Clotting can occur in the heart and arteries, but it is more common in the veins because here the blood is relatively slow moving. The leg or pelvic veins are the most common sites of

venous thrombosis, and these carry a risk of subsequent pulmonary embolism. Venous thrombosis is promoted under various circumstances, e.g. after childbirth, and following abdominal operations; it is one of the reasons for encouraging early mobility in surgical patients. Thrombosis may also result from some blood conditions (including anaemia), infections, venous stagnation (as in varicose veins), prolonged bed rest enforced by operation or illness, inflammation, and degeneration of the vessel wall. Venous stagnation may be prevented by limb exercises, or, clinically, by the use of elastic stockings or intermittent pneumatic compression of the limbs.

Common arterial clotting sites are the vessels of the heart, leading to coronary-thrombosis-induced heart attack (myocardial infarction, MI), and the brain's cerebral vessels, leading to a stroke (cerebral vascular accident, CVA). Pulmonary infarctions (caused by pulmonary embolism), MIs and CVAs have high mortality rates (see Liu *et al.*, 2001).

Deteriorating blood vessels in older people may promote thrombosis within the retinal artery, with the resultant loss of vision, or thrombosis of leg arteries, resulting in gangrene of the foot. As a result of research that established a link between long-haul flights and thrombosis, international airlines have come under pressure to do more to prevent passengers form developing blood clots due to the cramped conditions. The UK government has instructed airlines to issue health warnings with long-haul flight tickets informing passengers of the risks of developing potentially fatal in-flight thrombosis.

Blood clotting is a continuous process in blood vessels, since roughened surfaces are constantly being formed (fatty streaks have been identified upon autopsies of children as young as 6 years old). However, coagulation is always corrected homeostatically by the body's own clot-preventing (e.g. heparin) and clot-dissolving mechanisms (e.g. prostacyclins), i.e. heparin and prostacyclins are endogenous protective mechanisms against intravascular thrombosis.

The clinical correction of clotting hyperactivity involves the administration of anticoagulants, which prevent clotting, or factors that enhance thrombus dissolution.

Anticoagulants

Heparin, a fast-acting anticoagulant, inhibits the conversion of prothrombin to thrombin. The liver, mast cells and tissues secrete heparin. Damage to blood vessels may cause the liver to reduce its secretion, and so remove this inhibitor to the clotting process. Heparin administration is useful in preventing postoperative thrombosis, and is vital for patients on haemodialysis, and those who are undergoing open-heart surgery and some other operations, in order to prevent potentially fatal clot formation. Heparin is ineffective if it is given orally, since the digestive system's proteolytic enzymes break it down, so it has to be administered intravenously (into the veins) to have an effect. It is extracted for clinical use from the lungs and guts of slaughtered cattle.

Prostacyclin (a prostaglandin) is also an endogenous anticoagulant that is secreted from the lining of healthy vessels. It inhibits platelet aggregation, and is thus a potential anti-thrombotic agent for clinical use. The drug dipyridamole enhances the action of prostacyclins.

Vitamin K antagonists (e.g. warfarin, phenindione, dicoumarol) are given orally to patients susceptible to thrombosis as a preventive measure. These drugs work by lowering the concentrations of prothrombin and clotting factors II, VIII, IX and X in plasma.

Various calcium-binding compounds may be added to sample blood as anticoagulants (e.g. ethylenediaminetetraacetic acid (EDTA) and acid citrate dextrose (ACD)) to prevent clotting in donated blood, blood banks and laboratories. These compounds reduce the ionic calcium in plasma, and so prevent the conversion of prothrombin into thrombin.

Nonsteroidal anti-inflammatory drugs (e.g. aspirin, phenylbutazone) prolong the bleeding time by inhibiting TXA2 (see The platelet phase above). Blood clotting may be inhibited by preventing the production of normal clotting factors, or preventing the normal function of clotting factors.

It is important that people taking anticoagulants are monitored carefully for bleeding, and have regular prothrombin time measurements for blood tests. Many drugs, including aspirin, should not be taken during anticoagulant therapy, unless prescribed specifically. Discharge planning by the nurse should include education about the drug and its effects, especially for bleeding patients. Patients need to carry an anticoagulant card, and to tell all healthcare professionals they deal with that they are taking anticoagulants. Where possible, they should avoid hazards at work and during leisure activities.

Thrombus dissolution

Thrombus dissolution therapy involves the administration of fibrolytic enzymes (e.g. streptokinase, urokinase), which promote endogenous plasmin production. Streptokinase was the first thrombolytic agent to be identified (in 1982) for dissolving clots in the coronary arteries. It is also now used extensively for removing pulmonary and deep-vein clots. Streptococcal bacteria produce this enzyme.

Haemophilia

Haemophilia affects 0.01% of the population (Huether and McCance, 1996). It is frequently called the 'bleeding disease' because people with haemophilia are at risk of excessive bleeding if accidental blood vessel damage occurs, or if they are subjected to factors that precipitate bleeding. An overindulgence of alcohol or penicillin may produce internal haemorrhage. In haemophilia, the gene necessary for the production of specific clotting factors is lacking, defective or not expressed. This gene is on the X sex chromosome, and the condition occurs predominantly in males (see Figure 20.19). Patients with the disorder are prone to repeated episodes of severe and prolonged bleeding at any site, particularly into muscles and joints with little evidence of trauma.

Haemophilia A is the most common type of haemophilia; it is associated with the absence of (or an abnormal) clotting factor VIII. Haemophilia B is known as 'Christmas disease'; it is a result of the inactivation of clotting factor IX (also known as Christmas factor).

Correction of bleeding conditions

Short-term correction for uncontrolled bleeding involves the application of thrombin, a fibrin spray, or a rough surface, such as gauze, as these encourage clotting at a wound. Long-term control involves the administration of the deficient aetiological factor, e.g. factor VIII for the treatment of classical haemophilia A. Major injuries and operations require special measures, such as plasma transfusions and the administration of concentrated anti-haemophilic factors, in order to reduce or control the symptoms.

BLOOD GROUPINGS

People are classified into one of several blood groups. This depends on the presence or absence of genetically determined antigens, the erythrocyte membrane, and antibodies called agglutinins or isoantibodies in the plasma.

The ABO system

The ABO grouping is based upon two antigens (in blood groups these are referred to as agglutinogens) called A and

B O X   1 1 . 2 6   B L O O D   G R O U P S

There are over 35 blood groups. The groups are designated letters (e.g. MNSc), or they are named after the person who identified them (e.g. Lewis, Duffy, Kidd). Although these groups are of immense importance in forensic medicine, only two principal blood group systems, the ABO and rhesus systems, are important clinically. This is because transfusion of an inappropriate type of blood can promote clumping (agglutination) of red cells in the recipient, and consequently should be avoided at all cost.

B O X   1 1 . 2 7   A B O   A G G L U T I N I N S

The anti-A and anti-B agglutinins are antibodies of the IgM type (see Chapter 13). They appear at, or just after, birth, and they exist throughout life, although their production may decline or disappear during old age. Their occurrence in the blood is not understood, since they are produced even in the absence of contact with the non-self antigen.

B, and two agglutinins called anti-A (alpha, α) or anti-B (beta, β). The agglutinogens are attached to the membrane of the erythrocytes, and the agglutinins are found in the plasma.

The four blood groups associated with the ABO system are groups A, B, AB and O. Their frequencies exhibit ethnic variation, but in England they are 43%, 8%, 3% and 46%, respectively. People of group A have the A agglutinogen group; group B people have B agglutinogens;

group AB people have both A and B agglutinogens; and group O people do not possess either agglutinogen (Figure 11.19). If you follow the simple rule that the group is named after the agglutinogens present, then you will be able to predict which plasma agglutinins (if any) will also be present. This is because there are only two agglutinins, anti-A and anti-B, and these interact with opposing agglutinogens A and B, respectively. It is essential to have different agglutinins and agglutinogens in order to prevent auto-cross-reactions that would cause agglutination and haemolysis, as shown in Figure 11.19(b). This reaction could be fatal if the clump of erythrocytes blocked a blood vessel to a vital organ, such as the heart.

Inheritance of the ABO blood groups

Exercise

Before reading this section, familiarize yourself with the terms 'genotype', 'phenotype', 'alleles', 'allelic variation', 'homozygous' and 'heterozygous' (see Chapter 20).

Chromosome 9 contains the alleles A, B and O that determine the ABO blood group. Alleles A and B are co-dominant to each other; both are dominant to the recessive allele O. Thus, there are six genotypes that determine the four blood group phenotypes of the ABO system (Figure 11.19a). Blood group A is derived from homozygous dominant A (i.e. alleles AA) or heterozygous A (i.e. alleles AO) genotypes. Group B is derived from either the homozygous B (i.e. alleles BB) or the heterozygous B (i.e.

B O X   1 1 . 2 8   C R O S S - M A T C H I N G   B L O O D ,   A N D   B L O O D   T R A N S F U S I O N S

Before the patient receives a transfusion of blood cells, a specimen of blood is obtained for cross-matching with that of the donor. Stringent procedures are followed in identifying the patient's blood to ensure that the transfused blood is compatible. Mistakes do still occur, however, and nursing vigilance and adherence to checking procedures and policies is essential safe practice.

These principles are important when considering the essentials of successful blood transfusions. It is important to remember, however, that it is the effect of the recipient's plasma agglutinins on the donor's erythrocyte agglutinogens that may cause problems. This is because of the vast numbers of red blood cells (i.e. 5 million/mm^3) with their attached antigens that are transferred. The donor's plasma agglutinins are ignored, since the greater volume of fluid of the recipient soon dilutes them. Thus, agglutination will occur whenever recipient agglutinins and donor agglutinogens of the same type are mixed. Such blood is said to be incompatible; Figure 11.19(c) shows which transfusion combinations can be successful. For example, blood group A can be transfused into its own blood group. However, it cannot be

transfused into blood group B, since the recipient has plasma anti-A agglutinins, which would react against the donor's agglutinogens, i.e. agglutination will occur. Group A can also be a donor to blood group AB, since AB people do not possess either anti-A or anti-B agglutinins. Group AB individuals are known as 'universal recipients', as they can receive blood from any other blood group. Blood groups A, B and AB cannot be donors for blood group O because O recipients have agglutinins anti-A and anti-B, and the A, B and AB groups possess at least one agglutinogen. Conversely, group O individuals are 'universal donors': they can give blood to any other blood group, since they do not have agglutinogens A or B on their surface, and antibody–antigen reactions will therefore not be initiated.

The use of the term 'universal' has fallen into disuse nowadays, however, since this term means all possible circumstances, and takes no account of blood group systems other than the ABO. Usually, blood of the same group within the ABO system will be used to prevent any possibility of mixing incompatible bloods.

(a)

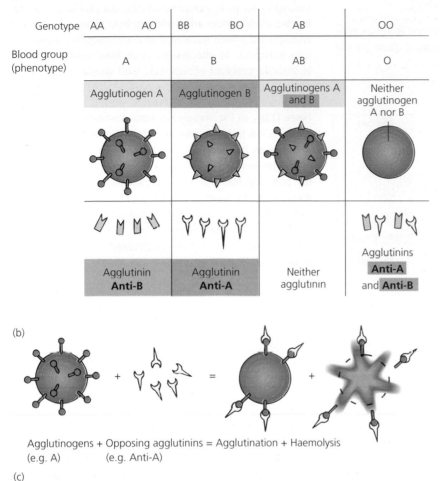

Figure 11.19 (a) Blood grouping. The blood group depends upon the presence of antigens (agglutinogens) on the surface of red cells. This is determined by alleles A, B and O. The plasma contains antibodies (agglutinins) that will react with 'foreign' agglutinogens, i.e. a reaction takes place when the agglutinogens are of the same variety of agglutinins.

Q. What are the frequencies within the UK population of blood groups: A, B, AB and O?

(b)

Agglutinogens + Opposing agglutinins = Agglutination + Haemolysis
(e.g. A)   (e.g. Anti-A)

(b) Cross-reactions (incompatible transfusions) occur when the plasma's agglutinins (antibodies) encounter complementary erythrocyte agglutinogens (antigens). The result is extensive clumping (agglutination) of the affected red cells, and subsequent haemolysis.
Q. Distinguish between agglutinogens and agglutinins.
Q. Which antibodies are present in blood group A?

(c) ABO transfusion combinations.

(c)

	Donors			
Groups	A	B	AB	O
Group				
Recipients A	✓	✗	✗	✓
B	✗	✓	✗	✓
AB	✓	✓	✓	✓
O	✗	✗	✗	✓

Key: ✓ = Compatible transfusion   ✗ = Incompatible transfusion

alleles BO) genotypes. People of blood group AB have both alleles A and B. Group O people are homozygous for O alleles, which are incapable of coding for agglutinogens.

The rhesus blood group and its inheritance

The rhesus system is so called because it was first identified in the rhesus monkey. People are classified as having rhesus-positive (Rh-negative) or rhesus-negative (Rh-positive) blood, according to the presence or absence of the rhesus antigen. About 85% of the UK population is rhesus positive, i.e. they possess the rhesus agglutinogen (called the rhesus or D factor) on the surface of the red cells. The remaining 15% of the population are rhesus negative, i.e. they do not possess the rhesus agglutinogen. The dominant rhesus (D) gene found on chromosome 1 controls the presence of the agglutinogen. Thus, the possible genotypes responsible for determining the rhesus groupings are:

- homozygous dominant (alleles DD) and heterozygous (Dd): these people will be rhesus positive;

- homozygous recessive (dd): this genotype is not capable of coding for the rhesus agglutinogen, so these people will be rhesus negative.

Scientists experimenting with the possibility of interconverting blood groups are investigating the problem concerning the availability of adequate supply of stored blood. Early attempts have been successful in converting blood group B into group O. In the future, such interconversions may abolish the problem of regional blood shortages.

	Father	Mother
Parents' genotype	DD	dd
Gametes	D and D	d and d
Offspring genotype	Dd Dd	Dd Dd
Offspring's blood group (phenotype)	Rh+ Rh+	Rh+ Rh+

	Father	Mother
Parents' genotype	Dd	dd
Gametes	D and d	d and d
Offspring genotype	Dd Dd	dd dd
Offspring's blood group (phenotype)	Rh+ Rh+	Rh− Rh−

(a)

Figure 11.20 (a) The inheritance of rhesus-positive (Rh+) offspring. There is a 75% chance of producing a rhesus-positive child from a rhesus-positive father and a rhesus-negative (Rh-) mother, because the father could be homozygous dominant (DD) or heterozygous (Dd). Thus, both possibilities have to be taken into consideration when calculating the probability of producing a rhesus-positive child from these two parental phenotypes. (b) Pregnancy and rhesus incompatibility.

Q. What accounts for the symptoms of haemolytic disease of the newborn (HDNB), and how can this be prevented?

Q. Why is the firstborn baby unlikely to have HDNB?

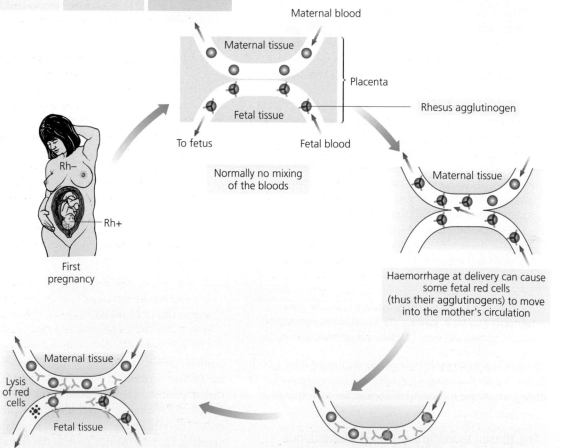

Maternal blood

Maternal tissue

Placenta

Fetal tissue

Rhesus agglutinogen

To fetus

Fetal blood

Normally no mixing of the bloods

Rh−

Rh+

First pregnancy

Maternal tissue

Haemorrhage at delivery can cause some fetal red cells (thus their agglutinogens) to move into the mother's circulation

Maternal tissue

Lysis of red cells

Fetal tissue

Second pregnancy
Maternal agglutinins being of the IgG variety can pass over the selectively permeable placenta. This causes antibody–antigen complexing and its subsequent consequences (HDNB; see text for details)

Maternal agglutinin production in response to the above 'antigenic insult'

(b)

Unlike the ABO system, the plasma of rhesus-negative people does not normally contain rhesus antibodies (agglutinins). However, transfusion of rhesus-positive erythrocytes into a rhesus-negative recipient may stimulate a response in the recipient with the release of anti-D (anti-rhesus) agglutinins. These agglutinins cause agglutination and haemolysis of the transfused cells. When considering transfusions, therefore, the rhesus factor must also be taken into consideration in order to minimize the risks of incompatible transfusions and their fatal outcomes.

Using Figure 11.19, explain the rationale of the following:

- Blood group A can donate to groups A and AB, and receive blood from groups A and O.
- Blood group O can donate to all other groups, but can receive blood only from group O.
- Blood group B can donate blood to group B and AB, and receive blood from groups B and O.
- Blood group AB can donate only to group AB, but can receive from all other groups.
- Blood group O negative is used as a universal donor in UK accident and emergency departments when a patient has had a significant blood loss.
- Blood group O positive cannot donate blood to group O negative.

Complications may occur if a rhesus-negative mother bears a rhesus-positive fetus, which is possible since the genotype of the fetus may be different to that of the mother. Genetically, there is a 75% chance of this occurring if the father is rhesus positive (Figure 11.20(a)).

Under normal circumstances in pregnancy, there is no mixing of fetal and maternal bloods, although the two circulations are in very close proximity within the placental unit. During childbirth, however, severe contractions of the uterus wall may squeeze some fetal rhesus-positive erythrocytes into the maternal circulation (Figure 11.20(b)). The fetal agglutinins passed into the maternal circulation do not pose a risk to the mother, as the large maternal blood volume dilutes their effects many-fold.

Maternal anti-D agglutinins are not produced in significant amounts against this 'antigenic insult' until after the delivery, and so the first infant is not affected. The small agglutinins (gamma immunoglobulins, IgG), however, are capable of crossing the placental membranes and entering the blood of subsequent fetuses. If the fetus is rhesus positive, then the anti-D antibodies will cause a transfusion reaction. This is referred to as haemolytic disease of the newborn (HDNB). This disease can be monitored in utero by amniocentesis, which samples amniotic fluid (for bilirubin assessment), and by fetoscopy, which obtains fetal blood samples for blood analysis. Both processes carry a risk of miscarriage, however.

Without treatment, such cases may result in stillbirths or neonatal death soon after delivery. Premature delivery may be induced after 7–8 months of development. Before this time, and in severe cases, the fetus can also be treated successfully by intrauterine transfusions. Neonates with HDNB have anaemia coupled with jaundice because the resultant rhesus antibody–antigen reactions cause excessive haemolysis (resulting in anaemia), and the metabolized pigment (now bilirubin) becomes deposited in the skin, mucous membranes and the eyes (leading to jaundice).

Correction after birth depends upon the severity of the condition. It may involve an exchange transfusion, whereby the neonate's entire rhesus-positive blood is replaced with rhesus-negative blood. The transfused blood will eventually be replaced by the baby's own rhesus positive blood, by which time the signs and symptoms of anaemia and jaundice will have disappeared. Milder forms of jaundice may not require an exchange transfusion, and principles of correction will then involve the application of artificial ultraviolet (UV) light. The UV light converts the fat soluble bilirubin into water soluble biliverdin, which is excreted in the urine.

There is no equivalent haemolytic disease of the newborn with reference to the ABO system. This is because the anti-A and anti-B antibodies are of the IgM type, and so are too large to pass through the placental membranes. However, problems can occur if there is damage to the maternal–fetal placental unit.

Rhesus immunization

If a risk of HDNB is known, the potential problem is avoidable by rhesus immunization, i.e. administration of anti-D. Anti-D destroys any fetal cells that may have passed into the maternal blood before they have time to stimulate the mother's own immune response. Anti-D is given in the following cases:

- when a rhesus-negative woman has become reactive (sensitized) to rhesus-positive blood cells, and who has given birth to a rhesus-positive baby;
- to prevent sensitization of a rhesus-negative woman before giving birth;
- to a rhesus-negative women having an abortion, unless it is shown that the fetus is rhesus negative;
- to a rhesus-negative woman who has not become reactive to rhesus-positive blood cells, following an incident during pregnancy that may lead to bleeding across the placenta (the afterbirth) or of the fetus;
- to prevent sensitization of a rhesus-negative woman who has been given, for any reason, blood components containing rhesus-positive red blood cells.

Anti-D should not be injected intravenously since it may cause a severe reaction. Injection should be intramuscular, so that the antibody enters the blood at a much slower rate. Care should be taken to draw back the plunger of the syringe before injecting, in order to be sure that the needle is not in a blood vessel. Injection should be within 72 h whenever possible, to have the best effects; however, if an incident occurs during pregnancy, then the injection should be given at the time of the incident to be most effective. After 72 h, the mother's immune system may begin to respond significantly to any fetal blood cells.

The use of anti-D may interfere with the response of other vaccines, especially MMR (measles, mumps and rubella) and varicella (chickenpox) vaccines. Such vaccinations should be given at least 3 weeks before, or at least 3 months after, anti-D.

BOX 11.31 ANTI-D DOSAGES

As a preventive measure before birth, 500 IU anti-D is given at 28 and 34 weeks to potential at-risk mothers following an incident during pregnancy and up to 20 weeks, the recommended dose is 250 IU. After this period, the recommended dose is 500 IU. Following birth, 500 IU is usually administered. For women given blood components containing Rh-positive cells, the recommended dose is 125 IU/ml of red cells that has been injected.

Summary

1 Blood is the fluid that, under normal circumstances, is contained within the cardiovascular system. Its main components are plasma and erythrocytes.

2 Additional components found in smaller concentrations are other cellular elements – leucocytes and thrombocytes – and non-cellular materials dissolved in the plasma. The latter include organic substances (nutrients, enzyme, hormone, urea, etc.) and inorganic substances (cationic and anionic electrolytes).

3 All components of blood must be maintained within their homeostatic parameters to maintain blood volume (hence blood pressure), interchange materials vital to maintain intracellular homeostasis, and combat pathogenic infection.

4 Deviations in the homeostatic ranges of blood constituents, together with the presence of abnormal constituents (e.g. cytoplasmic chemicals, such as cardiac-specific enzymes),

make serum analysis one of the most important clinical diagnostic tools.

5 Wound healing involves a number of homeostatic responses at cellular and biochemicals levels.

6 Haemostasis (blood clotting) is a homeostatic mechanism that prevents the loss of blood when a blood vessel is damaged. It involves the activation of both extrinsic and intrinsic pathways.

7 Intravascular thrombosis is a result of the activation of the intrinsic clotting mechanism.

8 Thrombocytes (platelets) have an essential role in activating the enzyme-controlled clotting cascade.

9 Different blood groups are associated with genetically determined differences in antigens on erythrocyte membranes and antibodies in blood serum.

10 The ABO and rhesus blood grouping systems are used to classify blood donated for transfusion.

Review questions

1 What is erythropoiesis?

2 Which hormone controls the production of red blood cells?

3 Which nutrients in the diet are required for the production of healthy red blood cells?

4 Describe the structure of haemoglobin. What is its function?

5 Define the term 'anaemia'. What are the common causes of anaemia? What are the signs and symptoms of it?

6 Iron-deficiency anaemia is very prevalent, and affects people of both sexes and of all age groups. As a nurse, which of your patient groups are most at risk of developing this condition, and why? How can you assist clients in preventing the development of this condition?

7 What is leukaemia? Which cells are affected?

REFERENCES

Browne, A., Lachance, V. and Pipe, A. (1999) The ethics of blood testing as an element of doping control in sport. *Medicine and Science in Sports and Exercise*, **31**(4): 497–501.

Clancy, J. and McVicar, A.J. (1996a) Homeostasis: the key concept in physiological control. *British Journal of Theatre Nursing* **6**(2): .

Clancy, J. and McVicar, A.J. (1996b) Shock: a failure to maintain cardiovascular homeostasis. *British Journal of Theatre Nursing* **6**(6): .

Clancy, J. and McVicar, A,J. (1997) Wound healing: a series of homeostatic responses. *British Journal of Theatre Nursing* **7**(4): 25–33.

Clancy, J and McVicar, A.J. (eds.) (1998) Nursing Care: a homeostatic casebook, London: Arnold.

Collier, M. (1996) The principles of optimum wound management. *Nursing Standard* **10**(43): .

Department of Health (1996) *The NHS Performance Guide 1995–1996*. London: HMSO.

DeCruz, G. (1998) The case of a man with a surgical wound. Case study cited in Clancy and McVicar (1998).

Flanagan, M. (1996) A practical framework for wound healing assessment 1: physiology. *British Journal of Nursing* **5**(22): 1391–7.

Flanagan, M. (1997) Wound healing and management. *Primary Health Care* **7**(4): 31–9.

Hinchcliff, S.M, Norman, S.E. and Scober, J.E. (1998) *Nursing Practice and Health Care*. London: Edward Arnold.

Huether, S.E. and McCance, K.L. (1996) *Understanding Pathophysiology*. London: Mosby.

Johns, A. (1998) Overview of bone marrow and stem cell transplantation. *Journal of Intravenous Nursing* **21**(6): 356–60.

Liu, M., Counsell, C., and Sandercock, P. (2001) Anticoagulation for preventing recurrence following ischaemic stroke or transient ischaemic attack. The Cochrane Library, Issue 1. Oxford: Update Software.

McVicar, A.J. and Clancy, J. (1997) The physiological basis of fluid therapy. *Professional Nurse* **12**(8).

Norfolk Health (1996) *Wound Care Guidelines*. Unpublished work.

Provan, D. and Weatherall, D. (2000) Haematology. Red cells II: acquired anaemias and polycythaemia. *Lancet* **355**(9211): 1260–8.

Silver I.A. (1994) The physiology of wound healing. *Journal of Wound Care* **3**(2): 106–9.

Smith, M.E. (1998) Facing death: donor and recipient responses to the gift of life. *Holistic Nursing Practice* **13**(1): 32–40.

FURTHER READING

Baugh, R.F. (2000) Platelets and whole blood coagulation. *Perfusion* **15**(1): 41–50.

Clancy, J. and McVicar, A.J. (eds) (1998) *Nursing Care: a homeostatic casebook*. London: Arnold.

Hutten, B.A. and Prins, M.H. (2001) Duration of treatment with vitamin K antagonists in symptomatic venous thromboembolism. The Cochrane Library. Oxford: Update Software.

Chapter 12

The cardiovascular system 2: the heart and circulation

INTRODUCTION: RELATION OF THE CARDIOVASCULAR SYSTEM TO CELLULAR HOMEOSTASIS

The cardiovascular system consists of the heart and the blood vessels of the body. The relation of this system to cellular homeostasis is that it delivers nutrients, oxygen, hormones, etc. to the cells of the body, and removes 'waste' products of metabolism from them, so preventing toxicity. The cardiovascular system, however, requires the co-operative functioning of other systems in order to maintain blood composition and so preserve intracellular homeostasis. For example, the digestive and excretory organs are instrumental in maintaining the homeostatic constitution of blood, and the autonomic nervous system and endocrine system co-ordinate cardiovascular (and other system) functions. Each co-operative component is a homeostatic control system, and a disturbance in one results in malfunction of another as a consequence of the interdependency of organ system function, as discussed in Chapter 1.

Cardiovascular function must be adaptable if adequate blood flow to the tissues is to be maintained during the varying metabolic demands, that occur during surgery, trauma, times of distress and when resting or exercising, since there is only a limited volume of blood available in the body. Blood may be directed to where it is needed most, and away from the less active areas, but at all times there must be an adequate blood flow to the most vital organs (brain and heart), since these high-priority tissues are particularly sensitive to reduced blood supply.

The cardiovascular system, therefore, provides the transport 'hardware' that keeps blood continuously circulating to fulfil intracellular homeostatic requirements. The heart (= 'cardio-') is the transport system's pump; the delivery routes are the hollow blood vessels (= 'vascular') leading from, and eventually back to, the heart (Figure 12.1). The blood is the transport medium.

The essential principles underlying the homeostasis of blood composition were described in Chapter 11. This chapter describes:

- specific aspects of the heart, including its size, location, functional anatomy, coronary circulation, conduction system and related electrocardiography, the cardiac cycle, and cardiac output;

- the functional anatomy of the arterial, capillary and venous systems, the routes of circulation, and the homeostatic control of blood pressure;

- some common examples of cardiovascular homeostatic failures and their principles of correction;

- developmental changes regarding the cardiovascular system.

Exercise

Reflect on your understanding of how cardiovascular function aids the maintenance of intracellular homeostasis.

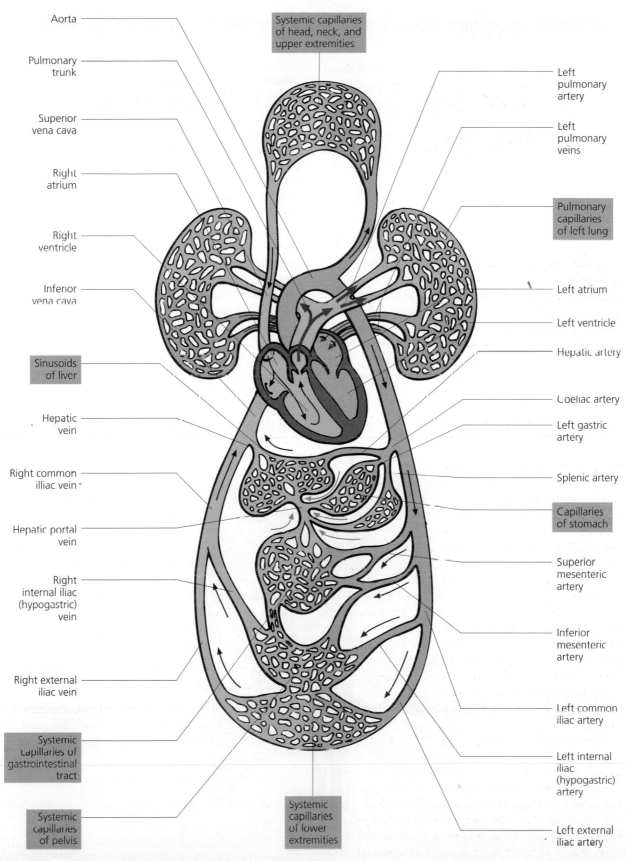

Aorta

Pulmonary trunk

Superior vena cava

Right atrium

Right ventricle

Inferior vena cava

Sinusoids of liver

Hepatic vein

Right common iliac vein

Hepatic portal vein

Right internal iliac (hypogastric) vein

Right external iliac vein

Systemic capillaries of gastrointestinal tract

Systemic capillaries of pelvis

Systemic capillaries of head, neck, and upper extremities

Left pulmonary artery

Left pulmonary veins

Pulmonary capillaries of left lung

Left atrium

Left ventricle

Hepatic artery

Coeliac artery

Left gastric artery

Splenic artery

Capillaries of stomach

Superior mesenteric artery

Inferior mesenteric artery

Left common iliac artery

Left internal iliac (hypogastric) artery

Systemic capillaries of lower extremities

Left external iliac artery

Figure 12.1   Circulatory routes. Black arrows show systemic circulation; thick red arrows in the pulmonary blood vessels show pulmonary circulation; thin green arrows indicate hepatic portal circulation.

Q. Describe the route taken by blood as it moves from the right atrium to the kidneys and back to the right atrium.

OVERVIEW OF THE ANATOMY AND PHYSIOLOGY OF THE CARDIOVASCULAR SYSTEM 1: THE HEART

The main role of the heart is to promote the flow of blood throughout the body in one direction. It also produces a hormone that is important in maintaining blood volume hence blood pressure. Flow of blood is promoted by the generation of a pressure gradient, and the pumping action of the heart is responsible for elevating blood pressure sufficiently to maintain an adequate blood supply to the tissues.

The volume of blood removed from the heart by this pumping action must match the volume of blood entering the heart during the 'filling' phase of the pump cycle, otherwise the heart will become congested (see Box 12.17). This in turn relates to the physical activity being performed by the body: an increase in activity reduces the time taken for blood to circulate around the body, so the heart must pump more blood per unit time. The heart, then, has to be versatile, with a variable pumping rate according to the needs of the body. The control of the heart pump is described later. This section outlines the basic structure and functioning of the heart in relation to the unidirectional flow of blood through it.

Heart size and location

Figure 12.2 shows that the heart is located obliquely (since the heart tips slightly to the left) between the lungs, and is enclosed within the medial cavity of the thorax, called the mediastinum. It lies anterior to the vertebral column and posterior to the sternum. The heart weighs approximately 250–350 g; its size is often compared with the person's closed fist to demonstrate the approximate, but variable, dimensions. The heart's broad 'base', formed by the upper chambers, or atria, is about 9 cm wide, and projects superiorly and posteriorly towards the right shoulder, extending some 12–14 cm within the second or third intercostal space. The organ is fixed by vessels at its base, thus allowing its more pointed apex to move upwards on contraction. The apex, formed by the tip of the lower chambers, or ventricles, of the heart (particularly the left ventricle), is directed inferiorly and anteriorly towards the left hip. It rests on a muscle called the diaphragm, which separates the thoracic and abdominal regions of the body's

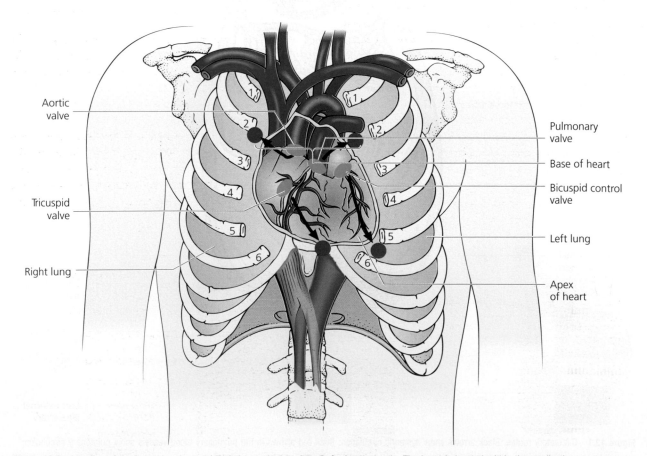

Figure 12.2 Location of the heart, heart valves ● and auscultation sites ● for heart sounds. The heart is located within the mediastinum, which is the middle region of the thoracic cavity.

trunk. The apical heartbeat, produced by contraction of the heart muscle, can be felt on the left side of the chest about 8 cm from the sternum between the fifth and sixth intercostal spaces. Approximately two-thirds of the heart is located to the left of the sternum.

The upper border of the heart, formed by the atrial chambers, is where the great vessels called the aorta, vena cavae and pulmonary artery enter and leave the heart.

Functional anatomy of the heart

The heart is a four-chambered structure enclosed within a supportive and protective membrane called the pericardium. The walls of the heart are comprised mainly of a specialized form of muscle called cardiac muscle (or myocardium). The chambers of the heart are separated by walls of tissue called septa. Communication between the atria and ventricles is provided by valve structures.

The pericardium

The pericardium ('peri-' = around) is a membranous sac comprised of two layers: the fibrous pericardium and the serous pericardium (Figure 12.3). The former is a tough, dense connective tissue layer, which protects the heart and anchors it to the diaphragm, great vessels and sternum. Although the fibrous pericardium holds the heart in position, it is flexible enough to allow sufficient movement, so that the heart can contract vigorously and rapidly when the need arises. The serous pericardium is a thinner, more delicate membrane, which forms a double layer around the heart. The outer (or parietal) layer lines the inner surface of the fibrous pericardium. The inner (or visceral) layer (also called the epicardium, meaning 'upon the heart') is attached to the muscle layer of the heart. Between these two serous layers is the pericardial cavity, which is a thin potential space containing a film of watery fluid. The tension produced by this film holds the two

layers together. The fluid also prevents friction between the membranes when the heart contracts.

The heart wall

The wall of the heart consists of three layers: the epicardium (a component of the pericardium), the myocardium ('myo-' = muscle), and the endocardium ('endo-' = inner) (Figure 12.3).

The myocardium
The myocardium forms the bulk of the heart wall. Upon contraction, it is responsible for pumping blood into the vessels of the circulatory system. The structure of cardiac muscle is discussed later. The external surface of the myocardium is lined by epicardium, and the internal surface by endocardium.

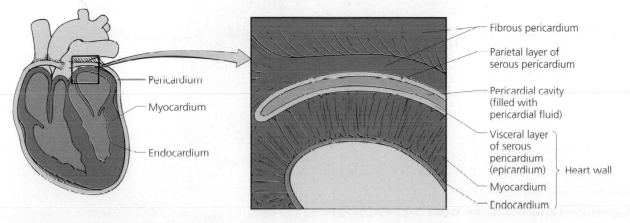

Figure 12.3 The pericardial layers and the heart wall.

The endocardium

The endocardium is continuous with the endothelial lining of blood vessels leaving and entering the heart, and also covers the valves between the heart chambers. It is a smooth, glistening, white sheet of squamous endothelium, which rests on a thin sheet of connective tissue. Its smooth surface prevents activation of the blood-clotting cascade. The presence of fat, calcium or fibrin deposits roughens the endocardium and enhances the likelihood of blood clotting.

Exercise

Reflect on your understanding of the clotting mechanism described in Chapter 11. Identify the clotting pathway (intrinsic or extrinsic) that instigates the common coagulation pathway to promote intravascular thrombosis.

The heart chambers

The heart's interior is divided into four hollow chambers that receive circulating blood. The two upper chambers are called atria (singular = atrium), and the two lower chambers are called ventricles (Figure 12.4). An internal partition divides the heart longitudinally and forms the interatrial and interventricular septa (singular = septum), which separate the two atria and two ventricles, respectively. The interatrial septum possesses an oval depression called the fossa ovalis. This structure corresponds to the location of the foramen ovale ('foramen' = window), an opening in the fetal heart that diverts blood away from the lungs since the placenta, rather than the lungs, provides the route for gaseous exchange (see Box 12.3).

Each atrium is separated from its respective ventricle by an atrioventricular valve. The atria are the receiving chambers for blood returning to the heart from the circulation. They are small and thin-walled, since they need to contract only minimally to push the blood a short distance to the ventricles (very little pressure is generated within the atria during their contraction). Flow into the ventricles is also encouraged by gravity. The ventricles are the discharging chambers, and form the actual pumps of the heart; accordingly, ventricular walls are thicker than atrial walls since they must generate a greater pressure to promote adequate output. However, the muscular wall of the right ventricle is thinner than that of the left, since the right ventricular pump is responsible for circulating blood in the

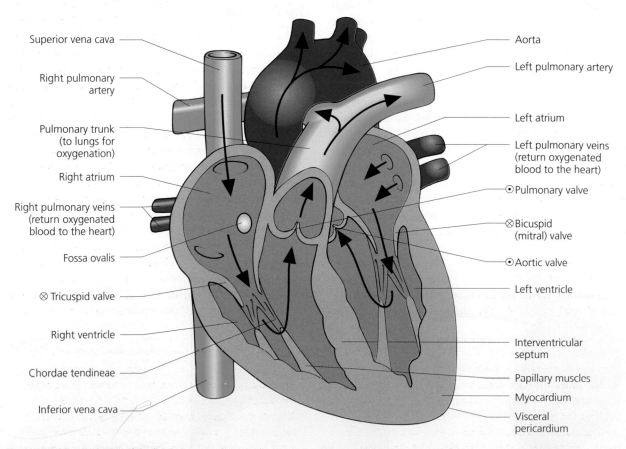

Figure 12.4 Frontal section of the heart.

⊗ Atrioventricular (AV) valves (tricuspid and bicuspid). ⊙ Semilunar valves (pulmonary and aortic).

Q. Describe the path of blood flow through the heart.

low-resistance circulation of the lungs, whereas the left ventricular pump is responsible for circulating blood to the rest of the body and must generate a much higher pressure to maintain this.

The heart valves

Blood flow through the heart and the circulatory system must be unidirectional if haemodynamic efficiency is to be maintained. Valves in the heart (and in the larger veins; see later) maintain this one-way flow. There are four heart valves: the paired atrioventricular and semilunar valves (Figure 12.4). These open and close passively in response to differences in blood pressure on the two sides of the valve.

The atrioventricular valves
The atrioventricular (AV) valve between the right atrium and the right ventricle is often called the tricuspid valve because it contains three cusps or flaps. Similarly, the AV valve between the left atrium and the left ventricle is the bicuspid (or mitral valve) because it consists of two cusps (and because of its resemblance to a bishop's mitre). The cusps are fibrous connective tissue covered with endocardium that extends from the chamber walls; their pointed ends project into the ventricles. White collagen fibres called the chordae tendineae, or 'heart strings', anchor the cusps to small papillary muscles within the ventricles.

The tendineae keep the valve flaps pointing in the direction of blood flow, so that the AV valve opens when blood is passed from atrium to ventricle. At this point, the papillary muscles relax and the chordae tendineae slacken, allowing the valves to open (Figure 12.5(a)). Upon ventricular contraction, however, blood is pumped out of the ventricle into an artery; any blood tending to pass back towards the atria drives the valve cusps upwards until they close the opening. Papillary muscles also contract, which tightens the chordae tendineae and prevents the flaps from inverting into the atria (Figure 12.5(b)).

The semilunar valves
The semilunar valves are so-called because of their half-moon shaped cusps. Aortic and pulmonary semilunar valves are located at the bases of the large arteries, the aorta and pulmonary artery, which leave the left and right ventricles, respectively. Their role is to encourage unidirectional flow from ventricle to artery. The mechanism of action is different from that of the AV valves. Upon ventricle contraction, the semilunar valves are forced open, and their cusps become flattened against the arterial wall as blood is ejected (Figure 12.5(c)). Upon ventricular relaxation, pressure within the ventricle falls; blood is no longer propelled forward, but begins to flow backwards. This causes the cusps to close, which prevents backward flow into the ventricles (Figure 12.5(d)).

A heart murmur is an abnormal rushing or gurgling noise heard before, between or after the normal heart sounds, or a sound that masks the normal heart sounds (Criley, 1999). Most murmurs indicate a valve disorder. Certain infectious diseases of the endocardium can damage heart valves, which are made up of this tissue. Endocardial damage can be congenital or acquired. The acquired forms cause inflammation (ischaemia), degenerative or infectious alterations of valve structure and hence function. The usual cause of acquired valve dysfunction is inflammation of the endocardium, secondary to acute rheumatic fever (hence why most patients are now elderly following rheumatic fever in childhood), which usually follows a streptococcal infection of the throat. These bacteria stimulate an immunological response, in which antibodies attack the bacteria but inflame the connective tissue of the heart valves. This can cause the cusps of the valve to stick together, thus narrowing their openings (a process called stenosis). Subsequent damage to the edges of the cusps impairs closure, and backward flow occurs. The valve is now said to be 'leaky' or incompetent. Although stenosis (Figures 12.6 (b) and (c)) and incompetence (Figures 12.6 (b) and (d)) may coexist, often one predominates.

In both instances, the pumping efficiency of the heart declines and, as a consequence, the workload of the heart is increased. However, severe valve deformity is required to cause serious impairment. In such cases, the heart ultimately becomes weakened, which can cause heart failure. It is the mitral valve that is usually affected, since pressure differentials developed by the left ventricle are greater than those across the tricuspid valve are. Mitral incompetence occurs in 10–15% of the population (Nagle and O'Keefe, 1999). Valve dysfunction is treated with

---

BOX 12.2 NORMAL HEART SOUNDS AND HEART MURMURS

When listening to a person's heart with a stethoscope, one does not hear the opening of the valves, since this is a silent, relatively slowly developing process. Valve closure is more sudden, however, and the sudden pressure differentials that develop across the valve produce vibrations of the valve and the surrounding fluid. The sounds given off travel in all directions through the chest; these are best heard at the surface of the chest in locations that differ slightly from the actual location of the valves (see Figure 12.2).

When ventricles first contract, the closure of the AV valves produces a long, booming sound, since the vibration is low in pitch and is of relatively long duration. This is the first heart (or Korotkoff) sound, and is described as 'lubb'. The second heart sound – 'dupp' – is caused by the closure of the semilunar valves at the beginning of ventricular relaxation. This sound is a relatively rapid 'snap', since valve closure is extremely fast, thus the surroundings vibrate for only a short period of time.

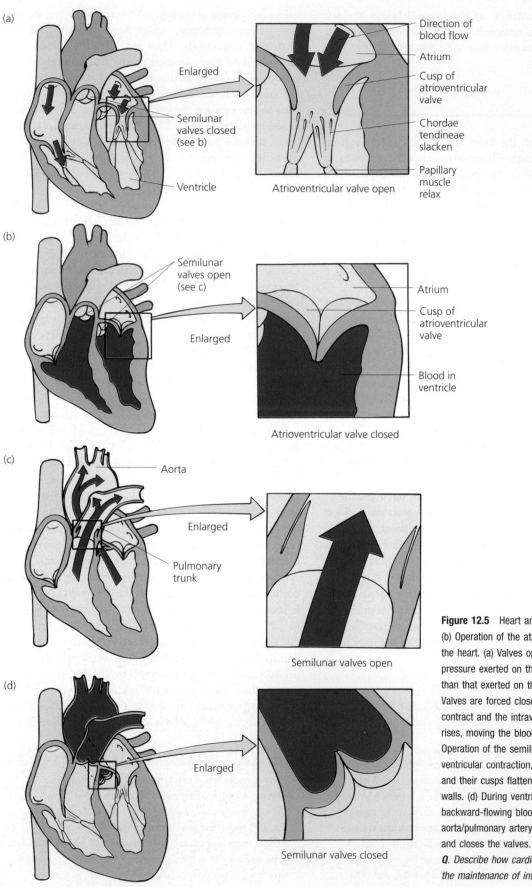

(a) Enlarged

Direction of blood flow

Atrium

Cusp of atrioventricular valve

Chordae tendineae slacken

Papillary muscle relax

Semilunar valves closed (see b)

Ventricle

Atrioventricular valve open

(b) Semilunar valves open (see c)

Enlarged

Atrium

Cusp of atrioventricular valve

Blood in ventricle

Atrioventricular valve closed

(c) Aorta

Enlarged

Pulmonary trunk

Semilunar valves open

(d) Enlarged

Semilunar valves closed

Figure 12.5 Heart and valve action. (a) and (b) Operation of the atrioventricular valves of the heart. (a) Valves open when blood pressure exerted on the atrial side is greater than that exerted on the ventricular side. (b) Valves are forced closed when the ventricles contract and the intraventricular pressure rises, moving the blood upwards. (c) and (d) Operation of the semilunar valves. (c) During ventricular contraction, the valves are open and their cusps flatten against their arterial walls. (d) During ventricular relaxation, the backward-flowing blood in the aorta/pulmonary artery fills the valve cusp and closes the valves.

Q. Describe how cardiovascular function aids the maintenance of intracellular homeostasis.

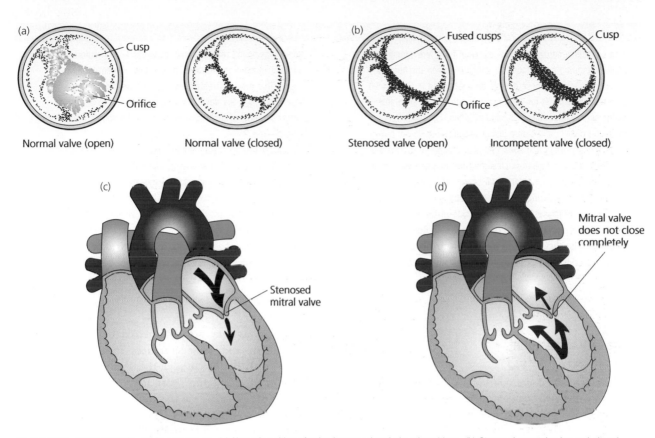

Figure 12.6 Valve stenosis and incompetence. (a) Normal position of valve in opened and closed positions. (b) Stenosed opened valve and closed incompetence valve. (c) In mitral stenosis, the valve is unable to open sufficiently during left atrial emptying, resulting in improper filling of the left ventricle. The left atrial wall has to work harder, hence its muscle wall thickens (hypertrophy). (d) In mitral incompetence, the valve does not close properly. During left ventricular emptying, some blood is returned to the left atria.

cardiac glycosides (e.g. digoxin), diuretics (e.g. bendroflu-azide), dietary salt restriction and antibiotics (e.g. penicillin) until the faulty valve needs to be replaced surgically with a synthetic or animal (usually pig) heart valve (Heuther and McCance, 1996).

Path of blood flow through the heart

The right atrium receives deoxygenated blood (i.e. blood that has given up some of its oxygen as it passes through tissues) from all parts of the body except the lungs. Blood enters the atrium via three vessels:

- the superior vena cava, which returns blood from structures above the heart (i.e. head, neck and arms);

- the inferior vena cava, which returns blood from structures below the heart (i.e. the trunk and legs);

- the coronary sinus, which collects blood from most of the vessels supplying the heart wall.

Relaxation of the atrium muscle enlarges the chamber and creates a suction pressure that draws blood into the right atrium (the entrances of the above vessels are not

guarded by valves). This atrium delivers blood to the right ventricle upon opening of the tricuspid valve. The right ventricle then pumps blood to the lungs via the pulmonary 'trunk' vessel through the opened pulmonary (semilunar) valve. Simultaneously, the tricuspid valve closes to prevent back flow. The pulmonary trunk divides into right and left pulmonary arteries, which take the blood to the right and left lungs, respectively. Oxygenation of blood takes place in lung tissue, and the blood is transported to the left atrium via the four pulmonary veins (two from each lung). Blood flows into the left atrium upon atrial relaxation, which again creates a suction pressure. Most of the blood passes passively through the opened bicuspid valve into the left ventricle. The rest of the blood then passes actively through the valve via the contraction of the left atria. Shortly after this, the ventricles contract, pumping blood into the aorta through the opened aortic (semilunar) valve. Simultaneously, the mitral valve closes to prevent back flow. From the aorta, some blood passes into the first branch of the aorta – the coronary arteries while the remainder is carried into the aortic arch, thoracic aorta and abdominal aorta. Vessels branching from the aorta transport blood to all body parts to sustain intracellular homeostasis (Figure 12.1).

Most congenital cardiac imbalances result from teratogenic influences during early stages of pregnancy when the heart is developing. Some of these defects are mentioned in Chapter 20. Such defects account for approximately one-half of all infant deaths arising from congenital abnormalities. The most frequent are septal defects and patent ductus arteriosus (a vessel between the pulmonary artery and aorta that allows blood to bypass the lungs in the fetus). Failure of closure of the foramen ovale soon after birth results in an atrial septal defect (ASD), commonly referred to as a 'hole in the heart' (Suddaby and Grenier, 1999).

Since blood passes from the right side of the heart to the lungs for oxygenation, cardiac defects involving right-to-left shunts (e.g. tetrology of Fallot, transposition of aorta and pulmonary arterial trunk) prevent complete oxygenation of the blood. Significant defects cause cyanosis (a blue coloration of the skin and mucous membranes due to low oxygen content of blood). This may be treated initially with oxygen therapy depending upon the severity of the cyanosis, and later with corrective surgical techniques to abolish the shunts and/or vessel abnormalities.

Conditions comprising left-to-right shunts (e.g. patent ductus arteriosus, patent foramen ovalis, septal defects) increase pulmonary blood flow and lead to congestive heart failure if not corrected. Correction involves controlling the consequential pulmonary oedema, providing respiratory support, and restricting fluids. Frusemide, a loop diuretic, may be prescribed if the imbalance does not correct itself, in order to reduce blood volume and cardiac congestion. Surgical correction may be necessary.

Coronary circulation

The heart chambers are continuously bathed with blood, which provides nourishment to the endocardial cells. The myocardial and pericardial cells, however, are too far away to receive nutrients from this blood source. Nutrition is provided by a number of blood vessels, which comprise the coronary circulation. Numerous vessels pierce the myocardium and carry blood to the vicinity of the myocardial and pericardial cells. This arrangement is essential, since the oxygen consumption of the heart muscle is greater than that of any other tissue because of its constant pumping action. At rest, the oxygen consumption is 8 ml/100 g of heart tissue per minute. The supply of blood via the coronary circulation accounts for one-twentieth of the total output from the heart, even though the heart represents only 1/200 of the body's weight. The main coronary vessels – the right and left coronary arteries – branch from the aorta just superior to the aortic valve. They lie on the heart's surface (the epicardium), encircling the heart in an atrioventricular groove. These vessels reminded early anatomists of a crown, or corona, hence the name (Figure 12.7(a)). Their branches and sub-branches penetrate deep into the cardiac muscle.

The right coronary arterial branches are the marginal artery, which supplies the lateral part of the right side of the heart, including the right atrium, and the posterior interventricular artery, which extends to the apex serving the posterior ventricular walls.

The left coronary arterial branches are the left anterior descending branch, which serves the interventricular septum and the anterior wall of both ventricles, and the circumflex branch, which supplies the left atrium and the posterior left ventricular wall.

Coronary vessels deliver most blood when the heart is relaxed. They are largely ineffective during ventricular contraction, as they are compressed by the contracting myocardium, and their entrances from the aorta are blocked partly by the cusps of the opened aortic valve.

Having supplied the heart tissue, blood is collected from the left ventricle via the cardiac veins, which merge to form the coronary sinus. This empties into the posterior aspects of the right atrium. The sinus is comprised of the great cardiac vein, the middle cardiac vein, and the small cardiac vein (Figure 12.7(b)).

Blood from the right side of the heart is collected via the anterior cardiac vein, which empties directly into the anterior aspects of the right atrium. Blood returning to the atrium will have very little oxygen – less than any other venous blood in the body, since the active heart muscle extracts more oxygen from the blood it receives than do other tissues.

Factors that influence coronary blood flow are:

● *The demand of cardiac muscle for oxygen*. The removal of oxygen from the coronary circulation at rest is approximately three times greater than in normal circulation; in times of increased oxygen demand (e.g. exercise, the stress of impending surgery), the additional oxygen required is supplied by an increased coronary blood flow. The change in blood flow is directly proportional to the oxygen requirements. The mechanism is intrinsic to the tissue (i.e. the tissue regulates it), but the metabolic stimulus to provide the additional blood has yet to be identified.

● *Neural mechanisms*. The autonomic nervous system indirectly affects coronary blood flow. Parasympathetic stimulation decreases the heart rate, resulting in a decreased cardiac oxygen consumption, therefore decreasing coronary flow. Conversely, sympathetic stimulation increases the heart rate and myocardial contractility, increasing oxygen consumption, and increasing coronary flow.

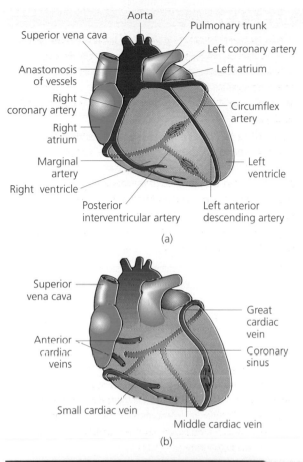

(a)

(b)

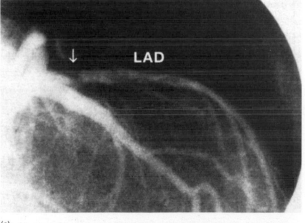

(c)

Figure 12.7 Coronary circulation. (a) Arterial supply. (b) Venous drainage. (c) Left coronary arteriogram — injection of left coronary artery. (Weir, J. and Abrahams, P.H. (1997) *Imaging Atlas of Human Anatomy*, 2nd edn. Published by Mosby-Wolfe, an imprint of Times Mirror International Publishers Ltd. Reprinted with permission.)

- *Aortic pressure.* This is the principal factor that determines the rate of blood flow to the cardiac muscle, since the aortic pressure is produced by the heart itself. Any increase in aortic pressure generated by the contraction of the heart results in increased coronary blood flow.

The conduction system

Before considering the conduction system of the heart, it is important that you understand the anatomy and functioning of cardiac muscle, and its differences from skeletal muscle (see Chapter 17).

Myocardial muscle fibres have anatomical features that reflect their unique function of pumping blood. Otherwise, their structure is similar to skeletal muscle cells. Both are striated in appearance, and their contractions are associated with the sliding filament mechanism (see Chapter 17). Cardiac fibres, however, are small, fat and branched, and usually have one nucleus, whereas skeletal muscle cells are taller and cylindrical, and have many nuclei. Adjacent cardiac cells are interconnected via intercalated discs and cross-bridges, unlike the independent skeletal muscle fibres. The intercalated discs contain anchoring structures (called desmosomes) that prevent separation of adjacent cells upon their contraction, and minute gap junctions that allow direct transmission of electrical impulses (depolarization) across the whole heart. The structure of cardiac muscle allows the entire myocardium to behave as a single unit or 'functional syncytium', but also ensures that the organ is contracted in different planes, unlike the linear contraction observed in skeletal muscle fibres.

Compared with skeletal muscle, myocardial cells also have more mitochondria, constituting 25% of the volume of the muscle fibres (2% in skeletal muscle). This is because heart muscle cells require more ATP for their continual demands of contraction. Both muscle types use a variety of 'fuel' molecules for respiration, although cardiac cells are more adaptable and can readily switch metabolic pathways to use whatever nutrient is available. The main problem associated with myocardial insufficiency, therefore, lies with a lack of oxygen, not fuel molecules.

The orderly and co-ordinated myocardial contraction, which produces efficient emptying of the heart chambers, is controlled by an intrinsic regulatory mechanism – the cardiac conduction system. This is comprised of a number of patches (called nodes) and conducting fibres of specialized muscle tissue called:

- the sinoatrial (SA) node;
- the atrioventricular (AV) node;
- the atrioventricular (AV) bundle (or bundle of His), and its left and right bundle branches;
- the Purkinje fibres (Figure 12.8(a)).

BOX 12.4 CORONARY ARTERIAL DISEASE

Ischaemic heart disease is a homeostatic imbalance that reflects myocardial oxygen insufficiency, arising from a narrowed or occluded coronary artery. Some people with the disease have no signs or symptoms; others experience angina pectoris (chest pain), and some suffer a heart attack (myocardial infarction). Atherosclerotic plaques may cause narrowing and occlusion, or plaques alone may become complicated by a thrombotic narrowing (see Box 12.7). If the narrowing progresses slowly, a collateral (alternative) arterial supply grows, effectively acting as a homeostatic control to replace the malfunctioned vessel. If, however, a sudden severe narrowing or occlusion occurs, the collateral circulation has insufficient time to develop, and consequently myocardial infarction may occur.

Angina pectoris literally means 'choked chest'. It may result from a variety of causes:

- Increased physical demands on the heart that cannot be met by the coronary circulation.
- Stress-induced spasms of the coronary arteries.
- Hypertension, which increases excessively the oxygen demands of the heart.
- Fever, which elevates cardiac activity and hence its oxygen needs.
- Hyperthyroidism (i.e. excessive release of thyroid hormones), which increases cardiac activity.
- Aortic stenosis.
- Atherosclerosis.

Myocardial infarction

A myocardial infarction, or 'coronary', occurs when the coronary arteries become completely occluded, cutting off blood flow to the tissue beyond the occlusion, which results in the death of the myocardial tissue. A thrombus or embolus (i.e. a homeostatic failure of the clotting process) may cause occlusion in one of the coronary arteries. The after-effects depend partly on the size and location of the necrotic area. In chronic ischaemic heart disease, small infarcts may give rise to myocardial weakness, angina, 'silent' myocardial infarction, or heart failure. If the ischaemic heart disease is acute, then one or more large arteries are occluded, and the atheroma is usually complicated by thrombosis. Consequently, a large infarct results, and death may occur as a result of acute heart failure, ventricular fibrillation (see Figure 12.10(a)), rupture of the ventricular wall, or pulmonary or cerebral embolism (leading to respiratory or cerebral failure). See the case study of a man with chest pain: myocardial infarction in Section 6.

Risk factors

Some risk factors for coronary arterial disease (CAD) are:

- modifiable by altering the diet, i.e. managing conditions have a direct link to CAD, e.g. diabetes mellitus. People who are overweight can reduce weight; those with high cholesterol may reduce their blood cholesterol levels;
- modifiable by changing other lifestyle habits, e.g. stopping smoking, changing type A personality behaviour, adopting a moderate exercise programme (which actually reverses the process of CAD);
- not modifiable (i.e. beyond our control). These factors include genetic predisposition, age and gender. Adult males are more

likely than adult females to develop CAD, but after the age of 70 years, the risks are roughly equal. The nurse's role in health education and health promotion is vital as a preventive measure and in minimizing the re-occurrence of CAD;

- controllable with medication, e.g. hypertension.

Diagnosis

Electrocardiograph (ECG) analysis (see Box 12.6) and serum cardiac-specific enzyme levels are used to diagnose CAD. Cardiac catheterization with coronary angiocardiography is an invasive procedure used to visualize the coronary arteries and assess the degree of the occlusion (Figure 12.7(c)). It is also used to:

- measure pressures in the chambers of the heart and blood vessels;
- assess cardiac output (the quantity of blood ejected by the left ventricle per minute) and diastolic properties of the left ventricle;
- measure the flow of blood through the heart and blood vessels, and the oxygen content of the blood;
- assess the status of heart valves and conduction system;
- identify the exact location of septal and valve defects;
- inject clot-dissolving drugs (e.g. streptokinase) into a coronary artery to dissolve an obstructing thrombus.

The procedure involves inserting a long, flexible radio-opaque cardiac catheter into a peripheral vein (for right heart catheterization) or peripheral artery (for left heart catheterization), and guiding it under X-ray observance. A radio-opaque dye is then injected into the blood vessels or heart chambers.

Treatment

Failure of myocardial homeostasis requires clinical intervention to re-establish it. Vasodilator drugs (e.g. glyceryl trinitrate) are given for angina to increase coronary flow, or beta-blockers (e.g. propranolol) may be used to reduce the oxygen requirements of the myocardium. The patient who has had an infarction may be given cholesterol lowering drugs (e.g. Colestipol hydrochloride, and simvastatin) and/or clot dissolving agents (e.g. streptokinase, and reteplase). Alternatively the patient may require a coronary bypass operation to remedy cardiac integrity, i.e. if a large area of the myocardium is affected and/or major vessels are occluded.

Coronary arterial bypass grafting

This is a surgical procedure in which the patient's own long saphenous veing or internal mammary artery is used for the graft. The vein is removed at the same time as the bypass surgery and grafted on to the aorta and coronary arteries to bypass the area of obstruction. The grafted blood vessels is sutured between the aorta and the unblocked portion of the coronary artery.

Percutaneous transluminal coronary angioplasty (PTCA)

This non-surgical procedure involves inserting a balloon catheter into an artery of an arm or leg, then gently guiding it into a coronary artery. The angiograms are taken to locate fatty plaques, the catheter is advanced to the point of obstruction, and a balloon-like device is inflated with air to squash the plaque against the vessel wall. A special device resembling a spring coil (called a 'sten') is placed permanently in the artery to keep the artery patent (open), thus permitting blood to circulate. This is inserted in order to prevent the recurrence of the stenosis of the opened arteries.

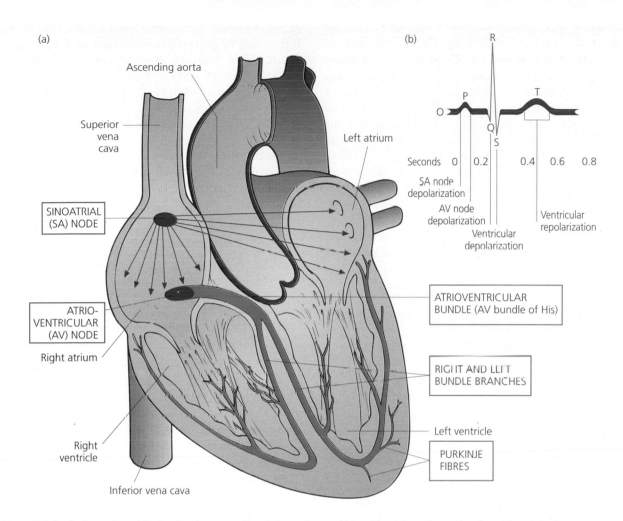

Figure 12.8 Conduction system of the heart and corresponding electrocardiogram. (a) Location of the nodes and bundles of the conduction system. Arrows indicate the flow of action potentials through the atria. (b) Normal electrocardiogram of a single heartbeat.

Q. Describe what is meant by the 'vagal brake'?

Q. Compare the intrinsic rhythm of the SA node with that of other components of the heart's conduction system.

The specialized myocardial cells of the nodes are self-excitatory, i.e. they spontaneously and rhythmically generate the electrical activity that results in their contraction. The resting rate of self-excitation of the SA node of an adult is faster than other members of the conducting system, hence it is called the pacemaker. The impulse that will eventually cause the heart to contract is therefore initiated within the SA node tissue located in the right atrium, just below the opening of the superior vena cava. The impulse spreads from the SA node to atrial myocardial cells, causing their neural excitation and subsequent contraction. It then enters the AV node located at the base of the interatrial septum. This is the last region of the atria to be stimulated; its slower conducting properties give the atria time to empty their blood into the ventricles, before the ventricles begin their contraction. The atria therefore finish their contraction before the ventricles begin theirs, which facilitates unidirectional blood flow. Once through the AV node, the impulse travels quickly through the rest of the conduction system, beginning with the bundle of His. This extends down to the heart apex as the right and left bundle branches, which distribute electrical impulses over the medial surfaces of the ventricles. Ventricular contraction is stimulated by the Purkinje fibres, which emerge from the bundle branches and carry the neural impulses to the lateral ventricular myocardial cells.

Although the rate of the heartbeat is determined by the intrinsic properties of the SA node, this may be altered by the autonomic nervous system, or by blood-borne hormones such as thyroxine or adrenaline. The SA node's ability to generate impulses in the absence of such external stimuli is referred to as autorhythmicity, and results from spontaneous changes in the permeability of cell membranes to potassium and sodium (see Chapter 8). The gradual stimulation (depolarization) of the membrane reaches threshold, forming an electrical impulse (action potential), which is transmitted through the rest of the conducting system, resulting in myocardial contraction.

Following the action potential, the SA node cell membranes return to their initial resting value and are gradually stimulated again. This repetitive, self-excitatory mechanism causes the rhythmical and repetitive muscle contraction associated with heart activity. Although the SA node is the pacemaker, autorhythmicity is also displayed in other parts of the conduction system. For example, the AV node discharges at a rhythmical rate of 40–60 beats per minute, while the rest of the system discharges at a rate of 15–40 beats per minute (beats/min). In life, these tissues rarely have the opportunity to generate action potentials because they are stimulated by impulses from the SA node before they reach their own threshold levels. If, for some reason, the SA node is inactivated, the tissue with the next fastest autorhythmical rate (i.e. the AV node) takes over pacing. This site is then called an ectopic pacemaker; it may pace the heart for some period of time.

BOX 12.5 ECTOPIC BEATS

Stimulants, such as caffeine and nicotine, when used in excessive amounts may increase the excitability of the conduction system to such a degree that ectopic beats result in abnormal contractions. Other triggers of ectopic beats are electrolyte imbalances, hypoxia and toxic reactions to drugs, such as digitalis.

Exercise

Draw a labelled diagram of the heart, including its conduction system.

The electrocardiogram

The action potentials of myocardial cells are electrical changes that can be recorded as they move through the myocardium. This recording is known as the electrocardiogram (ECG). The recording varies according to the positioning of the monitoring electrodes or leads (see Box 12.6).

The ECG is recorded by placing electrodes on the arms and legs (limb leads) and at six positions on the chest (chest leads). The ECG amplifies the heart's electrical activity, and produces 12 different recordings from different combinations of limb and chest leads. Each chest and limb electrode records slightly different electrical activity, because it is in a different position relative to the heart (Figures 12.9). By comparing these records with one another, and with normal records, the practitioner can check specific nodal, conducting and contractile properties, and determine whether the heart is enlarged or certain regions damaged.

Coronary care nurses use cardiac monitors, which consist of three chest leads attached to the patient. The electrical readout is presented on a small screen by the bed, or may be conveyed to the central monitor. Cardiac monitors are used for observing the heart rate and rhythm. Although certain changes in the shape of the ECG waves and intervals can be seen on the screen (e.g. ST segment elevation), the cardiac monitor does not pinpoint areas of myocardial damage like the 12-lead ECG does.

Figure 12.8(b) illustrates the important features of an ECG analysed with the leads in one of the standard configurations (lead II right arm to left leg). The three clearly recognizable events, or waves, normally accompanying each heart cycle are:

1 A small P wave upward deflection. This corresponds to atrial electrical stimulation (depolarization). The upward swing of the P wave represents SA node depolarization; the downward deflection represents AV node depolarization. About 100 ms after the P wave begins, the atria contract (i.e. mechanical events follow electrical activity).

2 The QRS complex signifies ventricular depolarization. The complex begins as a downward deflection, continues as a large upright triangular wave, and ends as a downward wave at its base. Shortly after the QRS complex begin,s the ventricles start to contract. The relatively strong electrical signal reflects the comparatively larger mass of ventricular muscle compared with that of the atria.

3 The smaller, dome-shaped T wave is indicative of ventricular electrical recovery (or repolarization), and occurs just before the ventricles start to relax. The T wave is smaller and wider than the QRS complex because repolarization occurs more slowly than depolarization There is no deflection corresponding to atrial repolarization, since it occurs during the ventricular depolarization period and the electrical event is hidden by the QRS complex.

Extrinsic innervation of the heart

Although external nerve stimulation is not required for heart contraction, the autonomic nervous system modifies the activity of the intrinsic conduction system. The regulatory significance of this effect is discussed later. This section is concerned with the anatomy of the nerve supply to the heart. The general anatomy of the autonomic nervous system is outlined in Chapter 8.

The medulla oblongata of the brainstem contains two 'cardiac centres' that control autonomic nerve activity to the heart. The cardiac accelerator centre controls sympathetic nerve activity to the heart, and the cardiac inhibitory centre controls parasympathetic nerve activity to the heart (Figure 12.11).

(a)

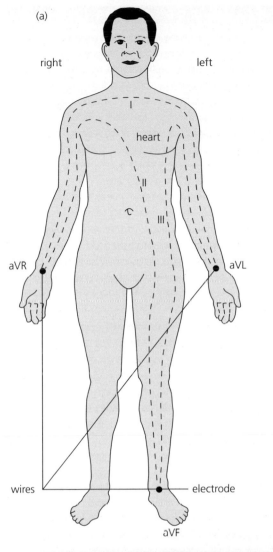

right left

heart

aVR aVL

wires — electrode

aVF

(b)

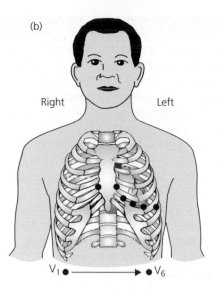

Right Left

V_1 ● ——→ ● V_6

Figure 12.9 A 12-lead electrocardiogram (EGC). (a) Limb leads. Bipolar: lead I measures voltage difference between left and right arms; lead II measures voltage difference between left leg and right arm; lead III measures voltage difference between left leg and left arm. Unipolar: aVR measures voltage difference between zero and right arm; aVL measures voltage difference between zero and left arm; aVF measures voltage difference between zero and left leg. (b) Chest leads. V_1, V_2: right ventricle; V_3, V_4: septum and part of left ventricle; V_5, V_6, rest of left ventricle. ● = lead positions. N.B. clavicles not shown. (c) sinus rhythm. The rate in this example is about 80 beats per minute. The P wave and QRS morphology are normal. The PR interval is normal (0.16 s). The QRS duration is normal. The frontal plane QRS axis is normal. An isolated T wave inversion in one of the inferior leads is normal.

(c)

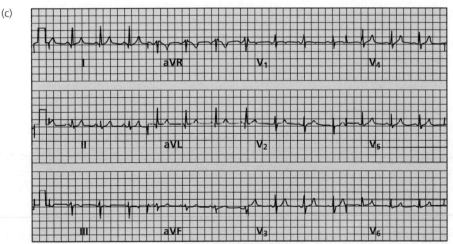

I aVR V_1 V_4

II aVL V_2 V_5

III aVF V_3 V_6

Sinus Rhythm Twelve-lead ECG

Neurons from both centres innervate collections of nerve cells (ganglia) within the heart wall, from which the neurons innervate the SA and AV nodes and some of the heart muscle. Sympathetic stimulation (as occurs in exercise and the stress response) accelerates the heart rate, and increases the force of myocardial contraction. Conversely, parasympathetic stimulation decreases the heart rate, but has little or no effect on the force of myocardial contraction.

BOX 12.6 ECG ANALYSIS, STRESS TESTING AND ARRHYTHMIAS

ECG analysis involves measuring voltage changes (i.e. the relative heights of the wave deflection) and determining the duration and temporal relationships between the various components. That is, small electrical signals associated with specific waves may mean that the mass of heart muscle associated with that wave has decreased, e.g. small P waves may represent atrial atrophy. Conversely, large electrical signals (large amount of depolarization) of specific waves may indicate heart muscle enlargement, e.g. larger-than-normal QRS complexes may indicate ventricular hypertrophy (as occurs in semilunar valve stenosis). An enlarged Q wave may indicate a myocardial infarction, and an enlarged R wave generally indicates enlarged ventricles. The size and shape of the T wave may be affected by any condition that slows ventricular repolarization. A flatter-than-normal T wave occurs when the heart muscle is receiving insufficient oxygen, e.g. in coronary arterial disease. An enlarged T wave may indicate hyperkalaemia (increased blood potassium levels), which may be a result of surgical or medical treatment, e.g. the unwanted side effects of certain drugs.

Reading an ECG also involves the examination of time spans between waves (called intervals or segments). For example, the PQ interval (also called the PR interval, because the Q deflection may not always be obvious) is the time between the start of atrial depolarization and the onset of ventricular depolarization. If this exceeds 0.2 s, it may indicate damage along the conduction system or within the AV node. In coronary arterial disease and rheumatic fever, scar tissue may form in the heart. As the impulse detours around the scar tissue, the PQ interval lengthens. The QT interval, i.e. the period required for ventricles to undergo a single depolarization and repolarization cycle, approximates to the duration of a ventricular contraction. A conduction imbalance, poor coronary blood flow, or myocardial damage may extend the interval.

Stress test

A stress test evaluates the heart's electrical response to the stress of physical exercise. During strenuous exercise (unlike when a person is at rest), the coronary arteries, if narrowed, are unable to meet the heart's increased need for oxygen, creating changes that can be noted on the ECG. These include ST segment elevation, and Q wave changes.

The ECG, together with other heart investigations, is therefore useful in diagnosing abnormal cardiac rhythms (arrhythmias) and in following the course of recovery from myocardial damage, as occurs in myocardial infarction. ECGs are also used to monitor fetal welfare.

Arrhythmias

The heart rate varies with changing activities. In exercise, an increased heart rate is considered quite normal, since the homeostatic set points are altered to accommodate the increased metabolic demands of the tissues to prevent intracellular homeostatic imbalances. However, if the heart rate is persistently and markedly increased or decreased at rest, but still in sinus rhythm (i.e. each P wave is followed by a QRS complex), this usually signals conduction malfunctions – sinus tachycardia (Figure 12.10(b)) and sinus bradycardia (Figure 12.10(c)), respectively. Sinus tachycardia is a heart rate beyond its homeostatic parameters ('tachy-' = fast); sinus

bradycardia is a heart rate below its homeostatic parameters ('brady-' = slow). Clinically, tachycardia and bradycardia refer to resting heart rates of >100 and <60 beats/min, respectively. A sinus tachycardia can be a physiological response to fever, exercise, anxiety or pain; it may accompany shock, left ventricular failure, cardiac tamponade, hyperthyroidism, pulmonary embolism; or it may be a response to sympathetic stimulating drugs. A sinus bradycardia may be normal in athletes; it may accompany hypothermia, or it may be caused by increased vagal tone due to bowel straining, vomiting or pain, or be a response to beta-blocking drugs.

The rhythm disturbances detected can indicate what course of action is necessary to re-establish homeostatic function. For example, if the pulse falls to as low as 40 beats per minute (as occurs in sinus bradycardia or complete heart block), and drugs fail to help the condition, this requires an insertion of an artificial pacemaker. This battery-driven device stimulates the ventricles at a set rate nearer to that of a healthy heart. The battery has to be replaced every 2 years.

In atrial flutter, the atria contract abnormally rapidly (about 200–300 times per minute) (Figure 12.10 (d)). The characteristic atrial 'saw tooth' waves occur at regular intervals, and at a rate of 240–400 per minute; only every second to fourth atrial impulse reaches the ventricles. Atrial flutter may arise as a result of heart failure, pericarditis, heart valve disease, pulmonary embolism or hypoxia. It is usually treated with propranolol or quinidine, or by direct current shock (cardioversion).

Atrial fibrillation (AF) is a rapid, irregular contraction of atrial fibres approximately 400–500 times per minute (Figure 12.10(e)). The arrhythmia may appear intermittently, or as a chronic rhythm. In AF, the pumping effectiveness of the heart is reduced by 20–30%, which is still compatible with life. The causes of this condition include congestive cardiac failure, mitral stenosis, post-coronary artery bypass or valve replacement surgery, pulmonary embolism, chronic obstructive lung disease, hyperthyroidism and hypoxia.

Ventricular fibrillation (VF) is a rapid, irregular contraction of the ventricular fibres (Figure 12.10 (f)). If the ventricles are fibrillating, they are useless as pumps. Unless the heart is defibrillated quickly, then the circulation stops and brain death occurs. Cardiopulmonary resuscitation is necessary. Defibrillation involves exposing the heart to strong electrical shocks that interrupt the chaotic twitching of the heart by depolarizing the entire myocardium, in the hope that the SA node will resume activities again and the normal (or sinus) rhythm will be re-established. Progressive defibrillation is as follows: DC shock 200 J, 200 J and 360 J, followed by adrenaline and DC shock 360 J, followed by lignocaine and DC shock 360 J.

The UK Resuscitation Council publish guidelines for managing all types of cardiac arrest.

Asystole occurs when the ventricles are at a standstill (i.e. no QRS complexes; Figure 12.10 (g)). The causes include myocardial ischaemia or infarction, aortic valve disease, hyperkalaemia and acute respiratory failure. A patient undergoing asystole requires cardiopulmonary resuscitation with the administration of adrenaline and atropine. Treatment is repeated if necessary

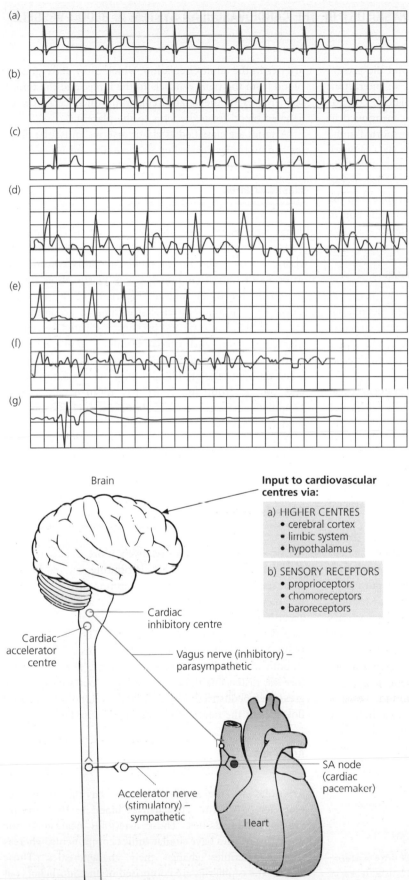

(a)

(b)

(c)

(d)

(e)

(f)

(g)

Figure 12.10 Cardiac arrhythmias. (a) Sinus rhythm (included for reference).

Q. What do the wave and interval components of the ECG represent?

Q. Describe what is meant by the term 'sinus rhythm'.

(b) Sinus tachycardia. The heart rate at rest is ≥100 beats/min.

Q. Identify the conditions that cause sinus tachycardia.

(c) Sinus bradycardia. The heart rate at rest is ≤60 beats/min.

Q. What is the treatment for this arrhythmia?

(d) Atrial flutter. The characteristic atrial 'saw tooth' waves appear at a regular interval and at a rate of 250—400/min.

Q. How many atrial impulses reach the ventricles?

(e) Atrial fibrillation (AF). Atrial waves are rapid, small and irregular.

Q. List three cause of AF.

(f) Ventricular fibrillation (VF). Ventricular rhythm is rapid and chaotic.

Q. Identify the treatment for a patient undergoing VF.

(g) Asystole. Ventricular standstill.

Q. Identify two causes of asystole, and the treatment for the condition.

Brain

Input to cardiovascular centres via:

a) HIGHER CENTRES
- cerebral cortex
- limbic system
- hypothalamus

b) SENSORY RECEPTORS
- proprioceptors
- chomoreceptors
- baroreceptors

Cardiac inhibitory centre

Cardiac accelerator centre

Vagus nerve (inhibitory) – parasympathetic

Accelerator nerve (stimulatory) – sympathetic

Heart

SA node (cardiac pacemaker)

Spinal cord

Figure 12.11 Neural pathways for controlling the heart rate.

Q. Compare the effects of parasympathetic and sympathetic stimulation on the heart's conduction system.

OVERVIEW OF THE ANATOMY AND PHYSIOLOGY OF THE CARDIOVASCULAR SYSTEM 2: BLOOD VESSELS AND CIRCULATION

The regulation of cardiovascular function and the preservation of intracellular homeostasis involve an interaction between the cardiovascular system, circulatory components, tissue fluid and other organ systems mentioned in the introduction to this chapter. Blood is transported in the systemic and pulmonary circulatory systems via a network of specialized vessels: arteries and arterioles transport blood away from the heart; capillaries exchange materials between blood and cells; and venules and veins return blood to the heart. This section examines the structure and function of these vessels that constitute the vascular system.

Structure and function of blood vessels

Blood vessel structure varies according to the function, but all vessels, except capillaries, have the same basic structure of three distinctive coats, layers or tunicae (Figure 12.12(a)): the tunica interna, the tunica media and the tunica externa.

The tunica interna – the innermost coat – consists of a single layer of flattened cells. This endothelial lining in vessels larger than 1 mm in diameter is supported by connective tissue dominated by elastic fibres (Figure 12.12 (a) and (c)). Capillaries are comprised only of this layer, with little or no elastic fibres, so as to aid the rapid exchange of water and solutes between the tissue fluid and blood plasma.

The tunica media – the middle coat – consists predominantly of smooth muscle fibres supported by a layer of collagen and elastin fibres.

The tunica externa – the outer connective tissue sheath – consists principally of elastin and collagen fibres.

The relative thickness and fibre composition of each layer varies according to the vessel's function (Figure 12.12 (a) and (c)). The middle layer shows the greatest variation. It is absent in capillaries, for example, but in large arteries close to the heart it is comprised mainly of elastin tissue. In addition to elastic properties, arteries (especially the arterioles) have contractile functions due to their smooth muscle layer being innervated by the sympathetic nervous system. Contraction squeezes the wall around the vessel, a process called vasoconstriction, since the muscle fibres are arranged in rings around the vessel. Conversely, when sympathetic stimulation is suppressed, the muscle fibres relax, causing the arterial lumen to increase in diameter, a process called vasodilation.

The arterial system

The characteristics of arteries are that they always transport blood away from the heart, and they usually carry oxygenated blood. The exceptions are the pulmonary arteries in the adult circulation, which carry deoxygenated blood from the right ventricle to the lungs, and the umbilical arteries in the fetal circulation, which carry deoxygenated blood from the fetus to the placenta.

Arteries are classified as elastic arteries, muscular arteries and arterioles, according to their size and function.

Elastic arteries

These large vessels have diameters of up to 25 mm. The aorta, pulmonary trunk and their major branches are elastic arteries. The tunica media contains considerably more elastic fibres than muscle fibres. Elastic fibres are also present in the other tunicae (Figure 12.12 (a) and (c)). These fibres facilitate arterial stretching to accommodate the extra blood volume and pressure instigated by ventricular contraction, and arterial recoiling upon ventricular relaxation Consequently, blood flows continuously, even when the ventricles are filling during the relaxation period and output from the heart has momentarily ceased. Despite their muscle content, elastic arteries have relatively ineffective vasoconstrictory powers.

Elastic arteries are the 'conduction arteries', since they conduct blood away from the heart to the muscular arteries.

Muscular arteries

Elastic arteries give rise to relatively more muscular arteries, sometimes referred to as 'distributing arteries' because these medium-sized vessels of 1–4 mm in diameter distribute blood to peripheral tissues. They are often named according to the tissue or part of the body that they supply (see *Blood vessel nomenclature* below). The vessels have a thick tunica media that contains considerably more smooth muscle fibres than elastin fibres. They are therefore less distensible than elastic arteries, but are capable of greater vasoconstriction and vasodilation, adjusting blood flow to suit the needs of the structures supplied.

Arterioles

Arterioles are the smallest arteries, having an average diameter of 30 μm. They deliver blood to the capillary vessels within tissues. Those arterioles nearest to the muscular arteries have similar tunica components, whereas smaller arterioles change their characteristics. Those nearest the capillaries are comprised of an endothelial coat and an incomplete layer of smooth muscle; these muscle

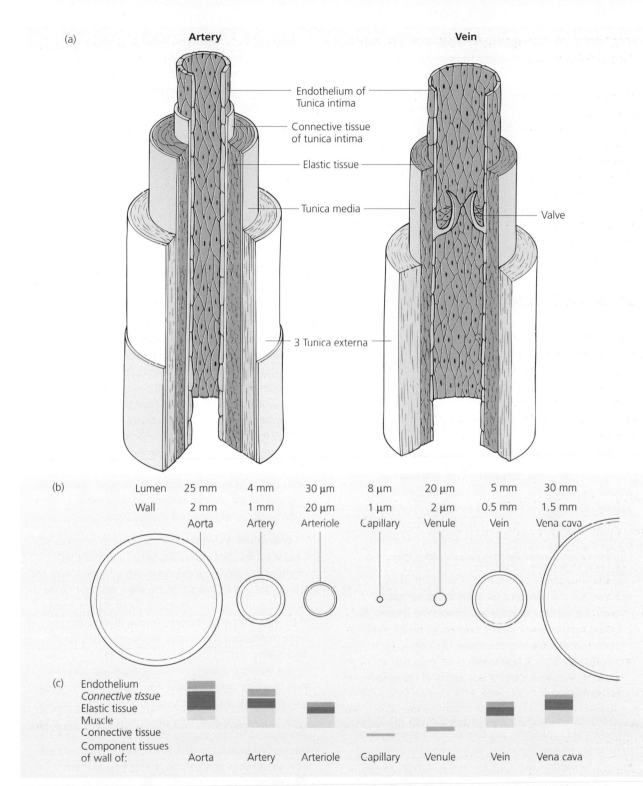

(a)

Artery   Vein

Endothelium of Tunica intima

Connective tissue of tunica intima

Elastic tissue

Tunica media

Valve

3 Tunica externa

(b)

Lumen	25 mm	4 mm	30 μm	8 μm	20 μm	5 mm	30 mm
Wall	2 mm	1 mm	20 μm	1 μm	2 μm	0.5 mm	1.5 mm
	Aorta	Artery	Arteriole	Capillary	Venule	Vein	Vena cava

(c)
Endothelium
Connective tissue
Elastic tissue
Muscle
Connective tissue
Component tissues
of wall of:

Aorta	Artery	Arteriole	Capillary	Venule	Vein	Vena cava

Figure 12.12 (a) Structure of blood vessels. (b) Variation in the thickness of the walls of blood vessels in the circulatory system. (c) Variation in components of the walls of the various blood vessels in the circulatory system.

Q. Identify the structure and composition of the walls of arteries and veins. How are they similar? How do they differ?

fibres enable the arteriolar diameter to be altered, and hence regulate blood flow through their dependent tissues (Figure 12.14). Relaxation of specialized regions – the precapillary sphincters (which consist of a few circular

muscle fibres) – close to the arteriolar capillary junction may cause the capillary bed to become fully perfused with blood. Partial sphincter contraction reduces blood flow, and total contraction causes capillary shutdown. Arteriolar

BOX 12.7 ARTERIOSCLEROSIS AND ATHEROSCLEROSIS

Several types of arteriosclerosis ('hardening of the arteries') exist, some more dangerous than others. Arteriosclerosis associated with ageing is a progressive, degenerate arterial imbalance, in which the artery walls gradually lose elastic and muscle fibres. These vessels become stiff, hard and relatively inelastic, and eventually their lumen is narrowed as they become infiltrated with collagen and calcium. Due to the lack of disensibility, atherosclerotic vessels are less able to change their radius and lumen size, hence blood pressure peaks are therefore much higher in the arteriosclerotic vessels. This exposes their walls to greater stresses, and increases the risk of cerebrovascular accidents and myocardial infarctions. The risks are elevated further if the patient is also hypertensive from additional factors.

Atherosclerosis

Atherosclerosis is a type of arteriosclerosis characterized by the deposition of lipids, cholesterol compounds, excessive smooth muscle and fibroblastic cells in the form of atheromatous plaques in the blood vessels walls. (Figure 12.13). Plaques grow and spread along the arterial wall, forming a swelling that protrudes into the lumen, thus compromising blood flow to the affected organs. The origin of plaques is debatable, although vascular 'fatty streaks', if not absorbed (a homeostatic control process), are thought to be precursors. Streaks are evident in autopsies of children as young as 6 years old, and may be of genetic and/or environmental origin. Arteries most commonly affected are those of the heart, brain, lower limbs and small intestine. Atherosclerosis is therefore an obvious cause of coronary artery disease (see Box 12.4), cerebral vascular accidents, and tissue ischaemia in peripheral vascular disease.

Atherosclerosis predisposes the person to other imbalances, such as:

● thrombosis. The endothelial lining over the plaque breaks down, and circulating platelets are activated and stimulate the clotting cascade; the developing thrombus (or emboli) may cause ischaemia and infarction (Figure 12.13 (b));
● aneurysm formation. A local dilation of the wall called an aneurysm weakens the arterial wall; rupture of this causes haemorrhaging.

Atherosclerosis has a multifactorial aetiology. The risk factors of smoking and hypertension may have their own adverse effects by damaging the endothelium (i.e. the inner lining of blood vessels). For instance, with smoking, nicotine increases platelet adhesion, and carbon monoxide may increase the permeability of the arterial endothelium, thus increasing plaque formation.

Research has also demonstrated a positive relationship between elevated serum cholesterol levels and the instance of atherosclerosis, especially associated with coronary arterial disease (Pradka, 2000).

Cholesterol is vital to the body, as cell membranes and steroid hormones are made from it. It can be synthesized by the liver from saturated fat; it is also obtained directly from our diets. Cholesterol is transported in the blood, mainly in combination with a protein soluble complex called low-density lipoprotein (LDLP or LDL). Excess cholesterol removed from tissues is transported in association with a different protein complex, high-density lipoprotein (HDLP or HDL). These biological processes are controlled by genes, and are common to us all. However, there is variation between people in the development of atheroma, because atheroma formation is promoted by environmental impacts on cholesterol metabolism (Clancy and McVicar, 1998):

● Cholesterol is delivered to the tissue to facilitate repair. Excessive or recurrent vessel damage due, for example, to smoking or hypertension will promote its deposition (Pradka, 2000).
● The uptake of large amounts of cholesterol or saturated fat from the diet promotes hyperlipidaemia, especially in the form of LDLP. Chemicals in tobacco smoke have similar effects, and reduce cholesterol metabolism (Pradka, 2000).
● Normally, there is a 2 : 1 ratio of HDLP to LDLP; this favours the removal of excess cholesterol from tissues. Exercise helps to maintain the ratio, but smoking reduces it and so removes the 'protection' afforded by it (Pradka, 2000).

Consequently, an inappropriate diet, smoking and a lack of exercise are important contributory factors that modify the underlying pathophysiology associated with atheroma (Clancy and McVicar, 1998). Such interactions are major risk factors in the incidence of coronary heart disease in the UK. Care is directed at the consequences of atheroma, but also at encouraging people to reappraise their lifestyle and so reduce the risk of heart disease.

The incidence of atherosclerosis increases with advancing years. It is more common in men than women, until the time of menopause; then the sex distribution of atherosclerosis becomes equal. Family history of arterial disease (both genetic and environmental factors), stressful lifestyle, personality type A (although the existence of such personalities is contested these days) characterized by aggressive restless behaviour, and diabetes mellitus are all associated with increased incidence of atherosclerosis.

and sphincter diameters are controlled by smooth muscle contraction, induced extrinsically by the sympathetic nervous system, or intrinsically (called autoregulation) in response to changes in tissue fluid composition. An example of the latter is the central nervous system ischaemic response, in which cerebral hypoxia (lack of oxygen in brain tissue) causes dilation of the cerebral arterioles.

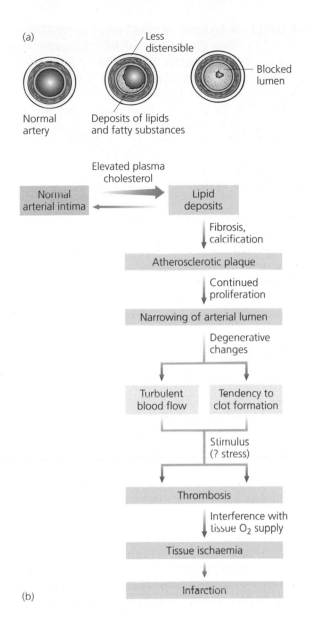

Figure 12.13 (a) Atherosclerotic vessel changes. (b) Mechanism producing atherosclerosis and tissue infarction.

Q. Explain how circulatory function is altered by atherosclerosis.

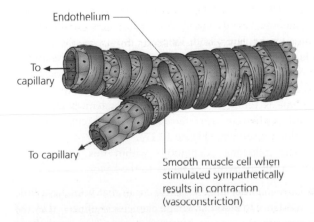

Figure 12.14 Structure of an arteriole.

Q. How do arterioles affect capillary blood flow?

Capillaries

Capillaries form the part of the circulation often referred to as the microcirculation, since they average only 8 μm in diameter. They are located close to almost all body cells, but their distribution varies according to the activity of the tissues they serve. For example, high-activity sites, such as muscle, liver, kidney, lung and nervous tissues, have a rich distribution, whereas lower-activity sites, such as tendons and ligaments, have a poor distribution. The skin's epidermis, the cornea of the eye, and cartilage tissue are devoid of capillaries, and cells of these tissues have very low rates of metabolism.

A typical capillary consists of a tube of endothelial cells sitting on a basement membrane. In most regions, this tube forms a complete lining, with the endothelial cells being connected by tight junctions; these are referred to as continuous capillaries. Fenestrated capillaries are located in those few areas where extensive fluid exchange occurs, e.g. in the kidney glomeruli, and in the brain's choroid plexus. Discontinuous capillaries are located in the liver (sinusoids), bone marrow and adrenal glands, where they form flattened, irregular passageways that slow the blood flow through these tissues to maximize the period of absorption and secretion across the capillary walls (Figure 12.15).

The prime homeostatic function of capillaries is to permit the exchange of metabolites and wastes between blood and tissue cells, thus they are sometimes called the 'exchange vessels'. For efficient exchange, it is necessary to have:

● *a short distance for substances to diffuse through:* the structure and location of capillaries is admirably suited for exchange, since they comprise a single layer of cells that are in close proximity to tissue cells. The thick walls of arteries and veins present too great a barrier for this process to be efficient;

● *a large surface area:* the total cross-sectional area of the capillaries throughout the body is many thousands times more than that of the aorta;

● *a steady but slow rate of blood flow:* the capillary flow velocity is about 700 times lower than that in the aorta because of the narrowness of these vessels.

Capillaries function as a part of interconnected networks known as a capillary plexus or capillary bed (Figure 12.16(a)). A single arteriole gives rises to dozens of capillaries, which in turn collect to form several venules. The capillary entrance is guarded by precapillary sphincters, which control flow, as discussed earlier. Blood flow in arteries is pulsate, related to the pulse in arterial blood pressure, but blood flow through capillaries between arterioles and venules is usually at a near constant rate. Blood flow can vary between individual capillaries, however. Each precapillary sphincter's cycle of alternate contraction and relaxation occurs perhaps a dozen times a minute. The activities of

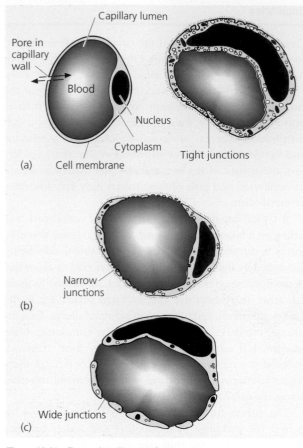

Figure 12.15 Types of capillary. (a) Continuous — connected by tight junctions (e.g. found in muscle). (b) Fenestrated — allows external diffusion (e.g. found in kidney glomeruli and brain choroid plexus). (c) Discontinuous — maximizes exchange of materials (e.g. found in the liver).

various sphincters within the tissue mean that blood may reach the venules by one route at a certain time, and by a different route at another time (Figure 12.16).

Other mechanisms that modify circulatory supply to capillaries include:

- *collateral circulation:* capillary networks may be supplied by more than one artery. The union of the branches of two or more artery supplies to the same region is called an arterial anastomosis. Such vessels could be considered an evolutionary homeostatic adaptation, since blockage of one arterial supply to a capillary bed, caused by disease, injury or surgery, is compensated for by another route of supply, thus guaranteeing a reliable blood supply to tissues. The alternative route of blood flow is known as a collateral circulation. Arteries that do not anastomose are known as 'end arteries'. Obstruction to an end artery interrupts the blood supply to the old segment of an organ, producing death (necrosis) of a segment (see Box 12.4).

- *arteriovenous anastomoses (AV shunts):* these vascular 'short circuits' result from a fusion of arterioles and venules, and are opened when the smooth muscle of arterioles contracts, causing the capillary bed to be bypassed. Relaxation of this muscular component encourages flow through the capillary bed, rather than through the anastomoses. Rates of blood flow through the low-resistance shunts can be very high, so they are found in tissues in which such rates are sometimes appropriate. In the skin, for example, they act as a thermoregulatory mechanism by facilitating the conservation or loss of body heat (see Chapter 16).

The venous system

The venous system is the collection or drainage system that takes blood from capillary beds (when blood has exchanged substances with tissue fluid) towards the heart (Figure 12.1). En route from the venous side of the capillary network, vessels increase in diameter, their walls thicken, and they progress from the smallest veins (venules) to the largest veins (vena cavae).

Venules

Capillaries merge to form venules, which range from 8 to 100 μm in diameter. The smallest post-capillary venules consist almost entirely of a lining endothelium with a few surrounding fibroblast cells. They are, therefore, extremely porous, e.g. inflammatory substances and leucocytes (white blood cells) move easily through their walls from blood to the site of injury via the process of diapedesis (see Chapter 13). As the venule approach veins, a sparse tunica media and tunica externa become apparent.

Veins

Venules merge to form veins. These vessels have the three tunicae found in arteries (see Figure 12.12(a)). Their walls are thinner, however, particularly the tunica media, since they have less elastic tissue and smooth muscle. Their lumens are larger for a given external diameter (Figure 12.12 (a) and (b)), and they offer less resistance to blood flow. This is important because the pressure of blood within the venous circulation is low and provides little force to circulate blood. Veins are, however; still distensible enough to adapt to variations in volume or pressure of blood passing through them. In fact, the thin walls and large lumen mean that about two-thirds of the total blood volume is found within the venous system at any time, which is why veins are referred to as the capacitance vessels or blood reservoirs (Figure 12.17).

The following adaptations within this low-pressure system aid the return of blood to the heart:

- *Large-diameter lumens.* These mean that veins have little resistance to blood flow. The diameter is influenced by the sympathetic nervous system, i.e. changes in sympathetic tone increase or decrease the pooling capacity of the vessel.

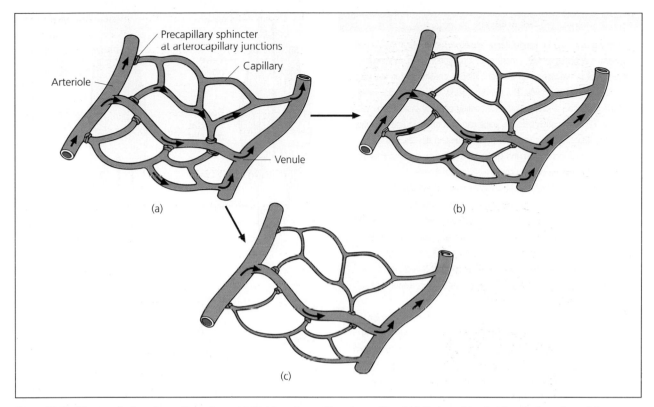

Figure 12.16 The organization of a capillary plexus. (a) Structure of a capillary plexus. (b) and (c) Two possible alterations in the pattern of flow through the capillary plexus as vasomotion occurs.

Q. *Arterioles provide the main means of varying resistance to blood flow through tissues. Identify three other factors that influence how easily blood flows through a vessel.*

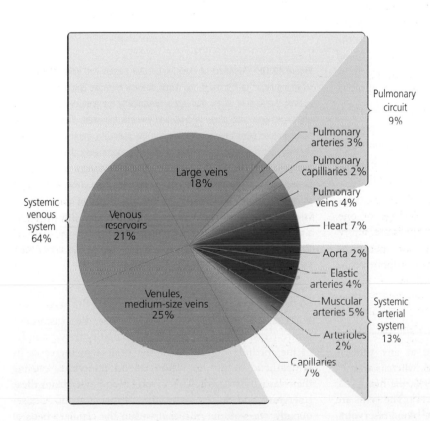

Figure 12.17 The distribution of blood within the circulatory system.

Q. *Why are veins called 'capacitance vessels'?*

BOX 12.8 VARICOSE VEINS

Valve damage may be congenital or acquired, as occurs if the venous system is exposed to high pressure for long periods, e.g. in venous hypertension, pregnancy, abdominal tumours, obesity, and in standing for long, extended periods. The resultant 'leaky' or incompetent valve allows back-flow of blood, causes a pooling of blood distal to the valve (Figure 12.18 (c)); such varicose veins can become long and tortuous. Consequently, fluid may leak into the surrounding tissues, producing oedema. The affected vein and tissue around it may become inflamed and painfully tender, and varicose ulcers may develop.

Areas in the vicinity of the varicose veins may ache because the diffusion of oxygen and nutrients following oedema is reduced. These veins are liable to haemorrhage if knocked, but the patient's main complaint is usually of their appearance. Veins close to the surface of the legs (especially the saphenous vein) are highly susceptible to varicosities. Deeper veins are not usually as vulnerable, because surrounding skeletal muscle prevents their walls from stretching excessively.

There is no cure for this condition, but an operation can be performed that strips outs the affected vein, with ligatures to the supplying veins. Non-surgical intervention includes wearing support tights or stockings, thus assisting venous return by maintaining pressure on the legs. Deep breathing also assists venous return. Preventive measures include sitting down at intervals throughout the day with the feet raised on a stool. Crossing the legs while sitting down should be avoided, since this stops blood flow through the vessel behind the knee.

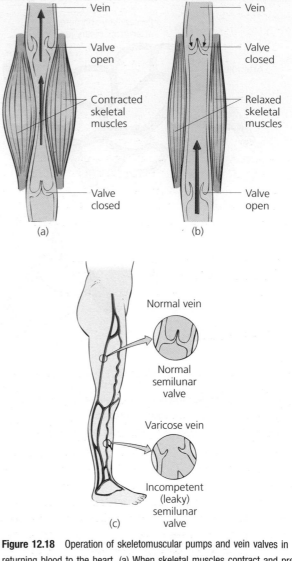

Figure 12.18 Operation of skeletomuscular pumps and vein valves in returning blood to the heart. (a) When skeletal muscles contract and press against the flexible veins, the valves proximal to the area of contraction are forced open and blood is propelled towards the heart. The back-flowing blood closes the valves distal to the point of contraction. (b) When skeletal muscles relax, the valves proximal to the muscle close to prevent backward flow. The distal valves open, creating an upward suction pressure and forcing blood upwards. (c) Varicose veins. Veins near the surface of the body (especially in the legs) may bulge and cause venous valves to leak. The enlarged vein is said to be 'varicose'. They may form a deep veing thrombosis (DVT) following pregnancy.

Q. How do varicose veins develop? What complications may arise from varicose veins?

- *Valves*. These are internal folds of the endothelial lining of large veins that resemble the semilunar valves of the heart in structure and function. They are present in the deep veins of the limbs; since the upward flow of blood is opposed by gravity, these veins are compressed by surrounding skeletal muscles (skeletomuscular pumps), which ensure unidirectional flow (Figure 12.18).

- *Large veins, such as the vena cavae*. These are responsive to the pressure changes in the thoracic cavity that occur during the respiratory cycle, thus assisting venous return to the heart by acting as a thoracoabdominal pump.

Venous sinuses

Venous sinuses, e.g. the coronary sinus, are specialized flattened veins consisting of tunica interna supported by surrounding tissues rather than other tunicae.

Blood reservoirs

Two-thirds of the total blood volume at any time is normally found within the systemic veins; whereas arteries contain about 13%, pulmonary vessels 9%, the heart 7%, and capillaries the remainder (Figure 12.17). The veins are known as the blood capacitance vessels or blood reservoirs, since they serve as storage depots for blood that can be moved quickly to other parts of the body if the need arises. For example, during strenuous exercise, the vasomotor centre ('vas-' = vessel, 'motor' = excitatory nerve supply) of the medulla oblongata of the brainstem increases its sympathetic output to venous blood reservoirs, causing their vasoconstriction. This diverts blood away from these reservoirs and so increases the cardiac output. Consequently, the volume of blood within the capillary beds of

BOX 12.9 HAEMORRHAGE AND ANEURYSM

Bleeding or haemorrhage causes a decrease in blood volume, and hence a decrease in arterial blood pressure. The nurse's role in assessing blood pressure changes is therefore a vital aspect of care. The in-built resultant homeostatic mechanism includes vasoconstriction of venous reservoirs to compensate for the blood loss by redistributing blood and helping to raise the arterial pressure again.

An aneurysm is a localized, permanent, thin, weakened section of the vessel wall that bulges outward, forming a balloon-like sack. Abdominal aortic aneurysms account for 75% of all aneurysms (Huether and McCance, 1996). Those occurring in the aorta are often caused by atherosclerosis, and are associated with hypertension (high blood pressure). Other common causes are syphilis, congenital blood vessel defects, and trauma. Elective surgery is the usual treatment, and can be very effective. If untreated, the aneurysm enlarges and the blood vessel wall becomes so thin that it bursts. If an aortic aneurysm ruptures, the results are disastrous unless immediate advanced life support and specialist surgery are available.

The Berry aneurysm, which affects vessels of the circle of Willis (an anastomosis of arteries at the base of the brain), results from a congenital vessel defect. Rupture leads to subarachnoid or intercerebral haemorrhage. This condition is also associated with hypertension. Signs and symptoms of a stroke occur when cerebral aneurysms leak. Clot-stabilizing drugs and a number of clinical measures are used to reduce intracranial pressure before surgical intervention.

skeletal muscles increases, enabling the tissues to obtain more oxygen and nutrients, and so manufacture ATP, necessary for the increased muscle contraction.

Routes of circulation

The heart operates as a double pump, since it has left and right ventricular pumps that serve two distinctive circulatory circuits – the systemic circulation and the pulmonary circulation (Figure 12.1). The systemic circulation routes oxygenated blood through a long-loop circuit, from the left ventricle of the heart (via the force created by the left ventricular pump), through the aorta and its branches, to all body cells other than those of lung tissue. Blood is returned to the right atrium via the vena cavae and coronary sinus. The roles of this circuit are to transport metabolites (e.g. oxygen and nutrients), and to remove 'waste' products of metabolism (e.g. excess carbon dioxide and water) from tissue cells.

The systemic circulation of the adult can be subdivided functionally, according to the organs supplied: the coronary circulation (discussed earlier), the renal circulation (see Chapter 15), the cerebral circulation (see Chapter 8), the cutaneous circulation (see Chapter 16), the skeletomuscular circulation (see Chapter 17), the hepatoportal circulation, and the pulmonary circulation.

The hepatoportal circulation consists of the hepatic artery, which supplies the liver with oxygenated blood, and the hepatic portal vein, which supplies nutrients directly from the digestive organs (this is deoxygenated blood). The hepatic vein drains blood from the liver into the inferior vena cava.

A portal vein is one that carries blood from one capillary bed directly to another, without passing through the heart and being redistributed by arteries. There are a few examples in the body, e.g. the vascular connection between the hypothalamus and the anterior pituitary gland (see Chapter 9), but the hepatic portal vein is the largest. This vein receives blood from veins draining the stomach, intestines and spleen (via the superior mesenteric vein and splenic vein), the pancreas (via the pancreatic vein and branches of the splenic vein), the colon (mainly via the inferior mesenteric vein) and the gall bladder (via the cystic vein).

The pulmonary circulation routes deoxygenated blood through a short-loop circuit from the right ventricle of the heart (via the force created by the right ventricular pump), through the pulmonary trunk, which bifurcates into the left and right pulmonary arteries, taking blood to their respective lungs. Within the lungs, gaseous exchange occurs (see Chapter 14). A pair of pulmonary veins eventually merge from each lung, routing blood back into the heart's left atrium. These vessels are the only veins (in the adult) that carry oxygenated blood. The role of the pulmonary circuitry, therefore, is to transport deoxygenated blood to the lungs for oxygenation and carbon dioxide excretion.

Blood vessel nomenclature

Blood vessel nomenclature is complex and outside the intentions of this book. Accordingly, blood vessels are only named in this book where appropriate, and chapters have only highlighted the important circulations and vessels associated with the homeostatic roles of particular organ systems. Suffice to say, the name of a blood vessel usually gives a clue to its appearance and/or distribution (Figure 12.19). Thus, if you becomes familiar with the major skeletomuscular and neural 'landmarks', there should be few surprises. You should note the following, however:

● The peripheral distribution of arteries and veins on the left and right sides are almost the same, except near the heart, where large vessels (i.e. the vena cavae and pulmonary veins) connect to the atria and other vessels (i.e. pulmonary trunk and aorta) connect to the ventricles.

● A single vessel may change its name as it passes specific boundaries, e.g. the aorta is subdivided into the ascending aorta, aortic arch, and thoracic and abdominal aorta. This makes accurate anatomical descriptions possible where vessels extend to the periphery.

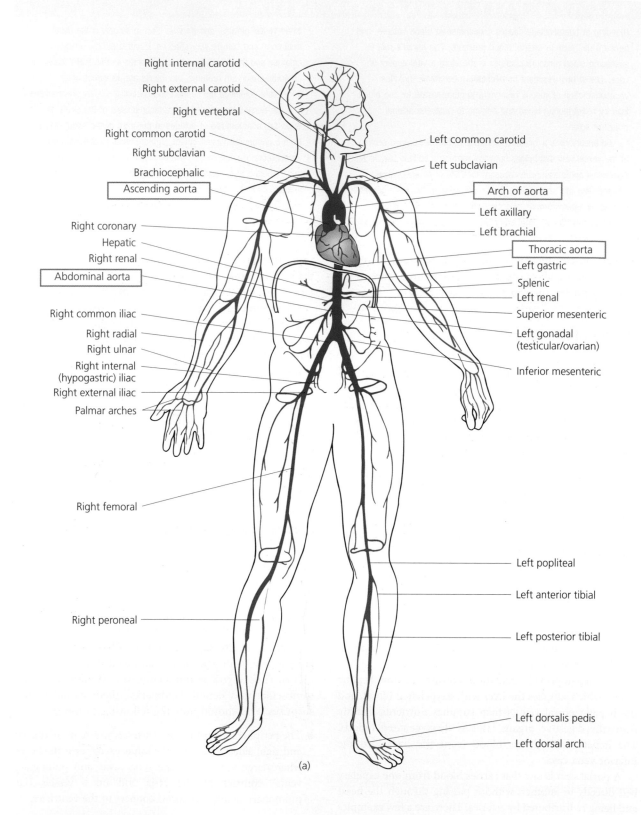

Figure 12.19 Major blood vessels of the systemic circulation. (a) Arteries; (b) veins.

Q. Describe the route taken by blood as it moves from the hepatic portal vein to the hepatic vein.

Q. Describe the route taken by blood as it moves from the left ventricle to the right external carotid.

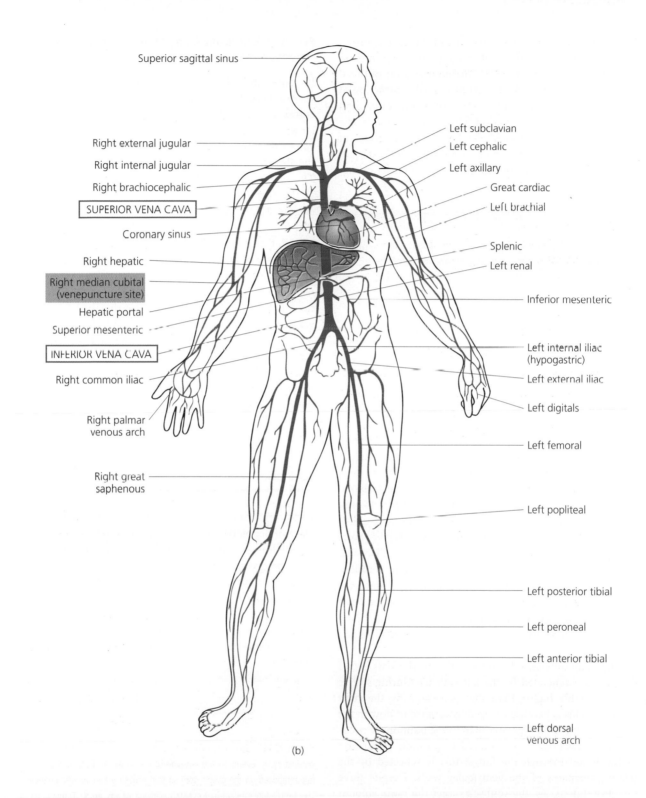

Superior sagittal sinus

Right external jugular

Right internal jugular

Right brachiocephalic

SUPERIOR VENA CAVA

Coronary sinus

Right hepatic

Right median cubital
(venepuncture site)

Hepatic portal

Superior mesenteric

INFERIOR VENA CAVA

Right common iliac

Right palmar
venous arch

Right great
saphenous

Left subclavian

Left cephalic

Left axillary

Great cardiac

Left brachial

Splenic

Left renal

Inferior mesenteric

Left internal iliac
(hypogastric)

Left external iliac

Left digitals

Left femoral

Left popliteal

Left posterior tibial

Left peroneal

Left anterior tibial

Left dorsal
venous arch

(b)

CARDIAC PHYSIOLOGY

The heart is an extremely active organ, beating approximately 30 million times, and ejecting some 2.1 million litres of blood, every year. The previous section outlined the physiological basis for the co-ordinated contraction of the heart, the structure and function of blood vessels, and the specific routes of circulation. This section examines the details of cardiac physiology associated with the events of each heart beat, the homeostatic control of cardiac output, and how cardiac parameters may be varied to meet changing peripheral demands.

Exercise

Re-familiarize yourself with the names of the chambers of the heart, and the names of the autonomic nerves that supply the heart and their origins in the brainstem.

Cardiac cycle

The cardiac cycle represents the events associated with the flow of blood through the heart during one heartbeat. Since alternate myocardial contraction and relaxation mainly achieve the movement of blood, the cycle employs the terms 'systole' (period of contraction) and 'diastole' (period of relaxation). Systolic contraction ejects blood from atria into adjacent ventricles, and from ventricles into the arterial trunks (i.e. pulmonary and aortic trunks). Diastolic relaxation is the period in which the heart chambers become filled with blood. Thus, the cardiac cycle is conveniently split into four phases: atrial and ventricular diastole, and atrial and ventricular systole. Since the sequence of events in the right and left sides of the heart is the same, we use the traditional approach of describing the cardiac cycle in terms of left-sided events (Figure 12.20).

The main difference from the right-sided events is that the pressure generated by the left ventricle during systole is considerably higher than that generated by the right ventricle. This is because the total resistance to flow in the systemic circulation is greater than in the pulmonary circulation, so less pressure is required to promote circulation of the blood through the lungs; this is reflected by the relative thickness of the ventricular walls. Despite these pressure differences, the ventricles eject the same amount of blood with each contraction.

Our explanation of the cardiac cycle begins with the heart in total relaxation, when both atria and ventricles are relaxed, and it is mid- to late diastole, i.e. the chambers are almost filled with blood.

Period of ventricular filling (mid- to late diastole)

Pressure within the heart is low at this point, so pulmonary venous blood flows passively into the left atrium. As blood enters, the atrial pressure becomes greater than ventricular pressure. Consequently, the atrioventricular (bicuspid) valve opens into the left ventricle, and blood passes from the atrium to the ventricle throughout the diastolic period. The semilunar (aortic) valve is closed, since the pressure in the aorta is greater than the left ventricular pressure (Figure 12.20, interval 1a). About 70–80% of the ventricular filling occurs during diastole. Towards the end of this period, the tissue of the SA node discharges spontaneously and a wave of electrical excitation spreads throughout the atria (i.e. atrial depolarization corresponding to the P wave of the ECG). The subsequent atrial myocardial contraction, or atrial systole, accounts for the final 20–30% of ventricular filling (Figure 12.20, interval 1b). The amount of blood within the ventricles at the end of ventricular diastole is called the ventricular end diastolic volume (VEDV). Atrial systole and ventricular diastole therefore occur simultaneously. Throughout diastole, the pressure in the aorta falls, since blood is moving throughout the systemic circuitry but is not being replenished by blood ejected from the left ventricle.

Ventricular systole

Following contraction, the atria go into diastole. The wave of depolarization is passed from the AV node to the conduction system provided by the bundles of His, and then progresses throughout the Purkinje system. This need for ventricular systole to be slightly delayed after atrial systole highlights the importance of the electrical resistance provided by the AV node. Ventricular depolarization (corresponding to the QRS complex of the ECG) induces ventricular myocardial contraction, or ventricu-

Figure 12.20 Summary of events occurring in the heart during the cardiac cycle. Events in the left side of the heart. An ECG tracing is superimposed on the graph (top) so that pressure and volume changes can be related to electrical events occurring at any point. Time occurrence of heart sounds is also indicated. Events of phases 1—3 of the cardiac cycle depicted in diagrammatic views of the heart.
Q. List the 'stages' of the cardiac cycle, and describe briefly the electrical events (as recorded by the ECG) that precede each mechanical event.

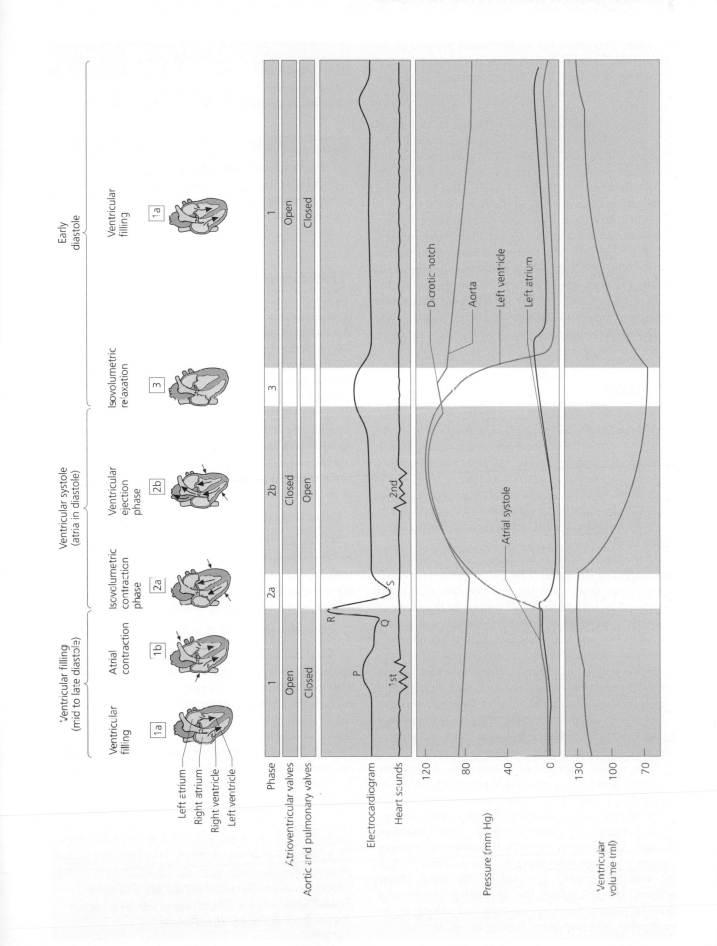

lar systole. This causes the left ventricular pressure to rise sharply, closing the atrioventricular (bicuspid) valve and preventing back-flow into the left atrium. For a split second, the ventricle is a completely sealed chamber; this brief period is sometimes referred to as the isovolumetric ventricular contraction phase (Figure 12.20, interval 2a), and is responsible for the rapid increase in the pressure within the ventricle. This phase ends as the ventricular pressure becomes greater than that in the aorta, when the semilunar (aortic) valve opens and ventricular ejection occurs (on the right side of the heart the right ventricle simultaneously ejects its blood into the pulmonary arterial trunk). The ejection is rapid initially, but then tapers off. The ejection of blood from the left ventricle (Figure 12.20, interval 2b) causes the pressure in the aorta to reach approximately 120 mm Hg (=15.8 kPa; 1 kPa = 7.6 mm Hg). The left atrial pressure rises slowly throughout the ventricular ejection period, because of the continued flow of blood into it from the pulmonary veins.

Early diastole

During this brief phase (i.e. following the T wave on the ECG), the ventricular myocardium relaxes, causing the left ventricular pressure to decrease to a value below the aortic pressure. This results in a backward flow of blood in the aortic trunk, which causes closure of the semilunar (aortic) valve. Closure of the aortic valve causes a very brief rise in the aortic pressure, known as the dicrotic notch (Figure 12.20).

After closure of the semilunar (aortic) valve, the atrioventricular (bicuspid) valve remains closed for a split second, thus once again the left ventricle is a sealed chamber. The ventricular blood volume at this phase of ventricular relaxation is referred to as the end systolic volume (ESV), and the relaxation phase as isovolumetric ventricular relaxation (Figure 12.20, interval 3). Pressure within the ventricle falls sharply. This stage ends when the left atrial pressure rises (as a result of atrial filling) above the ventricular pressure, thus causing the atrioventricular valves to open and the ventricular filling phase begins once again. Atrial pressure falls to its lowest point, and ventricular pressure begins to rise, completing the cycle.

At an average heart rate of 70 beats/min, each cardiac cycle takes about 0.8 s; atrial systole accounts for 0.1 s and ventricular systole for 0.3 s; the remaining 0.4 s is the period of total heart relaxation (diastole). There are two salient features to note about the cardiac cycle: blood flow through the heart is controlled entirely by pressure changes, and blood flows along pressure gradients through the available opening, provided by the valves. These pressure changes reflect the alternating systolic and diastolic periods, cause the opening and closing of the heart valves, and keep blood flowing in one direction.

Exercise

Find the four heart valves in Figure 12.4. Using Figure 12.5, describe when these valves open and close during the passage of blood through the heart, and how they ensure that blood flows in one direction. At what point on the chest is the heartbeat palpated most readily?

Cardiodynamics

Cardiodynamics investigates the movements of the heart and the forces generated by cardiac contraction. The stroke volume is the quantity of blood ejected into the systemic circulation with each left ventricular systole. Generally, this volume is related directly to the force of ventricular contraction. Since the stroke volume may vary during beats, the total cardiac output is of great clinical interest. Cardiac output is the quantity of blood ejected by the left ventricle each minute. It is expressed in litres per minute (l/min), and is calculated by multiplying the stroke volume (volume ejected per contraction) by the number of heartbeats (ventricular contractions) per minute, i.e.

Cardiac output (CO) = Stroke volume (SV) × Heart rate (HR)

The cardiac output, therefore, provides a useful indicator of ventricular homeostatic efficiency over a period of time. During 'normal' resting conditions, the average adult heart rate is 70 beats/min, and the stroke volume is 70 ml/beat, so the cardiac output is about 5 l/min:

CO = SV × HR = 70 × 70 = 4900 ml/min = 4.9 l/min

Since the average adult blood volume is about 5 l, this means that the entire volume of blood passes through the heart every minute. Cardiac output varies with the changing metabolic demands of the body, rising when the heart rate or stroke volume increases, and falling when the heart rate or stroke volume decreases. The output can increase up to 25 l/min in a normal, fit person performing strenuous exercise, and up to 35 l/min in a well-trained athlete. The increase above the resting cardiac output is termed the cardiac reserve.

BOX 12.12 CARDIAC
OUTPUT CHANGES DURING
PREGNANCY

Cardiac output rises by approximately 40% during pregnancy. A significant rise in cardiac output occurs during the first trimester. It peaks around 30 weeks, and is maintained for the rest of the pregnancy. The production of a reduced afterload in the myocardial fibres during left ventricular ejection is responsible for a fall in systemic vascular resistance, and therefore the rise in cardiac output. The rising levels of oestrogen and progesterone in pregnancy also contribute to the increase in cardiac output as they cause a fall in peripheral vascular resistance.

To understand how the cardiac output changes, we need to examine its contributory factors. For convenience, the regulation of the heart rate and stroke volume will be considered separately, although alterations in cardiac output usually reflect changes in both aspects of cardiac function.

Regulation of the heart rate

The resting stroke volume under healthy conditions tends to be relatively constant. However, when blood volume drops rapidly, e.g. following a haemorrhage, or when the heart is seriously weakened, as in myocardial infarction, the stroke volume declines, and the cardiac output and blood pressure are maintained by an increased heart rate. The sinoatrial node initiates contraction, and if left to it would set a constant heart rate of 90–100 beats/min. However, tissues require different volumes of blood flow under different conditions. Neural stimulation and endocrine activity during the stress response (see Chapter 22) influence the heart rate.

Neural mechanisms
The most important extrinsic influence affecting heart rate is the autonomic nervous system. The heart is innervated from the cardiac centres in the medulla oblongata of the brainstem by both sympathetic and parasympathetic divisions (Figure 12.11) via cardiac (or accelerator) and vagal nerves, respectively. When activated sympathetically, noradrenaline is released at its cardiac synapses (i.e. SA node, AV node and portions of the myocardium) and binds to beta-1 receptors. The sympathetic nervous system is activated when the person is exposed to physical stressors, e.g. exercise or hospital admission, and certain emotional conditions, e.g. sexual arousal, or the anxiety or fear associated with the outcome of a surgical operation. This excitatory neurotransmitter increases the heart rate and the force of myocardial contraction. The additional contraction prevents a decline of the stroke volume as would happen if only the heart rate was increased, since

the reduction of the diastolic period reduces the filling of the ventricle. By increasing the force of contraction, the ventricle empties more efficiently and so maintains, or even increases, the stroke volume.

Conversely, the activation of the parasympathetic neurons in certain emotional conditions, such as severe depression, and/or in normal circumstances when stress thresholds are not achieved, releases acetylcholine at their cardiac synapses. Acetylcholine binds to alpha receptors; it is an inhibitory neurotransmitter that hyperpolarizes the membrane of the sinoatrial cells by opening potassium channels, which stabilizes the membrane, reduces its rate of spontaneous depolarization in autorhythmic fibres, and so decreases the heart rate.

Both autonomic divisions are active under resting conditions, and so both acetylcholine and noradrenaline are normally released at the cardiac synapses. The predominant influence, however, is inhibitory, i.e. the parasympathetic nervous system (vagus nerve) exerts a 'vagal tone' or 'vagal brake' on the inherent rate of discharge of the SA node, which is about 100 beats/min, slowing the heart rate to 70–72 beats/min. With maximum stimulation by the parasympathetic division, the heart can slow to 20 or 30 beats/minute, or even stop momentarily. Conversely, during exercise the predominant influence is excitatory, and so sympathetic innervation dominates. With maximum sympathetic stimulation, the heart rate may reach 200 beats/minute in a 20-year-old. At such a high heart rate, the stroke volume is lower than at rest due to the very short filling time. The maximum heart rate declines with age. As a rule, subtracting the person's age from 220 provides a good estimate of their maximum heart rate.

The autonomic nervous system thus makes delicate adjustments in cardiovascular function to meet the demands of other systems.

The atrial reflex
The atrial (or Bainbridge) reflex involves a combination of intrinsic and neural (extrinsic) modifications of the heart rate, which consequently affect the cardiac output. Intrinsically, an increased return of venous blood to the heart, observed when lying down or during exercise, stretches the right atrial wall. This causes a greater cardiac output, because atrial stretch receptors respond by externally stimulating an increased sympathetic activity, thus causing the SA node cells to depolarize faster, and increasing the heart rate by 10–15%.

Endocrine control of the heart rate
Adrenaline and noradrenaline secreted from the medulla of the adrenal gland by its sympathetic activation mimic the cardiac effects of the excitatory neurotransmitter noradrenaline, and so quickly enhance the heart rate and the force of myocardial contraction. Exercise, stress and excitement cause the adrenal medulla to release more hormones. Endocrine secretions of the thyroid gland

(thyroxine), when released in large quantities, cause a slower but more sustained rise in the heart rate. A sign of hyperthyroidism (excessive thyroid hormone) is tachycardia. Endocrine secretions also enhance the cardiac effects of adrenaline and noradrenaline.

Intracellular and extracellular ionic homeostasis must be maintained for normal heart function, e.g. sodium and potassium are crucial for the production of action potentials in nerve and muscle fibres. It is therefore not surprising that ionic imbalances, as a result of hormonal actions becoming compromised, can quickly affect the pump effectiveness of the heart. In particular, the relative concentrations of potassium, calcium and sodium have a large effect on cardiac function. Hypernatraemia (excess blood sodium) inhibits the transport of calcium into cardiac cells, thereby reducing contractility, since calcium is the trigger for muscle contraction.

Hyperkalaemia (excess blood potassium) lowers the cells' resting electrical potentials, which may result in cardiac excitation and increased heart rate. However, large excess prevents repolarization (i.e. electrical recovery), and therefore restimulation of the membrane, leading to heart block and cardiac arrest. Hypokalaemia (insufficient blood potassium) produces a feeble heart beat thereby instigating life-threatening arrhythmia.

A moderate increase in extracellular and intracellular calcium speeds the heart rate and strengthens the heartbeat.

Other factors that influence cardiac function are age and gender, exercise and temperature.

Age and gender

The normal resting heart rates varies throughout the lifespan (Table 12.1). The resting heart rate of an adult female is 72–80 beats/min; this is higher than that of an adult male (64–72 beats/min), reflecting gender differences in heart size and hence stroke volume.

Exercise

Sympathetic stimulation increases the heart rate during exercise. The resting heart rate of a trained athlete is, however, substantially lower (about 40–60 beats/min) than

Table 12.1 Normal resting heart rate throughout the lifespan

Developmental age	Heart rate (beats/min)
Fetus (8–9 months gestation age)	140–150
Newborn	120–130
1 year	110
2–5 years	105–110
5–10 years	90–110
10 years to adult	60–90
Adult	60–80

Adapted from Whaley and Wong (1995).

in a less physically fit person, since the athlete has a well-developed myocardium that is better equipped to pump more blood per contraction. Similarly, the heart rate necessary to maintain an increased cardiac output during exercise will also be lower in a trained athlete.

Temperature

A raised body temperature, as occurs during fever or strenuous exercise, increases the heart rate by causing the SA and AV nodes to discharge more frequently. Conversely, a decrease in body temperature, such as that caused by prolonged exposure to a cold environment, depresses the heart rate.

Homeostatic regulation of the stroke volume

Remember that the stroke volume is the volume of blood pumped out of the ventricles per contraction, and thus represents the difference between the end diastolic volume (EDV), which is the amount of blood that collects in a ventricle during diastole or relaxation (left ventricular EDV is about 120 ml), and the end systolic volume (ESV), which is the amount of blood remaining in the ventricle after ventricular systole or contraction (left ventricular ESV is about 50 ml). The resting stroke volume, therefore, approximates to 70 ml:

SV (ml/beat) = EDV (120 ml) − ESV (50 ml) = 70 ml/beat

Consequently, a change in the EDV and/or the ESV will alter the stroke volume.

BOX 12.13 DRUGS AND THE HEART RATE

Drugs that increase the heart rate are called positive chronotrophic drugs ('chronos-' = time). These are sympathetic agonists, and include drugs such as isoprenaline, adrenaline and atropine. Drugs that decrease the heart rate are called negative chronotrophic drugs. These are sympathetic antagonists, and include drugs such as the beta-blockers, e.g. propranolol. This drug is also used to treat angina, thyrotoxicosis and anxiety states. Digoxin (foxglove) is a drug that slows and strengthens the heartbeat, and is used for cardiac irregularities.

BOX 12.14 SURGERY AND HYPOTHERMIC REDUCED HEART RATES

During surgical repair of certain heart abnormalities, it is helpful to slow the patient's heart rate by hypothermia, in which the person's body is deliberately cooled to a low body 'core' temperature. The hypothermia slows metabolism, which reduces the oxygen needs of the tissues, allowing the heart and brain to withstand short periods of interrupted or reduced blood flow during the surgical procedure (Clancy et al., 2001).

The end diastolic volume and the intrinsic regulation of stroke volume

The volume of blood within the ventricle at the end of diastole (EDV is also known as the preload) depends upon two interrelated factors:

- *The venous return:* i.e. the volume of blood entering the heart (and hence the ventricles) during ventricular diastole. This alters in response to changes in the cardiac output, the peripheral circulation, and other mechanisms that alter the rate of blood flow through the vena cavae (the main veins returning blood to the heart from all body tissues).

- *The filling time:* i.e. the duration of ventricular diastole. This depends entirely on the heart rate. When the heart rate exceeds 160 beats/min, stroke volume usually declines due to the short filling time. At such rapid heart rates, EDV is less, and the preload is lower. People who have slow resting heart rates usually have large resting stroke volumes, because filling time is prolonged and the preload is larger.

Exercise

What happens to the resting heart rate, EDV and stroke volume in a bradycardic patient?

The intrinsic control of stroke volume is illustrated by the responses of the heart to changes in venous return. If the venous return (hence venous pressure) is suddenly increased, more blood flows into the heart. Consequently, the increased EDV stretches the myocardium further. This additional stretch of the muscle fibres promotes a more forceful contraction when the myocardium is stimulated, and results in a greater volume being ejected. The 'more in – more out principle' is referred to as Frank Starling's law of the heart. In this way, venous return changes the ventricular EDV, and hence the stroke volume, and therefore cardiac output, since:

Cardiac output = Stroke volume × Heart rate

Cardiac output and venous return will then remain in balance. Factors that alter the venous return are discussed later.

The end systolic volume and autonomic regulation of stroke volume

The stroke volume is also altered by autonomic associated changes to the volume of blood left in the ventricle after systole. Sympathetic neurons, as discussed previously, release the neurotransmitter noradrenaline when activated, and also stimulate the secretion of adrenaline from the adrenal glands. These chemicals have two important effects on the heart: the heart rate is increased causing shorter filling times (i.e. reduction of end diastolic volume), and the force and degree of myocardial contractility are

BOX 12.15 INOTROPIC AGENTS AND MYOCARDIAL CONTRACTILITY

Substances that increase myocardial contractility are called positive inotropic agents, whereas those that decrease contractility are called negative inotropic agents. Positive inotropic agents, such as adrenaline and noradrenaline, often promote calcium in-flow during cardiac action potentials, which strengthens the force of the myocardial contraction. In addition, increased calcium levels in the extracellular fluid and the drug digitalis all have positive inotropic effects. Conversely, the inhibition of the sympathetic nervous system, via anoxia, acidosis, some anaesthetics (e.g. halothane) and increased potassium levels in the extracellular fluid, have negative inotropic effects. A class of drugs called calcium channel blockers exerts a negative inotropic effect by reducing calcium in-flow, thereby decreasing the strength of the heartbeat.

enhanced. When stimulated, the heart ejects more blood, consequently emptying the ventricle more efficiently and decreasing the ESV.

The interrelationship between these two factors is particularly noticeable during exercise, when sympathetic activity is pronounced. Thus, the increased venous return and the increased contractility of the heart act to produce a large increase in stroke volume (up to about 120 ml/beat).

Reducing the end systolic volume might be expected to reduce the end diastolic volume, as blood fills a more efficiently emptied ventricle. However, moderately increased heart rates during exercise actually cause the end diastolic volume to remain fairly normal due to the increased rate of venous return that is observed. However, heart rates above moderate levels reduce filling times, and decrease the end diastolic volume. Thus, stroke volume peaks at a heart rate of approximately 175 beats/min; further rises in heart rate are accompanied by a decrease in stroke volume. Conversely, parasympathetic neurons, via the inhibitory neurotransmitter acetylcholine, decrease the heart rate, thereby contributing to the decreased cardiac output.

Exercise

Reflect on your understanding of Frank Starling's law of the heart, and the chronotrophic and inotropic actions of drugs. Using a pharmacology textbook and/or discussing with an anaesthetist, identify some common drugs with these actions.

Afterload

Ejection of blood from the heart begins when the pressure in the right ventricle (about 25 mm Hg, i.e. approximately

3.29 kPa) supersedes the pressure in the pulmonary trunk (about 20 mm Hg, or 2.63 kPa), and the pressure in the left ventricle (about 95 mm Hg or 12.5 kPa) supersedes the pressure in the aorta (80 mm Hg, or 10.53 kPa).

At these points, the higher pressure in the ventricles causes blood to push the semilunar valves open. The

pressure that must be overcome before these valves can be opened is termed the afterload. At any given preload, an increase in the afterload causes stroke volume to decrease, and more blood remains in the ventricles at the end of systole. Hypertension and atherosclerosis increase the afterload.

BOX 12.16 CLINICAL ASSESSMENT OF THE CARDIAC OUTPUT

Cardiac output can be assessed by direct or indirect means. Indirect methods may include measuring related variables, such as the urinary output, or peripheral toe and limb temperatures. These variables are used to classify the cardiac output as being high, normal or low. However, a more accurate, direct and repeatable measurement, such as thermodilution, is required to monitor treatment in critically ill patients. Thermodilution involves inserting a triple-lumen Swan–Ganz catheter, with a thermistor (temperature sensor) located at its tip, into a peripheral vein, and advancing it to the right atrium. A bolus of cold saline of known temperature is injected into the catheter. As the saline and right atrial blood mix, the temperature changes; this is sensed by the thermistor, which records when the bolus passes its tip. The actual temperature recorded will depend upon the time taken for the bolus to reach the thermistor and the volume of blood into which the cold saline was dispersed. The data can then be used to calculate the cardiac output. Recent technology has largely superseded this method by using imaging techniques to assess the output. This methodology is non-invasive and also provides moment-to-moment evaluation of changes.

BOX 12.17 HEART FAILURE AND CARDIOMYOPATHIES

Heart failure

The venous return and the normal myocardial pumping activity largely determine the cardiac output. If the pumping is compromised (despite a satisfactory venous return), it may result in the cardiac output not being able to meet the metabolic demands of the body. In such circumstances, the terms heart failure, cardiac failure or pump failure are used. Since the heart has two ventricular pumps, it is possible to have left heart failure (as occurs in left-sided myocardial infarction, mitral or aortic valve incompetence, aortic stenosis and systemic hypertension), and right heart failure (as occurs in pulmonary diseases).

In left ventricular failure, the output is less than the volume received from the right heart. The left ventricle therefore becomes congested with blood, causing imbalances in:

- the chambers and vessels preceding the left ventricle, i.e. an increased volume, hence pressure, occurs in the left atrium, pulmonary veins, and capillaries. The latter may cause pulmonary oedema, which compromises gaseous exchange; if severe, this can be life threatening. A back-up of blood will also cause congestion of the right ventricle;

- the vessels and tissues after the left ventricle, i.e. the decreased cardiac output reduces tissue perfusion, the severity of which is related directly to the depressed cardiac output. Renal function may be impaired, causing fluid retention, which exacerbates the cardiac congestion. Other symptoms exhibited include:

  - *dyspnoea* (shortness of breath or difficulty in breathing) on exertion. This is due to low cardiac output failing to provide adequate oxygenation of the tissue cells, plus the increased venous return pooling in pulmonary circulation, causing pulmonary oedema resulting in a decrease in gaseous exchange;

  - *orthopnoea* (difficulty in breathing when lying down). This occurs due to the effects of the sudden increase in the venous return (which occurs when lying down) not being ejected from the left side of the heart. Blood pools in pulmonary circulation therefore restrict vital capacity. Sitting the patient up in bed or in a chair decreases venous return due to changes in hydrostatic pressure, and can relieve the condition. This position also improves chest expansion, hence vital capacity, therefore potentially improving gaseous exchange;

  - *paroxysmal nocturnal dyspnoea* (difficulty in breathing during the night);

  - *fatigue*, due to the lack of metabolites reaching the cells.

Correction is aimed at the underlying cause. Morphine sulphate is often administered to treat left heart failure accompanied by pulmonary oedema, because of its vasodilator effects, as well as its analgesic and opiate properties. An intra-aortic balloon is sometimes used to treat left heart failure. This device decreases afterload, decreases preload, increases coronary arterial perfusion, and increases systemic blood pressure. The mortality rate of left heart failure despite treatment is 60–80% (Huether and McCance, 1996).

In right heart failure, the right ventricular output is less than the volume returned from the systemic circulation; congestion therefore occurs behind the right ventricle in the systemic venous circulation. Consequently, oedema occurs at various peripheral sites, such as the feet, ankles and wrist, and the sacrum when lying, which may predispose the patient to the formation of pressure sores. The liver and spleen become distended, thus compromising their functions. Most commonly, right-sided heart failure occurs as a result of left-sided heart failure, because of the increased back pressure in the pulmonary circulation. Correction

BOX 12.17 CONTINUED

therefore begins with treatment of the underlying left heart failure or pulmonary disease. The goal is to reduce pulmonary hypertension and increase oxygen arterial content. Thus, oxygen is administered continuously. Diuretics (e.g. frusemide) in conjunction with restricted water and sodium intake decrease venous blood volume (preload). Myocardial contractility is increased with digoxin. Bed rest reduces myocardial oxygen demand, and promotes diuresis by increasing renal perfusion.

When both sides of the heart fail, the term 'congestive heart failure' is used.

Short-term homeostatic control mechanisms compensate in acute heart failure. Long-term homeostatic controls compensate in chronic heart failure. Acute failure, as occurs in myocardial infarction, means that the damaged ventricular myocardium cannot pump out its returning blood, leading to decreased cardiac output, heart congestion, and an increased right atrial pressure.

The decreased cardiac output induces a decreased arterial pressure, which stimulates the baroreceptor reflex and promotes appropriate vasomotor sympathetic activity (see main text). This precipitates an increased myocardial contractility and vessel vasoconstriction, which improves the arterial pressure. Increased venous return further increases atrial pressures, which increases the ventricular end diastolic volumes and thus the force of contraction (Frank Starling's effect). In addition, sympathetic activity redistributes blood flow away from non-essential organs (e.g. guts, kidney and skin) to vital organs (brain and heart).

In chronic heart failure, an additional compensatory mechanism occurs, i.e. the increased interstitial fluid volume (oedema) that is observed occurs at the expense of plasma volume, and so decreases cardiac output further. The renin–angiotensin system, sympathetic activity, and the secretion of aldosterone and antidiuretic hormone are activated by the reduced blood pressure (see main text). Such responses provoke the compensated heart failure mechanisms, i.e. by increasing blood volume, increasing venous return, and increasing the force of contraction (Frank Starling's effect), all of which aid the restoration of the cardiac output. In severe failure, these mechanisms can increase blood volume so much that the myocardium is pushed beyond its physiological parameters of contraction, resulting in ventricular congestion, and consequently an enlarged heart. A vicious circle of positive feedback ensues, which eventually, if not corrected, results in death. This is known as decompensated heart failure.

Correction involves the administration of drugs such as cardiac glycosides (e.g. digitalis) that increase the force of ventricular contraction, thus improving its emptying, thereby increasing cardiac output and improving renal function (Hood, et al. 2001). In addition, they decrease the heart rate, which extends the diastolic period, thus increasing myocardial oxygen supply (recall that, unlike other tissues, coronary blood flow is higher during diastole than during systole, when myocardial vessels may be crushed by the contraction).

Cardiomyopathies

Cardiomyopathy is a degenerative condition of myocardial cells, whereby the myocardium becomes thin and weak, the ventricles enlarge, and the muscle tone becomes incapable of maintaining an adequate cardiac output; consequently heart failure results. Cardiomyopathies frequently occur secondary to other imbalances, such as chronic alcoholism, coronary arterial disease, pathogenic infections, and multiple sclerosis. They also occur as primary imbalances, as there are several inherited forms of the condition. Correction is aimed at removing the underlying primary causal factor (e.g. avoiding alcohol in alcoholic cardiomyopathy). However, this is not always possible, as in the inherited cases, when correction necessitates a heart transplant.

CIRCULATORY PHYSIOLOGY

Having read the previous sections, you should now be aware that:

- the heart is a muscular pump;
- the arteries are the conduction and distribution vessels;
- the arterioles are precapillary resistance vessels;
- the capillaries are the exchange vessels;
- the veins are the blood reservoirs and drainage vessels.

In order to understand how the supply of blood to a tissue is regulated to maintain cellular, tissue and organ system homeostatic processes, we need to consider three interrelated physical aspects of circulation: blood flow, blood pressure and peripheral resistance. The latter two aspects influence the rate of blood flow. Changes in cardiac output and peripheral resistance collectively determine how blood pressure is regulated.

Blood flow

Blood flow is the quantity of blood that passes through a vessel in a given period of time. Blood circulates in the systemic and pulmonary circuits, and the rate of flow is dependent upon two factors: arterial blood pressure and the peripheral resistance (i.e. opposition to blood flow) provided by blood vessels and blood viscosity.

The flow rate of any fluid is proportional to the pressure applied to that fluid. Thus, fluid flows from high to low pressure regions, and the greater the pressure differential, the faster the movement. Flow only continues, however, if the pressure exceeds the opposing forces of resistance. Therefore, the rate of flow is inversely proportional to the resistance since for a given pressure, i.e. the higher the resistance, the lower the flow rate:

$$\text{Blood flow} = \frac{\text{blood pressure differential}}{\text{resistance to flow}}$$

The nature of the vessel's lining also influences blood flow. A smooth endothelial lining is associated with an even (or lamina) flow, whereas a roughened endothelium caused by calcium, fatty deposits, or thrombus formation, etc. causes irregular (or turbulent) flow. Lamina flow is silent, whereas turbulent flow may be heard using a stethoscope.

Initial pressure regulation occurs within the tissues themselves, since blood flow through capillaries is under local autoregulatory control, i.e. if peripheral tissues become ischaemic, then local arteries and precapillary sphincters dilate and so increase blood flow and oxygen availability. The central nervous system ischaemic response is of particular note. It occurs immediately to minimize the period of cerebral ischaemia, as brain cells can be damaged irreversibly if deprived of oxygen for only a few minutes.

Cells respond to ischaemic conditions by releasing carbon dioxide, lactic acid, adenosine, potassium and hydrogen ions, and other metabolites. These substances are responsible for the dilation of blood vessels. Consequently, the increased blood flow to the tissues aids restoration of oxygen levels to within the homeostatic range. This intrinsic mechanism is important for meeting the nutritional demands of active tissues, such as muscle, in times of strenuous exercise.

Blood pressure

Blood pressure is determined largely by the hydrostatic (water) pressure exerted by the blood on the walls of blood vessels. Blood circulates because the heart pump establishes a pressure gradient. The highest average pressure, created by the left ventricular pump, is observed in the aortic arch before its coronary branches, where it is about 95 mm Hg (12.5 kPa); the lowest average pressure is at the junction of the superior and inferior vena cavae, where it is about 3–5 mm Hg (0.39–0.66 kPa). Unless stated otherwise, the term 'blood pressure' refers to the pressure in the large arteries. The average pressure is most important, since the left ventricle pumps blood in a pulsating manner and tissue flow generally varies accordingly. The systemic arterial pressure in a resting young adult moves between about 120 mm Hg and 80 mm Hg (15.79 kPa and 10.53

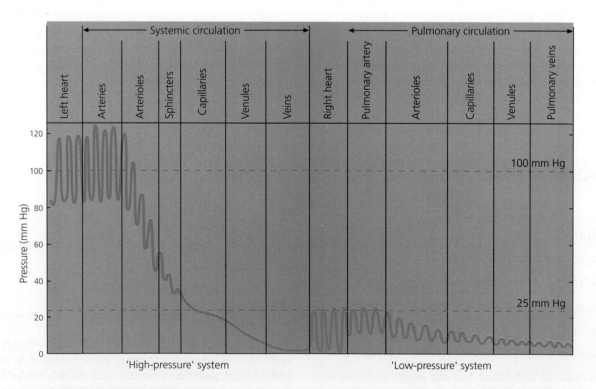

Figure 12.21   Blood pressure changes within the circulatory system. Note the gradual decline in circulatory pressures within the systemic circuit, and the elimination of the pulse pressure oscillations in the arterioles.

Q. Which blood vessels are known as (i) the distributing vessels, (ii) the precapillary resistance vessels, (iii) the exchange vessels?

kPa). The higher value is observed following ejection of blood from the left ventricle during systole, and is therefore called the systolic pressure. The lower value is that observed at the end of diastole, and is therefore called the diastolic pressure. Figure 12.21 illustrates how blood pressure declines unevenly throughout the cardiovascular system. The difference between the blood pressure at the base of the aortic arch and the right atrium represents the circulatory pressure. Bearing in mind the relatively small pressures of the venous system, arterial pressure approximates to the circulatory pressure.

Exercise

Suggest why the maintenance of arterial blood pressure is so important to intracellular homeostasis.

Peripheral resistance

Resistance refers to the impedance (or opposition) to blood flow created by the amount of friction the blood encounters as it passes through the vessels. The term 'peripheral resistance' is generally used, since most friction is encountered in the peripheral circulation. Resistance is related to blood viscosity, the length of the blood vessels, and the diameter of the blood vessels.

The viscosity (thickness) of blood depends mostly on the ratio of red blood cells to plasma (fluid) volume, and to a smaller extent on the a concentration of plasma proteins.

BOX 12.18 BLOOD VISCOSITY AND BLOOD PRESSURE IMBALANCES

Homeostatic imbalances, such as polycythaemia, dehydration and hyperproteinaemia, increase blood viscosity, resistance and pressure. Imbalances such as anaemia, haemorrhage and hypoproteinaemias decrease blood viscosity, resistance and blood pressure.

BOX 12.19 OBESITY AND HIGH BLOOD PRESSURE

High blood pressure (hypertension) and obesity frequently co-exist, both conditions attracting considerable morbidity. In dealing with a hypertensive patient whom the nurse considers overweight, it is important to establish the body mass index (see Chapter 5), whether the patient is aware that they are overweight, and whether the patient understands the types of problems that they be associated with this. Behavioural change is an extremely difficult undertaking, and patients need to be ready to change before advice is likely to be heeded. Once a patient is at this stage, having a strategy to assist weight loss is more likely to see an effective outcome (Holmwood, 2000).

The relationship between vessel length and resistance is simple: the longer the vessel, the greater the resistance. In a healthy person, the viscosity and length of vessels normally remains unchanged, and thus may be considered as constant variables.

In health, changes in the diameter of blood vessels provide the main means of varying peripheral resistance. The relationship between the diameter of blood vessels and resistance is also simple: the smaller the diameter, the greater the resistance to blood flow.

Normally, the peripheral resistance primarily reflects the resistance due to arterioles, in particular their diameter, and is influenced by neural and hormonal mechanisms, although tissues have varying degrees of intrinsic control. The vasomotor centre of the brainstem's medulla regulates arteriolar diameter via its sympathetic innervation. The normal background level of vasomotor activity sets the vasomotor or sympathetic tone of arterioles, which determines the peripheral resistance under resting conditions (Figure 12.22(a)). Thus, greater vasomotor sympathetic outflow increases the resistance due to arteriolar vasoconstriction (Figure 12.22(b)), and reduction in sympathetic output decreases the peripheral resistance by inducing vasodilatation (Figure 12.22(c)). Factors affecting vasomotor activity are discussed later in this chapter.

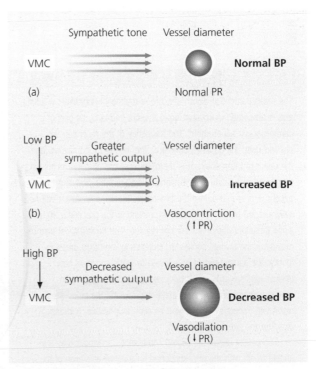

Figure 12.22 Vasomotor centre control of blood pressure via changing the peripheral resistance of arterioles. (a) Normal blood pressure, i.e. within homeostatic range. (b) Low blood pressure, i.e. below homeostatic range, results in vasoconstriction to increase the blood pressure. (c) High blood pressure, i.e. above homeostatic range, results in vasodilation to decrease the blood pressure.

BP, blood pressure; PR, peripheral resistance; VMC, vasomotor centre.

Normal blood pressure

There is no such value as a normal blood pressure reading for the population as a whole. However, there is a 'normal' value for any particular individual, but even that value will vary according to the different metabolic demands of night and day activities (i.e. circadian rhythms), and the developmental age. Multiple factors have an influence on blood pressure, and it is not surprising that people have significantly different but 'normal' blood pressure values. Thus, it is usual to refer to a 'normal range' of blood pressure rather than to a single value.

Common parameters affecting blood pressure include:

- *age:* there is a direct relationship between advancing years and increasing blood pressure (Table 12.2).

- *gender:* the average blood pressure of a 20-year old adult male is expressed as 120/80 mm Hg. Female values are slightly less, because women generally have lower blood pressures than men.

- *race:* in Western societies, blood pressure values tend to increase with advancing years; a contributory factor to this is the high levels of fat in the diet. This is not universal, e.g. South Sea Islanders show little, if any, increase in the mean blood pressure with increasing age. The elevation in blood pressure with age may be related to genetic and/or environmental factors, and is likely to be a result of arteriosclerosis (see Box 12.7).

Exercise

Suggest why, in general, there are gender differences associated with blood pressure.

Pulse and pulse pressure

The alternate expansion and elastic recoil of an artery with each left ventricular systole is called the pulse; the pulse rate is equivalent to the heart rate. The strongest pulse is in the arteries closest to the heart. It weakens progressively as it passes through the arterial tree, disappearing altogether within the capillary networks. The radial pulse is the most commonly used area to feel and monitor the pulse. In adults and infants over the age of 2 years, other areas include the brachial (arm), carotid (neck, a site frequently used in cardiopulmonary resuscitation) and

Table 12.2 Average blood pressures associated with developmental age

Age (years)	Systolic pressure (mmHg)	Diastolic pressure (mmHg)
Newborn	80	45
10	105	70
20	120	80
40	125	85
60	135	88

BOX 12.20 TAKING A BLOOD PRESSURE

The measurement of blood pressure is routinely undertaken in adults, and is advocated in children aged 8 years and over, as part of a cardiovascular assessment. The frequency of the recording will depend upon the patient's condition, the reason for admission, and the result of the reading. It is therefore essential that the technique is performed accurately, on the same arm each time, and that the patient is prepared before the procedure. Ideally, the patient will not have exerted himself or herself or smoked in the preceding 30 min, since these activities increase the reading. The patient must also be relaxed, since anxiety causes an increase in the blood pressure. Ideally, the patient should be allowed to settle into their new environment for at least 30 min before the procedure. In an emergency admission, this is inappropriate, and the blood pressure result will frequently be required as soon as possible, perhaps dictating the patient's treatment.

The patient should be seated comfortably, or lying if they are unable to sit, with the arm supported on a pillow at a level of the heart. Tight clothing should be removed (Figure 12.23). Arterial pressure is measured using a sphygmomanometer. This involves putting an appropriately sized inflatable cuff around the (usually) left upper arm to record blood pressure in the brachial artery (which is taken to be a measure of aortic pressure). A stethoscope is placed over the artery distal to the cuff. The cuff is inflated until a pressure is reached that exceeds the systolic value for the person's age, level of

fitness, etc., i.e. the pressure should be enough to compress completely the brachial artery and thus stop blood flow. The radial and brachial artery can be palpated as the cuff is inflated. The observer should be at eye level with the mercury and the thermometer, and the stethoscope placed over the brachial artery (just below the cuff). When the pulse disappears, the cuff is inflated a further 30 mm Hg (3.95 kPa). This will be sufficient to ascertain the systolic pressure, which may require cuff inflation to only 150 mm Hg.

The cuff is released slowly while listening for audible sounds that indicate flow of blood through the artery and the systolic and diastolic pressures. Upon deflating, the first (Korotkoff) sound is heard through the stethoscope. This 'tapping' sound is sharp and clear, and results from the movement of blood through the no-longer occluded vessel. The mercury column reading at this point corresponds to the systolic blood pressure (i.e. the force at which blood is pumped against the walls during left ventricular contraction). As the cuff pressure falls further, the sound changes to a 'blowing' or 'swishing' noise, then suddenly becomes muffled and faint. It then disappears, as blood movement beyond the previously sealed vessel is no longer impeded. This reading corresponds to the diastolic pressure (i.e. the force of blood in arteries during ventricular diastole).

Electronic equipment (e.g. Dynamap) for recording blood pressure is being introduced in many health authorities, but the mercury sphygmomanometer still predominates.

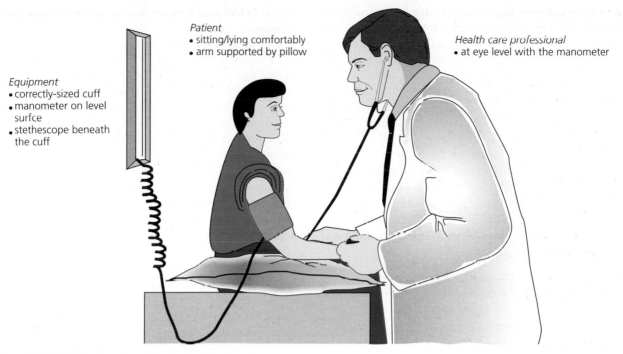

Equipment
- correctly-sized cuff
- manometer on level surfce
- stethescope beneath the cuff

Patient
- sitting/lying comfortably
- arm supported by pillow

Health care professional
- at eye level with the manometer

Figure 12.23 Conditions employed in measuring blood pressure.

Q. What is the equivalent in kPa of 150 mm Hg? (Use the conversion rate mentioned earlier in this chapter.)

popliteal (behind the knee) pulses (Figure 12.24). These are all sites where the artery lies superficially, and over a bony or firm surface, and so can be felt or palpated.

Apical pulse measurements (heard through a stethoscope placed over the apex of the heart) are advocated in children from birth to 24 months because during this period, the pulse rate is quite viable and can be influenced considerably by crying, activity and feeding. The apical pulse rate is also used in the assessment of adults with irregular heart rates and/or where measurements are pulse deficit is required. When assessing a person's pulse, three factors should be observed: rate, strength and rhythm.

The pulse rate is the number of beats in a 60-s period. The pulse rate is calculated most accurately by counting the beats felt within 60 s. Accuracy is particularly important, and is most difficult with patients who have a fast or irregular heartbeat. Pulse rates may vary as a result of age, level of fitness, posture, temperature, stage within the perioperative period, or change in health status.

Exercise

What terms are used to denote an abnormally fast heart rate and an abnormally slow heart rate?

Name a class of drugs that is used to decrease the heart rate.

Figure 12.24 Pulse points. Each pulse point is named after the artery with which it is associated.

Q. Explain what causes a pulse in an artery.

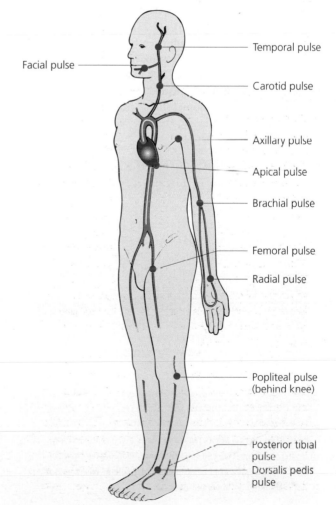

- Temporal pulse
- Facial pulse
- Carotid pulse
- Axillary pulse
- Apical pulse
- Brachial pulse
- Femoral pulse
- Radial pulse
- Popliteal pulse (behind knee)
- Posterior tibial pulse
- Dorsalis pedis pulse

The accurate recording and reporting of an abnormally fast or slow heart rate is essential. It will often indicate a sudden change in a person's condition that needs to be assessed and possible treated. Furthermore, extreme bradycardia and tachycardia result in inadequate filling of coronary arteries, which can lead to myocardial starvation and infarction. Also, a lack of oxygen to the brain initially leads to confusion and disorientation, and can give rise to brain damage.

The strength or volume of the pulse is important because it can give an indication of heart function, cardiac output and probable blood pressure. There is a clear relationship between palpable pulse sites and systolic blood pressures, e.g. the radial pulse is greater than 8 mm Hg, the femoral is greater than 70 mm Hg, and the carotid is greater than 60 mm Hg.

Exercise

Work out the kPa equivalent of pulse pressures of the radial, femoral and carotid pulses.

The rhythm of the pulse is the pattern in which the beats occur. In healthy people, the pattern is regular because the chambers of the heart are contracted in a co-ordinated manner. An irregular pulse may suggest an underlying disorder (see Box 12.23).

The pulse pressure comprises the difference between systolic and diastolic pressures; in a young adult male, this approximates to 40 mm Hg (5.26 kPa) (Figure 12.25). The pulse pressure provides information about the condition of blood vessels. Homeostatic imbalances, such as arteriosclerosis (hardening of the vessels) and patent

BOX 12.21 THREADY AND BOUNDING PULSES

A pulse that is weak and difficult to feel is often described as a 'thready' pulse. A thready pulse will usually be rapid, and may be obliterated by pressure on the artery, suggesting that the patient is dehydrated, bleeding or exhausted. In such cases, it may be necessary to feel the carotid or femoral pulse. Cardiac arrest should not be diagnosed simply because a radial pulse cannot be felt. In contrast, patients with infection, stress or anaemia, or after exercise, may have a very strong, 'bounding' pulse. An inconsistent pulse pressure within each beat may indicate Corrigan's (or 'water hammer') pulse, found in children with aortic valve incompetence.

BOX 12.22 CHILDREN'S PULSE RATE

In children, their pulse is regular; there is a slight acceleration during the inspiration and a slight deceleration during expiration. This is not usually from being present in young fit adults, and is not considered an important deviation.

ductus arteriosus (a vessel in the fetus), record higher pulse pressures.

The mean arterial pressure lies between the systolic and diastolic values (Figure 12.25), and is calculated by adding one-third of the pulse pressure to the diastolic pressure. Both the mean arterial and pulse pressure values become smaller with increasing distance from the heart. The former decreases because of the friction that blood encounters within blood vessels, the latter because vessels become less elastic. The pressure oscillations disappear in the arterioles (Figure 12.21), but arteriolar vessels containing precapillary sphincters cause the mean pressure to remain steady at about 25–30 mm Hg (3.29–3.95 kPa). As blood passes through the capillary beds, the pressure falls from 25–30 mm Hg at their arterial side to 15–18 mm Hg (1.97–2.37 kPa) at their venous side. The decline is necessary to slow the blood flow to aid capillary exchange of plasma constituents with tissue fluid (see later).

Exercise

Identify the common locations where the pulse point is felt most easily.

BOX 12.23 PULSE IRREGULARITY

A regularly occurring irregularity may be detected as a cyclical event that could be the result of a heart block.

An irregular irregularity is often the result of atrial fibrillation, and is the most common irregular cardiac rhythm. It occurs in 2–4% of the adult population over the age of 60 years.

An occasional irregularity may be perceived as a 'missed pulse' or 'dropped beat'. This is often the result of occasional ventricular ectopic (an 'extra beat', followed by a compensatory pause). This should be reported but might not be treated.

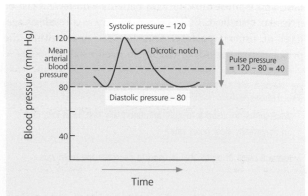

Figure 12.25 Arterial blood pressure: systolic, diastolic and pulse pressures.

Q. What are the primary determinants of blood pressure?

BOX 12.24 JUGULAR VENOUS PRESSURE AND CENTRAL VENOUS PRESSURE

Observation of the jugular vein in the neck gives a crude indication of the venous pressure, e.g. raised jugular venous pressure (JVP) may indicate cardiac failure. The central venous pressure (CVP) is the most frequently monitored venous pressure. This is the pressure in the central veins (the superior and inferior vena cavae) as they enter the heart. As the tip of the catheter used to measure CVP lies in the right atria, CVP is equivalent to right atrial pressure. The catheter is radio-opaque, and its position is confirmed by a chest X-ray. If the tricuspid valve is normal, the CVP equals the end diastole pressure in the right ventricle and, as such, is an index of right ventricular function. Impaired right ventricular function would lead to a back pressure that would raise the pressure in the atrium and hence give a higher CVP reading.

The volume of blood returning to the heart (venous return) is the other major determinant of the CVP. Changes in circulatory fluid volume and the venomotor tone will alter the venous return: An increase in a circulatory fluid volume or venomotor tone will increase the venous return and give a higher CVP reading, and vice versa. One of the major clinical advantages of measuring CVP is that it monitors the circulating blood volume, so it is used to manage fluid replacement therapy in hypovolaemia, which may occur after burns, haemorrhage or surgery. Sequential measurements give an indication of adequate fluid replacement therapy and also help prevent fluid overload.

Venous pressure

Whereas arterial pressure determines the rate of blood flow to tissues, venous pressure influences venous return to the heart, which in turn is an important determinant of the cardiac output. Venous blood pressure is less than one-tenth of arterial pressure. When a person is standing up, the venous pressure must overcome gravitational forces so that blood returns and flows within the inferior vena cava. This is made possible with the aid of three factors: valves, muscular pumps produced by muscle contraction in the limbs, and thoracoabdominal pumps, produced by pressure reductions in the thorax and pressure changes in the abdomen during breathing movements.

In exercise, the combined function of these factors is to increase venous return to its maximum, so as to enable an increase in cardiac output to a level required for the continuance of the exercise.

Homeostatic control of arterial blood pressure

Although variations in blood viscosity may affect blood pressure, such variations are not normally observed. The three principal factors influencing blood pressure are the cardiac output, the peripheral resistance, and the blood volume. (Figure 12.26). The factors are related by the equation:

Blood pressure = Cardiac output × Total peripheral resistance

Cardiac output

Cardiac output is the volume of blood ejected into the aorta each minute. Blood pressure varies directly with cardiac output, i.e. an increase in cardiac output increases blood pressure, and vice versa. Recall that:

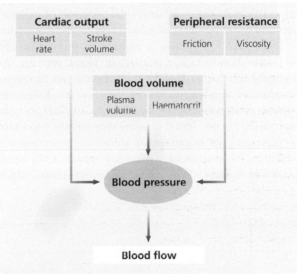

Figure 12.26 Factors influencing blood pressure and blood flow.

Q. What are the contributory factors of the cardiac output?

Q. How does the heart rate affect the cardiac output?

- cardiac output = stroke volume × heart rate, so changes in either will alter blood pressure;

- cardiac output is regulated partly by the cardiac accelerator and inhibitory centres of the brainstem's medulla via sympathetic and parasympathetic output, respectively.

- hormones (e.g. adrenaline, thyroxine), ions (e.g. potassium, sodium, calcium), physical and emotional factors (e.g. depression), temperature, gender and age all affect the heart rate, the heart's force of contraction (stroke volume) and, therefore, cardiac output.

Peripheral resistance

Peripheral resistance in a normal healthy person is the major opposition to blood flow through peripheral vessels, and is determined largely by the diameter of the vessels. Peripheral resistance is regulated by the activity of the sympathetic nervous system, which promotes constriction and dilation of arterioles (Figure 12.22), or by the release of vasoconstrictor hormones.

Blood volume

Blood pressure varies directly with blood volume.

The interrelationships between cardiac output, peripheral resistance and blood volume determine cardiovascular functioning, and their control stabilizes blood pressure to within its homeostatic parameters at rest and also during exercise, when these parameters are modified to increase blood pressure to its altered homeostatic set points. To maintain cellular homeostasis, blood pressure must be regulated tightly, since pressure changes (especially a decrease) influence the transport of metabolites and waste products of metabolism to and from cells.

Figure 12.27 illustrates a number of short-term and long-term homeostatic regulators of blood pressure. As discussed in Chapter 1, short-term controls act to restore homeostatic equilibrium quickly. If they fail, long-term controls must respond; if these fail to redress homeostasis, then illness occurs. Blood pressure controls are important in preventing its inappropriate elevation (hypertension), which can cause mechanical damage to vessels of the heart, brain and kidneys, or its reduction (hypotension), which

> ### BOX 12.25 IMBALANCES OF BLOOD VOLUME AND BLOOD PRESSURE
>
> The average volume of blood in a human body is 5 l. Homeostatic imbalances, such as haemorrhage, may decrease blood pressure by excessively decreasing the blood volume. Conversely, imbalances such as sodium retention (see Chapter 15) induced by aldosteronism (excess of the hormone aldosterone) increase blood pressure by promoting water retention and hence increasing blood volume. Accompanying the larger volume of blood is a greater stretch on the arterial wall, which in turn increases the elastic recoil, which contributes to the higher blood pressure.

can cause inadequate blood supply or ischaemia, and hence lead to necrotic changes to tissues. Short-term controls are neural responses; these adjust cardiac output and peripheral resistance to stabilize blood pressure and hence tissue blood flow. Various vasoconstrictor hormones support this action, but their effects are slower to be initiated. Long-term controls change the blood volume, which alters the cardiac output and hence blood pressure. These regulators are mainly hormonal responses, which again highlights the distinction between these two co-ordination systems: the nervous system responds and acts immediately to homeostatic imbalances, while the endocrine system is comparatively slower to respond and its courses of action are of a longer duration.

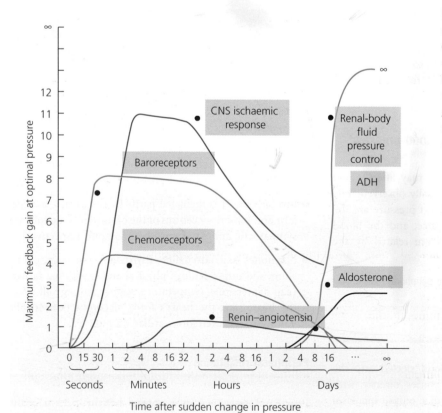

Figure 12.27 Arterial pressure control mechanisms at different times after the onset of an arterial pressure imbalance. Green boxes = short-term, blue boxes = intermediate and long-term controls.

Q. How do ACE inhibitors affect blood pressure? Using the BNF or a pharmacology textbook, name three commonly used ACE inhibitors.

Short-term homeostatic control of blood pressure

Neural mechanisms provide the immediate responses to changes in blood pressure and blood gas concentration. This immediacy prevents fainting due to an inadequate blood supply to the brain when a person stands upright very quickly (gravity causes a pooling of blood below the heart on standing, which reduces the cardiac output).

Reductions in cardiac output (including those imbalances that decrease blood volume) promote vasoconstriction of blood vessels, except those of the heart and brain, which can be considered a homeostatic adaptive mechanism that maintains blood flow to these vital organs. In these instances, blood pressure is controlled especially by sympathetic activity, which is stimulated by afferent information from stretch receptors (baroreceptors) within the circulatory system and/or chemoreceptors of vessels or higher centres in the brain. The latter detect changes in blood gas composition (oxygen, carbon dioxide) or blood pH (concentration of hydrogen ions). These reflexes are mediated by the brainstem's medulla vasomotor centre, and control arteriolar diameter (Figure 12.28).

Baroreceptor reflexes

Baroreceptors are specialized mechanoreceptors that respond to systemic blood pressure changes. Arterial baroreceptors are located mainly in the aortic sinus, carotid sinus, and within the large arteries of the neck and thorax; they monitor blood pressure at the beginning of the systemic circuit. Atrial baroreceptors monitor blood pressure at the end of this circuit. The atrial reflexes differs from the aortic and carotid reflexes in that they monitor stretch within the heart rather than in blood vessels. For example, an increase in right atrial blood pressure means that blood is arriving faster than it is being pumped out into the aorta. Atrial baroreceptors respond by stimulating the cardiac accelerator centre, which increases the cardiac output, which in turn removes the potential congestion in the right atrium, thus returning the atrial pressure to normal. In contrast, arterial baroreceptors are high-pressure receptors. When there is an increase in systemic blood pressure, they have a number of effects. First, they stimulate the cardiac inhibitory centre and hence parasympathetic vagal nerve activity, which depresses the heart rate and so reduces cardiac output. Second, they inhibit the cardiac accelerator centre, and so reduce sympathetic activity to the heart. This makes the influence of vagal nerve activity even more effective. Finally, they inhibit vasomotor centre activity, causing peripheral vasodilation, which reduces peripheral resistance. Collectively, such responses result in a compensatory decrease in blood pressure (Figure 12.28(a)).

Conversely, if there is a decrease in blood pressure, then arterial baroreceptors promote the opposite response by decreasing vagal nerve activity, and promoting sympathetic activity to the heart and blood vessels, causing an increase

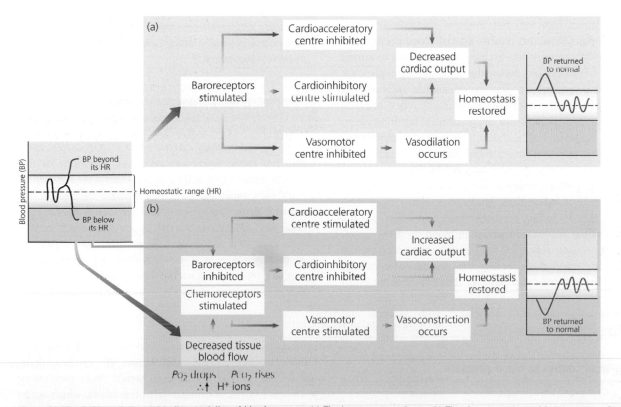

Figure 12.28 Reflexes that assist in the regulation of blood pressure. (a) The baroreceptor reflexes. (b) The chemoreceptor and baroreceptor reflexes.
Q. Which division of the autonomic nervous system causes an increased blood pressure?

in cardiac output and peripheral vasoconstriction. The consequence of such responses is a compensatory increase in blood pressure (Figure 12.28(b)).

The central role of baroreceptors is to protect the circulation against short-term (second-to-second) changes in blood pressure, such as those that may occur with changing posture. Figure 12.27 illustrates their immediacy of response to blood pressure changes, and their ineffectiveness in protecting against sustained blood pressure changes.

Chemoreceptor reflex

Chemoreceptors are located in the aortic arch, carotid sinus (specifically known as the aortic and carotid bodies), large arteries in the neck, and the central nervous system. They are sensitive to low levels of oxygen (especially those outside the central nervous system), and are even more sensitive to high levels of carbon dioxide (hypercapnia) and hydrogen ions (acidosis).

These imbalances are usually a consequence of low blood pressure and inadequate blood flow (Figure 12.28(b)). In such circumstances, chemoreceptors transmit impulses to the cardiovascular centres of the brainstem, which in turn increases blood pressure and blood flow to the heart to correct the imbalance.

The rate and depth of breathing are also increased, which facilitates gas exchange. The chemoreceptors are discussed in more detail in Chapter 14.

Higher centre control

Higher brain centres, such as the cerebral cortex and hypothalamus, although not involved routinely in blood pressure regulation, can modify arterial blood pressure via the medulla centre of the brainstem in response to strong emotions. For example, during the 'fight and flight' response and sexual excitement, the hypothalamus and cerebral cortex stimulate the vasomotor sympathetic reflex, bringing about vasoconstriction and an accompanying increase in arterial pressure. In addition, sympathetic stimulation causes the secretion of catecholamines (adrenaline and noradrenaline) from the adrenal medulla. These hormones mimic and prolong many of the sympathetic responses of Selye's general adaptation syndrome's alarm stage (see Chapter 22), including persistent vasoconstriction and the consequential protracted increase in blood pressure.

In depression and grief, the higher centres decrease the vasomotor sympathetic reflex; the resultant decrease in blood pressure can cause fainting. The hypothalamus also mediates the redistribution of blood flow and changes in cardiovascular dynamics associated with exercise and changes in body temperature.

Long-term control of blood pressure

Some hormones, e.g. adrenaline and noradrenaline, act as short-term homeostatic regulators of blood pressure by

> **BOX 12.26 CAROTID SINUS SYNCOPE AND CAROTID SINUS MASSAGE**
>
> Because of the anatomical position of the carotid sinus (i.e. close to the anterior surface of the neck), it is possible to stimulate the baroreceptors by putting external pressure on this region of the neck. Anything that stretches or puts pressure on the carotid sinus (e.g. hyperextending the head, wearing a tight collar, or carrying a heavy shoulder load) may slow the heart rate and cause carotid sinus syncope, i.e. fainting due to inappropriate stimulation of the carotid sinus baroreceptors.
>
> Physicians sometimes use carotid sinus massage to manipulate cardiac function. This involves carefully massaging the neck over the carotid sinus to slow the heart rate. Such a technique is useful in patients with paroxysmal supraventricular tachycardia, a type of tachycardia that origins in the atria.
>
> In chronic hypertension ('chronic' = persisting for some years), the baroreceptors seem to be reset to maintain pressure at a higher set point.

> **BOX 12.27 DRUG-INDUCED VASOCONSTRICTION**
>
> Drugs that mimic the action of the sympathetic nervous system (sympathomimetics, e.g. dopamine, adrenaline, noradrenaline) cause vasoconstriction. They also have varying effects on the heart. Adrenaline influences alpha and beta receptors, and affects both the heart and peripheral vessels. Noradrenaline mainly affects alpha receptors and the vascular system, causing an increase in peripheral resistance. Nicotine enhances the secretion of adrenaline from the adrenal medulla, and so causes vasoconstriction, hence its link with hypertension.

> **BOX 12.28 DRUG-INDUCED VASODILATION**
>
> Adrenergic blocking drugs inhibit the activity of catecholamines at the smooth muscle receptor sites and so cause vasodilation. For example, alpha-receptor-blocking drugs are used in the treatment of peripheral vascular decease in order to increase blood flow to ischaemic tissues. These drugs increase blood flow to the skin rather than to the muscles, and thus are sometimes used to assist in the treatment of varicose ulcers. Drugs can also affect the smooth muscle in the blood vessel wall directly, e.g. glyceryl trinitrate (GTN) is a potent vasodilator, as it relaxes the vascular muscle; GTN is particularly effective in the treatment of angina.

influencing cardiac function and peripheral resistance. Others hormones, e.g. angiotensin II, erythropoietin, aldosterone, atrial natriuretic factor and antidiuretic hormone (ADH), are longer-term regulators, which act by influencing blood volume and/or peripheral resistance (Figure 12.29).

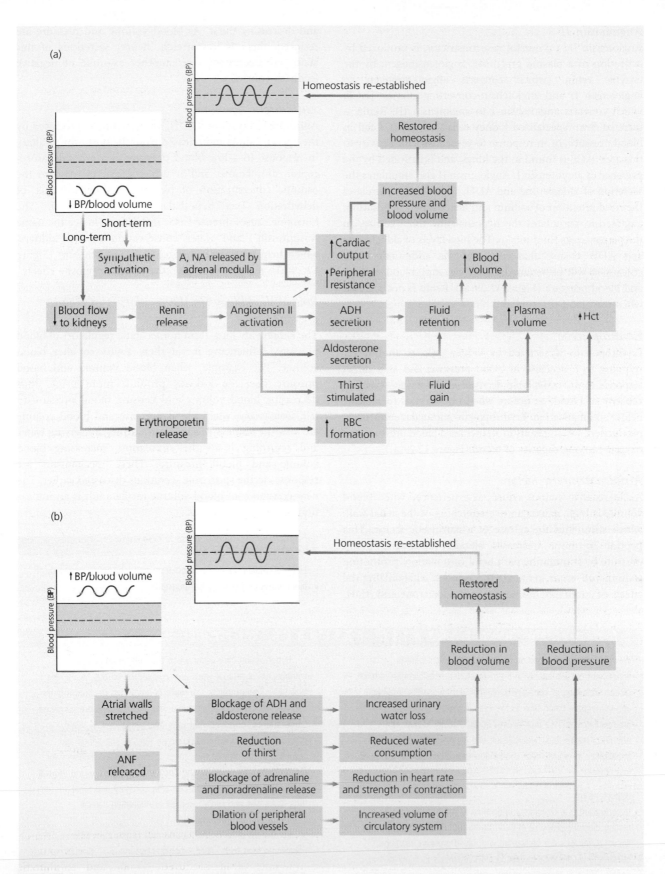

Figure 12.29 The homeostatic regulation of blood pressure (BP) and blood volume. (a) Factors that compensate for decreased blood volume and pressure. (b) Factors that compensate for increased blood volume and pressure.

A, adrenaline; ADH, antidiuretic hormone; ANF, atrial natriuretic factor; Hct, haematocrit; ↑ increased; ↓ decreased.

Angiotensin II

Angiotensin II, a powerful vasoconstrictor, is produced by activation of a plasma precursor, angiotensinogen, by the enzyme renin (which converts angiotensinogen to angiotensin I) and angiotensin-converting enzyme (ACE, which converts angiotensin I to angiotensin II). Renin is secreted from specialized kidney cells that detect a fall in blood pressure, or in response to vasoconstrictor activity to this area. ACE is found in the lungs, and is activated by the presence of angiotensin I. Angiotensin II also stimulates the secretion of aldosterone and ADH. Aldosterone stimulates the renal retention of sodium and hence water. In addition, angiotensin stimulates the hypothalamic thirst centre, so the person seeks fluid intake. The high levels of aldosterone and ADH ensure that much of the additional water consumed will be retained, hence elevating blood volume and blood pressure (Figure 12.29(a)). Renin is not secreted when the blood pressure and blood volume is high.

Erythropoietin

Erythropoietin is secreted by kidney cells as an indirect response to a decrease in blood pressure, and as a direct response to a considerable decrease in the oxygen-carrying capacity of blood, as occurs when one ascends to altitude before acclimatization. Erythropoietin stimulates erythrocyte production, which results in an increased blood pressure and oxygen-carrying capacity of blood (Figure 12.29(a)).

Atrial natriuretic factor

An increase in venous return, as experienced when blood volume is high, causes an overstretching of the atrial wall, which stimulates the release of a natriuretic factor. This peptide hormone decreases blood volume and blood pressure by stimulating peripheral vasodilation, promoting sodium and water losses via the kidneys, antagonizing the effects of adrenaline/noradrenaline, aldosterone and ADH,

and decreasing thirst. As blood volume and pressure are restored, there is less stretch, hence, secretions of this factor are decreased – yet another example of negative feedback control.

Antidiuretic hormone

Antidiuretic hormone (ADH, vasopressin) is produced by the hypothalamus and released from the posterior pituitary in response to a low blood pressure (via arterial baroreceptor stimulation) and/or an excessive increase in the osmotic concentration of plasma as a consequence of dehydration (via hypothalamic osmoreceptors). The hormone causes intense vasoconstriction (hence the name 'vasopressin') and water conservation by the kidneys, which help to reverse changes in blood pressure (Figure 12.29(a)). A high blood pressure has the opposite effects.

Role of the kidneys in the regulation of blood pressure

The kidneys are long-term homeostatic regulators of blood pressure, influencing it via their ability to alter blood volume. For example, when blood volume and blood pressure rise, the kidneys produce more urine, thus decreasing blood volume and causing blood pressure to fall. Conversely, when blood pressure and blood volume are low, the kidneys produce little urine, conserving water and returning it to the circulation, increasing blood volume and blood pressure. These mechanisms are responses to the endocrine secretions discussed earlier. The near constancy of blood volume in the adult is an indication of their effectiveness.

Exercise

List and explain briefly the short-term and long-term regulators of blood pressure following haemorrhage.

BOX 12.29 HOMEOSTATIC FAILURES OF THE CIRCULATION

We have already focused on imbalances in which there is insufficient oxygen supply to the myocardium (e.g. coronary arterial disease resulting in coronary ischaemia and myocardial infarction), and inadequate blood flow to the cells (e.g. atherosclerosis and arteriosclerosis). This box focuses on an inability to maintain arterial pressure (e.g. hypertension and hypotension), and further imbalances in which there is an inadequate blood flow to the cells (e.g. shock).

Hypertension

Hypertension is a circulatory imbalance in which a persistent resting diastolic pressure of over 90–95 mm Hg (11.84–12.5 kPa) occurs. Clinicians are concerned with blood pressure readings, because a significantly increased mortality exists in hypertensive people. The risk increases rapidly with increasing pressure, and the patient is most at risk from a cerebral vascular accident (CVA) or myocardial infarction (MI).

Hypertension may occur when the muscle and elastic components of arterial walls are replaced by fibrous tissue (see Box 12.7). Consequently, the walls of small and medium arteries become thick, hard and inflexible, and their lumens are narrowed. Large arteries, however, may lose their elasticity and dilate, resulting in an exacerbated pulsating flow. At the bends and branches of the arterial tree, there is an increased tendency for blood clotting, as platelets and fibrin are deposited. Blood vessels most commonly affected are cerebral, coronary and renal vessels, thus CVAs, MIs and renal diseases are common clinical manifestations of hypertension.

In 10–15% of all cases, hypertension results from other imbalances, and so is called secondary hypertension. Causes include:

● excessive renin release, as occurs with kidney damage, leading to excessive angiotensin generation, and hence an increase in peripheral resistance;

BOX 12.29 CONTINUED

● hypersecretion of aldosterone (Conn's syndrome) and cortisol, and hence an excessive blood volume, as occurs in people with:

– hypothalamic and/or pituitary tumours, which cause excessive release of adrenocorticotropic hormone (ACTH), the stimulant for the adrenal cortex hormones aldosterone and cortisol secretion;

– an adrenal cortical tumour that displays an excessive reaction to ACTH;

– failure in the negative feedback mechanisms that control ACTH and adrenal steroid release;

● hypersecretion of antidiuretic hormone (ADH) due to hypothalamic tumours, or a failure in the feedback mechanisms. Excessive release of ADH exerts its hypertensive effects by increasing peripheral resistance, and by promoting water retention.

Correction involves anti-hypertensive therapy aimed at the primary imbalance, or at compensation for the imbalance, for example:

● diuretic drugs (e.g. thiazides), which increase urinary sodium and water loss and so reduce blood volume;

● beta-blocker drugs (e.g. propranolol, methyldopa), which decrease heart rate, cardiac output, and hence blood pressure;

● angiotensin inhibitors, e.g. captopril inhibits angiotensin-converting enzyme (ACE) in the lungs and reduces the production of angiotensin II. Raised peripheral resistance is linked with hypertension, so drugs that produce vasodilation are useful;

● non-pharmacological treatments for hypertension are widely practised, and in most cases should be tried before starting a drug regime. Initiatives such as weight loss, salt restriction, decreasing alcohol intake and stopping smoking might help to relieve hypertension. Relaxation techniques and biofeedback decrease sympathetic activity, reducing cardiac output and promoting a decreased peripheral resistance, and have been successful in some cases. If hypertension is diagnosed and treated effectively (usually involving drug therapy), there is no reason why much of the cardiovascular-related disease cannot be prevented.

In 85–90% of people with hypertension, no obvious secondary cause can be determined, since it is almost certainly multifactorial and is likely to be produced by a combination of genetic and environmental factors. This form of hypertension is referred to as 'primary' (or essential) hypertension. See the case study of a young woman with secondary hypertension in Section 6.

Hypotension

Hypotension is a circulatory imbalance in which the patient has a sustained systolic blood pressure below 100 mm Hg (13.15 kPa). Acute hypotension is one of the most important indicators of circulatory shock (see Box 12.31). Chronic hypotension may be associated with:

● poor nutrition, resulting in anaemia and hypoproteinaemias;

● Addison's disease, i.e. an inadequate secretion of cortisol and aldosterone from the adrenal glands, leading to diminished blood volume and cardiac function;

● hypothyroidism, i.e. an inadequate secretion of thyroid hormones, leading to reduced cardiac function;

● severe tissue wasting, as occurs in cancer patients, resulting in lowered peripheral resistance and blood pooling.

Hypotension produces an inadequate blood supply to the brain, which may result in unconsciousness. Depending upon the cause, this may be brief (fainting) or prolonged, the extreme of which leads to death. Postural hypotension, which induces a transient loss of consciousness (called syncope), is common in older people, who suffer a temporary hypotension and dizziness when they rise suddenly from a lying or sitting position. This happens because of a decreased sensitivity of the baroreceptor reflex as a consequence of ageing.

When hypotension is the result of autonomic neuropathy, (e.g. due to poorly controlled diabetes mellitus) or overriding of autonomic reflexes during drug treatment for hypertension, the nurse may be asked to perform postural blood pressure recording. The blood pressure is recorded in the same arm, first with the patient lying down and then in a standing position. If a difference exists between the systolic pressures, the patient is said to have a postural fall in blood pressure (postural hypotension). It is particularly significant if the difference is 20 mm Hg (2.63 kPa) or more, and can indicate a large volume fluid loss.

Correction of hypotension is aimed at removing the underlying cause, and using anti-hypotensive drug therapy, including cardiac stimulants and vasoconstrictors.

Local regulation of blood pressure

Blood flow to tissues must be regulated tightly since it is responsible for:

● absorption of nutrients from the gastrointestinal tract;

● gaseous exchange in the lungs;

● transport of oxygen, nutrients, hormones, etc. to tissue cells throughout the body;

Explain how circulatory function is altered by (i) hypertension, (ii) hypotension, (iii) aneurysms and (iv) haemorrhage.

● the removal of waste products of metabolism from cells;

● processing of blood by the kidneys and other excretory organs.

BOX 12.30 PRE-ECLAMPSIA AND HELLP SYNDROME

Pre-eclampsia is the development of hypertension with proteinuria and oedema, or both, induced by pregnancy after the twentieth week of gestation.

Total peripheral resistance decreases by about 25% in normal pregnancy. In pre-eclampsia, the woman's total peripheral resistance increases – which appears to be the main cause for the elevation in blood pressure seen in this condition – and the normal cardiac output rise of 40% achieved in pregnancy rises even further. The failure of the total peripheral resistance to decrease is thought to be a consequence of the maternal circulatory system being unable to respond appropriately to the fetal trophoblast. The spiral arterioles of the placenta fail to dilate, and maternal blood is forced through these constricted arterioles, which consequently raises the blood pressure.

Management of this condition is possible when it is mild. If the condition becomes increasingly severe (i.e. the blood pressure continues to rise, proteinuria increases, and blood coagulation levels decrease) the only treatment is to deliver the fetus. The condition then usually resolves over 48–72 h.

Pre-eclampsia reflects itself in changes in the blood. Biochemical tests are performed regularly in women with pre-eclampsia. A rare condition that may present is haemolysis, elevated liver enzymes and low platelets (HELLP) syndrome. This presents with right upper quadrant pain, jaundice and nausea. The seriousness of HELLP should not be underestimated, and is considered to be an indication for delivery.

The flow of blood to specific tissues reflects the metabolic demands of that tissue. At rest, for example, skeletal muscles receive approximately 20% of the total blood volume each minute. During exercise, blood is redistributed from other areas (e.g. kidneys and abdominal organs), so that skeletal muscles receive a higher proportion of the (increased) cardiac output to cater for their increased metabolic demands (Figure 12.30).

Vasodilators produce local dilation of arterioles and relaxation of precapillary sphincters, the result of which is an increased flow of blood into the capillary beds. Vasoconstrictors have the opposite effect. This local regulation of blood pressure and flow is termed 'autoregulation'. It is the major regulator of regional blood flow in the brain, and as such is termed 'cerebral autoregulation'. Even though the total blood flow to the brain remains almost constant, regardless of the degree of physical or mental activity, blood distribution to various parts of the brain changes dramatically with different activities.

Velocity of blood flow

The speed at which blood flows varies throughout the systemic/pulmonary circulations and with the specific stages of the cardiac cycle. The greatest velocity is recorded in the aorta during ventricular systole. Furthermore, since velocity is related inversely to the cross-sectional area of blood vessels, the flow rate decreases as the aorta branches, being slowest within the capillary beds; this is essential, as the capillaries are the exchange vessels (Figure 12.31(a)). Flow speeds up again in the venous system as blood collects from the different tissues and is returned to the heart (Figure 12.31(b)).

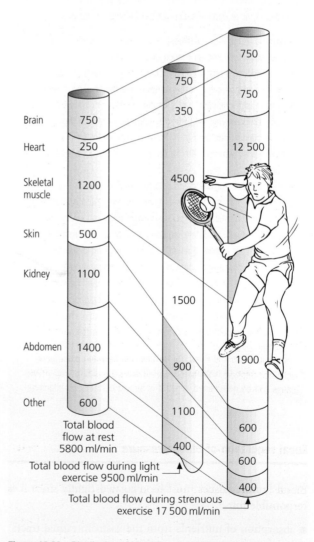

Figure 12.30 Distribution of blood flow to selected body organs at rest, during light exercise, and during strenuous exercise.

Q. Explain how an athlete's low resting heart rate does not compromise cardiac function.

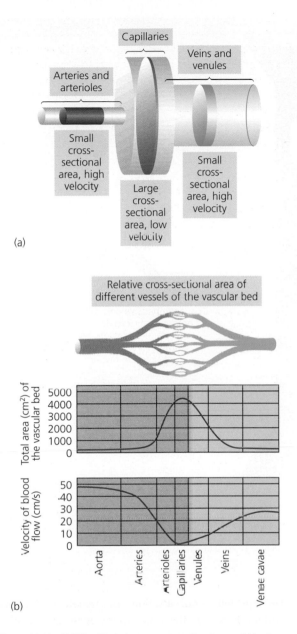

Figure 12.31 Relationship between cross-sectional area of blood vessels and velocity of blood flow. (a) Relative cross-sectional areas of arteries, capillaries and veins. (b) Relationship between blood flow velocity and total cross-sectional area in various blood vessels of the systemic circulation.

Tissue autoregulation – local regulation of blood flow

Tissue autoregulation of blood flow is independent of systemic control, but is proportional to the tissue's requirements, being regulated by local conditions. Flow is, therefore, increased automatically in response to:

- nutrients and oxygen levels falling below their homeostatic range, i.e. when they fail to meet the demands of the tissue;

- carbon dioxide levels above the homeostatic range. This is the most powerful trigger to autoregulation, and could be viewed as resulting from an accumulation of this metabolic product due to inadequate blood flow;

- the release of metabolically active substances from cells, such as lactic acid, kinins, prostaglandins, potassium and hydrogen ions, which will occur if blood flow to the tissue is inadequate;

- the presence of inflammatory chemicals, such as histamine, which promote the protective inflammatory response when the tissue is damaged.

These stimuli cause immediate arteriolar vasodilation and relaxation of precapillary sphincters, thus causing an increased blood flow to the tissues concerned. Autoregulation is considered to be both a short-term and a long-term regulator of blood flow, which acts to redress homeostasis in particular tissues. Cerebral blood flow in particular is regulated by one of the most precise autoregulatory mechanisms in the body. Brain tissue, however, is particularly sensitive to increased carbon dioxide (and the consequential decreased pH), although severely excessive carbon dioxide levels may remove the brain's autoregulatory response, resulting in severe brain damage. Oxygen deficit is a less potent stimulus, even though neurons are totally intolerant of ischaemic conditions. Oxygen deficit, however, increases the presence of many of the metabolites noted above, and the regulatory mechanisms protect the area from damage by responding to the changing levels of these metabolites.

Blood flow through capillary networks is intermittent, due to the contraction and relaxation of the smooth muscle fibres of the arterioles and precapillary sphincters of true capillaries.

Capillary dynamics related to cellular homeostasis

Body fluids are compartmentalized into intracellular and extracellular fluids. Extracellular fluid is subdivided further into plasma and interstitial (tissue) fluid. Within the extracellular fluid compartment, the exchange of fluid between plasma and tissue fluid is important since it brings nutrients into the proximity of cell membranes and aids the removal of substances secreted by cells ('wastes', hormones, etc.) in the opposite direction. Such exchanges are essential if solutes are to enter and exit intracellular fluid efficiently. In order to prevent excessive loss of fluid from plasma (which would induce hypovolaemia), or an excessive build-up of tissue fluid (oedema), a similar volume of fluid must be returned to plasma as was extruded from it.

The movement of water and some of its dissolved solutes between plasma and tissue fluid occurs at the

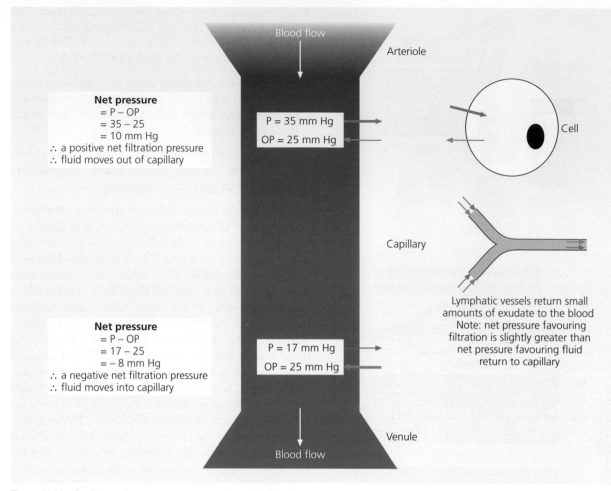

Figure 12.32 Capillary exchange processes.

OP, oncotic (osmotic) pressure due to plasma proteins; P, hydrostatic pressure within the capillary; ↓ direction of blood flow through capillary.

Q. Which components of blood do not pass into tissue fluid from the capillary?

Q. Describe how hypoalbuminaemia may cause oedema.

capillary level (Figure 12.32). Water is driven out of the plasma largely because the hydrostatic pressure of the arterial end of the capillary is higher than the osmotic (referred to as the oncotic or colloidal) pressure generated by plasma proteins. The hydrostatic pressure decreases along the length of the vessel as water is moved (exuded) into the tissue fluid, and eventually is exceeded by the plasma oncotic pressure. Proteins are largely retained within capillaries, due to their macromolecular size (although small proteins can be transferred across capillary membranes). Net pressure at the venous end of the capillaries thus favours the return of fluid into the capillary (a small volume of exudate is returned to the circulation via lymph vesselsthat drain the interstitial spaces).

Exercise

Identify the forces (i.e. pressures) that determine the exchange of water and nutrients between blood and tissue fluid across the walls of the capillaries.

Plasma protein concentration is, therefore, another important factor in the homeostatic maintenance of a normal circulatory blood volume.

Exercise: a change in cardiovascular homeostatic set points

A number of interrelated changes occur during a steady or low rate of exercise. For example, the oxygen consumption of exercising skeletal muscles is increased, facilitated by precapillary sphincter relaxation in these tissues as a response to their changing metabolic requirements. Consequently, blood flow increases (Figure 12.30), and blood is returned to the veins at an increased rate. The increased venous return to the heart results from a greater activity in the skeletal muscular 'pumps', which force blood along the peripheral veins. The accompanying increased breathing rate also increases blood flow into the vena cava via the suction pressure created by the thora-

BOX 12.31 SHOCK

Circulatory shock is any condition in which blood vessels are inadequately filled, thereby producing a tissue blood flow that is inadequate for cellular homeostatic requirements. The lack of cellular metabolites results in intracellular imbalances, e.g. insufficient oxygen produces hypoxia and promotes anaerobic respiration; the persistent build-up of 'waste' products causes cell death, and organ damage ensues. Shock is classified as hypovolaemic (due to low blood volume), cardiogenic (of cardiac origin), vascular (of blood vessel origin), neurogenic (of neural origin), or anaphylactic (as a consequence of an allergic reaction). Hypovolaemic shock ('hypo-' = low, '-volaemic' = blood volume) is the most common form of this imbalance. Causes include:

- severe acute haemorrhage;
- extensive superficial burns (when there is excessive loss of tissue fluid, leading to further exudation from the blood plasma);
- severe vomiting and diarrhoea (when excessive loss of gut fluid promotes further secretion from the blood plasma).

In hypovolaemia, there is:

- Increased heart rate, which acts to improve cardiac output and redress this homeostatic balance. The resultant rapid, 'thready' pulse is an initial sign of the condition (the 'thready' nature of the pulse reflects a diminished pulse pressure);
- intense vasoconstriction, which acts to re-establish blood volume by forcing blood from blood reservoirs (spleen, liver, etc.) into the circulation to enhance venous return, and by increasing peripheral resistance, both of which stabilize blood pressure. If blood loss continues, blood pressure drops sharply as compensatory mechanisms are exceeded; this is serious, and is a late sign of shock.

Figure 12.33 illustrates the homeostatic controls involved in redressing the blood volume after haemorrhage.

Cardiogenic shock (pump failure) results from a sudden reduction in cardiac output, as occurs in acute heart disease, such as myocardial infarction. In vascular shock, blood volume is normal and constant, and inadequate circulation results from a huge drop in peripheral resistance as a consequence of extreme vasodilation, leading to pooling in the large veins. Consequently, a decrease in venous return, cardiac output and arterial pressure results. The most common causes of this imbalance are loss of vasomotor (neural) tone, and septicaemia as a consequence of a severe Gram-negative bacterial infection, since bacterial toxins are potent vasodilators. Extensive peripheral vasodilation also occurs in anaphylactic shock, a dangerous allergic reaction (see Chapter 13).

Neurogenic shock may occur as a result of a sudden acute pain and/or severe emotional experience. Both stimulate a parasympathetic (vagal) slowing of the heart rate, thereby reducing the cardiac output and arterial pressure. Venous pooling of blood may reduce the venous return. These changes decrease cerebral flow, which may cause a temporary loss of consciousness (fainting), a phenomenon known as a 'vasovagal attack'. For further reading, see Clancy and McVicar (1996a).

---

coabdominal pumps. A greater venous return to the heart results in an increased cardiac output by mechanisms associated with Frank Starling's and Bainbridge's reflexes, and increased sympathetic activity. As long as the increased cardiac output can supply the increased demand, then arterial pressure will be maintained, despite the increase in muscle blood flow. Indeed, the increased cardiac output observed during exercise actually causes an increase in systemic blood pressure as a consequence of an elevated systolic blood pressure; diastolic pressure is little changed.

There are minimal alterations in blood flow distribution to accommodate low levels of exercise, although skeletal and cardiac muscles, together with the skin, exhibit a small increase. The increased skeletal muscular flow is via the release of local factors mentioned earlier, which relax precapillary sphincters at these sites. The increased skin blood flow is via hypothalamic-vasomotor centre responses to an increase in body temperature, which causes vasodilation of the skin arterioles and promotes the removal of the excess heat generated by the body. Severe exercise promotes additional physiological adjustments to accommodate the massive increase in the peripheral distribution of blood to skeletal muscles. In addition to metabolic factors, these include:

- sympathetic stimulation of the cardiac accelerator centre, which accounts for a cardiac output increase of up to 20–35 l/min, depending on the person's fitness;
- redistribution of blood flow to skeletal muscles via a shutdown of blood flow to 'non-essential' organs (e.g. kidneys, gut) by vasomotor sympathetic stimulation to their arterioles, and an increased blood flow to skeletal muscle, heart and lungs via reduced vasomotor sympathetic activity to their vasculature.

With training, cardiovascular fitness is improved by the increased myocardial bulk that develops. This increases the stroke volume and hence cardiac output; a trained athlete thus has a lower heart rate for a given cardiac output compared with an untrained person. Sebastian Coe, the famous 1500-m runner of the 1980s, claimed to have a resting heart rate of just 36 beats/min (compared with the adult average of 72 beats/min). This would still have been sufficient to maintain blood flow to his tissues, due to his large stroke volume. Such a heart rate associated with a non-athletic person, however, is clinically referred to as a bradycardia, since the accompanying lower stroke volume would be insufficient to deliver blood to the surrounding tissues.

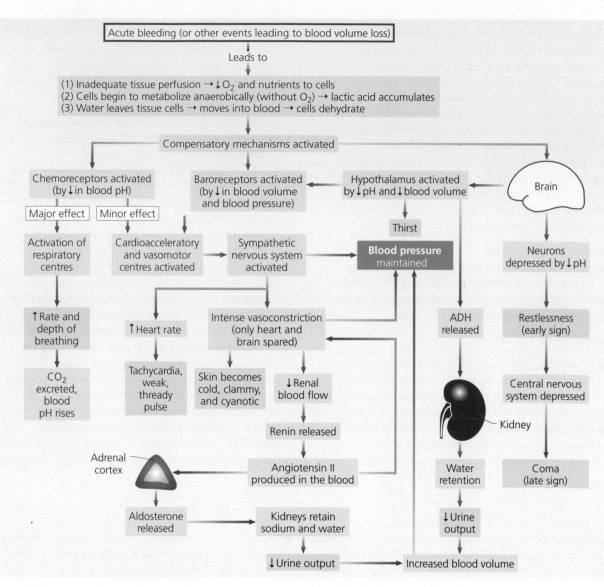

Figure 12.33 Events and signs of hypovolaemic shock. Conditions shown in boxes are clinical indications of shock.
Q. Define 'shock', and list the major types of shock.

Summary

1 The cardiovascular system is the body's transport network, and is adapted to maintain intracellular and extracellular homeostasis.

2 The cardiovascular system comprises a double circulation, i.e. pulmonary and systemic circuits. The pulmonary circuit oxygenates blood to within its homeostatic parameters. The systemic circuit delivers oxygen, nutrients, etc. to tissue cells throughout the body to maintain their intracellular homeostasis.

3 The heart has two ventricular pumps: the right pump supplies the pulmonary circuit; the left pump supplies the systemic circuit.

4 The heart wall comprises three layers (epicardium, myocardium and endocardium), and four chambers (paired upper atria and lower ventricles).

5 Valves ensure unidirectional flow through the heart and venous system.

6 The heart sounds 'lubb-dupp' correspond to the closing of the atrioventricular and semilunar valves, respectively, during the functional cycle of cardiac contraction. Heart murmurs are evidence of stenotic or incompetent valves.

7 Coronary vessels deliver blood to the myocardium. Their partial or complete occlusion compromises myocardial function, and leads to the homeostatic imbalances of angina and/or myocardial infarction.

8 The cardiac cycle describes the sequence of events that occurs with each heartbeat. The cycle consists principally of diastolic (relaxing and filling) and systolic (contracting and emptying) stages.

9 The cardiac output, a clinically important homeostatic parameter, is calculated by multiplying the heart rate by the stroke volume. Changes in either will change the cardiac output.

10 The heart rate is controlled intrinsically and modified extrinsically by the autonomic nervous system and the endocrine system. It varies according to age, gender, temperature and level of activity.

11 The stroke volume varies according to changes in the venous return, which alter the stretch within the chambers (Frank Starling's law), to the period of ventricular filling, and to autonomic neural activity.

12 Most blood vessels share a common structure, consisting of three tunicae (interna, media and externa). Their microstructure, however, is adapted for their specific homeostatic functions.

13 The path of blood flow is from the heart to arteries (elastic, muscular, distributing vessels), to arterioles (smallest arteries), to capillaries (exchange vessels), to venules (smallest veins), to veins (drainage vessels and blood reservoirs). The veins take blood back to the heart.

14 Blood flow is calculated by dividing the blood pressure differential between arterial and venous vessels by the peripheral resistance provided by the vasculature, particularly arterioles. Blood pressure provides the force necessary to produce blood flow along the vessels.

15 Arterial blood pressure is calculated by multiplying the cardiac output by the total peripheral resistance.

16 Arterial blood pressure is measured by a sphygmomanometer. It is expressed as systolic and diastolic values. Blood pressure increases with age and with homeostatic imbalances, such as arteriosclerosis, hypertension, etc., and decreases with imbalances, such as hypotension, shock, heart failure, etc.

17 Blood pressure is normally maintained within its homeostatic range via a number of short-term and long-term blood pressure homeostatic controls. These can be divided broadly into neural and endocrine mechanisms, respectively.

18 Cardiovascular homeostatic parameters are reset in 'normal' homeostatic adaptive states, such as exercise and pregnancy.

19 The medulla oblongata of the brainstem contains the cardiac centres and the vasomotor centres. These centres control cardiovascular function.

20 Cardiovascular malfunctions may be classified as cardiac (Figure 12.34) and circulatory (Figure 12.35) homeostatic imbalances. It cannot be overemphasized, however, that neither malfunction exists in isolation without compromising the other's homeostatic function, together with the homeostatic functions of other tissues and organs, because of the interdependence of organ system functioning. Consequently, a vast array of clinical problems, ranging from the less severe (e.g. temporary ischaemic pain), to the very severe (e.g. cerebrovascular accident, kidney failure, pulmonary failure), present themselves when cardiovascular function is impaired.

  If you had difficulties with this chapter, refer to Clancy and McVicar (1996b), which summarizes the basic physiology associated with this organ system.

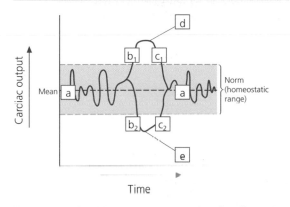

Figure 12.34 Cardiac output — an expression of cardiovascular function. (a) Cardiac output fluctuating within its normal homeostatic parameters. (b₁) Increased cardiac output as occurs normally, when the homeostatic parameters are reset (e.g. exercise), and abnormally, when indicating a homeostatic imbalance, such as right-to-left cardiac shunts (e.g. tetrology of Fallot, transposition of the great vessels), aortic stenosis (and its associated left ventricular hypertrophy), and tachycardia. (b₂) Decreased cardiac output, as occurs with homeostatic imbalances, such as the left-to-right cardiac shunts (atrial septal defects, ventricular septal defects, patent ductus arteriosus), cardiomyopathies, bradycardia, heart failure and incompetent valves. (c) Correction varies according to the imbalance, e.g. oxygen therapy for a cyanosed patient, drugs or pacemaker to correct conduction imbalances, and surgical techniques to correct structural defects. (d) Re-established homeostasis of cardiac output. (e) Homeostatic failure of cardiac output.

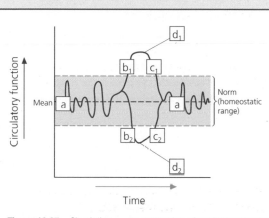

Figure 12.35 Circulation — an expression of cardiovascular function. (a) Circulatory function fluctuating within its homeostatic range. (b₁ Increased circulatory flow, as occurs normally with increased oxygen supply to the myocardium and muscle cells when the homeostatic flow parameters are reset, as in exercise, and abnormally, as occurs in hypertension. (b₂) Decreased circulatory flow, as occurs in the homeostatic imbalances of hypotension, ischaemic disease, myocardial infarctions, cerebrovascular accidents and thrombotic changes in vessels. (c₁) Clinical correction is dependent upon the underlying imbalance, i.e. anti-hypertensive therapy used in hypertension may be via diuretics, beta-blockers or relaxation therapies. (c₂) Clinical correction of the imbalance, e.g. hypotension is treated with anti-hypotensive drugs or by treating the underlying cause of the imbalance (e.g. hypothyroidism causes hypotension); myocardial ischaemia is treated with glycerol trinitrate, angioplasty or streptokinase therapy; tissue ischaemia is treated with peripheral vasodilators. (d) Continued imbalance because of the irreversibility of the underlying cause, e.g. (d₁) prolonged hypertension leading to cerebrovascular accident, myocardial infarction, renal failure, etc., or (d₂) prolonged hypotension leading to death due to cerebral ischaemia/infarction.

Review questions

1 Draw a simple diagram to show how the pulmonary and systemic circulatory pathways carry blood to and from the heart. Show the direction of flow of deoxygenated blood using a blue pen and that of oxygenated blood using a red pen.

2 Draw a simple diagram of the heart, labelling the four main chambers, four major vessels and the relevant heart valves. Identify the layers making up the wall of the heart and list the functions of each layer.

3 The heart is composed of muscle tissue that has special properties compared with skeletal and smooth muscle. Draw and label a diagram of a cardiac muscle cell. What are autorhythmic cells? Where are they found within heart tissue?

4 Explain how a nervous message spreads along a nerve cell by a wave of depolarization.

5 What is the heart aiming to achieve when it is working efficiently?

6 Try to visualize the route in which each message will travel throughout the heart muscle, bearing in mind that contraction of cells occurs immediately after they have conducted the impulse.

7 What is an electrocardiogram (ECG)? What does the QRS complex represent on an ECG?

8 What role do calcium ions play in muscle contraction?

9 Some drugs interfere with calcium ion release. What effect would these have on heart rate?

10 Rhythmic contraction of the heart establishes a pressure gradient throughout the vascular system, ensuring unidirectional flow of blood. What features do blood vessels possess that allow them to withstand such huge pressure fluctuations?

11 In which vessels does gaseous exchange occur? Why does it occur there?

12 In which blood vessels are valves found? What is the purpose of valves?

13 Some blood vessels are vasoactive. What does this mean?

14 Blood pressure must be kept within safe limits to allow the cells of the body to function efficiently. This can be achieved by altering the amount of blood that the heart pumps out and by altering the amount of peripheral resistance. What influences peripheral resistance?

15 Why do veins have thin walls and large lumens?

16 Consider how you would increase pressure in a hosepipe, then apply the same principles to the cardiovascular system.

17 Define the term 'arterial blood pressure'.

18 What do you understand by the terms 'systolic' and 'diastolic' blood pressure?

19 What is the function of baroreceptors, and where in the body are they located?

20 Describe the function and location of the vasomotor centre.

21 Why is venous return important in the control of blood pressure?

22 Identify other factors that may influence blood pressure.

Physiological rationale for cardiopulmonary resuscitation

23 Consider the steps involved in cardiopulmonary resuscitation (CPR) listed in Table 12.3 below. For each procedure, provide the physiological rationale for that particular action.

Table 12..3

Procedure
Assess environment and note time
Assess patient, including level of consciousness
Call for help
Assess other injuries
Position patient flat
Assess airway
Remove airway obstruction/finger sweep

Table 12..3 Continued

Procedure
Open airway using jaw-thrust or chin-lift technique
Assess breathing
Breathe exhaled air into patient (whilst pinching nose in adult/child)
Release nose pinch
Assess circulation by checking pulse (carotid in adult, brachial in infant)
Apply precordial thump ONLY If cardiac arrest is witnessed AND if ALS available
Place hands on sternum with arms straight and elbows locked
Commence external chest compression
Release pressure between compressions
Apply rhythmic compressions and ventilation at a ratio of 15:2 (or 5:1)
Continue until help arrives
Place patient in recovery position (should cardiopulmonary function return)

REFERENCES

Clancy, J. and McVicar, A.J. (1996a) Shock: a failure to maintain cardiovascular homeostasis. *British Journal of Theatre Nursing* **6**(6): 19–25.

Clancy, J. and McVicar, A.J. (1996b) The essentials of cardiovascular physiology. *British Journal of Theatre Nursing* **6**(4): 19–27.

Clancy, J. and McVicar, A.J. (1998) Homeostasis and nature–nurture interactions: a framework for integrating the life sciences: in Hinchliffe, S.S.M., Norman, S.E. and Schober, J.E. *Nursing Practice and Health*, 3rd edn. London: Arnold.

Clancy, J., McVicar, A.J. and Baird, N. (2001) *Fundamentals of Homeostasis for Perioperative Practitioners*. London: Routledge.

Colletti, C. (1999) Emergency! Pericarditis. *American Journal of Nursing* **99**(10): 35.

Criley, J.M. (1999) Bits and bytes of PA education. The physiological origins of heart sounds and murmurs: the unique interactive guide to cardiac diagnosis. *Perspective on Physician Assistant Education* **10**(3): 152.

Cucherat, M., Bonnefoy, E. and Tremeau, G. (2001) Primary angioplasty versus intravenous thrombolysis for acute myocardial infarction. The Cochran Library, Issue 1. Oxford: Update Software.

Holmwood, C. (2000) Overweight and hypertensive. *Australian Family Physician* **29**(6): 559–63.

Hood, W.B. Jr, Dans, A., Guyatt, G.H., Jaeschke, R. and McMurray J. (2001) Digitalis for treatment of congestive heart failure in patients in sinus rhythm. The Cochran Library, Issue 1. Oxford: Update Software.

Huether, S.E. and McCance, K.L. (1996) *Understanding pathophysiology* London: Mosby.

Nagle, B.M. and O'Keefe, L.M. (1999) Closing in on mitral valve disease. *Nursing* **29**(4): 32ccl–37ccl.

Pradka, L.R. (2000) Lipids and their role in coronary heart disease: what they do and how to manage them. *Nursing Clinics of North America* **35**(4): 901–91.

Suddaby, E.H. and Grenler, M.A. (1999) The embryology of congenital heart defects. *Paediatric Nursing* **25**(5): 499–504.

Whaley, L.F. and Wong, D.L. (1995) *Nursing Care of Infants and Children* St Louis: Mosby.

FURTHER READING

Blumenthal, J.A., Sherwood, A., Gullette, E.C.D., Babyak, M., Waugh, R., Georgiades, A., *et al.* (2000) Exercise and weight loss reduce blood pressure in men and women with mild hypertension: effects on cardiovascular, metabolic, and hemodynamic functioning. *Archives of Internal Medicine* **160**(13): 1947–58, 2068–9.

Ecord, J.S. (1999) Focus on peripheral pulmonary stenosis murmurs. *Neonatal Network – Journal of Neonatal Nursing* **18**(5): 65–6, 41–4.

Fleury, J. and Keller, C. (2000) Assessment. Cardiovascular risk assessment in elderly individuals. *Journal of Gerontological Nursing* **26**(5): 30–7.

Goh, T.H. (2000) Common congenital heart defects: the value of early detection. *Australian Family Physician* **29**(5): 429–31, 434–5, 462–3.

Hancock, E.W. (1999) ECG casebook. Mitral regurgitation with conduction defects. *Hospital Practice* **34**(9): 21–2.

Knight, M., Duley, L., Henderson-Smart, D.J. and King J.F. (2001) Antiplatelet agents for preventing and treating pre-eclampsia. The Cochrane Library, Issue 1. Oxford: Update Software.

Liu, M., Counsell, C. and Sandercock, P. (2001) Anticoagulation for preventing recurrence following ischaemic stroke or transient ischaemic attack. The Cochran Library, Issue 1. Oxford: Update Software.

Sowers, J.R. and Lester, M. (2000) Hypertension, hormones, and aging. *Journal of Laboratory and Clinical Medicine* **135**(5): 379–86.

Swierczynski, D. (2000) A taste of their own medicine. Diagnosis: heart murmur. *Men's Health* **15**(9): 62-4, 66.

Wigginton, M. (2001) Expanded ECGs: easy as V4, V5, V6. *Nursing* **31**(1): 50–1.

Yu, H.H., Pasternak, R.C. and Ginsburg, G.S. (2000) Lipid management for patients with CAD, part 1: what to expect, when to start: consider an aggressive strategy for prevention of cardiac events. *Journal of Critical Illness* **15**(5): 247–52, 262–4.

Chapter 13

The lymphatic system and immunity

INTRODUCTION

Relation of the lymphatic system to cellular homeostasis

Blood distributes oxygen and other metabolites to the body cells, and removes cellular waste products. Cells are bathed in tissue (interstitial) fluid, which acts as an intermediary fluid between blood and cells. The lymphatic system is an extensive, branched tubular network that aligns itself with the blood's circulation, and it is adapted for the prevention of tissue fluid accumulation. Excess fluid is returned back to the circulation, so the lymphatic system is important in the homeostatic maintenance of all body fluids. The system also acts as an intermediary between the digestive and circulatory systems, i.e. following absorption of a meal, it transports long-chain fatty acids and fat-soluble vitamins (A, D, E and K). In addition, the lymphatic system has immunological defence functions, filtering and destroying potential environmental hazards. Figure 13.1 summarizes the homeostatic functions of the lymphatic system.

BOX 13.1 WHY NURSES NEED TO UNDERSTAND IMMUNITY

An understanding of immunological homeostasis is important for nurses, since the human body's defences are continually operating to maintain intracellular integrity by waging warfare on harmful environmental agents. These noxious agents are in abundance in hospitals, even in the 'sterile' clinical areas of an operating theatre.

Of all the patients entering hospital without an infection, 10% will suffer a hospital-acquired infection. At any one time, about 20% of all patients in hospital are suffering from a hospital-acquired infection (May, 2000; Salvage 2000). Prevention of such an occurrence is a key nursing responsibility.

Nursing practice requires a swift response to dynamic changes associated with the patient's condition, e.g. as with the progressive nature of wound development, wound healing, and the stages of infection and fever. All need continued involvement in reassessing, modifying care plans, and implementing care according to the patient's changing needs. In relation to theatre, staff must constantly support, monitor and anticipate the side effects and complications of trauma caused by injury either outside the theatre or by surgery itself.

Aseptic technique is a procedure associated with specific tasks, such as wound dressing, but awareness of the importance of hand washing, cleanliness, and prevention of infection to yourself, others and vulnerable patients, is far more important in all nursing activities.

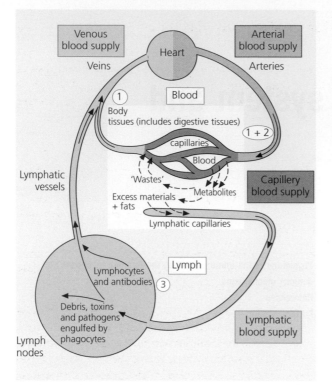

Figure 13.1 Summary of the homeostatic functions associated with the lymphatic system. 1, regulation of body fluids; 2, fat and fat-soluble vitamins (A, D, E and K) absorption; 3, defence functions.

venous blood supply; arterial blood supply; capillary blood supply; lymphatic blood supply.

Q. Using the text and this figure, describe the homeostatic functions of the lymphatic system.

Relation of the immune system to cellular homeostasis

The human body's external and internal (or immunological) defences act continually to maintain cellular homeostasis by combating harmful environmental agents. Agents that frequently trigger an immune response are:

- disease-causing organisms (pathogens or immunogens), e.g. bacteria and viruses;

- pathogenic surface receptors (antigens) (Figure 13.2);

- pathogenic secretions, e.g. bacterial toxins (also antigenic);

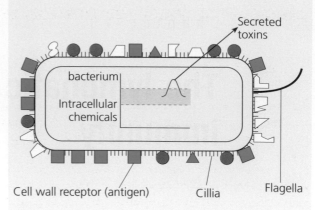

Figure 13.2 The immunogen is the bacterium, which may have many antigens (i.e. cell-wall receptors).

Q. Differentiate between the following: (i) immunogen, (ii) antigen and (iii) pathogen.

- environmental pollutants, e.g. dust particles (pollutants are in abundance, even, potentially, in operating theatre areas).

Resistance is comprised of complementary nonspecific and specific defence mechanisms. Nonspecific resistance is the immunity present at birth. It includes mechanisms that provide immediate but general protection against the invasion of a wide range of pathogens, such as bacteria, viruses, fungi and parasites. These defence mechanisms are the same for everyone, hence the term 'nonspecific'. They include:

- external physical barriers, such as the skin, and chemical barriers, such as the acidity of the stomach;

- internal (bodily) reactions, including the phagocytic response, which provide immunological surveillance against pathogenic microbes and microbial toxins.

Specific resistance is the immunity that is acquired during life upon exposure to harmful agents; it thus develops more slowly. It develops mostly after birth, when an individual becomes exposed to potential environmental hazards. The body system responsible for immunity is the lymphatic system. Specific immunity is the lymphocytic response. It involves activating specific lymphocytes (lymph cells), and stimulating them to release their secretions (cytotoxic substances and antibodies) in response to 'foreign' substances (antigens) entering the body.

Both nonspecific and specific immunities are adapted to maintain the equilibrium of the body's internal environment.

OVERVIEW OF THE ANATOMY AND PHYSIOLOGY OF THE LYMPHATIC SYSTEM

Lymphatic vessels and the lymphatic circulation

The lymphatic capillaries are thin, closed-ended vessels present in all body tissues, except in the spleen and in those areas not serviced directly by the circulation (e.g. cornea of the eye), the central nervous system, and bone marrow. The lymphatics of the skin travel in loose subcutaneous adipose tissue, generally following veins, whereas visceral lymphatics generally follow arteries, forming networks (called plexuses) around them. Lymph (the tissue fluid inside the lymphatics) is produced at a rate of about 1.5 ml/min throughout the body. The lymphatics merge, forming larger vessels, the largest of which drain into two large ducts called the right lymphatic duct and the thoracic duct.

These ducts empty their contents into blood within the neck region, at the junction of the left subclavian and jugular veins (Figure 13.3). By preventing tissue fluid accumulation, this drainage helps to ensure that a constant blood volume and composition is maintained. Approximately 2–4 l of interstitial fluid accumulate and return to the blood in 24 h. This results in a constant turnover of this fluid tissue. If, however, the return of lymph is blocked, as in the case of tumour compression, then tissue fluid accumulates (oedema) distal to the obstruction.

Return of lymph to the circulation

The flow rate of lymph is very slow compared with blood. Two factors control lymph flow rate, and hence its return to blood:

- *Tissue pressure.* When tissue fluid pressure (i.e. volume), rises above its homeostatic range, there is a greater formation of lymph, which enhances its flow rate.

- *Lymphatic pump.* Lymph vessels have valves that promote unidirectional movement towards the neck region, so lymph can be returned to the blood circulation. The flow of lymph is encouraged via the compression exerted by muscles and other tissues surrounding the lymphatic vessels. These muscles and tissues are referred to as the 'lymphatic pumps'.

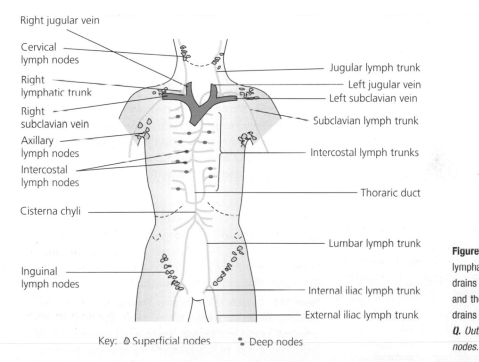

Right jugular vein
Cervical lymph nodes
Right lymphatic trunk
Right subclavian vein
Axillary lymph nodes
Intercostal lymph nodes
Cisterna chyli
Inguinal lymph nodes

Jugular lymph trunk
Left jugular vein
Left subclavian vein
Subclavian lymph trunk
Intercostal lymph trunks
Thoracic duct
Lumbar lymph trunk
Internal iliac lymph trunk
External iliac lymph trunk

Key: ○ Superficial nodes   • Deep nodes

Figure 13.3 The main vessels of the lymphatic system. The right lymphatic duct drains the right side of the head and neck, and the right arm. The thoracic lymphatic duct drains the rest of the body.
Q. Outline the clinical importance of lymph nodes.

BOX 13.2 LYMPHOEDEMA FOLLOWING SURGICAL REMOVAL OF BREAST CANCER

Upon surgical removal of the axillary lymph glands, e.g. in the treatment of breast cancer, the patient frequently has arm oedema (lymphoedema, see Box 13.5). The patient may experience problems such as heavy, painful arms and skin tightness and swelling, providing a further alteration of body image in addition to the breast surgery, and consequential loss of self-esteem. Management of the lymphoedema consists of skin care, massage and compression, advice on activities, exercise and psychological support.

Increased metabolic rate (such as experienced during exercise, illness and stress) increases the efficiency of lymphatic pumps. This is a homeostatic necessity, since an increased metabolic rate is associated with a greater blood flow to the highly metabolizing cells, resulting in greater tissue fluid formation. Consequently, a greater lymph formation results, producing a greater flow rate of lymph to maintain blood volume.

The lymphoidal system

In addition to fluid and solutes of the interstitium, lymph also contains specialized cells that form an important part of the mechanism by which the body defends itself against infection by microorganisms. The various organs that comprise the lymphoidal system may be classified as primary or secondary (Figure 13.4). The primary organs (bone marrow, thymus and fetal liver) produce the lymphocytes. These lymphocytes then migrate to the secondary organs (spleen, lymph nodes, and other lymphatic tissue throughout the body).

Lymph nodes

Lymphatic nodes are oval-shaped masses of lymphatic tissue encapsulated by dense, connective tissue. The organ consists of:

- *cortex:* contains B-lymphocytes aggregated into primary follicles. Following stimulation by an antigen, these follicles develop into a focus of active growth or proliferation, and are then termed secondary follicles. These follicles are in intimate contact with the antigen-presenting cells (see later);

- *paracortex:* contains T-lymphocytes;

- *medulla:* contains T- and B-lymphocytes.

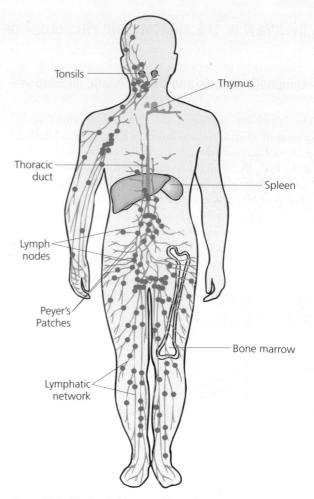

Figure 13.4 The lymphoid system. The various organs of the lymphoid system are classified as primary or secondary. The primary organs (bone marrow, thymus, fetal liver) are the sites where lymphocytes are produced. Lymphocytes generated in the primary lymphoid organs migrate to the secondary organs (mainly the spleen and lymph nodes, and various lymphoid tissues throughout the body).
Q. Which class of blood vessel transport blood in a manner similar to lymphatic vessels?

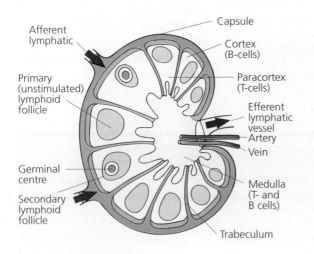

Figure 13.5 Structure of a lymph node. The organ consists of cortex, paracortex, medulla and connective tissue capsule. Lymphocytes and antigens (if present) enter the node through the afferent lymphatics. The lymph drains through the node (sinuses) and passes out of the medulla of the node through the efferent lymphatic vessel. The B-cells in the cortex are aggregated into primary follicles; subsequent to stimulation by antigen, they develop a focus of active proliferation (germinal centre) and are termed 'secondary follicles'. These follicles are in close contact with antigen-presenting dendritic cells. The paracortex contains T-cells, and the medulla contains both T- and B-cells. Each node has its own blood supply.
Q. Why are the spleen, thymus and gut-associated lymph nodes considered to be organs of the lymphatic system?

The roles of the T- and B-lymphocytes are described later. Each node has internal extensions of fibrous capsule, called trabeculae, which dip through the outer cortex and inner medullar regions of the node (Figure 13.5). Nodes can exist individually, located randomly, e.g. the urogenital and respiratory mucous membranes, or they can exist as multiple nodular complexes located at specific sites, e.g. the tonsils, Peyer's patches, appendix, spleen and thymus gland.

Afferent vessels transport lymph into the node sinuses (a series of irregular channels), after which it circulates into one or two outgoing (efferent) vessels located at the exit. Efferent vessels are wider than afferent vessels; they contain valves that open away from the nodes, and encourage the flow of lymph in one direction.

Nodular filtering action: a homeostatic function

Immunogens and antigens become entrapped in the lymph nodes as they filter the lymph passing through the lymphatic network during its passage from the periphery to the thoracic ducts. They are destroyed via:

- phagocytosis by macrophages;

- cytotoxic secretions (e.g. interleukin, interferon) produced and secreted by T-lymphocytes;

- antibodies produced and secreted by B-lymphocytes.

The thymus gland

The thymus is positioned in the upper thorax above and in front of the heart, between the lungs, and behind the sternum. It extends back into the root of the neck (Figure 13.4).

> ### BOX 13.3 THE THYMUS DURING THE LIFESPAN
>
> The size of the thymus increases until puberty. It begins to involute during adolescence, and by middle age it has returned to its size at birth. Despite this reduction in size during adulthood, evidence suggests that the thymus continue to function throughout life. However, the effectiveness of its lymphocytes in response to antigenic insults declines.

Structure of the thymus

The thymus is a bilobed gland encapsulated by fibrous tissue. Each lobe has a peripheral cortex and a central medulla. The cortex consists of small, medium and large, tightly packed lymphocytes; the medulla comprises mainly epithelial cells and diffused scattered lymphocytes. Internal capsular extensions (trabeculae) divide the organ into lobules, which consist of an irregular branching framework of epithelial cells responsible for the production of thymus secretions and lymphocytes.

Homeostatic functions of the thymus

The thymus is responsible primarily for the production and support of T-cells. Such cells originate in the bone marrow, where stem cells differentiate into specialized lymphocytes in a process called lymphopoiesis. The majority of these cells enter the thymus, where they develop in the cortex into stem T-lymphocytes. These undergo cell division (mitosis), and upon maturation move into the medulla. These mature cells remain in systemic blood, enter systemic blood, and are transported to lymphoidal tissue, or remain in the thymus gland, to become the future generations of T-lymphocytes.

Thymus epithelial cells also produce thymosin. This hormone is responsible for the maturation of the thymus and other lymphoidal tissue.

> ### BOX 13.4 DI GEORGE SYNDROME
>
> Children suffering from Di George syndrome are born without a thymus, and so are highly susceptible to those infections usually combated by T-cell-dependent immunity. Death may occur unless a healthy thymus graft is transplanted. Children born with B-cell deficiencies are subjected to infections usually combated primarily by antibody-mediated immunity (see later). These children require repeated injection of serum antibodies from healthy donors.

The spleen

The adult spleen is the largest collection of lymphoidal tissue in the body. It is approximately 12 cm long, 7 cm wide and 2.5 cm thick, and weighs about 150 g. The spleen is positioned in the left of the abdomen, lying between the stomach and diaphragm (Figure 13.4.).

Structure of the spleen

Anteriorly, the spleen's encapsulated surface is covered with peritoneum. The organ's oval shape is determined by structures that are in close proximity (Figure 13.6(a)). It contains a number of surface features including:

- a gastric impression (the organ's soft consistency enables its shape to change according to the stomach's contents);

- a renal impression;

- a colon impression;

- a smooth, convex diaphragmatic surface, which conforms to the concave surface of the adjacent diaphragm.

The organ is divided into an outer red pulp, which contains sinuses filled with blood, and a centrally located white pulp consisting of lymphatic tissue. The latter contains lymphocytes and macrophages. Entering and leaving the spleen are the splenic artery and vein, efferent

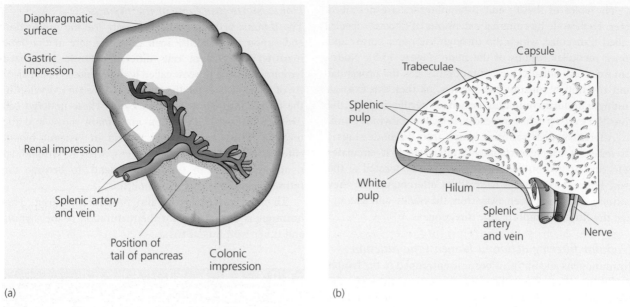

Figure 13.6 (a) The spleen. The oval shape is determined by the structures in close proximity to it. (b) Section of the spleen.

lymphatics, and a nerve supply (Figure 13.6(b)). Blood in the splenic artery flows into the spleen's sinuses. These have pores between the lining endothelial cells, allowing blood to come into close association with the splenic pulp cells.

Homeostatic functions of the spleen

The spleen performs the same functions for blood that lymph nodes perform for lymph, i.e. it is involved with:

- *phagocytosis:* as the spleen is part of the reticuloendothelial system, it has phagocytes that are involved with the breakdown of erythrocytes. The breakdown products bilirubin, iron and globin are released from haemoglobin, and are passed to the liver by splenic and portal veins. Leucocytes, thrombocytes and microbes are also phagocytosed in the spleen. The spleen has no afferent lymphatics, so it is not exposed to infections spread via the lymphatic system.

- *development of lymphocytes:* the spleen produces T-lymphocytes and, in particular, B-lymphocytes.

In addition to these immunological functions, the spleen acts as a blood reservoir, releasing blood on demand, e.g. following severe haemorrhage. This release is controlled by the sympathetic nervous system and is a homeostatic mechanism that helps to maintain the composition of body fluids.

Exercise

Before studying the next section, reflect on your understanding of the meaning of 'immunity', and the difference between the specific and nonspecific immune responses. Suggest why the spleen, thymus and gut-associated lymph nodes are considered organs of the lymphatic system.

PHYSIOLOGY OF THE LYMPHATIC SYSTEM: LYMPH FORMATION

Chapters 6 and 12 discussed how positive filtration pressures in blood capillaries cause the exudation (secretion) of fluid from plasma, resulting in the formation of tissue fluid, and how negative filtration pressures at the venous ends of capillaries ensure that tissue fluid is returned to the blood. The return, however, cannot compensate totally for the loss, thus there is a potential for the accumulation of tissue fluid. In addition, because capillary walls are slightly permeable to protein, there is a slow

but steady loss of small blood proteins to tissue fluid. These proteins cannot be returned to the circulation across capillary walls, since there is insufficient fluid pressure to move them in that direction.

The lymphatics drain the tissue fluid that is in excess of its homeostatic range, and so returns the proteins to the blood. The endothelial cells of lymphatic vessels are not bound tightly, but they overlap; the regions of overlap function as one-way valves. These permit the entry of fluid (and the exuded proteins) into the vessels, but prevent their return to the interstitial spaces. Accumulation of tissue fluid causes the tissues to swell; the increased tissue fluid pressure opens the endothelial valves further, so more fluid can flow into the lymph capillaries. The larger capillaries also contain semilunar valves. These are quite close together, and each causes the vessel to bulge, giving the lymphatic system a beaded appearance (Figure 13.4). As discussed earlier, these valves aid normal lymphatic flow. On its return journey to blood, lymph flows through one or more lymph nodes. Their homeostatic function is to filter the lymph of potential antigenic material, and then destroy pathogens and their toxins (described later).

The large thoracic duct receives lymph from vessels below the diaphragm, from the left half of the head, neck and chest, and empties into the venous system, close to the junction of the left internal jugular and left subclavian veins. The smaller right lymphatic duct ends at a comparable location on the right side. It drains lymph from the right side of the body above the diaphragm (Figure 13.3).

The lymphatic system is therefore a homeostatic mechanism for the maintenance of body fluid composition and volume. Clinical conditions that inhibit such a return may influence fluid distribution to such an extent that death can occur in less than 24 h if the balance is not restored.

Exercise

Describe the relationship between plasma, tissue fluid and lymph. Which factors promote the flow of lymph?

BOX 13.5 HOMEOSTATIC IMBALANCES OF THE LYMPHATIC SYSTEM

There are multiple clinical conditions associated with lymphatic homeostatic imbalances. This box considers two ways in which lymphatic function can be jeopardized: the spread of disease, leading to lymphatic infections and/or tumours, and lymphatic obstruction.

Spread of disease

Lymph capillaries drain tissue fluid, which may contain pathogens and tumour cells. If these are not phagocytosed, they may settle and multiply in the first lymph node they encounter, thus producing localized infection or tumours. Alternatively, subsequent to proliferation, they may spread to other lymph nodes, blood, or other parts of the body, using the body's transporting systems. Consequently, each new site of infection or (metastatic) tumour becomes a further source of infection or malignant cells via the same routes, thus producing infections or tumours elsewhere, such as in tonsillitis, appendicitis, glandular fever, lymphoma, thymoma and splenomas. Breast cancer frequently shows lymphatic spread.

Inflammation of the lymphatic vessels (lymphangitis) may cause the vessel to be visible in the superficial vessels as a red streak tracking to the next set of lymph nodes (e.g. from an infected toe to the nodes at the back of the knee).

Infections and tumours, and the presence of excessive amounts of abnormal material such as bacteria and their toxins, can cause lymph node and lymph organ enlargement (Figure 13.7). With a 'sore throat' or a 'cold', the cervical (neck) lymph nodes enlarge in response to the infection. Lay people often claim that their 'glands are up', but please note that lymph nodes are not glands, as they do not secrete or excrete secretions. Glands are 'up' because the nodes are actively producing defence mechanisms against the incoming antigens. The nodes only become swollen and painful when the immunogen (e.g. bacteria) has infected the node and the person's defence mechanisms are compromised.

The enlargement is reversed when the infection subsides (either naturally or by using clinical intervention, e.g. antibiotic therapy), and/or the tumour or abnormal particle is destroyed or moved on. Reinfections, new tumours or reintroduced abnormal particles, however, result in tissue fibrosis and a continued enlargement. Lymphatic organs that become chronically inflamed,

Figure 13.7 Lymphocytic structure and function: a homeostatic process. (a) Normal lymphocytic function and structure. (b₁) Hyperplasia of lymphatic tissue and organs. Tumours are examples of permanent failures of hyperplasia, e.g. lymphomas (Hodgkin's and non-Hodgkin's), thymoma (rare, but occurs in myasthenia gravis) and splenomas (hypersplenism). Pathogenic infections are examples of temporary hyperplasia, e.g. tonsillitis (bacterial infection), glandular fever (viral infection) and splenomegaly (secondary infected site). These are signs that the immune system is attempting to restore homeostasis. (b₂) Homeostatic failures associated with hypoplasia of lymphoidal tissue and organs, e.g. hyposplenism (missing or functionless spleen). (c₁) Clinical correction involves radiotherapy, chemotherapy, surgical removal (only cure for hypersplenism) or, more commonly, a combination of the above to remove permanent hyperplastic failures. Correction of temporary

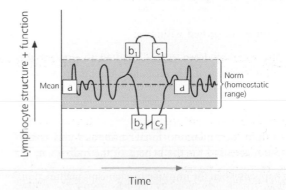

hyperplastic failures depends upon type of infection, e.g. antibiotic therapy for tonsillitis, rest for glandular fever. (c₂) Correction involves special immunization programmes.

BOX 13.5 CONTINUED

and are associated with abscess formation, may require surgical removal to reduce the incidence and severity of subsequent infections.

Cancerous lymph nodes, as well as feeling large, are firm, non-tender and fixed to underlying structures. In contrast, infected lymph nodes that are enlarged due to infection are not firm, are moveable, and are very tender. The cancerous nodes often become the sites of metastatic cancer.

Splenomegaly (enlargement of the spleen) usually occurs secondary to other conditions, such as circulatory disorders and infections, or cirrhosis of the liver. Hyperactivity of the spleen increases its phagocytic activities and leads to a reduced blood cell count (anaemia, thrombocytopenia and leucopenia). Surgical removal – splenectomy – is the only known cure for this condition.

Rupture of the spleen because of its soft consistency is quite common in traumatic injuries, such as broken ribs. Rupture causes severe intraperitoneal haemorrhage, and may lead to shock. Following diagnosis, the condition is stabilized with blood transfusion. Splenectomy is performed to prevent the patient bleeding to death.

Once bleeding has been controlled the person soon recovers. A common anxiety for the patient is 'How long can I live without my spleen?' Nurses can anticipate and prevent this anxiety by explaining that macrophages in other areas of the body (e.g. bone marrow, liver) take over, and that there is plenty of other lymphatic tissue to cope with the spleen's former immunological role.

A missing or non-functional spleen causes hyposplenism. This does not pose a serious problem, although hyposplenic people are more prone to microbial infection, so special immunization programmes are recommended.

Hypertrophy of the thymus is associated with autoimmune disease of the thyroid (thyrotoxicosis).

Lymphoidal tumours are classified as Hodgkin's and non-Hodgkin's lymphomas. Hodgkin's lymphoma, a malignant disease, is initially a homeostatic imbalance of cell division (hyperplasia) in the superficial lymph glands, which metastasize to other lymphoidal tissues throughout the body. Although white blood cell counts are elevated, the cells are immature. Specific complications include a deficiency of cell-mediated immunity and thus an increased susceptibility to microbial infections. This disease was formerly always fatal; however, isolated bouts of radiotherapy, or combined radiochemotherapy, have considerably improved the prospects of securing remission for long periods. The effectiveness of treatment depends largely on the stage of disease when the treatment is begun.

Non-Hodgkin's tumours occur in the lymphoidal tissue and bone marrow, and are classified as low grade or high grade. Low-grade lymphomas are well-differentiated tumours that progress slowly; death occurs usually after several years. High-grade lymphomas are poorly differentiated tumours that progress rapidly; death occurs in weeks or months.

Thymomas (thymus tumours) and splenomas (spleen tumours) are rare. Node and organ enlargement due to tumour growth usually necessitates surgical removal, since complications may arise due to growth interfering with the functions of adjacent structures.

Lymphatic obstruction

Tumours, depending upon their site and growth, can cause obstruction inside lymphatic vessels or inside nodes. In addition, if external to the lymphatic vessel, they may cause sufficient external pressure to restrict lymph flow. Surgery to remove lymph node cancers and to prevent metastases can also result in lymphatic obstruction. The accumulation of lymph as a result of the obstruction to lymph flow results in a swelling, called lymphoedema, the extent of which depends upon the size of the obstructed vessel. Lymphoedema also occurs as a consequence of local inflammation, and the subsequent lymphatic fibrosis, which enhances this condition. Other causes of lymphoedema include damage from surgery, radiotherapy or parasitic disease, such as filariasis (infestation with tiny thread-like worms).

PHYSIOLOGY OF THE IMMUNE SYSTEM: THE IMMUNE RESPONSES AND DEFENCE MECHANISMS

This section is concerned with:

● how the external defences are adapted to prevent the entry of environmental hazards into the body;

● how the internal defences operate following external defence failure;

● how immunization, monoclonal antibodies and transplantation are used for the benefit of the individual;

● what happens when the immune mechanisms malfunction.

Both external and internal defence mechanisms exhibit nonspecific (i.e. common) and specific responses. We mentioned in the introduction that nonspecific immunity is the body's natural resistance to disease. Its two roles are to prevent the entry of pathogenic agents into the body, and to prevent the spread of those agents that have successfully gained entrance to the body.

External defence mechanisms

The nonspecific components of the external defence mechanisms include (Figure 13.8):

● skin and mucous membranes

● digestive reflexes and secretions

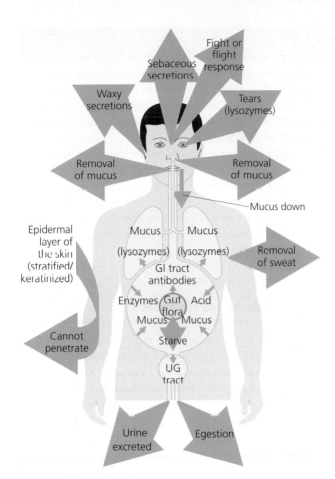

Figure 13.8 The physical and chemical barriers of natural immunity.
GI, gastrointestinal; UG, urogenital.

Q. Describe how the acid and alkali pH along the gastrointestinal tract is related to providing immunity.

- tears
- lysozymes
- urination and defecation
- memory and stress response.

Skin and mucous membranes

The skin and mucous membranes are the body's first line of resistance. Both act as physical barriers that prevent pathogenic agents from entering their target tissues. For example, the viruses that cause hepatitis must gain access to liver cells. These organisms, however, must first penetrate external barriers to enter blood, which then transports them to their target sites.

The intact skin is the most effective external barrier of the body. It provides a watertight barricade, protecting the internal organs (viscera) from infection. The effectiveness

becomes apparent only when there is widespread damage to the skin. For example, with serious burns, infection becomes a real danger, and infection prevention and control are major considerations in treating patients with burns.

New epidermal cells are continually being formed because the skin is constantly subjected to abrasion and injury. The epidermis is normally renewed every 15–30 days. This obviously relies on adequate nutrients in the microcirculation on the skin. If there is a reduced blood supply, the balance between cell breakdown and cell replacement is displaced in favour of cell death (necrosis), and erosion of the skin tissue occurs. If circulation is sluggish, or if local conditions promote vasoconstriction, then blood flow is reduced, further problems occur, and tissue breakdown occurs more quickly.

The skin contains two principal layers: the outer epidermis and the inner dermis. Together, they provide physical and chemical protection.

Physical factors

The epidermis is a stratified (layered) squamous epithelium; some of its cells contain the tough water-proofing protein keratin. The stratum corneum is the primary barrier to the loss of water and other hydrophilic (water-liking) substances from the body. The lipid matrix in which cells are embedded is not penetrated easily by hydrophilic substances (i.e. water does not pass through lipids). Also, proteins inside cells attract and hold on to those molecules. This restricts water loss from the body. Consequently, the surface of the skin is normally fairly dry, and only a small amount of water is lost from the surface each day. These characteristics make this tissue a formidable physical barrier for the entrance of potential pathogenic materials, and bacteria rarely penetrate the intact healthy epidermis.

Chemical factors

The epidermal surface contains sweat and sebaceous glands. Sweat and sebum secretions are acidic (pH 5.5) in nature, which discourages the growth of alkali-liking microbes whose enzymes cannot operate in such conditions. The acidic pH, however, encourages growth of microbes whose enzymes favour this environment. However, these organisms must still penetrate the stratified epidermis if they are to cause infection in the organs of the body. Sweat and sebum also contain bactericidal chemicals (i.e. chemicals that kill bacteria), antibodies and lysozymes, which contribute to the skin's functions of

BOX 13.6 INFECTIONS: A FAILURE OF THE EXTERNAL BARRIERS

When the epidermis and the blood vessels in the dermis are damaged by cuts and burns, the person is potentially exposed to pathogenic infection, in particular staphylococcal infections, since staphylococcus's (a type of bacterium) natural habitats include hair follicles and sweat glands. Other environmental pathogens may also seize the opportunity, e.g. it is common for tetanus-causing bacteria to be introduced into the circulation via gardening injuries. Since skin wounds are common, tetanus immunization programmes have been developed to prevent this type of infection.

When adhesive tape is removed from the skin, it removes the stratum corneum, thus making the skin much more permeable at that site. The use of detergents and organic solvents, such as white spirit and turps, also increases the permeability of the skin. These chemicals dissolve components of the lipid matrix between cells and allow fluid to enter the spaces, which act as channels for the diffusion of water-soluble substances.

Prolonged soaking in water changes the character of the skin's surface. The epidermal cells 'swell' as they take up more water, and the properties of the barrier change. Skin infections are therefore much more frequent in people whose skin is regularly soaked in water. Perhaps a contributory factor for this type of infection is the washing away of protective secretions.

protection and defence. Sebum, for example, inhibits the growth of certain bacteria, such as streptococcus, which are the main cause of sore throats.

Perspiration (sweating) actively removes some microbes from the skin's surface. Changing climatic conditions can, however, alter the skin's resistance to certain infections. For example, hot, humid environments, in which sweat evaporation is limited, encourage fungal infections, such as athlete's foot.

Skin derivatives, such as hair and nails, protect the epidermis from mechanical abrasion and consequential damage from hazardous stimuli. Ceruminous secretion (earwax) also acts as an external barrier to microbes.

The skin's interactive roles with the body's specific immune responses are discussed later.

Mucous membranes line those body cavities that are open to the external environment. The principal cavities concerned are the respiratory, digestive and urogenital tracts. Mucus is a viscous secretion that prevents membrane desiccation (drying out); its adhesive properties trap microbes, and so prevent their spread. In some regions, cilia remove the entrapped materials from the body. For example, respiratory epithelia move mucus (and inhaled noxious agents) to the throat. This stimulates coughing or sneezing reflexes to remove the mucoidal mixture to the external environment (unfortunately, this is also a highly effective way of spreading infection). Alternatively, the mixture is swallowed, and gastrointestinal secretions usually destroy any microbes present (see below).

The pH of mucus, and the presence of lysozymes and antibodies, contributes to epithelial defence functions. Mucous membranes, however, are less effective than the skin at inhibiting microbial penetration. Infection is therefore more frequent in body cavities that are open to the external environment. Common microbial infections of the respiratory, digestive and urogenital mucous membranes include colds, influenza, gastroenteritis and sexually transmitted infections.

Digestive reflexes and secretions

Information from our sensory taste buds and olfactory sensory receptors regarding the palpability of food will either enhance our desire to eat or lead us to reject it. In the digestive tract, the reflexes diarrhoea and vomiting (D & V) expel unwanted invaders and hence protect the epithelia.

After swallowing, the vomit reflex is a mechanism of rejection of food and its microbial content. The vomiting centre of the brain, located in the medulla oblongata, receives signals from receptors in the upper respiratory tract and the chemoreceptor trigger zone in the medulla oblongata itself. Receptors in the upper digestive tract monitor the volume and composition of ingested products, whereas cells in the medulla are sensitive to blood-borne chemicals, including drugs such as apomorphine.

The vomiting reflex triggers the relaxation of the stomach and retroperistalsis ('retro-' = reverse) of the small intestine. These events hold substances in the stomach. Simultaneously, the glottis closes, closing off the respiratory tract. Contractions of the abdominal muscles and diaphragm squeeze the stomach and expel its contents through the oesophagus and into the mouth. The pressure in the stomach drives the part of the oesophagus that usually lies in the abdomen up into the thorax, causing the cardiac sphincter function to be lost (see Figure 10.8). The vomiting reflex is accompanied by a generalized activation of sympathetic nervous system, which causes increased salivation, sweating, tachycardia and cutaneous vasoconstriction.

Irritation of the lower digestive tract causes secretion and contractile activity that promotes expulsion of irritants via the rectum, as in diarrhoea. Irritants include bacterial toxins (e.g. cholera toxin) and plant products used as laxatives (e.g. senna). Cells of the gastrointestinal epithelium are constantly shed, thus this epithelium must undergo constant renewal to sustain its homeostatic function. These cells, like food, are digested; the products are absorbed and used in cell metabolism. The rapid replacement of gastric cells in the stomach may be an important way to protect the stomach against erosion-producing ulcers.

Saliva

In addition to its digestive properties, saliva has defence functions, including:

- washing and cleansing the teeth, gums and mouth, thus removing food particles that otherwise would encourage bacterial growth and the consequential formation of acids, which may lead to dental caries, loss of teeth, or gum abscess;

- discouraging the growth of acid-liking microbes by inactivating their enzymes due to its slightly alkaline constitution (pH 7–8).

Gastric juice

Food (and the inevitable presence of microbes) is swallowed and passed to the stomach. In this region, gastric acid (pH 2–3) destroys alkali-liking microbes and bacterial toxins. Conversely, the stomach's pH encourages growth of acid-liking microbes.

Intestinal juice

The intestinal alkaline fluid (pH 7–8) destroys acid-liking microbes.

Digestive secretions therefore have important external defence properties by destroying (denaturing) microbial enzymes, and so promoting microbial death. Gastrointestinal tract infections such as gastroenteritis occur when these defence functions are overwhelmed.

Lachrymal secretions

Lachrymal secretions (tears) are continually secreted. Blinking spreads them over the eye surface. This continual washing action helps to dilute microbes and keep them from settling on the surface of the eye. Tears only become evident, however, when they are secreted in excess. Hypersecretion may be due to the presence of large microbial colonies or irritants on the eye surface, or when the individual is overcome by severe emotions.

Tears, together with their entrapped dust particles and microbes, are directed towards the nasal passageways via the lachrymal ducts. Respiratory and digestive defences then usually destroy pathogenic materials.

Lysozymes

Lysozymes are catalytic enzymes (nucleases, proteases, lipases, carbohydrases, etc.) that are capable of 'digesting' potential pathogens. Lysozymes are abundant in tissue fluids, tears, saliva and nasal secretions, so their effects are widespread.

Urination and defecation

Urine and faecal matter are potential media for the growth of pathogenic organisms. Frequent urination and defecation helps to prevent excessive growth of these colonies.

Memory and stress response

Once the individual has become conditioned to identify potential environmental threats, e.g. the expected presence of pathogenic microbes or corrosive acids, then memory and the stress response are involved in avoiding such potential hazards.

> **Exercise**
>
> Identify how each external defence mechanism attempts to prevent the entry of environmental hazards ('antigenic insults').

Internal defence mechanisms

When pathogenic agents penetrate the external defence mechanisms, they encounter a second line of defence: internal antimicrobial proteins, phagocytic cells, and the homeostatic reflexes associated with inflammation and fever. Blood and tissue fluid contain three main types of antimicrobial proteins that inhibit microbial growth:

- *Complement.* A group of normally inactive proteins (precursors) located in blood and on cell membranes make up the complement system. When activated, these proteins 'complement' certain immune, allergic and inflammatory reactions.

- *Transferrins.* These iron-binding proteins inhibit the growth of certain bacteria by reducing the amount of available iron.

- *Interferon.* Macrophages, lymphocytes and fibroblasts infected with viruses produce a group of proteins called interferons. These chemicals are released from infected cells and move to neighbouring uninfected cells, whereby they bind to surface receptors, stimulating the synthesis of antiviral proteins that interfere with viral replication. This inhibition of replication is essential since viruses can cause disease only if they replicate within body (host) cells. Interferons are an important defence against many different viruses.

External defences are mainly nonspecific. Nonspecific immune responses are also observed internally; these include the inflammatory and phagocytic responses to antigens. Internal defences also include the specific immune responses (called the lymphocytic response) that act against specific antigens. These will be described later. This section will discuss the process of inflammation.

Nonspecific responses: inflammation

Inflammation occurs when cells are damaged by antigenic components. This response has both protective and defensive roles, and acts to restore tissue homeostasis by neutralizing and destroying antigens at the site of injury. Inflammation is an internal defence mechanism representing a co-ordinated nonspecific response to tissue injury, i.e. the processes involved are the same in response to any antigenic insult or wound damage. The appearance of the inflamed area, however, depends upon two factors:

- *Strength of environmental hazard (or stimulus) applied*. The weakest stimulus produces a reflex vasoconstriction, causing the inflamed area to pale, whereas stronger stimuli produce vasodilation of capillary networks, then arterioles, bringing a flush to the tissue. The strongest stimulus produces a raised wheal around the lesion or wound. Such inflammation is usually associated with redness, pain, heat and swelling. The injured site may lose its functions, but this depends upon the actual site and the extent of the injury.

- *Pathogenicity*. Microbes with a greater pathogenicity (i.e. ability to cause disease) cause a greater degree of inflammation.

The body reacts in the same way regardless of whether a tissue is damaged via mechanical, thermal or chemical causes, or in response to a hypersensitive reaction or a pathogenic invasion. The tissue soon shows the four classic signs of inflammation (see Figure 11.16), which provide reassurance that normal homeostatic responses have been activated following injury (DeCruz, 1998). These signs are redness, increase in tissue temperature, swelling, discomfort and/or pain. An additional sign of loss of function may follow these responses. The first three responses are attributed to changes in the microcirculation in the injured tissue. The redness (erythema) is due to vasodilation of arterioles; heat is due to increased blood flow; and swelling (oedema) is due to an increase in the extravascular fluid content of the injured tissues. This post-traumatic oedema is promoted by an increase in the permeability of small blood vessels, and is termed an 'exudate'.

The permeability changes are in response to the secretion from the site of injury of cellular products of metabolism, such as:

- histamine, released from a type of white cell called mast cells (basophils), platelets, and damaged cells at the site of injury;

- serotonin and heparin, released from mast cells;

- kinins and prostaglandins, released from injured cells;

The vasodilator effects of histamine, kinins and prostaglandins also elevate the local temperature. This may act as a homeostatic defence mechanism, since it is likely to affect the functions of microbial enzymes.

BOX 13.7 FEVER ASSOCIATED WITH INFECTION AND INFLAMMATION

Fever commonly occurs during infection and inflammation. Many bacterial toxins elevate body temperature, sometimes by causing the release of fever-causing cytokines. Elevated body temperature intensifies the actions of interferons, inhibits the growth of some microbes, and speeds up body reactions that aid repair.

Exercise

Refer to Chapter 16 for a definition of fever and for details of how the hypothalamic thermostat is reset.

The role of the exudate is to promote the entrance of proteins and various phagocytic white cells into the wound from the plasma. Generally, the proteins in the tissue fluid create a colloidal osmotic pressure, promoting fluid leakage from plasma, resulting in the accumulation of tissue fluid (McVicar and Clancy, 1997). The increased blood flow to the area, and the accumulation of fluid in the soft tissues, eventually exerts pressure on sensory nerve endings, making the wound feel uncomfortable and/or painful (Flanagan, 1996). Specifically, proteins such as prothrombin and fibrinogen stimulate the clotting process – a homeostatic response discussed in Chapter 11 that creates a physical protective barrier between the external and internal environments of the body. The resulting clot thus acts to isolate the area and prevent the spreading of antigenic material.

The biochemical constitution of the exudate reflects the intensity and duration of the injurious agent, for example:

- serous exudate has a low protein content. Such exudate indicates that there is superficial and minimal damage, e.g. blistering of the skin;

- fibrinous exudate indicates damage of a more intense nature, since this type of wound requires the development of a protective fibrin clot. Such material must be removed to prevent the formation of a scar;

- haemorrhagic exudate has the same biochemical constitution as a fibrinous exudate, with the additional presence of red blood cells, indicating that the injury has damaged blood vessels;

- purulent exudates are wounds that contain pus (a mixture of living and dead cells of the body, dead microbes, cell debris such as proteinaceous fibres, and bacterial toxins). Such an exudate is detrimental to the healing process.

BOX 13.8 ABSCESSES AND ULCERS

If pus cannot be drained out of an inflamed area, the result is an abscess, i.e. an excessive build-up of pus in a confined space. Abscesses include pimples and boils. When superficial inflamed tissue is removed from the surface of an organ or tissue, the opening sore is called an ulcer. People with diabetes mellitus or advanced atherosclerosis are susceptible to ulcers in the tissues of the legs. These 'diabetic ulcers' develop because poor oxygen and nutrient supplies to the tissues cause them to become susceptible to very mild injuries and/or infectious processes. Stasis (venous) leg ulcers arise due to incompetent venous return, and may co-exist with diabetic ulcers in obese diabetic patients.

Exercise

Reflect on the function of leucocytes and blood coagulation role in wound healing, as detailed in Chapter 11.

Although the process of inflammation is considered beneficial, since it involves homeostatic responses that restore tissue integrity by neutralizing and destroying antigens locally at the site of injury, the patient may nevertheless feel generally ill. Signs and symptoms may include fever, loss of appetite, and tiredness. The process of wound healing may also instigate harmful effects, such as:

- oedemas to vital organs, such as the lungs, heart and brain. Cerebral oedema is a common cause of raised intracranial pressures in head injury patients;

- autolysis (self-destruction) of local body tissues, due to the release of lysozymes from the large numbers of phagocytes present in the exudate;

- complications caused by the lodging of the antigen–antibody complex (see later).

The next process of inflammation involves the removal of debris and microorganisms (DeCruz, 1998). Phagocytes, such as neutrophils and macrophages, dispose of damaged tissue cells, foreign material, and microorganisms via the process of phagocytosis. This process is facilitated by the presence in the exudate of other white cells, T- and B-lymphocytes and complement. The latter facilitates the phagocytic and lymphocytic responses to either prevent or fight infection, if present.

To summarize, neutrophils are attracted into the wound first, usually within a few hours of injury; they are soon followed by macrophages. The activity of lymphocytes essentially cleanses the wound bed. Macrophages secrete growth factors, prostaglandins and complement, and, since these chemicals promote healing, these cells are usually present during all stages of wound healing. Eosinophils, another type of white blood cell, become involved if the antigenic materials are coated with antibodies of the IgG and IgE classifications (see later). In clean wounds, the inflammatory phase lasts for about 36 h; in necrotic or infected wounds, the process is prolonged (Flanagan, 1996).

Antigenic materials, such as foreign protein, microorganisms and microbial toxins, which have accumulated and/or been presented to phagocytes at the site of inflammation, also stimulate the body's specific defences.

Nonspecific responses: phagocytosis

Microbes that have penetrated external defences must be kept in check by internal mechanisms. Phagocytosis is the body's first line of cellular defence against microbial invasion. The process is sometimes so efficient that microbes are removed as potential sources of infection before the lymphocytes have become aware of their presence.

Two broad classes of phagocytes exist: microphages and macrophages ('micro-' = small, 'macro-' =large).

Microphages

These phagocytes, called neutrophils and eosinophils, circulate and police the body by entering injured peripheral tissues. Neutrophils have the greater phagocytosing capacity, since they are more abundant and more mobile than eosinophils (see Chapter 11).

Macrophages

These phagocytes, called monocytes, are classified as 'wandering' or 'fixed' macrophages. The former migrate to areas of infection, and the latter are permanent residents of specific tissues, e.g. the reticuloendothelial (Kupffer) cells of the liver. The term 'fixed' is misleading, since these cells can be transported to nearby damaged tissue.

Phagocytic giant cells can be produced if several phagocytes accumulate together. This occurs in response to large and highly active antigenic material, and increases the capacity of such cells to destroy the material. Phagocytosis is greatly enhanced if the particles are coated (opsonized) with specific antibodies, and enhanced even further by certain components of the complement system.

Phagocytosis as a homeostatic process

Before phagocytosis begins, mobile microphages and macrophages must move through capillary walls (a process called diapedesis) to the vicinity of antigenic material. For convenience, the process of phagocytosis is divided into four stages (Figure 13.9).

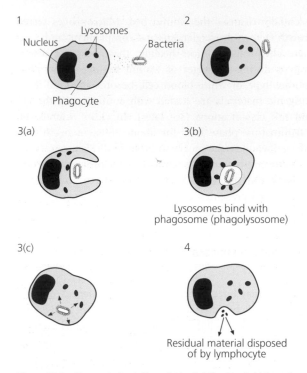

Figure 13.9 Phagocytosis. 1 Chemotaxis. 2 Adhesion. 3 (a) Ingestion; (b) intracellular digestion; and (c) intracellular absorption of useful products. 4 Disposal (exocytosis).

Q. Phagocytes move through capillary walls by squeezing between adjacent endothelial cells. Is this process known as (i) adhesion, (ii) chemotaxis, (iii) perforation or (iv) diapedesis?

Chemotaxis

Chemicals released from pathogens (e.g. bacterial toxins), lymphocytes (e.g. macrophage-attracting substances), and damaged tissue and surrounding tissues (e.g. histamines) attract phagocytes to the area by a process called chemotaxis. Microorganisms are not entirely defenceless against phagocytic cells. Some microbial toxins kill phagocytes, which contributes to the microbe's own homeostatic defences, e.g. some microbial toxins kill phagocytes.

Adherence

Adherence involves a firm contact being made between the phagocyte's plasma membrane and the antigen. Phagocytes have a number of membrane chemicals, which have sticky properties that aid microbial adherence. Complement also promotes this process. Adherence sometimes proves to be a difficult process, but it is facilitated by trapping the microbe against a roughened surface (e.g. a blood clot) or a solid surface (e.g. blood vessel). This activity is referred to as non-immune (or surface) phagocytosis.

Ingestion and intracellular digestion

Phagocytes employ cytoplasmic streaming to produce cell membrane projections called pseudopodia ('-podia' = feet), which engulf, or ingest, the material to be digested or phagocytosed. The engulfed antigen becomes surrounded by a membrane-lined vacuole, or phagosome, which becomes cytoplasmic bound. Lysosomes coalesce with it, forming a larger structure called a phagolysosome or a secondary lysosome. Lysozymes are released into the vesicle; these enzymes (lipases, proteases, nucleases, etc.) break down complex microbial components into simple molecules. These chemicals pass into the cytoplasm of the phagocyte to be utilized in its metabolism. Lactic acid, another component of lysosomes, provides the pH most suitable for lysosomal enzyme activity.

Some microbes (e.g. tuberculin bacilli) are not entirely defenceless to this process, since they may divide actively within phagocyte vacuoles and destroy phagocytes intracellularly. Others (e.g. HIV) remain dormant within phagocytes before exerting their effects. Problems can also arise if the phagocytosed antigens cannot be 'digested' (e.g. asbestos), thereby accumulating inside the cell.

Disposal

Inevitably, some microbial components cannot be degraded, since human genes cannot produce all of the enzymes necessary for total microbial destruction. Indigestible or residual material remains vacuolated within the phagocyte until they are ejected from the cell by exocytosis.

Some toxin-producing microbes are not necessarily killed by phagocytosis, but may become killers of the phagocytes themselves through secretion of toxins. Others (e.g. tuberculin bacilli) even divide within phagolysosomes and destroy the phagocytes inside the cells. Yet other microorganisms (e.g. HIV) remain dormant within phagocytes for long periods before exerting their effects. Further problems can arise if the phagocytosed antigen cannot be broken down (e.g. coal dust), thereby causing its accumulation inside the cells. These phagocytes then produce an abundance of lysosomes, which fuse with the phagosome in an attempt to destroy the particles. Eventually, phagocytic autolysis (literally 'self-destruction') occurs when lysozymes are released inside the cells.

An increase in cellular respiration accompanies the process of phagocytosis. Consequently, hydrogen peroxide is produced, which is toxic to many bacteria; it therefore

---

Exercise

Review the details associated with the nonspecific phagocytic response.

Make notes on the functions of complement in response to bacterial invasion.

Before considering cell-mediated and antibody-mediated reactions, use Figure 13.10 to familiarize yourself with the embryological origin of T- and B-cells, and use a nursing dictionary to familiarize yourself with the following terms: cytotoxic, cytokines, mast cells, interleukin, toxin, toxoid, antibody, passive immunity, active immunity, diphtheria, tetanus, poliomyelitis and meningitis.

contributes to the body's defence operations. Some bacteria counteract this effect by producing an enzyme, catalase, which converts peroxide into water and oxygen. Needless to say, this enzyme production is a useful homeostatic adaptation, which gives these bacteria a degree of resistance.

The specific immune response

In addition to surviving the above nonspecific defences, pathogens must also deal simultaneously with the specific (lymphocytic) immune responses if they are to be effective in producing infection or disease. In summary, the nonspecific mechanisms have common actions against all antigenic insults, whereas lymphocytic responses confer specific immunity against particular antigenic insults. Such responses have two closely allied components:

● A component involved in the production of specific T-lymphocytes, some of which attach themselves to antigenic materials to destroy them. This response is particularly effective against the antigens of fungi, intracellular viruses, parasites, foreign tissue transplants, and cancer cells. This is referred to as cellular, or cell-mediated, immunity, since it relies mainly on the secretion by these cells of cytotoxic chemicals and other substances, including lysozymes, macrophage-attracting substances, and interferon. The latter is released specifically when the antigen is a virus. It is important in controlling viral infections by preventing their replication inside host cells. Thus, since antibodies cannot enter cells, interferon succeeds where antibodies fail.

● A component involved in the production and secretion of specific antibodies into the circulation. Antibodies are produced by B-lymphocytes in an attempt to destroy specific antigens present in body fluids and extracellular pathogens that multiple in body fluid but rarely enter body cells (i.e. primarily bacteria). Thus, if antigen 1 penetrates the external defences, antibody 1 is produced against it, whereas if antigen 2 enters the body, antibody 2 is produced, etc. These cells confer humoral, or antibody-mediated, immunity, which is particularly effective against bacteria and viral antigens.

Often, however, the pathogen provokes both types of immune responses. Thus, lymphocytes have an essential role in identifying foreign or abnormal cells and antigens, and distinguishing these from normal cells and tissues. If they fail to do so, the consequences may be uncontrolled proliferation of bacteria, viruses and even aberrant cells of the body itself (i.e. cancer), or destruction of apparently normal cells (i.e. autoimmune disorders).

Before we consider cell-mediated and antibody-mediated reactions, we will discuss the origin of the cells involved, and the structures of antigens and antibodies.

Lymphocyte production and destruction: a homeostatic process

Embryological T-cells (responsible for cellular immunity) and B-cells (responsible for humoral immunity) are derived from bone marrow lymphocytic stem cells, which have originated from common stem cells within the bone marrow (Figure 13.10). The majority of lymphocytic stem

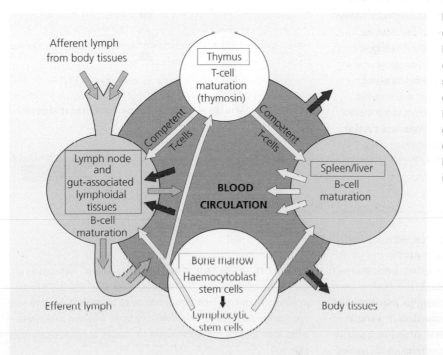

Figure 13.10 Lymphocyte development and circulation. Lymphatic stem cells from the bone marrow that mature in the thymus are called T-cells. Those that migrate to the spleen, liver and lymph nodes mature into B-cells. T-cells also migrate to the spleen and lymph nodes from the thymus. T- and B-cells circulate in the blood and lymph. T- and B-cells can be activated by pathogens, cells infected by cancers, interleukins and interferon.

cells migrate to the thymus gland, where they are processed into T-lymphocytes. Processing bestows immunological competence, i.e. cells develop the capacity and ability to differentiate into cells that perform specific immune reactions. Competence is endowed by the thymus shortly after birth, and for a few months post-delivery. Removal of the gland before processing impairs the development of cell-mediated immune responses.

Competent T-cells leave the thymus and become embedded in lymphoidal tissue of the fetal liver, spleen, lymph nodes and the gut-associated lymphoidal tissue (adenoids, tonsils, appendix, etc.). Thymosin, a hormone, and other thymus secretions stimulate further T-cell development.

The remaining lymphatic stem cells are destined to become B-cells. They are processed in the bone marrow, and then migrate to the lymphoidal tissue mentioned above. The presence of both T- and B-cells means that these tissues are now capable of stimulating both cellular and humoral immunities in response to antigenic insults. Consequently, the thymus gland and bone marrow sites are called the primary lymphoidal organs, whereas the above lymphoidal tissues are called the secondary lymphoidal organs.

In adults, lymphocyte production, (lymphopoiesis) is maintained in the bone marrow and lymphatic tissue. Lymphocytes have long lifespans compared with most body cells; approximately 80% survive for 4 years, and some live for 20 years or more. Cell production must match destruction to maintain the homeostatic functions of the immune system.

Antigens

Materials that induce specific immune reactions are called antigens. They are not usually normal constituents of the body. Sometimes, however, the distinction between self and non-self fails, and antibodies attack the body's own antigens in a variety of conditions known as autoimmune diseases (see Box 13.16). Antigens consist of a variety of chemicals. They are usually conjugated proteins, such as nucleoproteins, lipoproteins or glycoproteins, with molec-

ular weights in excess of 10 000. Others are lipids and polysaccharides.

Foreign cells, such as bacteria, viruses, fungi, and transplanted cells, are referred to as immunogens. The immune response against immunogens is a reaction to their cellular antigens. Immunogen antigens may be:

- plasma membrane receptors (Figure 13.2);

- cell surface structures, such as cilia, flagella, etc.;

- secretions, such as bacterial toxins;

- non-microbial antigens, such as incompatible blood cells, and transplanted tissues or organs, and allergic substances (called allergens), such as pollen grain, fur, feathers, wheat, food additives, etc. Allergens cause the production of specialized antibodies in hypersensitive or allergic immune responses (see Box 13.16).

Once past the body's nonspecific defences, antigens target the lymphatic tissue by one of three routes:

- Most antigens that enter the blood stream by an injured blood vessel locate themselves in the spleen.

- Antigens that penetrate the skin enter lymphatic vessels and pass to the lymphatic nodes.

- Antigens that penetrate mucus membranes lodge themselves in the mucosa-associated lymphoid tissue (MALT).

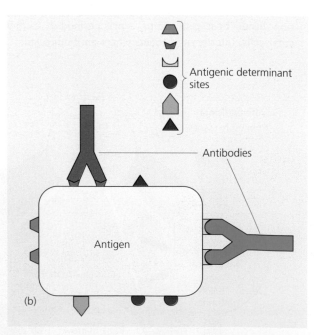

Figure 13.11 Relationship of an antigen to antibodies. The majority of antigens contain more than one antigenic determinant site (i.e. they are multivalent). However, most human antibodies are bivalent (i.e. they have two reaction sites that are complementary to the antigenic determinant sites). Each antibody has reaction sites for specific antigenic determinant sites only.

BOX 13.10 TISSUE TYPING AND IMMUNOSUPPRESSANT THERAPY

As discussed in Chapter 11, the antigens on erythrocytes are used to categorize the patient's blood group status. Antigens of other body cells (called histocompatibility antigens) are used to determine the patient's tissue type, which is controlled by the genes that are inherited from the biological parents. Transplanted tissues and organs from other people or animals thus possess non-self antigenic material, and recipients therefore produce a cell-mediated and antibody-mediated immune responses against transplanted antigens, which may cause transplant rejection. Tissue typing and immunosuppressant therapy minimize the possibility of rejection.

Tissue typing

Tissue typing involves matching the donor and recipient human lymphocytic antigens (HLA). Several hundred genes at the HLA loci on chromosome 6 determine histocompatibility antigens. Great variations of HLA therefore exist, since there are thousands of possible genetic, and thus antigenic, combinations; a complete match is extremely unlikely. The closer the HLA match between donor and recipient, the greater the likelihood of transplant success; a nationwide computerized registry helps in this process. Doctors select the most histocompatible and needy organ transplant recipients whenever donor organs become available. Despite national and international co-operation to match donors with recipients, immune rejection is still the main hazard in transplantation. Tissues with a similar genetic make-up are less likely to be rejected. Thus:

- autografts (grafts from the person's own body tissues) have no non-self antigens and are not rejected;
- isografts (grafting from individuals with 'identical' genetic make-up, i.e. identical or monozygotic twins) have little risk of rejection;
- allografts or homografts (grafting between members of the same species, but not genetically identical individuals) have a higher rate of rejection;
- xenografts or heterografts (grafting between species) have the highest rate of rejection.

Tissue typing can also be used to identify biological parents in paternity suits.

Immunosuppressant therapy

Immunosuppressant drugs are also of value in treating severe hypersensitivity states and autoimmune conditions, and to minimize the risk of transplant rejection. Subsequent to transplantation, patients receive immunosuppressant therapy in an attempt to prevent rejection. These drugs are aimed at T-lymphocytes, since these cells are the most active in rejection (Pace, 2000). Unfortunately, immunosuppressants are nonspecific, and suppression of the patient's natural defences to otherwise trivial pathogens may result in infection or disease, which may threaten life of the recipient. For example:

- Corticosteroids (e.g. prednisone, hydrocortisone) are used to prevent transplant rejections, in the treatment of severe allergies, and for autoimmune conditions. They operate by gradually destroying lymphoidal tissue, which directly depletes T- and B-cells. Their main action, however, is to decrease the activities of phagocytic cells. Thus, they may make the recipients more susceptible to infections.
- Cytotoxic drugs (e.g. methotrexate, 6-mercaptopurine) are used to inhibit replication of lymphocytes. In addition, they also inhibit mitosis of other cells, e.g. in the bone marrow, gastrointestinal tract, and skin cells. Consequently, these drugs can produce undesirable side effects, such as thrombocytopoenia, anaemia, leucopoenia, hair loss, skin disorders and gastrointestinal upsets.
- The drug cyclosporin inhibits secretion of interleukin-2 by helper T-cells, but has only a minimal effect on B-cells. Thus, the risk of rejection is diminished while retaining resistance to some diseases.
- Anti-lymphocytic serum (ALS) depletes T-cells, but also damages other lymphocytes, making the recipient more susceptible to infection. Immunizing horses or rabbits with human lymphocytes produces the serum. It has, however, a limited use in preventing the rejection of transplanted organs.

Non-self materials are classified according to whether they promote immunogenicity and/or reactivity. Immunogenicity is the ability to stimulate the production of specific antibodies and/or the proliferation of specific T-cells. Reactivity is the ability of the antigen to react specifically with relevant antibodies or cells it provoked.

Complete antigens possess both important features. Partial antigens (haptens) do not stimulate antibody production. Thus, such antigens have reactivity but not immunogenicity. The immune response to partial antigens depends upon their combination with other antigenic substances.

Antibodies target an antigen's exposed surface, known as the antigenic determinant site (Figure 13.11). The number of sites is known as the valence. Most antigens are multivalent, e.g. the antigen of individual microorganisms may have thousands of sites. Two sites are needed to induce antibody formation. Partial antigens have only one antigenic site, which explains why they do not individually stimulate antibody production.

Antibodies

Antibodies are produced and secreted in response to the presence of antigens (antigenic insults). They are found in all bodily tissues, although their greatest presence is within blood. Antibodies are very large proteins called gamma globulins; since they are a part of the immune response, they are often referred to as immunoglobulins (Igs). Major

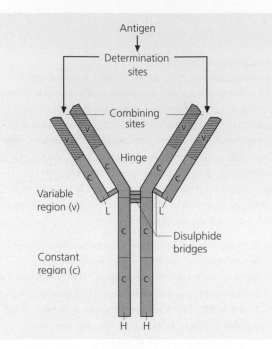

Figure 13.12 The antibody molecule and its combination with antigen. Antibodies consist of four polypeptide chains — two identical light (L) and two identical heavy (H) chains joined by disulphide bonds. The site at which the antibody molecule combines with the antigen is a relatively small area of the variable region. Both the light and heavy chains form this combining site. Flexibility at the hinge region permits the two combining sites to bind with antigens in different configurations. The shape of the combining site is complementary to a particular determination site on the antigen. Consequently, different antibodies recognize other determination sites on the antigen.

categories include IgG (Ig gamma), IgA (Ig alpha), IgM (Ig mu), IgD (Ig delta) and IgE (Ig epsilon).

Since antibodies are proteins, they consist of polypeptide chains. Most consist of two pairs, being comprised of a pair of 'heavy' chains (chains of more than 400 amino acids), and a pair of 'light' chains (consisting of 200 amino acids). The partner of each pair is identical, thus an antibody consists of identical halves, joined by disulphide (sulphur–sulphur) bonds (Figure 13.12). Each half consists of a heavy and a light chain, also held together by disulphide bonds. Within each chain there are two distinct regions:

- The constant region is identical in the number, type and sequencing of its constituent amino acids in all antibodies of the same class (i.e. IgG, IgM, etc.). However, this region differs between antibody categories, and is thus responsible for distinguishing between the different types of immunoglobulins and their biological functions.

- The variable region differs for each antibody, even for those of the same category, allowing antibodies to recognize and specifically attach themselves to particular

antigens. The combining site, at which the antibody molecule combines with the antigen, is located in a relatively small area of the variable region, and is formed by both the light and heavy chains.

Binding converts the normal T-shaped antibody molecule into a Y-configuration, and it is this transformation that activates the antibody. Each 'arm' of the Y-configuration contains a combining site; flexibility at the hinge region permits the two combining sites to bind with the antigens in different configurations.

The shape of the combining region will be complementary to the particular determination site on the antigen. Different antibodies will recognize different determination sites on antigens with different structures. This 'lock and key' binding of antibody and antigen sites gives immune responses their specificity. Most antibodies are single molecules (monomers) with just two combining

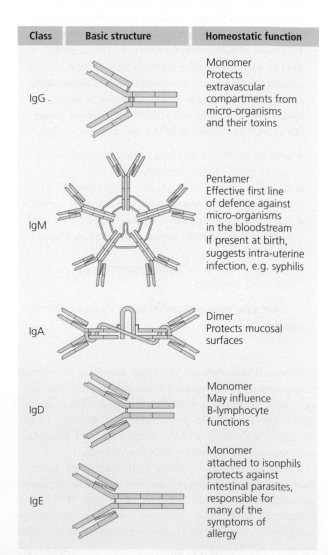

Class	Basic structure	Homeostatic function
IgG		Monomer Protects extravascular compartments from micro-organisms and their toxins
IgM		Pentamer Effective first line of defence against micro-organisms in the bloodstream If present at birth, suggests intra-uterine infection, e.g. syphilis
IgA		Dimer Protects mucosal surfaces
IgD		Monomer May influence B-lymphocyte functions
IgE		Monomer attached to isonphils protects against intestinal parasites, responsible for many of the symptoms of allergy

Figure 13.13 The structure and function of antibodies.
Q. Which antibodies can pass over the placenta?
Q. Describe the structure of an antibody.

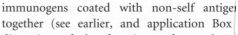
sites for the attachment of antigens; they said to be bivalent. IgM and IgA antibodies have a higher valency, because they are, respectively, pentamers (i.e. consist of five molecules joined together) and dimers (two molecules joined together) of the basic divalent unit.

The structures and homeostatic functions of immunoglobulins are summarized in Figure 13.13. The combining sites of the antibodies interact with antigens to form macromolecular complexes in a variety of ways, which neutralize, agglutinate, precipitate, lyse or opsonize the antigen (Figure 13.14). Others prevent the adhesion necessary for microbes to penetrate the skin and mucous membranes.

Neutralization

Bacterial toxins cause disease by binding to specific cells. Neutralization involves antibodies, called anti-toxins, including some IgGs, that bind to the determination sites of the toxin chemicals, thus neutralizing their toxicity. This interaction may alter the toxin's shape, thus removing its specific binding properties and preventing its interaction with cell membranes, or it may destroy the antigen by increasing its susceptibility to phagocytosis.

Agglutination

Specialized antibodies called agglutinins, which include some IgGs and IgMs, together with complement, cause

immunogens coated with non-self antigen together (see earlier, and application Box discussion of the functions of complement). This is referred to as agglutination; it makes bacteria more susceptible to phagocytosis.

Precipitation

Specialized antibodies called precipitants (including some IgGs and IgMs) react with soluble antigens via many cross-linkages to form a 'visible' insoluble precipitate, which is phagocytosed more readily.

Lysis

Some IgG and IgM antibodies called lysins attach to immunogen surface antigens and directly cause cellular rupture (lysis), hence causing their death. Alternatively, antibody–antigen formation enhances the fixation of complement, which also results in lysis.

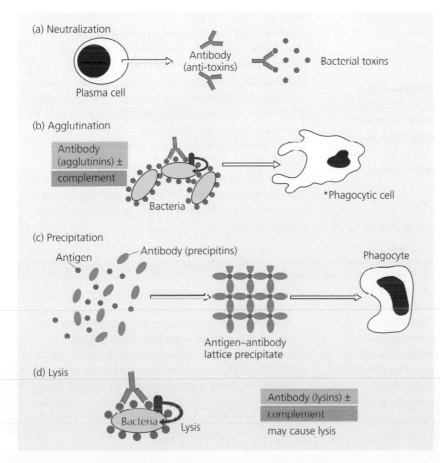

Figure 13.14 Antibody—antigen complexing.
Q. How does the antibody—antigen complex cause elimination of an antigen?

* Phagocyte cell Ga neutrophil, macrophages.
+ Presence.
– Absence.

(a) Neutralization

Antibody (anti-toxins)

Bacterial toxins

Plasma cell

(b) Agglutination

Antibody (agglutinins) ± complement

Bacteria

*Phagocytic cell

(c) Precipitation

Antigen

Antibody (precipitins)

Phagocyte

Antigen–antibody lattice precipitate

(d) Lysis

Bacteria

Lysis

Antibody (lysins) ± complement

may cause lysis

Opsonization

Microbes, such as bacteria, have structures ('slippery' plasma membranes) that, perhaps, are homeostatic adaptations to prevent phagocytosis. Opsonization is the coating of such microbes with antibodies (opsonins include some IgEs, IgGs and IgMs), and some complement proteins. This roughens their surfaces, enhancing the likelihood of adhesion and subsequent phagocytosis.

Prevention of bacterial adhesion

The IgAs present in mucus, sweat and digestive secretions coat bacteria, decreasing their capacity for attachment to body surfaces, thus minimizing their penetration of our external defences.

Exercise

You should be able to identify the specific immunoglobulins that are toxins, agglutinins, precipitins and lysins.

Activating the lymphocytic response: a homeostatic process

Very few antigens appear to bind directly to antigen-reactive T- or B-lymphocytes. Instead, some are presented to the lymphocytes on the surface of macrophages following phagocytosis; these are known as antigen-presenting cells (APCs; Figure 13.15). A much more important group of APCs is the non-phagocytic dendritic cells. These cell types are distributed widely throughout the body, and appear to trap the antigen, thereby preventing its spread. They then initiate local immune responses. Dendritic cells of the lymph nodes and spleen trap circulating antigens in the lymph and blood, and present them to the resident lymphocytes. Similarly, dendritic cells present in non-lymphoidal tissues trap the antigens; then the complex moves towards the lymphoidal tissues. The structure of the spleen and lymph nodes is such that the APCs and lymphocytes are in very close contact. Immunogen

BOX 13.12 CANCER AND MONOCLONAL ANTIBODY THERAPY

Cancer cells possess specific surface antigens characteristic of tumours. The immune system usually recognizes these as being non-self, and thus attempts to destroy them; this is called immunological surveillance. Although sensitized macrophages are involved in the response, there is general agreement that cell-mediated responses are especially involved in tumour destruction. Sensitized killer cells react with tumour-specific antigens, initiating their lysis. Some cancer cells, however, employ the phenomenon of 'immunological escape'. Explanations accounting for such an 'escape' include:

● Tumour cells shed their specific antigens, and therefore evade the initial recognition necessary for immunological surveillance.
● Decreased immune functioning makes people more susceptible to cancer, which supports the increased incidences of cancer observed with the use of immunosuppressive therapy in transplant patients, in people suffering from chronic distress, and in older people.

Scientists have been able to fuse individual B-cells with rapidly dividing tumour cells. The resultant hybridoma cells are plentiful long-term sources of antibodies specific against one antigen, hence the term 'monoclonal' ('mono-' = single). Such antibodies are of diagnostic importance in allergies, pregnancy, and diseases such as rabies, some sexually transmitted diseases, and hepatitis. They have also been used to detect cancer at an early stage, and to ascertain the extent of metastasis. The use of highly specific antibodies offers greater sensitivity, speed and specificity than conventional diagnostic tests. They are used independently, or in combination with radioactivity or chemotherapy, in the treatment of cancer. The clinical application of monoclonal antibodies to prevent cancers is an exciting discovery, since such antibodies selectively locate and destroy cancer cells, but cause little or no damage to surrounding healthy cells. This treatment, therefore, overcomes some of the major adverse effects of isolated chemotherapy and radiotherapy.

The use of monoclonal antibody vaccines may also prove to be useful in counteracting tissue and organ transplant rejection, and in treating autoimmune diseases. For further reading, see Kosits and Callaghan (2000).

BOX 13.13 THE COMMON COLD AND IgE

The common cold (clinically known as coryza) originates from a viral infection; several viruses are known to cause it. These viruses affect the mucous membrane of the nose, and trigger localized immune responses, leading to symptoms such as a running nose, coughing and sneezing. When the epithelium becomes inflamed in response to an infection, the swollen tissues and extra secretions obstruct the flow of air through the nasal passageways. This makes breathing difficult. The viral particles become attached to IgE, which results in lysis of basophils and the release of histamine (see Figure 13.23) and prostaglandins. These chemicals cause inflammation of the nasal passageways and excessive production of nasal secretions.

Allergens (i.e. antigens that stimulate an allergic reaction) also operate on IgE in this manner (see later). These protective symptoms of the cold are the means by which the viruses are passed on from one person to the next. Associated symptoms with a common cold include hyperthermia (raised temperature), chest infection and shortness of breath. These secondary complications are caused not by the virus, but by bacterial infection or by a hypersensitive response, such as occurs in asthma.

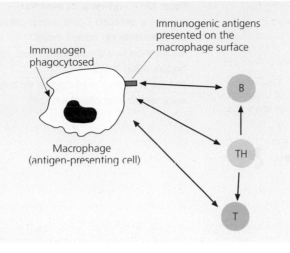

Figure 13.15 Lymphocyte response.

B, B-cells; T, T-cells; TH, T-helper cells.

Q A decrease in the number of T-cells would affect which type of immunity?

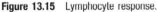

antigens, such as those associated with incompatible blood transfusions, transplanted organs, cancers, or 'self' antigens that have changed, also sensitize T-lymphocytes. A lymph node under antigenic stimulation shows T- and B-cell proliferation, and thus becomes enlarged in the process.

Upon contact with antigen, the macrophages secrete a chemical called interleukin-1, which is a cytokine (previously known as lymphokine, since it increases the activity of lymphocytes; see Killer T-cells below). This is responsi-

ble for promoting lymphoidal T- and B-cell multiplication. Proliferation stimulates further macrophage activity and hence further proliferation (i.e. positive feedback mechanism). Macrophages, dendritic cells, and T- and B-lymphocytes thus co-operate with one another to provide immunity against antigenic insults (Figure 13.16).

T-lymphocytes and cell-mediated immunity

There are thousands of different T-cells, but only those programmed specifically to react with the specific antigen present are activated. Sensitized T-lymphocytes divide, giving rise to clones, i.e. cells that are identical to one another and to their parent cells (Figure 13.17). The major difference is that the parent cells cannot destroy immunogens. Clones include:

- killer T-cells
- helper T-cells
- suppressor T-cells
- delayed hypersensitivity T-cells
- amplifier T-cells
- memory T-cells
- natural killer (NK) lymphocytes.

Killer T-cells

Killer (cytotoxic or null) cells become attached to immunogen antigens. They destroy foreign cells by secreting cytokines, cytolymphotoxins, interferons and

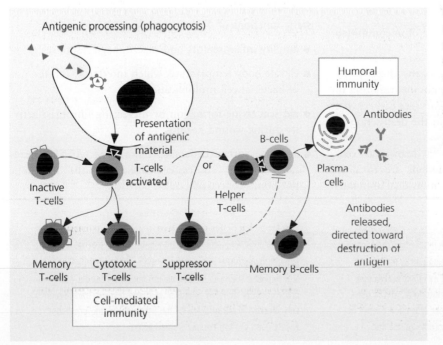

Figure 13.16 Interactions between macrophages, T-cells and B-cells. Non phagocytic dendritic cells also present antigenic material to activate the lymphocytic responses.

Q. Does complement activation (i) attract phagocytes, (ii) enhance phagocytosis, (iii) stimulate inflammation, or (iv) all of the above?

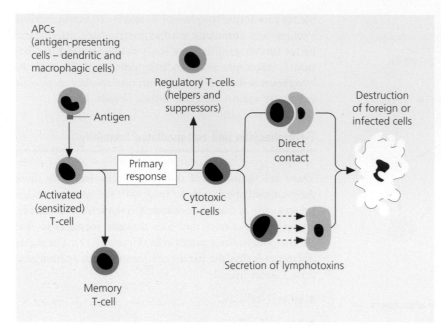

Figure 13.17 Cell-mediated immunity. Activated or sensitized T-cells undergo mitosis and differentiate into memory T-cells, regulatory (helper and suppressor) T-cells, and cytotoxic (killer) T-cells.

Q. A rise in the level of interferon in the body would suggest what kind of infection?

lysozymes (see earlier). Cytokines are powerful protein hormones; they give most of the protection provided by killer cells but act in a variety of ways. Cytokines include:

- *transfer factors:* recruit lymphocytes by transforming non-sensitized T-lymphocytes into sensitized T-cells;

- *macrophage-chemotaxis factor:* attracts macrophages, and thus intensifies phagocytosis of the antigen;

- *macrophage-activating factor:* directly increases the phagocytic activity of macrophages;

- *migration inhibitory factor:* prevents the migration of macrophages, and thus encourages their continued presence at the site of infection;

- *mitogenic factor:* induces rapid division of uncommitted or non-sensitized T-cells.

Cytolymphotoxins destroy immunogens directly, by producing 'holes' in their plasma membrane, resulting in their lysis. Interferons are antiviral agents (see earlier) that enhance killer cell activity, resulting in the destruction of the viral-loaded host cells.

The stimulation of killer T-cells is known as cell-mediated immunity, since their secretions are toxic to immunogens (foreign cells). Normally, individual immuno-gens/antigens stimulate both cellular and humoral immune responses. However, one type usually predominates, depending upon the invading immunogen. Some killer T-cell secretions promote nonspecific responses, and can result in the loss of 'self' tissue in the locality.

Helper T-cells

Helper T-lymphocytes assist plasma cells (those derived from B-lymphocytes) to secrete antibodies. In addition, helper cells secrete the chemical interleukin-2, which amplifies the proliferation of killer cells. Before this, however, interleukin-2 must be activated by interleukin-1, secreted from macrophages, thus demonstrating the inter-dependency of white cell types in controlling the homeo-static functions of defence. Interleukins also:

- amplify inflammatory and macrophage responses;

- elevate body temperature, which interferes with the rate of bacterial cell multiplication;

- aid scar tissue formation by increasing fibroblast activity during wound healing;

- promote adrenocorticotropic hormone (ACTH) secretion and the subsequent release of the metabolic hormones collectively called cortisol;

BOX 13.14 CYTOTOXIC THERAPY

Cytotoxic therapy is the use of cytotoxic substances to treat medical conditions. Interferons were the first cytotoxic substances found to be effective against human cancer. Interferon alfa is used for the treatment of kaposis sarcoma, a cancer that often occurs in people with acquired immune deficiency syndrome (AIDS). Its antiviral uses make it beneficial in the treatment of genital herpes and hepatitis B and C. Betaseron (an interferon) slows the progression of multiple sclerosis (MS) and lessons the frequency and severity of MS attacks. Of the interleukins, the one most widely used to fight cancer is interleukin-2.

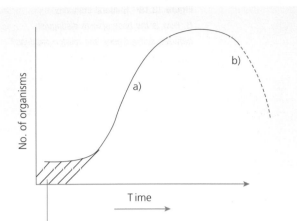

Basal level of organisms always in the human body
a) Increased number of pathogens during an infection
b) Decreased number of pathogens when convalescing

Figure 13.18 The multiplication of pathogens during an infection and when the patient is convalescing.

Q. Identify the ratio of killer cells to suppressor cells at the points labelled (a) and (b) on this figure.

● stimulate mast cell (i.e. cells that secrete histamine and other substances as a part of the response to antigens) production.

Suppressor T-cells

These lymphocytes restrain killer cell and B-cell activities, and so help to moderate responses. This is important, as it limits the effect of cytotoxic secretions on 'self' tissue in the locality. The interaction between suppressor and helper T-cells, therefore, regulates the immune response. The ratio of these cells can be used to indicate the presence or absence of infection, and the stage of infection. For instance, a 2 : 1 ratio of helper cells to suppressor T-cells occurs when there are no signs of infection. Early in the infection cycle, however, a higher ratio of helper cells (and hence killer cells, B-cells, and their antibodies) to suppressor cells exists, which promotes the removal of non-self antigens. Conversely, several weeks later, a high suppressor cells to helper cell ratio (and hence killer and plasma B-cells, and their corresponding antibodies) is observed, and the immunological response declines, since the person is recovering from the illness or infection.

Delayed hypersensitivity T-cells

These cells secrete various cytokines, including migration-inhibitory and macrophage-activating factors, in response to the presence of allergens. Destruction of the allergens at their site of entry means that these cells have key roles in delaying or preventing allergic (hypersensitive) reactions.

Amplifier T-cells

Amplifier lymphocytes somehow exaggerate the activities of helper cell, suppressor cell and B-cell descendants. There are specific amplifier cells for helper cells, and others for suppressor cells, etc.

Memory T-cells

Memory cells retain the ability to recognize previously encountered non-self antigens, so that second and subsequent exposures lead to a rapid 'secondary' immune response (Figures 13.19 and 13.20). Immunity of this kind is thus conferred for a long time, and often for life. Production of memory cells in response to administered antigen forms the basis of immunization programmes.

> **Exercise**
>
> Using Table 13.1, describe why children need to be immunized only once for measles, mumps, rubella and tuberculosis (see Box 13.18 for help).

Natural killer lymphocytes

Natural killer (NK) cells are similar to killer cells, in the sense that they lyse or break down target cells. The difference is that NK cells directly destroy those cells with altered surface membrane antigens without the need to interact with other lymphocytes or antibodies. NK cells are considered to be the first line of defence in specific immunity.

> **BOX 13.15 CANCER AND NK CELLS**
>
> Since it is believed that cancerous cells have abnormal surfaces, it is possible that secretion of interferon by NK cells plays a prime role in destroying virally infected or damaged cells that might otherwise form tumours. Cancer patients have a reduced number of NK cells; interestingly, the level of decrease corresponds to the severity of disease.

Specific and nonspecific defences are therefore co-ordinated by physical interactions, and by the release of chemical messengers. In addition to lymphocytic secretions, monocytes and macrophages also secrete monokines, such as the tissue tumour necrotic factor. This protein is responsible for:

● slowing down tumour growth;

● killing sensitive tumour cells;

● stimulating the production of granulocytes (white blood cells);

● promoting the activity of phagocytic granulocytes, called eosinophils;

● increasing T-cell sensitivity to interleukin chemicals.

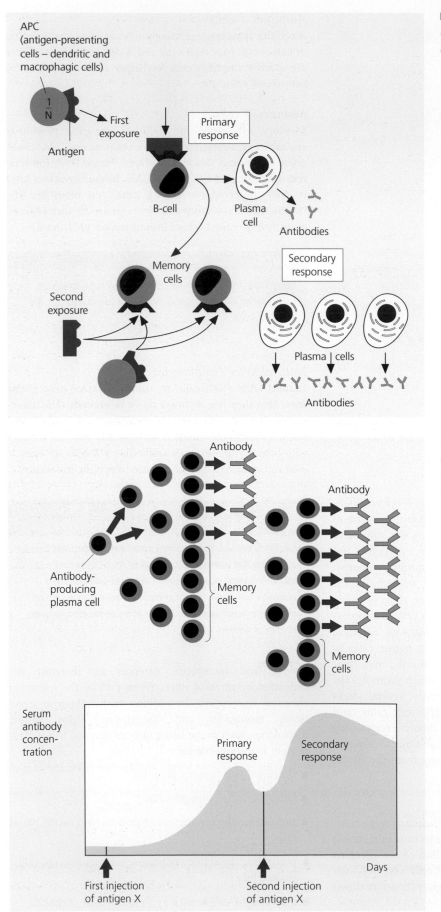

Figure 13.19 Humoral immunity.
Q. *How is the body able to distinguish between self-antigens and foreign antigens?*

Figure 13.20 The primary and secondary antibody responses and clones expansion.
Q. *Identify the principal differences between the primary and secondary immune responses.*

The skin and T-cell interactions

The skin's epidermal cells have active integrative roles with the body's specific immune responses. For example, when antigens penetrate the keratinized cell layer of the epidermis, they bind to cells called Langerhan cells. These cells present the antigenic material to epidermal T-helper cells, activating them. Langerhan cells also interact with epidermal suppressor T-cells, but usually the helper cells predominate, and instigate the destruction of the antigenic substances. If, however, Langerhan cells are destroyed, e.g. by ultraviolet (UV) radiation, or are bypassed, then these antigens react directly with suppressor cells, causing their predominance.

Humoral immunity: B-cells and antibody production

The body contains thousands of specialized B-cells, which carry (or express) on their surface antibody molecules that act as receptors for antigens. Each antibody is capable of responding only to a specific antigen. When a B-cell is exposed to an antigen, small B-lymphocytes (influenced by interleukin from activated macrophages) become larger plasma cells containing a mass of rough endoplasmic reticulum (Figure 13.16). These cells produce and secrete into the blood and lymph specific antibody (i.e. protein) of the same type as that expressed originally on the surface of the parent cell (even though B-cells remain in lymph). The antibodies then circulate to the site of antigenic invasion.

Within the plasma cell's lifespan (4–5 days to a few weeks), they are capable of producing approximately 2000 antibody molecules per second; their high metabolic rate explains their brief existence. Some B cells do not possess the genetic capability to differentiate. These remain as memory B-cells, which, together with T-memory cells, are programmed to recognize an original antigen on its second and subsequent invasion of the body. They are therefore responsible for stimulating the secondary immune response.

Exercise

Make notes on the specialized and distinctive roles of T- and B-lymphocytes.

Primary and secondary immune responses

Plasma cells initiate antibody production in the primary immune response. The speed of this response is determined by the time it takes for antigenic activation of the appropriate B-cell, and for that specific B-cell's multipli-cation and differentiation. Consequently, there is a gradual sustained rise in circulating antibody concentration, peaking about 1–2 weeks after the initial exposure. Antibody concentration subsequently declines, assuming that the person is no longer exposed to those antigens. The decline in antibody production parallels the death of the plasma cells, which have a limited lifespan due to their high rate of metabolism. If the person recovers from a microbial infection upon first exposure without having to use medication, then it is because the primary immune response has provided sufficient defence to aid recovery. If, however, the primary response has not provided sufficient defence, then an illness 'drags on', and using medication (such as antibiotics) facilitates recovery.

Memory B-cells may also differentiate into plasma cells, and become antibody producing, but only upon the second exposure to the original antigen. Memory cells have long lifespans, with some surviving 20 years or more. This secondary (anamnestic or memory) response occurs immediately on second contact with an antigen during this period, with antibodies being secreted rapidly in vast quantities. Peak values are higher and occur much more quickly than in the primary immune response. Figure 13.20 highlights the principal differences between primary and secondary immune responses. The secondary response is usually so swift that signs or symptoms of the illness are either very mild or absent, since the microbe is destroyed quickly and efficiently. The immediate antibody upsurge of the response may have pathological consequences, however, particularly if normal cells are also destroyed, since this could trigger a massive, widespread inflammatory response.

There is a lag phase between antigen exposure and antibody production. This depends largely on the pathogenicity of the organism concerned, the organism's mode of entry, and whether it is a primary or secondary immune response.

Exercise

Differentiate between the specific and nonspecific immune responses.

In summary, immunity is a set of reactions stimulated in response to the invasion of the body by non-self substances or antigens (Figure 13.21). The response is said to be:

- xenophobic, i.e. the body distinguishes between self and non-self antigenic materials;

- highly specific for different antigenic insults;

- adaptive, i.e. an antigenic invasion produces a response to the environmental (antigenic) insult;

- anamnestic, i.e. there is a memory component of the immune response, allowing both primary and secondary responses to occur.

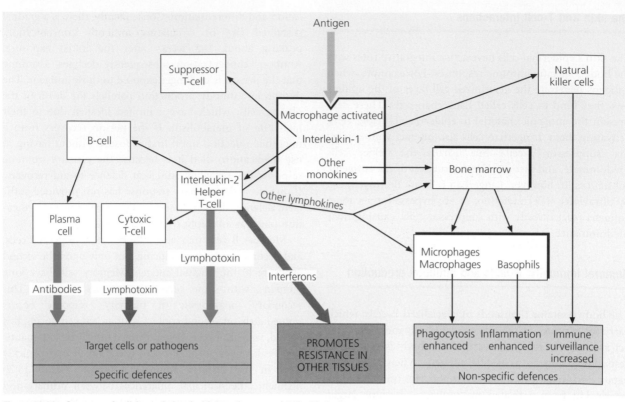

Figure 13.21 Summary of cellular and chemical interactions associated with the immune response.

Q. How would a lack of T-helper cells affect the humoral mediated immune response?

BOX 13.16 IMMUNE DEFICIENCY DISEASES AND HYPERSENSITIVE RESPONSES

Immune deficiency diseases

People who either lack, or have defective, immune system components are said to have immune deficiencies. Some of these are inherited viruses (see Box 13.4) and some, such as AIDS, are acquired via transmission (see the case study of a girl born with cytomegalovirus inclusive body disease in Section 6).

Acquired immune deficiency syndrome

Acquired immune deficiency syndrome (AIDS) develops subsequent to infection by human immunodeficiency virus (HIV). Typically, the initial infection stimulates antibody production. IgMs are produced up to 1 month following the humoral response, while IgGs appear approximately 1 month post-infection, and continue to rise throughout the remainder of the year; these antibodies are produced in response to HIV's core proteins (Figure 13.22). Interestingly, the inappropriately named 'AIDS test' identifies these antibody markers of HIV infection (perhaps it should therefore be referred to as the 'anti-HIV test', since it is not a test for AIDS, or even HIV). Eventually, however, HIV depresses the body's immune system, primarily by attacking helper T-cells, and thus inhibiting their central role in immunity. In this way, one homeostatic imbalance of T-cell deficiency leads to a failure of other interdependent homeostatic functions, for instance:

- a reduced antibody production, since helper cells stimulate immunoglobulins secretion by plasma cells;
- fewer killer T-cells, since helper cells secrete interleukin-2, which stimulates killer cell proliferation.

HIV also infects monocytes and macrophages. The virus mainly remains dormant in these cells, but it decreases the host cell's secretion of interleukin-1, which is needed for the stimulation of interleukin-2 release. Suppressor T-cells are relatively unaffected by HIV.

Overall, HIV infection grossly the impairs person's normal immune functions, and consequently normally harmless microbes can initiate potentially fatal infections; the impairment of the host's defences allows the development of cancer and opportunistic infections of various kinds. The appearance of an opportunistic (or indicator) disease signifies that the-person now has AIDS. The two most common diseases that kill AIDS patients are Pneumocystis carinii pneumonia (PCP) and Kaposi's sarcoma (KS). PCP is a rare form of pneumonia, caused by a protozoan; KS is a rare, malignant skin cancer. AIDS patients are also prone to infections of the central nervous system, which eventually produce neurological imbalances such as AIDS dementia.

To date, AIDS appears to be invariably fatal. At present, treatment consists of fighting infections as they occur,

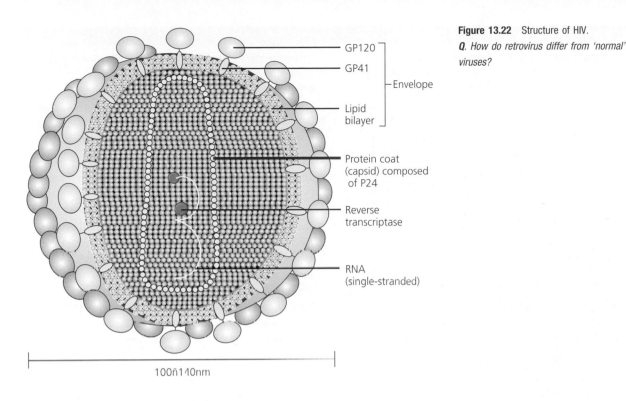

GP120 ⎤
GP41 ⎦ Envelope
Lipid bilayer ⎦

Protein coat (capsid) composed of P24

Reverse transcriptase

RNA (single-stranded)

100ñ140nm

Figure 13.22 Structure of HIV.
Q. How do retrovirus differ from 'normal' viruses?

BOX 13.16 CONTINUED

experimenting with antiviral medication, and, more recently, via the use of immune system stimulants.

The triggers for the conversions of an HIV infection to early symptoms of AIDS (called AIDS-related complex; ARC), and from ARC to AIDS, remain a mystery. Each transition has different signs and symptoms, due to different homeostatic imbalances. The presence of these imbalances at specific times may perhaps help to explain why HIV infection leads to ARC or AIDS. For further reading, see Haddad *et al.* (2001) and Darbyshire *et al.* (2001): these articles discuss the current treatments and educational support for people with AIDS.

Severe combined immunodeficiency

Severe combined immunodeficiency (SCID) is an inherited failure to develop cellular and humoral immunities, either as a consequence of a lack of both T- and B-cells, or because the cells are inactive. Consequently, even mild infections can be fatal. Bone marrow transplants from a compatible donor, usually a very close (i.e. genetically similar) relative, have been used to colonize the patient's lymphatic tissue with functional lymphocytes. Although the immunodeficient child cannot reject the bone marrow tissue, the bone marrow can reject the child, since it contains immunologically active lymphocytes that react against the child's tissues.

Hypersensitivity responses

Hypersensitivity occurs either because the body is exposed to an excessive amount of antigen, so the antibody is secreted in too high a quantity, or because the antibodies and T-cells are directed against the body's own tissues (called autoimmune diseases). There are four main types of hypersensitive reactions:

- type I (anaphylaxis) reactions;
- type II (cytotoxic) reactions;
- type III (antibody mediated) reactions;
- type IV (cell-mediated) reactions.

Type I reactions

An allergy is a hyperimmune response to an antigen (called an allergen in this case) to which most people have no noticeable responses. The symptoms of allergies, such as hay fever and asthma, following exposure to allergens (pollen, antibiotics, etc.) are dramatic and occasionally lethal. See the case study of a boy with hypersensitivity reaction: asthma in Section 6.

Type I reactions occur within a few minutes of being sensitized to an allergen, e.g. the chemicals in lextex gloves. Some people produce IgEs that bind to the surface receptors of mast cells and basophils (Figure 13.23). These cells are found in and underneath the mucous membranes in the nose, throat, eyes and lungs. Binding causes the person to produce an allergic response, since such an interaction causes cells to release the chemical mediators of anaphylaxis (e.g. histamine, serotonin, prostaglandins). These are responsible for increasing blood capillary permeability, increasing smooth muscle contraction, and increasing secretion of mucus. Consequently, the person may experience oedema, erythema or redness, breathing difficulties, and a runny nose, along with other inflammatory responses. Sensitive patients should therefore avoid histamine contained in foods.

Eosinophil (a type of white blood cell) counts are elevated during an allergic response, as a homeostatic adaptive response, since these cells are thought to exert anti-inflammatory effects by absorbing histamine.

Anaphylactic reactions, such as hay fever and bronchial asthma, may remain localized. Others are considered systemic, e.g. acute anaphylaxis may produce circulatory shock (in this case called anaphylactic shock) and asphyxia, both of which can be fatal without clinical intervention.

Some sensitized people can become accustomed to allergens if they are presented with them gradually and in increasing dosages, i.e. they become desensitized. Children often 'outgrow' allergies for this reason. Since only some people are allergic, this suggests that the tendency to produce IgEs in response to specific allergens may be determined genetically.

Type II reactions

Cytotoxic reactions involve IgG, IgM or IgA antibodies, which bind to antigens on body (mainly blood)cells. This interaction activates the complement system, which causes:

- mast cell secretion of histamine and kinins, which cause local vasodilation and an increased permeability of capillary walls.

They are also responsible for bronchoconstriction, which gives rise to inadequate gaseous exchange in the lung;

- the chemical attraction of neutrophils (a type of white blood cell) to the site of inflammation, enhancing phagocytosis by activating macrophages. Complement enzymes attached to the antigens and to antibodies identify the cells to be phagocytosed.

Affected cells are phagocytosed and/or destroyed. Recipient phagocytes lyse incompatible ABO blood transfusions (see Figure 11.19) promote such a reaction.

Drugs such as methyldopa may cause haemolytic anaemia in susceptible people, because the drug coats erythrocytes and promotes immune attack. Similarly, bacterial endotoxins, such as those released from salmonella, also cause erythrocyte haemolysis. Cytotoxic reactions may result in the chronic failure of transplanted organs, which may become necrotic due to thrombosis of the donated organ. This is caused by an antibody response to the endothelium of the donated organ's blood vessels, causing it to be damaged and resulting in the adherence of platelets and thrombus formation.

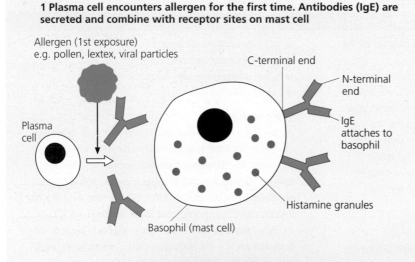

1 Plasma cell encounters allergen for the first time. Antibodies (IgE) are secreted and combine with receptor sites on mast cell

Allergen (1st exposure)
e.g. pollen, lextex, viral particles

Plasma cell

C-terminal end

N-terminal end

IgE attaches to basophil

Histamine granules

Basophil (mast cell)

2 Second exposure to allergen

Basophil's granules are exocytosed; histamine is released leading to inflammation of membranes of the upper respiratory tract resulting in mucus and tear secretion and bronchoconstriction

Pollen (allergenic determination sites) binds to the combining sites of the variable region (Fab) of the IgE; the IgE is activated and sends a signal to the basophil membrane

Figure 13.23 Immediate (type I) anaphylactic hypersensitivity, as occurs in hay fever, lextext allergy and the common cold.
Q. *Explain how histamine is released in response to pollen.*

BOX 13.16 CONTINUED

Type III reactions

Type III reactions cause antibody–antigen complexes to be deposited in various tissues, e.g. in joints, causing arthritis, in the heart, causing myocarditis, and in renal glomeruli, causing glomerulonephritis.

The complement system in the presence of IgG or IgM may also be activated. A localized type III reaction (Arthus reaction) occurs when antigens are injected: a local vasculitis and inflammatory response occurs as a result of immunoglobulins forming complexes with the injected antigens. This sometimes occurs in diabetic people who have developed IgG antibodies against an antigenic component of their insulin preparations.

Type IV reactions

Cell-mediated (delayed-type) reactions involve T-cells, and are often not apparent for a day or more. They become apparent when allergens bind to tissue cells, causing them to be ingested by macrophages; the antigens are then presented to the T-cells. Consequently, T-cell proliferation is responsible for the destruction of allergens. An example of a type IV reaction is a positive tuberculosis (Mantoux) skin test.

The symptoms of hypersensitive reactions can develop within minutes of the allergic or anaphylactic response. It is important to understand that hypersensitive reactions are normal homeostatic protective responses, which, if in excess (i.e. in severe cases), can result in extensive peripheral vasodilation, producing a fall in blood pressure, and possible circulatory collapse. Localized allergic reactions, such as those created by pollen exposure in hay fever sufferers, produce unpleasant but less severe symptoms.

Adrenaline administration counteracts some of the responses to histamine and antihistamine drugs. Treatment of severe anaphylaxis involves antihistamine and corticosteroid injections, in addition to respiratory and/or circulatory support.

Autoimmune diseases

Self-antigens do not normally initiate immune responses. However, our own body cells are sometimes destroyed by autoimmune responses. This type of reactivity may be important in the normal homeostatic control of body function, e.g. in wound healing by removing dead tissues and cells. At other times, autoimmune responses are less beneficial. When autoimmunity noticeably damages otherwise healthy tissues, it causes autoimmune diseases, such as:

- *diabetes mellitus:* autoantibodies may destroy the beta islets of Langerhan, thus causing the hypoinsulinism associated with type I or insulin-dependent diabetes mellitus;
- *Hashimoto's thyroiditis:* anti-thyroid antibodies may impair the activity of a person with thyroid gland;
- *myasthenia gravis:* autoantibodies interfere with the function of motor end plates at neuromuscular synapses, preventing the transmission of nerve impulses to motor muscles. They do so by decreasing the sensitivity of muscle membrane receptors to the neurotransmitter chemical acetylcholine, or by destroying the neurotransmitter itself. These patients have weak muscles that fatigue easily and eventually may become paralysed;
- *rheumatoid arthritis (rheumatoid disease:)* autoantibodies to certain immunoglobulins result in deposition of complexes within the synovial joints, eventually leading to destructive changes. Other tissues such as the lungs and blood vessels may also be affected.

BOX 13.17 IMMUNOLOGICAL COMPETENCE

Immunological competence is the ability to produce an immune response to an antigenic insult. Cellular immunity occurs from approximately the third month of gestation, but active humoral (antibody) immunity appears much later. The fetus, however, receives IgGs from the maternal circulation until delivery, although this is referred to as passive immunity, since it is not an immunological response of fetal tissue. In the seventh month of gestatory development, the fetus develops IgA and IgM immunological competence if exposed to the relevant antigens. The mother also provides IgAs in breast milk, post-natally. This passive immunity gives resistance for approximately 3 months after birth, until the liver eventually destroys the transferred antibodies. Since there is no anamnestic (memory) immune

response in the baby, during this period the infant is vulnerable to infection; routine primary immunization programmes are thus commenced at 2 months of age. This ensures the acquisition of active immunity against pathogens that have the potential to produce serious diseases, such as diphtheria, tetanus, poliomyelitis and meningitis. This active immunity is long lasting (see Table 13.1).

IgA, IgD and IgE antibody levels begin to rise 1 month after birth, and reach half the adult level by 3 years of age. During childhood, the antibody titres rise gradually towards adult levels, and the population of memory B- and T-cells increases progressively as one encounters different antigens, until their decline as a consequence of the ageing process (see Chapter 20).

Exercise

Discuss in broad terms the homeostatic failures associated with the immune system.

Table 13.1 Primary immunization programmes

When is the immunization due?	Which immunizations	Type
2 months	Polio	By mouth
	Hib	
	Diphtheria	
	Tetanus	One injection
	Whooping cough	
3 months	Polio	By mouth
	Hib	
	Diphtheria	
	Tetanus	One injection
	Whooping cough	
4 months	Polio	By mouth
	Hib	
	Diphtheria	
	Tetanus	One injection
	Whooping cough	
12–15 months	Measles	
	Mumps	One injection
	Rubella	
3–5 years (usually before the child starts school)	Measles	
	Mumps	One injection
	Rubella	
	Diphtheria	
	Tetanus	One injection
	Polio	By mouth
10–14 years (sometimes shortly after birth)	BCG (against tuberculosis)	Skin test followed by one injection if needed
School leavers 13–18 years	Diphtheria	
	Tetanus	One injection
	Polio	By mouth

Q. What is immunization, and how does it work?

Stress and immunity

It is generally accepted that distress depresses the immune responses. Interleukin-1, secreted from macrophages, stimulates the secretion of the hormone adrenocorticotropic hormone (ACTH) from the pituitary gland; this has a direct action on lowering antibody production, and stimulating the secretion of glucocorticoids from the adrenal glands. These steroidal hormones have anti-inflammatory effects, and their long-term secretion inhibits the immune response, lowering resistance to disease as a consequence (Figure 13.24). These inhibitory mechanisms are as follows:

1 Depression or cessation of the immune response. Glucocorticoids inhibit mast cell activity and so decrease the availability of histamine, the initiator of inflammation. Capillaries remain impermeable to protein, which this reduces the availability of fibrinogen, complement, and other cellular defences important in the inflammatory response. This inhibition can halt inflammation totally.

2 Inhibition of interleukin production and secretion. This depresses the stimulation of killer cell proliferation and other responses associated with interleukins.

3 Reduced number of phagocytes. This impairs phagocytosis, and the antigenic processing and presentation to lymphocytes.

4 Reduced number of lymphocytes.

Consequently, one becomes more susceptible to diseases ('diseases of adaptation', according to Selye's stress theory; see Chapter 22) when the immune system is depressed by chronic distress (known as 'unhealthy stress'). It appears, however, that some stress (i.e. eustress, or 'healthy stress') can enhance immune responses. Eustressful experiences

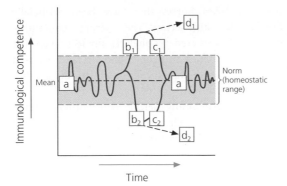

Figure 13.24 Immunological competence: a homeostatic process. (a) Normal homeostatic sensitivity and functioning of the immune system's component parts (i.e. cellular/humoral responses). (b_1) Hypersensitive immune response. This can be a temporary hypersensitive response to an overexposure to immunogen and non-immunogen antigens, e.g. as occurs in the secondary immune response, so that signs and symptoms are mild or do not appear, or it can be a pathological hypersensitive response reflecting a homeostatic imbalance, e.g. as occurs in allergies, tissue rejection following transplantation, and autoimmune diseases. (b_2) Hyposensitive immune response. This can be a temporary response that does not necessarily reflect an infection or illness, as occurs in acute bouts of distress, or a pathological response, as occurs with immune deficiency syndromes and chronic bouts of distress. (c) Normal function restored. (d_1) Terminal autoimmune allergic reaction (shock). (d_2) Terminal immunological deficiency syndromes, e.g. AIDS.

are, however, time dependent and generally short lived, before they become distressing, which could explain why most research has identified the association between distress, the loss of immunity and increased susceptibility to infectious disease. For further reading, see Schrader (1996) and Page and Ben-Eliyahu (1997).

The acquisition of immunity

Acquired immunity

Different people have different resistance and susceptibilities to infections, depending on the efficiency of their immunological responses. The subjectivity of a person's immunological response is governed by their unique genetic ability (inherited from our biological parents) to respond to harmful agents, and their environmental exposure to potential harmful agents.

An individual can acquire immunity to infectious diseases either naturally or artificially, both of which can be passive or active (Figure 13.25).

Passive natural immunity
Passive natural immunity is acquired before birth with the passage of maternal antibodies across the placenta, or after birth in breastfed babies with the passage of antibodies present in breast milk. The actual antibody transferred by the mother depends upon her active immunity. Passive immunity is short lived, since the child's lymphocytes are not activated, and the maternally derived antibodies are not replaced as they are metabolized.

Another important use of passive immunization is the prevention of rhesus incompatibility in pregnancy (see Box 11.30).

Active natural immunity
Active natural immunity involves stimulating or activating the body to produce its own antibodies. It is acquired via:

- *having the disease:* during an illness, B-lymphocytes differentiate into plasma cells, which produce and

Figure 13.25 Types of immunity.
Q. What defences, present at birth, provide the body with the defence capability known as the nonspecific response resistance?

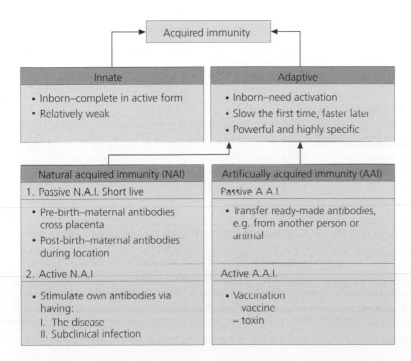

secrete immunoglobulins, usually in sufficient quantities to overcome the infecting antigenic material. Upon recovery and during convalescence, lymphocytes retain the ability to produce these specific antibodies against the antigens encountered previously, since there is a memory component associated with immunity;

- *having a subclinical infection:* in this situation, the infection is not severe enough to cause clinical manifestation of disease. It does, however, stimulate B-lymphocyte activity.

Passive artificial immunity
Passive artificial immunity is acquired by giving people ready-made antibodies using human or animal sera (see Box 13.18). Antibodies are obtained from convalescing

individuals, or from horses that have been artificially immunized. The anti-serum (i.e. serum containing antibodies) is administered prophylactically to prevent the development of a disease in people who are later exposed to the infection, or therapeutically after the disease has developed.

The antibody-containing serum from other species, however, can manifest itself as a dangerous hyperimmune response (anaphylactic reaction) in susceptible people. This has led to the removal of horse serum treatment (containing tetanus anti-toxins) in people infected with the tetanus organism (see also Box 13.16).

Active artificial immunity
Vaccines have been developed to protect people against diseases that can cause serious illness. Active artificial

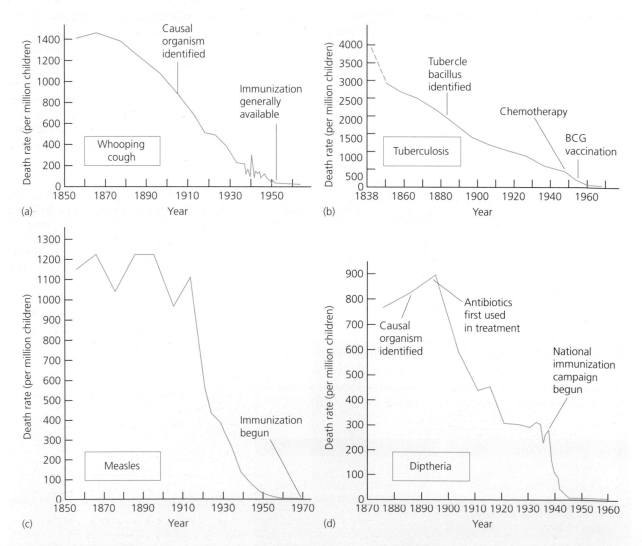

Figure 13.26 Graphs illustrating a reduced incidence of communicable diseases due to increased hygiene, housing, economic status and successful vaccination programmes. (a) Whooping cough: death rates of children under 15 years in England and Wales. (b) Respiratory tuberculosis: death rates of children under 15 years in England and Wales. (c) Measles: death rates of children under 15 years in England and Wales. (d) Diphtheria: death rates of children under 15 years in England and Wales.

Q. Suggest why some immunization programmes (e.g. whooping cough) confer life-long immunity and others (e.g. tetanus) relatively short-lived immunity.

immunity develops in response to the administration of dead, or live but artificially weakened (attenuated), microbes as vaccines, or of detoxified microbial toxins as toxoids. Vaccines and toxoids retain antigenic properties and therefore stimulate the immune response without causing disease.

Killed vaccines give protection against whooping cough, typhoid and cholera. Such administrations are given on two or three occasions, often with a booster dose after the initial programme of vaccination, because only small numbers of antigens are introduced on each occasion (Table 13.1).

Attenuated vaccines are those in which the organism has been cultured artificially to produce a strain that no longer has any pathogenic properties. However, the organism continues to divide within the body after it has been administered, and gives rise to a full immune response, closely mimicking that followed by a natural infection. Thus, often only one administration is required to give the protection of life-long immunity to the disease. Diseases prevented by this type of vaccine include mumps, rubella, tuberculosis and poliomyelitis.

Toxoids are preparations of bacterial endotoxins that no longer produce the disease: a chemical (e.g. formalin) is added that will render it harmless. The pathogens that cause tetanus and diphtheria both produce exotoxins, and protection is therefore achieved by the administration of toxoids.

Edward Jenner performed the first vaccination of this kind in 1796. He used the fluid extracted from cowpox blisters to confer immunity against the similar virus of smallpox. Modern immunization programmes have reduced the incidence of many serious diseases, including whooping cough, tuberculosis, measles, diphtheria (Figure 13.26), cholera, rubella, smallpox, typhoid and poliomyelitis. The success of these programmes means that some diseases, such as polio, no longer occur in the UK. In other countries where immunization is not so widely available, this is not the case. Since overseas travel is so popular now, there is a risk that these diseases could be brought back into the UK and spread to people who have not been immunized.

Immunization can confer either life-long immunity against infections, such as whooping cough and mumps, or short-lived immunity against certain other infections. Tetanus immunization, for example, is effective for just a number of years. Some immunity, however, may last for only a few weeks before revaccination is necessary.

The apparent loss of immunity to an infective microbe may result from contact with different microbial strains that are capable of producing the same clinical manifestations. Influenza viruses, for example, have rapid mutation rates, and even a slight mutation (i.e. change in the viral genetic make-up) produces different antigenic properties, hence we are constantly subjected to different bouts of influenza.

BOX 13.18 IMMUNIZATION PROGRAMMES AND CHILDHOOD IMMUNIZATION

Immunization prepares our bodies to fight against diseases in case we come into contact with them in the future. The anamnestic response forms the basis of immunization programmes, i.e. the initial immunization sensitises the body, so that if the immunogen is encountered in the future through infection, or a booster dose of the antigen is administered, then the body experiences the anamnestic response. Some immunizations have to be given more than once to build up immunity (protection) or to keep the level of antibodies 'topped up'. This 'top-up' is called a booster. Booster dosages are required because antibodies and memory cells have a limited metabolic lifespan, and therefore the antigen must be given periodically to maintain high antibody titres.

A child should not be immunized if he or she has:

- pyrexia;
- had a hypersensitive reaction to another immunization or after eating eggs;
- a bleeding disorder;
- been taking immunosuppressants (given after organ transplant or for malignant disease) or high-dose steroids;
- HIV or AIDS;
- had, or is having, treatment for cancer.

Specialist advice is needed before immunizing children who have had convulsions (fits) in the past.

All immunizations (except polio) are given with a small needle into the child's upper arm, buttock or thigh.

DTP-Hib vaccine

This vaccine protects against three different diseases – diphtheria, tetanus and pertussis (whooping cough) – and against infection by the bacteria Haemophilus influenzae type b (Hib). The vaccine is administered at 2–4 months; further tetanus and diphtheria boosters are given between 13 and 18 years. The DT part is administered as a booster at 3–5 years.

Diphtheria rarely occurs in the UK. The condition starts with a sore throat, and can progress rapidly to cause problems with breathing. It can damage the heart and the nervous system. In severe cases, it can be fatal.

Tetanus bacteria (tetani) are found in soil. They come into the body through a cut or burn. This is a painful disease that affects the muscles and can cause breathing problems. If untreated, it can be fatal.

Whooping cough (pertussis) can be very distressing. The patient becomes exhausted by extensive bouts of coughing, which frequently cause vomiting and choking. In severe cases, pertussis can be fatal.

Hib is an infection that can cause a number of serious conditions, including meningitis, pneumonia and blood poisoning,

BOX 13.18 CONTINUED

all of which can be dangerous if not treated quickly. Meningitis is an inflammation of the meninges or lining of the brain. It is a very serious condition, but if it is spotted and treated early, most children make a full recovery. The Hib vaccine gives protection against Hib meningitis, but it does not protect children against other bacterial types, such as meningococcal or pneumococcal meningitis, or viral meningitis. A baby with meningitis can become dangerously ill within hours. Early symptoms include fever, vomiting, irritability and restlessness. Refusing feeds is also common with colds and influenza. Other important signs to look for are a high-pitched moaning cry, difficulty in waking, pale or botching skin, and red/purple spots. Common signs in older children include stiffness in the neck, severe headaches, a dislike of bright lights, confusion or drowsiness, and red/purple spots.

Polio vaccine

This vaccine protects against the disease poliomyelitis. Polio is a virus passed in the faeces of infected people and of those who have just been immunized against polio. It attacks the nervous system and may cause long-term muscle paralysis. If the chest muscles are attacked, it can be fatal. Routine immunization has meant that the natural virus no longer causes cases of polio in the UK. The vaccine is administered at 2–4 months. A booster is administered between 3 and 5 years, and another booster is given between 13 and 18 years.

MMR vaccine

This vaccine protects against measles, mumps and rubella. Measles is a very infectious viral disease. It is immediately recognizable by its characteristic rash. The infection can cause a high fever. Approximately 7% of children who contract measles are at risk of complications, e.g. chest infections, fits and brain damage. In severe cases, measles can be fatal.

Mumps, another viral infection, causes swollen glands in the face. Mumps was the most frequent cause of viral meningitis in children under 15 years before immunization was commenced. The condition can cause swelling of the gonads (testicles and ovaries) and deafness.

If a pregnant woman contracts the rubella (German measles) virus in early pregnancy, it can harm the unborn baby after birth, although the condition is usually very mild and is not likely to cause the infant any problems.

BCG vaccine

This vaccine gives protection against tuberculosis (TB). TB is a bacterial infection that frequently affects the lungs. It may also affect the brain and bones. TB arguably no longer exists in the UK. However, there are between 5500 and 6000 cases a year, since TB is on the increase in Africa and in some Eastern European countries.

This vaccine is administered sometimes shortly after birth but more frequently at the age of 10–14 years, when a skin test is given to see if the person already has immunity to TB. If immunity is not present, the immunization is given.

Hepatitis B vaccine

Several types of hepatitis exist, and they all cause inflammation of the liver (see Box 10.29). This vaccine protects against hepatitis B, which is passed via infected blood and may be sexually transmitted. Some people are healthy carriers of hepatitis B; if a pregnant woman is a hepatitis B carrier, she can pass it on to her child. The child may not be ill, but has a high probability of becoming a carrier and developing liver disease in later years. Because of this risk, many pregnant women are tested for hepatitis B; babies born to infected mothers will be administered a course of vaccine to prevent them contracting hepatitis B and becoming a carrier.

Exercise

The Wakefield report of 2000 has, controversially, raised doubts over the safety of the MMR vaccine (Kawashima *et al.*, 2000). The researchers claimed that those children immunized with the MMR vaccine had an increased risk of developing autism later. It is generally accepted by immunology experts that the data of this report are far from being convincing, and the reader is directed to an article by Martin (2000).

Summary

1 The lymphatic system is associated closely with the cardiovascular system. It transports excess tissue fluid to the blood, helps defend the body against disease-causing microbes, and transports long-chain fatty acids absorbed from the gut into the blood.

2 Lymph is formed in blind-ended tubes that are closely associated with capillary networks. It then flows into lymphatic vessels that drain into the two major thoracic collecting ducts, which return lymph to blood at the junction of the subclavian and jugular veins.

3 Lymph flow is aided via the squeezing actions of surrounding skeletal muscles. low pressure in the thorax created by breathing movements, and the presence of valves.

4 Any condition that interferes with the flow of lymph results in the clinical condition called oedema.

5 Lymph nodes are clinically important, as they are the production centres for lymphocytes. They also contain macrophages, and so filter foreign particles present in the lymph.

6 The spleen resembles an enlarged lymph node, hence its similar function. It also acts as a blood reservoir.

Summary (Continued)

7 The body has a number of external defence mechanisms that provide formidable barriers against antigenic invasions.

8 Inside the body, the antigenic material encounters nonspecific defence mechanisms (phagocytic response) and specific defence mechanisms (lymphocytic responses). The phagocytic and lymphatic responses are extremely effective in protecting the body from pathogenic activity, and at promoting recovery from infection.

9 The phagocytic response consists of inflammation and phagocytosis.

10 Monocytes give rise to phagocytic macrophages.

11 The lymphocytic response is comprised of the cellular (T-cell) and the humoral (B cell) immune responses. T- and B-lymphocytes secrete cytotoxic substances and antibodies, respectively, in response to antigenic insults.

12 Stem cell lymphocytes originate in the bone marrow.

13 The thymus produces T-lymphocytes and a hormone thymosin (thymone), which stimulates other lymphoidal tissue to produce T-cells.

14 The bone marrow and other sites of the body produce B-lymphocytes.

15 The memory component of the immune response ensures a quicker and boosted response following subsequent detection of an antigen, resulting in the majority of situations presenting no signs and/or symptoms of a disease should the antigen enter the body once again.

16 Immunization gives protection against a variety of infections.

17 The two principal problems associated with homeostatic failure of the lymphatic system are lymphatic obstructions and the spreading of infections.

18 Knowledge of the location of lymph nodes and the direction of lymph flow is important in predicting the source of infection and the spread of cancers.

19 Homeostatic imbalances of immune responses involving abnormal immune system responses can be categorized as being problems arising from either inadequate or excessive sensitivity (Figure 13.24). The former includes the immune deficiency diseases, which result from inadequate humoral and/or cellular immune responses. Such an imbalance may be inherited or acquired. Excessive sensitivity involves homeostatic imbalances arising from the immune mechanisms responding too well or too often. Such imbalances result in allergies, tissue rejection following transplantation, or autoimmune diseases.

Review questions

The human body provides a warm and moist environment that is ideal for the growth of potentially pathogenic organisms. There are various entry points, such as the eyes, ears, respiratory passageways, and gastrointestinal and genitourinary tracts, which, without defensive mechanisms, would allow a constant bombardment of infection. The body can reduce the number of harmful substances that enter the body by three lines of defence.

First line of defence

The skin is the most visibly obvious defence in that (if intact) it can prevent entry of water and other substances.

1 Find out how the skin is waterproofed and what it secretes in order to inhibit bacterial growth.

2 Think about each of the other portals of entry listed above and discuss how each prevents the entry/growth of organisms. These methods could include structure, secretions, normal flora or even reflexes.

Second line of defence

If organisms get past the first line of defence, then the body has other nonspecific tricks up its sleeve.

3 Review the signs of inflammation, and link these symptoms to what is happening to the blood vessels in the region of disruption.

4 Look up phagocytes, pyrogens, interferons and the complement system, and become familiar with their modes of action.

Third line of defence

This is a highly specific system that we know as the immune response. It involves cells called B- and T-lymphocytes, which recognize foreign (non self) substances (known as antigens) and destroy them in a very efficient manner. This system mounts a response to an antigen it has met previously in a shorter period of time then it takes for an infection to become established. This occurs because the immune system has memory.

5 Distinguish between an antigen and a hapten.

6 Where does the production of lymphocytes occur?

7 Where do lymphocytes become immunocompetent?

8 Which type of lymphocytes are involved in the humoral immune response?

9 Describe the differences between what happens if an antigen enters the body and encounters a B-lymphocyte and if a T-lymphocyte is encountered.

10 Why do lymph glands in the neck swell and become painful in response to an upper respiratory tract infection?

11 What is the difference between plasma cells and memory cells?

12 What is the role of the T-helper lymphocytes? Bear in mind that these cells are the target of the human immunodeficiency virus (HIV), which results in devastation of the immune system.

13 Which of the B-cells produces antibodies?

14 Name the five classes of antibodies, and give their alternative names (abbreviated to Ig).

15 Why does passive immunity last for only a short time, yet active immunity usually lasts for much longer?

16 Find out the different types of allergic response and make short notes on each.

Review questions (Continued)

17 Define 'allergen', and give examples of common substances to which people may show an allergic response.

18 What are the signs of an allergic reaction?

19 Why do you not show the signs of an allergic reaction with the first exposure to an allergen?

20 Which cells are affected by IgE?

21 These cells will release chemicals that are described as vasoactive. Give an example of a vasoactive substance.

REFERENCES

Darbyshire, J., Foulkes, M., Peto, R., Duncan, W., Babkier, A., Collins, R., *et al.* (2000) Deciphering autoimmune disease in women. *Patient Care* **34**(7): 49–52, 54, 59.

DeCruz, G. (1998) The case of a man with a surgical wound. Case study cited in Clancy, J. and McVicar, A.J. (eds) (1998) *Nursing Care. A homeostatic casebook.* London: Arnold.

Flanagan, M. (1996) A practical framework for wound healing assessment 1: physiology. *British Journal of Nursing* **5**(22): 1391–7.

Haddad, M., Inch, C., Glazier, R.H., Wilkins, A.L., Urbshott, G., Bayoumi, A. and Rourke, S. (2001) Patient support and education for promoting adherence to highly active antiretroviral therapy for HIV/AIDS. The Cochrane Library. Oxford: Update Software.

Kawashima, H., Mori,T., Kashiwagi, Y., Takekuma, K., Hoshika, A and Wakefield, A. (2000) *Digestive Diseases and Sciences* **45**(4): 723–9.

Kosits, C. and Callaghan, M. (2000) Rituximab: a new monoclonal antibody therapy for non-Hodgkin's lymphoma. *Oncology Nursing Forum* **27**(1): 51–9.

Lesourd, B.M. (1998) Abstracts and commentaries. Nutrition and immunity in the elderly: modification of immune responses with nutritional treatments. *D.C. Tracts*, **10**(1): 13–14, 17–18.

Martin, J. (2000) Measles, mumps and rubella. *Practice Nurse* **20**(9): 552, 554–5.

May, D. (2000) Infection control. *Nursing Standard* **14**(28): 51–9.

McVicar, A,J. and Clancy, J. (1997) The physiological basis of fluid therapy. *Professional Nurse* **12**(8):.

Pace, B. (2000) JAMA patient page. Suppressing the immune system for organ transplants. *Journal of the American Medical Association* **283**(18): 2484.

Page, G.G. and Ben-Eliyahu, S. (1997) The immune-suppressive nature of pain. *Seminars in Oncology Nursing* **13**(1): 10–15.

Salvage. J. (2000) Now wash your hands ... hand hygiene remains the single most important means of preventing hospital-acquired infection. *Nursing Times* **96**(43): 22.

Schrader, K.A. (1996) Stress and immunity after traumatic injury: the mind-

FURTHER READING

Peto, T. and Walker, A. (2001) Zidovudine (AZT) versus AZT plus didanosine (ddl) versus AZT plus zalcitabine (ddC) in HIV infected adults. The Cochrane Library. Oxford: Update Software.

Palmer, J. (2000) Organ transplants. *Physiotherapy Frontline* **6**(1): 16.

Chapter 14

The respiratory system

Introduction
Overview of lung anatomy, and general principles of lung functions
Physiology of the respiratory system

Regulation of the respiratory system
References

INTRODUCTION

Respiration is the utilization of oxygen by the body in the production of energy. Chapter 4 described how energy is produced from the breakdown of chemical bonds within fuels such as glucose, and is incorporated into other bonds within the chemical ATP; the energy then becomes readily available for cell processes. Much of the production of ATP is by aerobic metabolism, i.e. it requires the presence of oxygen, so the oxygen requirement of tissues will vary according to their energy needs. For example, cardiac muscle is very active and uses about 30 times as much oxygen per minute than the relatively inactive skin. This influence of metabolism on oxygen consumption is illustrated strikingly by skeletal muscle tissue, in which oxygen utilization may increase 15-fold during exercise.

Maintaining an adequate supply of oxygen is therefore essential to the metabolic homeostasis of cells and tissues. Tissue oxygenation occurs in four stages:

1 Oxygen is taken up from the air by blood.

2 Oxygen is carried by the blood.

3 Tissues receive adequate perfusion with blood.

4 Oxygen passes from the blood to cells.

Once within cells, the oxygen is utilized. As a result of the process, oxygen is incorporated into carbon dioxide molecules. If the carbon dioxide that is present in body fluids becomes excessive, then this is potentially problematic because it will combine with water to form carbonic acid, and so cause the generation of harmful hydrogen ions (see Chapter 4). Carbon dioxide therefore must be excreted to prevent an accumulation of hydrogen ions in body fluids. Its excretion entails:

1 Uptake of carbon dioxide by blood from cells.

2 Transportation of carbon dioxide by blood.

3 Transfer of carbon dioxide from blood to the air.

Ensuring that tissues are perfused adequately with blood is therefore essential for meeting the respiratory requirements of cells, and is one of the most important roles of the cardiovascular system. The processes involved are described in Chapter 12. This chapter describes the processes involved in exchanging gases with air, in transporting them in blood, and in exchanging them at cell level.

Much of respiratory functioning is underpinned by principles of physics, so you are recommended to become familiar with the fundamentals in the overview section below before reading later sections.

Exercise

You might find it helpful to refer back to Box 4.10 to review what happens to cells if oxygen needs are not met, e.g. in circulatory shock.

OVERVIEW OF LUNG ANATOMY, AND GENERAL PRINCIPLES OF LUNG FUNCTIONS

This section introduces the general principles of lung function. These are explained in more detail in a later section in the context of lung physiology and lung disorders.

The lungs are paired organs lying within the thoracic cavity. The left lung has two lobes, and the right has three. The left lung is smaller than the right because of space occupied by the heart (Figure 14.1). The lungs and chest wall are lined with serous membranes called the visceral pleural membrane and parietal pleural membrane, respectively. The narrow cavity between these two membranes forms the fluid-filled pleural space, which is an integral component of the breathing mechanism. The volume of fluid normally present is only of the order of 5 ml; the space is thus extremely thin – so much so that it is often referred to as a 'potential' space. Although small, the pleural space and fluid form a crucial component of the functional anatomy of the lungs. We discuss in a later section how pressure changes generated within this space by movements of the chest act to promote air movement into the lungs during breathing.

Exercise

If you are unfamiliar with the structure of serous membranes such as the pleurae, review Chapter 2.

The lungs are totally separated from the abdomen by a sheet of skeletal muscle – the *diaphragm* – which is dome shaped before lung expansion but flattens during breathing in (Figure 14.2). These actions of the diaphragm are essential to lung inflation and deflation.

The 'respiratory tree'

The macrostructure of the lung may be likened to that of a tree, in which the continuously dividing airways represent the branches. The general anatomy of the lung and its airways is shown in Figure 14.1.

The nasal cavity is a large cavity lined with a ciliated and glandular epithelium that filters and moistens the air on breathing in. The area is well supported with blood, and the epithelium is therefore also effective at warming the air. These processes are helped by projections – conchae – that increase the surface area of the epithelium. The processes continue within the throat cavities – the *pharynx* – at the back of the mouth. The pharynx has two components: the *oropharynx* forms what most people would consider to be the throat itself, and the *nasopharynx* is an extension of the throat upwards towards the nasal passages. The opening into the airways from the oropharynx is called the *glottis*,

BOX 14.2 SOME GENERAL TERMS USED IN RELATION TO THE RESPIRATORY SYSTEM

Respiration: relating to the production of energy by cells.

Internal respiration: the biochemical reactions taking place within cells that consume oxygen and produce carbon dioxide.

External respiration: the processes occurring within the lungs in taking up oxygen from air and releasing carbon dioxide into it. Much of this chapter explains the processes involved in external respiration.

Inspiration: the process of breathing in.

Expiration: the process of breathing out.

Dyspnoea: strictly speaking, an inadequate ventilation of the lungs, . It is similar, therefore, to the term 'hypoventilation', but it is used

more widely in the context of difficulty in breathing (uncomfortable, laboured, even painful), since this relates the problem more satisfactorily to the patient's experience and to the nurse's observation.

Apnoea: cessation of breathing, or breathing that is ineffectual in oxygenating blood.

Anoxia: not related strictly to the respiratory system per se, this term is used in relation to tissue oxygenation secondary to lung function. Basically, it means 'no oxygenation'.

Asphyxia: a physical means, e.g. choking, that prevents breathing from occurring, leading to anoxia.

(a)

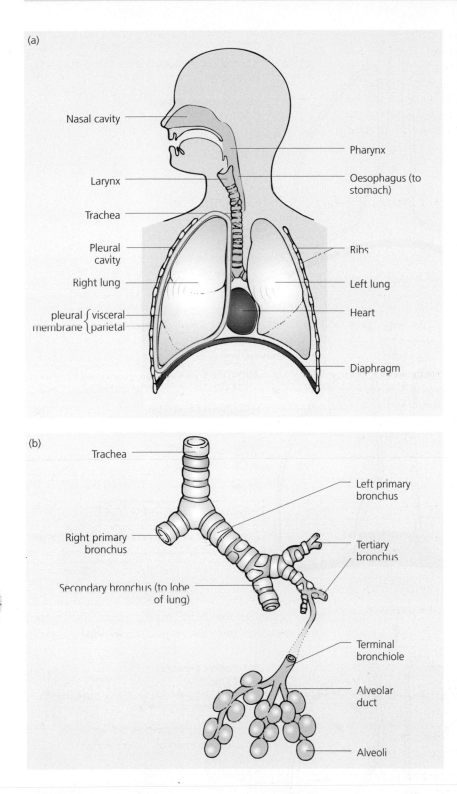

Figure 14.1   (a) Position of the lungs within the thoracic cavity. (b) The 'respiratory tree'. Pleural membranes shown on right side only.
Q. Which part of the 'respiratory tree' is affected by chronic bronchitis?
Q. What structure maintains the patency of the trachea?

(b)

which is closed off during swallowing by a small flap called the *epiglottis* ('epi-' = upon).

After the glottis, the air enters the *larynx*, a structure of cartilage and ligaments that forms the Adam's apple. The entire structure is supported by muscles that suspend the larynx from a small bone in the neck called the hyoid (see Chapter 3). Within the larynx are folds of cartilage that form the vocal cords. Air flowing over these cords causes them to vibrate and so produce sound: the voice. Their tension determines the tone or pitch of the sound; this can be altered by small muscles that pass from the cords to the cartilage of the larynx capsule. In men, actions of the sex steroid hormone testosterone causes elongation and thickening of the fibres during puberty, which is responsible for the larger larynx and the deeper voice tone that is produced.

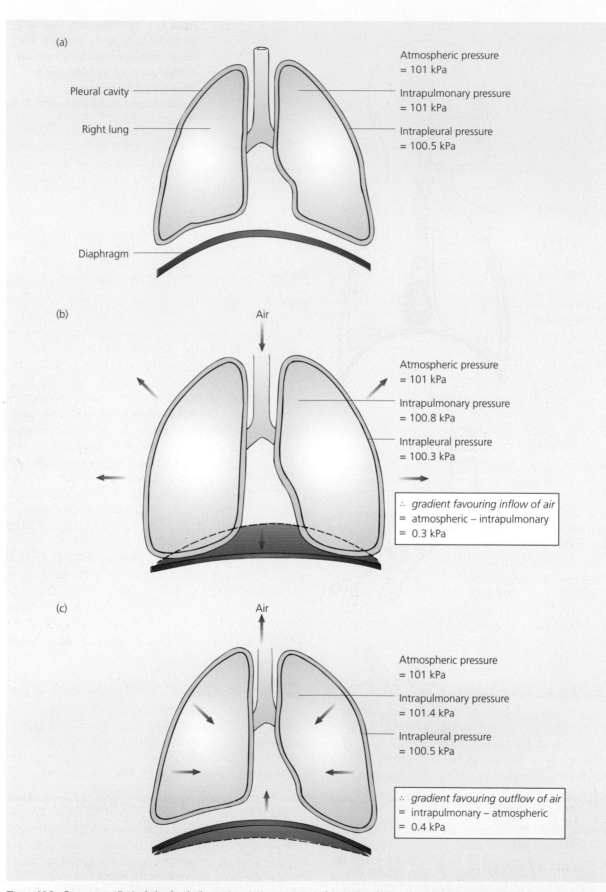

Figure 14.2 Pressure gradients during inspiration and expiration (a) at end of normal expiration, (b) during inspiration, and (c) during expiration.

Q. What is the relation between alveolar pressure and atmospheric pressure (i) during inspiration, and (ii) at end-expiration?

BOX 14.3 SPUTUM

Sputum is the mucus (usually mixed with saliva from the mouth*) that is removed from the airways by coughing. Mucus production is not unusual, but in health it is generally of a slightly thickened consistency, and is fairly colourless. The sputum is normally moved up to the throat by ciliated cells lining the airways, where it is swallowed.

If an infection is present, the mucus may be purulent (i.e. contains pus, the debris of dead micro-organisms and body cells). The amount, colour, consistency and odour of sputum vary with different lung disorders (Stockley et al., 2000). Colour and odour are influenced by the presence of micro-organisms or by the presence of blood. Infections can produce sputum of a characteristic colour. For example, Streptococcus pneumoniae produces rusty-coloured sputum, Staphylococcus aureus produces salmon-pink sputum, and Pseudomonas aeruginosa causes a greenish sputum.

Consistency and volume depend largely on the extent of infection, but also are influenced by the organisms present. For example, viral pneumonia produces scanty sputum, whereas bacterial pneumonia is much more productive. Obstructive airway conditions, such as chronic bronchitis, may cause production of a thick, stringy mucus on coughing. Early stages of such conditions may include a non-productive cough, but increased exertion with a worsening of the condition will be productive. The mucus may even contain casts of lining tissues that have been sloughed by the exertions of coughing.

---

*Some organisms are present within the mouth, and so may contaminate a sputum sample that is to be analysed for its micro-organisms. If this is of concern, then a sample may be obtained directly from the trachea.

From the larynx, the inspired air enters the *trachea*, a tube of fibrous and muscular tissue some 12 cm in length and 2.5 cm in diameter, and lined with a ciliated and mucus-producing epithelium. The trachea is strengthened by 16–20 C-shaped rings of cartilage, which prevent it from collapsing; the absence of cartilage posteriorly prevents friction rub with the oesophagus during swallowing. The trachea divides into two branches known as the left and right *primary bronchi* (singular = bronchus).

The primary bronchi are generally similar in structure to the trachea, but with a smaller diameter. One primary bronchus goes to each lung, where it divides into smaller *secondary* and *tertiary bronchi*. Each secondary bronchus supplies a lobe of a lung (i.e. there are three secondary bronchi on the right side, and two on the left). Cartilaginous structures become less well defined in these smaller bronchi, which later divide into numerous, even smaller branches, called *bronchioles*. Although less than 1 mm in diameter, these divide further, and thus continue the extensive network of branches of the 'tree'.

Bronchioles do not contain cartilage but consist of smooth muscle. They terminate in *alveolar ducts* that open into minute clusters of cup-shaped or globular sacs called *alveoli* (singular = alveolus) (Figure 14.3). Each alveolus is of the order of 0.3 mm in diameter and is supported by elastic tissue. Alveoli are richly supplied with blood capillaries, and the barrier formed by the capillary endothelial cells and the alveolar epithelial cells forms the surface across which gas exchange occurs between the lung and blood. Being globular and extremely numerous (there are about 300 million in total), alveoli provide a huge surface area for gas exchange between the alveoli and the blood: it has been estimated that the surface area of a pair of adult lungs is approximately 70 m^2.

Since only the alveoli provide the gas exchange surfaces within the lung, it follows that much of the structure of airways does not participate in this exchange. Thus, the nasal cavity, pharynx, trachea, bronchi and bronchioles comprise a 'dead space' for gas exchange. However, these airways will be filled with air during inspiration, which

BOX 14.4 ASPIRATION

Aspiration is the suction of fluids or objects into the airways during breathing in. Small particles will normally provoke a cough or sneeze reflex, the force of exhalation being sufficient to remove the objects. Fluids and larger particles are more hazardous. Aspiration of these normally does not occur because of reflex protection of the airway, e.g. by closure of the epiglottis. The risk, therefore, is greatest when there is an altered state of consciousness, or when neural reflexes are depressed, e.g. with drug abuse, trauma or anaesthesia.

Medium-sized particles may lodge in the trachea or penetrate down to the primary or secondary bronchi, in which case they tend to be lodged in the right lung. This is because the left-sided positioning of the heart makes the right bronchus larger and more

vertical than the left. Such particles are difficult for the lungs to remove by a cough reflex*. The larynx may prevent the passage of large objects deep into the lungs (although this is not always effective). In contrast, fluids pass easily through the larynx, and may pass deep into the lungs should aspiration occur, perhaps even to the terminal airways. Here, they can cause serious inflammation. An example is the aspiration of stomach acid that has refluxed out of the stomach perhaps during surgery.

---

*Striking someone on the back, or standing behind the person and squeezing up on to their diaphragm (known as Heimlich's manoeuvre), increases the force of expiration and may be sufficient to remove the object. These are potentially dangerous manoeuvres and must be used with caution if trauma to tissues is to be avoided.

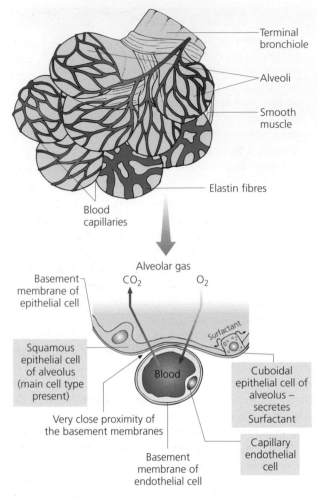

Figure 14.3 Alveoli and the alveolar-capillary membranes.
Q. How is gaseous exchange accomplished at the alveoli-pulmonary capillary interface?

means that only a proportion of the air breathed in will enter the alveoli, where it mixes with the alveolar gas that was left in the lung following the previous expiration, including the gas that filled the dead space structures upon breathing out. The mixing of air with alveolar gas means that the gas composition is altered only slightly, which has an important role in the homeostatic regulation of gas concentrations in blood leaving the lung by preventing large fluctuation.

BOX 14.5 BRONCHIOLITIS AND BRONCHIECTASIS

Bronchiolitis is a condition in which inflammation causes obstruction of the bronchioles. It is more common in children, secondary to an upper respiratory tract infection, but it can occur in adults due to inhalation of toxic vapours. Treatment is with appropriate antibiotics, anti-inflammatory steroids, and chest physical therapy.

Bronchiectasis is a long-standing dilation of the bronchi. It usually occurs in conjunction with other respiratory disorders, and is a consequence of long-term inflammation. The airways can become balloon-like, and heavy scarring affects smaller airways in the vicinity. Lung collapse (atelectasis) may also occur. Blood supply to these areas may increase as part of the inflammatory response, which leads to the presence of blood in sputum, the fluid brought up out of the lungs by coughing. This is called haemoptysis. The occurrence of scarring makes this condition difficult to treat. Antibiotics may be administered to prevent infection, and physical chest therapy used to remove secretions. Bronchodilator drugs may also help improve lung ventilation.

BOX 14.6 THE RESPIRATORY SYSTEM IN CHILDREN

The respiratory system becomes functional at birth (see Box 14.24), and it should not be surprising to find that it remains functionally 'immature' for some time after birth. The lungs undergo considerable development during childhood, notably a change in size and an increased complexity of the alveoli.

The respiratory system in infants

As might be expected, the airways differ in size and calibre when compared with older children or adults:

● The airways are shorter and narrower than in older children/adults.
● The upper airway is narrow, reduced further by the posterior displacement of the tongue (an adaptation for suckling).
● The cartilaginous rings of the trachea are less well developed, so the trachea is more prone to collapse.
● Overall, airway resistance is some 15 times greater in infants than in adults.

The support for ventilation is also less efficient in infants:

● The chest wall is softer and more pliant, and so is prone to be sucked in by the lowering of air pressure within the lungs during breathing in.
● Accessory muscles are less well formed, so breathing efforts are less sustainable.
● Alveoli are less numerous at birth (25 million alveoli compared with about 300 million at 8 years old).

The respiratory system during childhood

Development of the respiratory system during childhood consists basically of increased length of the airways (although the calibre changes little until approaching puberty), and increased number of alveoli (see above).

The main features, then, of the respiratory system in children is a respiratory tree that is functionally less efficient, and with narrow airways. These factors make children especially vulnerable to conditions that increase airway resistance further, such as bronchiolitis (see Box 14.5) and asthma (see Box 14.13).

General principles of lung function

At rest, an adult breathes in about 500 ml of air (7–8 ml/kg body weight) with each breath. This is referred to as the *tidal volume*. With a normal breathing rate at rest of about 10–12 breaths/min, about 5–6 l of air are breathed in (and out) each minute. This is sufficient to meet the needs of cells of the body at rest, which use about 250 ml of oxygen per minute. During exercise, however, oxygen requirements of tissues may be as high as 4 l/minute. To meet this increased demand, the volume per breath is increased, as is the breathing rate, with the result that the volume of air breathed is increased to perhaps 80 l/min. Lung function, therefore, must be adaptive according to metabolic needs. In fact, control of lung function ensures that the average gas composition of arterial blood supplying the tissues is held almost constant, even during exercise, i.e. the lungs are the effector organs that act to maintain blood gas homeostasis.

The gas composition of blood leaving the lungs reflects the composition of gas within the alveoli, since it is here that the exchange of oxygen and carbon dioxide takes place. Breathing facilitates the process by determining the alveolar gas composition.

Analysis of the gas in alveoli after breathing in shows that it has become enriched in oxygen and depleted of carbon dioxide. This is not surprising, since inspired air is comprised of approximately 21% oxygen and only 0.03% (effectively 0%) carbon dioxide. The remaining proportion (about 79%) is almost entirely nitrogen. Upon breathing in, the inspired air will mix with a relatively large volume of gas left in the lung, so the 'dilutional' effect that the air has on lung gases will not be pronounced. Even so, the changes in gas composition in alveoli during inspiration are sufficient to generate the necessary pressure gradients to promote oxygen diffusion into the blood and carbon dioxide from the blood.

Clearly, the volume remaining in the lungs at the end of a normal expiration will be an important influencing factor on the gas composition produced upon breathing in and therefore on gas exchange. It is referred to as the *functional residual capacity* and is an important factor in respiratory disorders.

Gas composition apart, gas exchange will be influenced by the barrier provided by the alveolar membrane. Our lungs provide a large surface area, and as thin a barrier as possible, for adequate gas exchange to occur between blood and environment. Protection of these delicate surfaces from airborne particles is provided by mucus produced by goblet cells in the lining of the airways. This mucus traps particulate matter in the air; other cells possess masses of cilia, which waft the mucus and trapped particles in the direction of the throat, where they are swallowed (see Box 14.3). The lining cells also

---

BOX 14.7 THE RESPIRATORY QUOTIENT

Chapter 4 described how the production of energy from glucose produces the same amount of carbon dioxide as the oxygen consumed. However, a proportion of our energy production also comes from the metabolism of fats (which produce less carbon dioxide per volume of oxygen used). The volume of carbon dioxide produced divided by the volume of oxygen used gives a parameter called the respiratory quotient. Thus:

$$\text{Volume of } CO_2 \text{ produced/volume of } O_2 \text{ consumed} = 220 \text{ ml/min}/250 \text{ ml/min} = 0.88$$

The respiratory quotient is a useful index that is sometimes used in medicine to assess which metabolic fuel predominates; for carbohydrate alone, the value is 1, and for fats it is 0.7. The above value reflects a mixed metabolism of fats and carbohydrate.

BOX 14.8 GAS PRESSURES AND PRESSURE GRADIENTS

Gas molecules are free to move. Their random movement brings them into contact with other structures, e.g. air molecules collide with our skin. The impacts produce the gas pressure, and will depend upon the density of the gas molecules and the speed at which they are moving, i.e. compressing additional molecules into an enclosed chamber, such as a gas cylinder, will raise the gas pressure, and heating it will raise it even more as energy is passed on to the molecules, so they move more rapidly.

Gas pressures used to be measured in terms of millimetres of mercury, written as 'mm Hg', i.e. the height of a thin column of mercury that can be maintained by such a pressure. Modern units of measurement utilize the Pascal (Pa): 1000 Pa (1 kPa) is equivalent to 7.6 mm Hg. It is now unusual for the unit mm Hg to be used with reference to respiratory functioning, although blood pressure measurements are still referred to in these units. This inconsistency of units used is likely to remain for some time, although mercury sphygmomanometers used to measure arterial blood pressure are gradually being replaced by electronic methods.

Gases move from one point to another according to pressure gradients. This principle operates even with a gas mixture, such as air. While the gas within the lung exerts an overall pressure, the movement of oxygen and carbon dioxide between blood and lung is influenced by the pressures they exert individually. The individual pressures of oxygen and carbon dioxide in the lungs are referred to as their *partial pressures* (see later). For now, it is important to note that the diffusion of oxygen and carbon dioxide across lung membranes will occur only if the gradient of their individual partial pressures is appropriate. Lung function is concerned especially with maintaining gradients that are conducive to adequate gas exchange.

moisten the inspired air, which prevents dehydration of the airways. Further protection is produced by the immune system. Macrophages are able to penetrate the airways, while antibody production makes it difficult for organisms to pass into the tissues (antibodies are also responsible for hypersensitive reactions, such as asthma; see Chapter 13).

As a final point in this overview, if a major role of the lung is to provide adequate oxygen for tissue function elsewhere in the body, then the process would be self-defeating if the lungs themselves were to utilize much of the oxygen taken in simply to sustain the muscle activity necessary for breathing. In fact, the energy requirements of the lung are relatively small: during a normal resting breathing cycle, the lungs and associated muscles consume less than 1% of the total uptake of oxygen. The low energy requirements are facilitated by the anatomy of the lung, described in more detail in the next section.

PHYSIOLOGY OF THE RESPIRATORY SYSTEM

Inspiration and expiration

Breathing movements are referred to as inspiration (breathing in) and expiration (breathing out). Inspiration requires inflation of the lungs, and expiration requires deflation. Although this appears a simple process, inflation or deflation can occur only if the appropriate air pressure gradients are generated that will move gases in and out of the lungs (Figure 14.2).

Inspiration

If we place a finger over the end of an empty syringe and try to withdraw the plunger, we can feel the suction produced inside the syringe. In other words, if the volume of a container is increased, then the pressure of gas within it will decrease. Lung inflation works on this principle, and occurs when the thoracic cavity is expanded by contraction of external intercostal ('inter-' = between, '-costal' = rib) muscles, which raise the rib cage upwards and outwards, and by contraction of the muscular diaphragm, which flattens the 'dome' of this muscle sheet (Figure 14.4). When we are at rest, contraction of the diaphragm alone may be all that is required to provide adequate ventilation of the lungs; this is called *diaphragmatic breathing*. Both mechanisms are necessary during even mild physical activity, however, and severe respiratory effort may even involve accessory muscles, such as the sternocleidomastoid muscle of the neck region, in order to raise the rib cage more effectively (Figure 14.4). The extra muscle contraction will, of course, increase the energy expended simply to maintain the appropriate level of breathing, but this still represents only up to about 3% of the total oxygen consumption, so breathing remains energy efficient.

Expansion of the thoracic cavity lowers the pressure within the lung. More precisely, the expansion lowers the pressure within the fluid-filled pleural cavity, which in turn

BOX 14.9 POSITIONING AND BREATHING MOVEMENTS

The functioning of the diaphragm is impeded if the abdominal organs are pressed against it. An upright position of the body facilitates the role of the diaphragm, and so simply sitting up a patient who has respiratory problems can make breathing much more comfortable and effective. Gravity effects may also help to reduce fluid accumulation as a consequence of pulmonary oedema (see Box 14.22).

BOX 14.10 DISTURBANCE OF THE PLEURAL SPACE: PNEUMOTHORAX AND PLEURAL EFFUSION

Pneumothorax is the presence of air or gas within the pleural space. It arises as a consequence of ruptured pleural membranes. In open pneumothorax, a penetrating wound of the chest allows air to be sucked into the pleural cavity during inspiration, and is expelled again on expiration. Lung inflation will be impaired. In tension pneumothorax, air from a penetrating wound, or alveolar gas via a ruptured visceral pleura (sometimes arising spontaneously from unknown causes), enters the pleural space on inspiration, but is trapped by the ruptured membrane acting as a valve. The accumulation of air/gas will cause the lung to collapse (atelectasis), which is life threatening.

An accumulation of fluid within the pleural cavity is called pleural effusion. The extra fluid usually originates from blood vessels or lymphatics in the area, and usually occurs because of high blood pressure (e.g. in congestive heart failure) or because of inflammation. Haemothorax is an accumulation of blood within the pleural cavity as a consequence of the rupture of blood vessels.

Pleural effusion compresses the lung and prevents normal inflation. The fluid usually accumulates at the base of the lung because of the effects of gravity, and may be drained by insertion of a catheter.

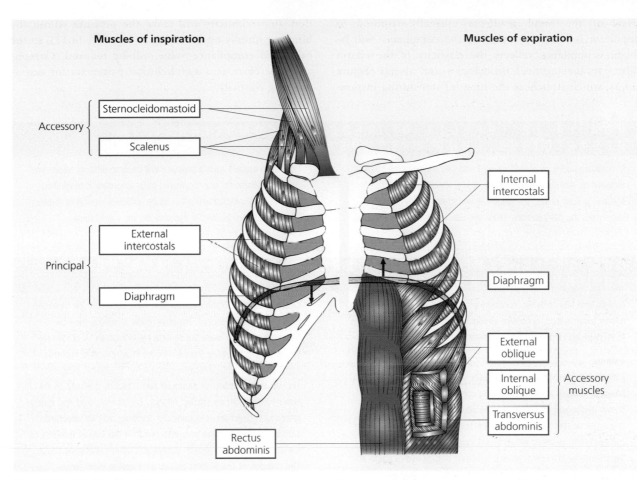

Figure 14.4 Muscles of inspiration and expiration.
Q. Which are the main muscles involved in normal inspiration?

'pulls' the lung outwards (remember that the lungs are not attached directly to the chest wall), thus lowering pressure within the airways. Figure 14.2 shows that the subatmospheric pressure generated is very slight, producing a gradient between the alveoli and the air of only 0.3 kPa. This gradient is not sufficient to generate even a breeze in air, yet it is sufficient at rest to draw some 500 ml of air into the lungs. Inflation at such low pressure gradients suggests that the resistance to air flow within the lung must be very low. This is, indeed, the case, and results from the way in which the airways divide. Thus, although the airways decrease in diameter as they divide, the large increase in the number of branches actually increases their total cross-sectional area. Consequently, it is the nasal cavities and the pharynx that normally provide the main site of airway resistance, especially if there is inflammation and excess mucus due to a cold. A low airway resistance is physiologically important: if it was high, the energy expended in muscle contraction to generate the large pressure gradients necessary to inflate the lungs would be excessive. The fatigue observed in people with chronic obstructive problems is an illustration of the importance of having a low airway resistance.

BOX 14.11 ORAL CARE

Oral care is an important part of nursing care, not least because failure to maintain oral hygiene is distressing for the patient who cannot self-care adequately. Oral hygiene also has implications for nutrition (Jones, 1998). Difficulties in inflating the lung due to an increased airway resistance may cause a patient to resort to mouth breathing, since this circumvents the resistance provided by the nasal passages. Mouth breathing can result in a drying of the oral mucosa and tongue surface, producing considerable discomfort. Mouth care becomes very important. If oxygen therapy or artificial ventilation are involved, the gas is moistened to reduce the consequences for oral hydration, but even this might not be adequate to prevent drying of the oral mucosa.

Air entering the alveoli causes them to expand and stretch. The ease with which the lung can be inflated is referred to as *lung compliance*; it is calculated as:

Compliance = change in lung volume/change in lung pressure

Thus, if the lung could be inflated without causing a large increase in pressure within it (clearly beneficial in view of the small gradients normally required to maintain inflation; see above), the compliance will be high. Compliance reflects the elasticity of the elastin fibres in the terminal bronchioles and alveoli (Figure 14.3), which stretch as the lung inflates during inspiration. Poor elasticity will make the pressure within the lung rise rapidly on breathing in (see Box 14.12), so the calculated compliance value will be reduced. Compliance, therefore, is a useful clinical parameter for assessing lung elasticity.

BOX 14.12 EFFECTS OF REDUCED COMPLIANCE IN RESTRICTIVE LUNG DISORDERS

In conditions such as asbestosis and silicosis, elastin in the lungs is replaced by scar tissue; collectively, this is known as pulmonary fibrosis. In such cases, the lungs will not stretch easily on inspiration, the gas pressure inside will rise rapidly, and maintaining inspiration against such a pressure will become difficult. Restrictive disorders, therefore, are considered to be disorders of inspiration. Inadequate inspiration will not produce sufficient change in alveolar gas composition, leading to hypoxaemia and hypercapnia.

BOX 14.13 EFFECTS OF INCREASED AIRWAY RESISTANCE: OBSTRUCTIVE AIRWAY DISEASE

Asthma and bronchitis are common examples of disorders in which airway inflammation, excessive airway secretions, and/or constriction of bronchioles increases airway resistance (see Brewin, 1997).

Asthma

Asthma is a condition associated with spasmodic contraction of the bronchial smooth muscle, producing symptoms of shortness of breath (dyspnoea), cough, wheezing and, often, distress as a consequence (which exacerbates the breathing difficulty). The most common form is called atopic or extrinsic asthma; this is a hypersensitive immune response to environmental agents, such as pollen or dust particles. This form is found mainly, but not exclusively, in children, who are more susceptible to obstructive problems because of the structure of their airways (Box 14.6). The bronchospasm episode normally resolves in a relatively short period of time, but occasionally there is a second episode several hours later. The first-phase bronchospasm is produced by histamine and parasympathetic nerve activity to the airways, whereas the second phase is a complex response to prostaglandins, thromboxanes and leukotrienes (these are all examples of eicosanoids; see Chapter 9). Inflammatory responses will also be observed, which exacerbates the increased airway resistance. Therapy is directed at reducing airway resistance through use of bronchodilator drugs, or preventing a response by using drugs to impair the release of histamine or to reduce inflammation, and avoiding causative factors. A poor response to bronchodilators during an asthma episode produces a state of status asthmaticus, a serious situation that will probably necessitate the use of oxygen therapy until it resolves.

Intrinsic asthma is promoted by factors such as stress or exercise, and is found more typically in adults. In this case, the bronchospasm is thought to result from an imbalance between parasympathetic nerve activity to the airways (which promotes bronchoconstriction) and sympathetic nerve activity (which promotes bronchodilation). Therapy is again preventive (by avoiding the causative factor) and drug-induced bronchodilation.

Bronchitis

Bronchitis is an inflammatory condition of the airways, usually as a consequence of infection or the presence of an irritant, such as cigarette smoke. Bronchospasm and fluid secretion are observed. With repeated incidences, hypersecretion of mucus may be observed, and the bronchial muscle hypertrophies. A productive cough lasting for more than 3 months in a year, and occurring 2 years in succession, indicates progression to chronic bronchitis. The chronic condition in particular has a profound effect on the airway resistance, as smaller airways become blocked and mucus retention encourages infections. Air trapping may be observed. With time, the condition may also result in the loss of integrity of the airway wall, with loss of elastin and other connective tissue. The collapse of tissue then makes air trapping even worse, leading to the condition emphysema. Long-standing bronchitis is debilitating, and the progression to emphysema is severely disabling. Bronchodilator drugs, chest physical therapy, and oxygen therapy as required may help to improve breathing, but the chronic state is irreversible. Prevention of progression is crucial, and health education is prominent in the care of this condition.

Airway resistance in obstructive conditions

People overcome the additional resistance by increasing the inspiratory effort. Expiration, even at rest, necessitates the use of muscular contraction in order to generate an intrathoracic pressure that is sufficient to force gases out of the lung. Obstructive airway disease, therefore, increases the energy required to maintain breathing movements. The problem is exacerbated because the extra force exerted on the airways during expiration compresses them, or moves mucus to form plugs, and so may increase the resistance further. For this reason, obstructive disorders are considered primarily to be disorders of expiration. In extreme situations, especially in emphysema, the compression on the airways may even result in air trapping within the lung, exacerbating the problem of reduced gas exchange (see Box 14.19).

Breathlessness is a very unpleasant experience for people with these conditions. Establishing a sound therapeutic relationship is essential to reduce anxiety and promote compliance and adherence to therapies (e.g. see Conway, 1999).

Expiration

In contrast to the active process of inspiration, expiration at rest is passive. The naturally high elasticity of lungs means that if inspiration stops and the inspiratory muscles relax, the lungs will simply recoil like a piece of stretched elastic and so expel the gases. This passive nature of expiration helps to keep oxygen use to a minimum during breathing. It can only be effective, however, if the resistance to air flow is extremely low, since only a small pressure gradient is developed between the lung gases and the air outside (Figure 14.2).

If necessary, e.g. during exercise, the expiratory effort can be increased through compressing the lungs by contracting the internal intercostal muscles, which lower the rib cage and move it inwards, and also by contracting accessory muscles, such as the rectus abdominis muscle of the abdomen, that help to lower the rib cage even more effectively (Figure 14.4). Expiration is then considered to be an active process. Such processes are important if breathing rate and depth are to be increased during exercise. Being able to move large breaths in and out of the lungs is also a reflection of the low airway resistance, and in fact can be achieved consciously, even at rest. Indeed, forced expiration of a maximally inhaled breath at rest provides a useful means of clinically monitoring airway resistance, since, for a given resistance, a predicted rate of gas flow should be attainable in health (see Box 14.14, and *Spirometry* below).

Surfactant

There is a potential danger that on breathing out, the walls of the alveoli may touch and adhere to each other. The danger lies in the fact that alveolar membranes must be kept moist to avoid dehydration, and contact between wet surfaces produces powerful adhesion because of the phenomenon of surface tension. Respiratory movements are inadequate to overcome such adhesion forces, so the collapse of alveoli in this way must be prevented. Alveoli do not, in fact, deflate totally following expiration. In addition, they are also coated with a detergent-like chemical – a phospholipid called surfactant – which is secreted by cuboidal epithelial cells of the alveoli (Box 14.15 and Figure 14.3) and that acts to lower the surface tension within the alveoli.

BOX 14.14 PEAK FLOW RATES

The simplest means of assessing airway resistance is to use a peak flow meter. With this, the person is asked to inhale deeply and then to breathe out through the meter as hard as possible. The meter measures the maximum flow rate of gas through it. Values are compared with standards for age, body size and gender, and provide information regarding airway resistance (see Box 14.21).

Problems in making peak flow measurements include:

- the mouthpiece size may not be ideal for the patient;
- the patient may not be using maximal respiratory effort, or a maximal inspiration;

- values will vary between attempts, thus some values will be a more accurate reflection than others. It is usual to take more than one reading and to record the maximum value (not the average, because such values are likely to overestimate rather than underestimate airway resistance).

Since peak flow rates standardized for body size, age and gender relate to airway resistance, they provide an indication of an underlying change in that resistance, e.g. as a consequence of smoking. A more accurate means of monitoring airway resistance is to use more sophisticated equipment (see *Spirometry* below).

BOX 14.15 SURFACTANT IN PREMATURE BABIES

Surfactant chemicals are phospholipids, predominantly lecithin and sphingomyelin, that are secreted by cells within the alveoli. Surfactant is not produced in quantity by the lungs until about the thirty-fourth week of fetal development. Before this, lecithin and sphingomyelin are present in small but equal amounts. After the thirty-fourth week, there is a surge in production, particularly of lecithin, which will eventually be present in double the amounts of sphingomyelin. The lecithin, therefore, is especially important as a surfactant chemical.

Surfactant enables alveoli walls to separate when an infant first inhales, and enables alveoli walls to separate should contact occur during expiration movements.

The lack of adequate surfactant in premature babies is a major factor in their survival (Wilson, 1998). Because of this, babies born very early will be placed in an environment in which the oxygen pressure is increased. This will raise the oxygen pressure in the alveoli that are functioning, and help to maintain oxygenation of the baby's blood until other alveoli become patent. Nevertheless, the likelihood of survival will be increased if the alveoli can be opened more effectively, and researchers are currently developing artificial surfactants that can be administered by inhalation and will maintain alveolar patency until the intrinsic surfactant is produced in adequate quantities.

If premature delivery is anticipated, then dexamethasone (a steroid) may be administered to the mother, as this has been found to accelerate the production of surfactant.

Respiratory distress syndrome of the newborn is a serious condition in premature babies that involves anatomical defects such as small alveoli and poorly developed chest structures, coupled with poor production of surfactant. Mortality rates in this condition are high.

To demonstrate surface tension, place a piece of glass or a flat, rigid plastic sheet on a wet kitchen surface. Now try (carefully) to lift it. Notice the powerful adhesion produced by surface tension in the thin layer of water between the glass and top. Now place a droplet of water onto a dry piece of glass. Notice how it forms a globule. The surface molecules are held in place by surface tension, producing the globular shape. Now add a little detergent. The drop disperses: surface tension is reduced by the detergent in much the same way as surfactant reduces it in the alveoli.

Pulmonary and alveolar ventilation, and dead space

We discussed earlier how a volume of lung gas will remain, after breathing out, within the 'dead space' provided by the major airways. This gas will re-enter the alveoli during the next inspiration, followed closely by the fresh air. Thus, at the end of inspiration, a portion of the inspired air will have mixed with this 'old' gas in the alveoli, but a proportion will also have filled the major airways. These parts of the respiratory tree do not exchange gases with the blood (hence the term 'dead space'). For a normal adult tidal volume of 500 ml, about 150 ml of the inspired air will fill the dead space, and only 350 ml will enter the alveoli. In some disorders, non-functioning alveoli increase the volume of this dead space (see Box 14.16).

The volume of air breathed into the lungs per minute is called the *pulmonary ventilation rate* (sometimes referred to as the respiratory minute volume), while that entering the alveoli each minute is called the *alveolar ventilation rate*. The

BOX 14.16 DEAD SPACE

Dead space can be envisaged either as being the volume of gas contained in non-exchanging parts of the lung, or as being that volume of inspired air that does not take part in gas exchange. Although apparently the same thing, there is a difference in these definitions: the first identifies an *anatomical* dead space, while the second identifies a *physiological* dead space. The anatomical dead space makes the assumption that all alveoli take part in normal gas exchange with the blood. This is usually the case, and the anatomical and physiological dead spaces are equal. A pathological disturbance of alveolar function may interfere with gaseous exchange, however, and the alveoli affected will thence become part of the dead space, i.e. the physiological dead space will then exceed the anatomical dead space, so the influence that the dead space has on lung gas composition after inspiration will be exaggerated.

Dead space is an important consideration in calculating the needs of patients (see Box 14.17).

presence of a dead space means that it cannot be assumed that pulmonary ventilation gives a measure of the ventilation of the alveoli, yet this latter is clearly a more important parameter since this will determine the gas composition in the alveoli and hence gas exchange there (see Box 14.17).

Refer to Box 14.17.

What would the alveolar ventilation be in someone with double the inspired volume (i.e. 1000 ml) but half the breathing rate (i.e. 5 breaths/min)? How would you advise someone who is very anxious?

BOX 14.17 EFFECTS OF DEAD SPACE ON ALVEOLAR VENTILATION

Consider these normal values:

Volume inspired per breath = 500 ml
Breaths/min = 10
Pulmonary ventilation = breath volume × breathing rate = 500 ml × 10 = 5000 ml/min (5 l/min)

Volume inspired per breath − dead space volume = 500 ml − 150 ml = 350 ml
Breaths per minute = 10
Alveolar ventilation = 350 ml × 10 = 3500 ml/min (3.5 l/min)

Thus, alveolar ventilation at 3.5 l/min is considerably less than the pulmonary ventilation of 5 l/min.
Now, suppose that the volume inspired is halved (to 250 ml), but the breathing rate is doubled (to 20 breaths/min):

Pulmonary ventilation = 250 ml × 20 = 5 l/min, i.e. unchanged.
Alveolar ventilation = (250 − 150) × 20 = 100 ml × 20 = 2 l/min, i.e. much reduced.

Thus, a person who is taking shallow, rapid breaths may seem to be achieving a reasonable lung ventilation, but in fact may be experiencing a decreased alveolar ventilation, poor gas exchange, and blood gas disturbance.

The influence of dead space on alveolar ventilation has implications for the use of mechanical ventilation therapies, because the tubing used will increase the dead space and therefore will have to be taken into account in calculating the depth and rate of ventilation. A tube inserted into the trachea will tend to reduce the anatomical dead space, since the oral/nasal cavities are bypassed.

BOX 14.18 ASSISTED VENTILATION

Ventilation may be assisted for two main reasons. First, breathing movements in respiratory disorders may not be sufficient to produce adequate alveolar ventilation, leading to lack of oxygen and an excess of carbon dioxide. Under such circumstances, oxygen therapy might be used to improve the composition of alveolar gas. Second, if independent breathing is not possible, then artificial means of ventilation will be used.

Oxygen therapy

One way to maintain adequate alveolar gas composition in respiratory disorder is to use an enriched mixture of inspired gas. Pure oxygen is toxic and produces severe inflammation of the airways, so the patient may be encouraged to breathe a gas mixture of air and oxygen, or perhaps a mixture of oxygen and carbon dioxide. In this way, the alveolar oxygen composition can be made to be near normal, even though the tidal volume is inadequate to provide normal alveolar ventilation.

The enriched gas mixture (from a gas cylinder or piped source) might be applied by free flow through a nasal tube or through a face mask. A face mask may be very uncomfortable, while gas pressure within the nasal tubing or face mask may also be disconcerting. It is important for nurses to be aware that breathing difficulties are extremely distressing to the patient, and that both methods may add to the anxiety experienced by patients who are already feeling breathless. Feeding and speech may also be affected adversely, which adds to the patient's frustration.

Artificial or mechanical ventilation

The most extreme form of assisted ventilation is that involving what was once referred to as an 'iron lung'. In this, the thorax is encased within a sealed chamber, and pressure changes within the chamber are used to produce the movements of the chest required for breathing. The method is used when paralysis of the chest arising from neck trauma or spinal cord dysfunctioning prevents the respiratory muscles from functioning.

Other methods are used to facilitate breathing by pumping air or a gas mixture into the lungs of an unconscious patient (a conscious person would work against the artificially induced movements). The patient is connected to a ventilator by tubing, the end of which may pass into the trachea. The machine pumps into the lungs a preset tidal volume of air/gas, at a preset rate, and so replaces the normal respiratory movements. There are a number of variations to the precise method used (see Tan and Oh, 1997).

In *continuous positive airway pressure* (CPAP), positive airway pressure is maintained throughout the breathing cycle. Maintaining airway pressure ensures a positive end-expiration pressure (PEEP), which increases the patency of alveoli and helps to prevent their collapse. It may also help to redistribute fluid into the tissue fluid space from the alveoli. There is a risk that the elevated pressure may induce barotrauma ('baro-'= pressure) by decreasing the output from the right side of the heart (and hence cardiac output from the left side). Hyperinflation also decreases the compliance of the lungs, making them harder to inflate (i.e. the work of breathing is increased), and increases the risk of pneumothorax (see Box 14.10).

Bi-positive airway pressure (BiPAP) is a modification of CPAP in which two airway pressures are applied, with synchronization during the breathing cycle. This ensures PEEP but also allows a reduction in pressure during the expiration (but not sufficient to allow alveolar collapse if this is a risk), which helps to reduce the risk of barotrauma and decreased compliance. The pressure is increased again during inspiration, which helps to inflate the alveoli.

Intermittent positive pressure ventilation (IPPV) pumps air or ventilation gas into the lungs by applying a positive pressure, but allows expiration to occur passively by recoil, as in normally functioning lungs. The risks of the method relate especially to the applied pressure and volume administered. If excessive, then pneumothorax may occur (see Box 14.10).

High-frequency ventilation (HFV) reduces some of the risks associated with applied pressure by administering very small volumes at high frequency. The pressure changes are not so large. The intention is to alter the composition of lung gases, including those within the dead space, so that small volumes can achieve the necessary 'dilutional' effect on the functional residual capacity.

Spirometry: pulmonary gas volumes and capacities

We have stated already that the volume of air inspired per breath at rest is called the tidal volume and that this averages about 500 ml in an adult. Even at rest, we can consciously increase the volume breathed in, or further deflate the lung, so it is clear that the alveoli are not inflated fully after normal inspiration, nor are they deflated maximally after expiration, i.e. there are inspiratory and expiratory *reserve volumes* (Figure 14.5). In addition, the lung contains a volume of gas even after maximal expira-tion has occurred, as deflation of the alveoli is incomplete and some gas fills the dead space, i.e. there is a *residual volume* of gas within the lungs (about 1.5 l in adults). Consequently, the gases within the lung into which the inspired air will pass when we breathe in will be the volume represented by the expiratory reserve plus the residual volume: this is the *functional residual capacity* (FRC; about 2.5 l in an adult), and is equal to approximately half the maximum capacity of the lungs (called the total lung capacity). Thus, the normal resting operation of the lung occurs with the lung being always about half inflated. The FRC is an important clinical parameter (see Box 14.19).

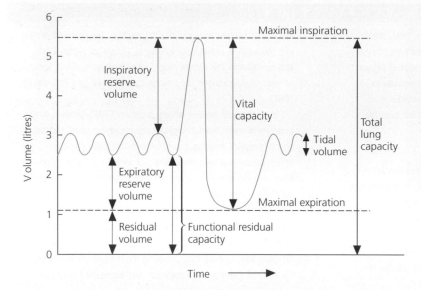

Figure 14.5 Spirometer recording (spirogram) of principal lung volumes and capacities in an adult. Note that the zero line cannot be ascertained directly.

Q. Define and give the average volumes in millilitres of the following: (i) tidal volume, (ii) vital capacity, (iii) inspiratory reserve volume, and (iv) residual volume.

Q. Which of the lung volumes/capacities given below cannot be determined directly using a simple spirometer: (i) tidal volume, (ii) vital capacity, (iii) inspiratory reserve volume, (iv) residual volume?

BOX 14.19 FUNCTIONAL RESIDUAL CAPACITY IN OBSTRUCTIVE AIRWAY DISORDERS

The importance of the FRC is illustrated by considering the consequences if it is increased. In chronic obstructive airways disease (COAD), the severity of the increased resistance prevents adequate expiration, leading to an increased FRC and, consequently, an overinflated lung with decreased inspiratory reserve. Air breathed into the enlarged FRC is then less effective at altering the gas composition, so the oxygen content of alveolar gas declines and that of carbon dioxide increases. Similar changes occur in the blood. These conditions, such as chronic bronchitis (see Box 14.13), can be debilitating. The problem is exacerbated because there is a reduced capacity to increase the breath volume during physical exertion, with the result that the patient fatigues easily (Truesdell, 2000).

Any inflammation in COAD may become so severe that areas of tissue become weakened or even necrotic. In emphysema, the airways may collapse during expiration, thus exacerbating the resistance problem and elevating the FRC further. Loss of functioning alveoli in this condition also increases the physiological dead space. Emphysema is an extremely debilitating, life-threatening condition.

BOX 14.20 RESIDUAL VOLUME AND PREGNANCY

The developing baby pushes up on the mother's abdominal organs, which tends to compress the diaphragm. While this can make breathing a little uncomfortable, it also acts to reduce the residual volume of gas left in the lungs after expiration (and in turn decreases the functional residual capacity). Thus, the air breathed in has a slightly greater influence on alveolar gas composition, which facilitates greater gas exchange. Alveolar ventilation is also enhanced through the actions of progesterone to relax the smooth muscle of the airways.

These changes are important, particularly with respect to carbon dioxide excretion, because the mother's lungs must adapt to excrete the load coming from her tissues and those of the baby. The actions of progesterone to raise the sensitivity of receptors (central chemoreceptors; see later) to carbon dioxide are also important in this respect.

If we inflate the lungs maximally and then breathe out maximally, the volume of gas expired from the lungs represents the maximum volume of gas that can possibly be expelled from the lung in a single breath; this is called the *vital capacity* (about 4 l in an adult). If we add the vital capacity to the residual volume (Figure 14.5), then this gives the *total lung capacity* (about 5.5–6 l in an adult). The residual volume cannot be measured directly, but an indirect method may be used by determining the effect of the residual gases to dilute an inert marker gas, such as helium after inspiration. The degree of dilution can then be used to calculate the residual volume.

Lung volumes and capacities are measured using a machine called a (re)spirometer. There are various kinds of spirometer, some of which are portable and may provide only some of the information (e.g. the vital capacity may be determined using a 'vitallograph' – see Figure 14.6). Full spirometric assessment (Figure 14.5) requires a more sophisticated spirometer, as found in lung function rooms in some larger hospitals.

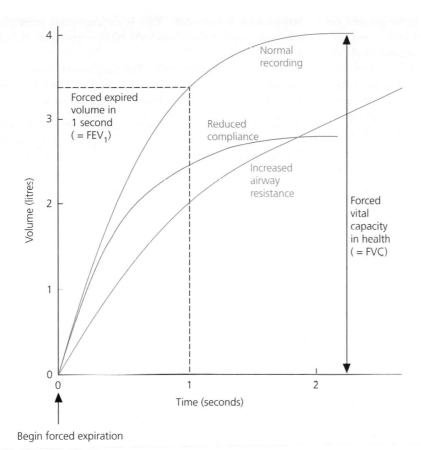

Figure 14.6 'Vitallograph' traces of vital capacity measurement to illustrate the use of FEV$_1$ as a diagnostic tool. Note that FVC varies between individuals, especially in disease states. Note the change in FEV, and in the FVC in respiratory conditions. See Box 14.21 for explanation. Values stated are examples for this illustration.

Q. How does long-term smoking affect the FEV$_1$?

BOX 14.21 USE OF A SPIROMETER TO MEASURE FORCED EXPIRATORY VOLUME AND TO ASSESS AIRWAY RESISTANCE

Box 14.14 notes that measurement of the peak flow rate during expiration provides a measure of airway resistance. In performing the test, the person breathes out forcibly the vital capacity, filled when the maximal inspiration was made before the test. Spirometers enable clinicians to measure the vital capacity, and to look in more detail at the peak flow rate.

If a person breathes in maximally and then breathes out forcibly to completion, then the entire vital capacity will be breathed out. Because it has been done forcibly, the volume measured is usually referred to as the forced expiratory volume (FEV). In health, more than 80% of the vital capacity should be expelled in the first second; the volume expired is referred to as the FEV$_1$, and the proportion of vital capacity as the FEV%. With increased airway resistance, this proportion falls, according to the severity of the condition (Figure 14.6).

Another significance of expressing the FEV$_1$ as a percentage (or as a ratio, where 80% = 0.80) is that even if the vital capacity is severely reduced because of a restrictive condition (i.e. pulmonary fibrosis), a normal airway resistance will mean that the FEV, may be a normal proportion of it. Spirometry therefore provides a means of monitoring any progress in both obstructive and restrictive disorders.

It can be seen, therefore, that the various lung capacities and volumes provide an indication of the relationships between various airway components and lung function. Ultimately, however, there must be gas exchange across the respiratory surface (see below).

Exchange of gases between alveoli and blood

Partial pressures

The exchange of oxygen and carbon dioxide between the alveoli and blood is a simple process of diffusion, and is influenced mainly by two factors:

- The thickness of the barrier formed by the alveolar membrane and the blood vessel wall (Figure 14.3). The cells of these membranes are flattened, so that the barrier is exceedingly thin (about 0.4 μm), and blood cells are brought into close proximity to the lung gases. The gases, however, still have to traverse across the intracellular fluids of the cells that form the membranes, and across the interstitial fluid between them (although this is minimal). Much of the resistance to gas diffusion is therefore caused by fluid, and the barrier problem relates to the solubility of oxygen and carbon dioxide in water during the exchange process.

● The pressure gradient between the alveolar gas and gas dissolved in blood. Up to now, we have considered only the total pressure of gases within the lung and in the air. In order to understand the exchange of individual gases within the mixture found in the lung, it is important that you understand the concept of partial pressures, since it is these individual pressures that form the gradients that promote the diffusion of individual gases.

As the name implies, partial pressures are those pressures generated by individual gases within a gas mixture. Each gas within a mixture exerts its own pressure, determined by the relative proportions of the gases; the sum of all the partial pressures must be equal to the total pressure of the gas mixture. For example, 21% of air is comprised of oxygen. At normal atmospheric pressure (at sea level), the total air pressure is about 101 kPa (760 mm Hg), so the partial pressure of oxygen will be 21% of this, i.e. about 21 kPa (160 mm Hg). The air also contains nitrogen, carbon dioxide and small quantities of other gases. Each of these will exert its own partial pressure, and the sum of these individual pressures, with oxygen, will equal 101 kPa.

In the lungs, the partial pressure of an individual gas within a mixture produces the driving force for its movement into or out of blood independent of other gases within the mixture (Figure 14.7). Note that gases dissolved in a fluid also exert a pressure. The amount dissolved will be determined by that pressure since this 'drives' the gas into solution. Gases vary in their solubility, however, so the quantity of gas dissolved will relate to both its partial pressure and its solubility (assuming temperature is constant). This is an important principle when we consider (in a later section) how gases are carried by blood.

Analysis of alveolar gases after inspiration shows that the partial pressure of oxygen averages 13.3 kPa (100 mm Hg Table 14.1(a)). This is lower than air because:

● alveolar gas into which the air passed contains a higher proportion of carbon dioxide. The partial pressure of carbon dioxide within the alveoli averages 5.3 kPa (40 mm Hg) after inspiration. It does not fall to zero, even though air is virtually free of carbon dioxide, because of the large volume of gas remaining in the lungs after expiration has finished;

● alveolar gas is saturated with water vapour (which will also exert a partial pressure).

Remember that the partial pressure depends upon the relative proportions of the gases – change the proportion of oxygen and its partial pressure will also change. The average partial pressures of alveolar gases, pulmonary arterial blood, pulmonary venous blood and air are compared in Table 14.1(b). Notice that the partial pressure of oxygen is relatively high compared with that of carbon dioxide.

The higher partial pressure for oxygen in alveolar gas is important because oxygen is poorly soluble in water, so its diffusion will be facilitated by the high pressure. In contrast, the solubility of carbon dioxide is much higher than that of oxygen, and adequate diffusion of the gas from the blood into the alveoli takes place with much lower partial pressure gradients.

BOX 14.22 PULMONARY OEDEMA AND GAS DIFFUSION

An accumulation of fluid within the alveoli significantly increases the barrier to gas diffusion, especially of oxygen, as this gas is poorly soluble in water. Ordinarily, the alveoli are kept relatively 'dry' because the low pressure in the pulmonary capillaries is exceeded greatly by the osmotic effect of the plasma proteins in blood passing through them (see Chapter 6 for an explanation of capillary–tissue fluid movements). This fluid barrier is increased if:

● pneumonia occurs – inflammatory exudate from lung cells fills the alveoli;

● pulmonary hypertension occurs, e.g. secondary to congestive heart failure – the increased blood pressure exceeds the osmotic action of the plasma proteins, causing exudation of fluid from plasma;

● an increased permeability of the pulmonary capillaries occurs, leading to leakage of plasma proteins and the formation of exudate from the capillaries. This can occur as a consequence of cardiovascular shock, or after severe trauma, and is referred to as (adult) respiratory distress syndrome (ARDS). The mechanism of ARDS remains poorly understood, and mortality rates are high when it occurs.

Collectively, the occurrence of fluid within the alveoli is referred to as pulmonary oedema (Seigh, 1999) The best means to remove the accumulated fluid is debatable. Gravitational effects or diuretic drugs may be used to reduce pulmonary hypertension (but may compromise cardiac function if this is the primary disorder). Reducing inflammation is indicated where appropriate, but in ARDS this is of limited benefit because of the profound changes to the structure of the barrier. Colloid infusions may be used to increase the osmotic pressure of plasma, thus withdrawing fluid from the lungs by osmosis, but they may also increase blood viscosity and impair blood flow through the lungs.

Treatment of pulmonary oedema will usually entail providing an oxygen-enriched breathing mixture, in order to raise the pressure of oxygen within the alveoli, and so promote better transfer of the gas through the fluid barrier.

(a) Gas pressures in solution

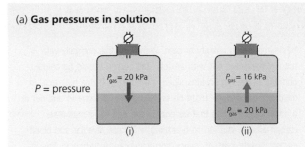

P = pressure

(i)   (ii)

(b) Partial pressures

Let the total pressure of a gas = 20 kPa. If 66.6% of the gas is oxygen, then the (partial) pressure due to oxygen (Po_2) will be $20 \times 66.6/100 = 13.3$ kPa. If 33.4% of the gas is carbon dioxide, then the (partial) pressure due to carbon dioxide (Pco_2) will be $20 \times 33.4/100 = 6.7$ kPa

In solutions,

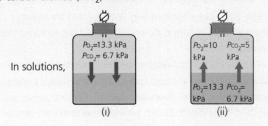

(i)   (ii)

(c) Representative values for lung/blood gas exchange after inspiration

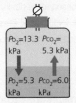

Figure 14.7 Partial pressures of gases. (a) Gas pressures in solution: (i) gas diffuses into solution, until pressures in the solution and above the solution equilibrate; (ii) reducing the gas pressure above the solution now favours diffusion of the gas out of the solution, until the pressures equilibrate again. (b) Partial pressures: (i) as above, oxygen and carbon dioxide will enter the solution, until the pressures above and in the solution equilibrate; (ii) if the pressures of oxygen and carbon dioxide above the solution are now reduced, both gases will tend to diffuse out of the solution, until pressures equilibrate again. (c) Representative values for lung/blood gas exchange after inspiration. The partial pressure gradient for oxygen favours diffusion of the gas into the solution (blood), while the gradient for carbon dioxide favours diffusion out of the solution into the gases above it (lung), i.e. gas exchange in the lung is promoted by the respective partial pressure gradients for oxygen and carbon dioxide.

Q. Why does oxygen diffuse into blood from the lung, and carbon dioxide from the blood into the lung?

Table 14.1(a) Representative partial pressures of gases in air (dry), inspired air (wet) and alveolar gas after inspiration

	Air (dry) kpa	Inspired air (wet) kPa	Alveolar gas after inspiration kPa
Oxygen	21.2	19.9	13.3
Carbon dioxide	0.03	0.03	5.3
Nitrogen	79.8	77.5	76.2
Water vapour	0	6.3	6.3
Total	100.9	100.9	100.9

Atmospheric pressure is taken to be 100.0 kPa. Note how the saturation of inspired air with water vapour changes the values for other gases – the sum of the pressures must remain the same.

Table 14.1(b) Representative partial pressures and gas composition of blood entering the lungs (mixed venous blood) and leaving the lungs (pulmonary venous blood)

	Po_2 kPa	Pco_2 kPa	Volume O_2 ml/100 ml	Volume CO_2 ml/100 ml
Mixed venous blood	5.3	6.0	14	52
Pulmonary venous blood (systemic arterial blood)	13.3	5.3	19.7	48
Change	+8.0	−0.7	+5.7	4.0

Net changes as blood passes through the lungs are shown. Note that the changes in oxygen and carbon dioxide content of blood as it passes through the lungs are produced by disproportionate changes in their partial pressures. The reason for this is that carbon dioxide is much more soluble than oxygen.

From Table 14.1(b), it can be seen that the partial pressures of oxygen and carbon dioxide present in blood leaving the lung (i.e. in pulmonary venous or systemic arterial blood) are the same as those of the gases in the lung alveoli after inspiration. In other words, equilibration between the blood and alveolar gas occurs. It must be stressed, however, that the values shown for alveolar gases are averages. Ventilation is not the same throughout the lungs, nor is the rate of blood flow in relation to the ventilation, so regional variations are observed in the composition of blood leaving these areas.

Regional disturbances in the ventilation or blood perfusion of the lung are among the most common causes of low blood oxygen content (hypoxaemia; 'hypo-' = less than normal, '-aemia' = of the blood). The term that is used is 'ventilation/perfusion ratio'.

BOX 14.23 PARTIAL PRESSURES AND BLOOD COMPOSITION DURING HYPERVENTILATION AND HYPOVENTILATION

Normal ranges for arterial blood oxygen values (partial pressures): birth, 1.1–3.2k Pa; 5–10 min after birth, 4.4–10.0 kPa; 1 day, 7.2–12.6 kPa; adult, 11–14.4 kPa.

Normal ranges for arterial blood carbon dioxide values (partial pressures): newborn, 3.6–5.3 kPa; adult, 4.5–6.4 kPa.

In hyperventilation, the rate of alveolar ventilation is greater than appropriate for the rate of metabolism at that time. The composition of alveolar gases alters more on inspiration, becoming much richer in oxygen (since more air is entering it) and more deficient in carbon dioxide (air is effectively 0% carbon dioxide). The partial pressure of oxygen is thus increased, and that of carbon dioxide is decreased. Arterial blood is normally saturated with oxygen, so the enrichment of lung gases with oxygen has little effect. However, the carbon dioxide depletion removes the gas from blood so efficiently that arterial blood carbon dioxide content falls. This disturbance of homeostasis will produce an alkalosis, but will also make cerebral blood vessels constrict (so that less carbon dioxide is washed out of the brain, thus restoring the carbon dioxide homeostasis in this tissue). This constriction will, in turn, impair oxygen delivery to the brain, so a person who is hyperventilating will tend to feel dizzy and may even faint.

In reality, hyperventilation induced consciously is impossible to maintain in normal health, since the blood gas changes will promote self-correcting responses. However, hyperventilation can be maintained in anxiety or pain. With pain, this normally will require analgesia, but with anxiety, the person should be calmed and encouraged to breathe slowly and deeply. If this fails (e.g. in children), the patient might be encouraged to breathe in and out of a paper bag: the gas that collects in the bag will accumulate carbon dioxide and, on re-breathing, will raise alveolar and blood carbon dioxide content, hence correcting the disturbance. This in itself will improve the way that the person feels, and so will have a calming effect.

In hypoventilation, the alveolar gases become depleted in oxygen and enriched in carbon dioxide, since the volume of air entering the alveoli is insufficient to maintain the normal composition. The lower partial pressure for oxygen means that arterial blood oxygen content may decrease, and the higher partial pressure of carbon dioxide will make blood content of this gas rise.

The onset of allergy-induced hypoventilation (asthma) can be extremely rapid, and if severe can quickly produce such a profound dyspnoea as to require immediate attention. Fear and anxiety are natural in these circumstances, but they serve to exacerbate the problem. Oxygen therapy, reassurance and bronchodilator drugs may be used to improve ventilation, but calming reassurance is also important.

Hypoventilation is also observed in obstructive and restrictive airway disorders, and in the inhibition of breathing observed with brainstem trauma, drug overdose and excessive opioid analgesia.

Ventilation/perfusion ratio

At rest, an adult breathes in (and out) about 5 l of air per minute. The rate of blood flow through the lungs is about 5–6 l/min at rest, so the ratio of ventilation/perfusion averages between 0.8 and 1.0. This near matching of gas and blood movements within the lungs ensures optimal oxygenation of blood and adequate removal of carbon dioxide. However, variation in the ventilation/perfusion ratio between regions of the lung means that regional oxygenation may be less, and carbon dioxide may be removed more or less efficiently.

Variation in the ratio arises largely because of the distribution of blood within the lungs, although it is also the case that ventilation of alveoli is uneven. Blood flow to the base of the lung is enhanced by gravity (note the anatomical position of the lung relative to the heart; Figure 14.1), whereas the perfusion of alveoli at the apex is reduced (in the upright position) since blood pressure in the pulmonary arteries is only of the order of 25/8 mm Hg, which will barely maintain blood flow against gravity to the lung apex.

Table 14.2 Regional variation in the rates of ventilation and blood perfusion in the lungs. Partial pressures indicate values at the end of inspiration

	Ventilation (l/min)	Perfusion (l/min)	V/Q	PO_2 (kPa)	PCO_2 (kPa)
Zone*					
Apex	0.24	0.07	3.3	17.5	3.7
Base	0.82	1.29	0.63	11.8	5.6
Whole lungs	5	6	0.83	13.3	5.3

Ventilation/perfusion ratios (V/Q) are shown, as are the regional partial pressures of oxygen and carbon dioxide. Average values for the lungs as a whole are shown for comparison.
*Zonal values between apex and base are not included, but they will contribute to values for the whole lung.

Q. What is meant by the ventilation/perfusion ratio? What would happen to gas exchange if the ventilation/perfusion ratio of the whole lung was to decrease?

BOX 14.24 LUNG PERFUSION AND INFLATION AT BIRTH

Before birth, the lungs are not functional as such, so much of the blood returning to the right side of the heart is shunted directly across to the left side, into the left atrium, via a perforation of the septum between the left and right atria called the foramen ovale. Of the blood that is ejected from the right ventricle towards the lungs, much is shunted directly from the pulmonary arterial trunk into the aorta, via a vessel called the ductus arteriosus. During fetal life, when gas exchange occurs in the placenta, the lungs receive only about 10% of the blood returning to the right side of the heart; 90% passes into the left atrium and aorta without passing first through the lungs.

Oxygenation of the baby's tissues is promoted at birth by some precise mechanisms (refer to the structure and function of the heart discussed in Chapter 12):

- At birth, the fetal lungs are either collapsed or partially filled with amniotic fluid, which is rapidly absorbed.
- The alveoli are inflated with air by a reflex initiation of inspiration. This occurs because respiratory centres of the brainstem (see Chapter 8) are stimulated by the rising concentrations of carbon dioxide in the blood caused by the loss of placental gas exchange.
- Oxygen uptake across the lung raises the partial pressure of oxygen in pulmonary venous blood, which stimulates closure of the ductus arteriosus. Having closed, the ductus arteriosus will atrophy into a ligament (the ligamentum arteriosum) during the succeeding months.

- The foramen ovale closes because more blood is arriving in the left atrium from the lungs (producing a pressure gradient between the left and right atria that favours closure).
- The closure of the ductus arteriosus and foramen ovale ensures that all blood from the right side of the heart now perfuses the lungs.
- Pulmonary blood flow is facilitated by a decreased pulmonary vascular resistance prompted by the rising oxygenation within the lung alveoli.

Persistence of embryological features

The importance of circulatory and respiratory changes are clear. A persictently low partial pressure of oxygen as a consequence of inadequate gas exchange (e.g. in infant respiratory distress syndrome) prevents adequate closure of the ductus arteriosus. Blood then flows from the aorta (in which pressure is increased at birth) into the pulmonary artery and lung, at the expense of the rest of the systemic circulation causing pulmonary hypertension. Inadequate closure of the foramen ovale (producing a 'hole in the heart') means that some blood will continue to be shunted from the right to the left side of the heart, without undergoing gas exchange. If severe, this will be life threatening, and even a small residual defect may become apparent years later when oxygen needs increases in the growing child.

Nevertheless, the cardiovascular changes at birth are not instantaneous or complete, and it may be weeks or months before final closure of the foramen ovale or ductus arteriosus takes place. For further reading, see Aloan and Hill (1997).

In this way, the ventilation/perfusion ratio actually increases vertically through the lung, and has an effect on the gas composition of blood leaving these areas, as shown in Table 14.2. Thus, regional variations in the ventilation/perfusion ratio within the lung will result in blood of differing gas composition leaving those areas. Subsequent mixing of blood produces the final composition found in pulmonary venous (i.e. systemic arterial) blood. Clinically, the term 'shunt effect' may be used to indicate that a lung is exhibiting a diminished ventilation/perfusion ratio (see Box 14.24).

Some correction of mismatch is possible physiologically, e.g. localized hypoxaemia as a consequence of reduced ventilation of an area of the lung (resulting in a low ventilation/perfusion ratio) causes vasoconstriction, which directs blood from this area to areas of high ventilation/perfusion ratio, and thus facilitates gas exchange.

Exercise

Refer to Box 14.28 for normal values for blood gases. Notice how the oxygen values change during the first day after birth as circulatory functions change and lung function becomes increasingly effective.

BOX 14.25 SHUNT EFFECTS

The significance of ventilation/perfusion matching is that areas of the lung may pathologically exhibit diminished ventilation or perfusion; the resultant mismatch will then alter the final composition of pulmonary venous blood. Ventilation/perfusion mismatches are among the commonest causes of lung-induced oxygen deficiency in blood (hypoxaemia).

If no gas exchange occurred at all (assuming life could still survive), then blood leaving the lungs would be depleted in oxygen and enriched in carbon dioxide; in fact it would have the same composition as mixed venous blood entering the lungs. It would be as though blood had missed the lungs completely, and the term

'shunt' was introduced as a consequence. Clearly, a 100% shunt is not compatible with life, but a less extensive shunt might be acknowledged in certain circumstances, e.g. 20% shunt refers to a blood composition leaving the lungs that would occur if 20% of blood had not passed through it. This might occur in a newborn infant if the ductus arteriosus or fenestra ovalis have not closed (Box 14.24 this is an example of an anatomical shunt). With a collapsed lung, blood does pass through the lungs, but the loss of gas exchange function in those lung areas will provide a physiological shunt that may still be expressed as a 'shunt effect'. The greater the shunt effect, the greater the implication for blood leaving the lungs.

Such a response is limited, however, and will not be effective if large areas of the lung are affected, as occurs in a collapsed lung, for example, or if there is considerable pleural effusion that prevents normal inflation of the affected part of the lung.

Gas carriage by blood

The carriage of gases by the blood is facilitated by the pigment haemoglobin present in red blood cells.

Structure of haemoglobin

Haemoglobin begins to be synthesized in the early stages of differentiation of the red blood cell, when the cell still has a nucleus (and is called a reticulocyte; see Chapter 11). The haemoglobin will eventually fill the cell, which loses its nucleus and becomes an erythrocyte ('erythro-' = red). A molecule of haemoglobin consists of four molecules of the protein globin, and four molecules of the pigment haem (Figure 14.8). The globin molecules within a haemoglobin molecule are not all identical, however, because of slight differences in their amino acid composition.

The types of globin are given Greek letters to distinguish them. Over 90% of the haemoglobin of children and adults (known as HbA) contains two molecules of alpha globin and two molecules of beta globin. In the remainder (HbA$_2$), the beta globin is replaced by delta globin, but functionally this type of haemoglobin is similar to HbA. Changes in the proportion of HbA$_2$ are diagnostic, e.g. it is increased in the blood disorder thalassaemia.

In contrast, some two-thirds of the haemoglobin of a fetus has two alpha and two gamma globin molecules in its molecule, and is referred to as HbF. This difference in the globins compared with the adult type has a significant effect on the relationship between haemoglobin and oxygen, and is an important adaptation to uterine life, as is discussed later. There is also a higher overall concentration of haemoglobin in the fetus (17 g/100 ml compared with 12–14 g/100 ml in adults). This will reduce to adult values within about 3 months after birth.

The haem molecule is a complex structure. It is an example of a group of organic chemicals called porphyrins. Each haem molecule has an iron ion at its core, so a haemoglobin molecule contains four ions of iron, each of which can combine reversibly with an oxygen molecule.

Exercise

In considering the structure of haemoglobin, it is worth revisiting what happens to the components when red blood cells are destroyed (see Chapter 11). Read the relevant section again, especially in relation to jaundice. What is the difference between physiological jaundice in the newborn, and pathological jaundice in a person with cirrhosis of the liver?

There are 200–300 million molecules of haemoglobin in each mature red blood cell, which means that each 100 ml of blood contains approximately 13–15 g of haemoglobin. This amount, together with the properties of the pigment, ensures that the blood can transport adequate amounts of respiratory gases. This is particularly so for oxygen, as this gas is poorly soluble in blood plasma; carbon dioxide is also carried dissolved in plasma, and also as bicarbonate ions produced by its chemical reaction with water. Haemoglobin deficiency (anaemia) therefore has greater implications for oxygen carriage than for the transportation of carbon dioxide.

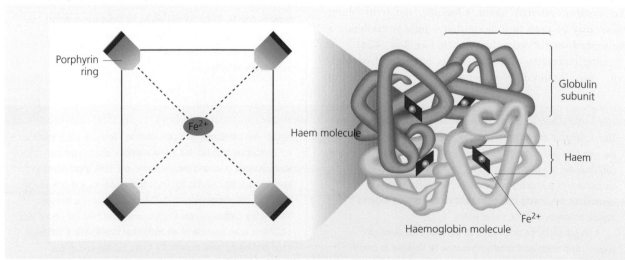

Figure 14.8 A molecule of haemoglobin, showing four molecules of globin and four molecules of haem. The haem molecule consists of a porphyrin ring surrounding an iron ion (as Fe^{2+}).

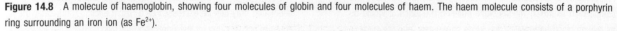

Q. Describe the structural relationships between the Fe^{2+}, globin and haem subunits of haemoglobin.

Carriage of oxygen

Oxygen is carried mainly in association with haemoglobin, i.e.

$$Hb \quad + \quad O_2 \quad \leftrightarrow \quad HbO_2$$

Haemoglobin + oxygen $\leftrightarrow$ oxyhaemoglobin

When fully saturated with oxygen, haemoglobin at a normal concentration of 15 g/100 ml of blood will carry about 19 ml of oxygen per 100 ml of blood. Only another 0.3 ml of the gas per 100 ml of blood will be transported dissolved in the plasma (remember that oxygen is poorly soluble in water). Thus, almost 99% of oxygen carried by oxygenated (arterial) blood is transported as oxyhaemoglobin; this is a measure of the importance of having sufficient pigment. Functionally, the bond between the pigment and oxygen must be reversible, otherwise the gas will not be released in the tissues. It is the local partial pressure of oxygen that is the determining factor: within the lungs it is relatively high; within the tissues where oxygen is utilized it is relatively low.

In the lung, haemoglobin rapidly picks up oxygen to form oxyhaemoglobin, and blood leaves the lungs with its haemoglobin virtually saturated with oxygen. This near saturation of haemoglobin is illustrated by the 'plateau' phase of the

---

BOX 14.26 MEASUREMENT OF HAEMOGLOBIN SATURATION USING PULSE OXIMETRY

Pulse oximetry is applied widely as a non-invasive means of observing the oxygen saturation of blood (Vines *et al.*, 2000). Blood in the fingertips is usually observed by this method and, in the warmth, approximates to arterial blood (the fingers use little oxygen, and blood supply to them is very good when the environment is warm). The plateau phase of the oxygen–haemoglobin curve means that a saturation of 95% (normal = 97–98%) has little meaningful consequence for oxygen carriage, and even 90% saturation represents a substantial carriage of oxygen.

The method does have limitations, for example, a reduction in blood flow to the area may reduce the value irrespective of lung function.

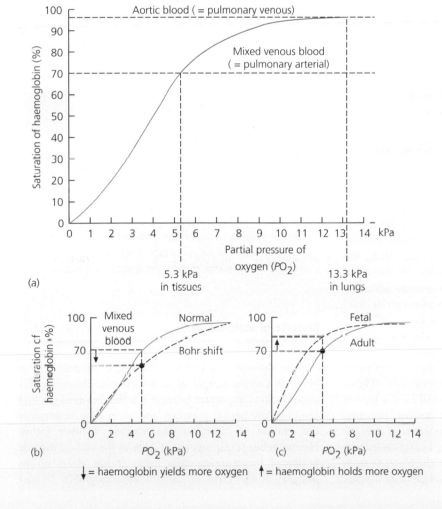

(a)

(b)

(c)

$\downarrow$ = haemoglobin yields more oxygen $\uparrow$ = haemoglobin holds more oxygen

Figure 14.9 Oxygen carriage by haemoglobin. (a) At normal pH 7.4, PCO_2 = 5.3 kPa, temperature = 37°C. (b) Shifted curves due to increased acidity, temperature or PCO_2 (Bohr shift) aids unloading. (c) Shifted curve for fetal haemoglobin aids loading.
Q. Which of the following conditions in the red cell shifts the O_2 dissociation curve to the right: (i) rise in PCO_2, (ii) reduction in temperature, or (iii) reduction in pH?
Q. What happens to oxygen—haemoglobin formation when CO_2 is given off by the blood in the lungs?

oxygen–haemoglobin dissociation curve (Figure 14.9(a)). Within the tissues, the low partial pressure of oxygen causes the gas to dissociate from the haemoglobin.

Releasing oxygen into the tissues causes blood to become considerably darker in colour than arterial blood. Consequently, venous blood draining the tissues is often said to be 'deoxygenated' – yet analysis shows that it still contains considerable amounts of oxygen: the haemoglobin of venous blood returning to the heart is still about 70% saturated with oxygen. An important feature of the association between oxygen and haemoglobin is that when oxygen usage is increased, e.g. in exercising skeletal muscle or in cardiac muscle, the steep slope of the dissociation curve at low partial pressures of oxygen ensures that the extra oxygen is unloaded rapidly from the pigment (Figure 14.9(a)).

The relationship between haemoglobin and oxygen is thus complex but very special, as it enables oxygen loading in the lungs, and unloading in the tissues.

Factors influencing the relationship between oxygen and haemoglobin

The relationship of haemoglobin with oxygen can be shifted under conditions found locally in highly active tissues: increased partial pressure of carbon dioxide, increased acidity, and increased temperature. Here, the position of the dissociation curve shifts to the right, referred to as the Bohr shift after the person who first noted it (Figure 14.9(b)). This means that for a given (low) partial pressure of oxygen, more of the gas is offloaded from the haemoglobin. The enhanced release of oxygen helps to maintain the increased metabolism.

In contrast, fetal haemoglobin has a dissociation curve toward the left of that of adult haemoglobin (Figure 14.9(c)). This means that the pigment will have a greater saturation with oxygen for a given partial pressure. Although this may seem detrimental in terms of unloading oxygen within the fetal tissues, it is in fact an important aid in the loading of oxygen across the placenta from maternal blood, which has already lost some of its oxygen.

These examples illustrate how the position of the dissociation curve in relation to partial pressures of oxygen has important physiological implications. One further example of note is the adaptation observed at high altitude, when a person is exposed chronically to an atmosphere with a low partial pressure of oxygen. Under these circumstances, the release of oxygen from haemoglobin is enhanced by elevation in red blood cells of the substance 2,3-diphosphoglycerate (2,3DPG). This combines reversibly with haemoglobin, and causes it to release its oxygen by shifting the dissociation curve to the right. As with the Bohr shift, this facilitates tissue oxygenation. This adaptive measure helps to maintain an adequate oxygenation of tissues, even under conditions of low atmospheric partial pressure of oxygen, and so performs an important homeostatic function that enables people to live more easily at high altitude.

Carriage of carbon dioxide

Carbon dioxide is a highly soluble gas, yet only 7% in blood is carried simply as dissolved gas. However, this component is important because it is the dissolved gas that produces the partial pressure, and so in time determines the amount of carbon dioxide carried in other forms. Haemoglobin transports about 23% of the carbon dioxide produced by respiring cells (after it has given up its oxygen) in the form of carbaminohaemoglobin (Figure

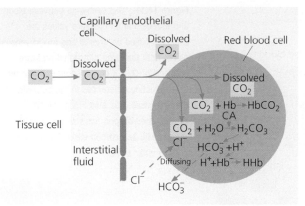

Figure 14.10 Carbon dioxide carriage: loading in tissues. Note that the amount of CO_2 dissolved determines the formation of carbaminohaemoglobin ($HbCO_2$) and also bicarbonate ions (in the presence of carbonic anhydrase (CA) enzyme). Note also the importance of deoxygenated haemoglobin (Hb).

Q. Describe how bicarbonate ions and haemoglobin act as buffers to control blood pH (refer to Chapter 6 for help).

14.10). About 70% of carbon dioxide carried by blood is found combined with water to form bicarbonate ions. The formation of bicarbonate ions from carbon dioxide is promoted within red blood cells by the enzyme carbonic anhydrase (Figure 14.10). Carbonic acid is formed initially; this dissociates weakly into bicarbonate and hydrogen ions (see Chapter 5), thus raising their concentrations within the red blood cells.

The hydrogen ions must be buffered. This is achieved by their combination with deoxygenated haemoglobin:

$$H^+ \quad + \quad Hb^- \quad \rightarrow \quad HHb$$

Hydrogen ions + haemoglobin → 'reduced' haemoglobin

The elevated concentration of bicarbonate ions favours their diffusion out of the blood cells and into the plasma. The disturbance in the electrical balance of plasma produced by the diffusion of bicarbonate ions out of red blood cells is corrected by the influx of chloride ions into the blood cells (called the chloride shift).

Blood therefore is an efficient transporter of carbon dioxide. To summarize, carbon dioxide loading of blood within the tissues results in the gas being dissolved in plasma, forming carbaminohaemoglobin, and forming bicarbonate. The transformation of the gas into other forms facilitates the further removal of carbon dioxide from cells.

When blood reaches the lung, the processes are reversed:

1 Carbon dioxide gas dissolved in plasma and within blood cells diffuses into the alveoli, reducing its partial pressure in blood.

2 As the partial pressure in blood decreases, carbon dioxide will be released from carbaminohaemoglobin, which will diffuse into the alveoli.

3 As carbon dioxide is removed from blood, the carbonic anhydrase enzyme in the red blood cells promotes the reformation of carbonic acid from bicarbonate and hydrogen ions, producing yet more gas for excretion:

$$HCO_3 \quad + \quad H^+ \quad \rightarrow \quad H_2CO_3 \quad \rightarrow \quad CO_2 \quad + \quad H_2O$$

| Bicarbonate ions (diffuses into red cells) | + hydrogen ions (released from HHb) | → carbonic acid | → carbon dioxide (diffuses into alveoli) | + water |

As bicarbonate ions diffuse into the red blood cells, chloride ions move out back into the plasma so that electrical balance is maintained.

Carbon dioxide carriage by blood is thus very different to that of oxygen. At physiological values, the relationship between the partial pressure of carbon dioxide and the volume of gas being carried cannot be considered to be reminiscent of the oxygen–haemoglobin dissociation curve. Rather, the relationship is virtually linear, and a slight change in partial pressure of carbon dioxide in arterial blood represents a pronounced change in the amount of carbon dioxide carried in its various forms. It is therefore not surprising to find that the control of lung function is very sensitive to changes in the partial pressure of carbon dioxide.

Gas exchange between blood and tissues

The exchange of gases between blood and the tissues also requires the presence of favourable pressure gradients (Figure 14.11). The partial pressure of oxygen within cells is relatively low (about 5.3 kPa) since cells utilize oxygen in metabolic processes This is considerably lower than that of the oxygen dissolved in arterial blood perfusing the tissues (13.3 kPa), so a substantial gradient exists for oxygen transfer into the cells.

Cells continually produce carbon dioxide through metabolism, and its partial pressure in intracellular fluid will be higher than that of arterial blood (6.0 kPa and 5.3 kPa, respectively). Equilibration will occur, so venous blood leaving the tissue will now have an average partial pressure of carbon dioxide of 6.0 kPa, i.e. it has gained carbon dioxide. Again, note the small pressure gradients required to transfer adequate amounts of this soluble gas. Such a small gradient, however, leaves little scope for adaptation to an increased partial pressure of carbon dioxide in arterial blood arising as a consequence of poor cardiac or lung function; the carbon dioxide content of intracellular fluid will rise as a consequence. This in turn will generate more carbonic acid (i.e. hydrogen ions) and eventually disturb cell homeostasis. This problem is normally avoided by the homeostatic regulation of the partial pressure of carbon dioxide in arterial blood, which facilitates removal of the gas from cells.

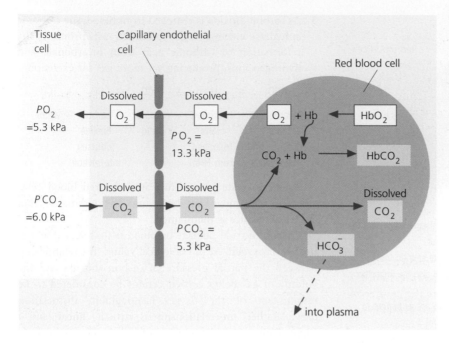

Figure 14.11 Gas exchange between blood and tissues. Partial pressure values are averages based on arterial and mixed venous blood. Note the large diffusional pressure gradient for O_2 but only a small gradient for CO_2, reflecting differences in the solubility of the two gases. See also Figure 14.10.
Q. How does oxygen leave blood to enter tissue cells, and carbon dioxide leave tissue cells to enter blood?

REGULATION OF THE RESPIRATORY SYSTEM

Neural control of the respiratory system

Breathing movements are largely involuntary, although they can be changed consciously, and are controlled by the rhythmical discharge of nerve impulses from 'respiratory centres'. These are located in the brainstem, and impulses pass from them down the spinal cord. Some impulses are then relayed via nerves arising in the IIIrd–Vth cervical segments of the cord, which form the left and right phrenic nerves and innervate the diaphragm (Figure 14.12). Other impulses are relayed to nerves exiting from the IIIrd-VIth thoracic segments of the cord; these form the intercostal nerves, which innervate the internal and external intercostal muscles. Further spinal nerves innervate the accessory muscles of inspiration and expiration.

The respiratory centres of the brainstem are illustrated diagrammatically in Figure 14.12. Breathing movements result from an integration of nervous activity from these centres.

- *Inspiratory/expiratory centres of the medulla area.* Impulses to the inspiratory and expiratory muscles originate from these centres, but they are controlled by the apneustic and pneumotaxic centres.

- *Apneustic and pneumotaxic centres of the medulla area.* The apneustic centre excites the inspiratory centre; to cause inspiration to cease at the end of breathing in, the centre must be inhibited at appropriate moments in the

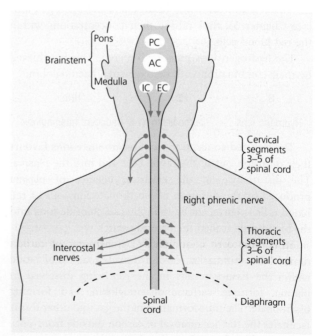

Figure 14.12 Respiratory centres and innervation of the thoracic muscles.

AC, apneustic centre; EC, expiratory centre; IC, inspiratory centre; PC, pneumotaxic centre.

Q. Which areas of the brain control normal quiet (i.e. diaphragmatic) breathing?

Q. Explain why respiratory adaptations are necessary when the body is experiencing (i) hypoxia, (ii) hypercapnia, (iii) acidosis, and (iv) exercise.

BOX 14.29 RESPIRATORY DEPRESSION BY OPIOID ANALGESICS

When administered orally or intravenously, opioid analgesics such as morphine have their main effects on receptors located within the brainstem, where they interfere with the pain-gating mechanisms (see chapter 21). A side effect of such drugs is to depress respiratory centre functioning and so cause dyspnoea and possibly hypoxaemia (Bailey, 1997). If severe, the problem can become life threatening and an antagonistic drug (e.g. naloxone) must be administered. This is quick acting but will modulate the analgesia produced by the opioid. The problems are reduced by using intraspinal routes of opioid administration (where spinal cord receptors are the targets); these are increasingly popular methods.

respiratory cycle. Such inhibitory impulses originate from inputs from stretch receptors present in the lung, intercostal muscles and diaphragm (which pass to the brainstem via the vagus nerve). The role of stretch receptors is illustrated by the Hering–Breuer reflex, in which overinflation of the lungs causes a cessation of activity in the nerve cells that stimulate the contraction of inspiratory muscles. Impulses from the apneustic centre also stimulate directly the expiratory centre when we wish to make a forced expiration, which in turn stimulates contraction of internal intercostal muscles and the accessory muscles of expiration.

The pneumotaxic centre of the pons area acts to inhibit the apneustic centre and so aids cessation of inspiration and the start of expiration.

Factors that modulate respiratory rhythm

The respiratory centres receive modulating neural inputs from chemoreceptors, and from higher brain centres, perhaps, but not necessarily, stimulated by sensory information from around the body (Figure 14.13).

Chemoreceptors

An essential role of the lung is to maintain arterial blood gas homeostasis. As part of this process, blood gas composition is monitored continuously by chemoreceptors that respond to changes in either oxygen or carbon dioxide (and acidity) content.

The oxyhaemoglobin curve in Figure 14.9a shows that a change in the partial pressure of oxygen from the normal 13.3 kPa to about 10.5 kPa has little effect on the volume of oxygen carried by blood, since the haemoglobin remains well saturated with oxygen. This lower partial pressure normally still represents an adequate pressure gradient to drive the diffusion of oxygen from blood into cells, and does not provide a powerful drive to increase breathing.

For carbon dioxide, however, an increase in its partial pressure from 5.3 kPa to 6.4 kPa would represent a similar percentage increase (about 20%) in carbon dioxide content, leading to a subsequent retention of the gas in the tissues and a resultant increase in the acidity of body fluids. It is, therefore, not surprising that even small changes in the partial pressure of carbon dioxide provide a stimulus to change lung function, whereas only a relatively substantial decrease in that of oxygen will promote a noticeable response.

The respiratory chemoreceptors are found centrally and peripherally.

Central chemoreceptors

These receptors are found in the brainstem (hence the term 'central') and do not actually monitor blood gases;

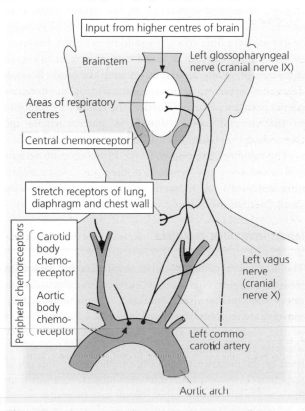

Figure 14.13 Sensory (afferent) input into respiratory centres of brainstem.

Q. Which of the factors in blood is the most important control of ventilation: PCO_2 or PO_2?

instead, they monitor the acidity of the cerebrospinal fluid bathing the brain This is separated from the circulatory system by the blood–brain barrier, which is actually a secretory epithelium (e.g. the choroid plexus; see Chapter 8). The epithelium is impervious to hydrogen ions in the blood, but is freely permeable to carbon dioxide. Thus, if the partial pressure of carbon dioxide is elevated in arterial blood, the gas will diffuse into the cerebrospinal fluid, form carbonic acid, and so increase the acidity of the fluid.

Central chemoreceptors do not monitor oxygen concentrations. Also, being outside the circulatory system, their responses to an elevated blood carbon dioxide content will be relatively slow. They appear to be involved in modulating the basal respiratory rhythm.

Peripheral chemoreceptors

These chemoreceptors are found in the walls of the aortic arch, and at the point where each of the common carotid arteries in the neck divides into its internal and external branches (an area called the carotid body). Changes in the partial pressure of carbon dioxide (and therefore the acidity) of arterial blood stimulate these receptors and impulses are relayed to the respiratory centres of the brainstem (Figure 14.13).

Peripheral chemoreceptors respond rapidly to changes in the partial pressure of carbon dioxide in arterial blood, and will quickly adjust breathing movements. They also respond to a modest decrease in the oxygen content of arterial blood, but small reductions in the partial pressure of oxygen have little effect. It would be incorrect, however, to assume that changes in blood oxygen have only a weak involvement in the regulation of lung function. If small degrees of hypoxaemia are accompanied by an increased partial pressure of carbon dioxide, the respiratory response to the elevated carbon dioxide is potentiated as the chemoreceptors become sensitized.

The rapidity of responses to the stimulation of peripheral chemoreceptors means that they are able to adjust lung function from moment to moment in response to small fluctuations in blood carbon dioxide content.

Inputs from other receptors

Thoracic receptors that modulate inspiration and expiration were noted earlier. Numerous other receptors influence respiratory movements when stimulated – some only acutely: muscle/joint receptors stimulated in exercise, chemoreceptors of the nasal mucosa, larynx and trachea stimulated by airborne irritants, and touch receptors of the pharynx stimulated by the presence of food. All produce reflex changes in respiratory movements. Exercise-induced changes are discussed below, but the other stimuli may promote:

- sneezing: a short inspiration followed by a forced expiration with the glottis open;

- swallowing: inhibits breathing movements;

- coughing: short inspiration followed by a series of forced expirations against a closed glottis. Sudden opening of the glottis releases the high pressure developed in the airways and carries away the irritants;

- hiccuping: spasmodic contractions of the diaphragm with the glottis closed.

The respiratory centres of the brainstem also receive impulses from higher centres of the brain. We can therefore alter breathing movements voluntarily, control expiration in singing or speech, inspire deeply with spasmodic expirations in weeping and laughing, prolong expiration in sighing, inspire deeply in yawning, and produce rapid movements in fear and excitement. The functions of many of these responses are not understood.

Respiratory adaptations to exercise and altitude

Exercise

Oxygen consumption and carbon dioxide production in heavy exercise may each be of the order of 4 l/min compared with 200–250 ml/min at rest. Increased oxygen demands during exercise, and increased carbon dioxide excretion, are met by increasing the alveolar ventilation rate through increased breath volume and breathing rate. In this way, 100 l or more of air may be inspired per minute (compared with about 6 l at rest).

An increased breath volume is made possible because the inspiratory and expiratory reserve volumes of the lungs are utilized. This results from a modification of outputs from the respiratory centres, and must also include an overriding of afferent impulses from stretch receptors within the thorax so that greater inflation can be achieved.

Efficient ventilation during exercise is also facilitated by a reduction in airway resistance. Mouth breathing is utilized, which bypasses the nasal cavity, and the smooth muscle of the bronchioles is relaxed to dilate the terminal airways; this is induced by the actions of the sympathetic nervous system (and adrenaline), which is stimulated during physical activity.

As a result of respiratory changes, the average gas composition of arterial blood does not alter during exercise, which helps to maintain cellular homeostasis, although venous composition will change as tissues use more oxygen and produce more carbon dioxide. It is still unclear what promotes the increased ventilation, but the response must result from a stimulation of receptors somewhere in the body. Suggestions include nerve impulses from muscle or joint receptors, from chemoreceptors within the pulmonary circulation and from potassium-sensitive receptors, since potassium ion concentration in blood rises sharply during exercise.

Altitude

The atmospheric pressure falls on ascending from sea level, which means that the partial pressure of oxygen in the air also decreases. This, in turn, will lower the partial pressure of oxygen in alveolar gas and hence in arterial blood and tissues. Eventually, hypoxaemia and hypoxia result. Note, however, that arterial carbon dioxide content will be unaffected since even at sea level its partial pressure in air is negligible. Thus, any increased ventilation promoted by the hypoxaemia will remove too much carbon dioxide from blood (i.e. it will represent a hyperventilation, Box 14.23), so the breathing response will quickly be reversed, leaving the person feeling breathless.

With adaptation, the hypoxaemia begins to exert a dominant influence on breathing movements, and the body begins to tolerate the consequential decrease in carbon dioxide content. Adaptation occurs because the blood–brain barrier maintains a normal pH of the cerebrospinal fluid in spite of changes in the concentration of carbon dioxide (see Chapter 6 for a discussion of buffers), so the central receptors are not stimulated. Thus, any influence of hypocapnia on lung function is counteracted, and the stimulation of the peripheral chemoreceptors by the hypoxaemia can now be expressed as an increased lung ventilation.

Other adaptations to altitude include an elevation in the 2,3DPG content of red blood cells (see earlier), which facilitates the unloading of oxygen in the tissues, and an increased red blood cell count (hypoxaemia stimulates the release of the hormone erythropoietin, which stimulates production of red blood cells by bone marrow). The additional red cells make more haemoglobin available to carry oxygen. Total lung capacity may also be increased.

BOX 14.30 VENTILATION THERAPY DURING CHRONIC OBSTRUCTIVE AIRWAY DISEASE

A person with chronic obstructive airway disease (COAD) will have undergone central adaptation to modulate breathing, but in the opposite way to that of a person at altitude (see text). Thus, the acidity of cerebrospinal fluid will be maintained normal in spite of elevated carbon dioxide concentrations in blood, so the elevated carbon dioxide content of blood becomes a new set point, about which breathing movements are regulated. Care must be taken not to remove carbon dioxide too rapidly from blood, since returning the blood gas composition to its previously normal carbon dioxide content will now be interpreted by the receptors as hypocapnia.

To reduce the hypoxaemia caused by the COAD, but still leave an elevated carbon dioxide, requires the use of only a slightly enriched oxygen mixture (perhaps 28% compared with 21% in air). In this way, some hypoxaemia remains and continues to stimulate breathing, but the carbon dioxide content remains at the elevated value, now considered by the body to be normal. The acidity of the tissues may require control by other means, e.g. by increasing the buffering capacity of blood.

Summary

1   The carriage of oxygen (O_2) and carbon dioxide (CO_2) to and from tissues, and the exchange of these gases with air, is vital for life.

2   A person at rest takes in, and breathes out, 5–6 l of air each minute. Physical exercise may increase this to 80–100 l/min, by increasing the depth of each breath and the rate of breathing. Such changes in lung ventilation ensure that the gas composition of systemic arterial blood remains almost constant.

3   The amount of energy required to maintain breathing movements is minimized by low airway resistance and a high compliance (elasticity).

4   The vital capacity represents the maximum volume of gas that can be taken into the lungs, and expired from them, in a single breath. The vital capacity is used clinically to assess airway resistance and compliance.

5   Gas exchange occurs across the lung alveoli; the rest of the airway comprises a 'dead space'. This space, together with the volume of gas left in the alveoli after expiration, constitutes the functional residual capacity (FRC). Inspired air mixes with the FRC gas and produces a slight enrichment of the O_2 content and a slight depletion of the CO_2 content.

6   Gases diffuse down pressure gradients. The air in the lung consists of a mixture of gases; the partial pressure exerted by each gas is physiologically more significant than the total pressure of the whole mixture. Lung ventilation ensures that the partial pressure gradients are conducive to the diffusion of oxygen into blood, and of carbon dioxide out of blood.

7   Alveolar gas composition and blood perfusion varies throughout the lungs, and the partial pressures of gases in systemic arterial blood represent the mean of those in the alveoli after inspiration.

8   Oxygen is poorly soluble in water, and is carried in the blood combined with the pigment haemoglobin. The O_2 is released from the pigment in tissues, where the partial pressure of O_2 is reduced by utilization of the gas. The release is facilitated by conditions associated with high rates of metabolism, such as high temperature and low pH; this is called the Bohr shift. Fetal haemoglobin has a slightly different structure to the adult form, which helps it to be saturated with oxygen at the partial pressures observed in the placenta.

9   Carbon dioxide is a soluble gas. It is carried from tissues dissolved in blood, or in combination with water to form

Summary (Continued)

bicarbonate ions. Some is combined with haemoglobin. The lower partial pressure of CO_2 found in the lungs promotes the conversion of bicarbonate to CO_2, the release of CO_2 from haemoglobin, and diffusion of the gas out of the blood.

10 Lung ventilation is controlled by neural activity from centres within the brainstem. The centres are modulated by neural inputs from various areas, in particular from chemoreceptors in the arterial system and in the brainstem. These especially

monitor pH, and so provide a means of evaluating the CO_2 content of blood and cerebrospinal fluid, since the gas forms carbonic acid in water. Other inputs originate from stretch receptors in the lung, from higher brain centres, and from joint receptors.

11 Some homeostatic set points are altered during exercise, and following ascent to high altitude, promoting the respiratory changes observed.

Review questions

1 The respiratory system must provide the cells of our bodies with a continual supply of oxygen and allow for the removal of waste products such as carbon dioxide. The visible movements of breathing are termed pulmonary ventilation. Follow the passage of air as it enters the nose/mouth and travels through the respiratory passageways to the alveoli of the lungs. Understanding the structure and function of the various parts is important. Distinguish between the conducting zone and the respiratory zone. Describe the 'dead space'. Could it be increased or decreased, and what would the consequences of this be?

2 What do (i) $PaCO_2$, (ii) PaO_2 and (iii) V/Q stand for?

3 How do gases get into the blood for transportation?

4 Why do these gases unload in the areas they are needed?

5 Explain the difference between internal and external respiration.

6 The elastic lungs are surrounded by the pleural membranes. Consider how these membranes help maintain dilated lungs.

7 The mechanism of breathing involves volume and pressure changes. Which muscles are used when inhaling and exhaling air? Where are the accessory muscles, and when might they be used?

8 We can control our breathing consciously, but which part of the brain controls our regular breathing, even when we are unconscious? What information does it respond to?

9 Define the following: (i) tidal volume; (ii) vital capacity; (iii) residual volume; (iv) inspiratory reserve volume; and (v) expiratory capacity. Can any of these be measured using a peak flow meter?

Breathlessness

People of all ages may experience shortness of breath. It is important for nurses in all branches to understand the reasons why a patient may become breathless, and how particular nursing interventions can relieve the symptoms.

10 Define the following terms: (i) breathlessness; (ii) dyspnoea; (iii) apnoea; (iv) tachypnoea; (v) orthopnoea; and (vi) hyperventilation.

11 Consider why a person may become breathless. (Clue: think about non-pathological causes such as running for a bus or eating too much, as well as pathological reasons, e.g. asthma. Don't forget that effective oxygenation of body cells involves the cardiovascular system in conjunction with the respiratory system.)

12 Consider your role in caring for a breathless patient. What would your assessment include? Think about the physiological rationale for these observations.

13 Identify what steps could be taken to assist the patient to breathe, and provide physiological rationale. (Clue: in addition to patient involvement, you may need to use other healthcare professionals and/or equipment.)

Effects of smoking

14 Smoking has various effects on the body, not only limited to the respiratory system. Cigarette smoke contains a cocktail of chemical ingredients including nicotine, which acts upon acetylcholine receptors in the neuromuscular junction. What is acetylcholine?

15 Nicotine causes a decrease in skeletal muscle tone, thereby giving the smoker a sense of relaxation. This could be seen as an advantageous effect of smoking. What other beneficial effects are there?

16 Why is smoking addictive?

17 Smoking is particularly hazardous in pregnancy. How does smoking affect the fetus? Why doesn't the placental barrier always prevent harmful substances from gaining access to the fetal blood supply?

18 Discuss why smoking has been linked with chronic health problems, such as lung cancer, coronary heart disease and peripheral vascular disease.

19 Despite increased knowledge about the harmful effects of smoking, many people continue to indulge in this habit. Consider which other factors often predict smoking behaviour. Is it appropriate for nurses to try to stop all patients from smoking? Think how your actions could influence a patient who would like to make the break.

REFERENCES

Aloan, C.A. and Hill, T.V. (1997) *Respiratory Care of the Newborn and Child*, 2nd edn. Philadelphia: Lippincott-Raven.

Bailey, P.L. (1997) Opioid-induced respiratory depression. *Current Reviews for Perianaesthesia Nurses* **19**(17): 171–80.

Brewin, A. (1997) RCN Continuing Education. Comparing asthma and chronic obstructive pulmonary disease. *Nursing Standard* **12**(4): 49–55.

Conway, A. (1999) Adherence and compliance in the management of asthma. *British Journal of Nursing* **7**:1374–6.

Jones, C.V. (1998) Nutrition. The importance of oral hygiene in nutritional support. *British Journal of Nursing* **7**: 74–83.

Seigh, P.J. (1999) Emergency! Pulmonary oedema: will you have to intubate? *American Journal of Nursing* **99**(12): 43.

Stockley, R.A., O'Brien, C., Pye, A. and Hill, S.L. (2000) Relationship of sputum colour to nature and outpatient management of acute exacerbation of COPD. *Chest* **117**(6): 1638–45.

Tan, I.K.S. and Oh, T.E. (1997) Mechanical ventilation support. In Oh, T.E. (ed.) *Intensive Care Manual*. Oxford: Butterworth Heinemann. pp. 246–55.

Truesdell, S. (2000) Helping patients with COPD manage episodes of acute shortage of breath. *Medical and Surgical Nursing* **9**(4): 178–82.

Vinca, D.L., Shelledy, D.C. and Peters, J. (2000) Current respiratory care, part 1: oxygen therapy, oximetry, bronchial hygiene. *Journal of Critical Illness* **15**(9): 507–10.

Wilson, D.F. (1998) Surfactant in paediatric respiratory failure. *Respiratory Care* **43**(12): 1070–85.

Chapter 15

The kidneys and urinary tract

INTRODUCTION

Chapter 6 described the distribution of water within the body, and the roles of the main constituents of the intracellular and extracellular fluid compartments. For health, the composition of these fluids must be appropriate for optimal cell functioning. The removal of 'waste' products of metabolism, and the maintenance of water and electrolyte balance, are predominantly the functions of the kidneys, frequently mediated by hormones. This chapter explains how the kidneys function, and identifies how changes in renal function act to maintain body fluid homeostasis.

The kidneys form the urine, which is then stored within the urinary bladder, and is eliminated from the body in a controlled process. This chapter therefore also considers the urinary tract and identifies the control of bladder emptying.

Some definitions

The terms 'excretion', 'secretion', 'urination' and 'defecation' frequently cause confusion and are worth defining before proceeding any further. *Excretion* is the removal of substances from the body in urine, faeces, sweat and expired gases: all contain substances that have been derived from body fluids. Note that the term refers primarily to a route of removal, not a process.

Secretion is the extrusion of substances and/or water across cell membranes. This may involve the release of substances from intracellular vesicles, as in the secretion of

hormones, enzymes, or neurotransmitters, or alternatively may involve the transport of substances using membrane carrier processes, e.g. into the forming urine, the forming sweat or the forming faecal stools.

Urination is the process of passing urine. Sometimes referred to as 'micturition', it relates to how the urinary bladder and the tube called the urethra facilitate the removal of urine from the body.

Defecation is the process by which faeces are passed from the body. Faeces contain various substances, such as bile salts and bile pigments, which have been added from body fluids during the formation of stools in the bowel, so defecation is a route for excretion. Faecal material also includes indigestible components, such as fibre, that have not come into contact with intracellular metabolism, so these materials cannot be considered as excretory products.

Elimination is identified as a need by models of care; it incorporates not only the biological aspects of excretion but also the psychosocial components that influence the ability of people to meet this need. The term covers both defecation and urination.

Why excrete?

Substances to be excreted fall into three categories:

- Metabolism produces a variety of 'waste' substances that cannot be utilized and that, if allowed to accumulate, will eventually disturb the body fluid environment and hence alter cell processes.

- The term 'waste' might also be used to describe substances produced by cells, which although functionally important, must be removed once their action is complete. Hormones, for example, must be removed from body fluids, or at least be inactivated, to stop their activities as required. Inactivation is carried out in the liver, and the products are usually excreted.

- In addition to products of metabolism, our body fluids are also continually influenced by substances absorbed from our diet. These may be in excess of body requirement, while some may not even be utilized at all. For example, dietary constituents such as water-soluble vitamins, minerals and water cannot be stored to any degree, therefore any excess must be removed from the body, while pigments and additives in food are frequently of no biochemical value.

Thus, the solutes dissolved in our body fluids are continually being added to via metabolism or dietary uptake. The maintenance of body fluid composition necessary for intracellular homeostasis therefore requires the rate of excretion of each substance to be equal to the rate at which it is added to the body fluids. In other words, excretion rates must be regulated homeostatically.

Excretory routes

The kidneys are usually viewed as being the only organs of excretion, but there are other routes by which substances are removed from the body. In summary, the routes and the substances excreted by them are:

- the kidneys (i.e. urine): metabolic products (e.g. urea, creatinine), electrolytes and water;

- the gut (i.e. faeces): bile salts, bile pigments, small amounts of electrolytes, and water;

- the lungs (i.e. expired gases): carbon dioxide and water vapour;

- the skin (i.e. sweat): electrolytes, water and some metabolic products (e.g. urea).

In general, then, the kidneys are the main routes for excretion, but in some instances they play only a minor role, e.g. in the excretion of carbon dioxide and bile pigments.

BOX 15.1 CHARACTERISTICS OF URINE

Inadequate or inappropriate kidney function will have consequences for body fluid volume and composition. Similarly, changes in hormonal functions or body fluid composition that are independent of renal pathologies will also promote a change in renal functioning. Thus, urine analysis is a valuable diagnostic procedure, and healthcare professionals should be familiar with the basic characteristics of urine (Cook, 1996).

It is usual to express urine volume as a rate of production, i.e. how long it has taken for the urinary bladder to accumulate the volume passed. The average rate of production in a climate such as that of the UK is 60 ml/h, but the rate will vary from about 30 ml/h in dehydration to 800+ ml/h in a very hydrated state. In a clinical setting, a rate of urine production of at least 30 ml/h is looked for, but it is important to note that urine produced at this rate should be deep yellow and concentrated. If it is not, or if production is at an even lower rate, then this is a cause for concern as it may be indicative of an advanced state of renal failure. *Oliguria* is a term used to describe inadequate urine production; *anuria* refers to little or no production at all ((100 ml/day).

Urine is characteristically yellow/amber because of the presence of pigments – called urochromes – derived from bile pigment. Colour will be influenced by urinary concentration (from a deep yellow to almost colourless). It may also be affected by pigments in food, e.g. it may be a reddish colour after eating beetroot. Fresh urine is clear, but it may sometimes be a little cloudy due to the presence of mucin secreted from the linings of the urinary tract.

The concentration depends on the state of hydration of the person. Very low rates of urine production in dehydration are associated with high concentration, while good hydration is associated with very dilute urine. On average, urine will be quite yellow, because people are usually slightly dehydrated.

Urine has a characteristic odour. On standing, it develops an unpleasant smell of ammonia as urea (a normal constituent) within it undergoes bacterial decomposition. Urine odour may also be affected by products in food, e.g. alcohol or the distinct smell after eating asparagus.

Urine contains various solutes, especially urea and electrolytes. There should, at most, be only a trace of blood cells, perhaps 100 red cells per millilitre of urine, compared with 500 million per millilitre of blood. An increase in the numbers present is indicative of structural damage to the kidney. Similarly, urine is normally almost protein-free and glucose-free, compared with concentrations of about 70 g/l and 5 mmol/l, respectively, in blood plasma. An increase may indicate underlying disease. The presence of haemoglobin (from red blood cells), protein and glucose in urine can readily be determined using a 'dipstick' method, in which tabs impregnated with enzymes promote a colour formation that relates to the substance concerned. Urea and electrolytes have to be measured in a sample sent to the laboratory.

The acidity relates to the urine composition, especially of hydrogen ions and bicarbonate ions. Urine pH is determined readily using a 'dipstick' method. The normal pH range is 6.8–7.8, i.e. slightly acidic to slightly alkaline, depending upon the acidity of blood at the time of urine formation.

OVERVIEW OF THE ANATOMY AND PHYSIOLOGY OF THE KIDNEYS

General anatomy

The kidneys are paired organs situated in the superior and posterior aspects of the abdomen wall, lying outside the peritoneum on either side of the vertebral column, and embedded in adipose tissue. Each weighs approximately 140 g and may be described as being bean-shaped (although some beans are kidney-shaped!). The right kidney lies a little lower than the left as a consequence of displacement by the liver. Each kidney receives blood via a branch of the abdominal aorta, called a renal artery, and nerve activity via efferent branches of the autonomic nervous system (Figure 15.1). Leaving each kidney is a renal vein, which drains blood directly into the inferior vena cava, afferent (or sensory) autonomic nerves, and a ureter, which transports urine to the urinary bladder for storage before urination.

The function of renal nerves has been debated for years. Certainly, activity in the efferent nerves can cause intense vasoconstriction following extensive haemorrhage as part of the homeostatic response to restore systemic arterial blood pressure, or during heavy exercise when blood is redirected toward exercising muscles. Nerve activity can also be recorded under less traumatic circumstances, however, and has been shown to influence the urinary excretion of sodium. Afferent renal nerves may provide sensory information that enables the function of each kidney to be matched. Despite their roles, transplanted kidneys (see Box 15.2) function well without them, which suggests that there may be means of compensating for their actions, especially in relation to electrolyte excretion.

A cross-section of the kidney reveals its gross anatomy (Figure 15.2). The outer surface is coated with a connective tissue capsule. Immediately under this is an outer layer – *cortex* – that is comprised of small lobules that extend into the deeper parts of the kidney. Within the cortex is an extensive vascular system that supports the initial stage of urine formation, by a process of filtration (see below). The filtrate is expressed into minute, blind-ended tubules called *nephrons* that eventually drain into an expanded space

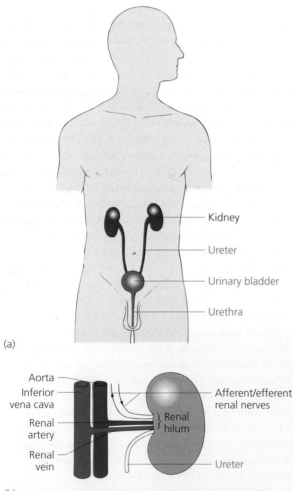

(a)

(b)

Figure 15.1   (a) Components of the urinary system. (b) Renal vessels and nerves.

Q. Describe the anatomical location of the organs that produce urine.

Q. Which blood vessels bring excretory waste products to the kidney?

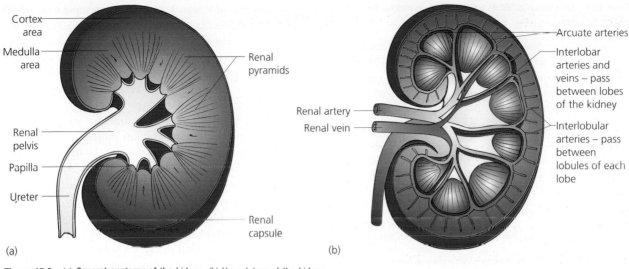

Figure 15.2 (a) General anatomy of the kidney. (b) Vasculature of the kidney.

Q. List the functions of the kidneys.

Q. Identify the two main layers of the kidney.

called the *renal pelvis*. From here, urine eventually drains into the ureters on the way to the urinary bladder. Between the cortex and pelvis, the tubules pass through deeper layers of kidney tissue; this inner area is referred to as the *medulla*. Many tubules actually pass from the cortex into the medulla and thence back out to the cortex again, before passing once more through the medulla and then draining into the pelvis. This contorted route is essential to the functions of the kidney.

The basic processes involved in urine formation

The kidney tubules (nephrons) are described in detail later. For now, we will consider simply the processes that take place in the nephrons that will determine the composition of urine that is finally produced (see Figure 15.3).

Urine formation begins with the filtering of blood plasma as it passes through the kidneys, i.e. a fluid is formed that contains water and solute molecules found in plasma other than those that are large, such as proteins (although smaller proteins may gain access); blood cells are also retained within the circulatory system. The composition of the filtrate will, therefore, be similar in many ways to that of plasma (Table 15.1); the process of its formation is considered in more detail when the filtering unit, called the glomerulus, is discussed later. The rate of excretion in urine of some substances, such as the metabolic waste substances urea and creatinine, is determined exclusively by how efficiently the kidneys are filtering. For most other substances, the composition of the filtrate is modified as it passes along the tubules by the cells that line the renal tubules.

The final urine is a complex solution of various ions and organic solutes, the majority of which are also found

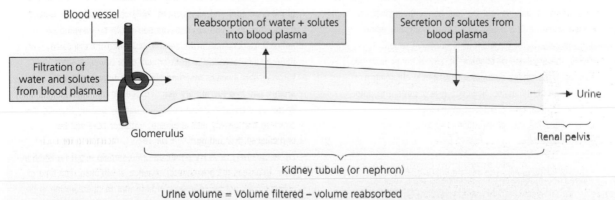

Urine volume = Volume filtered – volume reabsorbed
Solute excretion = Amount filtered – amount reabsorbed + amount secreted

Figure 15.3 Fundamental processes in the formation of urine.

Q. Differentiate between the following processes involved in the production of urine: (i) filtration, (ii) reabsorption, and (iii) secretion.

Table 15.1 Comparison of solute concentrations in plasma, the glomerular filtrate and urine

	Plasma (mmol/l)	Glomerular filtrate (mmol/l)	Urine (mmol/l)
Sodium	140	140	200
Potassium	4	4	50
Calcium	1.3**	1.3	5
Chloride	105	113	150
Bicarbonate	25	27	2
Glucose	4	4	Trace†
Urea	4	4	250
	(g/l)	(g/l)	(g/l)
Protein	70	0.2	Trace†

*These are only representative values – concentrations vary according to conditions (see text for details).
**Represents ionized, rather than total, calcium (approximately 50% of calcium in plasma is bound to proteins).
†Presence of glucose or protein in urine warrants further laboratory tests.

Q. Discuss the statement, 'the kidney is the ultimate regulator of homeostasis'.

in blood plasma, but not in the same proportions. 'Typical' urine composition is shown in Table 15.1 and for reference is compared with that of the plasma. While regulation makes any variations in plasma composition normally very small, this means that urine volume and concentration vary considerably according to the body's state of hydration, and also because the concentrations of many solutes may change independently, according to the need to excrete them. 'Typical' values for urine must therefore be considered only as a guide. The comparison is useful, however, because it illustrates how the concentrations of many electrolytes have become enriched in urine, as are those of urea. The latter accounts for a considerably greater proportion of the total solute concentration in urine than in plasma, which emphasizes the importance of urine as a route to excrete this substance.

One of the processes by which the composition of the filtrate is modified is reabsorption (Figure 15.3). This is a term used to describe the movement of solutes and water out of the lumen of the kidney tubules and back into the circulatory system, and so is distinct from absorption in the bowel, in which the uptake of substances into the blood plasma occurs for the first time. Some substances, such as sodium chloride, always undergo some reabsorption, which means that the amount excreted will always be less than the amount that was filtered. In some instances, the reabsorption of a substance is almost complete. For example, amino acids, small proteins or glucose filtered from the plasma will be conserved in this way, and so will be largely absent from urine. Altering the rate of reabsorption is an important means by which the kidneys are able to regulate the excretion of certain substances.

Another way in which urine composition is altered is by secretion (Figure 15.3). In the kidney, the term 'secretion' is usually used to indicate the addition of substances into the filtrate from cells lining the kidney tubules; these secretions then become constituents of the final urine. Secretion of certain substances into the forming urine also helps the kidney regulate the rate at which they are excreted. For example, the potassium that appears in urine has largely been secreted, since potassium ions filtered from the blood are almost entirely reabsorbed in the early stages of urine formation. An important contrast between reabsorption and secretion is that the rate of secretion can, if necessary, add so much of the substance to the forming urine that more of the substance can actually be excreted than could possibly be the case if variations in reabsorption alone were relied upon. This makes the excretion of substances such as potassium extremely efficient, and imbalances can be reversed quickly – very appropriate considering the effects of potassium excess on the heart (see Box 6.8). Similarly, some of the organic acid products of metabolism are secreted, which contributes to the

BOX 15.3 URINE COLLECTION

The concentration of solutes in urine is a frequently applied clinical assessment. It is a useful parameter, especially when assessing the capacity of the kidneys to conserve water. Alternatively, the presence or absence of, say, a hormone might be looked for. Under these circumstances, simply obtaining a urine sample will be adequate. However, it is important to note that the concentration of a substance in urine does not necessarily reflect the rate of excretion. The total amount excreted is calculated as:

Total excreted =
urine concentration of the substance × urine volume

The amount is usually expressed per unit time, depending on how long it took to produce the urine. In practice settings, this is often a 12- or 24-h collection; this helps to improve the accuracy

of measurement and assessment, as it compensates for periods during the day when urine production might be elevated or reduced. Depending on the setting, obtaining the urine may require catheterization (e.g. in critical care areas, or after surgery); this involves inserting a piece of tubing along the urethra and into the urinary bladder (see Box 15.14). Urine is encouraged to drain into a collection bag by placing the bag low down so that gravity aids drainage. Catheter care will be important in this setting.

Alternatively, a freely-produced urine sample might be taken in order to assess the presence or absence of infection. The time of collection will not be as important here, but for the clinician to be confident that the presence of infection derives from the bladder itself, a midstream urine (MSU) specimen is usually taken to reduce the risk of contamination from the urethra.

efficient excretion of these potentially dangerous substances.

To summarize, the amount of substance excreted by the kidney will be the net result of:

- how much was filtered from the blood plasma;
- how much was secreted into the forming urine by the cells of the kidney tubules;
- how much was reabsorbed by the tubule cells.

Regulation of body fluid composition by the kidneys seems to predominantly involve alterations in the secretion and/or reabsorptive processes, and not the rate of filtration.

Exercise

You might find it useful to refer back to Chapter 2 regarding transport and diffusion processes operative across cell membranes.

BOX 15.4 DIURESIS, ANTIDIURESIS AND NATRIURESIS

These three terms are frequently confused. *Diuresis* is an increased urine production. The term does not relate to the composition of urine, which may be rich in electrolytes or may be very dilute; rather, it simply notes the high rate of production.

Antidiuresis relates to a fall in urine production, usually as a consequence of increased water reabsorption. Again, the term does not relate to composition, although it is applied most widely to the reduction induced by antidiuretic hormone (ADH) and resultant increased urinary concentration.

Natriuresis refers to increased sodium excretion ('natrium' = sodium). This may occur in the presence or absence of pronounced changes in urine production, although urine production will normally be increased to some degree.

Diuretic drugs alter water reabsorption, usually by interfering with sodium reabsorption by the kidney tubules, and in doing so promote natriuresis as well as diuresis (see Box 15.10).

KIDNEY FUNCTIONS

Structural and functional aspects of the kidney

We discussed in the previous section how urine composition is the net result of filtration, reabsorption and secretion processes. In order for these processes to take place, the renal tubules are subdivided into segments of different anatomical arrangement and functions: the glomerulus/Bowman's capsule, the proximal tubule, the loop of Henle, the distal tubule, and the collecting ducts (Figure 15.4). Passage of urine to the bladder is completed by the ureters.

The glomerulus/Bowman's capsule

A filtrate of plasma is produced within the cortex of the kidney across microscopic filters, some 100–150 μm in diameter, called glomeruli (singular = glomerulus) (Figure 15.5(a)), of which there are over one million in each kidney. Each glomerulus is basically a tuft of blood capillaries that provides a large surface area for filtration; in an adult the total area for both kidneys is of the order of 2 m^2 (about the surface of a large bathtub). The filtrate from a glomerulus is produced into a cup-like receptacle called Bowman's capsule, from which a kidney tubule extends into the kidney mass. In some texts, a single glomerulus and its Bowman's capsule may occasionally be referred to by the old name of Malpighian corpuscle.

The filter itself consists of two layers of cells – the cells of the wall of the glomerular capillaries and the cells of Bowman's capsule – together with the basement membranes of protein fibres, which keeps the layers of cells in place (Figure 15.5(b)). Pores through both layers, together with the matrix of the basement membranes, allow the passage of smaller solute molecules (e.g. electrolytes, glucose) but prevent the passage of large molecules (e.g. plasma proteins) and blood cells. The rate at which fluid is passed across the glomeruli into the Bowman's capsule is called the *glomerular filtration rate* (GFR). For both kidneys, the total GFR is about 125 ml/min in young adults, which is about 180 l/day (see Box 15.6). This is a considerable volume, and requires the presence of a significant force to drive the process. This force is provided by the pressure gradient that exists across the filter, produced largely by the hydrostatic pressure of blood in the capillaries.

The driving pressure in the capillaries is, to a certain extent, counteracted by the osmotic pressure generated by plasma proteins (Figure 15.5(c)). This is the same situation as occurs in other capillary beds, as described in Chapter 6. However, the hydrostatic pressure in those capillaries declines along the vessel, until it is exceeded by the osmotic pressure due to proteins, with the result that most of the fluid exuded out of the capillary in the early stages is now drawn back into it again. This reversal of fluid movement does not occur in the glomerulus because

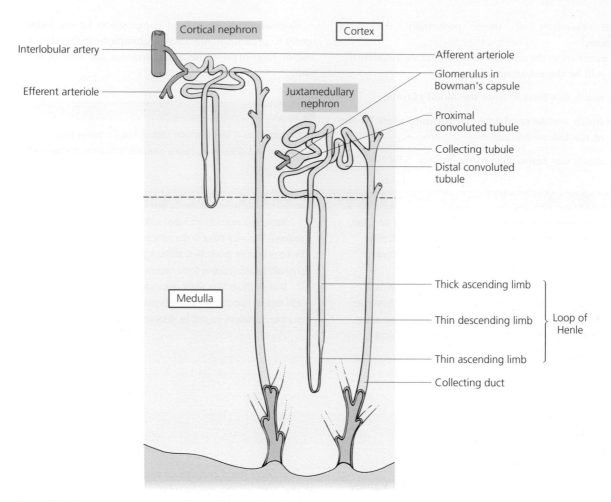

Figure 15.4 Anatomical segmentation of the renal tubule. Note the two types of nephron — one with a short loop, which does not extend into the medulla (cortical nephrons), and one with very long loops, which extend deep into the medulla (juxtamedullary nephrons).

Q. What is the basic structural and functional unit of the kidney?

Q. Describe the morphological features of juxtamedullary and cortical nephrons.

the hydrostatic pressure is maintained at a much higher value than in capillaries elsewhere. This occurs through the effects of an arteriole as blood exits the glomerulus (referred to as the efferent arteriole of the glomerulus), which is in addition to the conventional arteriole as blood enters it (the afferent arteriole). This blood vessel arrangement of arteriole–capillaries–arteriole is unusual, but it is essential for kidney function. In addition, the constrictor activities of sympathetic nerves on the efferent arteriole helps to maintain the glomerular capillary pressure and hence the filtration function of the kidney during moderate exercise, when blood flow to the kidney is reduced. In doing so, it helps to ensure that some kidney function is maintained whatever our daily activities.

The maintenance of a high rate of filtration also requires a high degree of blood flow to the kidney in order to ensure adequate volume to form the filtrate. Together, the two kidneys receive 1200 ml of blood per minute; this represents about 20% of the entire cardiac output. Of this blood, some 700 ml will be plasma, the remaining volume being occupied by blood cells. Thus, in a young, healthy adult, the kidneys filter out 125/700, or about 20%, of the plasma flowing through them. This is called the *filtration fraction*, and is a diagnostic factor that is used occasionally in renal assessment.

The rate at which glomerular filtrate is formed under normal circumstances is thought to be kept virtually constant under the precise control exerted by the kidney itself: it is autoregulated ('auto-' = self). The keeping of a near-constant filtration rate is important. Although substances such as ions could be excreted in normal amounts should the GFR decrease, because the kidney tubules could compensate by reabsorbing less or secreting more, other substances depend entirely upon filtration for their excretion and would be retained in the blood if the GFR decreased.

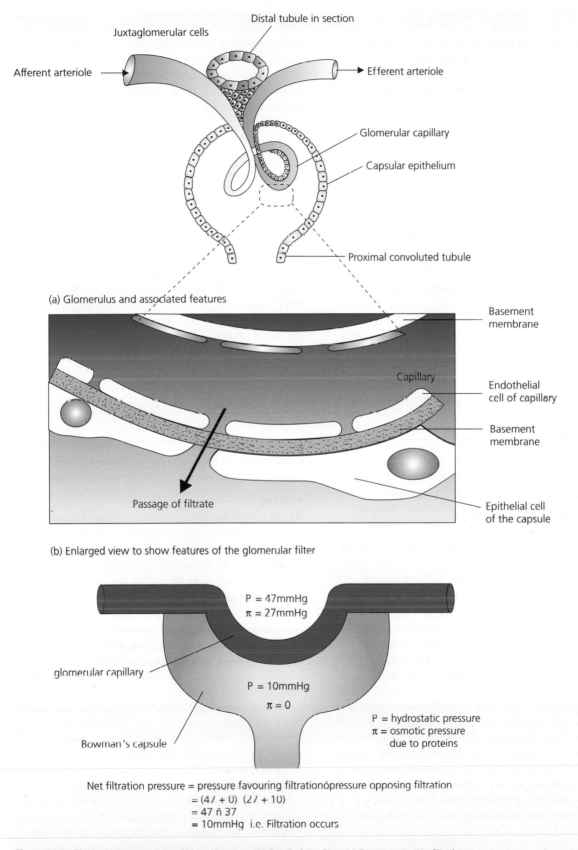

(a) Glomerulus and associated features

Juxtaglomerular cells

Distal tubule in section

Afferent arteriole

Efferent arteriole

Glomerular capillary

Capsular epithelium

Proximal convoluted tubule

Basement membrane

Capillary

Endothelial cell of capillary

Basement membrane

Passage of filtrate

Epithelial cell of the capsule

(b) Enlarged view to show features of the glomerular filter

P = 47mmHg
π = 27mmHg

glomerular capillary

P = 10mmHg
π = 0

P = hydrostatic pressure
π = osmotic pressure due to proteins

Bowman's capsule

Net filtration pressure = pressure favouring filtrationópressure opposing filtration
= (47 + 0) (27 + 10)
= 47 ñ 37
= 10mmHg i.e. Filtration occurs

Figure 15.5 The renal glomerulus. (a) General structure. (b) Detail of the filter. (c) Forces promoting filtration.

Q. Explain (i) why the overall diameters of the efferent and afferent arterioles are different; (ii) how this difference enables the afferent arteriole to control the volume of blood filtered in a given time.

Q. Describe the structure of the filtration barrier in the nephron, and discuss the forces that bring about glomerular filtration.

Glomerulonephritis is an inflammation of the glomeruli commonly caused by allergic responses to toxins, by drug abuse, by 'heavy' metal poisoning, or by renal infection that has spread to the kidneys from the lower urinary tract. There may also be a genetic component in some people. There are many kinds of glomerulonephritis, grouped according to which cell type within the glomerulus is affected. Symptoms include excessive urinary loss of blood cells and plasma proteins (haematuria and proteinuria, respectively) as a consequence of increased glomerular permeability. The condition can be acute or chronic, and can progress to renal failure.

Why filter so much?

The average rate of urine production in a temperate climate is about 60 ml/h (approximately 1 ml/min). If the kidneys filter at 125 ml/min, then over 99% of the filtrate must be reabsorbed to promote this rate of urine production. Even when we are very hydrated, and urine production is about 1200 ml/h (= 20 ml/min), over 80% of the filtrate will still have been reabsorbed. Such levels of reabsorptive activity are extremely expensive in terms of energy use, since water reabsorption occurs by osmosis linked to the active reabsorption of solutes. In fact, the kidneys account for about 10% of the body's resting oxygen consumption, yet represent only 0.4% of body weight. This helps to explain why the kidneys receive so much blood, but it appears very wasteful of energy. There are important advantages in having such a high rate of filtration:

● Without a high rate of filtration, the excretion of substances (e.g. creatinine) that are not transported by renal tubule cells would be low since little would be filtered from the plasma. Looked at in another way, novel substances produced by metabolism, or ingested in the diet, might not be excreted efficiently unless specific transport processes to secrete them into tubule fluid were present, which is unlikely to be the case.

Although the glomerular filtration rate is autoregulated so that it varies little on a moment-to-moment basis, it does alter with age and during pregnancy. At birth, the rate of glomerular filtration at birth is about 20% or so of the adult value, i.e. approximately 20–30 ml/min. It reaches the adult value within about 2 years, an indication of how soon renal function must mature if body fluid balance is to be maintained.

Ageing

The rate of filtration declines from about the age of 30 years, and typically may be reduced by as much as 50% or more by the time the person is 80 years old. Body fluid composition is still regulated by appropriate changes in reabsorption or secretion by the tubules, and urine composition will be normal. The excretion of creatinine and urea, which is dependent entirely on the amount filtered, may show signs of mild retention, although their production by metabolism will also reduce with age, so changes in plasma concentration will not normally be sufficient to be problematic.

Pregnancy

The rate of blood flow through the maternal kidneys increases by up to 50% during pregnancy. The cause of this is uncertain, but it produces a substantial increase in glomerular filtration rate and a subsequent fall in the concentration of those substances that are excreted in proportion to the filtration rate, such as creatinine and urea. The improved removal of these substances presumably facilitates their transfer across the placenta. Potentially disastrous consequences for solute and water excretion are prevented by an increased rate of reabsorption of most solutes by the kidney tubules. This adaptive mechanism is poorly understood.

In some people, the rate of decline of filtration is faster during ageing than is usual. The consequence is that eventually a rate of filtration is reached when substance excretion is compromised. In this case, the person will be diagnosed as having chronic renal failure. The consequences depend on the extent to which the GFR is reduced:

● Plasma urea and creatinine concentrations are moderately raised when GFR is about 25% of normal. This is referred to as 'renal insufficiency'.

● 'Renal failure' occurs with further reductions in GFR and is characterized by even more retention of urea and creatinine, and also of other solutes, especially ions. The patient may show symptoms of fatigue, anorexia, nausea and intense itching; the syndrome of renal failure may be referred to as 'uraemia' or 'azotaemia'. Strictly speaking, this latter term relates specifically to an observation of an increased plasma urea concentration.

● 'End-stage renal failure' occurs when GFR is less than 10% of normal.

See also 'acute renal failure' in Box 15.22.

● A high rate of filtration allows a high degree of flexibility in the regulation of solute excretion, particularly of sodium, and of water. This is observed with age in failing kidneys, (Box 15.6).

The consequences of renal failure upon body fluid homeostasis are described in Box 15.22.

Proximal tubule

The filtrate produced by the glomerulus enters the renal tubule from the Bowman's capsule into a segment called the proximal tubule. The modification of the filtrate composition and volume begins in this segment. The term 'proximal' describes its position, being close to the centralized structure, in this case the Bowman's capsule.

For most of its length, the proximal tubule is known as the proximal convoluted segment (or pars convoluta). The convoluted section is found in the cortical region of the kidney (Figure 15.4), but continues as a straight section, called the pars recta, which takes the proximal tubule toward the medulla region. The significance of the convolutions is that the twists and turns increase its length and therefore the surface area available for reabsorption and secretion. The surface area of the proximal tubule is increased further by the presence of finger-like microvilli on the inner surface of the tubule cells. The proximal tubule is also leaky to water, and its cells are rich in transport mechanisms, which makes the absorption of solutes and the resultant osmotic movement of water very prominent here. In fact, some 80% of the filtrate is reabsorbed by the time the filtrate has reached the end of the proximal tubule.

Analysis of the tubule fluid shows that some solutes, such as glucose, amino acids and small proteins, are absorbed even more efficiently – almost completely – by the proximal tubule. There is no secretion later of these substances, so the final urine is virtually free of them; this is important if these valuable nutrients are not to be wasted. Other waste solutes might be secreted into the tubule fluid by the proximal tubule cells, which promotes their excretion in urine. In general terms, however, the reabsorption of solutes and water by the proximal tubule occurs in the same proportion. Thus, although this section of the tubule reabsorbs the bulk of the filtrate, the osmotic potential of the fluid in the proximal tubule remains much the same as that of plasma. In contrast, the final excreted urine can be very dilute (with an osmotic potential considerably less than that of plasma) or very concentrated (with an osmotic potential far in excess of that of plasma); these diluting and concentrating processes are features of tubule segments beyond the proximal tubule.

Loop of Henle

Fluid enters the loop of Henle from the proximal tubule (Figure 15.4). This is a hairpin-like structure that carries the remnants of the filtrate deeper into the medullary region of the kidney via its descending limb and then back out into the cortex via its ascending limb. The loops of Henle penetrate the medullary region to varying degrees; about 15% of tubules have loops that extend very deep into the medulla (juxtamedullary nephrons), while most of the remainder do not penetrate it at all (cortical nephrons). The significance of this is seen from observations in the animal kingdom. For example, none of the loops of the aquatic beaver (which does not have problems of dehydration) penetrates the medulla, whereas those of desert rodents (which are faced with potentially major problems of dehydration) are all very long indeed. The loops clearly have a role in water conservation; their function is considered in detail later in relation to water homeostasis.

BOX 15.8 PRESENCE OF GLUCOSE IN URINE (GLYCOSURIA)

If the glucose-transporting sites in the proximal tubule are overloaded, then glucose begins to appear in quantities in the urine. Overload indicates that a threshold concentration for glucose has been exceeded, such that the normal transport processes in the renal tubule are saturated. Overload can occur in two ways:

● The amount of glucose being filtered by the glomerulus is excessive. This is observed in diabetes mellitus, when the raised plasma glucose concentration results in more glucose being filtered (the term 'mellitus' refers to the sweetness of the urine, and dates from days when physicians would taste urine to distinguish the disorder from others; happily, dipsticks have removed this necessity).

● The number of transport sites in the proximal tubule is reduced. Glomerular filtration rate is increased during pregnancy, but this should not produce a significant glycosuria, since transport sites in the proximal tubule should be able to cope with this excess simply by absorbing more glucose. However, there is a decrease in the number of transport sites in pregnancy, which seems to be the main cause of glycosuria when it occurs. In this case, the glycosuria is not indicative of diabetes mellitus, although this should not necessarily be ruled out. The reduction of transport sites, therefore, represents a lowering of the renal threshold for glucose.

One consequence of the presence of glucose in the renal tubule is that it acts to interfere with osmosis. This is why glycosuria is usually associated with an increased urine production rate (the term 'diabetes' is Greek for 'siphon'). Glycosuria also provides a nutrient-rich environment for bacteria, and so raises the risk of lower urinary tract infection.

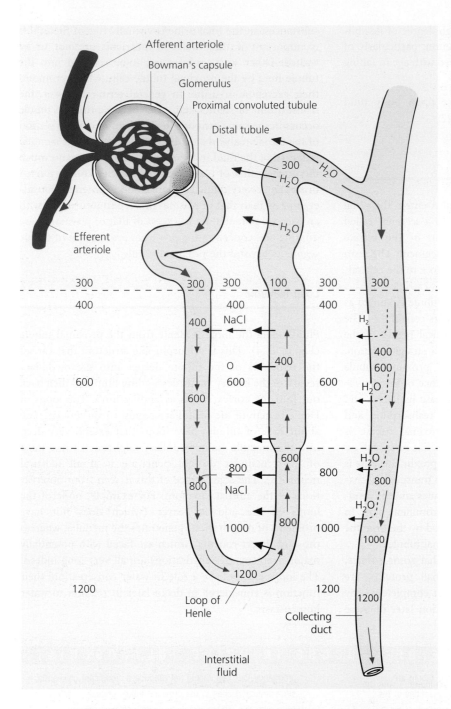

Figure 15.6 The loop of Henle counter-current multiplier mechanism in the production of a concentrated (i.e. hypertonic to plasma) urine. The numbers refer to osmotic concentration (blood plasma = 300; sodium chloride is the main solute involved) in the tubule fluid and in the interstitial fluid outside the tubule. The arrows indicate the movement of solute (in the loop of Henle) and water (in the distal convoluted tubule and collecting duct). The movement of water is along a concentration gradient for solute that is established between the tubule and interstitial fluid by the activities of the loop of Henle. See text for explanation.

The extent of the reabsorption of water by the distal nephron depends on the presence of antidiuretic hormone. The fluid dilution seen as the fluid leaves the loop of Henle will continue if the hormone is absent, so that the urine will have a high volume but low concentration, i.e. the process becomes one of urine dilution.

Q. What is the role of antidiuretic hormone in water balance?

Fluid leaving the ascending limb of the loop always has an osmotic potential less than that of plasma (Figure 15.6). Thus the activities of the loop are very different to those of the proximal part of the tubule. The dilution occurs because there has been reabsorption of electrolytes (mainly sodium chloride) without the simultaneous reabsorption of water; unlike the proximal tubule, this segment is almost impermeable to water, and is frequently called the diluting segment. The absorption of electrolytes causes their accumulation within the tissue fluid surrounding these tubule segments; this plays an important role in the final determination of urine volume and concentration.

The actions of the ascending limb are made more efficient through processes in the descending limb (Figure 15.6). As fluid passes through the descending limb, it becomes more concentrated as water is reabsorbed by osmosis into the concentrated tissue fluid, while solutes (mainly sodium chloride) diffuse into the tubule. This increases the concentration of electrolytes in the fluid arriving in the ascending limb, which makes the segment operate even more efficiently. For this reason, the loop of Henle is sometimes referred to as a 'counter-current multiplier': the descending and ascending segments pass in opposite directions, and the activities of both segments increase the effectiveness of the mechanism.

Distal tubule

The now dilute fluid leaving the ascending limb of the loop of Henle passes within the renal cortex into another convoluted section of tubule. This used to be called the distal convoluted tubule, and although the name persists, it is now doubtful that the segment forms a distinct anatomical part of the tubule. Rather, it seems to form a transition between the cells and processes of the ascending limb of the loop and later tubule segments. These latter tubule segments form part of a system in which a number of individual tubules join together and are referred to as 'collecting tubules'. The convoluted section of tubule, together with the collecting tubules, is referred to as the distal tubule.

By the time fluid leaves the loop of Henle, only about 15% of the filtrate volume remains; the other 85% has been reabsorbed along the proximal tubule and the descending limb of the loop of Henle. The dilution process instigated in the ascending limb of the loop continues along the distal tubule as solutes (again mainly sodium chloride) are reabsorbed in excess of water. Unlike the ascending limb, however, this is a section of tubule that has variable water permeability, so some water may follow by osmosis and does so in forming a concentrated urine (Figure 15.6).

Two important processes that occur in the distal tubule are the secretion of potassium ions and the secretion of hydrogen ions. Fluid entering the distal tubule is virtually potassium free; almost all of the potassium that is filtered from plasma by the glomerulus is reabsorbed by earlier segments. It has also become deficient in hydrogen ions, because many of these will have been reabsorbed in the proximal tubule. Potassium and hydrogen ions are then added to the tubule fluid by secretion from the cells of the distal tubule, loosely in exchange for sodium ions. The secretion of the ions in this segment makes this process the determinant of potassium excretion and of urinary acidification.

Collecting duct

A number of collecting tubules drain within the renal cortex into a common collecting duct, which descends back into the renal medulla (Figure 15.4). Solute and water reabsorption continues in this segment of tubule, but the main feature is that water permeability of the tubule wall is variable and can be controlled. This is the site of the mechanism that enables the kidney to switch from producing urine of high volume but low concentration to one of low volume and high concentration. Thus, if water permeability is low, then the dilution of tubule fluid that was first initiated in

---

BOX 15.9 THE URINARY TRACT IN PREGNANCY

There are 2 main aspects here: the influence of progesterone, and the compression from the growing uterus.

Progesterone
The release of this hormone is greatly increased during pregnancy. Among its varied actions, it acts as a relaxant of smooth muscle. In the urinary tract, this results in dilation of the renal pelvis and ureters. There is a risk that peristalsis in the ureters will be less effective in transferring urine to the bladder, so retention within the kidney pelvis may occur. Accordingly, urine will be routinely analysed at each antenatal visit, and will include tests for infection.

Compression
The enlarged uterus presses down on the urinary bladder, reducing its capacity. Bladder tension therefore rises much more rapidly during filling, leading to increased urinary frequency.

BOX 15.10 DIURETIC DRUGS

These drugs promote diuresis, and are known colloquially as 'water tablets'. *Osmotic diuretics* (e.g. mannitol) interfere with the uptake of water by osmosis in the proximal tubule. They are not reabsorbed themselves, and so remain in the tubule fluid, hence their effects. *Loop diuretics* (e.g. frusemide) are the most effective. These drugs inhibit the transport mechanism in the ascending limb of the loop of Henle, and in doing so prevent the build-up of electrolytes within the surrounding tissue fluid. As a consequence, the water reabsorptive functions of the distal nephron and collecting tubules/ducts are disrupted, and large volumes of urine are produced. Electrolyte excretion will also be high, in particular that of sodium chloride since this has not been reabsorbed effectively by the ascending limb. Loop diuretics are therefore an effective means of reducing the sodium and water content of extracellular fluid, hence their use to reduce blood volume in, for example, congestive heart failure or salt-induced hypertension.

In the distal tubule the secretion of potassium ions occurs loosely in exchange for sodium ions, and is therefore promoted when sodium reabsorption is increased in this part of the tubule. The delivery of sodium to the distal nephron is increased when loop diuretics are used to reduce salt reabsorption in the loop of Henle, and stimulates sodium reabsorption and hence potassium secretion in the distal tubule. The loss of potassium ions can be such that it causes a reduction in plasma potassium concentration (hypokalaemia), so dietary potassium supplements may be necessary in people who are taking loop diuretics.

Distal nephron diuretics act mainly on the distal tubule by reducing sodium chloride and water reabsorption there. These drugs, such as the thiazides, are less effective than loop diuretics, but because they act very late in the distal nephron, they do not have a major influence on potassium secretion. They are often referred to as 'potassium-sparing diuretics'.

the ascending limb of the loop of Henle, and that was also observed in the distal tubule, continues. If water permeability of the collecting duct is high, then the high concentration of solute within the tissue fluid in the kidney medulla (generated by the active reabsorption occurring in the ascending limb of the loop of Henle; Figure 15.6) will promote osmosis, and hence the reabsorption of water.

The collecting ducts eventually drain into the renal pelvis. From here, the urine is transported to the bladder by the ureter.

THE BLADDER AND CONTROL OF MICTURITION

The urinary bladder

The bladder is a hollow organ comprised largely of smooth muscle that lies within the pelvic girdle between the rectum and the symphysis pubis (Figure 15.7). In the female, it also lies anterior to the uterus and vagina. The bladder is outside the peritoneal lining of the abdomen, and as it inflates it extends between the peritoneum and the anterior body wall.

The bladder wall has three layers: an outer (or serous) layer, which is an extension of the peritoneum, a middle layer of smooth muscle, and an inner epithelial layer. The latter is composed of transitional epithelium, which means that the cells have the capacity to stretch, and so allow the bladder to fill without the epithelium rupturing. The muscle layer is subdivided into three layers: outer and inner layers of longitudinal muscle fibres, and a middle layer of circular muscle. This arrangement means that contraction causes the bladder to reduce both in length and diameter, thus emptying it effectively.

Most of the inner surface of the bladder is extremely folded. The folds are called rugae; they are important because they enable the bladder to fill without placing a high level of tension on the muscle wall. In contrast, the base of the bladder has a smooth triangular-shaped area, called the trigone, which lacks rugae. This area is formed between the points of entry of the ureters and the exit of the urethra (tube to the exterior), and forms a smooth

The ureters

Urine formed by the renal tubules passes down to the urinary bladder via the muscular ureters, assisted partly by gravity. The ureters are basically tubes about 25 cm long and 0.5 cm in diameter in adults that consist of smooth muscle arranged longitudinally and circularly; this arrangement allows them to undergo peristaltic contractions to move the urine away from the kidney.

funnel-like surface when the bladder is distended; this facilitates efficient emptying of the bladder.

Where the urethra leaves the bladder, the circular involuntary muscle layer is arranged so as to produce a functional sphincter – called the internal sphincter (Figure 15.7(c)) – which helps to keep urine stored within the bladder during filling. This sphincter is controlled by the autonomic nervous system, and we generally have little voluntary control over it. A second sphincter, the external sphincter, is formed from the striated muscle of the pelvic floor. This muscle is under voluntary control, and enables us to determine consciously when (and where) we will urinate.

The urethra

The urethra extends from the neck of the bladder. It opens to the exterior via the urethral meatus, or opening. No urine can enter the urethra until the internal sphincter has been relaxed. The urethra also passes through the external sphincter, which, unless relaxed, will prevent further progress of the urine.

In the female, the urethra is about 4 cm long and the meatus opens in front of the vaginal opening. In the male, the urethra is about 20 cm long and also passes through the prostate gland. Ejaculatory ducts from the testes empty into it (see Chapter 18), so the male urethra performs both an excretory and a reproductive role.

BOX 15.11 URINARY STONES AND HYDRONEPHROSIS

Calculi (urinary stones) normally consist of calcium and uric acid, i.e. substances with a low solubility (Pak, 1998). Deposition occurs when their concentrations in urine are abnormally high, particularly if urine pH is also appropriate. They may form anywhere within the urinary tract. Calculi result in blockage of the ureter, kidney pelvis, or tubules leading to urine retention, and kidney distension. They may even form within the bladder, where they interfere with bladder emptying. Stones may be removed by surgery, or may be disintegrated using ultrasound. The occurrence of stones is very painful, not least

because peristaltic contractions of the ureter increase in strength, and so increase the pressure within the kidneys.

Urethral obstruction, ureteral obstruction or tumours within the kidney may all cause an accumulation of urine within the renal pelvis (hydronephrosis). The renal pelvis dilates and enlarges, and the elevated pressure may even cause a reduction in blood supply to the tissue with resultant tissue breakdown. Treatment is aimed at removing the cause of the blockage and correcting the underlying disorder.

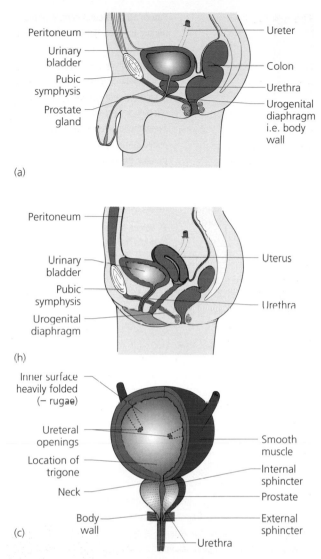

Peritoneum
Urinary bladder
Pubic symphysis
Prostate gland
Ureter
Colon
Urethra
Urogenital diaphragm i.e. body wall

(a)

Peritoneum
Urinary bladder
Pubic symphysis
Urogenital diaphragm
Uterus
Urethra

(b)

Inner surface heavily folded (– rugae)
Ureteral openings
Location of trigone
Neck
Body wall
Smooth muscle
Internal sphincter
Prostate
External sphincter
Urethra

(c)

Figure 15.7 *General anatomy of the urinary bladder: (a) male; (b) female; (c) detail of the male bladder.*

Q. What is the function of the internal lining of the bladder?

Q. How does the female bladder compare to that of the male?

Bladder emptying

The passing of urine is known as *urination* or *micturition*. It results from an interplay of the nervous control of the bladder and bladder sphincters. As the bladder fills with urine, the pressure within it rises but the muscle layers actively relax through actions of the sympathetic nerves to the bladder wall. The same nerve activity causes the internal sphincter to contract. The relaxation of the bladder wall means that the pressure inside the bladder rises only slowly as filling continues; this allows the bladder to accommodate more urine, and also means that we are little aware of the volume present. Eventually, a point is reached at which the accommodation begins to be exceeded, so addition of further urine causes a marked rise in pressure. A sensation of a 'full bladder' becomes more intense as the bladder

continues to fill. Micturition can still be suppressed at this stage, but it must occur if the bladder accumulates much more (the average capacity of the bladder of an adult is about 600–700 ml urine).

The contraction of the bladder is largely a reflex response to increasing wall tension, although practise can enable people to produce urine specimens to order (but they frequently cannot in anxiety-causing settings, such as clinics). The reflex operates through sensory nerve endings in the bladder wall, which influence nerve activity from the spinal cord to the bladder; if the bladder is very tense, there will also be activation of pain receptors. The sensory fibres enter into the spinal cord in the lower (eleventh and twelfth) lumbar segments (Figure 15.8), and when stimulated may cause an increase in parasympathetic nerve activity to the bladder. The main body of the bladder then contracts, and the internal sphincter reflexly dilates. At this point, relaxation of the external sphincter will allow micturition to occur. However, this is striated muscle over which we have a degree of conscious control, so we can prevent micturition unless the bladder is extremely full; the sphincter can even be closed once micturition is in progress.

Control of the external sphincter arises through the activity of the pudendal nerve, which enters/exits the lower lumbar area of the spinal cord. Sensory information regarding the tension of the bladder wall and the sphincters is relayed up the spinal cord to the sensory cortex of the brain, and final output to the external sphincter is generated from areas within the brainstem. The development of the ability to control the external sphincter is observed in young children, and encouraged by 'potty training'. The delay in maturation of the brainstem areas involved means that control is not normally established until about 1.5–2 years of age.

BOX 15.12 URINARY TRACT INFECTION

Cystitis is infection of the lower urinary tract, causing irritation and soreness on passing urine. Bladder discomfort and urinary frequency may be observed if the infection gains access to the bladder, whilst the connections with the kidneys make them susceptible to infection should this 'backtrack' along the ureter to the kidney. In backtracking, the infection will first reach the renal pelvis, producing inflammation, known as pyelonephritis. However, the infection is unlikely to be as localized as this, and infection of renal tubules, renal interstitial space (primarily in the medulla), and the renal pelvis may be observed. If the infection penetrates the renal cortex, then interstitial nephritis or glomerulonephritis may be observed (see Box 15.5). Infection in the kidney can be localized to other areas.

These conditions are not, however, caused only by infection from the urinary tract (Marchiondo, 1998). Pre-renal causes are possible, arising from the effects of antibody–antigen complexes secondary to infection elsewhere, or from the side effects of drugs. All of these kidney conditions are normally acute, but can lead to the loss of renal tissue and scarring. Acute renal failure may ensue, and in some instances may even progress to chronic renal failure.

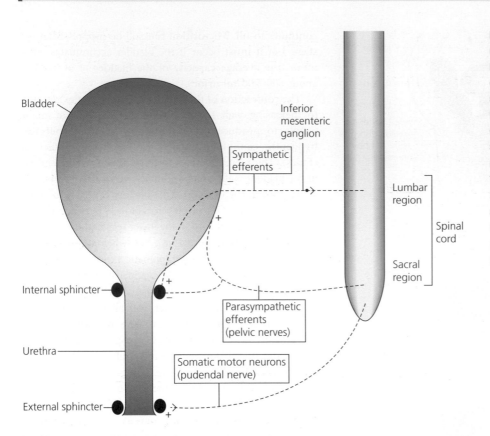

Figure 15.8 Neural control of the urinary bladder. Note that for the bladder to fill, parasympathetic efferent activity must decrease and sympathetic activity increase. For the bladder to empty, parasympathetic efferent activity must increase and sympathetic activity decrease. The pudendal nerve must also be inhibited to relax the external sphincter.

+, contraction when efferent nerves stimulated; —, relaxed when efferent nerves stimulated.

Q. Outline the neural processes involved in micturition.

BOX 15.13 URINARY INCONTINENCE, FREQUENCY AND RETENTION

Urinary incontinence

Urinary incontinence (see Norton, 1996) is the release of small amounts of urine at a time when it should be retained in the bladder. It results from a problem of controlling micturition, and has four main causes:

- *Irritation* of the internal surface of the bladder by infection or the presence of precipitates will make the bladder wall 'irritable' and more prone to contract. Cystitis is an inflammation of the urinary bladder that may cause frequent and even painful micturition.
- *Loss of muscle tone* in the external sphincter is sometimes observed with age. The stretching of the pelvic floor during, or any tissue trauma arising from, childbirth, and also the shorter urethra in the female (which places the internal and external sphincters in close proximity), means that this problem is more frequently observed in women. Immobility may cause a continence problem in both sexes. Stress incontinence is observed when an increase in abdominal pressure, perhaps through coughing or laughing, causes leakage of a small amount of urine through a weakened sphincter. Such potential for problems later in life provides a rationale for exercises to maintain the muscle tone of the pelvic floor.
- *Spinal cord trauma* often results in problems in controlling micturition, since the innervation of the sphincters exits from the lumbar/sacral regions at the lower part of the spinal cord. Cord

trauma in the cervical, thoracic or upper lumbar regions may disrupt transmission from brainstem to bladder, and so affect the ability to control the external sphincter.

- *Central nervous system disorder:* incontinence may be observed in dementia, probably because of a failure to promote normal conscious control of micturition.

Urinary frequency

Frequency (see Norton, 1996) relates to the urgency to pass urine when the urinary bladder is unfilled. Frequency may be observed as part of urinary incontinence. It might also be observed if the bladder is restricted (e.g. during pregnancy) or if the bladder is subjected to anxiety-induced nerve activity (in contrast, some people find it difficult to void urine when they are anxious, because they tense abdominal and pelvic floor muscles).

Urinary retention

Obstruction of the urethra will prevent adequate bladder emptying, and thus urinary retention. Apart from possible consequences to the kidney, this condition can also be extremely painful if it is severe enough to prevent micturition completely. Hyperplasia of the prostate gland is one such cause in males, where enlargement of the gland invades the area around the internal bladder sphincter. Where urinary retention is observed, a urinary catheter inserted into the bladder via the urethra will be necessary (see Norton, 1996, and Box 15.14).

BOX 15.14 CATHETERIZATION OF THE URETHRA

This is a widely applied technique to encourage free draining of the bladder if urinary retention is occurring. It is a useful method short term, e.g. after surgery, in which micturition is difficult, or long term in chronic illness, where it also helps the patient maintain skin integrity and dignity. In addition to enabling bladder emptying, a catheter also enables measurement of urine production rate; this is very useful in assessing renal function and/or hydration states after surgery.

A 'closed system' is used in introducing the catheter, by which the catheter is initially filled with sterile saline in order to reduce the likelihood of introducing infection. Nevertheless, infection is often problematic, so catheterization should only take place when absolutely necessary; the catheter should not remain in place longer than is necessary. Aseptic techniques are important when inserting the catheter, and when changing the urinary collection

bag or cleaning the area of the urethral meatus. Problems arising might include (Wilde, 1997):

● introduction of an infection through poor aseptic technique;
● reflux of urine into the bladder from a poorly positioned collection bag, or during bag changing;
● infection with urease-producing bacteria that convert urea in urine to ammonia. This reacts with other urine constituents to produce ammonium magnesium phosphate, which can encrust the catheter, causing pain on withdrawal and/or catheter obstruction, and even provide a site for microorganism growth;
● tissue damage (and pain) during insertion of the catheter;
● inflammation in response to the catheter composition. Solid silicone and hydrogel are usually used in catheter construction; both may promote local immune responses.

THE KIDNEYS AND HOMEOSTATIC CONTROL OF BODY FLUID COMPOSITION AND VOLUME

Renal clearance

Although the kidneys remove some of the solutes from blood plasma and excrete them in urine, for most substances this will not entail complete removal since they are continually added to plasma by metabolism or dietary means. However, the amount contained within a urine sample could be envisaged as coming from a discrete volume of plasma, which would be cleared entirely of the solute. This is then referred to as 'renal clearance', which can be defined as being *the volume of plasma that contains the amount of that substance excreted per unit time*. In reality, however, discrete volumes of plasma do not have their solutes removed entirely; so in relation to body fluid composition, the above definition means that the higher the clearance rate, the greater will be the effect to lower the overall plasma concentration of the substance. The significance of this concept is that if the clearance rate can be determined, then it gives a measure of how fast the substance is being removed from blood by the kidneys.

The clearance of a substance is calculated from the timed urine volume, the urinary concentration of the substance, and its concentration in blood plasma, using the equation:

Clearance of a substance (ml/min) = (urine concentration of the substance/plasma concentration of the substance) × urine volume (ml/min)

Clearance values can be determined for any substance found in urine. For example, the methodology is applied widely in pharmacology to determine how efficiently a

drug is removed from plasma after it has been administered, since dosages of a drug are calculated according to how long it remains at effective concentrations in blood. Thus, if a drug's clearance rate is low, then it may remain effective for a long period of time, so lower or more infrequent doses could be required. Pharmacologists will also need to know how much is removed from plasma by other routes, e.g. by liver clearance, but renal clearance will be an important part of the calculation.

Exercise

If urine concentration of sodium = 1.4 mmol/ml, plasma concentration of sodium = 0.14 mmol/l, and urine production rate = 1 ml/min, calculate the renal clearance of sodium using the equation above. What does this value mean?

Now assume that the amount of sodium filtered by the kidneys is 18 mmol/min. Using the value for sodium excretion of 1.4 mmol/min, calculate the percentage of filtered sodium that is being excreted. If the proportion is normally less than 1%, what does your calculated value tell you regarding the person's sodium intake?

Use of clearance methods to calculate the glomerular filtration rate (GFR)

The filtration of plasma by glomeruli is fundamental to urine production, and any clinical assessment of kidney function would be limited without knowledge of how well

A simple monitoring procedure utilizes the notion that, provided creatinine addition to plasma (from muscle) occurs at a fairly constant rate, then any change in the plasma concentration over time will reflect a change in its renal clearance, and hence in the GFR. A blood test repeated periodically will then identify whether glomerular filtration has changed, the extent of the change, and how quickly it has changed. This method is used widely to monitor the progression of chronic renal failure, in which there is a progressive reduction in the GFR. For example, if plasma creatinine concentration has doubled over a period of time, then the GFR will have decreased by about 50%.

the kidneys were filtering. Fortunately, clearance methodology also provides a technique to measure the rate of filtration by determining the clearance of a substance that is filtered freely by the kidneys, but that is neither reabsorbed nor secreted by the nephron. The excretion of such a substance is therefore determined by how efficiently it is filtered from the plasma. Creatinine is one such substance, and its use in measuring glomerular filtration rate is as follows:

Since none of the creatinine is reabsorbed by the tubules:

Amount of creatinine filtered from plasma per minute
= amount of creatinine excreted per minute in the urine.

The amount excreted or filtered is calculated as concentration × volume, i.e.

Plasma concentration of creatinine
× volume of glomerular filtrate/min
= urine concentration of creatinine × urine volume/min

Rearranging the equation gives:

Volume of glomerular filtrate/min = (urine concentration of creatinine/plasma concentration of creatinine)
× urine volume/min

This is a form of the clearance equation given above and, strictly speaking, measures the clearance rate of creatinine, which is then taken to equate with the GFR. The concentration of creatinine in a urine sample and plasma sample is measured easily, and the volume of urine formed per minute is calculated readily from noting the time interval between emptyings of the bladder, and dividing the total urine volume by the time in minutes. Thus, the GFR can be calculated without too much difficulty using a simple blood sample and a timed urine collection. For the method to work, however, the concentration of creatinine in plasma must remain constant during the entire urine collection period, as the equation assumes that an average value is used that is representative of it. This is not usually a problem with creatinine, but the clearance of creatinine has been criticized because the kidney tubule does, in fact, reabsorb and secrete small quantities of it, thus making it less acceptable that the total amount excreted is what was filtered during that time.

Because of this, other substances have been used clinically to monitor the GFR. Unlike creatinine, however, they are not normally found in body fluids and so have to be administered. The polysaccharide inulin is one such substance; this must be infused to keep its plasma concentration constant during the urine production period. A less time-consuming method is to inject intravenously a suitable substance such as ethylenediaminetetraacetic acid (EDTA), and then to estimate the filtration rate from the rate at which the concentration of EDTA in plasma declines during a period of an hour or so. The rate of disappearance provides an estimate of the GFR, but the lack of a urine sample or a constancy of plasma EDTA concentration prevents an accurate assessment of the actual value. However, the lack of a need for the patient to accumulate a urine sample or to receive inulin infusion makes this method much more convenient than using creatinine or inulin clearance.

Maintaining balance

Metabolic products: urea, creatinine and organic acids

We have seen in this chapter that for some products of metabolism, such as creatinine and urea, their excretion is determined largely by how much is filtered from the plasma, and less so by how much is reabsorbed or secreted by the tubules. The rate at which the kidneys filter is normally maintained constant, which would suggest that the concentrations of these substances in body fluids could fluctuate, depending on how much is being produced by the tissues. In practice, this is generally not a major problem if the glomerular filtration rate has not changed, because any increase in the plasma concentration will result in more being filtered, since the amount filtered is determined by the kidneys' filtration rate and the concentration of the substance in plasma. Thus, the concentrations of these substances in extracellular fluid do not change dramatically in health, unless their production is increased markedly. The process is limited, however, and regulation is not as precise as for those substances that are reabsorbed or secreted to varying degrees by the renal tubules. As a consequence, changes in plasma creatinine and urea concentrations are amongst the first consequences of the decline in renal function that is observed with age and in kidney failure.

Urea and creatinine appear to have relatively low toxicity, and only become a problem to tissues in renal failure when their concentration is very excessive. The metabolic products called organic acids, however, must be excreted much more efficiently because of the effect that acidity has on cell functions (see Chapter 4). These substances seem to be regulated simply by the effect that a change in their concentration in blood plasma has on secretion by kidney tubule cells. Thus, an increased concentration stimulates directly the transport of organic acid into forming urine by the cells of the proximal tubule. The transport processes are sensitive and efficient, so wide fluctuations of organic acid concentration in the extracellular fluid are prevented.

Water and electrolytes

For water and electrolytes, the amount excreted will depend upon, and be controlled by, how much is reabsorbed or secreted by the tubules. These processes provide much more flexible responses than those for metabolic wastes, and the remainder of this section looks at how kidney function is altered in response to homeostatic disturbances in water balance, sodium balance, potassium balance, calcium balance and acid/base status. The importance of regulating these parameters, and the kinds of receptor necessary to detect changes, were introduced in Chapter 6.

Regulation of water balance

We noted in Chapter 6 that the osmotic movement of water across cell membranes ensures that the osmotic pressure of intracellular and extracellular fluids remains in equilibrium. To maintain a constant cell volume and intracellular composition, it is therefore essential that changes in the osmotic pressure of extracellular fluid are detected, so as to promote a rapid change in renal water excretion in order to restore water balance.

The regulation of water balance is not, however, simply a question of increasing or decreasing urine volume. For example, the effect of overhydration is to increase body fluid volume and also to dilute it; this will be corrected more rapidly by the excretion of a large volume of urine that is more dilute than plasma (i.e. by excreting water more efficiently than solutes). Likewise, the effects of dehydration when plasma becomes more concentrated than normal will be corrected better by excretion of a small volume of highly concentrated urine (i.e. by excreting solutes more efficiently than water). The roles of the loop of Henle, distal tubule and collecting ducts in the process of water balance were noted briefly earlier. To understand how changes occur, the actions of these tubule segments need to be considered in further detail.

We noted earlier (Figure 15.6) that dilution of the tubule fluid begins in the ascending limb of the loop of Henle. Here, the abundant sodium and chloride ions are

Exercise

Review negative feedback processes, discussed in Chapter 1, and look at the principles of water and electrolyte homeostasis, introduced in Chapter 5.

extracted (by active transport) out of the fluid, but the osmotic movement of water with these salts is prevented by the tubule being virtually impermeable to water. Paradoxically, the diluting action of the limb occurs regardless of whether the kidneys are producing a dilute or a concentrated urine.

If the dilution process continues in the distal tubule and collecting ducts, then the final urine will be much less concentrated than plasma. The effect can be pronounced. Osmotic potential is measured in terms of osmolality (milliosmoles per litre; see Appendix A); whereas that of plasma is about 285 mosmol/l, that of urine may be as low as 50 mosmol/l (i.e. less than one-fifth that of plasma). Note, however, that dilution of tubule fluid can continue only if both the collecting tubules and collecting ducts have a low permeability to water, since water will otherwise be absorbed by osmosis into the highly concentrated tissue fluid in this region (generated by the loop of Henle). Looked at another way, allowing this section to become water permeable will promote osmosis, and so could act as a 'switch' to enable the kidney to now produce a low volume of concentrated urine. This is, in fact, how the mechanism operates, and urine can have a concentration up to about five times that of plasma (with an osmolality of 1400 mosmol/l).

The switch from producing a high-volume, dilute urine to a low-volume, concentrated one is produced by antidiuretic hormone (ADH; 'anti-' = against, 'diuretic' = promote urination), which determines the water permeability of the collecting ducts. Central to the determination of urine concentration and volume, then, is the degree to which ADH is released from the posterior pituitary gland. This depends upon the osmolality (i.e. level of hydration) of the plasma, and how much it has deviated from its homeostatic set point of about 285 mosmol/l (Figure 15.9). Any change in plasma osmotic pressure outside its homeostatic range is detected by specialized nerve cells called osmoreceptors within the hypothalamus.

An additional component to the urinary concentrating mechanism is the role of urea. When the kidneys are producing highly concentrated urine, water reabsorption out of the collecting ducts causes a considerable increase in the concentration of urea in the tubule fluid. Diffusion of urea out of the tubule fluid is therefore enhanced, which adds to the solute content of the tissue fluid. This promotes further osmotic movement of water, which acts to increase the concentrating capacity of the kidney. Urea is a product of protein metabolism, and it has been known for many years that people with a low protein intake have a reduced urine-concentrating ability.

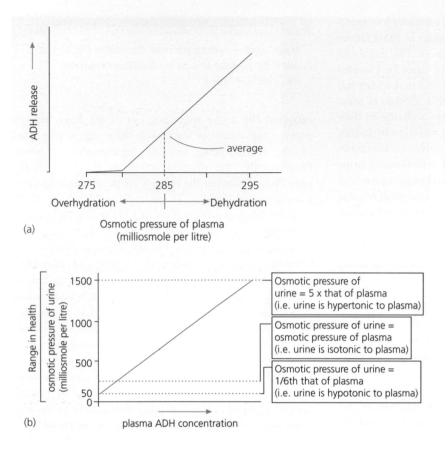

Figure 15.9 Antidiuretic hormone and water conservation by the kidneys. Note the narrowness of the range of values for osmotic pressure of blood plasma (a), and the capacity of the kidneys to produce a very dilute or very concentration urine, relative to plasma, according to the absence or presence of ADH (b).

Q. Why do the responses have to be sensitive?

Q. Why is the production of hypertonic urine when we are dehydrated so important?

BOX 15.16 EFFECTS OF DISORDERS OF ADH RELEASE/ACTIVITY ON KIDNEY FUNCTION

ADH is clearly central to the conservation of body water. This is illustrated by the effects of some (unusual) conditions. Syndrome of inappropriate ADH release (SIADH) induces overhydration because too much ADH is secreted relative to the state of hydration. Most commonly, this is the consequence of an ADH-secreting tumour, either within the pituitary gland or more commonly at a site somewhere else within the body (referred to as ectopic production of the hormone). Tumours do not exhibit the normal feedback controls on hormone release; in this case, ADH will continue to be produced even if the patient is well hydrated. The condition

induces hyponatraemia (low blood sodium concentration), and also cell swelling as a consequence of osmosis. Water intake must be moderated under these circumstances.

In contrast, diabetes insipidus (literally translated as 'siphoning of tasteless urine') is characterized either by a failure to release ADH or, more usually, as a failure of the kidney to respond to the hormone as a consequence of a lack of ADH receptors. In this condition, the patient will continue to produce large volumes of dilute urine, even when dehydrated, and will have a persistent thirst.

The mechanism of ADH release is very sensitive (Figure 15.9), but it is important to note that our need to excrete urea and electrolytes means that we must produce some urine, even if dehydrated. Zero urine production is not an option in health. The availability of drinking water is essential for survival but, provided that water is available to drink, the mechanism ensures that our water balance is maintained within the limits of ±2% of the homeostatic set

point. The response is relatively quick. For example, drinking a litre of water results in the excretion of the excess within 1–2 h.

Fluid balance charts

We have focused on the means by which the kidneys can act to regulate the volume and concentration of body fluids through the actions of antidiuretic hormone. Water balance will also be influenced by water gained and lost via other routes. Determination of the hydration status of a person must take these other aspects into account, and

Exercise

Drink a litre of tap water as quickly as possible. How long does it take for you to notice an increased rate of production of urine?

BOX 15.17 FLUID BALANCE IN INFANTS AND ELDERLY PEOPLE

Box 6.1 highlighted the fact that infants are more susceptible to fluid imbalance, partly because they have a relatively higher turnover of extracellular fluid, and partly because regulatory processes are immature. This latter point makes it difficult for babies to maintain fluid homeostasis if their hydration is not maintained by adequate fluid intake. Elderly people also have a problem in maintaining fluid balance, but this time partly as a consequence of ageing, which affects hormone production, release and actions, and partly because of inadequate dietary habits. Poor dietary habits often mean that dehydration predominates.

BOX 15.18 EFFECTS OF SURGERY ON FLUID BALANCE

Nil-by-mouth procedures will often mean that the patient is dehydrated before going into surgery (Jester and Williams, 1999). Surgery also makes additional excretory routes significant, e.g. fluid loss by dehydration during the operative procedure, blood loss or fluid lost through drains. Evaporative loss may also be high after surgery if the patient breathes heavily because of pain, stress or anxiety. Diarrhoea, vomiting or renal function problems complicate the picture further. Fluid gains come from infusions, so the infusion rates used must reflect the loss of fluid. Much of the fluid loss is difficult to assess, or even estimate, and vigilance will be necessary to ensure that the infusion rate used is appropriate (see Clancy et al., 2001).

balance charts are frequently produced in clinical areas. A daily water balance chart for an adult in a temperate climate might look like this:

Water input (ml)		Water output (ml)	
Drink	1500	Urine	1400
Food	800	Evaporation:	
Metabolic production	200	Lungs	500
		Skin	400
		Faeces	200
Total	2500 ml/day		2500 ml/day

As can be seen, most water loss in temperate climates, such as the British one, will be via urine (although sweat can form a significant route during hot weather). Water lost via sweat and respiration is termed 'insensible' loss, and the volume is largely unaffected by our state of hydration; urinary losses are referred to as 'sensible' losses because they do relate to water balance.

Assessment of insensible losses and the volume generated by metabolism will clearly be difficult, if not impossible, in a ward or home environment. A quick look at the balance table, however, shows that water drunk is the major component of water intake, while most lost from the body is in urine. Thirst is usually a late indication of dehydration, and so is often underplayed in biological terms. However, thirst is actually a major part of the mechanism by which body fluid osmotic pressure is normalized, provided that drinking water is available, and its onset should be taken seriously in patients, especially those who are particularly susceptible (see Box 15.17). A reasonable estimate of fluid balance can therefore be obtained using these parameters and an estimate of insensible loss; this is the basis of ward assessments of hydration state.

Regulation of sodium balance and extracellular fluid volume

Table 15.1 shows that apart from protein, blood plasma is basically a solution of sodium chloride with other electrolytes and various organic substances added. This means that sodium and chloride ions are the main contributors to the osmotic potential of plasma. Sodium chloride in our diet is absorbed almost entirely by the small intestine, and distributes throughout the extracellular fluid; it is prevented from accumulating in cells by the cell membrane Na^+/K^+ exchange pump. Any change in sodium and chloride concentration of the extracellular fluid will be detected as a change in the osmotic pressure of plasma, and will be corrected quickly by promoting a change in water balance by the mechanism described earlier. This is illustrated by the feelings of thirst promoted by eating salty foods.

A change in the sodium and chloride content of extracellular fluid will at most, therefore, alter the fluid's sodium and chloride concentration only transiently, but there will be a change in the fluid volume as a consequence of a change in water balance. Note that although the change in volume represents a change in water balance, this is quite different from the situation described in the previous section on water homeostasis, in which overhydration was not associated with a concomitant change in sodium balance. Thus, if the kidneys respond to the increased extracellular fluid volume simply by increasing water excretion, this will only cause the concentration of sodium chloride (and the osmotic pressure) of the extracellular fluid to increase, which will then promote water conservation again. Clearly, excess sodium chloride and water must be excreted together.

The simultaneous stimulation of sodium chloride and water excretion occurs when an increased extracellular fluid volume is detected. More precisely, the blood component of that fluid compartment is monitored by receptors associated with the circulatory system. The location of all of these receptors is still debatable, though some have been found in the atria of the heart and in the kidneys.

An increased blood volume promotes the urinary excretion of sodium (and water) through the actions of hormones (Figure 15.10). Two hormones that have been implicated in the response are aldosterone (a steroid from the adrenal gland) and atrial natriuretic factor (ANF, a peptide from the cardiac atria; 'natriuretic' = sodium-excreting). Aldosterone acts to stimulate the reabsorption of sodium by the distal tubule, but an expansion of blood volume decreases its release and so promotes sodium chloride excretion (with water). The change in hormone release is mediated by changes in the activity of the sympathetic nervous system and of the intermediary hormone angiotensin (see Chapter 9). ANF acts by inhibiting sodium reabsorption by the collecting tubules and ducts; its release is increased when blood volume in the heart is increased.

Both hormones have other actions, and neither can be said to be solely sodium regulating. In addition, the decrease in sympathetic nervous activity that occurs when blood volume is expanded (necessary to prevent an increased arterial blood pressure; see Chapter 9) also reduces renal sodium reabsorption. The control of sodium balance is therefore multifactorial.

The renal responses to blood volume changes are relatively slow. Figure 15.11 illustrates what happens when a person is given a higher dietary sodium intake. The renal excretion of sodium increases gradually over a period of days, during which time sodium will have accumulated (with water) in the extracellular fluid. The delay in response means that a change in sodium balance does not produce complete correction: people with high sodium intake will have a higher extracellular fluid volume (and possibly blood volume) than those with a low sodium intake. Conversely, going on to a diet that entails food (and hence sodium) restriction results in an initial net loss of

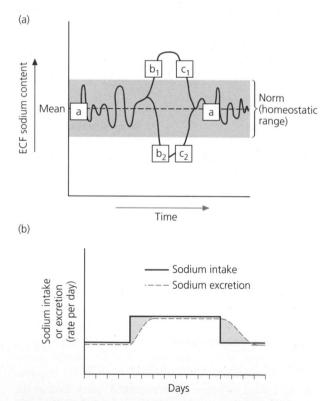

Figure 15.11 (a) The homeostatic regulation of sodium balance. [a] Homeostatic range for sodium content (and volume) of extracellular fluid (ECF). [b_1] Increased ECF sodium content resulting from dietary intake being in excess of excretion rate. [b_2] Decreased ECF sodium content resulting from excretion rate being in excess of dietary intake. [c] Restoration of ECF sodium content (and volume) to homeostatic norm by appropriate changes in sodium intake and sodium (and water) excretion. (b) The homeostatic response to an increased sodium intake is delayed. The delay in producing a new balance state can be seen to increase body fluid sodium content (shaded area) and volume, which increases blood volume. Reducing sodium intake results in excretion of the retained excess but again the response is delayed.

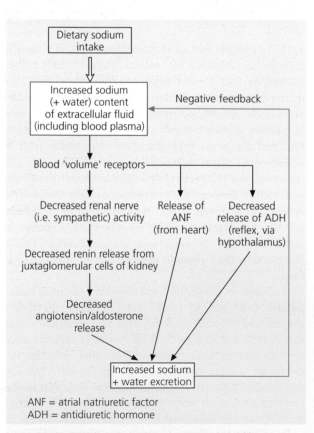

ANF = atrial natriuretic factor
ADH = antidiuretic hormone

Figure 15.10 Endocrine responses to an elevated blood volume, resulting in increased sodium and water excretion. ANF = atrial natriuretic factor; ADH = antidiuretic hormone.

Q. How might excess sodium (chloride) in extracellular fluid contribute to an increased blood pressure?

sodium and water until the new balance is established. Initial weight loss, therefore, may look promising but is only due to a reduction in body water content, rather than a loss of fat stores.

Sodium balance chart

As with water, there are times when a clinician may wish to assess the electrolyte balance of a patient. Again, urine is just one route for the excretion of electrolytes, so other routes must be taken into account. Urine losses of sodium dominate, however, so urine output of sodium relates closely to the sodium intake and provides a reasonable means of monitoring sodium balance. Note, however, that other routes assume greater significance if a patient has diarrhoea or if sweat rates are very high.

A typical adult's (UK climate) daily balance chart for sodium would look like this (note that individual values will vary with diet):

Sodium input		Sodium output	
Food	200	Faeces + sweat	20
		Urine	180
Total	200 mmol/day		200 mmol/day
	(≈ 9 g/day)		

The sodium content of foods can be altered if there are difficulties in excreting sodium, e.g. in renal failure. In

contrast, saline infusions, e.g. after surgery, can replace or supplement dietary intake, and sodium balance charts will need to take into account this new intake rate.

Potassium balance

We described in Chapter 8 how the concentration gradient of potassium ions across cell membranes is the main determinant of the resting electrical potential of the membrane. In nerve and muscle cells, the capacity to change the electrical potential is important because it provides the means of generating the electrical currents necessary to produce the nerve impulse and to induce muscle contraction. It is therefore essential that the resting potential (and hence potassium concentration) is maintained, since any fluctuations could have dramatic effects on the sensitivity of these cell membranes to stimulation. In particular, short-term fluctuations must be avoided, since the limited compensation that cells can make take some time to occur.

Potassium concentration in extracellular fluid is normally of the order of only 4 mmol/l (compared with 140 mmol/l for sodium), yet this low concentration is maintained. It is therefore not surprising that the potassium concentration of blood plasma is monitored very closely (by receptors in the adrenal glands). Unlike sodium, the regulation of potassium balance appears to

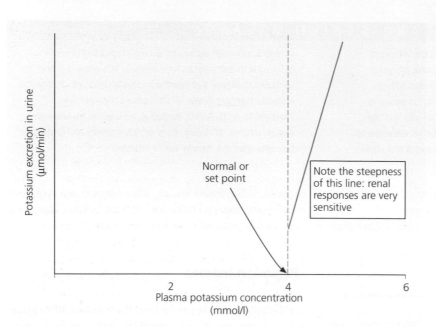

Figure 15.12 Potassium balance. The sensitivity of renal responses (and hence the narrowness of the homeostatic range) to changes in plasma potassium concentration is shown.

Q. How are sodium and potassium regulated in the body?

Q. Why is it important that blood potassium concentration has a narrow homeostatic range?

involve just one hormone; the increased potassium excretion observed when plasma potassium concentration is increased is due primarily to the actions of the aldosterone released from the adrenal gland. This hormone was mentioned earlier in relation to sodium balance; it acts by stimulating sodium reabsorption by the distal tubule, but in doing so it also promotes the secretion of potassium ions into the tubule fluid. The secretion of these ions makes the excretory response very rapid and quickly effective (Figure 15.12).

Potassium balance charts can be constructed along similar lines to those for sodium.

Calcium balance

Calcium ions have a number of functions. Inside cells, they are a trigger for muscle contraction, while outside cells their concentration determines the threshold electrical potential at which nerve and muscle cell membranes are stimulated (see Chapter 8). Regarding the latter, about 50% of the calcium found in blood plasma is bound reversibly to plasma proteins, but this component will not be physiologically active; it is the concentration (about 1.25 mmol/l) of the 50% of ions that are free that must be regulated closely. This concentration can change rapidly if the proportion bound to proteins is altered; this is dependent particularly on the acid/base status of the plasma, the regulation of which is covered in the next section.

Unlike sodium, potassium and chloride ions, which are absorbed almost entirely from our foods and are not stored by the body, calcium stores (as bone) are very large, and only some 50% of our dietary calcium may be absorbed. Calcium in bone is constantly being deposited, or resorbed into the extracellular fluid, and the concentration of calcium in that fluid must be seen to be a balance between the addition from intestine and bone, and the loss into bone and in urine (see Figure 9.11). The handling of this ion is therefore very different from that of the ions mentioned previously, and balance charts are difficult to construct.

The movement of calcium in and out of bone is controlled by the hormones calcitonin and parathyroid hormone, respectively (both are produced by the parathyroid glands). Parathyroid hormone is released when plasma calcium ion concentration decreases, and promotes bone resorption. In doing so, the hormone also releases phosphate ions from bone mineral; these are excreted through the actions of parathyroid hormone to inhibit phosphate reabsorption by the proximal tubule of the kidney, thus helping to maintain both calcium and phosphate homeostasis. Parathyroid hormone also increases indirectly the uptake of calcium from the gut by promoting the conversion (in the kidneys and liver) of inactive vitamin D to the active form. This role of vitamin D in calcium balance has prompted some authorities to now view it as a hormone rather than a vitamin.

Note that changes in renal calcium excretion have only a relatively small role in the regulation of plasma calcium ion concentration. This role, nevertheless, is important in the overall scheme.

Another hormone calcitonin is released when plasma calcium ion concentration is increased above normal. It promotes calcium uptake into bone, and also opposes the actions of parathyroid hormone. Together, the two hormones maintain a constancy of the plasma concentration (Figure 15.13).

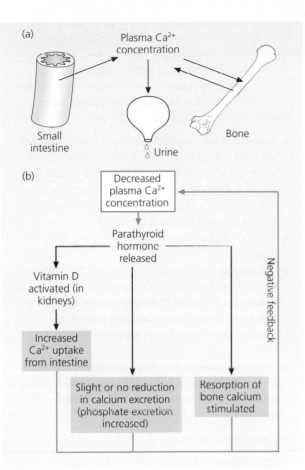

Figure 15.13 Calcium homeostasis. (a) Unabsorbed calcium in the intestine and also bone calcium provide a 'reservoir' that can be drawn upon if required. Note that plasma calcium concentration takes priority over bone calcium content. (b) Role of parathyroid hormone. Note that if Ca²⁺ concentration had been elevated, this decreases parathyroid hormone release and so stimulates calcitonin release. Responses are therefore reversed, and act to decrease calcium concentration.

Q. Which gland releases calcitonin?

Acid/base balance

The need to regulate body fluid pH (i.e. hydrogen ion concentration) was highlighted in Chapter 6. Hydrogen ions are produced continually through metabolism, either directly (from protein) or indirectly (from carbon dioxide; see chapter 6). Regulation is achieved by controlling hydrogen ion excretion by the kidneys, and carbon dioxide excretion via the lungs. Buffer chemicals help to prevent local fluctuation in acidity within the tissues.

The process is illustrated by the response to an elevated acid load. As the hydrogen ion concentration of plasma rises, it stimulates the peripheral chemoreceptors, and lung ventilation is increased; more carbon dioxide is exhaled than usual, which reduces the acid load from this source.

BOX 15.21 COMPENSATORY RENAL RESPONSES TO ACID/BASE DISTURBANCE

Excessive acidity of body fluids is referred to as an acidosis; this can be either respiratory or metabolic in cause. In respiratory acidosis, the problem is due to being unable to excrete carbon dioxide adequately via the lungs (e.g. chronic bronchitis, emphysema). In metabolic acidosis, there is acidity produced somewhere in the body that is in excess of the normal regulatory processes (e.g. ketoacidosis, lactic acidosis, or hydrogen ion retention through renal failure). Both forms produce different compensatory mechanisms when chronic, but neither is fully compensated for – the medium-/long-term homeostatic processes can only be considered to be partially effective.

In chronic respiratory acidosis, the kidney responds by excreting more hydrogen ions (hence the urine becomes more acidic) and by retaining bicarbonate ions, which increases the buffering capacity of the blood. The increased bicarbonate concentration will be detected in analysis by blood gas monitoring, but will not necessarily reflect the extent of the compensation. This is because carbonic acid (from carbon dioxide) breaks down to bicarbonate as well as to hydrogen ions. The base excess reading provided by the monitor allows for this, and provides an indication of how much compensation by the kidneys has occurred.

In chronic metabolic acidosis, more carbon dioxide will be excreted by the lungs as a compensatory response to reduce this source of acidity. The kidneys will also respond as above (unless, of course, renal failure is the cause of the acidosis). The main difference in the blood picture between chronic respiratory and chronic metabolic acidosis, therefore, is the carbon dioxide content.

Compensatory responses will also be observed in chronic metabolic alkalosis, and will be the opposite of the above. They will include an increased bicarbonate excretion in urine, and hence a reduction in the bicarbonate concentration of blood. As a consequence, there is likely to be the apparently paradoxical negative base excess ('base deficiency' would be a more accurate term, but 'excess' is the standard term used). Chronic respiratory alkalosis is unlikely to occur.

Overbreathing in anxiety and pain can induce acute respiratory alkalosis. In this case (and in acute acidosis), it is unlikely that compensatory responses will be seen, as these are slow to be established, taking several hours.

Should the elevated acidity still persist, then hydrogen ion secretion by the distal tubules of the kidneys will be increased, causing an increased acidity of the urine (urine pH is normally about 6–7, it but has a range of 4.5–8, i.e. acidic or alkaline according to needs). Bicarbonate reabsorption by the proximal tubule is also promoted; this additional bicarbonate will maintain the buffering capac-

BOX 15.22 BODY FLUID COMPOSITION IN ACUTE RENAL FAILURE

The relation of renal function to body fluid composition is illustrated most clearly by the consequences of acute renal failure (ARF). ARF is frequently observed if the kidneys have received poor supplies of blood, e.g. in some lengthy surgical procedures, or following severe haemorrhage (Seaton-Mills, 1999). ARF caused by poor blood supply is referred to as having a pre-renal cause. Often, the acute failure is associated with a breakdown of kidney tubule organization and function, referred to as acute tubular necrosis (ATN). The cause may be linked to the poor perfusion with blood, but it may arise without a pre-renal cause, e.g. because of sepsis or toxic chemicals.

ARF is a condition characterized by a sudden, rapid deterioration in renal function:

● Oliguria is observed (i.e. 30 ml urine/h or <400 ml/24 h). In some cases (although not this one), renal function can be so depressed as to cause anuria (0–100 ml urine/24 h). The lower limit for 'normal' function relates to the ability of kidneys to conserve water when we are dehydrated. Thus, urine production may be very low, but the urine will not be as concentrated as would be anticipated had the patient been very dehydrated. The patient's appearance also would not indicate dehydration of this magnitude.
● Uraemia – a raised blood urea concentration – is present. Urea (and uric acid) is especially dependent upon an adequate GFR for its excretion. Uraemia (and uricaemia) is often indicative of an inability to excrete the normal load.
● Potassium concentration is elevated in blood plasma. In the absence of a potassium infusion, hyperkalaemia is almost certainly due to an inability to excrete potassium normally. Failure to maintain electrolyte balance may lead to raised blood potassium sufficient to cause fatal cardiac arrhythmias (see the case study of a man with hyperkalaemia in Section 6); this is often the cause of death in ARF.
● An acidosis is present. The acidosis is of metabolic origin, and is due to a failure to excrete hydrogen ions. The acidosis causes respiration to be slightly elevated (Box 15.21).

Additional imbalances produced by the renal dysfunction will be:

● fluid overload: this is due partly to water retention and partly to an expansion of the extracellular fluid compartment as a consequence of sodium retention. Peripheral oedema might be observed. In severe cases, pulmonary oedema may occur;
● poor appetite, nausea and vomiting arising from the disturbed blood composition;
● changes in mental functioning, such as drowsiness and confusion, as a consequence of altered blood composition.

The specific goal of caring for a patient in ARF is to try to normalize as far as is possible body fluid composition by managing dietary input. In this way, a new homeostatic balance can be established so that input once again equals output:

● Restoration of fluid balance. Fluid intake is reduced, usually to 500 ml/24 h plus a volume equal to the previous day's urine output. This is to replace the water lost through residual renal function and that lost via insensible means (lungs, skin, etc.). Daily weighing is a crude means of assessing the amount of any fluid that might continue to be retained.
● Restriction of dietary sodium intake. This prevents further fluid shifts.
● Restriction of dietary potassium intake. With this electrolyte, ion exchange resins such as Calcium Resonium® can also be administered to promote K^+ secretion into the colon. A high calorie intake is also helpful because it promotes tissue anabolism, which helps to shift more potassium into the cells.
● Restriction of dietary protein. This is necessary to help reduce the production of urea and other nitrogenous products, and so help to compensate for the reduced excretion of these substances.

ARF usually has three phases:

1 *Oliguric phase.*
2 *Diuretic phase:* follows after perhaps several days, or even several weeks, and is usually indicative that the kidneys are recovering.
3 *Recovery phase:* the diuresis declines and homeostasis is re-established without the need for restricted dietary inputs.

Body fluid management can still be required even when the diuretic phase commences because the kidneys are initially unable to concentrate the urine. Strict monitoring is therefore essential throughout the course of ARF. Nursing care also includes psychological support and optimum nutrition (often as total parenteral nutrition).

About 60% of patients regain most or all of their renal function, but ARF is a life-threatening condition, and there is still quite a high mortality rate, despite new and sophisticated technological treatments. In some patients, ARF progresses to chronic renal failure. The problems therefore will worsen with time and a time may come when dialysis (or renal transplantation) will be necessary (Box 15.23). Anaemia may develop, since the kidneys are the source of erythrogenin (see Chapter 11), in which case blood transfusion may be required.

ity of plasma, and in chronic circumstances it may even be increased (Box 15.21).

While responses to changes in body fluid pH are pronounced, pH regulation seems to be governed largely by neural control of lung function, and by intrinsic processes within the kidneys: hormones do not appear to be involved specifically. The regulatory process has sufficient sensitivity to ensure that moment-to-moment changes in metabolic rate produce at most only slight, perhaps undetectable, changes in the extracellular pH. The acidity changes become more pronounced if there is an excessive change in acid production, e.g. during exercise when lactic acid from muscle cells adds to the acid 'load', but even then changes are not large.

BOX 15.23 DIALYSIS

Dialysis is an artificial means of replacing kidney function, although the intermittence of its application means that the control of blood composition cannot be as precise as that normally provided by the kidneys. Dialysis is used especially in cases of renal failure, when the disturbance in body fluid composition can be profound. In chronic renal failure, renal transplantation would be ideal but the reality is that patients will have a prolonged spell of dialysis before a donor becomes available, if at all. Dialysis may also be used in acute renal failure, until renal function improves, or to remove poisons quickly and efficiently. Two procedures are available (see Stark, 1997):

Haemodialysis

In haemodialysis, blood drains from a vein, usually in the arm, and is pumped to the dialysis machine. The blood passes over a selectively permeable membrane, on the other side of which is dialysate fluid. This fluid is a carefully prepared, balanced electrolyte solution that will also permit the withdrawal of water from blood by osmosis. The blood and dialysate fluid do not mix; solute and water exchange is by diffusion.

Haemodialysis can maintain a patient for many years, but there are psychosocial costs: the treatment is time consuming (6–8 h), and it must be performed regularly in an appropriate clinical unit, often entailing a degree of travelling for the patient. The treatment is not a perfect replacement for kidney functions. For example, it does not replace red blood cells, the synthesis of which is reduced in renal failure since the kidneys do not produce erythrogenin. Other complications include arteriosclerotic disease, partly because of poor calcium control but also because uraemia is not removed completely by dialysis.

Peritoneal dialysis

The principle here is to use the patient's peritoneum as the selectively permeable membrane for dialysis. The dialysate fluid is introduced into the peritoneal cavity at regular intervals. Exchange with blood occurs, then peritoneal fluid is drained slowly, bringing with it the solutes that had accumulated from blood. The method takes longer than haemodialysis (36–48 h), but it changes blood composition much more slowly, which may be an advantage in some patients.

Continuous ambulatory peritoneal dialysis (CAPD) is a variant that enables patients to take an active role in their dialysis – the treatment may take place at home (Macdonald, 1997). A permanent peritoneal catheter is put into place, and dialysate fluid is delivered from a plastic bag. After delivery, the bag can be rolled up under the clothing until drainage is necessary. Several treatments a day may be performed – more than if the patient has to attend a unit – so control of blood composition is often better. The method is clearly also less restrictive on lifestyle.

Summary

1 Metabolism and our diets provide excesses of substances, which, if retained in the body, will eventually disturb cellular and systemic functions. The main route for their excretion is via the urine.

2 Urine is initially formed in the glomeruli of the renal tubules as a filtrate of blood plasma. At this point, it contains all the solutes found in plasma, other than large proteins. The composition and volume of the filtrate is modified as it passes along the renal tubules by solute reabsorption and by secretion of solutes by the tubular cells.

3 The bulk (normally 99%+) of the filtrate is reabsorbed by the tubules, mostly by the proximal tubule. Separate renal handling of solute and water reabsorption by the loop of Henle, distal nephron, and collecting ducts means that the final urine can be more dilute or more concentrated than plasma, with consequential effects on plasma osmotic pressure. The process is controlled largely by antidiuretic hormone.

4 The urinary excretion of many metabolic products, such as urea, is determined primarily by the glomerular filtration rate. That of electrolytes and glucose is determined by how much is reabsorbed from the filtrate or how much is secreted into it.

5 Virtually all of the glucose and amino acids filtered by the kidneys is reabsorbed, and the urine is characteristically free of them.

6 Electrolyte excretion is controlled mainly by the actions of hormones on the kidneys. Homeostatic control of solute excretion is essential because of the pronounced effects that retention or excessive loss have on systemic functions. The means of detection of disturbance depends upon the physiological consequences of that disturbance, and renal responses vary accordingly.

Review questions

1 The kidneys have other functions as well as making urine. What are they?

2 Become familiar with the structure of the kidney, and be able to distinguish between the cortex and medullary regions.

3 The functional units of the kidney are called nephrons. Using the following terminology, draw and label a nephron: glomerulus, Bowman's capsule, glomerular filtrate, proximal convoluted tubule, loop of Henle, distal convoluted tubule, and collecting duct.

4 Where would you find the juxtaglomerular complex? What is its function?

5 The formation of urine requires three processes: filtration, reabsorption and secretion. Where do these processes occur along the length of the nephron, and which substances are involved? Which parts of the nephron are affected by antidiuretic hormone (ADH)?

6 Why may urinalysis be described as a window into the body? What substances are tested for in urinalysis? What is the significance of abnormal results?

7 What will happen to the colour of urine if you (i) drink lots of water, (ii) eat beetroot, (iii) have renal failure?

8 Define the following terms: (i) polyuria, (ii) haematuria, (iii) anuria, and (iv) oliguria.

9 Urine is normally considered sterile, although there may be odd stray organisms found. Microbiological analysis of a correctly collected specimen (midstream urine, MSU) can reveal the causative organism of a urinary tract infection (UTI). This information can be used to ensure appropriate treatment. Which organs are included in the urinary tract?

10 UTIs usually affect women rather than men. Why?

11 Identify the signs and symptoms of a UTI.

12 What factors can increase the risk of a UTI?

REFERENCES

Chrysant, G.S. (2000) High salt intake and cardiovascular disease. Is there a connection? *Nutrition* **16**(7–8): 662–4.

Clancy, J., McVicar, A. and Baird, N. (2002) Perioperative influences on water and electrolyte homeostasis. In: *Fundamentals of Homeostasis for Perioperative Practitioners*. London: Routledge. Chapter 3. (in print)

Cook, R. (1996) Urinalysis: ensuring accurate urine testing. *Nursing Standard* **10**(4): 49–52.

Jester, R. and Williams, S. (1999) Pre-operative fasting: putting research into practice. *Nursing Standard* **13**(39): 33–5.

Macdonald, J. (1997) Dialysis: continuous ambulatory peritoneal dialysis. *Nursing Standard* **11**(22): 48–55.

Marchiondo, K. (1998) A new look at urinary tract infections. *American Journal of Nursing* **98**(3): 34–9.

Matta, C. (2000) Encourage patients to shake the salt habit. *Practice Nurse* **19**(3): 122–5.

Norton, C. (1996) (ed.) *Nursing for Continence*, 2nd edn. Beaconsfield, UK: Beaconsfield Publishing.

Pak, C.Y.C. (1998) Kidney stones. *Lancet* **351**(9118): 1797–1801.

Seaton-Mills, D. (1999) Acute renal failure: causes and considerations in the critically ill patient. *Nursing in Critical Care* **4**(6): 293–7.

Stark, J. (1997) Dialysis choices: turning the tide in acute renal failure. *Nursing* **27**(2):41–8.

Wallace, M. (1998) Renal transplantation. *AORN Journal* **68**(6): 962–6.

Wilde, M.H. (1997) Long term indwelling catheter care: conceptualising the research base. *Journal of Advanced Nursing* **25**(6): 1252–61.

Chapter 16

The skin

INTRODUCTION

The skin is the largest organ of the body. Its functions and anatomy relate to its role in providing the main interface between the body and the external environment.

Functions of skin

Protection

Being in contact with the external environment, the skin is obviously the first line of defence against potential pathogenic organisms. The structure of the skin provides a physical barrier, and the bactericidal constituents of skin secretions also provide a degree of chemical protection. The impervious nature of skin, and its role as a physical barrier, also protects the body from chemical agents.

Excretion

The skin is not an excretory organ in the sense that it has a central role in the homeostatic processes involved in body fluid regulation, but sweat composition may vary in its sodium chloride content if we are sodium deficient. However, sweat contains various substances, including metabolic products, and the skin therefore is a route of excretion for these substances. Although normally a relatively minor route, the amount of substance lost from the body via sweat must be considered a component of total excretion. This is particularly the case for water and electrolytes. Thus, even in cool, temperate conditions, sweat accounts for almost 10% of the water output from the body, while in very hot weather, sweat secretion may rise to as much as 4 l/day and so exceed the total excreted by other routes, including in urine.

BOX 16.1 ITCHING

Itching (pruritus) is caused by local irritation of the skin that stimulates nerve endings. The sensory physiology of 'itch' is poorly understood. Pruritus might result from contact of the skin with irritant agents, from inflammation or infection of the skin, or perhaps from the deposition of 'waste' substances in the skin. The latter may arise because excretion of substances via sweat can be enhanced in renal failure. Although sweat will not compensate for body fluid disturbances in renal failure, there is an increased content of metabolic wastes in the secretion. Thus, a 'snow' of uric acid and urea may be apparent on the skin of patients, left behind when sweat evaporates. This deposition of crystals within the skin may cause intense itching.

Exercise

Refer to Chapter 15 and identify 'sensible' and 'insensible' water losses in the section on fluid balance. Why are evaporative losses from the skin considered to be 'insensible'?

Prevention of tissue dehydration

The structure of the intact epidermis makes the skin almost impervious to water (note that sweat secretion is via ducts from sweat glands and so is a physiological process). This property of the skin is essential for our existence, because it prevents evaporative water loss to the atmosphere. In contrast, surgical procedures or extensive burns breach the skin and expose underlying 'wet' tissues to the environment. This produces extensive loss of water by evaporation, and is a concern for care.

Support and shape

This is an obvious role of the skin. Support of the viscera is provided by muscles of the body wall, but is facilitated by the tough, durable nature of the overlying skin. Muscles, skin and adipose tissues also give rise to the body shapes associated with sexual dimorphism. Being the visible aspects of the body, skin also makes clear the effects of ageing on tissues. Loss of elasticity, which also occurs in other tissues and organs, is unfortunately readily apparent as the skin wrinkles with age.

Regulation of body temperature regulation

Our bodies continuously gain heat from metabolism, and (in the UK climate) usually continuously lose heat to the environment. Under very hot conditions, the body may gain heat from the environment. Maintaining an optimal temperature of the essential organs of the body is an important aspect of homeostasis, and controlling heat transfer across the skin is part of that regulatory process. The importance of skin in the regulation of body temperature is such that the topic is covered in a separate section later in this chapter.

ANATOMY OF THE SKIN

The skin consists of two principal parts (Figure 16.1(a)): the inner *dermis* ('derm-' = layer) and the outer *epidermis* ('epi-' = upon). Below the dermis lies a subcutaneous layer ('sub-' = below; 'cutaneous' = of the skin), sometimes called the superficial fascia since it also includes part of the connective tissue that covers muscles. Embryologically, the subcutaneous layer does not develop as part of the skin, but it is functionally linked with it and so will be considered in this context.

Epidermis

Cell layers

The epidermis is comprised of a type of tissue called a stratified squamous epithelium. This means that it has multiple layers (strata) of simple, flattened (i.e. squamous) cells that sit, ultimately, on a basement membrane of protein. There are various layers of cells (Figure 16.1(b)):

- The basal layer (= stratum basale) sits on the basement membrane, thus separating the epidermis from the dermis. The cells within the epidermis are generated by mitotic division within the basal layer, so this is often referred to as the germinal layer of the skin. Some of the daughter cells produced by mitosis maintain this layer, while others ascend toward the surface of the skin and form the following layers.

- A layer of 'prickly' looking cells (= stratum spinosum) lies above the basal layer. Within the stratum spinosum, the cells become irregularly shaped and develop protuberances that cause them to appear 'prickly', hence the name of this layer. The cell extensions interlock, and this is the start of the formation of a structure that will be tough and durable. Tactile nerve endings, called Merkel's discs (see Chapter 7), may also be present in this layer.

- A layer of cells that contain granules (= stratum granulosum) lies above the stratum spinosum. After the stratum spinosum, the cells continue to ascend and begin to flatten. They also begin to produce keratohyalin, a substance that will eventually be converted into the tough, waterproofing protein keratin. The compound is stored in the cells, hence this layer may be referred to as the granular layer. The nuclei of the cells within the layer begin to degenerate, and consequently metabolism declines.

- A layer of tough, hardened (i.e. cornified; = stratum corneum) cells lies above the granular layer, and at the skin surface. By this time, the cells are dead. This cornified layer gives the epidermis the toughness needed to provide a barrier against external physical stresses, and environmental agents such as bacteria and chemicals. The latter include water, as the epidermis is now impervious. In adults, the epidermis is 0.5–3 mm thick, depending upon site; this relates especially to the thickness of the cornified layer, and hence to the physical stresses placed on that area of skin. In view of its position as the outer layer, it is not surprising that cells are continuously lost from it during day-to-day living. The attrition is substantial, e.g. most of the 'house dust' in bedding is comprised of these cells.

(a)

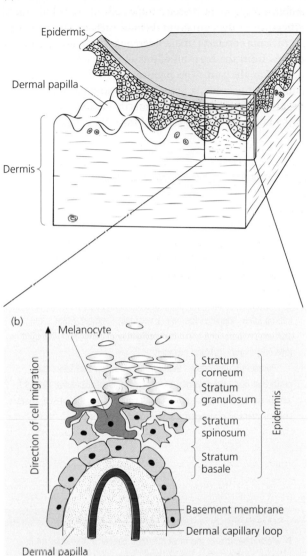

(b)

Figure 16.1 The epidermis. (a) General plan and relation to the dermis. (b) Cell layers.

Q. Which layer of skin is referred to as a stratified epithelium? Name the subdivisions of the layer.

Q. The skin is referred to as a 'labile' tissue due to its repair capabilities. What does this mean?

● Areas of skin that are exposed to considerable frictional stress, such as the soles of the feet, have a fifth layer between the granular and cornified layers. This is a 'clear' layer (= stratum lucidum). The cells produce a translucent substance that is intermediary between keratohyalin and keratin. This is called eleidin, and provides a degree of frictional resistance by cushioning and absorbing shearing stresses, e.g. during walking.

There are no blood vessels within the epidermis itself. The demands of the cells are met by blood vessels within the dermis that extend into the vicinity of the basal layer cells.

BOX 16.2 . AGEING AND THE EPIDERMIS

The thickness of the epidermis is determined by the rate of cell division in the basal layer, which must then be in balance with the rate of cell attrition from the cornified layer. Epidermal growth factor is a peptide that has been isolated and found to promote mitosis in epithelia, including the epidermis, although its precise role in the maintenance of the skin is unclear. One feature of ageing is that the rate of mitosis generally begins to slow down. As mitosis declines, the epidermis becomes thinner. In contrast, the epidermis of the soles of the feet of older people may be very tough, as the cornified layer becomes even more hardened.

BOX 16.3 EPIDERMAL WOUND HEALING AND SKIN GRAFTING

The germinal layer of the epidermis has to be highly proliferative in order to maintain the cornified layer. Being this active means that the epithelium regenerates very quickly if damaged.

Epidermal wound healing

We discussed wound healing in detail in Chapter 2. We noted that superficial injury is repaired largely by cell migration. In the epidermis, the cell layers are all derived from the germinal layer, i.e. there is no need for specific cell types to migrate from elsewhere, although lateral migration from adjoining epidermal layers may occur. Superficial wounds to the epidermis therefore heal very quickly, without a need for scarring, and tissue structure is soon reorganized.

Skin grafting

This entails removal of a section of skin and transferring it to another site (Francis, 1998; Donato *et al.*, 2000). It is used when there are areas of denuded skin (e.g. burns), where skin is inadequate to close a wound, or if skin has been removed (e.g. in excision of a tumour).

The graft is obtained from a suitable site using a razor or similar implement. The section of skin removed is predominantly epidermis. Remnant germinal cells will re-epithelialize the donor site, although great care must be taken to ensure that the raw, exposed dermis is maintained. The graft is transferred to the graft site, which must have an adequate blood supply to support the transplanted tissue.

Epidermal coloration: melanocytes

Interspersed among the cells of the basal and prickly layers are cells called melanocytes. Aggregates of melanocytes form nevi or moles. Melanocytes contain the pigment melanin (Figure 16.1(b)), and have extensions that pass between cells of the other layers. When melanin production is stimulated, that released from the processes will be taken up by other epidermal cells and will pigment most areas of skin. Skin pigmentation relates primarily to the amount of pigment present in the cells; there is little racial difference in the actual numbers of melanocytes present.

Melanin protects the underlying basal layer and the dermis from the harmful effects of ultraviolet (UV) radiation from the sun. The pigment is synthesized from the amino acid tyrosine, a process that is stimulated directly by the actions of UV light, and indirectly by melanocyte-stimulating hormone (MSH) released from the pituitary gland.

BOX 16.4 SKIN COLORATION

Blood supply

In the absence of large amounts of pigment, the skin is pinkish-white, and its colour is determined mainly by the visualization of blood within it:

- Drainage of blood away from the skin in shock causes it to take on a greyish colour.
- The skin will look flushed in hot weather, when blood flow to the skin is increased.
- The skin circulation is regulated by the sympathetic nervous system. When this is inhibited by emotional responses, it may cause 'blushing' as vessels dilate in localized areas.
- Cyanosis, observed when blood is deoxygenated, can also be observed through skin, or the nails.

Skin colour produced by blood is therefore an important indicator of wellbeing, and an important aspect of nursing assessment.

Albinism

Albinism is characterized by pigment-free melanocytes and hair. It occurs when a genetic deficiency prevents the synthesis of those enzymes necessary for the conversion of the amino acid tyrosine to the pigment melanin. Albinism is commonly, but not always, associated with Huntington's disease, a neurological disorder arising from an inability of cells to metabolize tyrosine appropriately. Visually, the hair is very fair – almost white – the skin is very pale, and there is a deficiency of pigment in the eyes (eye colour also involves melanin).

People who are albino therefore have a skin that lacks the protection normally provided by melanin against excessive UV light, which makes skin damage, including cancers (see Box 16.5), more likely if there is prolonged exposure to bright sunlight.

BOX 16.5 SKIN TUMOURS

There are various types of skin tumour:

- *Basal cell carcinoma:* this is the most common form of skin cancer. It arises from basal cells of the epidermis. UV light is a risk factor. The tumour has a slow growth rate, and generally does not metastasize beyond skin, but it can produce severe local destruction of tissue.
- *Squamous cell carcinoma:* sunlight is also an important risk factor for this tumour. There are two basic types: the tumour may become invasive and malignant, or it may be cornified, and rarely invasive or malignant, so forming a tumour in situ only.

- *Melanoma:* this is the most common cancer of the skin. As its name implies, it is a cancer of the pigmented melanocytes, especially occurring where the cells are aggregated in a mole. The main promoter seems to be overexposure of melanocytes to UV radiation, leading to a failure to control the cell cycle. The tumour is normally invasive and metastasizes.
- *Kaposi's sarcoma:* this is a malignancy arising from the endothelial cells of skin blood vessels. It is seen especially in immune deficiency state,s e.g. AIDS. The tumour can be rapidly progressive and multifocal. It normally first appears in the lower extremities but then progresses to the upper body.

BOX 16.6 RADIOTHERAPY AND THE SKIN

Radiotherapy for tumours may be by internal or external means. External application exposes the skin to relatively high doses of radiation. The intention of the treatment is to disrupt the cell cycle (see Chapter 2) of tumour cells, but in doing so this will also affect rapidly proliferating normal cells. These include oral, oesophageal and gastrointestinal mucosae, and also the skin. In the skin, local responses occur at the site of application, including reduced cell production and migration in the epidermis, skin thinning and even penetrating lesions of the epidermis or dermis (Porock *et al.*, 1999). The skin becomes more susceptible to irritation, so patients should avoid using lotions or ointments. Skin care is therefore an important feature of care for people undergoing such treatment, and skin assessment an essential part of nursing practice.

Other epidermal cells

Further cell types are found scattered within the epidermis, with the forbidding name of non-pigmented granular dendrocytes ('dendrite' = branch; the characteristics of these cells is that they are melanin-free and granulated, and they have branching processes). These are cells of the immune system. They remain inactive within the epidermis unless the tissue is damaged. They then interact with helper and suppressor T-lymphocytes in assisting immune responses (see Chapter 13), and so form part of the protective function of the skin.

Hair and nails: epidermally derived structures

A quick glance at Figures 16.2 and 16.3 gives the impression that hair and nails are part of the dermis, and simply protrudes through the epidermis, but closer examination of the diagram shows that their base sits within a sheath made of epidermal tissue. Hair and nails are made of the epidermal protein (keratin) and dead cells, and are produced by germinal cells at their base (the hair follicle and nail bed, respectively). These cells are more active than other cells of the epidermis, and require a better blood supply. It therefore makes sense that the follicles and nail beds extend deeper within the skin where blood flow is adequate.

Hair

One function of hair is to protect underlying skin or structures. For example, head hair helps to prevent the heating effect of the sun on brain function, and to reduce heat loss in the cold, while eyebrows protect the eyes from direct sun and from particulate matter in the air. In some areas, notably the surface of the eyelids and in the lips, the presence of hair would affect their delicate functions, so these areas are hairless. In other places, the hair has become sparse (over much of the skin; thought to reduce insulation and aid heat loss), or bristly (in the ears and nose; thought to facilitate functions as filters). However, even where hair is sparse there are touch receptors associated with hairs, and so hair also has a sensory role.

The hair shaft is visible externally. It consists of:

- an inner structure or medulla of granulated cells and air spaces;

- a cortex of melanin-pigmented cells (with extensive air spaces in those people with white hair);

- an outer cuticular layer of heavily keratinized cells (Figure 16.2).

Note that all of these cell types are modifications of those identified in the epidermis.

The hair root consists of the growing region of the hair and a protective sheath. The outer sheath originates from the basal and prickly layers of the epidermis, and the inner

---

BOX 16.7 SKIN CONDITIONS

Conditions associated with infection

Acne vulgaris is an inflammation of sebaceous glands in response to bacterial infection. The problem is particularly noticeable during puberty, when gland activity increases.

Warts are produced by a focus of cells that have divided excessively in response to infection by a virus called a papovavirus.

Cold sores are lesions produced by infection of skin with *Herpes simplex* virus (type I). This virus may lay dormant for long periods, with cold sores appearing only when the virus is 'triggered'. This activation may be in response to factors such as UV light, or the release of sex steroids.

Chickenpox and *shingles* are produced by the *Herpes zoster* virus. Varicella (chickenpox) occurs as a primary infection; zoster (shingles) is usually secondary. Zoster is characterized by pain localized to a single dermatome (an area of skin supplied by branches from a single spinal nerve), followed by vesicle eruptions. Calamine lotion or antiviral drugs offer some relief.

Inflammatory conditions

Acne rosacea is an inflammatory condition of adults; its cause is unknown. It is characterized by facial erythema (red patches) and pustules. Hypersensitivity of the sebaceous glands may occur causing a bulbous appearance.

Eczema is an inflammatory response of skin to chemical agents. The term is synonymous with dermatitis. The cause may be endogenous (e.g. in response to substances within sebum) or exogenous (e.g. allergic contact dermatitis, a type of hypersensitive immune response, or irritant dermatitis, a response that does not entail mediation by the immune system). Erythema (red patches due to blood vessels approaching the skin surface, a process called telangiectasis), scaly texture and itching are usually present, possibly accompanied with oedema and crusting. Scratching exacerbates the latter, so anti-itch preparations may be used to reduce the incidence. Long-term eczema can make skin texture leathery and thickened.

Lupus erythematosus (LE) is an inflammatory disease; its causes are unclear. In discoid (cutaneous) LE the skin, especially of the face, develops lesions that contain immunoglobulin deposits (the cause is unknown, but it may result from sensitization to an antigen). Skin blood vessels are usually prominent, producing red erythematous patches. Sensitivity to UV light is also common. Healing is frequently associated with scarring. In systemic LE, many organs are affected but skin lesions and erythematous patches are again apparent, especially of the face. Photosensitivity is also present.

Inherited conditions

Psoriasis is perhaps the best known example of an inherited skin condition, although most cases do not appear to have a familial link. Skin eruptions occur because mitotic divisions proceed too rapidly.

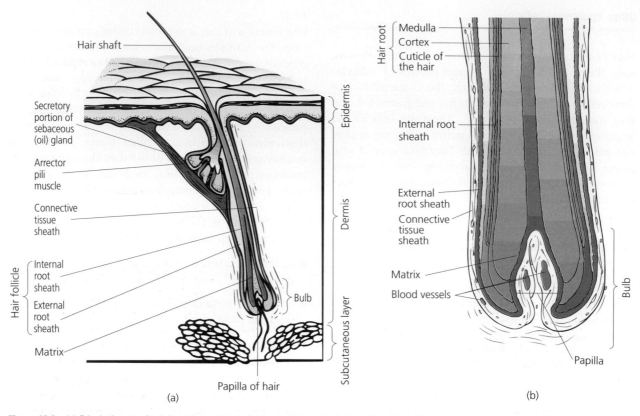

Figure 16.2   (a) Principal parts of a hair and associated structures. (b) Longitudinal section of a hair root.

Q. Describe the structure and functions of hair.

Q. Identify the glands associated with hair.

sheath derives from clusters of germinative cells, called the matrix, which produce new hairs after old ones are shed. About 70–100 hairs are shed from the scalp each day and will be replaced by growth from the matrix. A papilla of connective tissue is present below the matrix, and contains the blood vessels that supply the matrix cells. Collectively the root, matrix and papilla comprise the hair follicle (Figure 16.2(b)).

Sebaceous glands are also associated with hair follicles, although some are also found in hairless skin, such as the lips and eyelids. These glands secrete sebum, an oily mixture of fats, cholesterol, protein, and salts that helps to maintain the suppleness of hair and skin, and aids water-proofing of the epidermis. It also contains bactericidal chemicals. Sebum therefore helps to maintain the condition of the skin (the atmosphere is often drying) and contributes to the protective functions.

Small arrector muscles are also associated with follicles (Figure 16.2(a)). These are a genuine part of the dermis, and when stimulated cause the hairs to stand erect, a

BOX 16.8 HAIR LOSS AND EXCESS

Hair loss

Alopecia is the term used for hair loss. In men, hair follicles on the top of the scalp may be sensitive to male sex steroids (androgens). Typically, there is loss of hair along the frontal hairline, as well as over the scalp. Alopecia may also be observed in women, but there is not usually recession from the frontal hair. Again, androgens have been implicated (note that women produce male steroids from the adrenal gland; see Chapter 19), so the occurrence is more likely postmenopausally. Alopecia areata is the rapid loss of hair from patches of scalp, usually forming rounded, hairless areas. The cause is unknown, but it has been linked to stressful episodes, genetic susceptibility, immune factors and metabolic disorders, such as those of the

thyroid. There is usually permanent regrowth of hair, but this may take 1–3 months. Total hair loss can sometimes occur (alopecia totalis), usually in young people; regrowth is less likely in this form of alopecia.

Hair excess

Hirsutism is excessive hair growth, usually on the face and body. In men, recession of the frontal hairline is also commonly observed. The areas where the hair grows appear to be sensitive to androgens. The occurrence of hirsutism in women may be associated with excessive adrenal gland activity or underactivity of the ovaries (i.e. deficiency of oestrogens), which disturbs the normal oestrogen/androgen ratio.

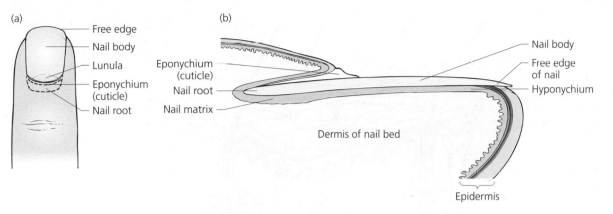

Figure 16.3 Structure of nails. (a) Fingernail viewed from above. (b) Sagittal section of fingernail and nail bed.
Q. Why are nails so hard?

BOX 16.9 NAIL CHARACTERISTICS

Nail formation may be influenced by infection. *Paronychia* is an infection of the cuticle. Inflammation, and sometimes abscess formation, occurs, and the shape of the nails may be affected. *Onychomycosis* is a fungal infection of the nail plate. The nail may be raised because of deposits underneath, and is usually discoloured.

Ageing causes the nails to become thickened and hardened. Older people who become unable to maintain toenail care may become disabled as a consequence. Poorly fitting shoes can exacerbate the problem.

Nail 'colour' is a useful observation for the health of the vascular system. For example, circulatory shock is associated with intense peripheral vasoconstriction, so the nails lose their pink colour. Similarly, a bluish tinge to the nail could indicate systemic hypoxaemia. Anaemia frequently makes the nails appear pale.

Thin or flaking nails could reflect a poor diet: remember that the nails are made primarily of protein (keratin), and they grow continuously from the nail root. Nails that have undergone altered rates of growth may be flecked with pale spots and patches, frequently in a lunar shape that reflects the production across the matrix at the base of the nail.

---

process called piloerection ('pili-' = hair). In animals, this is an important thermoregulatory mechanism; it also occurs during moments of anxiety and alarm (notice how a cat appears to grow in size when alarmed; this is a threatening or defence response). The sparsity of body hair in humans makes these roles much less effective, although the thermoregulatory action probably contributes (see later).

Nails

Fingernails and toenails consist of extremely hard, cornified epidermal cells. They provide protection for the tips of the fingers and toes, and also aid the manipulation of small objects.

The root of the nail is hidden within the nail groove at its base, and largely consists of a germinative matrix that produces cells that will comprise the main nail body (Figure 16.3). The proximal border of the nail and the epidermal cells of the nail groove are lined by a narrow band of epidermis called the cuticle (eponychium). The nail body typically appears pink because the underlying epidermis is thin, so the blood vessels of the dermis are visible. The white crescent (lunula) at the nail base is produced by the obscuring of the dermal blood by the thickened epidermal layer below this part of the nail body.

Dermis

The dermis is the subepidermal layer of the skin. It is composed largely of connective tissue, including collagen and elastin fibres. These protein fibres provide the skin with durability and elasticity. The spaces between the fibres contain many of the structures associated with the skin (Figure 16.4):

● blood vessels;

● nerves;

BOX 16.10 LANGER LINES

These are not actually visible, but relate to the orientation of collagen fibres within the dermis. Surgeons are aware of how the fibres are oriented in parts of the body, and so will often make an incision in the axis of the fibres, rather than across them. The incision will then be stretched to reduce the need to cut further. In this way, scarring is reduced, and the dermis is more likely to regain its structure afterwards.

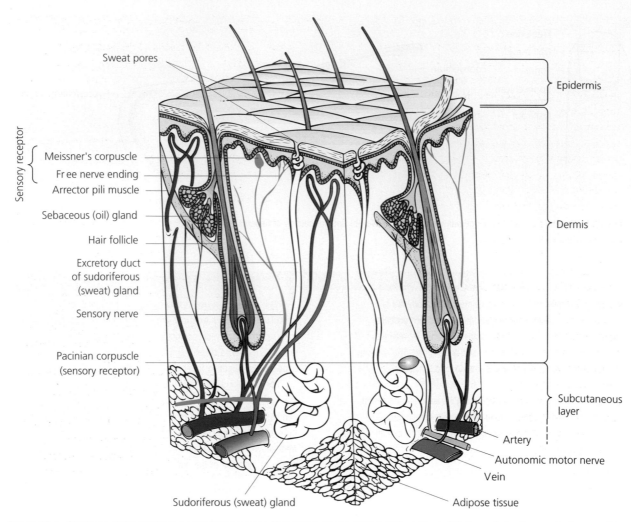

Figure 16.4 Structures of the dermis and subcutaneous layer. Note that hairs are derived epidermally, and that sweat glands are actually present in the subcutaneous layer. Not shown are the collagen/elastin fibres, which form the matrix of the dermis.

Q. Which tissues constitute the dermis, and what are their functions?

Q. List the functions of the subcutaneous adipose tissue.

- sensory receptors (including touch and pressure receptors, thermoreceptors and nociceptors);

- hair follicles (though these are epidermal in origin) and arrector muscles;

- ducts of subcutaneous glands (the glands themselves lie in the subcutaneous layer).

The upper region of the dermis has small projections called dermal papillae. These finger-like structures project into the epidermis. Such papillae contain touch-sensitive receptors (Meissner's corpuscles), and also loops of blood capillaries that supply the active layers of the epidermis. These loops are oriented vertically, and are visible as small pinpricks of blood when the epidermis is grazed.

Subcutaneous layer and glands

This layer consists of loose connective tissue, and adipose tissue. It attaches the dermis to the underlying tissues. The presence of relatively few collagen fibres means that the subcutaneous layer allows flexibility of movement of skin across the underlying tissue, which helps to prevent shearing injuries. The adipose tissue is useful because the subcutaneous layer is readily distended and so can accommodate storage of substantial amounts of fat, and because it provides a layer of insulation to reduce heat transfer from the body to environment (see later).

From a clinical perspective, the presence of loose connective tissue provides an ideal site for injections, since

BOX 16.11 BURNS

A classification of burns based only on the visible extent of surface damage to the skin is now considered too simplistic. The assessment must take into account the depth of injury, whether there is facial injury, whether there are breathing difficulties, and whether the site is prone to infection, e.g. in the perineal area.

Depth of injury is important because it influences the capacity for tissue regeneration. *Partial-thickness injury* (first-degree burn) may be superficial and influence only the epidermis, in which case healing will produce very good restoration of skin structure. Alternatively, there may be deep injury that affects some of the dermis (second- or third-degree burn), in which case wound healing and a degree of regeneration is likely, but some scarring may occur, if the area damaged is not too extensive.

Full-thickness injury (fourth-degree burn) includes the epidermis, dermis and subdermal tissues, such as muscle. This depth of damage will have destroyed any germinal cells and will require skin grafting.

Burns are also now classed as being major, moderate or minor. Assessment includes the area of injury, site, proportion of full-thickness trauma, recognition that children under 10 years have proportionately larger heads than adults (and very young children have immature immunity responses), and recognition that adults over 40 years exhibit poorer homeostatic control as a consequence of the ageing process.

Major burns are those in which:

● more than 25% of the body surface area (BSA) is damaged (more than 20% in children under 10 years and adults over 40 years); or

● more than 10% of BSA exhibits full-thickness injury; or
● the face, hands, feet, or perineal area are badly damaged; or
● there is inhalation injury; or
● there is pre-existing disease, such as poor peripheral circulation.

Moderate burns are those in which:

● 15–25% of BSA is damaged (10–20% in children under 10 years and adults over 40 years); or
● less than 10% of BSA exhibits full-thickness injury.

Minor burns are those in which:

● less than 15% of BSA is damaged (10% in children under 10 years and adults over 40 years); or
● less than 2% of BSA exhibits full-thickness injury.

A further complication of assessment is that electrical burns may be extensive internally, but may not be indicated by external signs.

There are a number of considerations in the intervention against burn injuries (Wiebelhaus & Hansen, 2001). In particular, wound healing must be promoted (including infection control), the flexibility of scar tissue, especially over joints, must be maintained, and fluid balance must be controlled. The effects on fluid balance arise because subepidermal 'wet' tissues are exposed, leading to excessive dehydration. Inflammation of the site also leads to oedematous exudate. The latter is derived from the blood plasma and, if severe, can induce hypovolaemia and shock. Intervention in this case must be aimed at preventing excessive disturbance of fluid balance, and maintaining blood volume and pressure.

BOX 16.12 ULCERATION OF THE SKIN

Ulceration of the skin occurs when areas are subjected to prolonged ischaemia, leading to cell death (necrosis) and tissue atrophy. Decubitus ulcers are commonly observed in people who are immobilized, e.g. people sitting for lengthy spells or confined to bed rest. Under such circumstances, the body weight acts on a point of skin, frequently the buttocks, sacrum or heels, and induces ischaemia. The problem is exacerbated if cutaneous circulation is poor anyway, as in older people or people with diabetes mellitus. In such cases, the skin may ulcerate without the additional effect of weight.

Intervention is aimed at preventing prolonged ischaemia, and by promoting wound healing if ulceration does occur. This latter process, however, can be very slow, since granulation of repair tissue is dependent upon a reasonable blood supply to the area. The management of such wounds continues to provoke debate, especially in relation to the need to maintain hydration, nutrition and oxygenation of the wound. Interested readers are referred to Clancy and McVicar (1997), Patten (2000) and Harding *et al.* (2000).

the volume of injectate is accommodated more easily and is therefore less painful.

The subcutaneous layer also contains two types of gland: sweat (sudoriferous) glands and ceruminous glands (in the external ear). The ducts of these pass to the skin surface via the dermis and epidermis. Mammary glands are specialized sudoriferous glands, but generally they are not considered as glands of the skin; they are described in Chapter 18.

Sweat glands

Sweat, or perspiration, is a mixture of water, salts and products of metabolism (e.g. urea, uric acid, amino acids, ammonia, lactic acid). The glands can be subdivided according to the type of sweat they produce, and therefore to their structure. *Apocrine glands* are simple, tubular structures found in the skin of the armpits (axillae), pubic areas, and the areolar areas of the breast. Their secretion is viscous because they contain metabolic substances such as fatty acids. These are also useful metabolic substrates for bacteria, and growth of such organisms produce body odour. Apocrine sweat also contains pheromones, particularly those that are sexual attractants. Antiperspirants prevent the release of such chemical messengers, which might seem detrimental to sexual attraction – but they also prevent bacterial growth and body odour, and so at least prevent the opposite sex being deterred!

Eccrine glands are distributed more widely, although they are absent from the lip margins, penis, labia minora and outer ear. They are simple, coiled tubular glands, and produce a thin, watery secretion. The main role of eccrine sweat is in temperature regulation, since the evaporation of sweat from the body surface has cooling properties. The composition of eccrine sweat can be varied, however, particularly in relation to its sodium chloride content; this will occur in sodium chloride deficiency when the body is conserving this electrolyte.

Ceruminous glands

These are modified sweat glands found within the skin of the auditory canal. Their secretions are mixed with sebum (from sebaceous glands in the dermis) to form a sticky, wax-like substance called cerumen (earwax). This provides a barrier to particulate matter, and so protects the tympanic membrane. Occasionally, the secretion of cerumen may be excessive and induces conditions that promote troublesome bacterial growth. Hearing will also be impeded if excessive wax is present (Box 16.13).

BOX 16.13 REMOVAL OF EXCESSIVE EARWAX

If earwax becomes excessive, the person may express a muffling of hearing in the ear, or even soreness, as the tympanic membrane becomes inflamed secondary to infection behind the wax. The patient may have the ears syringed to flush out the wax, possibly after a period of several days of softening the wax with a solution applied by dropper. Syringing should be performed using an appropriate ear syringe. An ear syringe has a high degree of inertia that prevents the contents from being expelled at great pressure with a resultant risk of damage to the tympanic membrane; the syringe also has a high volume. Warmed, sterile 'normal' saline is used, since the temperature behind the tympanic membrane will be about 37°C. A kidney dish is held in place against the neck to collect the flushings.

REGULATING BODY TEMPERATURE

Influence of temperature on cellular homeostasis

Metabolic reactions within a cell are influenced by temperature. The optimum temperature for metabolic processes to occur in man is about 37°C. Reactions are generally more efficient if energy is put into them, so temperatures that are suboptimal will reduce the rate of metabolism. In contrast, temperatures that are higher than optimal do not substantially raise the metabolic rate, even though more energy is available to influence the process; in fact, the reverse is eventually observed. This is because the additional heat energy breaks the weak hydrogen bonds between amino acids within enzyme molecules, which disturbs their three-dimensional shape. This denaturing of enzymes results in the loss of specific binding sites (see Chapter 4), with the consequence that their activities as catalysts are diminished. The temperature optimum is therefore a balance between the effects of heat to promote chemical reactions and the rate at which heat denatures enzymes (Figure 16.5).

Cells, and hence physiological systems, will function most efficiently if their temperature is held virtually constant at or close to the optimum. This requires a homeostatic process to balance the rate of heat production by metabolism with the rate of heat transfer between the body and the external environment (i.e. across the skin and respiratory surfaces). At rest, the brain and organs of the chest and abdomen generate some 70–75% of the total metabolic heat, and comprise the body 'core'. Only the temperature of this core is held near constant.

The surface area of skin in the adult is about 1.8 m², and provides the major site of heat transfer between the body and the external environment. The limbs provide the main sites for heat exchange because they have a large surface area relative to their volume. The ambient temperature in the UK usually means that the tissues tend to cool rather than overheat, so the skin in these areas will generally have a much lower temperature than that of the chest and abdomen. Controlling the rate of heat transfer across the skin is an essential component of the regulatory process.

Heat balance

The receptors necessary to detect a change in core temperature are located within the hypothalamus. Brain nuclei

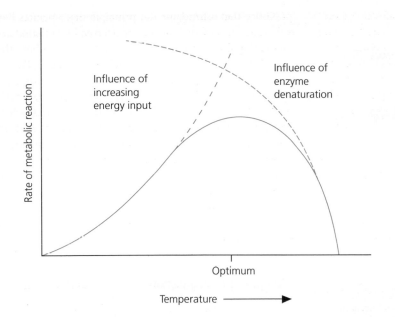

Optimum

Temperature ⟶

Figure 16.5 Influence of temperature on metabolic processes. The balance between the effect of energy (heat) put into the reaction and the thermal denaturization of enzyme (catalyst) structure determines the optimal reaction rate.

Q. *List four factors that determine the rate of metabolic reactions.*

BOX 16.14 MEASURING BODY TEMPERATURE

When body temperature is measured, it is usually the core temperature that is of interest. The tissues of the core are accessible by thermometer via the orifices of the body, namely the mouth, external ear (i.e. from the vicinity of the brain) and the anus (i.e. from the rectum). The core is usually close to the surface near the armpits, so this area can also give a reasonable measure of core temperature if other routes are not possible.

Body temperature is often measured using an electrical thermometer. This has a thermistor incorporated into the tip, the electrical resistance of which changes with its temperature. Such thermometers produce rapid readings and good reproducibility (Braun *et al.*, 1998). They also do not contain mercury, which is a toxic metal.

Recorded temperatures vary slightly according to site, e.g. in adults:

* oral temperature should be very close to 37°C (36.9–37.1°C);
* ear temperatures should be very similar to oral values, but note that values fall sharply if the thermistor is not close to the tympanum;
* rectal temperature is usually slightly higher than the oral value, about 37.5°C;
* axilla (armpit) temperatures are usually slightly lower than oral values, about 36.5°C.

---

within this area provide the monitoring process, and determine the homeostatic set point. Other temperature receptors are found within the skin, and also provide afferent input into the hypothalamus. These receptors (called Ruffini organs and Krause end bulbs) will detect a change in condition at the body surface, and so homeostatic processes can be instigated even before consequential changes in core temperature have occurred. Together, these central and peripheral thermoreceptors provide an efficient means of ensuring core temperature does not change markedly.

If the core temperature of the body is to be kept constant, then the homeostatic equation must hold:

Heat gained by the body = heat lost from the body

Heat gain is that produced by metabolism, although heat will also be gained if the environment is hotter than the body core (e.g. in a hot climate). Heat is lost from the

body if the environment is cooler than the core (the usual case in a temperate climate, such as in the UK), or if evaporation of water can be promoted, since this has a cooling effect (see below).

The physiology of temperature regulation therefore concerns the control of heat gain or loss, appropriate to needs.

Basic principles of heat transfer

Heat can be transferred to or from the environment by three main processes (see Figure 16.6):

* *Radiation.* Any physical body at a temperature above absolute zero (0° kelvin (K) – –273°C) will radiate energy. The wavelength of the energy that is emitted is related to the actual temperature of the body. For example, the sun

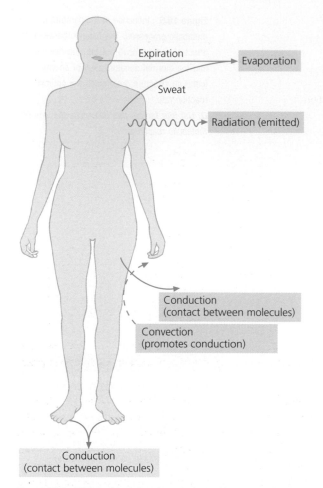

Figure 16.6 Routes of heat loss from the body. Note that heat *gains* by conduction and radiation will be promoted in hot environments.
Q. Discuss what is meant by the following terms with reference to heat transfer: (i) radiation, (ii) conduction, and (iii) evaporation.

Notice that a fundamental principle that operates here is that the rate at which heat is transferred by radiation and conduction is determined by the temperature gradient that exists between the skin and external environment. Thus, if the skin is warmer than the surrounding environment, then heat will be lost from it; the greater the difference, the faster the rate of transfer. If it is cooler, then heat will be gained from the environment. It is the immediate environment that is important here, i.e. the environment in contact with, or close to, the skin surface. Convection of air or water around the skin will introduce new environmental temperatures, and therefore could promote further heat transfer across the skin. Thus, convection may facilitate or even reduce heat transfer, but it is not a means of heat transfer per se.

Temperature regulation in cold climates

In cold or cool environments, the temperature gradient between the air and skin promotes heat loss from the body. Referring back to the equation above, the homeostatic regulation of the core temperature in cold conditions can utilize two strategies (Figure 16.7). First, the response may lower the temperature gradient between skin and air, and so reduce the rate of heat loss. Second, it may increase the rate of metabolic heat production to compensate for enhanced heat loss. Both strategies are applied, but it is convenient to examine each separately.

provides energy at a range of wavelengths, some of which constitute the 'visual' part of the light spectrum. In humans, the radiated energy is in the infrared (IR) region of the spectrum, and can be visualized only by using appropriate aids. Radiated heat is normally the main way by which heat is lost or gained by the body. The rate of transfer is determined by the temperature gradient between the skin and external environment.

- *Conduction.* Conduction is the direct transfer of energy between molecules that have made physical contact with each other. This will include contact between molecules within the skin and those of air or objects in contact with the skin. The rate of transfer is determined by the temperature gradient between the skin and external environment.

- *Evaporation.* Converting water into vapour requires energy (584 cal/ml = 2450 J/ml; this is called the latent heat of evaporation), so the evaporation of sweat from the skin, or of water from the oral cavity and respiratory tract, are effective means of removing heat from the body.

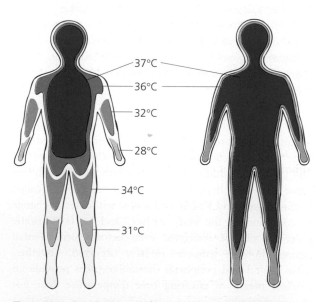

Figure 16.7 Temperature distribution in the body of a person at room temperatures of 20°C (left) and at 35°C (right). At 35°C room temperature, a core temperature of 37°C extends almost to the surface of the body. At 20°C room temperature, the core temperature is restricted to the trunk and head.
Q. Describe the homeostatic regulation of the core temperature when the body is subjected to cold environmental conditions and hot environmental conditions.

Decreasing the skin–air temperature gradient

The strategies used to reduce the temperature gradient between skin and air in a cool environment are the warming of air in contact with the skin, and the reduction of the temperature of the skin itself (Figure 16.8). Air warming can be widespread (e.g. by raising the central heating, or by moving to a warm area) or local to the skin surface. The latter involves the warming of air close to the skin, irrespective of the surrounding air temperature. This is achieved by externally insulating the body, or by physiologically stimulating arrector muscles of the skin that cause piloerection. Both trap an unstirred layer of air against the skin, which warms up rapidly because air has a low specific heat. The specific heat is the heat required to raise the temperature of 1 g of substance (e.g. air) by 1°C. The insulative effect of a layer of warmed air is reduced if air currents dislodge it, i.e. by convection currents, wind chill or fans.

If the body is in water, warming the water close to the skin requires a lot of heat since it has a high specific heat and thus requires a lot of energy to raise its temperature even by 1°C. This is one of the reasons why a person will develop hypothermia rapidly if they fall into a cold sea. However, if a thin layer of water can be confined (unstirred) at the skin surface, it can form an effective insulation layer. Specific heat can act to our advantage: water may require a lot of energy to warm up, but it also has to lose substantive amounts to cool. Thus, once the layer is warmed it cools very slowly; this is the basis of the wetsuit used in water sports.

Reducing the temperature of the skin is achieved by reducing the rate of blood flow to the skin. This is mediated by the activation of sympathetic nerves to the tissue. If conditions are extreme, then blood vessels in deeper subcutaneous tissues, especially in the limbs, will also be constricted. In this way, the parts of the body that are at the core temperature will contract in size (Figure 16.7). In freezing air, the skin may exhibit a paradoxical vasodilation through effects of cold on the blood vessels. Although not profound, this 'flushing' is sufficient to help

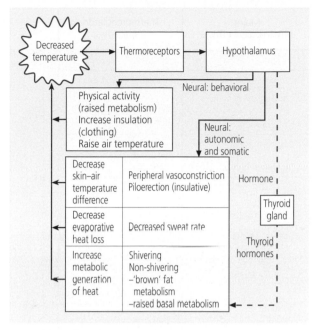

Figure 16.8 Flow chart of thermoregulatory responses to cooling. Note the range of effector mechanisms and tissues employed in the response.

protect the skin from freeze damage. Thus, people may have rosy cheeks even when the weather is extremely cold.

Altering the pattern of blood flow in the limbs is another means of facilitating heat conservation. Venous blood, having cooled near the skin surface (note that the blood supply to skin cannot be stopped entirely), drains into deeper veins that are in close anatomical arrangement with the arteries bringing warm blood into the limb from the core. The close proximity of the vessels, and the opposite direction of blood flow between them, means that the venous blood is warmed by the arterial blood, and so returns some of the heat directly to the core. This arrangement is called a counter-current exchange process.

The loss of heat from skin can be reduced even further by the deposition of fat in subcutaneous tissue, since this acts as an internal insulator that reduces the conduction of heat from within the body to the skin surface.

BOX 16.15 HYPOTHERMIA

Hypothermia is a core temperature below normal limits. It normally arises from prolonged exposure to cold environments, but a tendency toward hypothermia is also observed in people with lowered metabolism arising from deficient thyroid hormone secretion.

The effects of hypothermia on metabolic rate include a reduced heart rate, slowed reflexes, lethargy, and poor mentation (Figure 16.9). Neurological and cardiac functions decline with progressive hypothermia, eventually leading to death. Sometimes, however, the cold produces such a profound decrease in metabolism that survival may actually be enhanced (being metabolically inactive means that cold tissues become hypoxic much more slowly). There are numerous instances of apparently 'miraculous' recoveries in people suffering prolonged cold exposure; the principle of cooling is also used widely in surgery and transplantation.

With a person who is suffering from hypothermia, it is important to raise the body temperature *slowly*, because a sudden rise in blood temperature may promote physiological response to cause heat loss, thus negating the improvements. Cell functions also are not tolerant to sudden temperature changes. Blankets are ideal to prevent further heat loss, allowing heat produced by metabolism to accumulate within the body. Reflective blankets are even better, because not only do they insulate and reduce conduction losses, but they also reduce radiative losses by reflecting heat back onto the skin surface.

Major physiological effects	Thermoregulatory capabilities	°C
Death		
Proteins denature, tissue damage accelerates	Severely impaired	44
Convulsions Cell damage	Impaired	42
Disorientation		40
Systems normal	Effective	38
		36
Disorientation	Impaired	34
Loss of muscle control		32
Loss of consciousness		30
	Severely impaired	28
Cardiac arrest		26
Skin becomes cyanosed	Lost	24
Death		

Figure 16.9 Normal and abnormal body temperatures, and their physiological effects.

Q. Why is it essential that the body has a narrow range of body (core) temperature?

Q. Using information described in Chapter 23, outline how the body temperature fluctuates during a 24-h period.

Increasing the metabolic rate

Chapter 4 explained how most of the energy generated by cellular respiration is not harnessed by the cell, but is lost as heat. Raising the metabolic rate – thermogenesis – is therefore an efficient means of generating additional heat in cold conditions. The means of generating heat can be placed into two categories: shivering and non-shivering thermogenesis.

Shivering is a series of small, repeated, involuntary muscular contraction/relaxation cycles, which increase the metabolic rate of the tissue (Figure 16.8). When shivering, we may feel that the contraction cycles are out of control, but in fact they are being co-ordinated by the hypothalamus, cerebral cortex and cerebellum. Shivering is extremely effective and, if severe, can double a person's total metabolic rate. It is, however, impractical as a long-term solution because it drastically impedes lifestyle, and so is best viewed as a rapid but acute response to cold. Similarly, exercise is another excellent short-term measure to generate additional heat.

Non-shivering thermogenesis involves elevation of the basal metabolic rate, i.e. the rate at which cells generate

energy in the absence of extrinsic stimulation (see Chapter 5). This makes it much more effective as a long-term adaptation to cold conditions. It is especially notable in infants in whom temperature regulatory processes are immature. 'Brown' fat is utilized to provide additional heat in order to compensate for the relatively high heat loss that results from having a high surface area/volume ratio (see Box 16.16). This adipose tissue is found mainly between the shoulder blades and is coloured by the presence of extensive blood vessels (the more familiar white fat has poor vascularization). The tissue is supplied with sympathetic nerves, and it is these that promote metabolism of the stored lipid. Little of the released energy is incorporated into ATP, so almost all of the heat is released into the blood and carried into the core.

The capacity to generate additional heat without the inconvenience of shivering is an attractive mechanism for cold adaptation. Adults do not have brown fat reserves, however, and the evidence for non-shivering thermogenesis in adults in cold or cool climates is controversial. Some findings have implicated an increased release of thyroid hormones in the cold, which would alter basal metabolism throughout the body. This may be an important mechanism to those who live in polar regions, but may be of too slow onset to be useful to those exposed to fluctuating temperatures during a winter season in, for example, the UK.

BOX 16.16 SURFACE AREA/VOLUME RATIO IN INFANTS

Temperature regulatory mechanisms in neonates and infants are immature, and are compounded by the relatively large surface area/volume ratio, as this favours heat loss. The surface area of the skin is the route of heat loss (in cool environments), whereas body volume influences the capacity to generate heat through metabolism. The high ratio in babies means that newborns are very susceptible to environmental temperatures, and so require a protected environment. Heat loss is partially compensated for by a metabolic rate that is relatively higher than in children and adults (non-shivering thermogenesis; see text).

The comfort zone

As we have seen, air temperature that is considerably lower than that of the core temperature promotes responses to conserve heat, primarily by reducing heat transfer to the environment. However, air temperature that is similar to that of the core would also cause major difficulties. This is because heat is generated continually by metabolism, and in order to remain in homeostasis, some of this heat must be lost from the body, otherwise body temperature would rise. This would be made difficult by an absence of a temperature gradient. An air temperature of around 24–25°C will suffice to promote the loss of excess heat with little need to stimulate physiological mechanisms either to conserve it or promote loss. This is termed a 'comfort zone', and provides an ideal temperature for living/working and for inactive people in hospital.

Exercise

When would a room temperature of 24–25°C be uncomfortable? To answer this, think about factors such as inactivity, type of work, presence of fever, surgery, presence of pain, and excessive muscle activity in people with respiratory problems.

Temperature regulation in hot climates

An air temperature above the comfort zone means that the rate of heat loss to the environment will begin to decrease, so the balance between heat gained from metabolism and that lost from the body will be disturbed. Referring to the heat balance equation from earlier, metabolic rates are little changed in hot spells, although appetite may be reduced, and so heat loss from the body must now be promoted. This will be the case especially if metabolism is increased, e.g. by physical activity.

The strategies employed are to elevate the skin–air temperature gradient, and to promote sweat production. Again, both strategies will be used at the same time, but it is convenient to consider them separately.

Elevating the skin–air temperature gradient

In many ways, these responses are the opposite of those described above for cold environments. The air temperature close to the skin may be cooled by reducing insulation (e.g. removing clothing, reducing piloerection) and by introducing air convection, while skin temperature is raised by vasodilation within the skin, which effectively expands the core area into the periphery (Figure 16.7).

Some areas of skin, such as the hands, are very efficient at losing heat because they have a high surface area. A diagram of the cutaneous vasculature in these areas is shown in Figure 16.10. The feature to note is the presence of arterial-venous anastomoses, i.e. vessels that connect arterioles directly to venules. Dilation of these arterioles shunts blood directly into the venous system, bypassing capillaries, and so more blood per unit time can perfuse these areas.

Finally, the counter-current exchange process identified earlier that helps to conserve heat in the cold would be counterproductive in warm weather, and so must be made

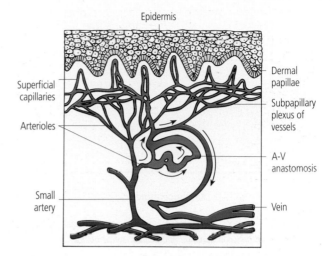

Figure 16.10 Arrangement of blood vessels in skin of the finger. Note the arterial-venous anastomosis. When patent, this will substantially increase the rate of blood flow through the skin (→).
Q. Identify two situations when you would expect the skin vessels to vasodilate.

less effective. This is achieved by directing venous blood draining the limb away from the deep veins (which lie adjacent to incoming arteries) to more superficial vessels, thus reducing the heat transfer from the arteries. This helps to explain why surface veins are more noticeable in warm weather, or if someone is hot from fever, or after exercise.

Sweat production

As air temperature rises and begins to approach the core temperature, the capacity for changes in cutaneous blood flow to sustain an appropriate temperature gradient declines. Under these circumstances, the evaporation of sweat from the body surface becomes the most effective means of removing heat from the body. Indeed, at very high air temperatures (>37°C), when the temperature gradient is actually reversed, heat gain from the air will be promoted and so evaporation is the only physiological response available for temperature regulation (Figure 16.11; Table 16.1). Sweating is mediated by autonomic (sympathetic) nervous activity, and secretion rates may be as high as 4 l/day. This figure is put into perspective if we consider that the average volume of urine produced in 24 h in a climate such as that of the UK is only about 1.5 l.

Note, however, that sweating will be effective at reducing body temperature only if it can evaporate from the skin surface. High atmospheric humidity reduces the effect since the more saturated with water the air becomes, the less likely it is that sweat will evaporate.

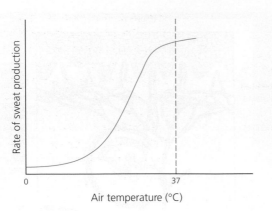

Figure 16.11 Influence of air temperature on the rate of sweat production.
Q. Differentiate between apocrine and eccrine sweat glands.

Table 16.1 The relative rates of heat loss via evaporative and non-evaporative means. Note the relative importance of evaporative heat loss at high air temperatures

Air temperature (°C)	20	25	30	35	40
Evaporative heat loss (% of total)	15	30	50	95	100
Non-evaporative heat loss (% of total)	85	70	50	5	0

Q. How does the process of evaporation promote heat loss?
Q. What would happen if air humidity was high?

BOX 16.17 SWEAT SECRETION IN SHOCK

Shock illustrates the role of the sympathetic nervous system in promoting sweat secretion. In circulatory shock, sympathetic activity is stimulated by the need to maintain blood pressure in the face of failing cardiovascular functioning. The symptoms of shock include a cool, pale skin as a consequence of increased peripheral resistance (see Chapter 12). Paradoxically, the patient will sweat. Clearly the sweating is not due to an elevated core temperature. It is, in fact, a secondary occurrence of the sympathetic outflow from the brain (ordinarily, such outflow would be observed in stress or exercise when losing heat by sweating would be entirely appropriate).

BOX 16.18 BODY TEMPERATURE REGULATION IN ELDERLY PEOPLE

Ageing reduces the basal metabolic rate, decreases the effectiveness of autonomic activity to the skin, reduces the capacity to shiver (and to co-ordinate it), and decreases the numbers of sweat glands in the skin. Physiological regulation of core temperature is therefore less precise, with the result that it is more likely to move outside the homeostatic range, and perhaps remain outside, depending on environmental conditions. Elderly people are therefore at much greater risk of hypothermia during cold spells (see Box 16.15), and hyperthermia in extremely hot weather (see Box 16.19), than younger people.

BOX 16.19 HYPERTHERMIA AND FEVER

Hyperthermia

Hyperthermia is an elevation of core temperature above normal limits. It may arise because of an inability to maintain an appropriate rate of heat loss (e.g. in hot climates) or because of elevated metabolism (e.g. transiently after heavy exercise, or chronically in excessive thyroid hormone secretion states).

Neural tissues are most susceptible to a change in core temperature, and nerve conduction velocity decreases at high temperatures as enzymes denature. Depending upon severity, the consequences are headache, mental confusion, delirium and lethargy (Figure 16.9). Disruption of integrative neural processes will also affect the control of other tissues already disturbed by the hyperthermia.

Fever

Hyperthermia arising from a fever (pyrexia) is an indication that pathogenic infection has occurred. In this case, the elevated temperature observed is a physiological response to the presence of substances (called pyrogens) released by the pathogens themselves, and/or by certain cells of the immune system that are activated by the infection. The pyrogens act on the hypothalamus to alter the set point, perhaps to 39°C or so, and hence even a normal body temperature will be recognized by monitoring areas of the hypothalamus as being too low. The person will then express feelings of being cold. Physiological mechanisms such as shivering and vasoconstriction in the skin are implemented that raise the core temperature to the new homeostatic mean (Figure 16.12), so the person appears pale. In clinical terms, this represents a hyperthermia, but note that it is induced physiologically.

As the pathogen is destroyed by immune responses, a point is reached when the amount of pyrogen released cannot sustain the new hypothalamic set point, and this then reverts to normal. The pyrexic temperature is now in excess of the homeostatic mean, and the person will feel hot. Heat loss is promoted by vasodilation in the skin and sweating, so the skin will appear flushed and clammy.

The advantage of such a process is that the pyrexia interferes with the metabolic enzymes of the pathogen, reducing its reproductive activities and making it more susceptible to attack by the immune system. The disadvantage is that our own metabolic processes are also affected and make us feel ill. The level of hyperthermia that necessitates treatment is debatable. Some authorities advocate a temperature of 38°C or above. Interventions usually involve paracetamol or nonsteroidal anti-inflammatory drugs such as aspirin, since these influence the actions of pyrogens.

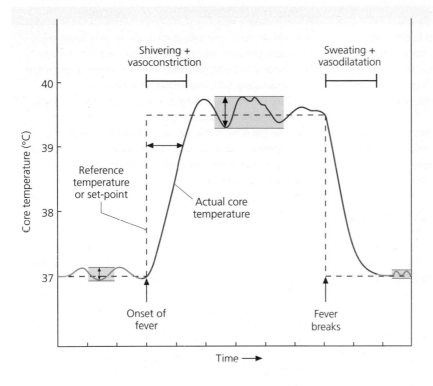

Figure 16.12 Time course of a typical febrile episode. The actual body temperature lags behind the rapid shifts in set points. Note that regulation is normally maintained during the fever but that it is less precise, so temperature fluctuations are generally greater than normal.

Q. Describe the physiological changes associated with pyrexia (fever).

Q. What chemical initiates pyrexia. Refer to Chapter 13 if you have difficulty in answering this question.

Factors that influence core temperature

If the temperature regulatory mechanisms are intact, then the core temperature is regulated extremely well, with very little variation about the set point (about 37°C), although very hot air temperature or high humidity may cause difficulties in maintaining heat loss, and may even promote a slight hyperthermia. The actual set point, however, is subject to slight variations within and between individuals, and core temperature changes accordingly, although only by perhaps 0.5°C or so.

Circadian rhythmicity

Body temperature displays a 24-h rhythmicity linked into the day–night cycle. However, it can be synchronized to match activity–rest cycles (see Chapter 23).

Sex differences

Generally speaking, there is little difference between the core temperature of men and women. In women, however, there is a slight decrease in body temperature a few days before menstruation, which is maintained during the preovulatory phase of the menstrual cycle. The change is less than 0.5°C, and appears to be associated with the low secretion of the hormone progesterone during this period. After ovulation, body temperature rises again; the correlation between this rise in temperature and ovulation is useful in family planning, although the smallness of the change may make it difficult to observe.

Age

We noted earlier that babies utilize non-shivering thermogenesis to elevate basal metabolism and compensate for excessive rates of heat loss. The core temperature in young children (37.5–38°C) is actually higher than that found in adults.

Summary

1 The skin is the largest organ of the body. Its functions are associated closely with it being the physical barrier between the body and external environment. It is protective but also has a vital role to play in the regulation of body temperature.

2 The skin consists of three layers: the epidermis, dermis and subcutaneous layers.

3 The epidermis forms the outer layer; it consists of cells that eventually form the tough keratinized outer surface.

4 Nails and hair are modified epidermal structures that project into the dermis, a layer of connective tissue that contains blood vessels, neurons and various other structures.

5 The subcutaneous layer contains the sweat glands, the ducts of which project through the dermis and epidermis. Sweat performs an important role in temperature regulation, but also influences fluid balance and provides a protective role.

6 Body temperature regulation is essential if the functioning of vital tissues is to be optimal, so the temperature of the body 'core' is controlled tightly.

7 Constancy of 'core' body temperature can be achieved only if heat generation from metabolism is balanced by appropriate rates of heat loss, particularly across the skin. Changes in heat exchange with the environment are the main responses to adverse environments, but changes in the metabolic rate may also play a role, particularly in cold environments.

8 The role of the skin in conserving or promoting heat loss is facilitated by its structure, by the influence of sympathetic nerves on its blood supply, and by the presence of sweat glands.

9 Hyperthermia and hypothermia usually represent states in which the capacity to regulate body temperature is inadequate or has been compromised. The exception is hyperthermia produced by fever. Fever is a physiological response to infection, and results from a resetting of the homeostatic set point. It probably helps to reduce the metabolic activity of the invading pathogen and so reduces the rate of spread of infection.

10 Factors such as circadian rhythmicity and ovulation influence 'core' temperature.

Review questions

1 The skin is the most visible part of the body. If it remains intact, it provides us with vital functions. What are these functions?

2 Observation of skin colour and condition forms a vital clue to the wellbeing of patients without the need for invasive tests. What causes the same person's face to appear pale one minute and flushed another? Why do you go pale if feeling unwell? What other situations may cause paleness?

3 What do the terms 'vasodilation' and 'vasoconstriction' mean?

4 Identify the layers of the skin, the epidermis, dermis and hypodermis. Find out which structures are found in each of these layers. If a region of skin is burned badly, it is referred to as a full-thickness burn. Why will the patient now feel no pain in that area? Consider the effects a large area of burned skin will have on the whole body, bearing in mind the functions you have identified. Make a list of the types of damage that can occur to the skin. Think about how the body deals with these situations to lessen their consequences.

5 How does the skin protect itself from the harmful effects of ultraviolet (UV) rays in sunlight? What are the advantages and disadvantages of sunlight to the skin?

6 What is keratin? What is its function?

7 How does the body ensure that internal organs remain at a constant temperature (vital for optimum cell functioning) even though the external temperature changes so dramatically?

8 What role does the skin play in thermoregulation?

9 Think about how the body generates and loses heat. Consider what your body does when you are in a cold environment. Define the terms 'evaporation', 'radiation', 'convection' and 'conduction'.

10 What is hypothermia? How may it affect body functioning? What treatment would the nurse offer?

11 What is hyperthermia? How may it affect body functioning? Which patient groups are particularly at risk of disorders of thermoregulation, and why?

12 What are febrile convulsions?

REFERENCES

Braun, S.K., Preston, P. and Smith, R.N. (1998) Getting a better read on thermometry. *Registered Nurse* **61**(3): 57–60.

Clancy, J. and McVicar, A. (1997) Wound healing: a series of homeostatic responses. *British Journal of Theatre Nursing* **7**(4): 25–34.

Donato, M.C., Novicki, D.C. and Blume, P.A. (2000) Skin grafting: historical and practical approaches. *Clinics in Podiatric Medicine and Surgery* **17**(4): 561–98.

Francis, A. (1998) Nursing management of skin graft sites. *Nursing Standard* **12**(33): 41–4.

Harding, K., Cutting, K. and Price, P. (2000) The cost-effectiveness of wound management protocols of care. *British Journal of Nursing* **9**(19 suppl): S6–27.

Patten, J. (2000) A case study in evidence-based wound management. *British Journal of Nursing* **9**(12 suppl): S38–49.

Porock, D., Nikoletti, S. and Kristjanson, L. (1999) Management of radiation skin reactions: literature review and clinical application. *Plastic Surgical Nursing* **19**(4): 185–92.

Wiebelhaus, P. and Hansen, S.L. (2001) What you should know about managing burn emergencies. *Nursing* **31**(1): 36–42.

Chapter 17

Posture and movement

Introduction
Overview of skeletal muscle anatomy and physiology
Muscle contraction

Control of posture and movement
References

INTRODUCTION

The skeletomuscular system enables us to maintain a posture against gravity, and to move in a co-ordinated way. Failure to maintain the contraction of appropriate muscles, the flexibility of joints, or adequate bone strength rapidly induces inadequate mobilization. This might be an inability to cope with, say, stairs or distance walking, or an inability to withstand gravity and therefore maintain an upright posture.

Lack of mobility can lead to a dependency on mobility aids or other people, in order to perform basic activities of daily living. Postural problems can become exacerbated with time, compounding the difficulty, and may lead to

further problems, e.g. difficulties in breathing may be experienced, and changes in cardiovascular and digestive functions become apparent.

Chapter 3 considered the supporting role of the skeleton, but also noted how the presence of joints within it means that maintaining a posture against gravity would not be possible without the actions of muscles to stabilize them. The muscles must also be capable of imparting movement; the control of posture and movement are part of the same mechanisms. This chapter considers how muscles associated with the skeleton enable posture to be maintained, and how they enable movements to be made.

BOX 17.1 MOBILIZING

Mobilizing is fundamental to many areas of practice. It has a number of beneficial actions. In addition to getting people moving again and encouraging independence, mobilizing:

- prevents loss of bone mass by helping to maintain the density of bone mineral (see Chapter 3);
- prevents loss of muscle protein, since muscle mass is influenced by the workload;

- prevents contractures from developing, and so helps to maintain joint flexibility;
- improves blood circulation through the limbs, and so reduces the likelihood of venous thrombosis (see also Chapters 11 and 12).

Dependency on others or on mobility aids, and the accompanying effects on body image, can have a severe influence on both physical and psychological wellbeing.

OVERVIEW OF SKELETAL MUSCLE ANATOMY AND PHYSIOLOGY

Muscles consist of cells that are capable of changing their length and shape. Three types of muscle tissue are found in the body: smooth, cardiac and skeletal. All utilize similar means of contracting, but have different cellular anatomies, rates of contraction and control mechanisms. Skeletal muscle is associated with the movement (or prevention of movement) of the skeleton, and so it is this type of muscle that we consider in detail in this chapter.

Most skeletal muscle lies immediately below the skin. There are over 600 muscles in the body. Some are tiny, e.g. those muscles that move the ossicles of the middle ear, whereas others are substantial, e.g. the gluteus maximus of the buttock. Studying fully labelled diagrams of the body musculature can be bewildering, as the reader is confronted with many muscle names, such as the levator palpebrae superioris. As with much of anatomical nomenclature, that of muscles is classical, and relates to various features of the muscle, for example:

- shape, e.g. the deltoid muscle of the shoulder is delta- or triangle-shaped;

- size, e.g. the gluteus maximus muscle of the buttock;

- location, e.g. the tibialis anterior lies in front of the tibia bone of the shin;

- attachments, e.g. the sternohyoid muscle is attached to the sternum and hyoid bones;

- number of 'heads' of muscle origin, e.g. the biceps muscle of the upper arm has two 'heads'('cep-' = head);

- movement type, e.g. levator indicates that a muscle lifts something;

- axis of muscle fibres relative to bone, e.g. transversus.

Clearly, there is no common approach to naming muscles. In fact, the situation is even more complex because frequently the nomenclature of muscles relates to one or more features, e.g. in the levator (= 'lifter') palpebrae (= 'lip') superioris (= 'upper') mentioned above, the name indicates both its position and action.

It is beyond the scope of this book to consider all muscles individually, and the interested reader is referred to the many available texts that do so. There are, however, some aspects of muscle structure and function that must be described if the role of muscle in determining posture and movement is to be understood. These are muscle architecture and general anatomy, muscle histology, and the mechanism of muscle contraction.

Muscle architecture and general anatomy

Generally speaking, each muscle has a wide central region, or belly, and two ends that attach to other tissues, usually bone or cartilage (Figure 17.1). Some muscles have more than one attachment at the same end, e.g. biceps and quadriceps. The connection to bone is provided by means of tough cords of connective tissue called tendons (Figure 17.1(a)). These are extensions of the connective tissue that forms an integral part of the structure of the muscle and bone, and they therefore provide continuity between muscle and bone.

The largest single tendon in the body is the Achilles tendon, named after the Greek hero, which attaches the large muscle of the calf (the gastrocnemius) to the heel bone (calcaneus; the technical name for the tendon is the calcaneal tendon). In some parts of the body, the tendons of muscles combine to form a larger sheet-like structure called an aponeurosis. Such structures are found, for example, in the abdominal wall and in the palms of the hands.

Muscles are covered in layers of dense, connective tissue called the deep fascia (there is also a superficial fascia, or subcutaneous layer, between muscle and skin; see Chapter 16). For many muscles, the deep fascia acts to separate them, and so facilitates their independent functioning (Figure 17.2(a)).

Below the deep fascia lie three distinct sheaths of connective tissue that provide support for the muscle fibres and whole muscle, and also convey blood vessels, lymphatic vessels and nerves into the muscle structure. These sheaths are:

- *the epimysium ('epi-' = upon, 'myo-' = muscle):* encloses the entire muscle;

- *the perimysium ('peri-' = around):* extends from the epimysium into the muscle, and encloses bundles of muscle cells, which are elongated cylindrical cells that lie parallel to each other. The length of skeletal muscle cells means that they are often referred to as muscle fibres (Figure 17.2(b)). Each bundle of muscle fibres is called a fascicle;

- *the endomysium ('endo-' = inner):* covers individual muscle fibres.

Muscle size and fascicle organization

Muscles vary considerably in size, according to how many muscle fibres are present, the diameter of individual fibres, and the length of the muscle belly. These are all features related to the role of the particular muscle. For a given muscle, its size is, to a large extent, predetermined because the length of the belly and the number of muscle fibres are developmental features. However, the amount of work a muscle is persistently required to do is also a determining factor (see Box 17.2).

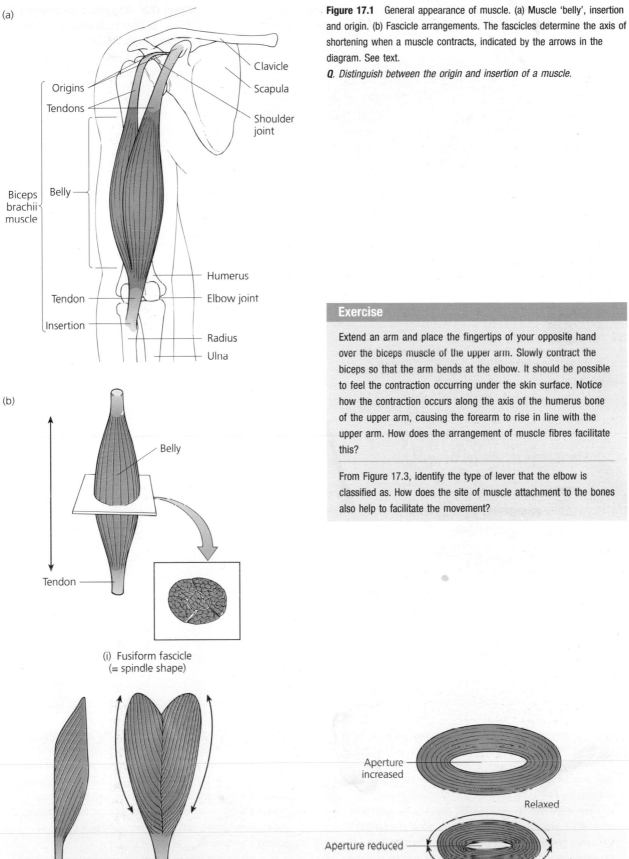

(a)

Biceps brachii muscle

Origins
Tendons
Belly
Tendon
Insertion

Clavicle
Scapula
Shoulder joint
Humerus
Elbow joint
Radius
Ulna

Figure 17.1 General appearance of muscle. (a) Muscle 'belly', insertion and origin. (b) Fascicle arrangements. The fascicles determine the axis of shortening when a muscle contracts, indicated by the arrows in the diagram. See text.
Q. Distinguish between the origin and insertion of a muscle.

(b)

Belly

Tendon

(i) Fusiform fascicle
(= spindle shape)

Unipennate   Bipennate

(ii) Pennate fascicle

Aperture increased
Relaxed

Aperture reduced
Contracted

(iii) Circular fascicle

Exercise

Extend an arm and place the fingertips of your opposite hand over the biceps muscle of the upper arm. Slowly contract the biceps so that the arm bends at the elbow. It should be possible to feel the contraction occurring under the skin surface. Notice how the contraction occurs along the axis of the humerus bone of the upper arm, causing the forearm to rise in line with the upper arm. How does the arrangement of muscle fibres facilitate this?

From Figure 17.3, identify the type of lever that the elbow is classified as. How does the site of muscle attachment to the bones also help to facilitate the movement?

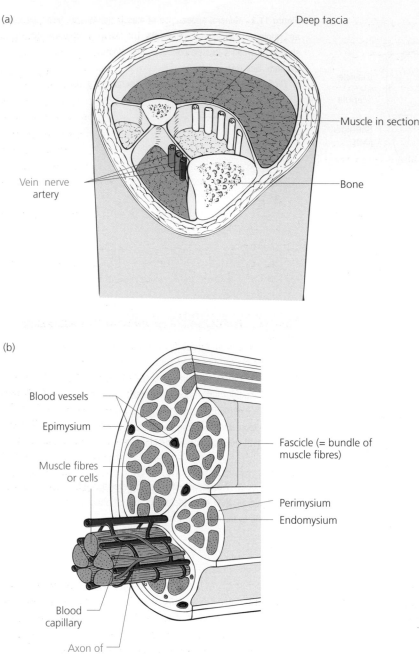

(a)

Deep fascia

Muscle in section

Vein nerve artery

Bone

(b)

Blood vessels

Epimysium

Muscle fibres or cells

Fascicle (= bundle of muscle fibres)

Perimysium

Endomysium

Blood capillary

Axon of motor neuron

Figure 17.2 Connective tissue sheathing of muscle. (a) Deep fascia between muscles. (b) Sheaths within a muscle.

Q. Name the connective tissue surrounding muscle fibres, separating them into fascicles.

BOX 17.2 WORKLOAD AND MUSCLE SIZE

The diameter of individual muscle fibres, and thus the muscle itself, may be altered by the work performed by the muscle. For example, regularly lifting heavy weights stimulates protein synthesis in the muscles used (e.g. the biceps of the upper arm), which will in time lead to a greater muscle mass. The strength of the muscle correlates with its cross-sectional diameter, so the increased mass should be viewed as being an adaptive response.

Conversely, someone who is immobile will use their muscles less frequently, with less load bearing, so the muscle protein content will fall accordingly. Such changes can be identified from urine analysis very soon after confinement. Similar processes also operate on smooth and cardiac muscle. For example, the heart enlarges if a person undertakes regular exercise, and so provides a greater stroke volume (and lower heart rate) than if little or no exercise is performed.

This influence of load on muscle mass is sometimes explained by the maxim 'use it or lose it'.

Understanding the relationship between workload and muscle mass helps in recognizing why postural muscles in the body are so substantial. Upon standing, such muscles must support the joints that are particularly subjected to the force of gravity. The bulk of these muscles provides a reminder of how significant this force is:

- The erector spinae muscles of the back (a group of muscles with several components) have to be substantial to stabilize the back and so facilitate an erect vertebral column and head.

- The gluteus maximus of the buttock has to be substantial to stabilize the hip joint against gravity, and so facilitate an erect posture.

- The quadriceps femoris of the thigh has to be substantial to stabilize the knee joint against gravity and so facilitate leg extension.

Exercise

The amount of work done (by a person or machine) is calculated as:

$$\text{Work} = \text{force} \times \text{distance}$$

An athlete who regularly lifts heavy weights exhibits a change in muscle bulk leading towards a 'Mr Universe' physique. Another athlete who regularly runs marathons may be super-fit but will have a very slim, wiry physique. From the discussion in the text, it should be clear that the muscle adaptation shown by the weight lifter is due to their performing more work. Yet a marathon runner will run 26 miles, so why don't their muscles enlarge? To answer this, we need to consider the weight that is being moved in a *single* muscle contraction. In the runner, this equates approximately with taking a single step.

How does the principle identified here relate to (i) the enlargement of the heart in response to arterial hypertension; (ii) rehabilitation following a myocardial infarction; (iii) physiotherapy following an injury?

The arrangement of fascicles and tendons influences the appearance of muscle (Figure 17.1(b)). For example, the fascicles may run in parallel to the long axis of the muscle, in which case the muscle is referred to as either a fusiform (spindle shaped; the muscle has a distinct belly) or a strap type. Fusiform types, such as the biceps of the upper arm, are generally able to generate a greater force of contraction than strap types, such as the rectus abdominis muscle of the anterior abdomen wall, because the muscle belly is more substantial. Note that the arrangement of fascicles will mean that the muscle fibres that make up a fascicle will also be in the long axis of the muscle. Thus, contraction will shorten the muscle along this axis.

Fascicles may also be arranged obliquely to the long axis of the muscle to give the muscle a feather-like appearance (Figure 17.1(b)). These are referred to as pennate-type muscles ('penna' = feather) and are generally stronger than strap or fusiform types. The direction of contraction will follow the fascicles, so pennate muscles will shorten in more than one axis. An example is the deltoid muscle of the shoulder, which is particularly important in maintaining the position of the shoulder girdle. The shoulder is a ball-and-socket joint, with a wide degree of possible movement, so a pennate type of muscle provides useful support here.

Finally, fascicles may be arranged in a circular pattern around an aperture (Figure 17.1(b)). Contraction of these muscles causes a change in aperture size. They are found around the mouth, for example, and also form the external sphincters around the anus and urethra.

Muscle arrangement in relation to associated bones

The contraction of a skeletal muscle will usually cause a bone to move, but normally only the bone to which one end of the muscle is attached will move. This is called the insertion end of the muscle; the stationary end is called the origin. The mode of movement varies, however, according to the particular situation, and sometimes the origin end becomes the insertion end. In other words, such terms are relative, but are useful when disorders of specific movements are considered.

Levers

The force of contraction developed by a muscle must be sufficient to move the load placed on it. That is, the muscle will have to work against the weight of the bone and tissues or materials associated with bone (i.e. tissues, body weight, or perhaps an object to be lifted). While the generation of adequate power is facilitated partly by the arrangement of fascicles within the muscle, the leverage provided by the position of muscle insertion relative to the joint to be controlled is also a determining factor.

By causing bones to move, skeletal muscles are utilizing a system of levers (Figure 17.3). The bone to be moved acts as the 'arm' of the lever, which will move about the joint or fulcrum. The resistance to be overcome is the load. The arrangement of muscle, lever arm and fulcrum varies (referred to as type 1, 2 or 3 levers), but a general feature is that the further the muscle insertion is away from the fulcrum, the greater the leverage will be. In this way, more power can be generated when the insertion is some distance from the joint than if the same muscle was inserted close to the joint. The movement will be slower, however.

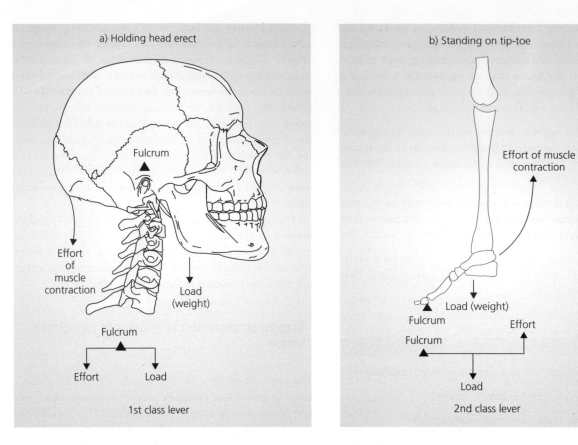

a) Holding head erect

Fulcrum

Effort
of
muscle
contraction

Load
(weight)

Fulcrum

Effort   Load

1st class lever

b) Standing on tip-toe

Effort of muscle
contraction

Load (weight)

Fulcrum

Effort

Fulcrum

Load

2nd class lever

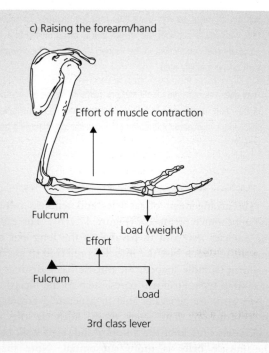

c) Raising the forearm/hand

Effort of muscle contraction

Fulcrum

Load (weight)

Effort

Fulcrum

Load

3rd class lever

Figure 17.3 Skeletomuscular levers. The three classes of lever are shown. These differ in the arrangement between the pivotal point (fulcrum), the position of the load (weight), and the direction of muscle contraction (effort) that is required to move the load.

Q. What is the function of the following muscles: (i) an agonist (prime mover), (ii) a synergist, and (iii) an antagonist?

Levers enable considerable forces to be generated. Without leverage, it would, for example, be difficult to stand from a squatting position unless we had a much greater muscle bulk. Levers also help us to lift considerable weights, again without the need for excessively bulky muscles.

Structure of muscle fibres

Skeletal muscle cells have numerous nuclei. This identifies that a skeletal muscle 'cell' is actually derived from a large number of cells that have fused to form a long fibre-like structure (Figure 17.4). Indeed, we noted earlier that 'muscle fibre' is a term used synonymously with 'muscle cell'. Many muscle fibres are as long as the muscle itself; as some muscles are very large, e.g. the quadriceps femoris of the thigh, then some fibres may be as long as 30 cm. The advantage of this differentiation is that the entire muscle fibre functions as though it were a single cell, so a muscle can be induced to contract rapidly and efficiently throughout its length.

Each muscle fibre is surrounded by a plasma membrane with some specialized functions. In order to distinguish it from that of other cells, it is called the *sarcolemma* ('sarco-' = flesh). Below this is a layer of cytoplasm (the *sarcoplasm*) within which can be seen organelles. Many organelles within the muscle fibre are identical to those found in cells elsewhere, since many of the metabolic activities of the fibre will be identical to those in other cells, but some are modified (Figure 17.4(a)). For example the *sarcoplasmic reticulum* is analogous to the endoplasmic reticulum of other cells (see

Chapter 2), but it extends into the fibre and helps to convey calcium ions for activation of the contractile process (see below). Before release, calcium ions are stored in distended areas of the sarcoplasmic reticulum called *cisternae*; these also take up the ions after the contraction has finished. The

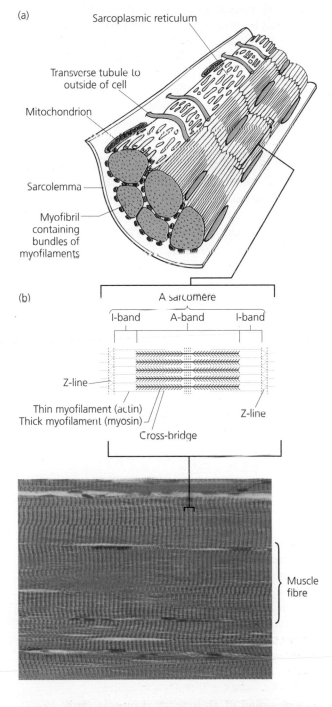

(a)

(b)

(c)

Figure 17.4 Muscle histology and microfilament arrangement. (a) Intracellular features. (b) Filament arrangement. I-band: striation due to actin filaments only. A-band: striation due to myosin and myosin/actin overlap. (c) Light microscopy photograph of a muscle fibre to show striations.
Q. Identify the scientific names of thin and thick muscle fibres.

sarcolemma also has tubular invaginations called transverse or T-tubules; these are responsible for conveying electrical signals from the sarcolemma to the cisternae when the muscle cell is stimulated, resulting in the release of calcium ions from the stores.

The inner core of the muscle fibre is comprised of numerous minute fibre-like structures called *myofibrils*. These run longitudinally inside the fibre, in close association with the sarcoplasmic reticulum and its cisternae. Each fibril consists of a precise arrangement of smaller, thread-like structures of protein called *myofilaments* (Figure 17.4(a)). Microscopically, the myofilaments appear as overlapping thick and thin threads: thick ones are composed of a protein called myosin, and thin ones of a protein called actin (Figure 17.4(b); see also *Details of muscle contraction* below).

The arrangement of myosin and actin shown in Figure 17.4(b) is precise and repeats along the length of the muscle fibre in distinct functional segments. Each segment of banding is called a *sarcomere* ('meros' = part). When viewed under the microscope, a banding pattern is apparent in each sarcomere: a pale band of actin only (the I-band), and a darker band where actin and myosin overlap (the A-band). Intermediate banding occurs, e.g. where myosin is found alone. The arrangement makes the fibre appear to have stripes of light and dark areas, so skeletal muscle is frequently referred to as striped or striated muscle (Figure 17.4(c)).

BOX 17.4 ALTERED MUSCLE FUNCTION DUE TO FIBRE DEFECTS

Muscle weakness due to fibre defects occurs if the fibre is deficient in protein filaments, if the sarcolemma structure prevents it from being electrically stimulated, or if there is a metabolic defect:

- *Protein deficiency*. Fibre protein is affected adversely in malnutrition and diabetes mellitus, when the protein is utilized as an energy substrate, and in prolonged immobility, when the lack of physical stress removes the need for muscles to produce a large force of contraction. Correction of muscle fibre disorder is directed at removing the underlying causes, and physiotherapy to maintain existing muscle.
- *Sarcolemma disorder*. *Myotonia* is a hyperexcitability of the sarcolemma, arising from a defect that makes it difficult for the membrane to repolarize after being stimulated. Without

adequate repolarization, the muscle demonstrates progressive weakness. *Duchenne's muscular dystrophy* is a sex-linked inherited defect in the gene for a sarcolemma protein called dystrophin. The lack of dystrophin leads to eventual wastage typical of this disorder. Another sarcolemma disorder, *periodic paralysis*, is poorly understood. It is characterized by intermittent episodes of muscle weakness. In some cases, the problem seems to be linked to hyperkalaemia.

- *Metabolic deficiency*. These problems are rare, and include defects in the breakdown of glycogen from muscle stores (to provide glucose for respiration) or in the formation of creatine phosphate (for ATP production). This group of disorders includes *toxic alcohol myopathy*, in which cramps and severe weakness arise as a consequence of alcohol abuse.

MUSCLE CONTRACTION

The contraction of a muscle necessitates the contraction of the muscle fibres of which it is comprised. Common processes are involved in contracting the individual fibres, but the behaviour of the whole muscle, and the actual tension developed within it as a consequence of contraction, can vary. This section considers initially the chemical events that occur when a muscle fibre contracts, then continues by exploring whole muscle responses.

Contraction of an individual muscle fibre

Sliding filament mechanism

Before reading this section, ensure that you are familiar with muscle fibre structure, as outlined above.

A muscle fibre contracts when it is stimulated by an associated nerve cell, and results from an interaction between the myosin and actin proteins. The interaction entails a movement of the actin protein filaments over the myosin. This process is usually referred to as the sliding filament theory of muscle fibre contraction. This is an unfortunate term, first because the filaments do not 'slide' in the conventional sense, but move via a ratchet type of mechanism, and second because the process has been studied so well that it has moved beyond the realms of 'theory'.

Figure 17.5 illustrates how the process is thought to operate. The interaction between the myosin and actin filaments is initiated when calcium ions are released from the cisternae into the sarcoplasmic reticulum and pass toward the centre of the fibre. When these ions reach the area of the myofilaments, they have two important actions.

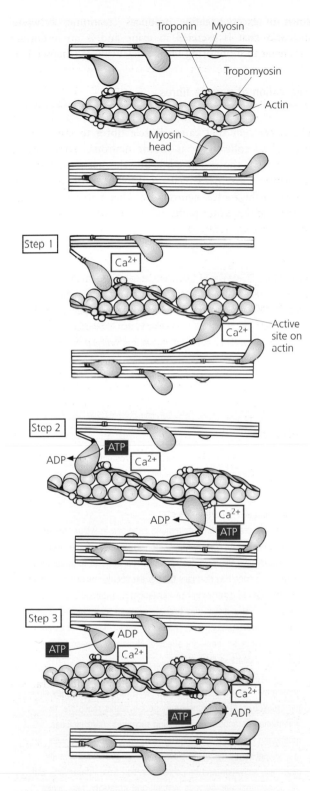

Figure 17.5 The sliding filament theory of muscle fibre contraction. Step 1, distortion of troponin/tropomyosin by calcium ions. Formation of bond between myosin head and active site on actin. Step 2, splitting of ATP by myosin to provide energy to move myosin/actin cross-bridges (actin is pulled along myosin), and then to break cross-bridge for new actin/myosin interaction. Step 3, movement of myosin heads to interact with next active site on actin.

Q. Describe the molecular interactions involved in muscle contraction.

Calcium ions cause a protein that is associated with the actin, called troponin, to distort its molecular shape. This in turn distorts another associated protein called tropomyosin. This latter response exposes sites on the actin molecule that can now interact with complementary sites, called the myosin heads, on the adjacent myosin filaments (step 1, Figure 17.5). The interaction forms chemical bonds between the myosin and actin that act to pull the actin filament over the myosin (step 2, Figure 17.5). The myosin heads then detach and move to the next active sites on the actin, and the process is repeated (step 3, Figure 17.5). In this way, the actin is pulled further along the myosin in a process analogous to a ratchet mechanism. The whole process is very rapid and as many as 100 repeat interactions can occur per second.

Calcium ions stimulate myosin to act as an enzyme that can split ATP and so cause the release of energy. It is this energy that is used to move the myosin heads to the exposed active actin sites, and also to break the myosin/actin bonds.

Within a sarcomere, the ratchet-like movement of the actin myofilaments occurs towards one end of the actin molecule. The other end of the actin (the I-band; Figure 17.4(b)) is attached to a proteinaceous structure called the Z-line, which lies transversely across the muscle fibre and marks the boundary of each sarcomere. As a consequence of the myosin/actin interaction, the Z-lines at each end of the sarcomere are pulled towards each other, so the sarcomere reduces in length. The shortening of all the sarcomeres in the muscle fibre means that the entire fibre shortens (Figure 17.6). Contraction ends when nerve activity ceases, and calcium ions are taken up again into the cisternae. The actin then moves back to its original position, i.e. the fibres and muscle are relaxed.

The role of ATP in this process is significant because repeated interactions between actin and myosin are relatively expensive in energy terms. Clearly, the reservoir of ATP within the fibre will be utilized rapidly, so more must be synthesized if the contractile process is to be sustained. Cellular respiration of glucose will be promoted to form more ATP (see Chapter 4), but in order to maintain a contraction lasting for several seconds, an alternative source of ATP is required. Muscle cells contain a substance called creatine phosphate; the phosphate part may be removed and combined with ADP to generate new ATP. Removal of the phosphate group leaves behind the creatine portion. Break-

BOX 17.5 CONTRACTURES

A contracture is a shortening of the muscle in the absence of an active contractile process. It arises as a consequence of muscle spasm or weakness as the result of a biochemical imbalance within the muscle fibres, e.g. in muscular dystrophy, or as a result of scar contraction in a joint following joint trauma. Prevention of contractures is important if mobility is to be retained or restored (see Box 17.8).

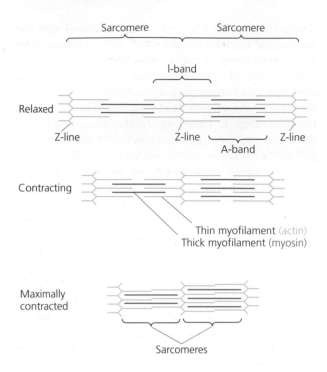

down of excess creatine produces creatinine, a 'waste' substance that is excreted in urine and is an important parameter in monitoring renal efficiency (see Chapter 12).

Innervation of muscle fibres

The nerve cells that cause muscle fibres to contract are referred to collectively as motor neurons. They pass to muscle from the spinal cord, but the nerve activity will frequently have been generated within the brain and passed to the motor neurons by other nerve cells. Those neurons of the motor pathways that lie within the brain or spinal cord are referred to as upper motor neurons, and

Figure 17.6 Shortening of sarcomere length during myofibril contraction. Note that myofilament lengths do not change, but the overlap between actin and myosin increases, drawing consecutive Z-lines together. Note that it is the I-band striation that is reduced.

Q. Describe the roles of actin and myosin in shortening the sarcomere.

BOX 17.6 ALTERED MUSCLE FUNCTION DUE TO PERIPHERAL NERVE DISORDERS

A failure of peripheral nerves to supply muscles, or to stimulate them, will result in muscle weakness and even paralysis. Nerve activity in these motor neurons derives from the central nervous system (CNS); CNS disorders are considered later in Box 17.14.

Disorders of peripheral nerves

1. Crushing the nerve, e.g. if an intervertebral disc prolapses, or if muscles of the lower back undergo spasm contractions, will affect associated muscle function and induce severe pain.

2. The most prevalent peripheral neural disorder is peripheral neuritis, or Guillain–Barré syndrome, arising from viral infection of nerve endings. The inflammation tends to track along the nerve cells, and even into the central nervous system. In doing so, there is ascending muscle weakness. Reflexes are absent in affected areas. As the weakness ascends, it may affect respiratory function and swallowing. Corticosteroid drugs may help to reduce the inflammation, but care is largely targeted at psychological support, monitoring for signs of breathing or swallowing difficulties, and the provision of ventilation or nasogastric feeding as necessary until recovery occurs (McMahon-Parkes and Cornock, 1997; Worsham, 2000). The patient will require rehabilitation therapy to regain mobility (see Box 17.8)

3. Motor neuron disease (MND) is a collection of disorders in which anterior horn cells (i.e. motor neurons) in the spinal cord and periphery are destroyed. The most common disorder in adults is amyotrophic lateral sclerosis (ALS), in which there is a progressive and ultimately fatal degeneration (Skelton, 1996). Muscle weakness and wasting occurs, and cramps may also be observed. The cause of ALS is not known; suggestions include

damage due to excess glutamate (an excitatory neurotransmitter in the anterior horn), autoimmunity, or damage from oxidative biochemical processes within cells.

Neuromuscular junction defects

Myasthenia gravis is an autoimmune condition in which the actions of acetylcholine as a neurotransmitter are inadequate because antibodies have removed post-synaptic receptors to it. In its early stages, the condition normally affects extraocular muscles, leading to difficulties in controlling eye movement and drooping eyelids (ptosis). Facial muscles may become involved, producing a mask-like expression. Speech and swallowing difficulties are apparent if the muscles of the neck are affected. Muscle weakness throughout the body appears in later stages.

Drugs that antagonize the enzyme acetylcholinesterase (e.g. neostigmine) can help to improve muscle function since they slow the breakdown of acetylcholine by post-synaptic receptors, thus potentiating its actions on remaining receptors. Care includes monitoring for side effects arising from drug interactions with (acetyl)cholinergic synapses elsewhere, e.g. abdominal cramps, diarrhoea, salivation and bronchial secretion from interactions with the parasympathetic nervous system, and irritability, headaches and insomnia from central nervous system actions (Cunning, 2000).

Muscle relaxants

The neuromuscular synapse also provides the opportunity for the development of muscle relaxant drugs. The actions of acetylcholine are blocked by drugs such as vecuronium or suxamethonium; these are used clinically to relax muscles before surgery.

are considered later in this chapter. The peripheral neurons to the muscles are referred to as lower motor neurons; these terminate at the muscle fibre in a structure referred to as the neuromuscular junction.

The neuromuscular junction

The neuromuscular junction is a form of synapse. A muscle fibre forms numerous synapses along its length with terminals from the same nerve cell. In this way, if the nerve cell is active, then impulses directed along the terminals will stimulate the entire fibre length almost simultaneously, thus ensuring that the whole fibre contracts. The synapse at the neuron/muscle fibre interface is shown in Figure 17.7. Its structure is somewhat different to that of a neuron/neuron synapse, detailed in Chapter 8, and it is called a *motor end plate* to distinguish it from such synapses. However, the end plate functions in much the same way as other synapses, and utilizes acetylcholine as the neurotransmitter chemical. Acetylcholine is released from the endings of the nerve cell by the arrival of an electrical impulse, and causes a depolarization of the sarcolemma. The electrical current generated within the sarcolemma is then transmitted to the T-tubules (see Figure 17.1), and initiates the release of calcium ions from intracellular stores that trigger the contractile process, detailed earlier.

The motor-unit

The previous section considered the activation of single muscle fibres by individual nerve cells. Often, a single nerve cell activates more than one muscle fibre; the number of fibres innervated by a single nerve cell is called a motor unit. The ratio of muscle fibres to nerve cells relates to the role of the muscle. Large motor units are found in the major postural muscles, such as the quadriceps of the thighs, and make the process of developing a considerable force of contraction more efficient, otherwise large numbers of nerve cells would be required to provide the necessary innervation of the tissue. In such muscles, a single nerve cell may innervate hundreds of muscle fibres. In contrast, small muscles, such as the pupillary muscles inside the eye, may have fibres that are innervated by individual nerve cells. These muscles do not generate a large force of contraction, and their role requires a more subtle control than that exerted on the major postural muscles.

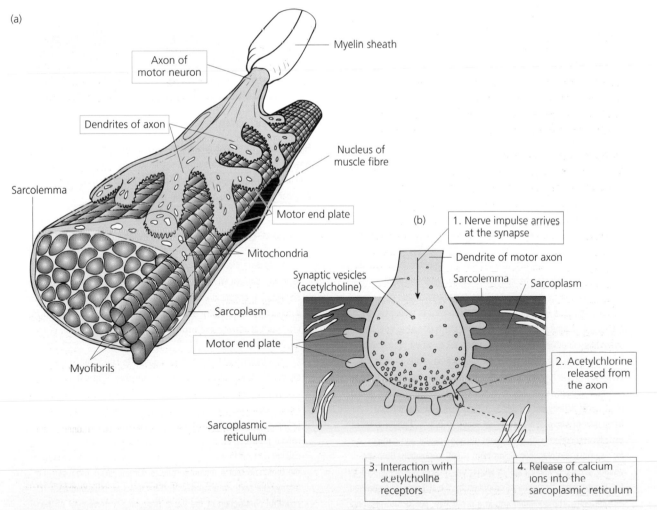

(a)

Myelin sheath

Axon of motor neuron

Dendrites of axon

Nucleus of muscle fibre

Sarcolemma

Motor end plate

Mitochondria

Sarcoplasm

Myofibrils

(b)

1. Nerve impulse arrives at the synapse

Dendrite of motor axon

Synaptic vesicles (acetylcholine)

Sarcolemma

Sarcoplasm

Motor end plate

2. Acetylchlorine released from the axon

Sarcoplasmic reticulum

3. Interaction with acetylcholine receptors

4. Release of calcium ions into the sarcoplasmic reticulum

Figure 17.7 Neuromuscular junction. (a) The motor end plate. (b) Detail of the synapse.

Q. Describe the roles of the components at a neuromuscular junction.

From a clinical viewpoint, motor units mean that loss of relatively small numbers of nerve cells can result in the loss of large numbers of functional muscle fibres. Fortunately, nerve cells can produce outgrowths and re-innervate nearby muscle fibres, although the improvement in muscle function may be limited.

Contraction of whole muscles

Having considered the activation and behaviour of individual muscle fibres, we will now consider features of whole muscle contraction produced when fibres are activated.

Twitch, treppe and tetany

Observation of the contraction of whole muscle identifies a variety of forms of contraction:

- *Twitch* is a momentary, spasmodic contraction produced by a brief, single stimulus (Figure 17.8(a)).

- *Treppe:* if a muscle is stimulated repeatedly, but is allowed to relax between stimuli, the contraction induced by each stimulus increases in intensity to a maximum (Figure 17.8(b)). This principle operates when athletes warm up.

- *Tetany:* if a muscle is stimulated repeatedly but is not allowed to relax fully between stimuli, the contractions induced by each stimulus are additive, so that each twitch summates to produce an intense, continuous contraction called a tetany (Figure 17.8(c)). This may be very painful (Box 17.7).

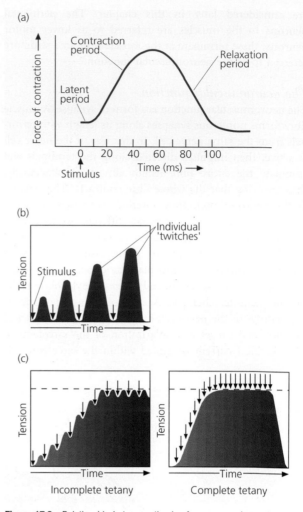

Figure 17.8 Relationship between stimulus frequency and muscle tension. (a) Twitch produced by a single stimulus. (b) Treppe produced by continued activation/relaxation. (c) Tetany induced by continued activation. *Q. What do you understand by the term 'tetany'?*

BOX 17.7 MUSCLE SPASM/CRAMP AND TETANUS

The strength of contraction of a muscle will depend on its rate of stimulation. It will also be influenced by the local chemical environment, since this will affect the sensitivity of the sarcolemma. The internal chemical environment is influenced by the length of time that a contracting muscle has had to spend in anaerobic conditions. Spasm and cramp occur when the excitability is increased to the point that nerve stimulation of the muscle induces a powerful contraction that is sustained, leading to hypoxia and consequently pain. Cramp is normally associated with a period of physical activity during which the muscle is subjected to a frequency of nerve stimulation that leads to tetany. Spasm is more usually associated with lower-level muscle activity and can occur, for example, simply when rising from a sitting position. Both are painful situations – nociceptors within the muscle are stimulated by the biochemical environment produced by the hypoxia and stressed muscle cells. The spasm/cramp is a protective device that prevents muscle damage occurring through its continued use.

Increasing blood supply to the area by the use of massage or local vasodilators will help to reverse any hypoxia, and will help to stabilize the chemical environment within the muscle. However, the sarcolemma will usually retain for a period of time a likelihood of increased sensitivity and excitability, making repeat spasm of the muscle more likely.

The threshold of stimulation required to cause the electrical changes (i.e. an action potential; see Chapter 8) in the sarcolemma is especially susceptible to calcium ion concentration in the extracellular fluid. Acute reductions in calcium concentration induced, for example, by hyperventilation during an anxiety 'attack' (which produces an alkalosis that facilitates the combination of calcium ions with blood proteins) may result in such a lowering of the threshold that a maximal muscle contraction is produced (i.e. tetany; see text). In alkalosis, this is often first observed as a powerful contraction of the hand, producing a movement of the thumb across the palm of the hand in a characteristic carpopedal

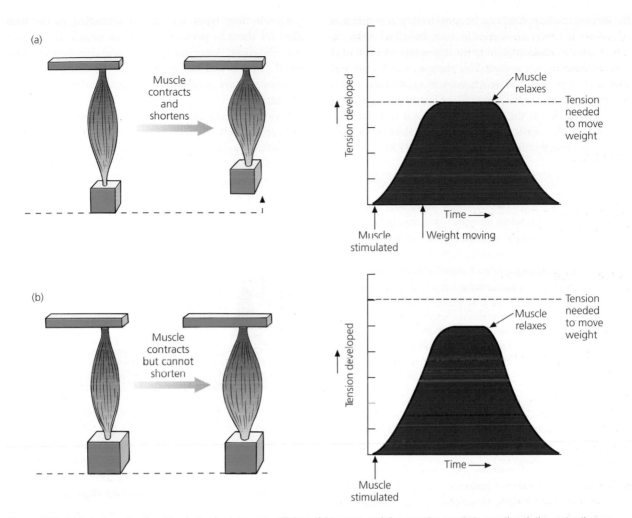

Figure 17.9 (a) Isotonic contraction. Muscle tension increases until the weight moves, and then remains constant, even though the contraction continues. (b) Isometric contraction. The weight cannot be moved: muscle tension increases during the contraction, but the muscle does not shorten. Note that in (a) the initial contraction before weight moves will also be an isometric contraction.

Q. Define the following terms with reference to contraction of the whole muscle: (i) twitch, (ii) isotonic, and (iii) isometric.

spasm. Before this, a person who has become alkalotic may report intense tingling in the fingers and hands, a prelude to muscle contraction.

Tetanus

Tetanus is a condition in which a toxin produced by infection with *Clostridium tetani* lowers the threshold for muscle excitation, making tetany likely even with very low rates of nerve stimulation. For reasons that are unclear, the condition affects some muscles more markedly than others; the condition is colloquially known as 'lockjaw' because of its effects on muscles of the face. The main danger is from tetany of the muscles of the chest, since this will cause respiratory arrest. Anti-tetanus injections are available; these contain antibody to the toxin, thus preventing its actions. The causal organism is common and lives in soil. It is important for health carers to recognize this, since anti-tetanus injections should be considered if a wound is open, and if there is no evidence that the patient has maintained a tetanus immunization programme.

Isotonic and isometric contractions

If an object is lifted, muscles of the arm must first generate the tension necessary to move the load. Once the object is moving, further tension need not be developed, and the muscle shortens as the skeletal joint moves. The contraction is said to be isotonic ('isos-' = equal, 'tonos' = tension) (Figure 17.9(a)).

Figure 17.9(b) shows an example of isometric contraction. In this example, the development of tension before the object can be moved occurs without moving the skeletal joint. Muscle length must therefore remain constant in spite of the contraction that is occurring. The actin–myosin interaction within the muscle fibres will still be acting to move the actin myofilaments; this is exhibited as a rise in muscle tension. The contraction is then said to be isometric ('metros' = length).

In lifting an object, then, both types of contraction will play a role in the movement. For lifting very heavy loads, the isometric component can be considerable; it is this that stimulates the increase in muscle mass identified earlier in this chapter as an adaptation to the imposition of additional workloads on muscle actions. This phenomenon is observed elsewhere, e.g. the increased heart size of athletes, which occurs in response to the frequency of isometric contraction by the ventricles in the initial stages of systole before the opening of the aortic and pulmonary valves. It is also applied in rehabilitation programmes (Box 17.8).

Exercise

Extend an arm and grip a reasonably heavy weight, such as a small bag of potatoes (but not too heavy – don't damage the muscle!). Place the opposite hand over the extended biceps muscle of the upper arm. Now lift the weight. Notice how the tension develops first in the muscle before it begins to shorten when the elbow bends. This is the isometric phase of contraction. As the muscle shortens, the muscle is in its isotonic phase.

Now place both hands on your thighs (i.e. on the quadriceps femoris muscle) whilst in a sitting position. Begin to stand. Can you detect the two phases of contraction during the process?

Maintaining muscle contraction: fatigue resistance

The maintenance of posture and physical activity may require muscles either to maintain a degree of contraction for a period of time, or to contract repeatedly over an extended period of time. Such muscles must therefore be resistant to fatigue. In contrast, some movements involve very rapid contractions maintained for only a short period of time. Types of muscle fibre have been identified that are suited best to these roles, but it is important to note that muscles will normally contain a mixture of fibre types; only the relative proportion of fibre types varies.

Muscle fibre types are named according to the time taken for them to perform a cycle of muscle contraction and relaxation. Accordingly, they are classified as slow-twitch (type I) and fast-twitch (type II) fibres (although subtypes are now recognized that have intermediate rates of contraction).

Slow fibres are relatively more frequent in muscles that are unlikely to have a major role in activities that necessitate rapid contraction/relaxation cycles. Those muscles that act to maintain posture against gravity, e.g. the quadriceps of the thighs, have a preponderance of slow fibres, and are therefore slow muscles. The muscle fibres will have an excellent blood supply, but they will

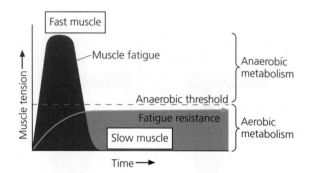

Figure 17.10 Fatigue resistance in muscles. Fast-twitch muscles rapidly exceed the anaerobic threshold during contraction. Slow-twitch muscles can maintain contraction below anaerobic threshold for long periods of time (but can exceed threshold, e.g. during exercise). *Q. Distinguish between the roles of slow and fast muscle fibres.*

Exercise

Refer to Chapter 3 and reflect on how walking aids impact on the position of the body's centre of gravity during movement. Using the examples of aids given in Box 17.8, consider how a person using these might maintain the position of the centre of gravity and so improve postural stability.

BOX 17.8 REHABILITATION OF AN IMMOBILE PATIENT

The aims of preventing contractures (see Box 17.5) are to restore as much normal movement as possible, to maintain muscle strength and joint flexibility, and to facilitate muscle co-ordination. A range of movement exercises are employed to support joint movement through appropriate planes:

- *'Passive exercise'*. This term is a misnomer, applied when a nurse/physiotherapist manipulates joints without assistance from the patient.
- *Active-assisted exercise*. This is performed by the patient with the assistance of the nurse/physiotherapist, and encourages normal muscle actions.

- *Active exercise*. This is performed solely by the patient. It encourages normal muscle action, and also the development of muscle strength.
- *Resisted exercise*. This is active exercise performed against resistance. In doing so, the isometric phase of muscle contraction is increased, which helps to increase muscle bulk and hence increase muscle power.

Mobility may necessitate the patient using aids such as a leg cast, a cane, crutches or calipers. Clearly, aids may not produce normal movements, or facilitate posture control, and the patient will require some training to walk efficiently and to maintain posture when aids have been removed.

also have a rich store of myoglobin, a haemoglobin-like pigment that provides a supplementary oxygen store. The fibres therefore have the capacity to maintain ATP production by aerobic metabolism (Figure 17.10), and are therefore resistant to hypoxia and hence to fatigue. This is useful if we have to remain standing for long periods of time.

Fast fibres increase in proportion in those muscles that are responsible for producing rapid movements, as in the movement of the eye or hand. Fast-type muscle fibres have lots of mitochondria but little myoglobin, so they cannot maintain contraction for long periods of time. They are not likely to predominate in the major anti-gravity muscles.

CONTROL OF POSTURE AND MOVEMENT

Introduction

Posture is the position of the body in space, and includes whole body orientation and the relative positions of body parts. The degree of tension observed in individual muscles will be appropriate for the maintenance of position of the associated joint. Movement results from a change of posture, and may or may not involve propulsion of the body from one point to another. Movement is produced by changes in the tension of muscles relative to others.

Agonistic, antagonistic and synergistic muscles

A muscle that primarily produces a movement is called an *agonist*; a muscle that opposes the movement is called an *antagonist*. The latter only opposes contraction sufficient to protect the joint involved, and does not normally prevent the movement from occurring (note the similarity in use of these terms in pharmacology, in which agonist drugs promote an action, and antagonistic drugs prevent or reverse it). The agonist muscle may act to flex (i.e. bend) or extend the joint; it is therefore referred to as a flexor or extensor type of muscle.

Consider the movement of the knee joint during walking. A number of muscles in the leg are involved, but the main ones are the quadriceps femoris ('quad-' = four; there are four parts to this muscle) of the thigh, and the hamstring muscles at the back of the thigh (Figure 17.11). Both sets of muscles have attachments with the top of the femur or bones of the pelvis, and with the tibia of the lower leg. The quadriceps is an extensor muscle in that its contraction extends the leg; the hamstrings are flexors, and cause the joint to bend during contraction. During walking, the knee extensor muscles will be agonistic as the leg is extended, and the flexors antagonistic. When the knee is flexed, the situation is reversed. The movement therefore requires cyclical stimulation/relaxation of the muscles involved.

By altering the position of a body part, or by causing a change in body orientation, the actions of an agonist could adversely influence additional joints nearby. These are stabilized by the simultaneous contraction of other muscles that, in terms of the movement produced, may be referred to as synergistic muscles. In the example of walking, there is a tendency for the body to be unbalanced, which is counteracted by the contraction or relaxation of muscles of the opposite leg, the back and the shoulders. Thus, what appears to be a relatively simple movement that we would normally take for granted requires complex responses throughout the muscular system.

The control of posture and movement therefore depends upon the regulation of the tension of all muscles appropriate to the desired joint position, or to the movement to be induced. This section is concerned with exploring how the activity of motor nerve cells is regulated. In doing so, it considers the kind of sensory information required, the involuntary processes involved in reflex movements, the integration required to produce voluntary movement, and the central nervous system centres involved in co-ordinating posture control.

Sensory information: proprioception

The brain must be 'aware' at all times of the spatial positions of the body parts, and of the orientation of the body in general, although we are not usually conscious of this information unless we need it. The senses were described in Chapter 7, and many are involved in the monitoring of posture. Vision is clearly of use in monitoring spatial positioning, yet closing our eyes or looking away does not prevent us from being aware of our posture

---

Exercise

Refer to figure 17.11. Why are the quadriceps muscles so much larger than the hamstrings? You might consider the effects of gravity on the knee joint when standing, and the role of the quadriceps as an extensor muscle that acts to extend (straighten) the leg.

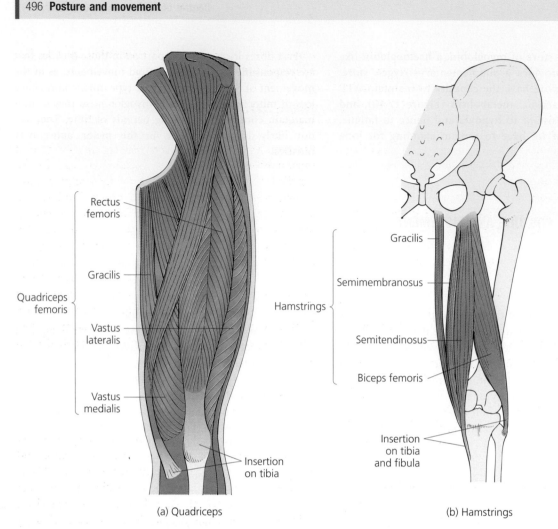

Rectus
femoris

Gracilis

Quadriceps
femoris

Vastus
lateralis

Vastus
medialis

Insertion
on tibia

(a) Quadriceps

Gracilis

Semimembranosus

Hamstrings

Semitendinosus

Biceps femoris

Insertion
on tibia
and fibula

(b) Hamstrings

Figure 17.11 Muscles controlling the knee joint. (a) Flexors, anterior view. (b) Extensors, posterior view.

Q. *What are the general rules applied to the nomenclature of muscles?*

Q. *What does the difference in bulk tell you about the roles of these two muscle groups?*

or the position of our hands, and blind people fare as well as visually-able people in this respect. Other receptors must be involved then.

Mechanoreceptors of the skin convey tactile information, and so the contact between, say, a foot and the floor can be monitored and the information used. However, most postural information is produced by a variety of receptors collectively called *proprioreceptors* (or proprioceptors; 'proprio-' = position). These receptors are the vestibular receptors, joint receptors, tendon receptors, and muscle 'spindles'. To be effective, they must be able to provide information even when the posture is unchanging, otherwise the brain will not be able to continue to identify the relative positions of parts of the body. This capacity to provide information when stationary is called a 'static' property of the receptors. They must also, of course, be capable of monitoring position change, the rate of change, direction of change, and any acceleratory component during the movement. These are called 'dynamic' properties.

Vestibular receptors

These receptors were introduced in Chapter 7 (The Senses). Readers should refer to that section and accompanying diagram before proceeding.

The vestibular (or equilibrium) receptors are found within the vestibular apparatus of the inner ear (Figure 7.2). They can generally be divided into the otolithic ('oto-' = ear, 'lith' = stone) organs and the semicircular canals.

The otolithic organs are comprised of distended structures called the utricle and saccule (Figure 7.2(b)), which contain masses of small calcium carbonate crystals lying on top of a jelly-like otolithic membrane (Figure 7.2(c)). Receptor hair cells project from cells in the area into this membrane. The rest of the utricle/saccule is filled with fluid called endolymph. If the position of the head alters, the fluid moves, but the denser otolithic membrane moves more slowly. The fluid therefore moves over the membrane; in doing so, it distorts the hair cells and generates electrical activity, which is transmitted to the brain via the vestibulocochlear nerve (cranial nerve VIII, which arises from the vestibule and cochlea). These receptors, then, provide information regarding the orientation of the head. The response is too slow, however, to convey dynamic information, so these are concerned largely with static equilibrium, i.e. the position of the crystals of these receptors enables the brain to be aware of the position of the head relative to gravity.

Dynamic equilibrium is monitored by receptors of the semicircular canals (Figure 7.2(b)). There are three canals in each ear, arranged at right-angles to one another in three planes. At the base of each canal there is a distended region – the ampulla – in which lies the crista, an elevated structure containing the receptor cells. The hair-like projections from these cells are inserted into a jelly-like covering called the cupula. When the head moves, the fluid currents produced within the canals cause a deflection of the cupula, which activates the receptors. Impulses generated pass to the brain via the vestibulocochlear nerve. Comparison of the information from each of the three cristae, and each ear, gives information regarding the direction and plane of head movement, whether it is rotational, and how rapidly it is moving. These receptors are therefore important if the position of the head changes rapidly.

By monitoring the position and movement of the head, the vestibular receptors are involved in helping us to maintain balance. In doing so, they promote the muscle contraction necessary for its maintenance.

Joint receptors

Joint receptors are nerve endings found within the cartilage and synovial capsules of joints. They respond to distortion of the joint and provide information regarding the position of the joint (a 'static' property), and the rate of change and acceleration during joint movement ('dynamic' properties). In doing so, the brain can determine accurately the change in orientation of the skeleton, and can predict where a limb will finish up after the movement is complete. Muscle contraction can therefore be modulated accordingly.

Tendon receptors

Receptors within the tendons of muscles are composed of small bundles of collagen fibres enclosed in a capsule and supplied with nerve endings. The tendon receptors (also known as Golgi tendon organs) are arranged in line with the muscle fibres, and so provide information regarding fibre tension. However, their precise role in posture and movement is unclear. It is likely that tendon receptors provide a protective function by prompting a sudden cessation of muscle contraction if excessive tension is being applied to the tendons. In this way, the tendons and muscles are prevented from damage or even separation from the bone. This action is observed, for example, when muscles apparently 'give way' if an object being lifted is too heavy.

Muscle spindles

Of all the proprioreceptors, it is the muscle spindles that are best situated to enable the brain to monitor and modulate the contraction of skeletal muscles. This is because the receptors are present within the muscles themselves. The spindle-shaped receptor is actually a collection of modified muscle fibres enclosed within a connective tissue capsule (Figure 17.12). The fibres are said to be intrafusal ('intra-' = inside, 'fusiform' = spindle-like) to distinguish them from the other muscle fibres. The connective tissue around the spindle connects the receptor to adjacent muscle fibres, so any stretching or shortening of the latter will also produce distortion of the spindle, and a change in intrafusal fibre length. Thus, these receptors monitor the length of the muscle spindles and in doing so monitor the length of the muscle fibres to which the receptors are attached.

The spindle fibres have sensory nerve endings associated with them that respond when the length of the intrafusal

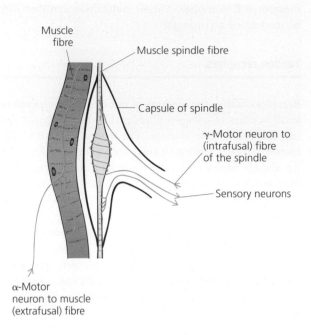

Muscle fibre

Muscle spindle fibre

Capsule of spindle

γ-Motor neuron to (intrafusal) fibre of the spindle

Sensory neurons

α-Motor neuron to muscle (extrafusal) fibre

Figure 17.12 Muscle spindle fibre and its innervation.
Q. What information does this type of receptor provide?

fibre is altered, and continue to do so for a period of time after. The nerve activity therefore conveys static information regarding spindle and muscle fibre length, but they also impart information regarding the rate of change should the muscle length alter, and so provide a dynamic component.

An important feature of muscle spindles is that the brain may act to modulate their sensitivity. Thus, the role of the spindles is supplemented by motor neurons to the fibres within them (these neurons are separate from those that supply the muscle fibres, and are classified as gamma-neurons or gamma-efferents). Activity within these nerve cells causes the spindle fibres to contract. The significance of this is explained later in relation to voluntary movements.

Muscle spindles and control of posture by involuntary reflexes

The importance of involuntary reflexes in postural control cannot be overemphasized. A reflex response is extremely rapid because it involves neural pathways that remove the necessity to process information by the brain, which would introduce a delay before the response was initiated. Many involve integration within the spinal cord, although those involving the cranial nerves pass via direct routes through the brain.

A reflex change in muscle contraction results from a sequence of events:

1 Stimulation of a sensory receptor.

2 Conduction of sensory activity to the central nervous system via sensory neurons.

3 Activation of motor neurons to promote an appropriate response.

Collectively, these events form a *reflex arc*. A monosynaptic arc is an arc in which the sensory neuron synapses directly with the motor cell, i.e. there is only one synapse involved. Some reflexes utilize one or more interneurons, and so involve more synapses (which slows the reflex). The fundamental elements of a reflex were illustrated in Chapter 8 in relation to a withdrawal reflex in response to pain. This is a reflex that entails a change in posture, which removes the limb from the source of the

---

BOX 17.10 REFLEXES IN INFANTS

Some reflexes are apparent soon after birth, including the feeding reflex, the grasping reflex, and the positive supporting reaction, seen as an extension of the legs when firm contact is made on the soles of the feet. Many reflexes become modified as the baby grows. For example, the reflex changes in position of body and limb induced by stimulating the vestibular apparatus of the ear must remain operative in the child and adult during involuntary head movement, but must be suppressed during voluntary movement of the head.

---

pain, but it does not explain the responses of muscles elsewhere that act to stabilize the body's new position once the reflex is instigated. These further reflexes are stretch reflexes; they play a vital role in helping us to maintain our posture. The knee jerk is an example of such a reflex; this is used clinically to assess reflex functioning (see Box 17.11).

The knee jerk is a rapid, reflex extension of the knee joint that involves the contraction of the quadriceps femoris muscle of the thigh. It is activated by tapping the patellar tendon, which attaches the quadriceps muscle to the tibia bone of the shin (Figure 17.13). Tapping the tendon stretches the muscle fibres of the quadriceps, including the fibres within its muscle spindles. The sensory nerve endings of the spindles are activated, and impulses pass along the sensory neurons to the spinal cord. Here, the neurons synapse directly with the motor nerve cells that convey impulses back to the muscle fibres of the quadriceps, causing them to contract. Simultaneously, the nerve activity to the antagonistic muscles (i.e. the hamstrings) is inhibited, which relaxes these muscles so that the movement is not impeded. The result is that the knee is extended as a little kick.

BOX 17.11 CLINICAL USES OF THE STRETCH REFLEX

Stimulating a stretch reflex (or tendon reflex) is simple. A small tendon hammer can be used to direct an impact on various tendons of the body, especially where the tendon passes over a joint. The tendon of the quadriceps (at the knee), the tendon of the biceps (at the elbow), and the tendon of the gastrocnemius (the Achilles tendon at the heel) all provide a means of testing for the presence of the reflex and its efficiency. Such tests provide an indication of the functioning of the sensory and motor nerves

to the muscle and/or spinal cord connections (Riggio and Jagoda, 1999).

The placement of electrodes over the nerves also enables a calculation of conduction velocity for the nerve pathway (from the time delay between tapping the tendon and recording the nerve activity), although this requires the use of sophisticated equipment and is not usual in general clinic practice.

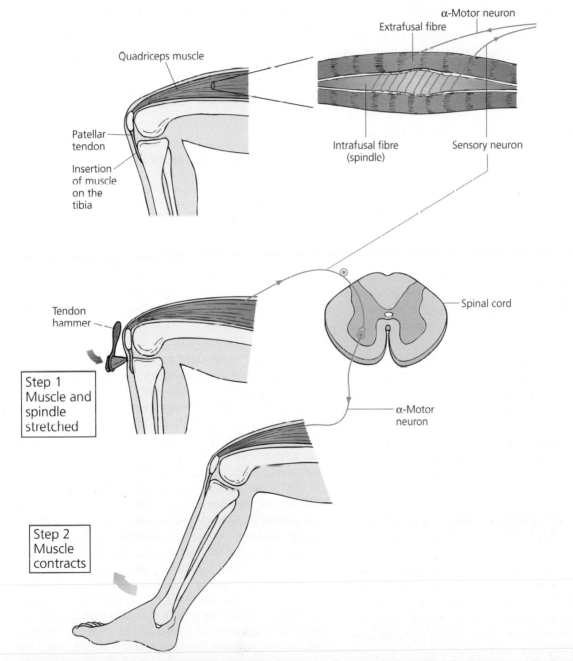

Figure 17.13 The stretch reflex, as illustrated by the knee jerk. Step 1: when a reflex hammer strikes the patellar tendon, the muscle spindle fibres stretch, resulting in a burst of activity in the afferent fibres that synapse on motor neurons inside the spinal cord. Step 2: an immediate reflexive kick is produced by the activation of motor units in the stretched muscle.

Q. Describe the role of muscle spindles in the reflex response.

The knee jerk is a demonstration of the way that spindle receptors act to keep muscle length constant. If a muscle is stretched, then contraction returns it back to the original length. The knee jerk is an artificial situation, but the reflex it demonstrates is illustrated in the following examples:

● Upon standing, gravity acts to flex the knees, hips and intervertebral joints. The activities of the muscle spindles in the relevant extensor muscles that are stretched by these effects of gravity help to prevent us from crumpling into a heap, and so are vital if we are to maintain an upright posture unconsciously.

● Consider a situation in which a person is standing by a supermarket shelf, contemplating what to buy, when another shopper bumps into them. The unexpected and involuntary change in posture alters the length and tension of various muscles, and the resultant reflex responses to spindle activation play an important role in the quick return to stability. Other synergistic and postural muscles will also be activated because of the stimulation of other proprioreceptors (e.g. the vestibular apparatus), and because of reflexes instigated by spindles within the muscles themselves. The interactions of spindle sensory neurons and motor neurons in the spinal cord are shown schematically in Figure 17.14. By involving interneurons, the reflex response can simultaneously promote contraction of appropriate muscles in another limb, and relaxation of antagonistic muscles (which facilitates the shortening of the agonistic muscle). The stretch reflex thus makes a powerful contribution to the maintenance of posture.

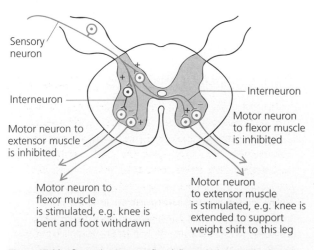

Sensory neuron

Interneuron

Interneuron

Motor neuron to extensor muscle is inhibited

Motor neuron to flexor muscle is inhibited

Motor neuron to flexor muscle is stimulated, e.g. knee is bent and foot withdrawn

Motor neuron to extensor muscle is stimulated, e.g. knee is extended to support weight shift to this leg

Figure 17.14 Crossed-extensor reflex. Influence of the same stimulus to promote the flexor response on the same side, and to stimulate extensors on the opposite side. The opposite leg will be extended to support the change in body position.

● When an object is thrown for us to catch, or when we intend to lift an object, we unconsciously appraise the forces required, based on object size, composition, etc. An appropriate muscle tension is generated, but if we have under- or overestimated, then control of the situation is lost. If the object is heavier than anticipated, then muscles in the arm will be stretched, activating the spindles and reflexly stimulating further muscle contraction.

In all three examples, the reflex response is produced independently of passing sensory information to the brain. The brain, however, must be aware of how the initiation of reflexes has altered the relative positions of parts of the body. Thus, apart from synapsing with motor neurons, the sensory neurons from the spindles will also synapse with ascending neurons within the cord that convey information to appropriate areas of the brain and so keep it 'informed'.

Muscle spindles and control of voluntary movement

Individual muscles are contracted during voluntary movement as a consequence of nerve activity generated in the brain and transmitted to them. The contraction is of the muscle fibres themselves; consequently, the contraction will tend to passively shorten the spindles within the muscle. From the previous discussion, the reflex response to this reduced spindle tension is to cause muscle relaxation and so return muscle fibre and spindle length to as it was before. In this way, the muscle spindles tend to act to oppose any voluntary changes in muscle contraction (and also relaxation). The role of spindles in the reflex maintenance of posture could therefore potentially act to restrict movement by preventing the necessary muscular changes. A mechanism is necessary to modulate the actions of spindles, and this is provided by the activities of the motor innervation of the spindles identified earlier.

We noted earlier that the intrafusal fibres of the spindles are associated not only with sensory nerve cells but also with gamma-efferent neurons. The latter are motor neurons, and their activation will cause the spindle fibres to contract (remember that the spindle fibres are modified muscle cells). During voluntary movement this occurs in time with the surrounding muscle fibres. In this way, the spindle receptors are modulated and do not sense a change in muscle contraction, so muscles can be contracted or relaxed voluntarily without inducing the (involuntary) stretch reflex. It is worth reflecting for a moment on the complexity of this process. What it means is that every muscle movement must be accompanied by a precise contraction/relaxation of the spindle fibres within the agonistic, antagonistic and synergistic muscles involved. Apart from simultaneously controlling the motor activity to each of the 600-plus muscles of the body, the brain must therefore also control the co-activation of their many muscle spindle fibres if a controlled, smooth movement is to occur.

The central nervous system and the control of posture and movement

It is clear from the preceding discussions that the control of individual muscle contraction involves a complex integration of sensory information and the activation of appropriate motor neurons to the muscle and to the muscle spindle receptors. The brain receives a bewildering array of information regarding every aspect of posture, and also moment-to-moment updates on how the position of body parts and body orientation is changing. Motor neuron output must strike a balance between that produced by reflex responses to changes in muscle/tendon activity, and that produced by motor output from the brain.

Clearly, the control of posture and movement is of a complexity of the highest order; much of the brain is concerned with that control. This section considers some of the parts of the brain involved. We described brain architecture in Chapter 8, and readers are referred to that chapter for supplementary material.

Sensory input to the brain

Sensory information from the muscles, tendons and joints, together with that from various mechanoreceptors in the skin, passes to the somatosensory ('soma' = body) areas of the cerebral cortex, or to the cerebellum. The main tracts of spinal cord neurons that convey this information are the posterior spinothalamic tracts (i.e. in the posterior aspect of the cord and passing to the thalamus, and thence to the cerebral cortex), and the spinocerebellar tracts (from cord to cerebellum).

Neurons of the spinothalamic tracts ascend the dorsal columns of the cord and synapse with neurons in the dorsal column nuclei of the medulla oblongata (see Chapter 8). From here, projections cross over to the other side of the medulla, pass to the thalamus via a tract called the medial lemniscus, and then are relayed to the cerebral cortex. The cross-over in the medulla means that information from one side of the body passes to the opposite side of the brain.

BOX 17.12 TREMORS

A tremor is a series of rapid muscle contractions that represent an oscillation in the control of tension in pairs of agonistic and antagonistic muscles. Many people exhibit a slight tremor, particularly if a limb is extended, and especially if being watched. This postural or intention tremor probably arises from the cerebellum of the brain, but is not associated with other neurological abnormalities and is not considered to relate to any underlying pathology.

The tremor observed in Parkinson's disease is an example of a tremor that occurs at rest. It is produced by oscillations in the activity between the basal ganglia and cerebral cortex of the brain (see Box 17.14), which determine the final output to the muscles. This tremor disappears during voluntary movement, presumably because other pathways in the brain are activated that override the oscillation.

BOX 17.13 SENSORIMOTOR DEVELOPMENT

Neurons are responsible for the functions we associate with the brain, such as sensory processing, motor co-ordination, memory and reasoning. For these facilities to develop in infants, the process of myelination (to increase nerve cell conductivity and insulation) must progress, the cells must become more organized, and intercellular communication must be established by the development or maintenance of appropriate synapses. Motor and sensory function matures earlier than 'higher' cognitive functions, such as memory, reasoning and judgement. This early sensorimotor development is illustrated in the ability of the young child to eventually assume an upright posture, to walk, to acquire basic speech, and to gain voluntary control of the urinary and anal sphincters.

The 'maturation' process of neural integration can take many years to complete (see Sheridan, 1997). Sensorimotor maturation is observed in the continuing development of motor skills. Gross motor control improves most rapidly, and is enhanced by physical activity. It is almost complete by the end of childhood. Fine motor skills (e.g. eye/hand and arm/leg co-ordination) improve more slowly, and development continues into the teenage years. A slight sex discrepancy is apparent, with boys developing a greater grip strength and tending towards better arm/leg co-ordination than girls, who exhibit better control of balance and rhythmic movement. There is a considerable overlap in the acquirement of these skills, however.

Areas of the somatosensory cortex can be identified that receive information from particular parts of the body (Figure 17.15(a)). More grey matter is devoted to the face and hands than to the entire trunk, which relates to the complexity and volume of information from those parts.

The spinocerebellar tracts ascend the lateral aspects of the cord to the medulla, where they pass to the cortex of the cerebellum via tracts called the cerebellar peduncles. Many of the neurons will again have crossed over, but this time within the cord, and so most of the information from one side of the body will have been conveyed to the opposite side of the cerebellum.

Sensory information from the vestibular apparatus of the ear passes to the brain via a cranial nerve and not via the spinal cord. The vestibular component of the vestibulocochlear nerve sends fibres to the vestibular nuclei of the medulla, and to the cerebellum. Some information is conveyed from the medulla to the superior colliculi of the midbrain, which are areas involved in co-ordinating eye movement (see Chapter 7).

Exercise

The text mentions various parts of the brain. The motor cortex and cerebral nuclei are parts of the forebrain, the midbrain nuclei are part of the midbrain, and the cerebellum is part of the hind brain. Refer to Chapter 8 for explanations of these terms.

In this way, sudden head movement detected by the vestibular receptors induces changes in eye position (called vestibulo-ocular reflexes) that help us to maintain appropriate vision.

Motor output from the brain

The mass of sensory information received by the brain is constantly monitored, integrated and relayed to those areas that determine the motor output from the brain. This output originates from various parts of the brain: the motor cortex, the basal ganglia and the cerebellum.

Motor cortex and pyramidal pathways

The motor cortex is an extensive part of the cerebral cortex. It occupies parts of the frontal and parietal lobes of the cerebral hemispheres, and lies immediately anterior to the somatosensory cortex (see Chapter 8). Like the somatosensory cortex, the motor cortex can also be 'mapped' (Figure 17.15(b)). The complexity of controlling hand and facial movements is reflected in the disproportionate areas involved in their co-ordination.

Much of the neural output to muscles comes from the motor cortex and passes out of the brain via the pyramidal pathway. This output largely passes down the spinal cord via the lateral and anterior corticospinal tracts (Figure 17.16). The lateral tracts are characterized by the crossing over (decussation) of the upper motor neurons within the

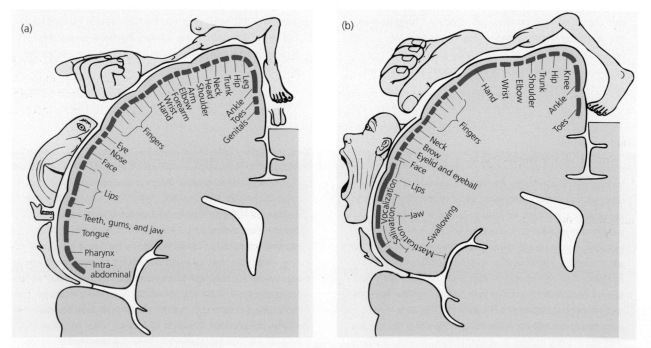

Figure 17.15 Topographical analysis of the sensory and motor areas of the cerebral cortex. (a) Somatosensory cortex, right hemisphere. (b) Motor cortex, right hemisphere.

Q. Identify the area associated with sending information to the jaw muscle when we are taking a meal.

medulla. Here, the tracts are known as the 'pyramids', which gives the pathways their name. The nerve cells continue down the cord and eventually synapse with lower motor neurons to the muscles. The anterior tract fibres also cross over, but this time within the grey matter of the cord, where they also synapse with lower motor neurons. The crossing over means that muscles located on one side of the body are controlled by neurons from the opposite side of the brain.

Some output passes to the nuclei of various cranial nerves within the brainstem for transmission via cranial nerves to muscles of the face and neck. These form the corticobulbar tracts. They do not project to the spinal cord, or pyramids, at all, but they are still considered to be part of the pyramidal pathways because they originate within the motor cortex of the brain.

Basal ganglia and extrapyramidal pathways

The basal ganglia are a number of paired masses of grey matter within the cerebral hemispheres; collectively, these are called the cerebral nuclei. Some midbrain nuclei, however, are linked functionally with the cerebral nuclei, and are usually considered as components of the basal ganglia. The names of the nuclei reflect their appearance to early anatomists, or their position. Major nuclei are identified in Figure 17.17.

The presence of identifiable structures in the control of posture and movement has enabled researchers to determine some of their roles. In general terms, the basal ganglia are involved in the subconscious production of gross intentional movement, rhythmic movements such as walking, and the positioning of the body before producing an intended movement. Much of the nerve activity generated is relayed first to the motor cortex, where it is modulated further before passing to the muscles via the pyramidal pathways (see above). The interactions between the ganglia and the cortex are extremely complex. There are numerous interconnections (excitatory and inhibitory), some of which even form 'circular' pathways, so that neural activity feeds back to the grey matter from where it came.

Not all of the neural output from the basal ganglia passes initially to the cortex for modulation. Some of it leaves the brain from the basal ganglia for direct transmission to muscles via extrapyramidal pathways. These include all those motor tracts that are not part of the pyramidal pathways. They normally originate in the brainstem components of the basal ganglia and are named according to their site of origin:

- The *rubrospinal tracts* ('rubro' = red) originate from the red nuclei of the midbrain. Fibres cross over and descend in the lateral aspects of the cord.

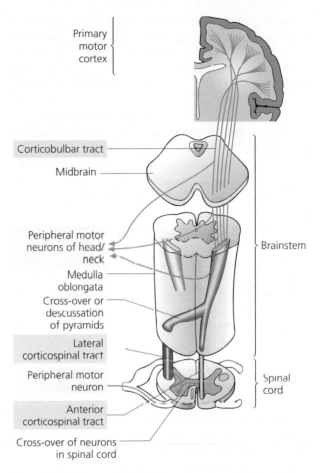

Figure 17.16 The pyramidal tracts from the motor cortex to muscles. The major tracts of neurons are identified.

Q. Distinguish between the pyramidal and extrapyramidal pathways.

- The *tectospinal tracts* ('tectum' = roof) originate from the superior colliculi of the tectum area of the midbrain, which receives input from the eyes. This tract is therefore part of the pathway that controls movement in response to visual stimuli.

- The *vestibulospinal tracts* derive from the vestibular nuclei of the medulla, and are influenced by input from the vestibular receptors of the inner ear.

The cerebellum

Observations indicate that the cerebellum assists the outputs from the motor cortex and basal ganglia by controlling the timing and sequence of muscle contractions. The cerebellum therefore has a vital role in the precise control of fine movements, e.g. in writing, buttoning clothing, hitting a tennis ball, and placing the foot during walking (i.e. without stamping).

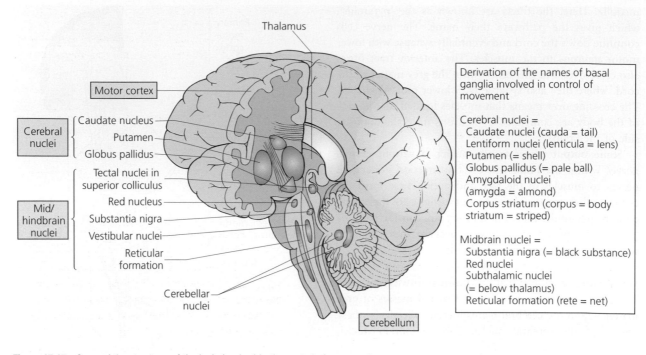

Figure 17.17 within image area labels: Thalamus, Motor cortex, Cerebral nuclei { Caudate nucleus, Putamen, Globus pallidus }, Mid/hindbrain nuclei { Tectal nuclei in superior colliculus, Red nucleus, Substantia nigra, Vestibular nuclei, Reticular formation }, Cerebellar nuclei, Cerebellum

Derivation of the names of basal ganglia involved in control of movement

Cerebral nuclei =
  Caudate nuclei (cauda = tail)
  Lentiform nuclei (lenticula = lens)
  Putamen (= shell)
  Globus pallidus (= pale ball)
  Amygdaloid nuclei (amygda = almond)
  Corpus striatum (corpus = body striatum = striped)

Midbrain nuclei =
  Substantia nigra (= black substance)
  Red nuclei
  Subthalamic nuclei (= below thalamus)
  Reticular formation (rete = net)

Figure 17.17 Some of the structures of the brain involved in the control of movement.
Q. Discuss the importance of movement and posture to health.

BOX 17.14 ALTERED MUSCLE FUNCTION DUE TO CENTRAL NERVOUS SYSTEM DISORDER

Trauma

Although protected by the cranium, the position of the cerebral cortex and cerebellar cortex at the surface of the brain make these structures susceptible to damage from head trauma, or from subarachnoid or subdural haemorrhage (see Chapter 8). Both cortices have central roles in the co-ordination of movement. The movement disorder will depend on the location and the extent of the haemorrhage.

Metabolism

Deeper structures, such as the basal ganglia, are less susceptible to direct physical trauma, but will be affected by localized hypoxia resulting from cerebrovascular haemorrhage (stroke), circulatory restriction (e.g. at birth leading to cerebral palsy), or restricted respiration (e.g. asphyxia, or drug-induced dyspnoea). Glucose deficiency during hypoglycaemic episodes may also induce temporary disorder, as energy requirements of neurons are not met. The uncoordinated movements of a person with diabetes mellitus having a hypoglycaemic episode (who will also be exhibiting behavioural change, such as aggression) should not be mistaken to be resulting from alcohol abuse.

Imbalance of excitatory and inhibitory pathways

Disturbance in the balance of excitatory to inhibitory neuronal pathways will disrupt the integration necessary to produce controlled movement. Parkinson's disease (unknown pathogenesis; onset peaks in the early 60s) arises as a consequence of the loss of dopamine as a neurotransmitter within the pathway between the substantia nigra (a midbrain nucleus) and the corpus striatum

nucleus of the cerebrum. The imbalance produced between the inhibitory neurons (which utilize dopamine) and excitatory neurons (which utilize acetylcholine) results in poor co-ordination of motor output, leading to hypertonia (see Box 17.15), expressed as muscle rigidity and a tremor at rest, and akinesia (slowness of movement and occasional freezing). The akinesia may also affect speech and swallowing. The person may also report sudden onset of extreme fatigue. As postural muscles become involved, there will be postural disequilibria (stooped posture on standing, and involuntary flexions of the head). Treatment is mainly with drugs that replace dopamine, or anticholinergics to reduce the excitatory pathway activities (Roy and Redfern, 1998). Support and rehabilitation may be necessary to improve mobility (see Box 17.8).

Huntington's disease (chorea) is an autosomal dominant, inherited disorder (see Chapter 20) with an onset typically at 40–50 years. Neurons that utilize gamma-aminobutyric acid (GABA) as an inhibitory neurotransmitter, and are found within the pathway between the substantia nigra and other basal ganglia (the caudate and putamen nuclei) and the cerebral cortex, degenerate leading to an imbalance of pathway activities. This produces hyperkinesia (exaggerated, involuntary movements) typical of chorea: the face and arms begin the movement, but eventually the whole body is affected. Cognitive problems also develop. The condition is untreatable.

Loss of nerve tracts

Multiple sclerosis is an immune disorder in which neurons are demyelinated, normally commencing in early adulthood. The pathogenesis is unclear, but it may be a response to viral infection.

BOX 17.14 CONTINUED

Plaques are produced, primarily within the white matter of the central nervous system. Loss of neurons in the corticospinal tracts produces muscle stiffness, slowness and weakness. The lower limbs are usually affected more severely, with involvement of the bladder. Loss of neurons in the brainstem affects the cranial nerves, which produces facial/neck weakness. The condition may also involve other parts of the brain producing ataxia (see Box 17.15) and even paroxysmal attacks of abrupt movements. Sensory function may also be affected, e.g. of the eye. Pain is common.

Multiple sclerosis is episodic in its early phases. Steroids may be helpful in reducing the rate of plaque formation. However, the condition is progressive, and care is supportive and rehabilitative (Campion, 1997).

Cerebral degenerative conditions such as Alzheimer's disease and Creutzfeldt–Jakob disease also produce movement problems. However, these are not normally considered to be disorders primarily of posture and movement, and are considered in Chapter 8 (see Box 8.9).

BOX 17.15 TERMS USED TO DESCRIBE DISORDERED VOLUNTARY MOVEMENTS

Clinical terminology in relation to movement and movement disorders is extensive and complex. Below are some of the more common terms:

● *Hypokinesia:* collective term for poor production of movement. *Paresis* is a related term used to signify weakness, and *paralysis* ('-plegia') signifies no movement. Hypokinesia arises through disorders associated with upper or lower motor neurons.
● *Akinesia/bradykinesia:* slowness of movement; often reflects a disorder of the extrapyramidal pathway.
● *Dystonia:* maintenance of abnormal posture through inappropriate muscle contractions.
● *Dyspraxia/apraxia:* inability to perform voluntary movements in the absence of paralysis, sensory loss, poor co-ordination or postural disorder. True dyspraxia arises from a failure of communication between the cerebral hemispheres.
● *Hyperkinesia:* production of abnormal involuntary movements, e.g. spasms (paroxysmal hyperkinesia), or of the face trunk and extremities (tardive hyperkinesia).
● *Ataxia:* poor fine co-ordination of movement; usually signifies a cerebellum disorder.
● *Hypotonia:* decreased muscle tone. Characterized by little resistance to passive stretch of the muscle, indicative of depressed muscle spindle functions. This usually means poor motor output control, so it is frequently observed as a consequence of trauma to the pyramidal tracts (e.g. spinal cord

injury) or to the cerebellum (e.g. cerebrovascular accident). Other symptoms include ease of tiring and weakness, but the damage may even make it difficult to rise from a chair or to use stairs. With time, the lack of motor output to the muscles causes the muscles to atrophy.
● *Hypertonia:* excessive muscle tone, noticeable when the muscle is stretched passively. Often arises as a consequence of trauma to the primary motor areas of the cerebral cortex, or to spinal cord tracts (which causes uneven excessive contractions – spasticity), or as a consequence of elevated muscle spindle sensitivity (causing more even but excessive contractions – rigidity). *Dystonia* is a condition in which damage to basal ganglia prevents the normal control of agonistic and antagonistic muscles, leading to sustained, involuntary twisting movements.
● *Clonus:* form of hypertonia, in which stretch reflex responses spread to other muscles. Often seen in spasticity.

Upper motor neuron syndromes promote the following disorders:

● *Paraparesis/paraplegia:* weakness of the lower extremities.
● *Hemiparesis/hemiplegia:* hypokinesia of the upper and lower extremities on one side.
● *Quadriparesis quadriplegia:* weakness of all four extremities.
● *Diplegia:* paralysis of both upper and lower extremities.

Lower motor neuron syndromes promote *flaccid paresis/paralysis* and *hyporeflexia/areflexia* (i.e. depression or absence of reflexes).

Summary

1 The skeletomuscular system provides the support and mobility required for the performance of basic activities of living.
2 Skeletal muscles support the skeleton and provide the capacity to move joints. They are comprised of bundles of muscle fibres, called fascicles, and are activated by associated motor nerves. Muscle fibres are cells that became fused together during differentiation. Each fibre acts as one cell, and stimulation contracts the entire fibre.
3 Under the microscope, muscle fibres exhibit a striated pattern that repeats along the fibre. Each 'segment' is called a

sarcomere, and the striations result from the arrangement of protein filaments within it.
4 Muscle fibre contraction involves an interaction between the actin and myosin protein filaments. Molecular cross-bridges between the proteins cause the actin to slide over the myosin, pulling the ends of the sarcomere together and shortening the fibre. The process requires the presence of calcium ions, released into the cytoplasm of the muscle fibre as a consequence of nerve stimulation.

Summary (Continued)

5 The neuromuscular junction exhibits the properties of a synapse, utilizing the release of the neurotransmitter acetylcholine, which induces a change in the electrical property of the muscle fibre. Each muscle fibre within a muscle is innervated, but the numbers of fibres, called a motor unit, that are innervated by branches from a single motor neuron varies from muscle to muscle. Large postural muscles have large motor units, which aids the efficiency of maintaining protracted periods of contraction.

6 Muscle fibres capable of maintaining contraction for long periods of time must utilize aerobic metabolism in order to withstand fatigue. These are called slow fibres. In relative terms, fast fibres produce a much faster contraction and relaxation, but rapidly exceed aerobic capacity and therefore fatigue quickly.

7 The arrangement of muscles in relation to the joints provides a system of levers that facilitates movement by reducing the force of contraction necessary to move the joint.

8 The degree of contraction produced by a muscle must be appropriate to the situation. This means that all of the 600-plus muscles of the body must be controlled individually. Control is provided by reflex action and by co-ordination of the neural output from the brain.

9 Sensory information is provided by the proprioceptors, or positional receptors. These are found in the joints, tendons of muscles, in the muscles themselves, and in the inner ear (balance or equilibrium receptors). They provide continuous information regarding the position and movement of joints, of tension in muscles, of muscle length, and of head position in relation to gravity.

10 Muscle spindle receptors are of particular importance, as they not only monitor muscle length but can also act to control that length. This is possible because they consist of modified muscle fibres and can be induced to contract or relax according to the activity of their own motor innervation. Thus, spindle length can be varied independently of the rest of the muscle, and in doing so can reflexly induce muscle contraction or relaxation but also facilitate voluntary movements. Muscle length, therefore, is determined by the neural activity in the motor nerve cells that innervate its fibres, and also by the motor nerve cells that innervate the spindles. This dual innervation provides a high degree of control, and also emphasizes the complex nature of motor co-ordination provided by the brain.

11 Much of the brain is involved in receiving sensory information from around the body, and in motor control. The latter areas are the motor cortex of the cerebrum, the basal ganglia, and the cerebellum of the hindbrain. Interactions between these areas occur, involving complex excitatory and inhibitory neural pathways, before the final activity is conveyed to the appropriate peripheral motor neurons.

12 Output from the motor cortex passes to the spinal cord or cranial nerves via the pyramidal pathways. The output that passes directly from the basal ganglia without passing first to the motor cortex comprises the extrapyramidal pathways.

Review questions

1 Physical activity is an important component of a healthy lifestyle for all age groups. How does exercise improve health? What effects does it have on the musculoskeletal system, the cardiovascular system, the respiratory system and the digestive system, and on mental health?

2 What role does exercise play in weight control?

3 How much exercise is recommended? Is this the same for everybody?

4 What are the hazards of exercising?

5 Examine your daily activity habits. Do you include exercise in your daily routine? What motivates you to do exercise, and what factors act as barriers? As health promotion is an important part of your role, do you think you could successfully promote physical activity in your patients?

Problems with immobility

6 Immobility of patients is a problem common to all branches of nursing. Give reasons why the following people might be immobile: (i) adult; (ii) child; (iii) a patient with a mental health disorder; and (iv) a patient with a learning disability.

7 Immobility may have serious consequences on a person's wellbeing as problems arise in specific body systems. Some of these problems may even be fatal. Below are some of the major complications of immobility; for each complication, (i) provide a definition; (ii) describe how immobility causes the complication; and (iii) make brief notes to indicate how a nurse can help to prevent the complication.

Cardiovascular complications: deep vein thrombosis; orthostatic hypotension; decreased tissue perfusion.

Respiratory complications: hypostatic pneumonia; pulmonary embolus.

Urinary complications: urinary tract infection; renal calculi; incontinence.

Musculoskeletal complications: osteoporosis; muscle wasting; foot drop; contractures.

Gastrointestinal complications: constipation.

Skin complications: pressure sores.

Psychosocial issues: loss of self-esteem; frustration; boredom; isolation.

REFERENCES

Campion, K. (1997) Multiple sclerosis. *Professional Nurse* **13**(3): 169–72.

Cunning, S. (2000) When the Dx is myasthenia gravis. *RN* **63**(4): 26–31.

McMahon-Parkes, K. and Cornock, M.A. (1997) Guillain Barré syndrome: biological basis, treatment and care. *Intensive and Critical Care Nursing* **13**(1): 42–8.

Riggio, S. and Jagoda, A. (1999) The rapid neurological examination 2: movement, reflexes, sensation, balance: know the signs that lead to the site of the pathological process. *Journal of Critical Illness* **14**(7): 368–72.

Roy, S. and Redfern, L. (1998) Parkinson's disease. *Nursing Standard* **12**(22): 49–56.

Sheridan, M.D. (1997) *From Birth to Five Years: children's developmental progress*. London: Routledge.

Skelton, J. (1996) Caring for patients with motor neurone disease. *Nursing Standard* **10**(32): 33–6.

Worsham, T.L. (2000) Easing the course of Guillain Barré syndrome. *RN* **63**(3): 46–50.

Chapter 18

The reproductive systems

Introduction: relation of reproduction to homeostasis
Overview of the anatomy and physiology of the human reproductive systems
Reproductive physiology

Physiology of birth control
References
Further reading

INTRODUCTION: RELATION OF REPRODUCTION TO HOMEOSTASIS

All organ systems of the body operate as homeostatic controls to maintain the wellbeing of the body, providing the person is not genetically and/or environmentally compromised. At the cellular level of organization, reproduction may be regarded as a homeostatic process in which cells divide once they have reached their optimal size. Growth beyond this would mean that the cell would be unable to obtain sufficient levels of nutrients to sustain intercellular homeostasis, or to remove toxic chemicals, as the cell membrane (i.e. surface area) grows at a slower rate then the rest of the cell (i.e. volume) that it supports. Cellular reproduction is therefore necessary to maintain the appropriate growth, development, specialization, and repair of human tissues, thus contributing to a person's wellbeing.

At the organism level of organization, reproduction may be regarded as a homeostatic control adapted for the survival of the species (Figure 18.1). The human reproductive system is dormant until the onset of puberty, when there seems to be a trigger that activates the genetic code responsible for the production of hormones for the initiation and continuation of this developmental stage.

Although the common purpose of both sexes is to produce offspring, their functional roles are quite different. The male role is to manufacture up to half a billion gametes (sperm) per day, which are mixed with glandular secretions, creating a mixture called semen. This fluid leaves the male system by the process of ejaculation. The complementary roles of the female are to manufacture and mature female gametes (oocytes, i.e. immature 'eggs' or ova), and subsequently to release (ovulate) one potential ovum per month (although sometimes one from each ovary are released simultaneously). These gametes travel to the Fallopian tubes (oviducts). Upon sexual intercourse, the male and female gametes may fuse (= fertilization). This fusion produces a new cell called the zygote. The zygote contains all the genetic information required to produce another human. A pregnancy is initiated if the zygote derivative implants into the lining of the uterus (womb). Thus, although the female and male are equal partners in the fertilization process, it is the female's uterus that provides a life-support system until birth. During this period (= gestation), the female's homeostatic parameters are reset to provide a suitable environment for prebirth development, and nutritional support via breast milk for the newborn until it is able to take a mixed diet.

The intentions of this chapter are to present an overview of the anatomy and physiology of the male and female reproductive systems, and to give a detailed account of the physiological processes and hormonal mechanisms responsible for the homeostatic regulation of reproductive function. The physiology underpinning birth control will also be discussed, and boxed applications identify common male and female homeostatic imbalances, with their principles of correction identified.

Figure 18.1 Cellular and sexual reproduction: homeostatic devices. (a) Reproductive function fluctuating within its homeostatic range. On a cellular level, this reflects that cellular reproduction matches cellular loss. On an organism level, this reflects that the population size is sustainable, e.g. by its food supplies. (b_1) Increased reproductive capacity. On a cellular basis, this reflects that cell reproduction is greater than cellular losses, e.g. following injury when cells are reproducing to replace lost or damaged cells. Alternatively, it could indicate some underlying pathology, such as tumour growth or hypertrophied organs. On an organism basis, this reflects that the human population number has increased beyond its capabilities of maintaining such a population explosion. (c_1) Homeostatic 'controls' that correct the cellular disturbance, as occurs normally during post-healing periods and when cancers are destroyed by the body's anti-cancer agents or via clinical interventions using chemotherapy, radiotherapy, surgery and/or laser therapy. Homeostatic 'controls' that correct the population explosion, e.g. limited food supplies accompanied by the survival of the fittest. (b_2) A decreased cellular reproduction. (c) Correction of underlying pathology or natural changes. (d_1) An increase in cellular reproduction that

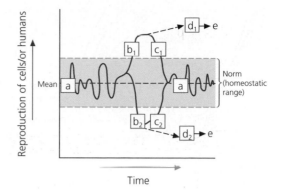

is beyond control as occurs, for example, in certain cancers, or population explosion living beyond human resource level. (d_2) A decreased cellular reproduction that is beyond control, as occurs normally with the ageing process, or abnormally in pathological wasting conditions, such as anorexia nervosa. A severe decrease in the population as occurs in natural disasters, such as war, famine, etc. (e) Death at a cellular or human level.

OVERVIEW OF THE ANATOMY AND PHYSIOLOGY OF THE HUMAN REPRODUCTIVE SYSTEMS

The human reproductive system consists of:

- a pair of primary sex organs (gonads) that produce, store and nourish the developing gametes. The gonads are involved in the initial transport of the gametes (i.e. sperm and potential ova), and function as endocrine tissue to produce hormones that co-ordinate activities specific to the different sexes;

- a diverse range of other structures, such as ducts that transport gametes, accessory glands that secrete fluid into ducts, and external genitalia associated with the sexes.

The various functions of the male and female reproductive tracts are summarized in the tables accompanying Figures 18.2 and 18.3.

The male reproductive system

The male reproductive system is adapted for:

- the production of spermatozoa;

- the transportation of sperm to the female reproductive tract;

- producing hormones that control the development of the secondary sexual characteristics, such as enlargement of the larynx, development of the male form, and body, pubic and facial hair.

The primary sex organs are called the testes (singular = testis). These produce the male gamete – the spermatozoa – in a process called spermatogenesis. This process is

BOX 18.1 SEXUAL DIFFERENTIATION FROM UTERO TO PUBERTY

During embryonic development, the most important sex hormone is the male sex hormone testosterone. Until the seventh week of gestation, the initial reproductive structures of the male and female are the same. Soon after this, the gonads of a genetically male embryo begins to produce testosterone. This causes the primary male sex gonads to develop into two testes, which produce sperm. The lack of testosterone causes the two female gonads to develop into ovaries, which will produce immature ova.

Throughout fetal life and childhood, the testes secrete low levels of testosterone and the ovaries secrete low levels of oestrogens. Between the ages of 8 and 12 years, the gonads start to secrete more sex hormones. This triggers sexual maturation, or puberty. In girls, puberty commences at about 10 years; in boys, it begins at about 11 years. Puberty last for 2 or 3 years, and is complete when the person is capable of reproduction.

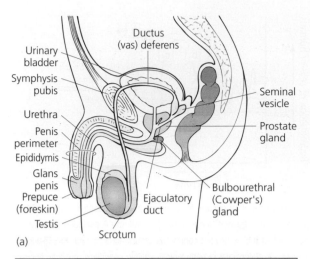

(a)

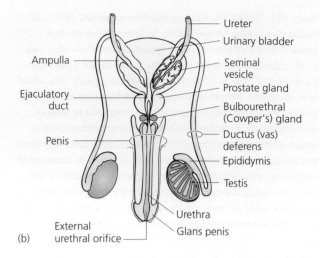

(b)

Structure	Homeostatic function
Testes	Produce sperm and sex hormone
Accessory organs	
Vas deferens, urethra	Carry sperm out of the body
Glands – seminal vesicles, prostate, Cowper's	Contribute the majority of fluid within semen
Scrotum	Houses the testis outside the pelvic cavity – essential for viable sperm production
Penis	Organ of copulation and excretion

Figure 18.2 The male reproductive system: (a) sagittal view and (b) posterior view.

Q. Identify the accessory sex gland that contributes fructose to the seminal fluid.

Q. What accessory glands contribute the majority of the seminal fluid?

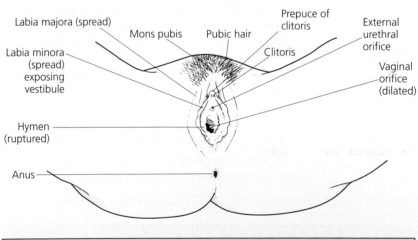

Figure 18.3 External genitalia of the female (the vulva).

Q. Name the location of the erectile tissue found in the female.

Structure	Homeostatic function
Mons pubis	Cushions the pubic symphysis during sexual intercourse
Labia majora	Enclose and protect other external reproductive organs
Labia minora	Form margins of vestibule; protect openings of vagina and urethra
Clitoris	Gland is richly supplied with sensory nerve endings
Vestibule	Space between labia minora that includes vaginal and urethal openings
Vestibular glands	Secrete fluid that moistens and lubricates vestibule

controlled by the release of a gonadotropin hormone called follicle-stimulating hormone (FSH) from the anterior pituitary gland (see Figure 9.8). The testes store sperm until they are either released from the body or broken down into their component parts and then recycled to contribute to intracellular homeostatic mechanisms. The testes also contain endocrine cells, which produce and secrete the male hormones (androgens). This process is regulated by the release of a gonadotropin, luteinizing hormone (LH), from the anterior pituitary. Testosterone is the main androgen produced by the testes.

The accessory reproductive organs consist of the scrotum, ducts, glands and penis. These protect the sperm and aid its transport outside the body (Figure 18.2).

Structure of the testes

The paired oval-shaped testes, or testicles, originate from a location close to the developing kidneys near the posterior abdominal wall of the embryo. They develop from the embryonic tissue, which also gives rise to the urinary system; indeed, the urethra of the male provides a common route for the exit of sperm and urine from the body. The testes descend through a channel called the inguinal canal into their sac-like scrotum during the seventh month of gestation, following contraction of specialized muscular tissue called the gubernaculum (Figure 18.4). The testes are thus suspended outside the abdominal pelvic cavity. This means that their temperature is 2–3°C below the core body temperature of 37°C. Sperm development will only progress normally at this cooler temperature. The testicular venous plexus also contributes to the cooler temperature of the testes, since it coils around the testicular artery and functions to absorb heat from arterial blood, thus cooling it before it enters the testes.

Each oval-shaped testis is surrounded by the tunica albuginea, a connective tissue capsule that extends inwards, dividing it into compartmentalizing lobules. Each lobule contains one to four seminiferous tubules, which produce sperm. These sperm-producing factories are continuous with other tubules (the ductus efferentia, epididymis, vas deferentia and urethra) that provide the distribution route for sperm exiting from the body (Figure 18.5(a)). A cross-section of the seminiferous tubule reveals that it contains immature sperm cells at various stages of development (Figures 18.5(b–c)). The most immature cells, called the spermatogonia, are located peripherally; the fully mature spermatozoa are located centrally within the tubule lumen. In between these two locations, the cells are of advancing maturity, and are called primary spermatocytes, secondary spermatocytes, and spermatids, respectively.

Embedded between the developing sperm cells are the Sertoli or sustentacular cells. Their homeostatic functions are to:

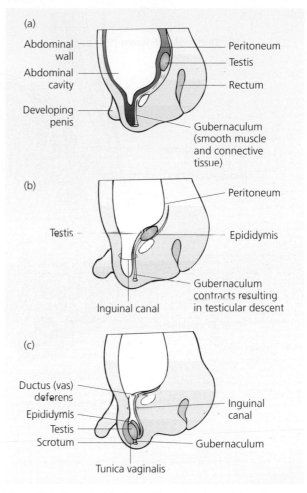

Figure 18.4 Descent of the testes. The testes descend from the posterior abdominal wall into the scrotum during fetal development: (a) 6-month-old fetus; (b) 7-month-old fetus; (c) at birth.
Q. Normally, the testes descend before birth. In which homeostatic imbalance is there a failure of this descent?
Q. Which hormone is responsible for the differentiation of the external genitals of the male?

- support, nourish and protect developing spermatogenic cells;

- phagocytose degenerating spermatogenic cells;

- control the movement of spermatogenic cells;

- control the release of sperm into the lumen of the seminiferous tubules;

- secrete chemicals that maintain testicular homeostasis, e.g. the hormone inhibin depresses FSH production and hence spermatogenesis; and androgen-binding protein helps prevent androgen hormones (e.g. testosterone) from going beyond their homeostatic parameters, and also facilitates the actions of the androgens. These secretions provide negative feedback loops, which maintain reproductive function within its homeostatic parameters (see later, and Figure 18.14).

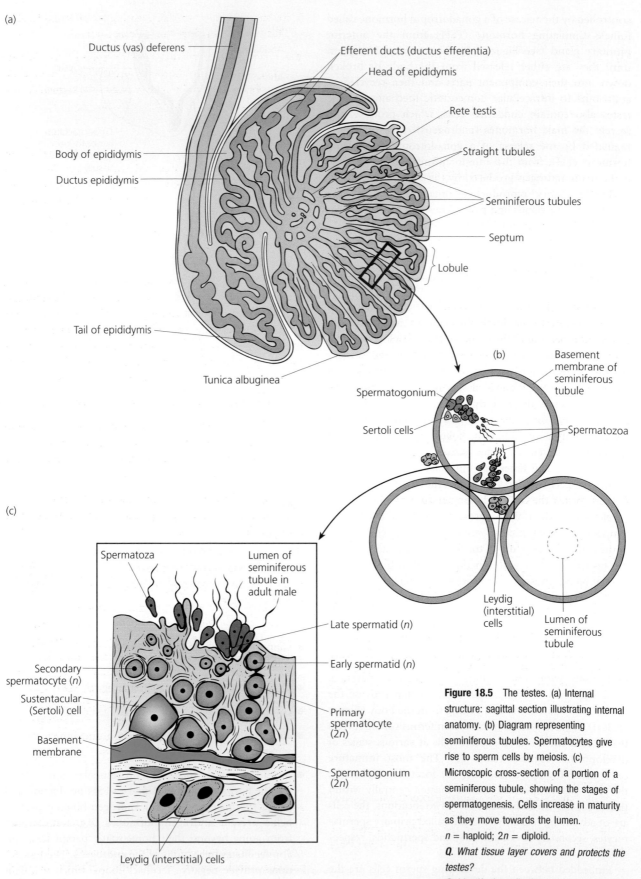

(a)

Ductus (vas) deferens

Efferent ducts (ductus efferentia)

Head of epididymis

Rete testis

Body of epididymis

Straight tubules

Ductus epididymis

Seminiferous tubules

Septum

Lobule

Tail of epididymis

Tunica albuginea

(b)

Basement membrane of seminiferous tubule

Spermatogonium

Sertoli cells

Spermatozoa

Leydig (interstitial) cells

Lumen of seminiferous tubule

(c)

Spermatoza

Lumen of seminiferous tubule in adult male

Secondary spermatocyte (n)

Late spermatid (n)

Early spermatid (n)

Sustentacular (Sertoli) cell

Basement membrane

Primary spermatocyte (2n)

Spermatogonium (2n)

Leydig (interstitial) cells

Figure 18.5 The testes. (a) Internal structure: sagittal section illustrating internal anatomy. (b) Diagram representing seminiferous tubules. Spermatocytes give rise to sperm cells by meiosis. (c) Microscopic cross-section of a portion of a seminiferous tubule, showing the stages of spermatogenesis. Cells increase in maturity as they move towards the lumen.

n = haploid; $2n$ = diploid.

Q. What tissue layer covers and protects the testes?

Q. Identify the cells that produce sperm and androgens.

Cryptorchidism is an undescended testis at birth. It occurs in about 3% of full-term babies and about 30% of premature infants (Kennedy et al., 1998). This condition may cause hormonal imbalances; therefore such infants require early treatment by surgery or by testosterone injections, which stimulate the descent of the testes. If untreated, spermatogenesis is inhibited permanently; an undescended testis left in the abdomen may undergo malignant changes.

Testicular cancer is 30–50 times greater in people with a history of late descended or undescended testes (Kinkade, 1999); most cancers arise from the sperm-producing cells. Testicular tumours represent 1–2% of male malignancies, and it is the commonest cancer affecting men aged 20–24 years (Kinkade, 1999). Nurses should encourage monthly self-examination of the testes, since an alteration of or an enlarged testis, although not necessarily a malignancy, should be reported to the patient's GP as soon as possible. As with all cancers, correction is most effective when diagnosis is made early in the development of the tumour, and necessitates removal of the cancerous tissue.

Exercise

Discuss why it is important that the testes descend before birth.

Accessory organs of the male reproductive system

Accessory organs of the male system comprise the duct system, various secretory glands, and the penis.

After production, the sperm are moved from the seminiferous tubules to the straight tubules (Figure 18.5(a)). The latter lead to a network of ciliated ducts called the rete testes ('rete' = net), which empty into the ductus efferentia. From here, the sperm are transported through a duct system averaging 8 m in length. In order of transit, the sections of this system are called the epididymis, the vas deferens (sperm tube), and the urethra (Figure 18.2(b)).

The duct system

The epididymis

From the rete testes, the spermatozoa enter the head, body and then the tail of the epididymis via the ductus efferentia. It takes about 2 weeks for the sperm to transit the epididymis. The homeostatic functions of this region are to:

- absorb excess fluid from the lumen, and secrete nutrients into the lumen, so as to provide a suitable environment

for sperm maturation, i.e. ensuring motility and fertility. This process is referred to as 'capacitation';

- act as a temporary storage site for sperm until they are either released into the vas deferentia when the male is sexually aroused and ejaculates, or broken down chemically, and their constituents recycled.

The vas deferens

The vas deferens (ductus deferens) is about 40–45 cm long. It begins at the epididymis and ends behind the urinary bladder, where it expands to form the ampulla region from which the ejaculatory ducts emerge. These ducts penetrate the muscular wall of the prostate gland, and upon contraction empty their contents into the urethra (Figure 18.2(b)).

The urethra

The urethra extends for a distance of about 15–20 cm from the urinary bladder to the tip of the penis. This terminal portion of the male system, together with the penis, serves both the urinary and reproductive systems, as it conveys urine and semen to the exterior. Thus, these structures form a common part of the urogenital tract. Figure 18.6(a) shows that the urethra has three anatomical regions:

- *prostatic urethra:* passes through the prostate gland;

- *membranous urethra:* a short segment that passes from the prostatic urethra to the penile urethra, and penetrates the urogenital diaphragm and the muscular floor of the pelvic cavity;

- *penile urethra:* extends from the distal border of the urogenital diaphragm to the external orifice at the tip of the penis.

Nonspecific urethritis (NSU) is a condition in which the urethra becomes inflamed. This impedes the flow of urine, and a burning pain accompanies urination; there may also be a pus-containing discharge. NSU affects both sexes, and can result from trauma (e.g. the passage of a catheter), chemical agents (e.g. alcohol), and nonspecific microbes. Bacterial agents can pass from an infected mother to infant during birth, and infect the eyes of the infant. Many infections remain untreated, as symptoms in the male are mild and females are usually asymptomatic. Bacterial NSU responds to antibiotics (e.g. tetracycline).

Accessory sex glands

The accessory glands of the male reproductive tract include paired seminal vesicles, paired bulbourethral (Cowper's) glands, and a single prostate gland (Figure 18.2). They contribute approximately 95% of the fluid contained in

(a)

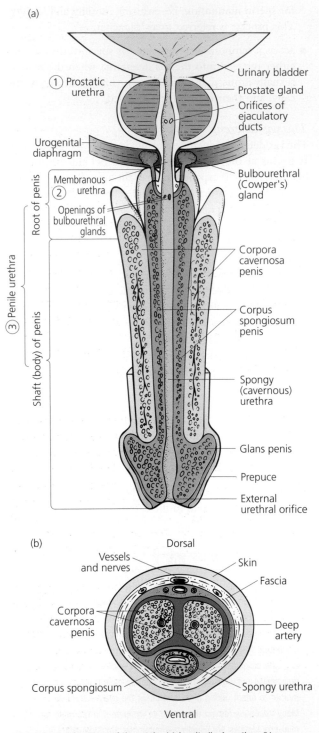

Figure 18.6 Structure of the penis: (a) longitudinal section; (b) transverse section. 1–3 denotes anatomical regions of the urethra.
Q. Which tissue forms the erectile tissue in the penis?

semen (the fluid conveyed and expelled from the urethra via peristalsis during ejaculation). The seminiferous tubules and the epididymis produce secretions that contribute a small percentage to semen. Collectively, the secretions activate sperm in the semen by providing nutrients for their motility, and act as a buffer mechanism, thus counteracting the acidic environments of the urethra and the female tract.

The seminal vesicles
The seminal vesicles are located on the posterior wall at the base of the bladder. They secrete a viscous alkaline fluid, which accounts for approximately 60% of semen volume. This fluid contains chemicals such as fructose, prostaglandins and ascorbic acid, which contribute to the life (viability) of the sperm. Fructose provides the essential fuel necessary to initiate and maintain the beating of the sperm tail (flagella). Prostaglandins are thought to:

● decreases the viscosity of the mucus plug, which guards the entrance to the uterus (i.e. the cervix) of the female;

● stimulate antiperistalsis of the female reproductive tract, and so aid transportation of sperm to the site of fertilization in the fallopian tubes;

● stimulate the release of the hormone relaxin and certain enzymes that enhance sperm motility;

● stimulate a seminal chemical called plasmin, which has bactericidal properties. Together with other unidentified chemicals with antibiotic properties, this may help to prevent urinary tract infections, and thus must be considered a part of the homeostatic external defence mechanisms;

● stimulate clotting factors (e.g. fibrinogen) in semen, which cause its coagulation after ejaculation, helping to retain it within the female tract;

● stimulate the enzyme fibrinolysin, which liquefies the coagulant mass about 5–20 min after it clots, so that the sperm can swim out and begin their journey within the female tract;

● stimulate ascorbic acid to act as a cofactor in some metabolic reactions within the sperm's cytoplasm.

The prostate
The prostate, a large gland positioned just below the bladder, secretes a thin, milky, alkaline secretion that accounts for 14–30% of semen. It contains fibrinolysin and acid phosphatase, enzymes that are important in promoting maximum motility of the sperm.

The bulbourethral glands
The bulbourethral (Cowper's) glands are inferior to the prostate. They are so called because of their shape, and because they secrete their fluid directly into the urethra. They release a thick, clear, alkaline mucus just before ejaculation; this neutralizes traces of acidic urine that reside in the urethra, and lubricates the end of the penis before and during sexual intercourse. The female reproductive organs, however, provide most of the lubricating fluid for intercourse.

BOX 18.4 PROSTATISM, PROSTATIC HYPERTROPHY AND PROSTATIC CANCER

Prostatism is a male urinary tract problem associated with lesions of the prostate. Symptoms include difficulty in micturition, a poor urinary stream, and urinary frequency with nocturia (micturition during the night).

The prostate gland is susceptible to infection, enlargement and benign/malignant tumours. Benign prostatic enlargement or hypertrophy (BPH), is a common problem in older men. Approximately 51% of men aged 60–69 years have prostatic hypertrophy (Heuther and McCance, 1996). Since the prostate surrounds the urethra, its enlargement can obstruct the flow of urine, resulting in secondary homeostatic imbalances of the bladder, uterus and kidneys. BPH can be managed successfully with drugs (e.g. finasteride). Correction involves partial removal of the enlarged tissue or total removal of the gland. However, if the patient cannot tolerate surgery, a permanent indwelling catheter is inserted with appropriate care, including:

● selecting the appropriate length (i.e. shorter in female) and bore size of catheter and balloon;
● ensuring that the catheter bag is positioned lower than the bladder, that the drainage tubing is free of kinks, and that

the drainage outlet is not touching any potential contaminants;
● controlling fluid intake to reduce the risk of constipation and of concentrating the urine, which can be a potential cause of bladder irritation;
● providing psychological support, since the catheter in situ affects body image;
● meatal hygiene to minimize encrustation.

Prostatic cancer is a common and leading cause of cancer death in men. However, it rarely occurs before the age of 50 years (Heuther and McCance, 1996). Since testosterone stimulates an increased growth rate of the cancer, and oestrogens inhibit growth, treatment may involve surgical removal of the testes, or the administration of drugs that are testosterone antagonists or oestrogenic agonists. Although drug administration does not stop the cancer, it may slow growth. Radiotherapy is also an option. Palliative measures are aimed at relieving urinary bladder outlet, colonic obstruction, spinal cord compression and pain. Treatment and prognosis depend upon the extent of the disease. See also the case study of a man with prostatic hyperplasia in Section 6.

The penis

The cylindrically shaped penis is a urogenital organ. Its shape facilitates the introduction of sperm into the female reproductive tract during sexual intercourse (copulation or coitus); therefore, the structure is a necessity for the perpetuation of the species. It is also the male organ of urinary excretion since it conveys urine through the urethra to the external environment.

The penis and the scrotum constitute the male external genitalia. The penis consists of an attached root and a free body (shaft) that ends in an enlarged sensitive tip, called the glans penis, over which the skin is folded doubly to form a loosely fitted retractable case (the prepuce or foreskin) (Figure 18.6(a)). Internally, the penis comprises the spongy urethra and three cylindrical masses or bodies (corpora) of spongy erectile tissue. All three masses are enclosed by a fibrous connective tissue (fascia) and loose-fitting skin

BOX 18.5 PARAPHIMOSIS, HYDROCOELE AND INGUINAL HERNIA

The penis may be subjected to numerous sexually transmitted infections and structural abnormalities. *Paraphimosis* is a condition in which the foreskin (prepuce) fits so tightly over the glans penis that it cannot retract. This can occur in catheterized patients, and results in severe discomfort. It is treated by manual reduction. Circumcision (excision or cutting of the prepuce) may be necessary once the inflammation subsides. Mild paraphimosis causes the accumulation of dirt or organic matter under the foreskin, resulting in severe infection. Severe paraphimosis can result in urinary flow obstruction; it may result in death in an infant born with the condition. After puberty, failure to achieve a penile erection occurs; although this does not affect sperm production, it may cause infertility since normal intercourse may not be possible.

A common cause of scrotal swelling in the male is the accumulation of fluid called a *hydrocoele*. The cause of chronic hydrocoele is unknown. Acute hydrocoele occurs in association with mumps or acute infections of the epididymis of the testes, or as a

result of local trauma such as an inguinal hernia. Treatment is only necessary if the hydrocoele compresses the testicular circulation, or if the scrotum becomes enlarged, uncomfortable or embarrassing. A surgical incision is made through the wall of the scrotum. The sac is resected or, after opening, sutured to collapse the wall. Nursing care involves applying an ice pack to the scrotum to reduce the oedema and bruising. A scrotal support is worn postoperatively.

An *inguinal hernia* occurs because the intestines are pushed through a weakened area of the abdominal wall that separates the abdominal pelvic cavity from the scrotum. Such hernias usually occur upon lifting heavy objects, although they can also be formed congenitally. Inguinal hernias are much more common in men and femoral hernias more common in women, although they do occur in either sex. Correction involves external supports that prevent organs from protruding into the scrotum and aspiration (or drawing) of fluid, but the more serious hernias require surgical repair, thus require perioperative nursing care.

(Figure 18.6(b)). The two larger, uppermost cylinders form the corpora cavernosa; the smaller, lower one, which contains the urethra, is the corpus spongiosum.

The male sexual act

During sexual arousal, increased parasympathetic nerve activity causes vascular spaces or sinuses within the spongy erectile tissue of the penis to vasodilate and become engorged with blood. The expansion compresses the veins draining the penis, so most blood flowing into it is retained, enlarging the penis and causing it to become rigid. The resultant erection permits the penis to perform a penetrating role during sexual intercourse.

Ejaculation is a sympathetic reflex that also causes the bladder sphincter to close, and so prevents the mixing of urine and semen in the urethra (which could immobilize the sperm), and prevents semen entering the bladder. Ejaculation occurs when peristaltic contractions from the testes spread to the epididymis, vas deferens and accessory glands simultaneous to the closing of the bladder sphincter. Muscles in the penis contract, and the semen is discharged. The penile flaccid state returns when the arteries constrict and pressure on the veins is relieved.

The female reproductive system

The female reproductive system is adapted for:

● oogenesis, i.e. the production of ova;

● receiving sperm;

● providing a suitable environment for fertilization and for prebirth development (see Chapter 20);

● producing hormones that control the development of secondary sexual characteristics, such as pubic hair, and the provision of the feminine form.

The female reproductive system, therefore, has a greater variety of tasks than the male system, which is involved only in sperm production and ejaculation. This is reflected in the increased complexity of the female reproductive organs.

The primary female sex organs are the paired ovaries. The accessory reproductive organs consist of the uterine (Fallopian) tubes, the uterus (womb), the vagina, and the external genitalia that comprise the vulva (Figure 18.7(a)). In addition, the mammary glands have a significant role in female reproduction (see later and Chapter 20).

BOX 18.6 INFERTILITY AND STERILITY IN MALES

Male infertility is the inability of the man to bring about conception. Male sterility is the inability to produce potent spermatozoa. A decreased sperm production (oligospermia) can result from disruption of seminiferous tubule function. The decrease may be temporary, as occurs with acute infections (the leading cause of infertility), or permanent, as occurs occasionally when a baby is born with undescended testes (cryptorchidism), or has a physical deficiency or obstruction of the reproductive ducts (the leading cause of sterility). A reduced reproductive capacity in males may also be due to factors that cause structural abnormalities of the sperm. Thus the number, motility and shape of the sperm can give a hint of fertility, and are used clinically to assess the degree of infertility. Normal values are as follows:

Volume of semen ejaculated: 2–6 ml.
Sperm count: 60–150 million/ml.
Shape: 60–80% should have the normal appearance.
Motility: 50% should be motile after incubation for 1 h at 37°C.

The vast number of sperm is required since only a small percentage survive and eventually reach the site of fertilization; although only one sperm fertilizes an ovum, fertilization requires the combined action of large numbers to chemically break down the barrier produced by the follicular cells surrounding the ovum. The volume and number will be progressively decreased if the man has had frequent ejaculations.

Sperm can be frozen and stored at −70°C; their motility and fertilizing potential reappears when thawed. This process is used when artificial insemination by husband or donor is required. It may also be used for men who are undergoing chemotherapy, since this type of treatment may cause infertility.

Undersecretion of gonadotropin-releasing hormones and gonadotropins (FSH and LH) can lead to sterility in either sex, since functional gametes will not be produced. The depression of hypothalamic secretion of gonadotropin-releasing hormones may be a consequence of dietary disturbances, distress or anaemia. In males, fatigue, alcohol abuse and emotional factors are more common causes of impotency (i.e. inability to perform sexual intercourse). High testicular temperatures decrease sperm production and thus are also associated with sterility. Pituitary, gonad and adrenal gland tumours may also cause infertility by secreting abnormal types and amounts of gonadotropin or sex hormones.

(a)

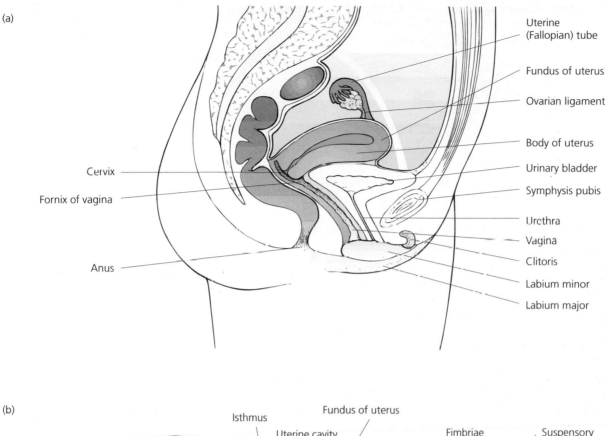

(b)

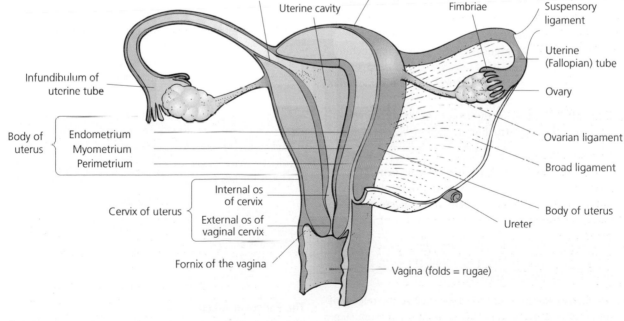

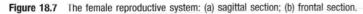

Figure 18.7 The female reproductive system: (a) sagittal section; (b) frontal section.

Ovaries

The paired ovaries are structures about twice the size of almond nuts. One lies on each side of the pelvic cavity. Their position is supported by ovarian ligaments, which anchor them medially to the uterus, suspensory ligaments, which anchor them laterally to the pelvic wall, and broad ligaments, which anchor them to the posterior wall of the pelvis (Figure 18.7(b)).

Each ovary contains a hilus where nerves, blood, and lymphatic vessels enter/exit. Just as the testes are adapted for sperm and hormonal production in the male, the

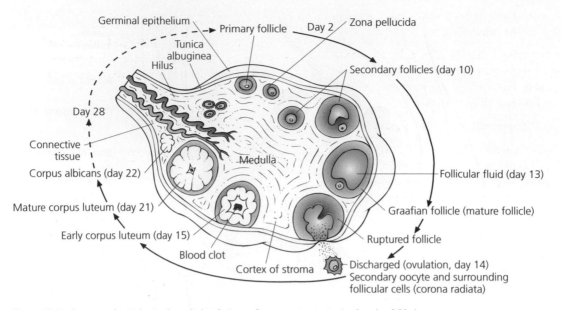

Figure 18.8 An ovary. Approximate times in brackets are for an average menstrual cycle of 28 days.
Q. What structures in the ovary contain endocrine tissue, and what hormones do they secrete?

ovaries are adapted for the production of oocytes (cells that develop into mature ova following fertilization) and hormones (progesterone, oestrogens and relaxin). Therefore, they contain germ cells, distributed as a germinal epithelium found as a surface layer of cuboidal cells in the outer cortex of this organ (Figure 18.8). Other structures include the tunica albuginea, that is a capsule of connective tissue immediately encloses the general epithelium, and a stroma, a region of connective tissue deep to the tunica albuginea in the outer cortical and inner medullar regions.

The cortical region of the ovary contains the ovarian follicles. As the menstrual cycle proceeds, the follicles progressively change their structure, as follows.

1   In the early stages of the menstrual cycle, primary follicles consist of a couple of external layers of epithelial cells and a primary oocyte. The inner layers comprise the granulosa cells.

2   Secondary follicles develop fluid-filled spaces around the granulosa cells. The spaces unite to form a central fluid-filled cavity or antrum.

3   A Graafian follicle is observed just before the release of the oocyte at ovulation. This is the most mature stage of follicular development. The oocyte is now referred to as a secondary oocyte.

4   A corpus luteum (= 'yellow body') develops after ovulation. This consists of the Graafian follicle minus its secondary oocyte and encasing granulosa cells. The corpus luteum degenerates into the corpus albicans (= 'white body'), unless fertilization takes place, in which case it is retained for a while as the corpus luteum of pregnancy.

Like the testes, the ovaries originate from embryonic tissue close to the posterior abdominal wall near the developing kidneys. During development, they descend to locations just below the pelvic brim, where they remain attached to the lateral pelvic wall.

Exercise

Identify and describe the structure of the primary sex organs of the female, and state the equivalent in the male.

BOX 18.7 OVARIAN CYSTS

Ovarian cysts are benign enlargements on one or both ovaries, or within the corpus luteum. The cyst, a fluid-filled sac, develops from a follicle that fails to rupture completely, or from the corpus luteum that fails to degenerate. They rarely become dangerous, and often disappear within a few months of appearance. If they remain and cause pain, then surgical removal corrects the problem. (See also Crayford *et al.*, 2000.)

The Fallopian tubes

The two Fallopian tubes (oviducts, or uterine tubes) transport the secondary oocyte (or the fertilized ovum if fertilization has taken place) to the uterus. The oviducts are attached to the uterus at its superior outer angles, which lie in the upper margins of the broad ligaments. Each tube is about 10 cm long and has three distinct regions:

• *isthmus:* the narrow, thick-walled portion that joins the uterus;

- *ampulla:* the intermediate, dilated portion that makes up about two-thirds of the tube's length;

- *infundibulum:* the funnel-shaped, terminal component that opens into the peritoneal cavity surrounding the ovary. The opening has a fringe of finger-like projections, called the fimbriae (Figure 18.9).

The wall of the Fallopian tube consists of three layers:

- *internal mucosa:* contains cilia adapted to aid the movement of the ovum and to provide it with nutritional support. This layer is in direct contact with the peritoneum of the pelvic cavity, and is continuous with the cavity of the uterus, and hence with the vagina;

- *muscularis layer:* the middle region comprising inner circular, and outer longitudinal, muscle sublayers responsible for the peristaltic movements that move the fertilized ovum into the uterus;

- *serosa:* an outer serous connective tissue membrane.

Approximately once a month, a secondary oocyte (immature ovum) ruptures from the surface of the ovary near the infundibular region of the Fallopian tube in a process called ovulation. The oocyte is swept into the tube by suction pressure generated by the ciliated epithelium of the infundibulum. It is then propelled along the Fallopian tube by ciliary action, supplemented by peristaltic contractions of the muscularis layer. Fertilization usually occurs in the ampulla of the uterine tube (at this point, the secondary oocyte becomes an ovum, and then with the sperm nucleus fusion forms a zygote), and may occur at any time up to 24 h after ovulation. The resultant zygote divides by mitosis, producing a specialized structure, the blastocyst, which descends into the uterus over the next few days. If unfertilized, the secondary oocyte disintegrates, and the remains leave the female tract. The details of fertilization are discussed in Chapter 20.

Exercise

See Chapter 20 for the details of fertilization. Describe the path of spermatozoon and secondary oocyte exit from their respective reproductive systems, clearly identifying how the gametes are moved along the Fallopian tubes.

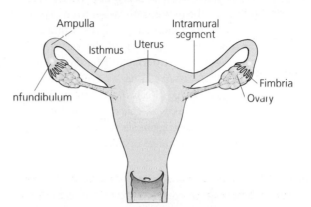

Organ	Homeostatic function
Ovary	Production of egg cells and female sex hormones
Uterine tube	Conveys egg cell toward uterus; site of fertilization; conveys developing embryo to uterus
Uterus	Protects and sustains life of embryo during pregnancy
Vagina	Conveys uterine secretions to outside of body; receives erect penis during sexual intercourse; transports fetus during birth process
Vulva	Protection, sexual arousal
Mammary glands	Produce milk

Figure 18.9 The Fallopian (uterine) tubes and uterus.

BOX 18.8 PELVIC INFLAMMATORY DISEASE

Pelvic inflammatory disease (PID) is a collective term used to include any extensive bacterial infection of the pelvic organs, especially the uterus, Fallopian tubes or ovaries. The external opening of the female tract makes this a susceptible area to infection by pathogens (e.g. gonococcal bacteria). Spreading of inflammation is also common.

Salpingitis (inflammation of the Fallopian tubes), for example, spreads readily and causes peritonitis (inflammation of the peritoneum), a potentially serious problem. Endometriosis, another benign condition, is the presence of functional endometrium tissue outside the uterus. The displaced tissue can occur in many different locations, although it is most often found in or on pelvic and abdominal organs. The tissues develop and regress influenced by the normal events of the menstrual cycle;

symptoms include premenstrual pain or unusual menstrual pain (dysmenorrhoea) caused by the displaced tissue being shed during menstruation.

The infection causing PID may spread to other tissues, including the blood, where it may cause septic shock and death. The infection may be very distressing for the patient. The hospitalized patient is maintained on bed rest. Local warmth may be applied to the abdomen to provide comfort externally. Healthcare professionals provide support in explaining how PID occurs and how it can be controlled see Best, 2000).

Early treatment with antibiotics (tetracycline or penicillin) is essential to stop the PID spreading. To prevent recurrence, sexual partners must also be treated with antibiotic combinations (Stones and Mountfield, 2001).

The uterus

The uterus is located between the bladder and rectum, and is the site of menstruation (if fertilization has not occurred), implantation, embryo-fetal development and labour. A female who has never been pregnant has an inverted pear-shaped uterus that is about 7.5 cm and 5.3 cm at its widest and narrowest parts, respectively (Figure 18.9). Anatomically, the uterus is divided into an expanded superior body called the fundus, a constricted isthmus, and an inferior narrow neck region called the cervix, which opens into the vagina at its external orifice, the cervical os (Figure 18.7(b)). The cervix can be felt readily by inserting a finger into the vagina; it feels like the tip of the nose. The space within the uterus is called the uterine cavity. Three pairs of suspensory ligaments stabilize the position of the uterus and limit its range of movement.

BOX 18.9 CERVICAL CANCER

Cervical cancer is a relatively common disorder that kills about 2000 women in the UK each year (Shepherd *et al.*, 2001). The condition begins with cervical dysplasia, i.e. an abnormal change in the shape, growth and number of cervical cells. If the dysplasia is minimal, cells may regress to normal, but if severe it may progress to cancer. Depending on the progression of the disease, cervical cancer may be detected in its early stages by a Pap smear. Treatment may consist of tissue removal by cutting out (excising) the lesions, by hysterectomy (removal of the uterus or womb), and/or by radiotherapy, chemotherapy and laser therapy to destroy discrete areas of tissue.

Histologically, the uterine wall can be divided into three main layers: an inner endometrium, a muscular myometrium and an outer serosa or perimetrium.

Exercise

The suffix '-metr-' means uterus. Can you remember the meanings of the following prefixes: 'endo-', 'myo-' and 'peri-'?

The endometrium is a mucous membrane consisting of three distinctive layers:

- *stratum compactum:* a compact surface layer of ciliated epithelium;
- *stratum spongiosum:* a spongy middle layer of loose connective tissue;
- *stratum basale:* a dense inner layer attached to the underlying myometrium.

The superficial functional zone of the endometrium (layers 1 and 2, sometimes collectively referred to as the stratum functionalis) nourishes the developing embryo, and is sloughed off following delivery, or during menstruation if fertilization has been unsuccessful, in response to low levels of the sex hormones oestrogens and progesterone.

The thick myometrium layer forms the bulk of the uterine wall, and its thicker upper fundic and thinner lower cervical regions are good examples of structural adaptations to function: to expel a fetus, the fundic region contracts more forcibly than its cervical counter part, dilating the cervix to encourage childbirth. The myometrium contains three layers of involuntary muscle fibres that extend in all directions, giving the uterus great strength.

The uterine cavity is directed downwards and opens at the cervical canal at the internal os. The lower region of the cervical canal (or external os) opens into the vagina.

The vagina

The vagina is a thin-walled, muscular, tubular organ lying between the urinary bladder and the rectum. It extends from the cervix to the external genitalia. On average, it is about 7.5–9 cm long. The fornix – the region where the vagina attaches itself to the cervix – is an important anatomical landmark for the positioning of the contraceptive diaphragm (see Figure 18.17). The vagina is a distensible organ that serves as a passageway for menstrual flow and for childbirth, hence it is often called the birth canal. It is the receptacle for the penis (and semen) during sexual intercourse, thus its wall is composed mainly of involuntary smooth muscle, and its folded lining is lubricated with mucus to aid its role during intercourse. The vaginal secretions are acidic (pH 3.5–4.0) and provide a hostile environment for microbial growth and for sperm. The alkaline semen acts to neutralize this acidity to ensure sperm survival. However, this is only partly successful, since most sperm die due to the effects of the acidic pH on their enzymes before the neutralizing process.

The external genitalia

The external genitalia (vulva) lie immediately external to the vagina. The vulva is comprised of a number of components: the mons pubis, labia majora, labia minora, and the components of the vestibule and the clitoris (Figure 18.3).

The mons pubis is an elevated, rounded fatty-tissue area that cushions the underlying pubic symphysis during sexual intercourse. During puberty, it becomes surrounded by pubic hair. From the mons pubis, two elongated pigmented fatty folds of skin, called the labia majora (the homologue of the male scrotum), extend downwards, enclosing and protecting other external genitalia. On the outside, these folds contain numerous hairs, sweat and sebaceous glands; inside, there are two delicate hair-free skin folds, the labia minora. These contain sebum-producing cells and function to protect the opening of the urethra and vagina. They also enclose the vestibule, which comprises:

- the hymen, a folded mucous membrane that partly closes the vaginal orifice in young girls, and females who have not had penetrative sex;

- the vaginal orifice;

- the external urethral orifice;

- the opening of the mucus-secreting paraurethral (Skene's) glands (the homologue of the male prostate);

- the mucus-secreting greater vestibular (Bartholin's) glands (the homologue of the male bulbourethral glands).

The role of the mucous glands is to lubricate the area, thereby facilitating intercourse.

The clitoris

The clitoris looks small externally, but it is much larger that it appears. This organ is composed of two layers of erectile tissue (corpora cavernosa), and it is the homologue of the male glans penis. The junction of the labia minora folds forms its hood, a layer of skin called the prepuce or foreskin. The clitoris is richly innervated with sensory nerve endings, therefore, like the penis, it is capable of enlargement upon tactile stimulation; this contributes to female sexual arousal.

The perineum

The perineum is a diamond-shaped, muscular region found in both sexes between the external genitalia and the anus.

The female sexual act

The phases of female sexual arousal resemble those of the male, i.e. involving erection, lubrication and orgasm. During arousal, parasympathetic activation leads to the erectile tissue of the clitoris and other parts of the female genitalia becoming engorged with blood. Parasympathetic impulses also cause the lubrication of the vagina, which facilitates intercourse. During intercourse, rhythmical contractions of the clitoris and vaginal walls produce stimulation that eventually leads to orgasm. Female orgasm is accompanied by peristaltic contractions of the uterine walls, vaginal walls and the perineum muscles. The pleasurable sensation experienced with the contractions is analogous to that produced by male ejaculation.

The mammary glands

The mammary glands are accessory organs of the reproductive system present in both sexes.

The mammary glands are modified sweat (sudoriferous) glands, and they are actually a part of the skin. The breast extends from the second rib to the sixth rib, and from the sternum to the armpits (axillae). It overlies, and is connected to, the pectoralis major muscles (Figure 18.10). Slightly below the center of each breast is a ring of pigmented skin, the areola, which surrounds a central protruding nipple. Large areolar sebaceous glands give this region a slightly bumpy appearance; these glands secrete sebum to lubricate the areola and nipple during breast-feeding. Exposure to cold, tactile or sexual stimuli stimulates the smooth muscle fibres in the areola, causing the nipple to become erect.

BOX 18.10 EPISIOTOMY

Clinically the perineum is of importance to females because of the danger of it being torn during childbirth. To avoid this, an incision (called an episiotomy) may be made in the perineal skin and underlying tissues just before delivery. After delivery, the incision is sutured to promote healing and prevent later vaginal prolapse (downward displacement). The perineum is innervated extensively, so the laceration is likely to be very painful. Sitting, and defecation may all become more difficult. Constipation should be avoided, and aperient and high-fibre diets are encouraged. Scrupulous hygiene is also required to avoid infection. Pelvic floor exercises are encouraged soon after delivery to improve blood flow to the area, which minimizes infection risk and maximizes the healing process (Gould, 1990).

Exercise

Draw and label the male and female reproductive tracts.

BOX 18.11 DEVELOPMENT OF THE MAMMARY GLANDS

When a child reaches puberty, the male glands remain underdeveloped, while the surge of ovarian hormones (oestrogens and progesterone) in the female stimulate further gland development of the mammary glands. The male breast may appear enlarged because of the accumulation of fatty tissue. During puberty, some males experience gynaecomastia, a condition in which the breasts enlarge temporally as a result of a hormonal imbalance.

The female breasts only become functional following pregnancy, since their role is to produce and secrete milk in order to provide a source of nourishment to the newborn. The size of the breast is determined by the amount of fat surrounding this glandular tissue, and is not related to its functional capacity.

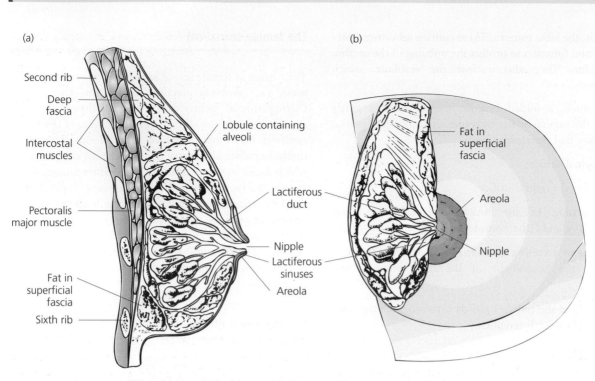

Figure 18.10 The anatomy of the mammary glands: (a) sagittal section; (b) anterior view (partially sectioned).

Q. Identify the roles of the female hormones involved in development of the breast during pregnancy and lactation.

BOX 18.12 AREOLA: A MARKER OF FIRST PREGNANCY

In Caucasians (white people), the areola changes colour from delicate pink to brown early in the first pregnancy, a fact that is useful in diagnosing a first pregnancy. Although it never returns to its original colour, the colour intensity decreases after lactation has ceased. In darker skinned women, there is no noticeable colour change.

BOX 18.13 FIBROCYSTIC DISEASE AND MALIGNANCIES OF THE BREAST

Fibrocystic disease of the breast is the most common cause of breast lumps in females. One or more cysts (fluid-containing sacs) and thickening of the alveoli occur. The condition is common in women aged 30–50 years, and is possibly due to an excess of oestrogens or a deficiency of progesterone in the postovulatory phase of the menstrual cycle. The condition usually causes one or both breasts to become lumpy, swollen and tender a week before menstruation.

Malignancies of the reproductive tract and related organs, especially the breast, account for the majority of cancer cases amongst women. In the UK, breast cancer affects up to 1 in 12 women, and kills about 16 000 women annually (Bailey, 2000). In 1998, genes (e.g. BRCA1 and BRAC2) responsible for a small number of inherited breast cancers were identified. Mammary cancers often spread (metastasize) to the ovaries, producing ovarian cancers. Ovarian cancers can also occur independently. Breast cancer has one of the highest fatality (death) rates of all cancers affecting women. It often goes undiscovered, since its associated pain becomes evident only when the cancer is quite advanced. Corrective measures of breast cancers depend on the size and type of cancer, but usually involve a combination of:

- surgical approaches – lumpectomies and mastectomies ('-ectomy' = cutting out). The axillary nymph nodes may be removed if metastasis is suspected. The operation obviously has implications for body image, sexuality, self-esteem and relationships;
- radiotherapy;
- cytotoxic drugs after the excision;
- administration of tamoxifen and raloxifene (oestrogen antagonists), since some cancers are oestrogen dependent. Before the menopause, the ovaries may be removed; postmenopausally, the steroid aminoglutethimide may be given, which inhibits the conversion of androgens into oestrogens.

The healthcare professional's role in planing and implementing care may include the reduction of emotional stress, fear and anxiety, since the patient's major problems include the fear of coping with the diagnosis, the treatment, its side effects and prognosis, the change to the body image, etc. (see also the case study of a woman with breast cancer in Section 6).

Internally, each breast consists of 15–25 irregularly shaped lobes radiating around the nipple, each of which is separated from the others by a sector or wall of connective tissue that forms the suspensory ligaments of the breast. In each lobe, smaller lobules called alveoli are present in which are found the milk-secreting cells. During lactation, milk is passed from the alveoli glands to the lactiferous ducts. These enlarge to form the lactiferous sinuses just before their openings on the surface of the nipple. The milk accumulates in the sinuses during 'nursing'. In non-pregnant, non-nursing females, the breasts and the duct system are underdeveloped. The homeostatic control of lactation is described in Chapter 9. Suffice to say, from puberty onwards, and especially during pregnancy and for a short time after delivery, oestrogens stimulate the development of the duct system and progesterone stimulates the development of the alveoli regions. Initiation and maintenance of lactation involve two hormones, prolactin and oxytocin, released from the pituitary, which stimulate milk production and control milk let-down, respectively.

REPRODUCTIVE PHYSIOLOGY

Gametogenesis

Gametogenesis is a general term that refers to the production of gametes by the gonads. Spermatogenesis and oogenesis are the specific terms for the production of spermatozoa by the male testes and ova by the female ovaries, respectively. Gametogenesis involves mitotic and meiotic divisions of cells. You should therefore review the mechanism of cell division discussed in Chapters 2 and 20, since it is our intention at this point only to review a few key concepts.

Humans reproduce sexually by producing gametes by meiosis, a reduction division that ensures that the chromosome number in the gametes is halved to 23 (the haploid number). The fusion of male and female gametes produces a zygote, containing 23 pairs of chromosomes (the diploid number), one partner of each pair from the sperm cell and one from the ovum. The zygote divides by a duplication division called mitosis to ensure that cells derived from it contain the diploid number of chromosomes. Consequently, just before cell division, the zygote and subsequent daughter cells must duplicate their DNA.

Spermatogenesis

Spermatogenesis is the sequence of events that occurs in the seminiferous tubules of the testis and leads to the formation of spermatozoa. It involves mitosis, meiosis and a process called spermiogenesis. As discussed previously, histological investigation of the seminiferous tubules reveals that the majority of the cells comprising the tubule walls are at various stages of cell division (Figure 18.5(c)). These cells, collectively called spermatogenic (sperm-forming) cells, develop into mature spermatozoa via a number of cell divisions and transformations.

Mitotic division of spermatogonia

The undifferentiated spermatogenic cells in direct contact with the germinal epithelium of the testis are called the spermatogonia. These stem cells divide continuously by mitosis until puberty; consequently, all the spermatogenic cells in a young male are undifferentiated spermatogonia, and each contains 23 pairs (i.e. diploid number) of chromosomes, the usual number for human cells. During early adolescence, certain hormones (gonadotropins and steroidal androgens) stimulate mitotic divisions of the spermatogonia. Some of the new cells give rise to daughter cells to provide a reserve supply of the germ cell line, while others migrate towards the lumen of the tubule, where they enlarge and become primary spermatocytes. The latter are destined to become mature sperm via the processes of meiosis and spermiogenesis (Figure 18.11).

Meiosis

Meiosis involves two successive divisions (see Chapter 20). During the first meiotic division, the chromosome pairs of the primary spermatocytes separate so that each forms two haploid secondary spermatocytes. Each secondary spermatocyte in turn gives rise to two spermatids via the second meiotic division. The chromosomes during this second stage act much as they do in mitosis, i.e. the DNA is duplicated to ensure that daughter cells have an identical number of chromosomes to the parent cell.

Spermiogenesis

Spermiogenesis is the final stage of spermatogenesis, in which spermatids differentiate into mature spermatozoa. This transformation involves streamlining the non-motile spermatid by shedding most of its superfluous cytoplasmic baggage and providing a tail.

Each day, spermatogenesis produces several thousand spermatozoa. Subsequent to their production, they migrate

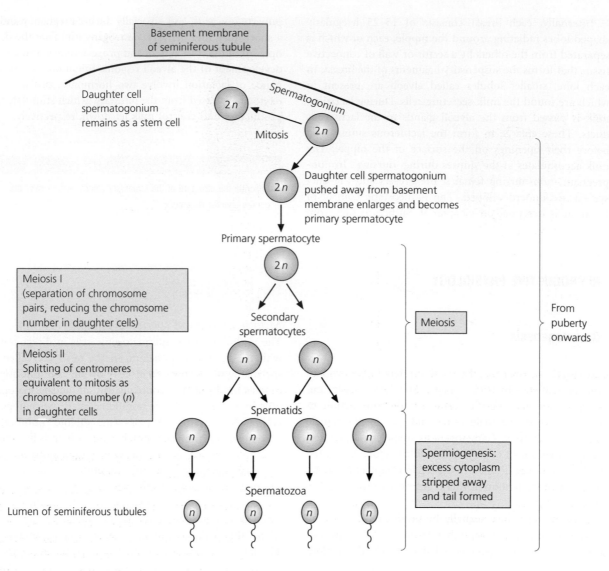

Figure 18.11 Flow chart of events of spermatogenesis. 2*n* = diploid; *n* = haploid.
Q. What do the terms 'diploid' and 'haploid' mean?

to the epididymis stores. Over the next 18 h to 10 days, they undergo further maturation, a process called capacitation. After this, the sperm are either expelled via ejaculation or broken down chemically and their constituents recycled. Sperm are also stored in the sperm tube (vas deferens) where they can retain their fertility for up to several months. Once ejaculated, however, they have a life expectancy of about 48 h within the female reproductive tract.

Exercise

Write brief notes on the distinguishing features of meiosis and mitosis.

The structure of spermatozoa

The mature spermatozoon is a tiny (approximately 60 μm long) tadpole-shaped structure consisting of three distinct

regions: a flattened head, a cylindrical body or midpiece, and an elongated tail (Figure 18.12). The head is composed primarily of a nucleus, which contains 23 densely packed chromosomes. Its anterior tip forms the acrosomal cap, which contains hydrolytic enzymes (e.g. hyaluronidase) with roles in fertilization. A very short neck attaches the head to the midpiece. The latter contains a central filamentous core with a large number of mitochondria arranged in a spiral. These organelles provide energy (ATP) for the contraction of protein filaments in the tail; the resultant propulsive forces move the sperm at a rate of 1–4 mm/min.

A mature spermatozoon lacks many of the usual cell organelles, including endoplasmic reticulum, Golgi body, lysosomes and cytoplasmic inclusions. It also does not contain glycogen or other energy reserves, so it must absorb nutrients, primarily fructose, from the surrounding seminal fluid.

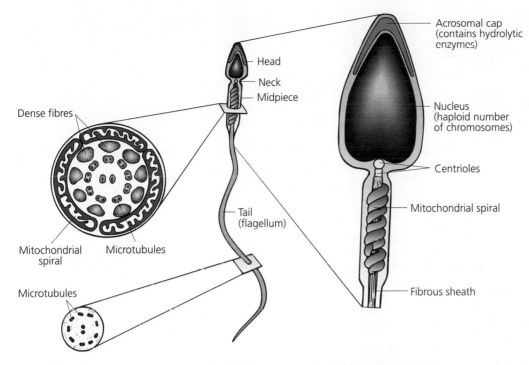

Figure 18.12 Schematic diagram of a sperm cell, showing its internal structure and parts, including the head, midpiece and tail.
Q. Which organelle would be highly represented in the (i) acrosomal cap and (ii) midpiece of the sperm?
Q. Which sugar is used to give the sperm energy to 'swim' to the site of fertilization?

BOX 18.14 SPERMATOGENESIS

Spermatogenesis occurs from puberty and throughout life. However, with advancing years, there is a decline in sperm production since there is a significant atrophy of the testes with a depletion of the germinal and Sertoli cells.

Oogenesis

The female homologue of spermatogenesis is called oogenesis. As discussed previously, sperm production in males begins at puberty and generally continues throughout life. Gamete production in the female, however, is quite different. The first meiotic division of the undifferentiated oogonium, which produces the primary oocytes, begins before birth.

Figure 18.13 illustrates how the female fetal oogonia, which are diploid at this stage, multiply rapidly by mitosis to produce a reserve of germ cells. Subsequently, oogonia enter a growth phase; gradually, primordial ovarian follicles appear, and the oogonia are transformed into primary oocytes, surrounded by a single layer of flattened follicle cells called the corona radiata. Many primordial follicles deteriorate before birth; those remaining occupy the cortical region of the immature ovary. By birth, a female's life supply of primary oocytes is approximately 750 000. These cells are 'stalled' in the early stages of the first meiotic division, and will not complete meiosis and produce functional female gametes until stimulated to do so by hormonal changes following puberty.

Once the menstrual cycle is established, a small percentage (6–7%, i.e. about 500 cells) of the primary oocytes begin their growth and developmental cycles each month. Thus, as in the male, nature has provided a generous supply of sex cells. The number of primary oocytes is continually being degenerated. Only one oocyte per month (or perhaps one from each ovary) completes the first meiotic division, which ends when two haploid daughter cells, called a secondary oocyte and the first polar body, are produced. The secondary oocyte only undergoes the second meiotic division following fertilization by a sperm cell; this division produces a haploid ovum and the second polar body. The first polar body may or may not divide again.

The ovum, then, is only one of the daughter cells produced from the primary oocyte. The mature ovum occurs only as a brief stage of oogenesis, as the haploid nuclei of ovum and sperm soon combine (now called a zygote) to restore the normal diploid number of chromosomes. The polar bodies are often referred to as the 'nuclear dustbins', since their DNA is destroyed. Details of conception, and embryonic and fetal development are given in Chapter 20.

Exercise

Distinguish between the following developing cells: primary oocytes, secondary oocytes, polar bodies, ova and zygotes.

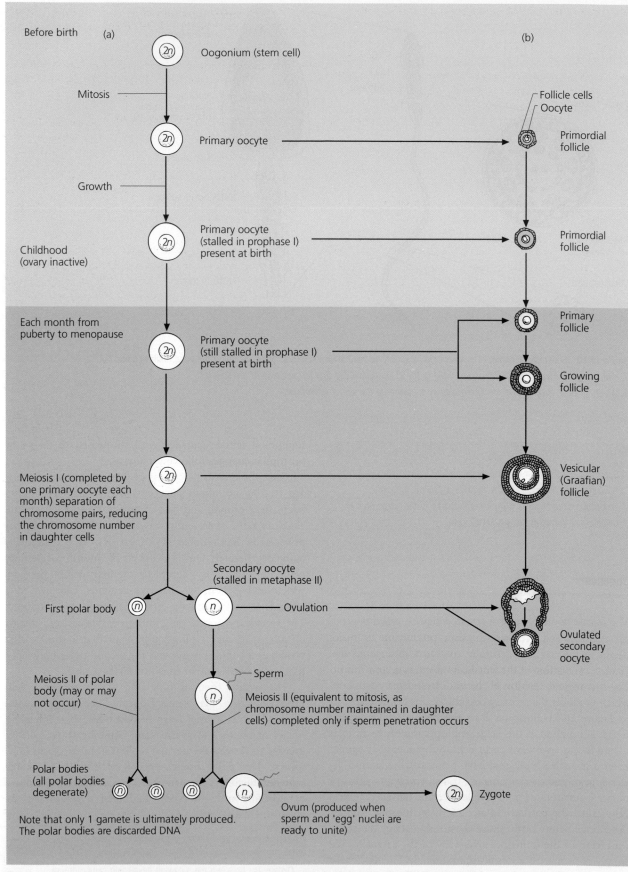

Figure 18.13 (a) Flow chart of events of oogenesis: 2*n* = diploid; *n* = haploid. (b) Follicle development in the ovary.

Q. How does the age of the primary spermatocyte in the male compare with the age of a primary oocyte in a female?

Hormonal regulation of gametogenesis in the male

The production of sperm clearly does not require the refinement associated with ova production. Nevertheless, the control of spermatogenesis has two important aspects: development of spermatozoa from spermatogonium cells must be stimulated, and the spermatozoa must undergo a 'maturation' process, without which they are incapable of independent life.

Spermatogenesis is controlled by interplay between testosterone and the gonadotropin hormones, a relationship sometimes called the hypothalamic-pituitary-testicular axis. Another gonad hormone, inhibin, may also be involved.

Clusters of interstitial cells between the seminiferous tubules, called cells of Leydig, secrete the male sex steroid testosterone in response to luteinizing hormone (LH) from the anterior pituitary gland (Figure 18.14). Testosterone is essential for the growth and maintenance of the testes, and also for the maturation or capacitation of spermatozoa in the epididymis. The gonadotropin, follicle-stimulating hormone (FSH), and also to some degree LH, stimulates Sertoli (sustentacular) cells. These cells lie amongst the developing spermatogonia, and secrete nutritive substances and chemicals that promote spermatozoa development. For example, an androgen-binding protein is released, which facilitates the binding of testosterone to spermatogenic cells. In this way, FSH helps to make the spermatogenic cells receptive to the stimulatory effects of testosterone.

The whole process of spermatogenesis, therefore, depends on the presence of appropriate concentrations of the pituitary gonadotropins and the male sex steroid. The release of these hormones is kept in check by negative feedback. Thus, as testosterone is released beyond its homeostatic range, it inhibits the release of LH and FSH by acting on the hypothalamus to suppress the secretion of gonadotropin-releasing hormone (GnRH) (Figure 18.14). As LH release declines, the secretion of testosterone will consequently be reduced. Testosterone already present in the blood is metabolized, the concentration of the hormone decreases, and inhibition by negative feedback becomes less effective. Consequently, when the blood concentration of this steroid is below its homeostatic range, LH release increases again, and so on.

A second control component is also present, in that the Sertoli cells exert a degree of control on the rate of spermatogenesis. These cells release another hormone, called inhibin (a peptide), when the sperm count goes beyond its upper homeostatic limit. Inhibin directly inhibits the release of FSH from the pituitary, and probably also inhibits the hypothalamic secretion of GnRH. When the sperm count falls below its lower homeostatic limit (20 million/ml of semen), inhibin secretion is prevented and spermatogenesis is stimulated again.

Spermatogenesis is thus controlled by tight negative feedback loops (Figure 18.14) involving the following hormones:

- gonadotropin-releasing hormones from the hypothalamus, which stimulate the release of gonadotropins from the pituitary;

- pituitary gonadotropins (FSH and LH), which stimulate spermatogenesis and the secretion of testosterone and inhibin;

- testicular hormones (testosterone and inhibin), which exert negative feedback controls on the secretion of hypothalamic releasing hormones and the pituitary gonadotropins.

The names of the gonadotropins are derived from their functions in the female, but the hormones are chemically identical in both sexes. In males, LH is sometimes called interstitial cell-stimulation hormone (ICSH), in recognition of its role in promoting testosterone secretion from the interstitial cells of the testes.

Testosterone exerts a number of actions in addition to the capacitation of spermatozoa, including:

- promoting the descent of the testes in the fetus towards the end of the gestation period;

- regulating the development of the male accessory sex organs;

- controlling the development and maintenance of the secondary sexual characteristics, such as the growth of facial, axillary and pubic hair, enlargement of the larynx, and provision of masculine muscular development;

- being partly responsible for promoting a number of behavioural characteristics associated with adolescence.

Removal of the testes does not usually lead to a loss of secondary sexual characteristics, however, since there is an increased output of androgen steroids from the adrenal cortex. The testes also produce female sex hormones, but their function in males is unclear.

Table 18.1 summarizes the major male reproductive hormones.

Hormonal regulation of the female reproductive cycle

Changes occur periodically in the female between the onset of menses (the menarche) and its cessation (menopause or climacteric). Menstruation is the visible external sign that cyclical changes to the endometrium are occurring. This section discusses the hormonal regulation of the menstrual and ovarian cycles.

The menstrual cycle involves cyclical changes within the endometrium and mammary glands in a non-pregnant female in response to changing levels of ovarian hormones (Figure 18.15). Each month, the endometrium is prepared

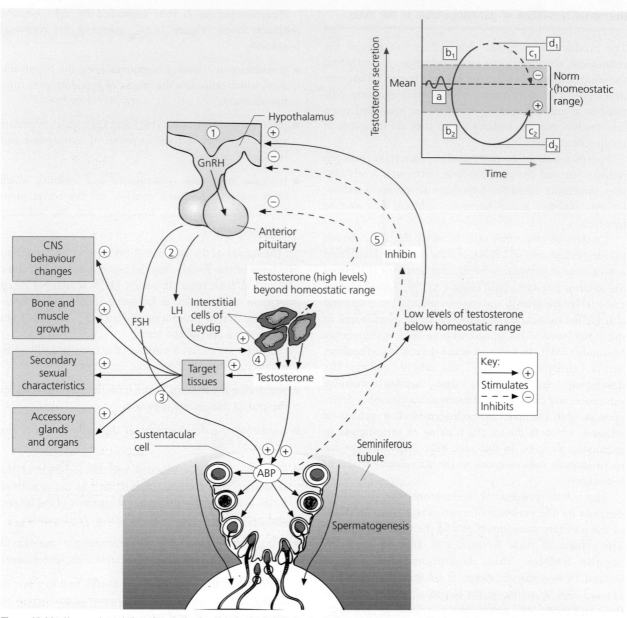

Figure 18.14 Hormonal regulation of testicular function by the hypothalamic-pituitary-testicular axis. 1 The hypothalamus releases gonadotropin-releasing hormone (GnRH). 2 GnRH stimulates the anterior pituitary to release the gonadotropins FSH and LH. 3 FSH acts on the sustentacular cells, causing them to release androgen-binding protein (ABP). 4 LH acts on the interstitial (Leydig) cells, stimulating their release of testosterone. ABP binding of testosterone then enhances spermatogenesis. 5 Rising levels of testosterone and inhibin exert feedback inhibition on the hypothalamus and pituitary. (a) Testosterone fluctuating within its homeostatic parameters. (b_1) Hypersecretion of testosterone. (c_1) Correction of imbalance via natural negative feedback (e.g. inhibin) or via clinical removal of the underlying pathology causing the imbalance (e.g. removal of testicular cancer). (b_2) Hyposecretion of testosterone. (c_2) Correction of imbalance via natural negative feedback stimulated by LH. (d_1) Irreversible clinical hypersecretion, e.g. hypothalamic and pituitary tumours. (d_2) Irreversible genetic disorders that result in low levels of testosterone.

Q. Which pituitary hormone stimulates the secretion of the male hormone testosterone?

Q. Which male hormones inhibit secretion of FSH and LH by the anterior pituitary gland?

Q. What do the abbreviations FSH and LH mean?

to receive a fertilized ovum. The development of this lining is essential for embryonic and fetal development during the period of pregnancy (gestation). If fertilization does not occur, part of the endometrium is shed as the menstrual flow (menses).

The ovarian cycle involves changes that occur in the ovaries during the menstrual cycle. These include the maturation of a secondary oocyte, its release at ovulation, and the development and degeneration of the corpus luteum (Figure 18.15). The hormonal control of the events of both

Table 18.1 Major reproductive hormones

Hormone	Functions	Source
Male		
GnRH	Controls pituitary secretion of FSH and LH	Hypothalamus
FSH	Increases testosterone production, aids sperm maturation	Pituitary gland (controlled by hypothalamus)
LH	Stimulates testosterone secretion	Pituitary gland (controlled by hypothalamus)
Testosterone	Increases sperm production, stimulates development of male primary and secondary sex characteristics, inhibits LH secretion	Interstitial endocrinocytes (Leydig cells) in testes (controlled by LH)
Female		
GnRH	Controls pituitary secretion of FSH and LH	Hypothalamus
FSH	Causes immature oocyte and follicle to develop, increases oestrogen secretion, stimulates new gamete formation and development of uterine wall after menstruation	Pituitary gland (controlled by hypothalamus)
LH	Stimulates further development of oocyte and follicle, stimulates ovulation, increases progesterone secretion, aids development of corpus luteum	Pituitary gland (controlled by hypothalamus)
Oestrogen	Stimulates thickening of uterine wall, stimulates oocyte maturation, stimulates development of female sex characteristics, stimulates lactiferous ducts of the mammary glands inhibits FSH secretion, increases LH secretion prior to ovulation	Ovarian follicle, corpus luteum (controlled by FSH)
Progesterone	Stimulates thickening of uterine wall, stimulates formation of alveoli regions of the mammary glands	Corpus luteum (controlled by LH)
hCG	Prevents corpus luteum from disintegrating, stimulates oestrogen and progesterone secretion from corpus luteum	Embryonic membranes, placenta
Prostaglandin	Initiates parturition (labour)	Endometrium
Relaxin	Relaxes symphysis pubis and dilates uterine and cervix	Corpus luteum
Prolactin	Promotes milk production by mammary glands after childbirth	Pituitary gland (controlled by hypothalamus)
Oxytocin	Stimulates uterine contractions during labour, induces mammary glands to eject milk after childbirth	Pituitary gland (controlled by hypothalamus)

FSH, follicle-stimulating hormone; GnRH, gonadotropin-releasing hormone; hCG, human chorionic gonadotropin; LH, luteinizing hormone.

Q. Do the gonadotropins derive their name from their functions in the male or female?

cycles is influenced by hormones of the hypothalamic-pituitary-ovarian axis: the gonadotropin-releasing hormones from the hypothalamus, the gonadotropin hormones (LH and FSH) from the anterior pituitary, and the steroidal oestrogens and progestins from the ovary (Figure 18.16).

The occurrence of the first menstrual flow is an indication that the uterus has begun to undergo cyclical development of its endometrium. The complete menstrual cycle becomes established with the eventual onset of ovulation. The menstrual cycle, therefore, is a sequence of changes to the reproductive tract of a non-pregnant female, and is controlled by interplay of the ovarian steroids and gonadotropin hormones. From a functional viewpoint, the uterus is anatomically most suited to carry one developing fetus, although multiple births are not uncommon. The cycle normally promotes the release of a secondary oocyte from an ovary; this becomes a mature ovum if it is fertilized. The product of fertilization (the zygote) develops into the early embryo, which must implant in the endometrium for a pregnancy to occur. The hormones involved in controlling these events, therefore, must:

- promote the development of a new endometrium;

- promote ovulation at a time when the endometrium is sufficiently developed for implantation to occur;

- promote further nutritive development of the endometrium, and prevent its shedding, in order to support the early embryo should implantation occur.

The processes involved are illustrated in Figure 18.15. The menstrual cycle typically has a duration of 28 days, although there is individual variation, and it is subject to many environmental influences. Conventionally, timing begins at the onset of menstrual bleeding, when the endometrium that developed in the previous cycle begins to be shed; this lasts for about 5 days. During this time (and just before it), the release of ovarian steroids is diminished; it is the lack of these that causes the endometrium to be shed. In addition, as ovarian steroid release is reduced, the negative feedback they exert on the anterior pituitary weakens, and increasing amounts of gonadotropins are secreted, stimulating development of the next cycle.

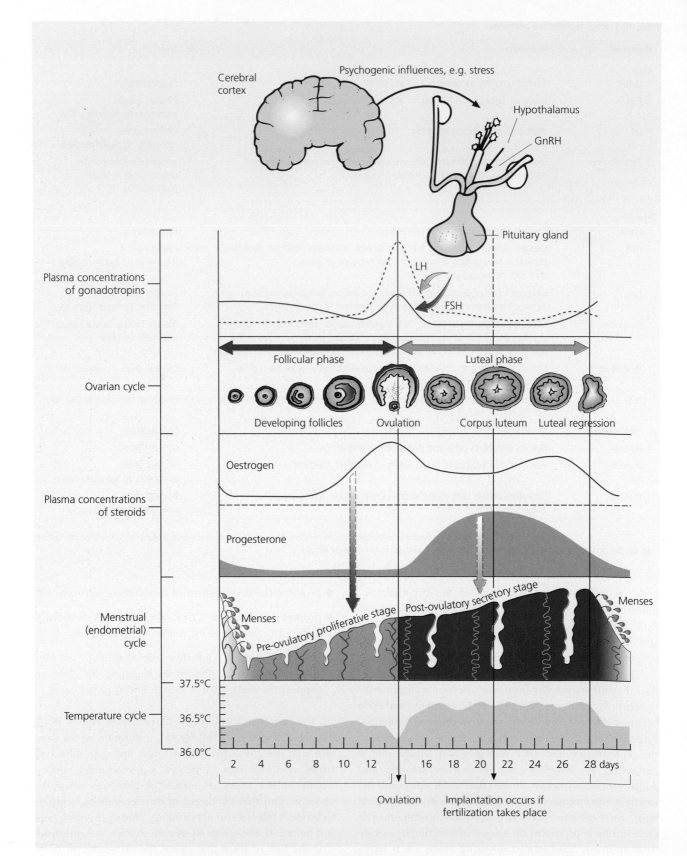

Figure 18.15 The female reproductive cycle. The diagram illustrates the interrelationship of cerebral, hypothalamic, pituitary, ovarian and uterine functions throughout a usual 28-day cycle. Note that the LH surge causes ovulation. The low levels of steroids initiate menstruation.

Q. *Which hormones are responsible for regulating the preovulatory, ovulatory and postovulatory phases of the menstrual cycle?*

Q. *Which hormones are responsible for regulating the growth of the corpus luteum and the surge of LH mid-cycle?*

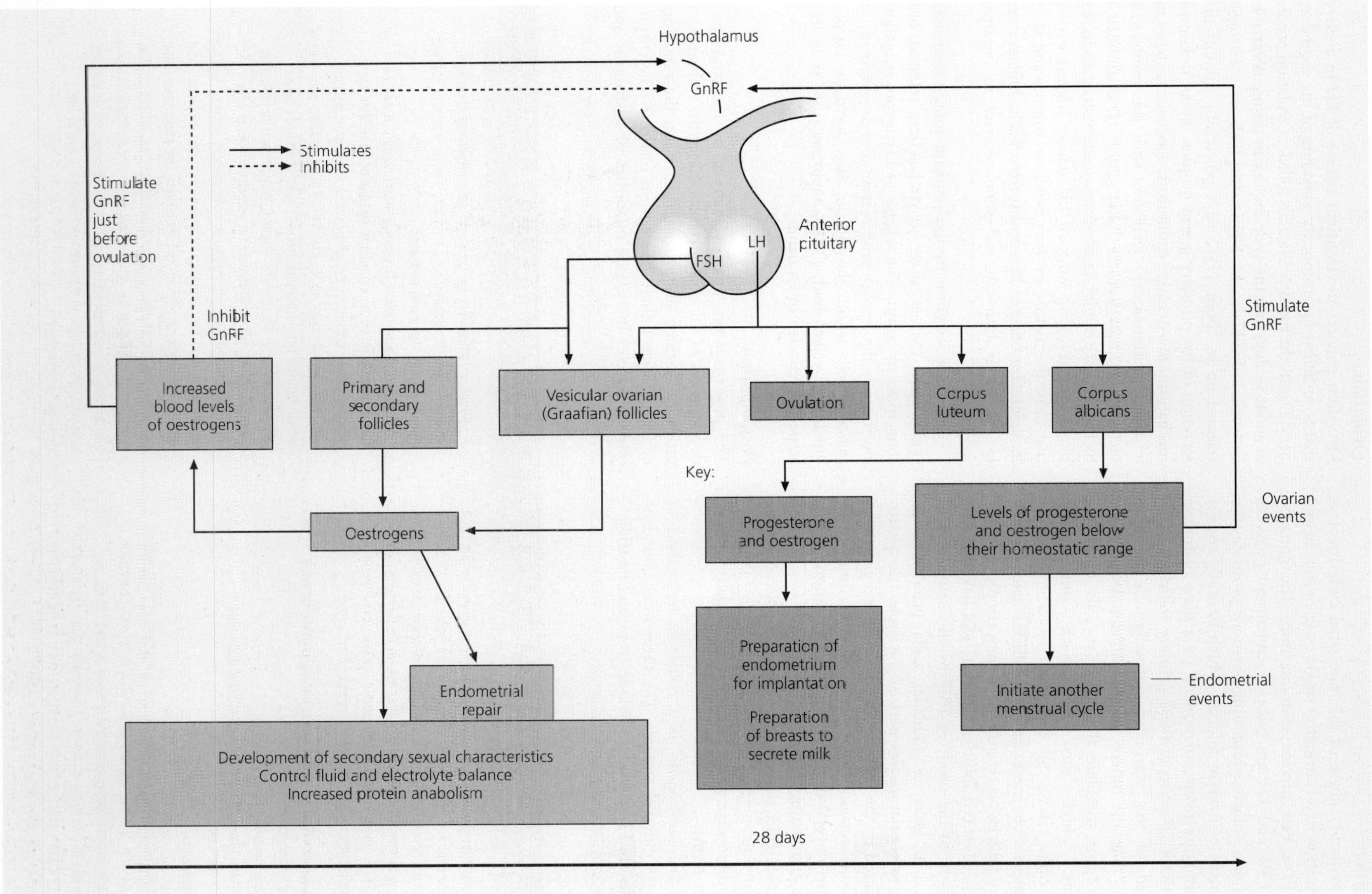

Figure 18.16 Functional aspects of the hypothalamic-pituitary-gonadal axis in females during the menstrual and ovarian cycles.

Q. Using your knowledge of the hypothalamic-pituitary-gonad axis, suggest potential sites of endocrine tumours that may give rise to female pseudohermaphroditism (see Chapter 9 for help).

Preovulation

The preovulatory phase of the menstrual cycle involves the maturation of a (normally) single ovarian follicle and growth of a new uterine endometrium. The gonadotropins FSH and LH are released concurrently. As its name implies, follicle-stimulating hormone promotes the development of ovarian follicles, which basically consist of an immature ovum surrounded by a mass of follicle cells. Perhaps 20 or so of these primary follicles will be stimulated in this way, but normally one is more advanced than the others. As the follicles develop, the gonadotropins stimulate the follicular cells to secrete oestrogens, which then feed back and inhibit gonadotropin release by the pituitary. Thus, further development for most of the follicles (now called secondary follicles) is retarded, and they atrophy and die. The most advanced follicle, however, will have become independent of the need for FSH by this stage, and so continues to grow as follicular cells proliferate. In addition to regulating this part of the cycle, the oestrogens released by the follicles also promote the growth of a new endometrium, i.e. a new stratum functionalis (functional layer) develops from the stratum basalis (basal or germinating layer).

The role of the follicular oestrogens is reflected in the name sometimes given to this part of the cycle – the follicular or proliferative phase (although 'preovulatory phase' is a better term).

Note that 'oestrogens' is a collective term used to describe six different steroids. The three most abundant oestrogens are 17-beta-oestradiol, oestrone and oestriol.

Ovulation

Ovulation requires the transient release of LH in a surge that is sufficient to prompt the shedding of the secondary oocyte from the mature Graafian follicle. Ovulation occurs at about 14 days into the cycle, but again timing is variable between individuals. As Figure 18.15 shows, oestrogen released up to about 11-12 days powerfully inhibits the secretion of the pituitary gonadotropins. By an unknown mechanism, this negative (inhibitory) feedback switches to a positive (stimulatory) feedback, with the result that secretion of pituitary stores of LH (and FSH) is stimulated by the presence of high concentrations of oestrogens in the blood. The resulting surge of LH release triggers events that cause the mature ovarian follicle to rupture and shed its secondary oocyte. The positive feedback influence on LH release is transient and soon reverses to negative feedback.

Oestrogen secretion by the remnant follicle decreases slightly once the secondary oocyte has been released, but soon picks up again. The release of LH before ovulation also triggers the further proliferation and development of follicular cells within the follicle; these form the corpus luteum (= 'yellow body'). The importance of LH in this respect is reflected in its name.

Postovulation

The post-ovulatory phase is marked by the continued development of the endometrium under the influence of progestins, principally progesterone, from the remnants of the Graafian follicle (the corpus luteum). The corpus luteum secretes increasing quantities of oestrogens and

---

BOX 18.15 PREMENSTRUAL SYNDROME, OVULATORY PAINS AND DYSMENORRHOEA

Premenstrual syndrome (PMS) is a term usually reserved for the severe physical and emotional distress that can accompany the premenstrual phase of the menstrual cycle, although sometimes it overlaps with menstruation. PMS is also known as premenstrual tension (PMT). The causes of PMS remain unclear, but Frye and Silverman (2000) suggest the following may play a role:

- excessive levels of oestrogen, with effects on fluid balance, breast development, etc.;
- inadequate levels of progesterone;
- inadequate levels of the neurotransmitter dopamine;
- vitamin B6 deficiency;
- hypoglycaemia.

Current treatments focus on relieving the symptoms of PMS, which include oedema, breast swelling, abdominal distension, backache, constipation, fatigue, depression and anxiety (Aiken, 2000). Prostaglandin-suppressing drugs are commonly used. Diuretics and vitamin B6 administrations have also been found to be helpful in some women (Barnard *et al.*, 2000)

Ovulatory pains may be caused if pain-producing chemicals released from the ruptured follicle irritate the peritoneum, causing a sharp pain in the lower abdomen.

Dysmenorrhoea refers to painful menstruation. It can be classified as primary or secondary dysmenorrhoea. Primary dysmenorrhoea occurs in the absence of associated pelvic pathology. It is thought to be caused by an excessive secretion of certain uterine prostaglandins, since these chemicals cause painful spasms of the uterine muscle. Vasopressin (antidiuretic hormone, ADH), which stimulates myometrial activity and leukotrienes, and thus increases smooth muscle activity, has also been indicated in the aetiology of dysmenorrhoea. Prostaglandin antagonists, such as aspirin and ibuprofen, are sometimes used to relieve the symptoms. Oral contraceptives that inhibit uterine contractions may also be administered. Secondary dysmenorrhoea can be due to a narrowing (stenosis) of the cervix or to various inflammatory conditions. Correction involves treating the underlying pathology.

progesterone. Up to this point, progesterone release from the ovary has been only slight. The significance of its release after ovulation is that it promotes the secretory activity of glands within the endometrium, the vascularization of the superficial layer of the endometrium, and glycogen storage within the endometrium cells. These actions prepare the endometrium to receive the embryo, should the secondary oocyte be fertilized. The activities peak about 1 week after ovulation, which is about the time an embryo could be expected to arrive in the uterus after passage along the Fallopian tube. The importance of the corpus luteum and progesterone is reflected in the names for this phase of the cycle – the luteal or secretory phase (although 'postovulatory phase' is a more correct term).

The release of progesterone has an additive effect on the negative feedback actions of oestrogens on the anterior pituitary gland. LH (and FSH) release eventually decreases to levels at which the hormone is incapable of maintaining the corpus luteum. If pregnancy has not occurred, this degenerates into the corpus albicans (= 'white body'), and secretion of oestrogens and progesterone declines sharply. Consequently, the endometrium cannot be sustained and it is shed – and so the next menses begins. As ovarian steroid release diminishes, the secretion of gonadotropins increases again, further ovarian follicles begin to develop, and a new cycle is initiated.

Should the secondary oocyte be fertilized, and the early embryo implants in the endometrium, then the release of the ovarian steroids increases and initiates the maternal

---

BOX 18.16 PSEUDOHERMAPHRODITISM

The phenotypic sex of the newborn depends upon hormonal cues received by tissues during development, i.e. it is not dependent entirely on the genetic sex of the individual – although the two are usually associated. Pseudohermaphroditism is a condition in which a person's genetic and anatomical sexes differ. Although such cases are relatively infrequent, the most common cause of female pseudohermaphroditism is adrenal genital syndrome (adrenal hypertrophy), in which an excessive secretion of androgens exists. This can occur in the female fetus or in the mature female; in the latter case, the androgens gradually transform the female appearance into a male form. An absence of menstruation (amenorrhoea) occurs, causing sterility. Other causes of female pseudohermaphroditism include androgen drug abuse, pregnant females exposed to androgen drugs, maternal pituitary and/or

adrenal endocrine tumours, and the genetic condition known as XY females.

Male pseudohermaphroditism occurs in response to an undersecretion of androgens. A common cause is testicular feminization syndrome. This homeostatic imbalance involves a defect in the cellular receptors that respond to androgens. Consequently, embryonic and adult tissues cannot respond to the existing normal levels of these male hormones, and the person develops and remains physically female. However, the menstrual cycle does not appear (amenorrhoea), the uterus is absent, and the vagina ends in a blind pocket. The genetic condition known as XX males also exists.

Correction involves hormonal therapy and surgery to produce a sexually functioning male or female.

BOX 18.17 INFERTILITY AND STERILITY IN FEMALES

Homeostatic imbalances associated with infertility or sterility are common, and most are attributed to problems with the female reproductive system. An infertile female has a low ability to produce functional ova and/or support a developing embryo/fetus. Physiological (functional) infertility and sterility have multifactorial aetiologies. Sexually transmitted diseases, for example, may damage reproductive structures, and thus abolish the reproductive capacity. In addition, developmental structural abnormalities of the reproductive system and physiological problems affecting hormonal and neural regulation of reproductive function can cause sterility (i.e. an inability to become pregnant).

Menstruation reflects the health of the endocrine glands that control the process, and imbalances of the female reproductive system frequently involve menstrual disorders. Endocrine disorders can cause amenorrhoea. An undersecretion of gonadotropin-releasing hormones and gonadotropins (FSH and LH) can lead to sterility, since functional gametes will not be produced. An undersecretion of oestrogens by the ovaries, and the depression of

hypothalamic secretion of gonadotropin-releasing hormones, has a similar effect, and may be a consequence of dietary disturbances, distress or anaemia. In females, these factors, together with abnormal congenital ovarian and uterine development, a change in body weight, or continuous rigorous athletic training, can also cause amenorrhoea.

Correction involves treating the underlying disorder or condition. The use of fertility drugs involves stimulating the hypothalamic-pituitary-ovarian axis. Clomiphene, for example (usually administered with human chorionic gonadotropin), is thought to block oestrogen receptors in the hypothalamus. Consequently, the levels of FSH and LH are raised (since the negative feedback mechanism is inhibited) to induce ovulation. Multiple ovulation (super-ovulation) sometimes occurs, resulting in multiple pregnancies. Gonadotropin administration has also proved successful as a fertility treatment. However, the administration of gonadotropin-releasing hormone has so far proved ineffective in fertility treatment.

physiological changes associated with pregnancy. In this case, the functional integrity of the corpus luteum must be maintained for a few weeks in the absence of adequate LH. A hormone called human chorionic gonadotropin (hCG), which is released from the implanted embryo, brings this about. By the time secretion of hCG has diminished, the developing placenta will be secreting steroids (oestrogens and progesterones) at a rate appropriate to maintain the pregnancy. In addition to maintaining the endometrium, progesterone and oestrogens also prepare the mammary glands for lactation. Relaxin, a hormone secreted by the placenta towards the end of pregnancy, relaxes the pelvic ligaments and the pubic symphysis to aid the dilation of the uterine cervix to facilitate delivery. Pregnancy, therefore, is an altered state of health in which the homeostatic set points are reset.

The female gonadal steroids clearly have potent physiological actions, and their release cannot continue unchecked. The secretion of gonadotropins and steroids therefore fluctuates with time, and utilizes negative feedback to establish a physiologically appropriate range of values. The onset of menopause is signalled by the climacteric, when the release of steroids is insufficient to maintain the usual menstrual cycles, which therefore become less frequent. The climacteric typically begins between the ages of 40 and 50 years, and occurs due to a failure of the ovary to respond to the pituitary gonadotropin hormones. The details of menopause are discussed in Chapter 20.

Table 18.1 summarizes the major female reproductive hormones.

Exercise

Discuss the similarities and differences between the timing of oogenesis and spermatogenesis.

PHYSIOLOGY OF BIRTH CONTROL

Most adults, whether for physiological, logistic, financial and/or emotional reasons, practise some form of birth control during their reproductive years. Methods of birth control in the extreme case include the removal of the gonads and the uterus, but more usual methods are sterilization, and mechanical and chemical contraception. Although research is making progress in its search for a male chemical contraceptive, so far the burden of birth control lies predominantly with women, since most methods are directed at females (Figure 18.17). All methods are used to avoid unwanted pregnancies, and each has potential risks and benefits, which must be analysed carefully on an individual basis. Interested readers should read other texts to consider the pros and cons of such methods, as we provide only a brief overview here.

Surgical methods

The surgical removal of the testes (castration), the ovaries (oophorectomy) and the uterus (hysterectomy) are all absolute and irreversible methods, and are performed only if the organs are diseased. The removal of the gonads (testes and ovaries) has adverse effects because of their important endocrine roles. Premenopausal women undergoing a hysterectomy do not experience an artificial menopause straight away, since the ovaries are not removed. However, if an oophorectomy is performed at the same time, then the artificial menopause will be experienced a few days after the operation. After a simple hysterectomy, pregnancy is impossible and menstruation will cease. However, a women's femininity or enjoyment of sex should not be altered.

In contrast, sterilization in either sex denies the provision of functional gametes for fertilization, but maintains the endocrine function of the gonads. One means of male sterilization is a vasectomy, in which segments of the vas deferens are removed or destroyed by heat (a process called cauterization), thus making it impossible for spermatozoa to pass from the epididymis to the distal portions of the male reproductive tract. The cut (cauterized) ends do not reconnect, and scarring eventually forms a permanent seal; such vasectomies are irreversible, making them unsuitable for men who still plan to have children but want to select the time. Vasectomies, however, can be reversible in a modified procedure that involves blocking the cut ends of the vas deferens with silicone plugs, which can later be removed.

Vasectomies do not impair normal sexual function, since the epididymal and testicular secretions account for only about 5% of semen. Spermatozoa continue to develop in the epididymis until they are broken down chemically and recycled, and men may remain fertile for up to 8 weeks after the vasectomy. The duration of fertility depends upon the frequency of ejaculation. During this period, there is obviously a need for extra contraceptive methods. The man is usually required to go back to the clinic twice with a specimen of their ejaculate to check for the absence of sperm before an assurance of sterility can be given.

Female sterilization is generally achieved by ligating the Fallopian tube, which prevents the secondary oocyte and sperm meeting. The procedure may be reversed, although this cannot be guaranteed. There is no impairment of sexual performance or enjoyment.

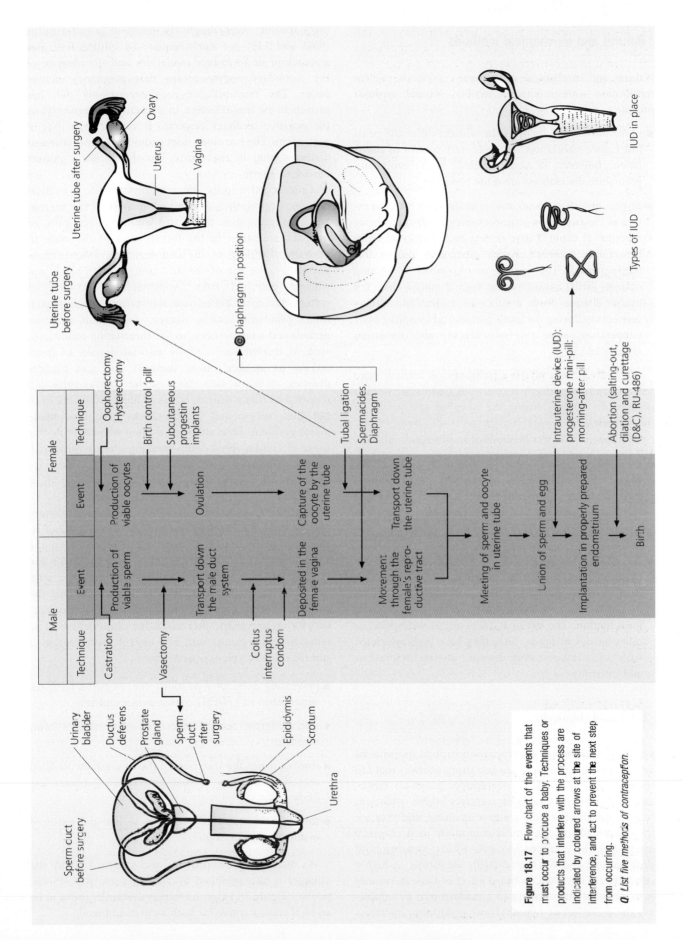

Figure 18.17 Flow chart of the events that must occur to produce a baby. Techniques or products that interfere with the process are indicated by coloured arrows at the site of interference, and act to prevent the next step from occurring.

Q. List five methods of contraception.

Male			Female		
Technique	Event		Event		Technique
Castration	Production of viable sperm		Production of viable oocytes		Oophorectomy Hysterectomy
Vasectomy	Transport down the male duct system		Ovulation		Birth control 'pill'
					Subcutaneous progestin implants
Coitus interruptus condom	Deposited in the female vagina		Capture of the oocyte by the uterine tube		Tubal ligation Spermacides, Diaphragm
	Movement through the female's reproductive tract		Transport down the uterine tube		
	Meeting of sperm and oocyte in uterine tube				
	Union of sperm and egg				Intrauterine device (IUD): progesterone mini-pill: morning-after 'pill'
	Implantation in properly prepared endometrium				
	Birth				Abortion (salting-out, dilation and curettage (D&C), RU-486)

Sperm duct before surgery
Urinary bladder
Ductus deferens
Prostate gland
Sperm duct after surgery
Epididymis
Scrotum
Urethra

Uterine tube after surgery
Ovary
Uterus
Vagina
Uterine tube before surgery

Diaphragm in position

IUD in place
Types of IUD

Natural and mechanical methods

Natural and mechanical contraceptive methods prevent fertilization without altering fertility. Natural methods include:

- *coitus interruptus:* involves the withdrawal of the penis just before ejaculation. The voluntary control of ejaculation, however, is never assured, since involuntary premature ejaculations are quite common;

- *rhythm or fertility awareness methods:* these take advantage of the fact that a secondary oocyte is fertilizable for a period of about 3 days during each menstrual cycle; the couple therefore avoids intercourse during this fertile period. The period is recognized by noting changes in the consistency of vaginal mucus, since the mucus changes from a sticky to a clear and stringy consistency during the fertile period, and by noting body temperature, since this rises slightly after ovulation (Figure 18.15).

The effectiveness of these techniques is limited, since few women have perfectly regular cycles, and some woman occasionally ovulate during the so-called safe period of menstruation.

Mechanical (barrier) methods of contraception include:

- *the condom:* prevents the deposition of sperm in the vagina. This method has become the most common form of birth control in recent years, to reduce the incidence of sexually transmitted diseases;

- *the diaphragm:* stops sperm from passing into the cervix;

- *the intrauterine device (IUD):* thought to change the uterine lining so that it produces a substance that destroys either the sperm, thus preventing fertilization, or the products of the fertilized ovum by preventing implantation. The use of IUDs is not as widespread as other barrier methods, since they have been associated with pelvic inflammatory diseases, uterine perforations and infertility.

Chemical methods

Chemical methods of contraception include spermicidal agents (foams, creams, jellies and suppositories) that kill spermatozoa, and oral contraceptives based on reproductive hormones. Oral contraceptives inhibit ovulation. Many contraceptive pills are now available, and they are in widespread use. The most commonly used chemical method is the combination pill, which contains both progesterone and oestrogens (with the former in higher concentrations). The combined effect of these hormones is to decrease the secretion of gonadotropins by inhibiting the secretion of hypothalamic gonadotropin-releasing hormone. Accordingly the levels of gonadotropins (FSH and LH) are not adequate to initiate follicular maturation or to induce ovulation, and the absence of the secondary oocyte means that pregnancy cannot occur. The mini-pill, or progesterone-only pill, has proven to be less effective in preventing pregnancy, as the negative feedback response is weaker than that of oestrogens. The hormone does promote the formation of a mucus plug in the cervix, but this is not a perfect barrier to sperm.

Contraceptive pills are administered in a cyclical fashion, beginning 5 days after the start of the menses and continuing over the next 3 weeks. Placebo pills, or no pills, are taken in the fourth week of the cycle to promote shedding of the endometrium. Despite their popularity, the use of the oral contraceptive pill is not without potential risks. Approximately 40–45% of women taking it experience side effects ranging from minor problems, such as nausea, weight gain, irregular periods and amenorrhoea, to life-threatening conditions, such as thrombosis (and its associated risks of heart attacks or strokes), liver tumours and gall bladder diseases. A major side effect of the contraceptive pill reported by many women is loss of libido. Refinement of pill composition and health checks have now made major problems rare, although women who combine this form of contraceptive with smoking and/or other risk factors associated with heart attacks and strokes are obviously increasing their chances of developing these conditions.

Norplant®, launched in 1993, is a revolutionary contraceptive for women. The method involves administering a potent synthetic progesterone-related hormone (levonorgestrel) via six flexible tubes, each about the size of a match-stick, inserted under the skin of the upper arm. Norplant has a 98.5% reliability, second only to the combined contraceptive pill. It provides reversible protection for up to 5 years, after which the capsules have to be removed and replaced with new ones if contraception is still required. Norplant operates by:

- preventing 50% of ovulations (i.e. negative feedback suppression of LH/FSH release is incomplete);

- thickening the cervical mucus, so sperm cannot swim through;

- slowing down the transport of the successfully ovulated secondary oocytes, so that fertilization becomes less likely;

- thinning the endometrial lining, so that the fertilized ovum cannot develop.

As discussed previously, the secretion of FSH by the pituitary is also inhibited by another gonadal hormone, inhibin (Figure 18.14). Inhibin may eventually prove to be an ideal contraceptive for both women and men.

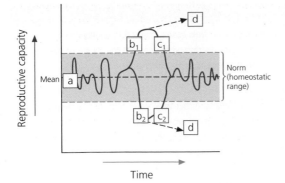

Figure 18.18 Reproductive capacity, a homeostatic function. (a) Reproductive capacity fluctuating within its homeostatic range. This corresponds to the acquisition of 'normal' requirements for gametogenesis and the absence of factors (e.g. emotional) that may diminish the desire to have sexual intercourse. (b_1) Increased fertility, which accompanies increased spermatogenesis (high sperm counts) or increased monthly ovulations. The latter can occur naturally, as in the case of twinning, or artificially, as a result of the in vitro fertilization (IVF) programme, producing 'super-ovulation'. (c_1) Contraception (either reversible or irreversible) encouraged to decrease the number of conceptions and potential offspring. (b_2) Decreased fertility, as occurs (i) temporarily in females, accompanying distress or anaemia; in males, accompanying high testicular temperatures, fatigue or increased alcohol intakes; and in both sexes, accompanying malnutrition, fever, radiation or infection (STDs); (ii) permanently, i.e. as a result developmental structural abnormalities (e.g. male and female hermaphroditism and cryptorchidism), and physiological neural and hormonal mechanisms (e.g. hyposecretion of the gonadotropins). (c_2) Correction of the underlying pathology, e.g. surgical removal of tumours, surgical correction of hermaphroditism, hormone administration in hyposecretion imbalances. (d) Irreversibility of homeostatic imbalance as occurs with certain cancers.

Q. Describe the major male and female homeostatic imbalances mentioned in this chapter that may be associated with infertility and sterility.

Abortion

Abortion is the expulsion of the products of conception from the uterus. There are many forms of abortion, but they can be classified broadly as spontaneous (naturally occurring) and induced (intentionally performed).

Induced abortions may be performed as a form of contraception when the birth control methods discussed above have not been practised or have failed, although this is highly controversial. Procedures include vacuum aspiration (suction), surgical evacuation (scraping), and the use of saline solution or drugs. The latter interfere with the hormonal actions necessary to maintain pregnancy. For example, RU-486 (mifepristone) acts by blocking the quieting effects of progesterone on the uterus. It is taken in the first 7 weeks of pregnancy in conjunction with prostaglandins to induce uterine contractions and a miscarriage. The drug has a 96–98% success rate. Similarly, anti-hCG vaccine inhibits the actions of chorionic gonadotropin, and therefore stimulates menstrual flow instead of maintaining pregnancy.

BOX 18.19 CONTINUED

invade body organs; the signs of organ degeneration (such as brain changes) mark the appearance of the tertiary stage. The antibiotic penicillin interferes with the ability of dividing bacteria to produce new cell walls, and is still the treatment of choice for all stages of syphilis. Very few new cases of syphilis occur in the UK now.

Gonorrhoea

Gonorrhoea is caused by the bacterium *Neisseria gonorrhoeae*. This STD affects primarily the mucous membranes of the urogenital tract, rectum and, occasionally, the eyes, throat and lower intestines. Transmission is by direct contact, usually sexual, although bacteria can be transmitted to the eyes of the newborn through the birth canal. Administration of 1% silver nitrate solution to the baby's eyes prevents infection. Symptoms vary depending on the sex of person. Most infected women experience few symptoms, and medical treatment is not sought. Consequently, these carriers may spread the infection. The most common symptom in males is urethritis, accompanied by painful urination and pus discharge from the penis. If untreated, gonorrhoea in males can lead to urethra constriction and inflammation of the entire duct system; in females it may lead to sterility. Correction involves antibiotic therapy (e.g. procaine penicillin), although strains are becoming increasingly resistant to these antibiotics, and gonorrhoea is becoming

increasingly prevalent. New cases reported to genitourinary medicine clinics are decreasing in line with the Health of the Nation target (Department of Health, 1992).

Genital herpes

Many people are unaware that they suffer from genital herpes. *Herpes simplex* II is the organism responsible for most herpes infections below the waist, including genital blisters on the prepuce and glans penis in the male, and the vulva and sometimes the vagina in females. *Herpes simplex* I is responsible for the majority of infections above the waist, e.g. cold sores.

The painful lesions of the reproductive organs observed in genital herpes are usually more of a nuisance than a threat to life. If a pregnant woman suffers symptoms at the time of birth, a Caesarean section is strongly advised to prevent complications in the newborn, since congenital herpes can cause severe malformations. Unlike syphilis and gonorrhoea, genital herpes is viral; the virus remains inside the body, and the person may be subjected to recurrent symptoms several times a year.

Treatment involves management of the symptoms via the administration of antiviral agents (e.g. aciclovir), analgesia and saline compresses. Sexual abstinence for the duration of eruption prevents sexual transmission.

Summary

1 Cells are reproduced by (i) mitosis, a duplication division that occurs in all body (somatic) cells and ensures that the diploid number of chromosomes is sustained, so that homeostatic functions can proceed within their normal parameters; and (ii) meiosis, a reduction division that occurs in the gonads and ensures that gametes have the haploid number of chromosomes, so that the diploid number (essential for normal embryonic/fetal development) is restored at fertilization.

2 Reproductive organs have specialized exocrine tissues adapted to produce, maintain and transport gametes, and endocrine tissue adapted to produce steroidal hormones.

3 Primary sex organs include the male testes and the female ovaries. These organs produce spermatozoa (a process called spermatogenesis), secondary oocytes (oogenesis), and sex hormones. Accessory organs include the internal and external reproductive organs.

4 At puberty, hypothalamic gonadotropin-releasing hormone stimulates the production and secretion of gonadotropins (FSH and LH) by the pituitary gland. These hormones are important in gametogenesis and in the production of the male sex hormones (androgens) and female sex hormones (oestrogens and progesterone).

5 In males, mature spermatozoa are produced in the seminiferous tubules and collect in the epididymis, where they are stored until they are broken down chemically and recycled or released into the vas deferens upon ejaculation. The vas continues as the urethra at the base of the bladder; this latter

part provides the exit route for both sperm and urine at the tip of the penis.

6 The seminal vesicles, prostate and Cowper's glands (and, to a small extent, the seminiferous tubules and the epididymis) add secretions to the sperm cells to produce the semen.

7 Testes descend via the inguinal canal into the scrotal sacs before birth. Cryptorchidism is an imbalance that reflects undescended testes. Inguinal hernia is a dropping of a portion of the intestines into the inguinal canal.

8 The penis is the male copulatory organ with specialized tissue (corpora cavernosa and corpus spongiosum) that becomes engorged with blood when sexually aroused, producing a rigid and erect structure necessary for the insertion into the vagina during sexual intercourse.

9 In the female, gametes are produced and matured in ovarian follicles at puberty under the hormonal influence of pituitary FSH. Adequate FSH release signals the onset of menarche (the first menstrual flow).

10 The mature (Graafian) follicle releases the secondary oocyte (and some of its surrounding follicular cells) at ovulation. These cells are taken to the uterus via the Fallopian tubes. The trigger to ovulation is an LH surge from the pituitary caused by a transient positive (stimulatory) feedback mechanism produced by oestrogen, the release of which is relatively high at this point within the menstrual cycle.

11 LH converts the follicle cells remaining in the ovary after ovulation into the corpus luteum, a body that secretes steroid

Summary (Continued)

hormones (progesterone and oestrogens). These hormones suppress FSH and LH release by negative feedback, in order to prevent further follicular development, and to promote further development of the endometrium.

12 The uterine cycle (average 28 days) begins with menstruation (up to the fifth day). Following this, steroids (from the preovulatory follicles and the postovulatory corpus luteum) prepare the uterus for implantation of the fertilized ovum. If fertilization does not occur, the corpus luteum becomes the corpus albicans, which then degenerates and is recycled. Consequently, steroid secretion from the ovary decreases, removing their inhibitory action over the gonadotropins; their subsequent release is associated with the next menstrual cycle.

13 The vagina is the female copulatory organ. The hymen guards its entrance in virgins. Bartholin's glandular tissue secretes a lubricant in anticipation of, and during, sexual intercourse. The external genitalia of the vulva are comprised of the mons pubis, labia majora and minora, clitoris and vestibule.

14 During sexual arousal, the engorgement of blood in the clitoris causes its erection.

15 Fertilization occurs high in the Fallopian tubes. The fusion of sperm and ovum nuclei produce the diploid zygote.

16 Contraceptive methods are designed to prevent gamete formation or prevent the sperm reaching the secondary oocyte. Methods are classified as being natural, mechanical and chemical.

17 Homeostatic imbalances of male and female reproductive tracts are divided into anatomical and physiological abnormalities, both of which may be responsible for infertility or sterility in either sex (Figure 18.18).

Review questions

The male reproductive system

1 List the functions of the male reproductive system.

2 Draw a labelled diagram of the male reproductive organs.

3 Identify where spermatogenesis takes place.

4 What factors affect spermatogenesis, i.e. influence male fertility?

5 How does meiosis differ from mitosis?

6 Distinguish between the sustentacular cells and the interstitial (Leydig) cells. Which of these (if any) are described as germinal cells?

7 What happens to spermatozoa that are produced but not ejaculated?

8 What are the functions of testosterone?

9 The prostate enlarges with age. What symptoms would indicate this?

10 What is a TURP?

11 Discuss the physiological mechanism that enables the normally flaccid penis to become erect.

12 Can patients with a spinal injury achieve ejaculation?

The female reproductive system

13 List the functions of the female reproductive system.

14 Draw a labelled diagram of the female reproductive organs.

15 Oogenesis occurs in stages. When and where does each stage occur?

16 What are polar bodies, and why are they produced?

17 What are the functions of oestrogens? Why do its levels fluctuate during the menstrual cycle?

18 What is fertilization? Where does it occur?

19 What is an ectopic pregnancy?

20 Which uterine layer is shed during menstruation?

21 Why is vaginal pH acidic? How do ejaculated spermatozoa manage to withstand this potentially hostile environment?

22 How may fertilization be prevented?

REFERENCES

Aiken, C. (2000) The impact of the cyclical symptoms of PMS. *Practice Nurse* **19**(4). 148, 150–2.

Bailey, K (2000) The nurse's role in promoting breast cancer. *Nursing Standard* **14**(30): 34–6.

Barnard, N.D., Scialli, A.R., Hurlock, D. and Berton, P. (2000) Diet and sex-hormone binding globulin, dysmenorrhea, and premenstrual symptoms. *Obstetrics and Gynecology* **95**(2): 245–50.

Best, K. (2000) How to minimize PID risks. *Network* **20**(1): 7.

Crayford, T.J.B., Campbell, S., Bourne, T.H., Rawson, H.J. and Collins, W.P. (2000) Benign ovarian cysts and ovarian cancer: a cohort study with implications for screening. *Lancet* **355**(9209): 1060–3.

Frye, G.M. and Silverman, S.D. (2000) Women's health. Is it premenstrual syndrome? Keys to focused diagnosis, therapies for multiple symptoms ... fifth in a series. *Postgraduate Medicine* **107**(5): 151–4, 157–9.

Gould, D. (1990) Ectopic pregnancy: causes and outcomes. *Nursing Times* **93**(14): 53–5.

Heath, D. (1988) Osteoporosis. *Prescribers Journal* **28**(4): 121–9.

Heuther, S.E. and McCance, K.L. (1996) *Understanding Pathophysiology*. London: Mosby.

Hinchcliff, S.M and Montague, S.E. (1996) *Physiology for Nursing Practice*. London: Baillière Tindall.

Kennedy, W.A. II, Huff, D. and Snyder, H.M. III (1998) The value of testis biopsies in cryptorchidism. *Contemporary Urology* **10**(4): 46–7, 50, 53–4.

Kinkade, S. (1999) Testicular cancer. *American Family Physician* **59**(9): 2539–44.

Lambing, C.L. (2000) Osteoporosis prevention, detection and treatment: a mandate for primary care physicians. *Postgraduate Medicine* **107**(7): 37–41.

Meston and Frolich (2000) The neurobiology of sexual function. *Archives of General Psychiatry* **57**: 1012-30.

Shepherd, J., Weston, R., Peersman, G. and Napuli, I.Z. (2001) Interventions for encouraging sexual lifestyles and behaviours intended to prevent cervical cancer. The Cochrane Library, issue 1. Oxford: Update Software.

Stones, R.W. and Mountfield, J. (2001) Interventions for treating chronic pelvic pain in women. The Cochrane Library, issue 1. Oxford: Update Software.

Tortora, G.J. and Grabowski, S.R. (2000) *Principles of Anatomy and Physiology*, 9th edn. New York: J. Wiley & Sons.

FURTHER READING

Challen, V. (1998) Prostatic cancer screening – does it fulfil the criteria for medical screening?

Radiography **4**(2): 115–20.

Cook, N. (2000) Clinical: health promotion. Testicular cancer: testicular self-examination and screening. *British Journal of Nursing* **9**(6): 338–43.

Peate, I. (1998) Clinical. Cancer of the prostate 2: the nursing role in health promotion. *British Journal of Nursing* **7**(4): 196, 198–200.

Section Five

Influences on homeostasis

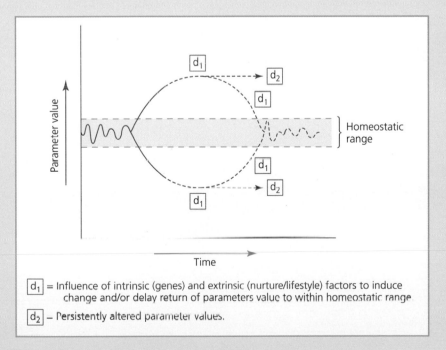

d_1 = Influence of intrinsic (genes) and extrinsic (nurture/lifestyle) factors to induce change and/or delay return of parameters value to within homeostatic range.

d_2 = Persistently altered parameter values.

Chapter 19

Nature–nurture: an individualized approach to health and healthcare

Introduction
Integrated approaches to health and healthcare

References
Acknowledgement

INTRODUCTION

In exploring body functioning, previous sections of this book have largely considered how tissues and organs respond to change and to need. In some cases, the change process itself has been identified as being necessary for wellbeing, e.g. in the cell membrane processes that are responsible for the generation of an action potential (nerve impulse), or in the hormonal responses that promote sexual maturation. In other circumstances, it is the application of negative feedback principles that is important, i.e. responses that counteract change so that parameters remain within an optimal homeostatic range. Illness arises because the capacity of the body to maintain homeostasis is compromised, and so change occurs to the internal environment that is inappropriate to body function at that time, and that, in all likelihood, will be persistent.

Examples of homeostatic imbalances or failure that underlie physiological and mental disorders have been identified in the various chapters, and others are identified in Section 6. But what causes these problems, and what are the implications for health and healthcare?

Recent approaches to healthcare:

- recognize that people are individuals. Providing healthcare that is based solely on common biological change is unlikely to be fully effective for all patients, partly because people vary biologically, but also because psychological and sociological variations can be profound and so will have an impact on the therapies;

- place an increased emphasis on the psychosocial influences on human behaviour and health. The focus has

moved towards understanding how the environment acts on the individual, and hence how this interaction can be manipulated. The biological disturbances produced by such interactions will also be important here (e.g. see Box 19.1).

These are principles embraced by holism. Human beings are complex, so it could be argued that considering

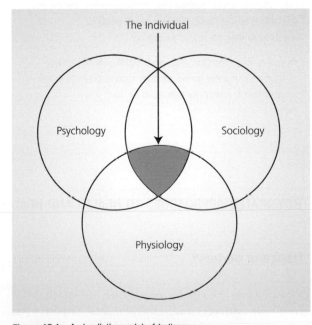

Figure 19.1 A simplistic model of holism.
Q. What does the term 'holism' mean to you?

aspects of biopsychosocial wellbeing is itself being divisive, but in practical terms providing effective care requires the healthcare professional to have the appropriate psychological, sociological and biological information necessary to make decisions (Figure 19.1). Clearly, all three disciplines will underpin the care given.

In trying to explain the biological aspects of health, this book so far has used a systematic format to identify how body systems are constructed and how they function. In doing so, it has also identified how changes in one system can induce profound alterations in the functioning of others, and how psychosocial perspectives may also impact on biological functioning. This latter interactional approach to health (and healthcare) is expanded upon here as an introduction to the remaining chapters of the book, which consider biological functioning in a more holistic framework.

BOX 19.1 SMOKING AS AN EXAMPLE OF AN INTERACTIONAL APPROACH TO HEALTH

Smoking frequently commences as a social or psychosocial phenomenon, but it is a habit that has been known for some 30 years to be associated with long-term health risks. Nicotine in tobacco smoke is a drug that acts as both a stimulant and a sedative. Its stimulant properties arise from the release of adrenaline and through the actions of nicotine on the central nervous system. They include:

- raising heart rate by 10–20 beats/min;
- raising arterial blood pressure by 5–10 mm Hg;
- raising the concentrations of blood glucose and free fatty acids;
- enhancing memory and alertness;
- improving cognition.

Its sedative properties also relate to its actions on the central nervous system:

- reducing stress perceptions;
- reducing aggressive responses to stressful situations;
- suppressing appetite.

Nicotine is also addictive. Smoking is a widespread behaviour, but it is considered to be the single most important, preventable health risk. Cigarette smoke contains over 2000 chemicals, and the risk to health is multisystemic. Smoking has been shown to substantially raise the risk of developing:

- cancer (lung, laryngeal, oral, oesophageal, bladder, kidney, pancreas): cigarette smoke contains approximately 20 known carcinogens, collectively referred to as 'tar';

- chronic lung disease (chronic bronchitis, emphysema): this probably results from adaptive responses to the long-term presence of irritants from the smoke. Responses include increased numbers of goblet cells in the airways, increased mucus secretion, and loss of the cilia that normally produce the 'mucus staircase' that removes mucus from the airways. The accumulated mucus provides a medium for bacterial growth;
- coronary heart disease (atherosclerosis): the causative factors are unknown, but there is suggestion that the release of free fatty acids raises the low-density lipoprotein form of cholesterol and so lowers the high-density to low-density lipoprotein ratio, leading to the deposition of cholesterol in the walls of blood vessels (see Chapter 5: Box 5.5). The presence of substantial amounts of carbon monoxide in cigarette smoke (and in the blood of frequent smokers) is also thought to have a role through its effect on the carriage of oxygen by blood (see Chapter 14: Box 14.27);
- stroke: possibly linked to long-term cardiovascular adaptations (e.g. hypertension), but may also be linked to atheroma formation.

Smoking by pregnant women increases the risk of underweight babies and premature delivery. In such cases, the placenta size is usually smaller than usual. Placental blood flow is likely to be reduced, hence slowed fetal growth.

Changes in skin tone are also apparent in frequent smokers, often resulting in excessive facial wrinkling.

INTEGRATED APPROACHES TO HEALTH AND HEALTHCARE

Nature or nurture?

Discussions on the relative importance of biological (i.e. genetic or nature) and environmental aspects (i.e. nurture) have, for many years, provoked heated academic debates, especially in relation to human development. This is particularly the case when considering the factors that influence cognitive and behavioural changes, since both genetic and environmental contributions to psychological development are well recognized. The discussion should also extend to physical factors, since lifestyle interactions undoubtedly induce homeostatic disturbance (e.g. see Box 19.1). The exact means by which the environment can influence psychological and physical functions are increasingly the subject of research, and there is now greater emphasis on prevention through health education. Breakthroughs in gene research are expected to facilitate further developments in this respect[1].

Interactions and psychological functions

Childhood and adolescence are viewed as being the main formative periods of our lives, evidenced by the complexity of psychophysiological development during these periods, although behaviour and personality remain labile throughout life.

Our mental faculties have a biological basis, since there are sites within the brain that have roles in, for example, emotion, aggression, sexual behaviour, cognitive functions and memory (see Chapter 8). The functioning of synapses in neural networks requires the activation of appropriate genes within brain neurons, not only for the existence of the neural components of the brain but also to promote neuronal growth and to enable a cell to produce the features necessary for neurochemical transmission at synapses. The observable characteristics produced by the activities of such genes in neural cells might be behavioural or cognitive, so there is a genetic basis to all aspects of psychological function. For example, 'intelligence' is currently considered to be primarily genetic, with 60–80% being accounted for by heredity. The remaining proportion identifies the importance of psychosocial interactions on brain development.

A genetic component helps to explain the apparent familial occurrence of some psychological disorders. By implication, gene mutation should be capable of inducing behavioural disturbance by altering neurological structure and functioning. Putative genes have been identified, but the situation is complicated by the likelihood that behavioural traits are characteristics that involve numerous genes, which increases the complexity of investigation.

Genetic involvement could also help to explain how behavioural disorders are associated with specific neurochemical imbalances, such as an underactivity of neural pathways that utilize the neurotransmitters serotonin and noradrenaline in depressive behaviour (see Box 19.2). Pharmacological therapies target this 'nature' component of behavioural disorders, and are an important tool.

Nevertheless, current pharmacological therapies may not reverse a disorder, and may only provide a means of managing it. Psychotherapy is an alternative method that utilizes the lability of neural connections (referred to as 'neuroplasticity') in order to promote appropriate pathways and thus modify behaviour. How such 'environmental' interactions influence the expression of genes and behaviour has not been elucidated. It is clear, however, that to consider only the relative contributions of either genes or environment on psychological function is to take too narrow a perspective. Much of brain function reflects an interaction of both, and this is reflected in clinical approaches to disorders of mental health (see Box 19.2, and also the mental health case studies in Section 6).

BOX 19.2 DEPRESSION AS AN EXAMPLE OF AN INTERACTIONAL APPROACH TO HEALTHCARE

Psychological and sociological studies have made a considerable impact on the understanding of behaviour, yet the continued use of pharmacological therapies, whether as primary or secondary interventions, provides a reminder that the brain is a biological structure. The lack of psychological equilibrium in depression represents a disturbance of the internal environment of the brain, and the promotion of an optimal neural environment has failed. Clinical intervention aims to reverse the disturbance; this is illustrated by the therapeutic approaches used in the treatment of depression.

Depression is characterized in its extreme by a dysphoric mood, or a loss of interest or pleasure. The majority of studies indicate that the activities of monoamine neurotransmitters (noradrenaline and serotonin in particular) are reduced in depressive states, resulting in a functional imbalance between certain neural pathways of the brain. The aim of clinical intervention is to either artificially correct the neurochemical imbalance by using drugs, or to reverse the neurological change that resulted in the imbalance by using psychotherapy to re-establish neurological balance.

Pharmacological therapies largely involve the administration of drugs that either inhibit the uptake of neurotransmitter from the synapse, and so prolong its action (tricyclic antidepressants and serotonin-uptake inhibitors), or maintain the presence of neurotransmitter for longer by preventing its breakdown by enzymes (monoamine oxidase inhibitors). The efficacy of these drugs in acute care is well established, but they do not remove the psychosocial cause of the disturbance.

Life events and a lack of social support have long been known to act as precipitating factors in the aetiology of depression. Cognitive behavioural therapy has been found to be as effective as pharmacological intervention for acute treatment, and may even be associated with lower rates of relapse.

Both treatments are therefore concerned with re-establishing neurological homeostasis, and an integrated approach should be taken that utilizes the best of each. See Case 3 in Chapter 26.

---

[1]The human genome was published in February 2001. One surprise is that there seem to be just 30 000 or so genes in human cells. This is far fewer than the original estimates of 100 000 plus. Early estimates assumed a principle usually operated of one gene–one protein; as the number of genes is actually much lower, this suggests that there are as-yet unrecognized ways by which the genetic blueprint is manipulated in cells to produce the diversity required in the human body. It has also stimulated further debate on the role of environmental interactions, particularly in such complex areas as human behaviour.

Interactions and physical functions

The success of heath education programmes to reduce physical disorder also indicates that the environment (i.e. lifestyle) has an influence on genetic expression throughout the body. Some of these influences, e.g. diet, exercise and drug abuse, are well documented. Others are only poorly understood (although the situation is changing rapidly), e.g. the extrinsic factors involved in the development of many cancers. Health education programmes are less apparent in such instances, but scientists increasingly recognize causative or modulating agents, and so preventive approaches may be available one day.

Numerous examples are provided in this book. The interactional approach to health and healthcare in the context of physical functioning is illustrated in Box 19.3.

Systems theory

General principles

The principle of interaction between the body and the external environment is founded within an established concept called systems theory. This concept has applications in many branches of science, such as engineering, behavioural science and ecology. The term 'system' is used here in a conceptual context, and not literally in terms of, say, organ systems within the body.

Systems theory views all things, living or not, as components of a wider whole that is comprised of further systems. Its main aspects are:

- Every order of systems, except the smallest, is comprised of subsystems.

- All but the largest operate within a suprasystem.

- Every system has an arbitrary boundary that distinguishes it from its environment.

- The environment of a system is everything external or internal to its boundary. The environment may be immediate or distantly removed.

The boundaries between the various levels are considered to be 'permeable', i.e. each level interacts with the one below or above it. Thus, systems represent levels of interaction. Such interactions mean that living systems have a tendency to vary, and so move to a greater degree of heterogeneity. The important term here is 'tendency'. A system may counteract change, provided that certain conditions are met. In other words, a steady state can be maintained, or the change controlled, in spite of continuous interaction with other systems. In order to negate this tendency for heterogeneity, living systems must operate

BOX 19.3 DYSPNOEA AS AN EXAMPLE OF AN INTERACTIONAL APPROACH TO HEALTHCARE

A balance between lung ventilation and lung perfusion is essential for health (see Chapter 14: Box 14.23). Chronic cardiopulmonary disorders therefore frequently arise from heart disease, such as cardiomyopathies or myocardial infarction, or from lung diseases, such as chronic obstructive airway disease or pneumonia. These might be considered to be the primary problems. A common cause of heart disease is the presence of atheromatous plaques within the coronary circulation, and that of lung disease is infection or environmental pollutants, such as cigarette smoke. In both cases, there are strong lifestyle or environmental links (see examples in the appropriate chapters). Acute pulmonary disorders are also possible, especially with regard to asthma or pneumonia. Once again, both usually have environmental risk factors.

Poor lung ventilation and/or perfusion causes dyspnoea (poor blood oxygenation and difficulties with breathing) and results in difficulty in maintaining the normal gas composition of arterial blood, and hence of the tissues elsewhere in the body. The management of dyspnoea includes some or all of the following:

- *Pharmacological methods*, including the administration of bronchodilators to improve ventilation, steroids to reduce inflammation, mucolytics to loosen mucus secretions, and anti-anxiety drugs to reduce the work of breathing and to reduce the risk of bronchospasm.

- *Physical techniques*, including:
  - positioning of the patient: a semi-prone position uses gravity to reduce pressure from the abdomen on the diaphragm, and hence on the lungs;
  - 'pursed-lip' breathing, to maintain alveolar expansion during breathing out, or 'diaphragmatic breathing' to reduce the work of breathing and to reduce air trapping as a consequence of airway compression during forced exhalation;
  - chest physiotherapy, to remove secretions (and suctioning to facilitate expectoration if necessary);
  - cough control, to facilitate removal of secretions.
- *Psychosocial therapies*, including relaxation and meditation to reduce anxiety and the work of breathing. Reduced anxiety will improve the disposition of the patient, and may also reduce the need for other interventions.
- *Oxygen therapy*, to facilitate oxygenation of alveolar gases; this is a clear example of environmental change impacting upon physiological parameters.

Thus, the aetiology of disorders that promote dyspnoea often have an environmental component, and the clinical interventions used to alleviate dyspnoea include both biological and environmental factors.

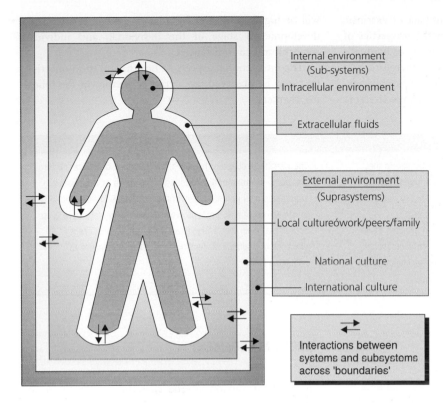

Figure 19.2 Systems theory and health. The individual represents a system with identifiable subsystems, which relate to intra- and extracellular environments. The sociocultural environment, in which the individual lives, provides a number of suprasystems. Note the interactions across boundaries between the suprasystems and subsystems. These will influence the health of the individual.
Q. Which structures within the human body form our link to the environment?

using feedback by detecting change and promoting an appropriate response of the appropriate magnitude. In other words, by utilizing processes identical to those that were discussed in Chapter 1 as underpinning homeostasis.

If we view the human body as a system, then sub- and suprasystems can be identified (Figure 19.2). Thus, organs comprise the body subsystems, which in turn are comprised of further subsystems, i.e. tissues and cells. Cells are comprised of organelles, which consist of chemical molecules and ions. The individual lives within an immediate social suprasystem comprised of the family unit/peers/workmates (all of these form systems themselves). These, in turn, have a position within the larger suprasystems that comprise the local and wider communities.

From the healthcare point of view, it is the interactions with the immediate environment that are of particular relevance, although the influences of the economic and political climates on that environment are also recognized as sources of illness. The application of this model, however, requires a definition of 'environment'. If we take

a broad definition, then an individual's environment consists of the physical, chemical, social, emotional and spiritual circumstances in which the individual lives.

Systems theory and homeostasis

Interactions between the individual and the external environment act to change the internal environment of that individual, which is why intrinsic homeostatic processes are so important, since they prevent those changes from becoming destabilizing and causing biochemical change incompatible with wellbeing. In acting to prevent or reverse the effects of extrinsic influences on the internal environment, healthcare professionals are also demonstrating homeostasis in action. In fact, we can identify processes analogous to homeostasis at all system levels, even, for example, in government socioeconomic policies directed (we hope!) at maintaining or promoting the wellbeing of society.

Systems theory and homeostasis therefore provide a working framework for health and healthcare. Placing holism into a conceptual framework does not mean losing the sense of person, but presents us with the means of viewing the health–ill-health continuum.

The impact of extrinsic factors on the internal environment of an individual may be influenced by the degree to which they act upon the individual, and the degree to which the individual is capable of responding to the

Exercise

Various models of care have been developed during the last 40–50 years. Many of these take an 'interactional' stance, and the viewpoints expressed in this chapter are a development on those expressed in the Roy Adaptation Model. Interested readers are directed towards the work of Andrews and Roy (1991).

imposed change. In other words, the impact of extrinsic factors on health will depend partly on the properties of the factors themselves, but also partly on the individual's innate capacity to respond to them. It is therefore also important to note that our ability to maintain psychophysiological equilibrium in the face of environmental stressors will be highly subjective because of genetic variation, the developmental stage of the individual, and individual sociocultural circumstances.

The interactional aspects of health, and the subjectivity that may be observed, are explored further in the following chapters.

Summary

1 According to systems theory, individuals are subjected to the impact of environmental change (from physical, psychological and social perspectives), but the individual will act to negate any detrimental consequences of such change.

2 Homeostasis is a concept that explains how we are able to do this. Systems theory and homeostasis provide an interactional framework that gives structure to nature–nurture considerations on the basis of wellbeing and healthcare practices.

The remaining chapters highlight the influence of nature–nurture (i.e. gene–environment) interactions. The issue of the relative importance of a genetic or environmental basis to health is likely to remain debatable. Perhaps what is more important here is to accept that each has a significant role, and to encourage practices of maintaining health or providing healthcare to recognize both.

REFERENCES

Andrews, H.A. and Roy, C. (1991) Essentials of the Roy Adaptation Model. In: Roy, C. and Andrews, H.A. (eds) *The Roy Adaptation Model: the definitive statement.* Norwalk, CT: Appleton-Lange.

ACKNOWLEDGEMENT

An extended version of the material presented in this chapter is available in McVicar, A. and Clancy, J. (1998) Homeostasis: a framework for integrating the life sciences. *British Journal of Nursing* 7(10): 601–7.

Chapter 20

Genes in embryo development and ageing

INTRODUCTION

The human body is comprised of billions of cells, each being specialized for its role within a tissue and hence in overall body function. Specialization of function occurs largely during the differentiation of cells in the embryo, and is controlled primarily by the genetic information encoded within the cell, although the expression of that information is influenced by the environment within the uterus. Differentiation is a complex and poorly understood process, but it can be envisaged as resulting in the generation of cells of distinct structure and activity. Differentiation and the maintenance of cell function are promoted by the activities of enzymes, which must be present at the appropriate time.

The specificity of enzyme action results from the three-dimensional shape of these proteins, since the reactants of a chemical reaction must combine with precise 'active' sites within the protein structure (see Chapter 4). The variety of enzyme structures results from variations in the number of amino acids present, the types of amino acids present, and the sequencing of those amino acids. Here lies the importance of the genetic code within the cell's nucleus, since cells construct proteins according to the 'blueprint' encapsulated within DNA. The process of protein synthesis is described in Chapter 2, and you should familiarize yourself with this process, and the nature of the genetic code, before continuing with this chapter.

Chromosomes

The majority of genes in a cell are located on *chromosomes* ('chromo-' = colour, 'soma' = body), which are the molecules of DNA within the cell. There are 46 molecules of DNA within a human body cell (i.e. one that is not a sex cell), hence there are 46 chromosomes. The 46 chromosomes are comprised of 23 pairs, because one member of each pair is inherited from each parent. Sex cells therefore contain only 23 chromosomes, i.e. just one member of each chromosome pair.

The chromosomal make-up of a cell is called its *karyotype*. Karyotyping is useful because it identifies if there is a chromosomal defect (e.g. too many or too few chromosomes, or fragmented chromosomes). It does not, however, give information about the genetic make-up of a cell – the *genome* – since this relates to the presence or absence of specific genes within the chromosomes. Chromosomes differ in size and according to their broad role within the body. Two of the chromosomes are called *sex chromosomes*, as they are involved in the development of the sexual characteristics of the fetus (but with some involvement in other functions). The remaining 44 are called *autosomes* (Figure 20.1) and are concerned mostly with the non-sexual functioning of the body. The autosomes are numbered according to their size: pair 1 is the largest, pair 22 the smallest.

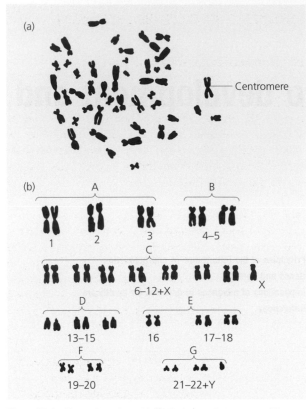

(a)

Centromere

(b)

A — 1, 2, 3 · B — 4–5

C — 6–12+X

D — 13–15 · E — 16, 17–18

F — 19–20 · G — 21–22+Y

Figure 20.1 Human karyotype. (a) Chromosomes from a normal human diploid cell. (b) Karyotyping of chromosomes from a male.
Q. How does the female karyotype differ from that of the male?

Most of the chromosomes are indistinguishable between males and females. The exception is the pair of sex chromosomes. In females, the karyotype is referred to as XX, i.e. there are two X chromosomes. In males, there is only one X chromosome; the other member of the pair is considerably smaller and is called the Y chromosome (i.e. the male karyotype is XY). This difference has implications for the inheritance of certain disorders, as they are linked to these particular chromosomes and the disorder typically is observed in males. Autosomal and sex-linked inheritances are considered later.

Are genetic disorders inherited or acquired?

The activities of genes are evident throughout life, and scientists are increasingly identifying genetic causes of ill-health. A number of inherited disorders are recognized (approximately 3000, although most of these are rare). Many readers will have heard of the commoner ones, such as cystic fibrosis and Duchenne's muscular dystrophy. A feature of inherited disorders, of course, is that they are usually present from birth, although some inherited genes become problematic later in childhood or even adulthood, because gene expression may be 'masked' for a while. However, recent advances are now beginning to identify how genetic disturbances can also be acquired during life. Thus, disorders such as cancer and heart disease are now known to have genetic components that become problematic because the genetic code is altered during life. Even with these disorders, it is clear that some people inherit certain genes that give them a greater likelihood of developing the condition.

In relation to ill-health, therefore, two significant aspects are the genes that we inherit that either influence embryo development or give a propensity to later acquired conditions, and the genetic changes that we acquire during the lifespan. Acquired genetic changes not only contribute to specific adulthood diseases, but also are evident in the ageing process.

Specific disorders are noted in various chapters of this book, and are not discussed in depth here. Rather, this chapter considers the main stages in tissue specialization during embryo development, the inheritance of characteristics, and how acquired gene changes seem to be an important factor in the declining function associated with ageing.

BOX 20.1 THE HUMAN GENOME PROJECT

The entire collection of genes within a body cell is called the *genome*. It comprises those genes for the various characteristics of that person. The ability of science to identify genetic coding wherever it lies within a chromosome has made possible the identification of the genetic coding of the entire human genome. Much of the human genome (95%) is considered to be 'junk' DNA, functionless leftovers from the evolutionary process, but within the genome will be the genetic coding of the genes that make up the remaining 5%. The Human Genome Project commenced in the late 1980s as a collaborative venture between various countries, although commercial projects joined the endeavour. June 2000 saw the announcement that the identification of the genome is effectively complete, and February 2001 saw its publication. Thus, the complete human 'blue print' is effectively identified. The questions to be answered at the time of writing are:

- The genome project identified 30 000 or so genes – much less than the anticipated 100 000 plus. How does the relatively small number of genes enable the synthesis of such a vast array (100 000–150 000) of proteins found in the human body?
- Exactly where are the genes within the genome? Many have been identified but some remain to be identified or to be linked to a given characteristic.
- Now genes are being identified, what are their roles in health and ill-health?
- Are the activities of certain genes influenced by environmental factors or ageing, and if so can this be manipulated?
- Can a commercial company claim ownership of genes that their laboratories have identified and/or classified? This argument places business and scientists in academia in opposition, and is still under discussion.

EMBRYO DEVELOPMENT, AND THE ROLE OF GENES AS MEDIATORS OF TISSUE DIFFERENTIATION

The following section outlines the processes of moving from a fertilized egg cell to a formed fetus. Critical steps that are actioned by genes during differentiation and lead to tissue specialization are highlighted. It should be noted, however, that although recent research has identified some of the genes that are essential in these processes (called 'homeobox' genes; Mark *et al.*, 1997), other crucial genes remain to be identified. The normality of these (and other) genes and of their expression is vital to the whole process.

Stages of embryo development

It is convenient to consider the milestones of tissue differentiation in two substages: the early embryo before implantation, and the later embryo after implantation.

Differentiation of the early embryo

Fertilisation normally takes place within the Fallopian tubes of the uterus to produce the stage called the *zygote*. This must travel along the tube to the body of the uterus, which normally takes a few days. During this time, the zygote develops into early embryological stages called a *morula* and a *blastocyst*.

The morula

Cell division begins immediately after the ovum and sperm nuclei have fused. The cells divide approximately every 12 h, eventually producing a ball of 64 cells. This stage is called the morula (= mulberry, as the appearance is likened to this fruit) (Figure 20.2). There is no increase in overall size, however, as the cells (which therefore must decrease

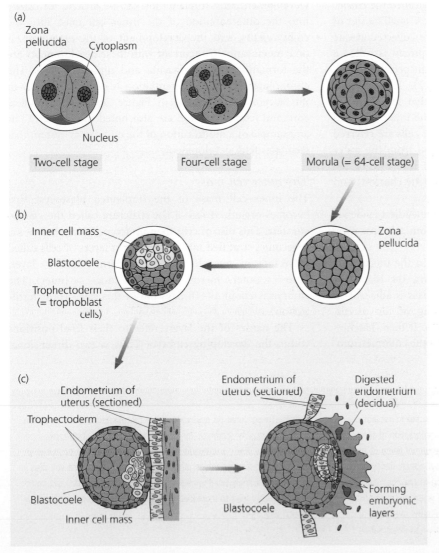

(a)
Zona pellucida · Cytoplasm · Nucleus

Two-cell stage · Four-cell stage · Morula (= 64-cell stage)

(b)
Inner cell mass · Blastocoele · Trophectoderm (= trophoblast cells) · Zona pellucida

(c)
Endometrium of uterus (sectioned) · Trophectoderm · Blastocoele · Inner cell mass · Endometrium of uterus (sectioned) · Digested endometrium (decidua) · Blastocoele · Forming embryonic layers

Figure 20.2 Pre-implantation development. (a) Development of the morula from the zygote. (b) The blastocyst (in section). (c) Implantation.

Q. Discuss the events leading to the formation of the zygote.

Q. Distinguish between the morula and blastocyst stages of development.

in individual size) remain encapsulated within the protein coat, called the zona pellucida, that was present when the oocyte was shed from the ovary. This coat continues to provide protection for the morula as it is wafted along in fluid within the Fallopian tube.

The cells within the morula appear very simplistic. While some genes are undoubtedly active within the cells, a cell can actually be removed from the morula without affecting the future development of the embryo. The cells, therefore, do not yet have a predetermined 'destiny': the developmental genes have still to be activated.

Exercise

You might want to refer to the later section on genetic screening, since this identifies how gene analysis of cells from the morula have an impact on inheritance.

The blastocyst

By the time the morula reaches the uterus, it will have been transformed. Some cells will have migrated to the outer surface, leaving a fluid-filled cavity called the *blastocoele* ('-coele' = space or compartment). A small cluster of cells, called the *inner cell mass*, will have collected at one side of the cavity. This stage of development is called a *blastocyst* ('blast-' = a simple, as-yet unspecialized cell, '-cyst' = fluid-filled mass) (Figure 20.2). The developmental significance of the blastocyst is that cells within it have now shown a degree of identity. The inner cell mass is destined to become the embryo (these cells are referred to as 'embryoblasts'), while cells derived from the outer surface will eventually be incorporated into one of the membranes that surround the embryo (the chorion) and form part of the placenta.

The blastocyst, therefore, provides the earliest evidence of functional specialization resulting from selective gene activation/deactivation.

Two or three days after arrival within the uterus (i.e. around the sixth day after fertilization), the blastocyst orientates itself so that the inner cell mass is adjacent to the surface of the endometrium lining of the uterus, usually in the upper areas of the uterus. It then 'hatches' from the zona pellucida, and adheres to the endometrium.

At this point, the cells that form the outer layer of the blastocyst begin to secrete enzymes, which digest the immediate endometrial cells and so initiate implantation (Figure 20.2). This action explains the name – *trophoblasts* – given to these cells ('troph-' = nutrition) and that given to the cell layer – the *trophectoderm* ('ecto-' = outer, 'derm' = layer). Note, however, that the trophectoderm bears no relation to the embryonic *ectoderm* mentioned later. The two terms are confusing, but a general rule of thumb is that any reference to tissues in a fetus, infant, child or adult as being 'ectodermal' in origin will usually be referring to the ectoderm, not the trophectoderm.

Implantation is completed by about the eleventh day after fertilization. Developmental changes occurring within the implanted blastocyst now gain in momentum, not least because fuels for metabolism become available from the digested cells of the endometrium.

Differentiation of the later embryo

Development after implantation can be divided for clarity into the differentiation of the inner cell mass into the embryo/fetus, and the development of the extra-embryonic membranes. Concurrent with these developments are the formation of the placenta and umbilical cord. The chronology of tissue differentiation is described briefly in this section, and detailed in Figure 20.3. The umbilical cord and fetal circulation are also noted in Chapter 12 as an example of a modification of the circulatory system that facilitates fetal development.

The inner cell mass

The inner cell mass of the implanted blastocyst first becomes organized into a flat structure called the *embryonic disc*. This disc of cells then undergoes gastrulation, i.e. it becomes stratified into three distinct layers of cells called the ectoderm, mesoderm and endoderm ('derm' = layer, 'ecto-' = outer, 'meso-' = middle, 'endo-' = inner). The embryo is about 14–18 days old at this stage (post-fertilization).

The names of the layers refer to their final positions within the developing embryo. Thus, a two-dimensional

BOX 20.2 EMBRYO IMPLANTATION

It is pertinent to note here that many blastocysts fail to implant. The process of implantation involves chemical interaction at the interface between the blastocyst and the endometrial lining of the uterus. Science is beginning to understand how adherence takes place. It will be a while before the contribution of the chemicals involved is understood fully but, interestingly, scientists working to improve the success of in vitro fertilization methods suspect that chromosomal abnormalities might be involved when implantation

fails. These could be assessed at the morula stage to aid selection of 'high-quality' embryos for transfer to the uterus. This move towards routinely examining chromosomes in embryos produced in vitro introduces an ethical dilemma, since the procedure will also identify routinely whether the embryo is male or female, and could conceivably lead to increased pressure on the government to allow sex selection.

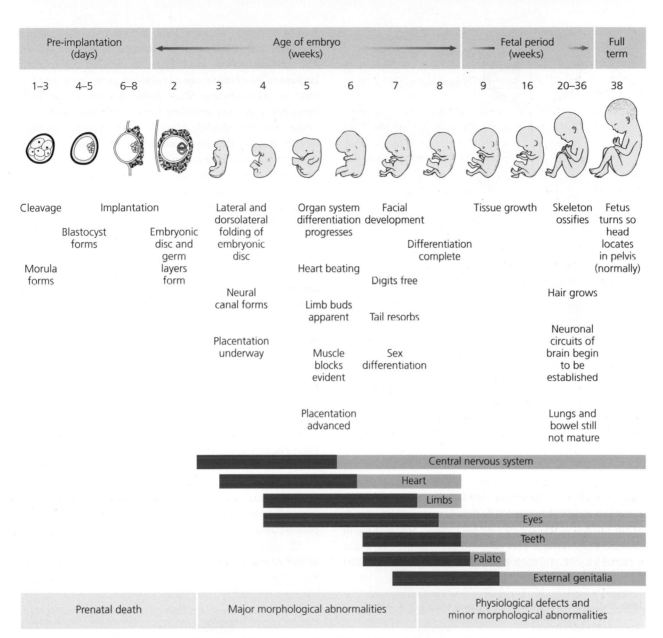

Figure 20.3 Embryo/fetal development. Chronology of tissue differentiation. Horizontal bars at the bottom of the figure provide examples of developmental susceptibility to teratogenic agents.

Q. Distinguish between the embryo and fetal stages of development.

Q. Discuss the role of genes and the environment in the initiation of each stage of human development.

Q. How may congenital malformation arise?

structure is transformed into a three-dimensional one by the curling over of the ectoderm, with the result that the endoderm and mesoderm form concentric tube-like layers within it (Figure 20.4). This process represents the second phase in tissue differentiation. Clearly, further gene activity has been initiated to produce such changes. The phase should not be underestimated, since this seemingly simple act lays down the basic body plan: if you imagine a cross-section through the adult abdomen, you can envisaged which tissues the cell layers are destined to develop into (Table 20.1):

- The bowel and associated structures are derived from the endodermal tube.

- The epidermis of the skin is formed from the embryonic ectoderm.

- The skeleton, skeletal muscle layers, and blood are structures found between the skin and bowel, and are derived from the mesoderm.

- The perforations at each end of the tube-like structure eventually become the mouth and anus, so the ends of the tube are set to become the 'head' and 'tail' ends.

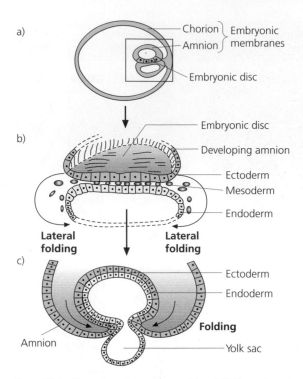

a)

Chorion ⎫ Embryonic
Amnion ⎰ membranes

Embryonic disc

b)

Embryonic disc

Developing amnion

Ectoderm

Mesoderm

Endoderm

Lateral folding   **Lateral folding**

c)

Ectoderm

Endoderm

Folding

Amnion

Yolk sac

Figure 20.4 The embryonic germ layers. (a) and (b) The embryonic disc. (c) Folding to internalize the endoderm. (Mesoderm not shown). *Q. Name the three germ layers. To what organs do the layers give rise (use Table 20.1 if you have difficulty in answering this question)?*

hollow structure is eventually reflected in the cerebral ventricles and spinal canal of the central nervous system. The nervous system must begin to develop early, partly because of its ultimate complexity and partly because of its role in co-ordinating fetal tissue functions. Similarly, further gene activation will ensure that the heart and circulation also develop early, since it is this system that must ensure adequate delivery of nutrients and oxygen to tissues in order to support the rapid growth that is taking place. The early development of the nervous and circulatory system, and the need for continued development throughout the embryo/fetal period, makes these systems especially susceptible to developmental disorders (see Box 20.3).

Recent evidence suggests that the development of the embryo entails the genetic activation of the synthesis of chemicals, collectively called morphogens, by embryological cells. These chemicals determine which parts of the embryo will form the 'head' end and the body segments, and ultimately determine organ development (Lemaire and Kessel, 1997; Mark *et al.*, 1997).

Thus, within just 3 weeks of fertilization, gene activities have established the general plan of the body, and specific tissues and organs have started to develop. Tissue differentiation continues during the following weeks, and the embryo becomes increasingly humanoid in shape (Figure 20.3). The final process is sex determination, which occurs from about the seventh week, and is mostly complete by the end of the eighth week. This early period is the time during which the embryo is particularly susceptible to environmental agents that could cause errors in gene expression. It is also a period when the mother may not even be aware that she is pregnant.

All organs are basically defined by the end of 8 weeks of embryonic development, although their functions may

The embryo still has some way to go before these organ systems have differentiated. The first sign of a specific organ being formed is the appearance of a raised neural plate in the ectoderm surface. This collection of cells then becomes a neural groove and then a neural tube (Figure 20.5). This

Table 20.1 Structures produced by the three primary germ layers

Endoderm	Mesoderm	Ectoderm
Epithelium of digestive tract (except the oral cavity and anal canal) and its associated glands	All skeletal, most smooth and all cardiac muscle	Nervous tissue
	Cartilage, bone and other connective tissues	Epidermis of skin
Epithelium of urinary bladder, gall bladder and liver	Blood, bone marrow and lymphoid tissue	Hair follicles, arrector pili muscles, nails, and epithelia of sebaceous and sudoriferous glands
	Endothelium of blood vessels and lymphatics	
Epithelium of pharynx, external auditory tube, tonsils, larynx and airways of the lungs	Dermis of skin	Lens, cornea and optic nerve of eye, and internal eye muscles
	Fibrous and vascular coats of eye	Inner and outer ear
Epithelium of thyroid, parathyroid, pancreas and thymus glands	Middle ear	Neuroepithelium of sense organs
Epithelium of prostate and bulbourethral glands, vagina, vestibule, urethra and associated glands	Epithelium of kidneys and ureters	Epithelium of oral and nasal cavities, paranasal sinuses, salivary glands and anal canal
	Epithelium of adrenal cortex	
	Epithelium of gonads and genital ducts	Epithelium of pineal gland, pituitary gland and adrenal medulla

Q. What do the prefixes 'endo-', 'meso-' and 'ecto-' mean?

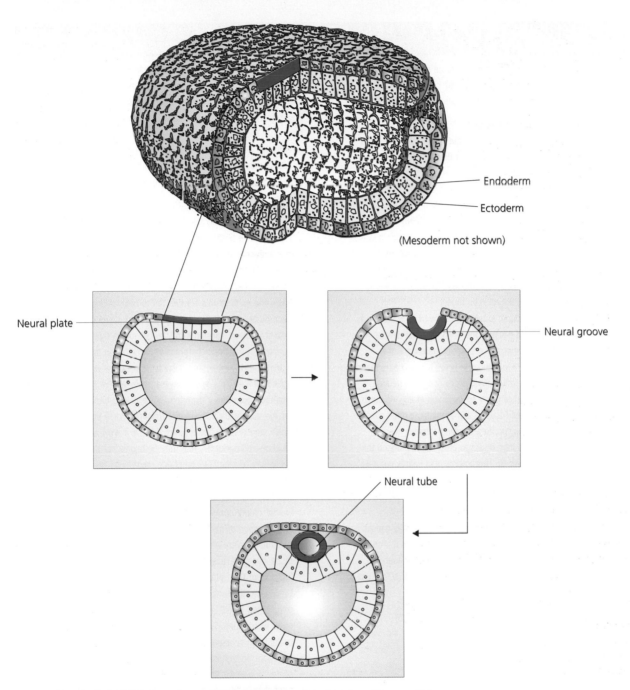

Figure 20.5   The first (visible) signs of organ development in the embryo: formation of the neural tube.
Q. From which embryonic germ layer is the neural tube derived?

be only rudimentary. The embryo is now considered to be a fetus. Further development of the fetus primarily entails growth and the functional maturation of the organs laid down during the embryonic period. This does not mean that the fetus is now no longer susceptible to abnormalities of development, but the risk does decline.

Sex differentiation
There are a number of congenital disorders of sex development (see later), and it is worth noting here how sex differentiation occurs. Tissue that can form both male and

female gonads develops at the same site within the abdomen of the embryo. These are, of course, non-functional, and it would be incorrect to consider the embryo a hermaphrodite. Rather, the embryo has bipotential in that it may become male or female. Associated with the undifferentiated gonadal tissue are two sets of ducts called the Wolffian and Müllerian ducts (named after the people who first identified them) (Figure 20.6). If a Y chromosome is present, then male sex determination is triggered by activation for a short period of genes on this chromosome. These in turn stimulate certain genes on the

BOX 20.3 ABNORMALITIES OF NEURAL AND CARDIAC DEVELOPMENT

The lists presented here are not intended to be comprehensive but provide examples of how congenital disorder can have a profound effect on the neural and cardiovascular systems.

Abnormalities of neural development

Spina bifida is an incomplete closure of the neural arch of one or more vertebrae. In its most severe form a fluid-filled sac (called a myelomeningocoele) protrudes through to the skin, usually in the lumbar region. This thin protection afforded to underlying spinal neurons is usually inadequate, leading to infection, damage, and resultant paralysis. Spina bifida is a congenital condition but its incidence has decreased dramatically in recent years since it was recognised that folic acid deficiency was a major contributing factor (Wald 1991). Supplemention of this vitamin in the mother's diet early in pregnancy is now recommended to reduce the risk of the embryo developing this neural tube defect.

Microcephaly is an abnormal smallness of the head in relation to the rest of the body, caused because the brain does not develop fully.

Hydrocephalus occurs when there is an interference in the circulation of cerebrospinal fluid within the brain. It produces a raised pressure of the cerebrospinal fluid that acts to compress neural tissue. Such cranial hypertension may be observed at any life stage, e.g. as a consequence of head trauma, but in infants it often arises because there is poor connection between the ventricles (these spaces form the fluid which then drains to other spaces around the brain and spinal cord; Chapter 8). Hydrocephalus in infants normally induces an enlargement of the head because the sutures of the skull are not closed. The rise in intracranial pressure presents itself by drowsiness and vomiting, and neurological dysfunction.

Cri du chat syndrome is a congenital condition and is caused by absence of one of the arms of chromosome number 5. The widespread loss of genes that this produces causes profound abnormalities, both physical and mental. The name refers to a cat-like cry in infancy.

Abnormalities of cardiac anatomy (see also Box 12.3)

The fetal circulation exhibits adaptations for intrauterine life, when the lungs are inoperative and nutrient exchange occurs across the placenta (Stables 1999a). Blood is conveyed to the placenta via two *umbilical arteries* in the umbilical cord, and returns in an *umbilical vein* that links to the hepatic portal vein and joins with the inferior vena cava via the *ductus venosus*. Within the heart,

most blood passes directly from the right to left atrium via the *foramen ovale* in the septum between them. That which does enter the pulmonary artery (from the right ventricle) largely drains into the aorta via the *ductus arteriosus*, and so relatively little passes to the lungs. These fetal features close at or soon after birth, thus establishing the child/adult pattern of circulation.

Congenital abnormalities may arise that cause problems after birth (Stables 1999b; Suddaby & Grenier 1999). For example,

- *Septal defects*. A *persistent foramen ovale* allows some blood to pass from the left to the right atrium (pressure changes in the left atrium at birth promote this reversal in blood flow), leading to a reduced cardiac output. If mild this may not have immediate consequences for the infant, but it may influence growth during childhood. A *ventricular septal defect* occurs when the ends of this septum fail to fuse as they grow towards each other when the heart chambers are developing. This results in blood passing from the left to the right ventricle during systole (since the pressure is higher in the left). Cardiac output will decrease, and there will be excessive volume in the right ventricle. This latter may cause excessive growth of this chamber, pulmonary hypertension, and long-term consequences for the pulmonary valve, which might become stenosed.

- *Valve stenosis* is when a heart valve is narrow or fails to function appropriately. This may be congenital or develop secondary to other problems (e.g. ventricular septal defect). It has consequences for the passage of blood through the heart, and may promote excessive pressure in the heart chamber that cannot empty normally.

- *Transposition of the great vessels* is when the insertion of the pulmonary artery and aorta into the right and left ventricles, respectively, is reversed. The aorta now takes deoxygenated blood from the right ventricle and directs it to the body tissues, by-passing the lungs. The pulmonary artery now directs oxygenated blood arriving from the lungs back to the lungs. In other words there is a separation of the pulmonary and systemic circulations. Babies born with this problem will usually be reliant on the little bit of blood mixing that continues to occur for a while through the foramen ovale and the ductus arteriosus, which do not close immediately after birth. Corrective surgery will be necessary very early on.

X chromosome, which act to promote the differentiation of the gonadal tissue into testes, which then begin to produce the male sex steroid hormone testosterone and a peptide hormone called Müllerian inhibition substance (MIS). These hormones promote the appropriate duct system: testosterone stimulates the differentiation of the Wolffian ducts into the vas deferens and associated structures of the male reproductive tract, and external genitalia develop accordingly; MIS causes the Müllerian ducts to degenerate.

In the absence of a Y chromosome, the early gonadal tissue will not be activated to produce testosterone, so the

Wolffian ducts regress and atrophy. Likewise, MIS is not produced, so the Müllerian ducts persist and develop into the Fallopian tubes and uterus of the female tract. The undifferentiated gonads develop as ovaries, and the embryo becomes female.

In rare cases, the activities of the Y chromosome cannot be expressed (fully), and the baby develops as a female with no, or at most rudimentary, testes. This situation may arise because the Y chromosome fails to activate the appropriate genes on the X chromosome. Alternatively, it may be that the early gonadal tissue fails to

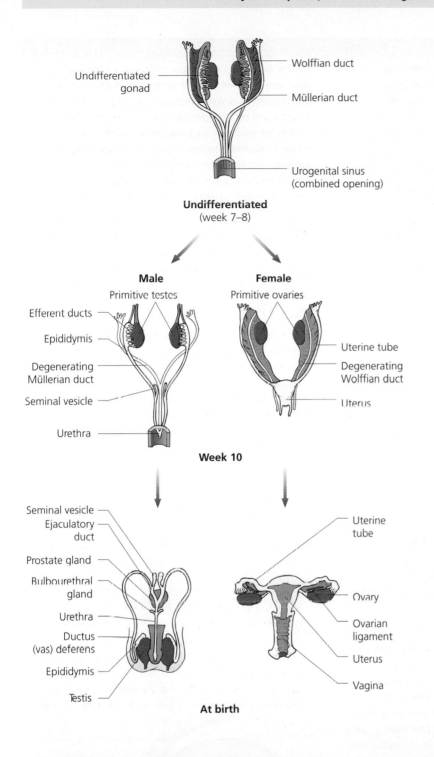

Figure 20.6 Differentiation of the sex organs.
Q. Discuss the role of the sperm in determining the sex of the offspring.

BOX 20.4 RESEARCH ON HUMAN EMBRYOS

The Human Fertilisation and Embryology Authority (est. 1991) works on behalf of the government to advise on developments in genetic and embryological research and practices. The principles operated are enshrined in the Human Fertilisation and Embryology Act of 1990. Regarding human embryos:

1 research on human embryos must be licensed with the Human Fertilisation and Embryology Authority, and must not involve embryos more than 14 days old. This conforms to the period when the nervous system begins to differentiate, i.e. when the embryo begins to develop a recognizable organ system;

2 researchers are forbidden to produce identical individuals by genetic replacement (i.e. by cloning; see Box 20.9);

3 researchers must not attempt to produce an embryo by combining the egg or sperm of a human with those of another animal.

Points 2 and 3 highlight how rapidly research methods and capabilities have progressed during the last 10–15 years.

BOX 20.5 BIRTH WEIGHT

Various factors, such as race and gestational age, affect birth weights, and there are accepted 'norms'. The term 'weight for gestational age' is usually applied. Body weights outside the normal range frequently result from maternal behaviours, or are consequences of maternal ill-health, i.e. gene expression, rather than the genes themselves, is altered.

Excessive stimulation of fetal growth produces birth weights in excess of the norm. Maternal diabetes mellitus induces increased insulin release in the fetus, with subsequent deposition of food stores. Excessive birth weight has obvious implications for labour, e.g. cephalopelvic distortion (CPD) or obstructed labour.

Low birth weights reflect either inadequate placental blood flow, which restricts nutrient supply to the fetus (e.g. the effects of nicotine from smoking), or depressed metabolism (e.g. in fetal alcohol syndrome, and possibly from carbon monoxide in cigarette smoke).

Very low-weight-for-age babies are more susceptible to neonatal difficulties (Agustines *et al.*, 2000). Recent studies have also suggested that there may be a link between low birth weight and increased risk of ill-health later in life, which suggests that tissue development as well as growth might have been adversely affected. This is a controversial topic, and interested readers are referred to a review paper by Scrimshaw (1997).

secrete adequate testosterone, or perhaps the male reproductive tract tissue fails to develop adequately under the effects of the testosterone. The situation introduces a potential dilemma in that genetically the person is XY, i.e. male, but phenotypically they are female.

Extra-embryonic membranes

Screening programmes for embryological disorders can be implemented quite early (11–16 weeks) in pregnancy. The methods basically entail obtaining samples of fetal tissue so that chromosomal and biochemical analyses can be performed. Information is provided in Box 20.6, but to understand how tissue can be sampled, it is important to first consider the development of the membranes that support and provide for the growing embryo/fetus. There are four membranes that develop from embryological tissue:

● The *chorion* develops from the trophectoderm of the blastocyst, and eventually increases in size until it lines the uterine cavity. Parts of the chorion will be incorporated into the placenta (see Chapter 18). The remaining three membranes develop as outgrowths of cell layers of the actual embryo.

● The *amnion* develops from ectoderm of the embryonic disc, and distends to encompass the developing embryo (Figures 20.4 and 20.7). It secretes amniotic fluid, which provides support for the growing fetus, helps to maintain a constant temperature, and acts as a shock absorber during maternal movement. The fluid is also swallowed by the fetus, and a dilute urine excreted into it, which facilitates the functional development of the bowel and kidneys. Its volume at term is 1–1.5 l; the amnion will have grown outwards to meet the chorion and so line the uterine cavity.

● The *yolk sac* grows from the endoderm, and also incorporates migrated mesodermal cells. It projects into the cavity enclosed by the growing chorion, and helps in the nutrition of the embryo (Figures 20.4 and 20.7). Blood vessels develop from the mesodermal cells, which are also responsible for early synthesis of red blood cells. The sac is evident only early in embryo development, and it

eventually becomes incorporated into the developing 'body stalk' that attaches the embryo to the developing placenta and is destined to become the umbilical cord.

● The *allantois* is another endodermal sac. It originates close to the base of the yolk sac (Figure 20.7). It also contains mesodermal cells. Blood vessels that develop from these cells help to establish the vascularization of the chorion/placenta. The membrane is eventually incorporated into the umbilical cord, although a part of it is incorporated into the growing fetal bladder.

The chorion and amnion are the most developed of these membranes. Together, they are the membranes that 'burst' in the first stage of labour; the 'waters' are amniotic fluid released from the cavity.

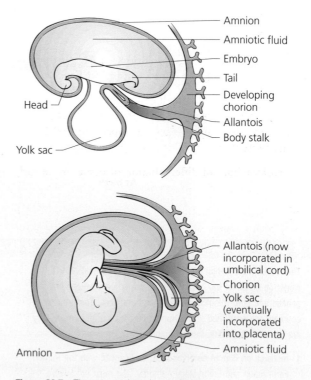

Figure 20.7 The extra-embryonic membranes.
Q. What is the purpose of amniotic fluid?

BOX 20.6 SCREENING METHODS

Fetal testing

This falls under two broad categories: examination of fetal cells, and imaging of the fetus. *Cell sampling* enables examination of fetal tissue for chromosomal abnormalities. Two main methods are used: amniocentesis and chorionic villus sampling (Stranc, *et al.*, 1997). Both convey increased risk of miscarriage and so are not performed until considered safe to do so. *Amniocentesis* is not usually performed until the sixteenth week. About 20 ml of amniotic fluid is aspirated following a transabdominal insertion of a needle. The fluid contains cells of the amnion membrane and also cells shed from the fetus. The risk of spontaneous abortion is about 1 in 100.

The fluid itself is also of value in screening, e.g. alphafetoprotein (AFP) or the enzyme acetylcholinesterase may be measured, since these are elevated in various abnormalities of development, especially neural tube defects. However, detailed ultrasound scanning of the fetal spine, which is more conclusive, is now possible, and so has largely superseded the chemical screening method.

Chorionic villus sampling entails taking a sample from the chorion at the edge of the placenta, using a hollow needle and suction. This membrane originated from the embryological cells that formed the outer layer of the blastocyst stage of development. Chorionic villus sampling is normally performed from 8 to 12 weeks. The risk of spontaneous abortion is about 2 in 100.

Ultrasound imaging is now detailed enough to enable close examination of the developing fetus, and is beginning to supersede cell sampling as a screening tool. The imaging of the spinal cord was mentioned above, but other measurements are utilized as indicators of development, e.g. the thickness of the nuchal (neck) fold of the fetus and the biparietal diameter of the fetal skull.

Maternal testing

The risk of miscarriage as a consequence of obtaining fetal cells through amniocentesis or chorionic villus sampling makes maternal testing an attractive alternative. This entails assessing chemical markers in maternal blood samples. For example, the AFP that is released from the fetus into the amniotic fluid enters the mother's circulation. Its secretion is increased if there is incomplete neural tube closure in the embryo, so raised concentrations in the maternal blood may be indicative of such a defect (Kubas, 1999). In contrast, the maternal serum AFP concentration may be reduced if the baby has Down's syndrome. The test is not conclusive, however, and other tests are required to raise confidence in the assessment.

The level of confidence of the screening is increased by the concomitant presence of a lower-than-normal concentration of unconjugated oestriol and a higher-than-normal concentration of human chorionic gonadotropin (hCG). Together with the AFP test, these tests constitute the 'Bart's triple test', which is commonly applied as a diagnostic aid during pregnancy in women at risk. However, the level of confidence provided by this test is still not especially high – of the order of 60–70% (Wald *et al.*, 1999) – and false positive and false negative results are possible. The triple test may therefore be combined with other parameters, e.g. another protein called inhibin A (to produce a 'quadruple test') or, increasingly, with fetal data obtained by imaging (see above) in order to raise the level of diagnostic confidence still further.

Genetic and environmental factors in congenital disorders

Congenital disorders are caused by errors of development or function; they usually have an impact on health, and they are present at birth. Such disorders arise from:

- *dysplasia:* failure of differentiation of tissue in the early embryo, usually due to genetic causes;

- *defect:* failure of further development of tissue, which may have a genetic cause or may arise through the influence of environmental factors e.g. drug abuse by the mother;

- *deformation:* altered tissue size or shape arising as a consequence of the effects of physical forces on tissue growth, e.g. poor brain growth in a fetus with hydrocephalus (see Box 20.3).

Tissue differentiation and development therefore depend largely on two factors: the expression of genes, and the genetic complement of the embryo. Note, however, that the majority of cases of congenital abnormality have no known attributable cause – this is an area that is still poorly understood.

Gene expression

Agents that induce physical problems in the newborn are referred to collectively as *teratogens*. These include mutagens, which alter genetic structure, and agents that alter the expression of genes. There is a tendency to look at teratogens as being agents introduced in some form into the body. Various agents are known to influence tissue differentiation, including toxins produced by certain bacteria that increase the risk of congenital problems, and numerous chemicals that are relatively harmless to the mother but may influence embryo/fetal cells. Some examples are given in Table 20.2.

A deficiency of essential substances may also be teratogenic. For example, studies have shown that the incidence of spina bifida can be reduced dramatically by ensuring that the maternal diet contains adequate folate, a vitamin of the B group (see Box 20.3). Folate has a particular role in maintaining neural functions, and it should not,

Table 20.2 Selected teratogenic influences on embryo/fetal development. It should be noted that these influences raise the risk; the occurrence of problems is not certain, or even likely in many instances

Teratogenic influence	Possible effects on fetus or newborn
Drugs taken by mother	
Androgens	Masculinization of fetus
Anaesthetics	Depression of fetus, asphyxia
Antihistamines	Abortion, malformations
Aspirin	Persistent truncus arteriosus, abnormal heart
Diuretics	Polycystic kidney disease
Heroin and morphine	Convulsions, tremor, neonatal death
Insulin shock	Fetal death
LSD (lysergide; lysergic acid diethylamide)	Chromosomal anomalies, deformity
Nicotine (from smoking)	Stunting, accelerated heart beat, premature birth, organ congestion, fits and convulsions
Oestrogens	Malformations, hyperactivity of fetal adrenal glands
Streptomycin	Damage to auditory nerve
Thalidomide	Hearing loss, abnormal appendages, death
Maternal infection	
Chickenpox or shingles	Chickenpox or shingles, abortion, stillbirth
Syphilis	Miscarriage
Cytomegalovirus (salivary gland virus)	Small head, inflammation and hardening of brain and retina, deafness, poor mental development, enlargement of spleen and liver, anaemia, giant cells in urine from kidneys
Hepatitis	Hepatitis
Herpes simplex	Generalized herpes, inflammation of brain, cyanosis, jaundice, fever, respiratory and circulatory collapse, death
Mumps	Fetal death, endocardial fibroelastosis, anomalies
Pneumonia	Abortion in early pregnancy
Poliomyelitis	Spinal or bulbar poliomyelitis, acute poliomyelitis of newborn
Rubella (German measles)	Anomalies, haemorrhage, enlargement of spleen and liver, inflammation of brain, liver, and lungs, cataracts, small brain, deafness, various mental defects, death
Scarlet fever	Abortion in early pregnancy
Smallpox	Abortion, stillbirth, smallpox
Syphilis	Stillbirth, premature birth, syphilis
Toxoplasmosis (protozoan parasite infection)	Small eyes and head, mental retardation, cerebral oedema (encephalitis), heart damage, fetal death
Tuberculosis	Fetal death, lowered resistance to tuberculosis
Typhoid fever	Abortion in early pregnancy

Q. Differentiate between mutagens and teratogens.

Q. Using this table and Figure 20.3, identify the critical periods of gestation in which administering the drug thalidomide to a pregnant woman would cause (i) major changes in limb formation, (ii) minor changes in limb formation, and (iii) no changes to limb formation.

perhaps, be surprising that it has a profound role in neural development. Retrospect is much easier than foresight, however, and the protective effects of folate have been recognized only recently.

Genetic complement

Genetic changes can occur while the embryo is in utero, either spontaneously or because of an extrinsic agent (e.g.

radiation) that acts as a mutagen. In most cases, however, the genetic complement of an embryo is determined by the genes inherited from the sperm and ovum at fertilization, and so disordered development arises when inherited, mutated genes are expressed, or when genes are in excess or are absent because of chromosomal defects.

Inheritance is a large topic, and to appreciate how the genes that inherited may or may not affect development it is necessary to explore it in detail. The next section considers the many aspects of inheritance.

THE FUNDAMENTALS OF INHERITANCE: GENES, ALLELES AND CELL DIVISION

Terminology

Like all branches of biology, genetics has its specific terminology. First, then, some general definitions. Collectively, the entire gene composition of the DNA of an individual is called the *genome*. The genome provides the full genetic blueprint of an individual.

The genes of an individual are largely responsible for observable or measurable characteristics called the *phenotypes*. Such characteristics are normally expressed as physical ones, but, as outlined in Chapter 2, the activities of genes are also observed at the biochemical level of cell activity. The term 'phenotype' therefore could be applied to characteristics ranging from a particular protein, to cell organelles, to tissue types, to organ function, to external features of the individual. Some characteristics are produced by a single gene, while others involve several genes. The gene(s) responsible for a given phenotype comprise the *genotype* for that characteristic.

The occurrence of chromosomes in pairs has major implications. This is because each set of 23 chromosomes within a cell is inherited from one parent and so must contain the blueprint for an individual; each chromosome within a pair will usually carry genes for the same characteristics. There must therefore be a duplication of genes: if a chromosome contains genes inherited from the mother that provide the code for, say, eye colour, then there will be a complementary set of genes on the other member of the chromosome pair inherited from the father. Thus, most phenotypes of an individual reflect the net effects of pairs of genes, and the genotype will be written to reflect this (e.g. for a gene A, the genotype might be written as AA, rather than simply A). Pairs of chromosomes are said to be *homologous* chromosomes ('homo-' = same) in recognition that each member of the pair will carry genes that are complementary for the same characteristics.

It is important to be aware of this, because although a pair of genes may produce a single given characteristic, they may not necessarily have precisely the same genetic coding, either to each other or to those of another individual (Figure 20.8). Thus, each member of the gene pair may introduce variation into the characteristic produced. Since the pair of genes may not be identical, the two forms are called allelomorphs, or *alleles* for short. As a general rule, if reference is made to a gene for a particular characteristic (e.g. 'the gene for cystic fibrosis'), this will normally refer to the allele that is mainly responsible for that characteristic.

If the genetic codes of a pair of alleles are identical, then both will cause the cell to produce the same protein (Figure 20.8). Accordingly, the individual is said to be

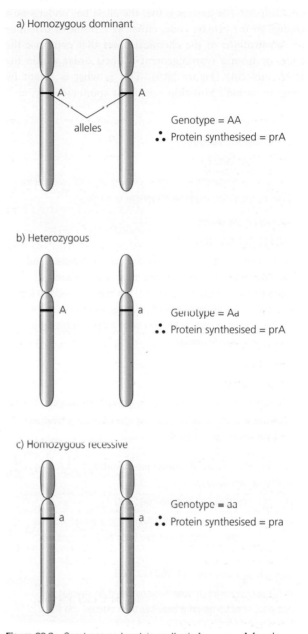

Figure 20.8 Genotypes and protein synthesis for a gene A found on a (hypothetical) chromosome. (a) Homozygous dominant: genotype is AA, therefore protein synthesis is prA. (b) Heterozygous: genotype is Aa, therefore protein synthesis is prA. (c) Homozygous recessive: genotype is aa, therefore protein synthesis is pra.

Q. *Define the terms 'homozygous', 'heterozygous'; 'dominant' and 'recessive'.*

homozygous for the characteristic that is produced. If the two alleles are slightly different, then the individual is said to be *heterozygous* ('hetero-'– different) for that characteristic.

Alleles and cell function

How can one allele have a different genetic code to its counterpart? The answer is that the allele has undergone a change to the genetic code, either as a result of deletions or substitutions of the chemical bases that comprise the code, or from a rearrangement of their order within the DNA molecule (Figure 20.9). This is what is meant by 'gene mutation'. Mutation can occur spontaneously, or it

(a) Consider this sentence:

THE OLD CAT WAS TOO FAT

This is an understandable sentence. By analogy, if this was genetic code, its translation would be acceptable to a cell.

Rearranging the words:

THE FAT CAT WAS TOO OLD

In this genetic code, the translation would still be acceptable, but the meaning of the original sentence (by analogy a protein synthesized by the cell) has been lost. The function associated with that sentence is no longer available, but has been replaced with the new one, which may or may not be to a cell's advantage, or may even be a disadvantage.

Alternatively:

THE OLD CAT WAS TOO FTA

The original meaning has been lost, and been replaced with a nonsensical sentence. By analogy, this new code (i.e. protein) will not have any action in the cell.

(b) Using this principle to illustrate gene mutation, the following is a piece of genetic code:

GCA ACC CAG CUU CAC UCA UCC GGC ACG

In the next sequence, a gene mutation called a substitution has occurred, in which a base at one point has been changed into another:

GCA A*A*C CAG CUU CAC UCA UCC GGC ACG

In the next sequence, a gene mutation called an insertion has occurred, in which an extra base has been inserted into the sequence:

GCA ACC *G*CA GCU UCA CUC AUC CGG CAC G..

Compare these to the original above. Which of the two mutations is likely to be most effective as far as changing cell function is concerned? To answer this, you might want to refer to Table 2.3 and 'translate' these codes into a sequence of amino acids.

Figure 20.9 Gene mutation. The base sequence (i.e. genetic code) of DNA is 'read' in groups of three bases; each group represents an amino acid. In this way, a cell constructs a protein of a specific amino acid sequence (see Chapter 2). (a) Genetic code in the form of a simple English sentence highlights the principle of gene mutation. (b) An example of gene mutation by substitution or insertion of a base (i.e. a 'letter' in the three-letter word).

may result from the actions of certain environmental agents, such as radiation, toxins or viruses. The consequence of mutation is that the altered genetic code potentially might induce a cell to synthesize novel proteins, and the actions of the new protein, or alternatively the absence of the 'normal' protein, may change cell and tissue function and consequently alter the phenotype (Figure 20.10).

Dominant and recessive alleles

It is likely that we all have within our DNA mutated alleles that are capable of producing disordered functioning. So why are the dysfunctional changes not always observed? The explanation is that the alleles are usually paired with a 'normal' counterpart that exerts dominance over the mutated one, which is then said to be recessive. The cell therefore synthesizes the 'normal' protein, and the altered allele is ineffective (Figure 20.3). In writing the genotype, it is usual to show the dominant allele as a capital letter and the recessive one as a lower case letter (e.g. Aa). Of course, if both alleles are of the recessive mutation (e.g. genotype aa), there is no 'normal' form to dominate cell function, so the recessive alleles can express themselves. Most genetic disorders involve a recessive allele, so two copies of the allele will be necessary for the condition to be expressed.

It is still poorly understood how one allele assumes dominance over another, but it is clear that occasionally dominance is incomplete, in which case both alleles are active to some extent. In some instances, mutated alleles may even be dominant to the 'normal' form, in which case having just one copy of it will alter cell or tissue functioning.

When mutated alleles are expressed, the consequences for the individual's wellbeing will depend on the extent of their influences on cell and tissue functioning:

- The characteristic produced may not be altered markedly because many other genes also have an influence on it, i.e. it is a 'polygenic' phenotype (see below).

- The changes induced may be benign (see Box 20.7).

- Some genes are vital to basic cell processes. Thus, a single mutated gene may give rise to serious inherited conditions, such as cystic fibrosis, sickle cell anaemia, haemophilia and Duchenne's muscular dystrophy.

Although alleles can vary, many are actually going to be identical in all people. For example, the ability of cells to generate ATP from glucose will involve much the same genetic code in everybody, otherwise the vital proteins could not be synthesized and life will not be possible. Nevertheless, the difference in people's appearances is a clear indication of how variable some alleles may be. In healthcare, the tendency is to consider only those gene mutations that cause ill-health through disruption of normal embryo development. This forms the focus of this

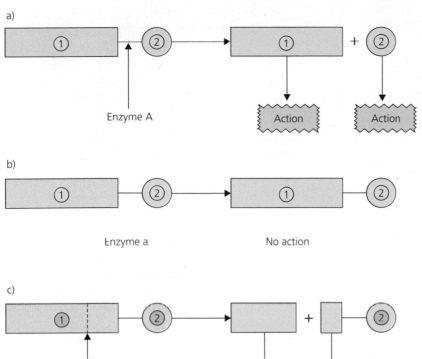

a)

b)

Enzyme a

No action

c)

?

Enzyme a

Partial or different actions

Fig. 20.10 Schematic representation of consequences of gene mutation. (a) Action of enzyme A to catalyse production of chemicals 1 and 2. (b) Gene mutation (homozygous recessive) induces production of enzyme a. Chemicals 1 and 2 are not produced, and the cell loses the actions associated with them. (c) Alternative gene mutation (homozygous recessive) induces production of enzyme a, which, although unable to produce chemicals 1 and 2, catalyses the original molecule into two similar molecules. These may have a partial action similar to that of chemicals 1 and 2, or may have different actions in a cell. *Q. Why are some mutations lethal?*

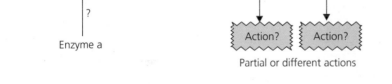

BOX 20.7 BENIGN GENE MUTATIONS

The consequences of altered genes do not have to be detrimental to health. For example, try to roll your tongue lengthways. If you can do this, then you have inherited two copies of the appropriate recessive gene. Similarly, is your ear lobe rounded, or does it taper to the side of the neck? This also relates to inheritance of a gene mutation. Other examples are even more readily apparent - the breadth of variation between physical appearances results from 'gene mixing', but basically entails the inheritance and expression of various genes that will differ between people because of genetic variation.

part of the chapter, and instances are cited below, but it is also important to recognize that gene variation can be a positive influence, as it may enable adaptation to a changing environment, e.g. an individual may have an inborn resistance to HIV infection.

Polygenic phenotypes

Many phenotypes represent complex integrated functions and result from the net effect of the activities of a number of genes, rather than a single gene, which are not necessarily all found on the same chromosome. The net appearance of such polygenic phenotypes will depend on how many of the alleles of the functional group are mutated and expressed – the more variations present, or the more crucial the genes that are affected, the greater the likelihood of an altered phenotype.

The net expression of the numerous alleles is additive. For example, skin pigmentation results from the expression of several genes, but as an illustration we could consider just two (i.e. two pairs of alleles). The inheritance is summarized in Figure 20.11. If both pairs are homozygous for the recessive alleles, then skin colour is 'white'. If both are homozygous for the dominant form, which increases the amount of the melanin pigment present, then skin colour is 'black'. If one gene pair is heterozygous and the other homozygous, then an intermediate skin colour will be produced.

Lethal alleles

Occasionally (thankfully rarely), a mutation of an allele can occur that has such a drastic influence on tissue functions that life is impossible. Such alleles are called lethal alleles; they may be dominant or recessive. One protection we have against such mutations is the presence in DNA of numerous 'back-up' copies of some of the most vital genes.

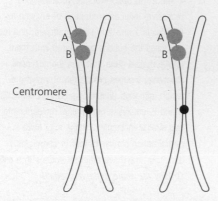

Consider a pair of cofunctional autosomal alleles, A and B on homologous chromosomes

A
B

A
B

Centromere

Homologous chromosomes – genotype written as AABB, i.e. homozygous A, homozygous B

If A and B determine skin colour:

Possible genotype	Phenotype (i.e. skin colour)
AABB	'Black' due to dominant A, B alleles
AaBB	'Black' due to dominant A, B alleles
AaBb	'Black' due to dominant A, B alleles
Aabb	Intermediate as only 1 dominant allele present
AAbb	Intermediate as only 1 dominant allele present
aaBB	Intermediate as only 1 dominant allele present
aaBb	Intermediate as only 1 dominant allele present
aabb	'White' as both alleles recessive

Figure 20.11 Effect of allelic variation on a phenotype determined by more than one gene.

Q. Define the term 'allele'.

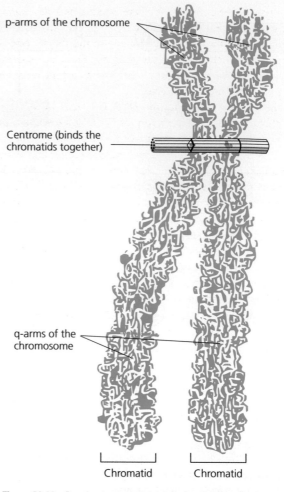

p-arms of the chromosome

Centrome (binds the chromatids together)

q-arms of the chromosome

Chromatid   Chromatid

Figure 20.12 Drawing to show the detail of a chromosome. Notice how the structure has a coiled appearance. A chromosome is comprised of two (identical) DNA molecules, each forming one chromatid.

Gene transmission during cell division

Forming the chromosomes

Cell division is concerned with the production of new cells. In doing so, the DNA in a cell must be assorted so that the new 'daughter' cells contain the appropriate amount and the correct genetic code. During much of the time that a cell is actively performing its functional role, the DNA forms an almost amorphous mass within the nucleus. In order for the cell to manipulate the DNA during cell division, this must first be packaged into units that can be moved easily around the cell. An analogy would be trying to assort 46 strands of wool that are tangled together within a ball (strands of DNA within the cell nucleus): assortment is much easier if the strands have first formed 46 individual small balls (i.e. the DNA molecule coils around and folds in on itself, and so becomes shorter and fatter). It is these small packages of DNA that are the chromosomes; they become visible under a microscope only when cells are undergoing cell division.

To form the chromosome, the DNA molecule duplicates; this is necessary because a fundamental aspect of cell division is that each new cell will require a faithful copy of the original DNA. The duplicated DNA takes on a characteristic 'X' shape (Figure 20.12), with each half of the chromosome being comprised of a single molecule of DNA. The two molecules of DNA in each chromosome represent the copies formed in the duplication process, and are joined together near the central point (the *centromere*).

Each half of the chromosome is referred to as a *chromatid*. The centromere is not exactly central, so the two arms of each chromatid are not equal in length: the shorter one is referred to as the p-arm, the longer one as the q-arm. Reference to the p- or q-arm is used when a gene location on a chromosome is identified.

The process of duplicating DNA is crucial in forming the chromosome. The structure of DNA was described in Chapter 2, but it is important to remember that it consists basically of two strands of structural molecules, and pairs of molecules, called bases, that connect the two strands together rather like the rungs of a ladder. If a molecule of DNA is 'unzipped' (via the actions of certain enzymes) to expose the constituent bases of each strand, it is a relatively straightforward process for a new set of complementary bases to combine with those that have been exposed (see Chapter 2). New strands complete the process; as a result, two molecules of DNA, identical to the original, will have been produced. Complementary pairing of bases ensures that the process of attaching new bases is not random, so the new DNA molecules, and hence the genetic code contained within it, are conserved.

Cell division by mitosis

Mitosis is fundamental to tissue growth and cell replacement. The general process is relatively simple:

1   As a cell prepares to divide, its molecules of DNA are duplicated and the chromosomes are formed, each being comprised of the two duplicates, or chromatids, as explained above.

2   The membrane around the nucleus breaks down, and the chromosomes align within the cytoplasm across the centre of the cell (Figure 20.13).

3   The chromosomes are held in place by the attachment of their centromeres to an array of protein fibres called a *spindle*. This latter is produced by small organelles called *centrioles* that are found in all cells but that only produce the spindle when the cell is dividing. The spindle fibres are secured at opposite ends, or poles, of the cell.

4   The pair of chromatids that make up each chromosome (i.e. the duplicates of the original DNA molecule) separate, and the spindle fibres draw them to the opposite poles of the cell (Figure 20.13). Thus, 46 chromatids will accumulate at each pole of the cell. In this way, each pole will have 46 molecules of DNA of identical structure to the 46 DNA molecules of the original cell.

5   A nuclear membrane forms around each cluster of chromatids, and an intervening cell membrane develops between the two new nuclei. Thus, two 'daughter' cells have been produced from the single 'parent' cell,

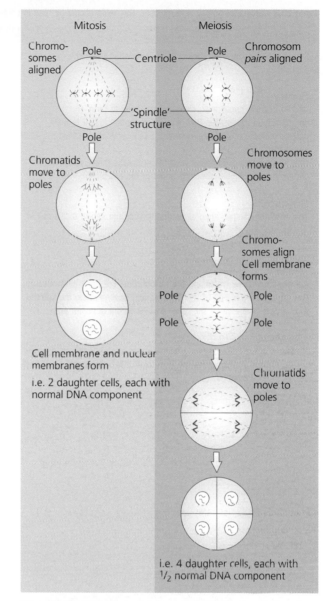

Figure 20.13 Comparison of chromosomal behaviour in mitosis and meiosis. Refer to Table 20.3 for details. Both processes are shown at the metaphase stage to begin with.

Q. Identify the tissues within the female and male where meiosis takes place.

and each will be genetically identical to it. The term *diploid* is used to indicate that the cells have the usual complement of chromosomes.

Each stage of mitosis has a characteristic name (Table 20.3), but such names serve to confuse readers unfamiliar with the process, and it is suggested that they are used only for reference; it is more important to understand the significance of the behaviour of the chromosomes during cell division. Thus, mitosis provides new cells with a genetic blueprint identical to the original, so the new cells should have the same structure and functions as the originals.

Table 20.3 Stages of mitosis and meiosis. This table should be read in conjunction with Figure 20.13

Mitosis	Meiosis
Before cell division, each molecule of DNA within the cell is duplicated.	Before cell division, each molecule of DNA within the cell is duplicated.
Prophase DNA in nucleus condenses, shortens and coils to form 46 chromosomes. Duplicated DNA molecules remain joined to their partner molecules by the centromere. Each duplicate is called a chromatid. Late in prophase, the nuclear membrane breaks down, releasing the chromosomes. Spindle structure forms in the cytoplasm.	*Prophase I* DNA in nucleus condenses, shortens and coils to form 46 chromosomes. Duplicated DNA molecules remain joined to their partners molecule by the centromere. Each duplicate is called a chromatid. Late in prophase, the nuclear membrane breaks down, releasing the chromosomes. Spindle structure forms in the cytoplasm.
Metaphase The 46 chromosomes align at random across the centre of the cell.	*Metaphase I* The 46 chromosomes align independently in their 23 pairs across the centre of the cell. Segments of chromosome may be exchanged between each member of the pair (called crossing over).
Anaphase **Centromeres break, releasing the chromatids. For each chromosome, one chromatid (i.e. one of the DNA copies) passes along the spindle to one pole of the cell – the other passes to the opposite pole.**	*Anaphase I* **A member of each pair of chromosomes passes along the spindle to one pole of the cell, the other member to the opposite pole. Centromeres still intact.**
Telophase Nuclear envelopes form around each cluster of chromatids, and a new cell membrane forms across the equator of the original cell. Each new cell has 46 chromatids.	*Telophase I* A new cell membrane forms at the equator of the original cell – a temporary phase for the chromosomes, which soon enter the meiosis II phase. Each temporary cell has 23 whole chromosomes.
	Prophase II/Metaphase II New spindles form in each of the two new cells. Chromosomes align at the equator of the cell.
	Anaphase II Centromeres break, releasing the chromatids. This stage is analogous to the anaphase in mitosis. One chromatid from a chromosome passes to one pole of the cell, and the other passes to the opposite pole.
	Telophase II Nuclear envelopes form around each cluster of chromatids, and a new cell membrane forms across the equator of the original cell. Each cell contains 23 chromatids.
Result **Two new cells, each with 46 chromatids (molecules of DNA), i.e. the same as the original.**	*Result* **Four new cells, each with 23 chromatids (molecules of DNA), i.e. half that of the original.**

Cell division by meiosis

Meiosis is the form of cell division that occurs during the production of the sex cells (gametes), a process described in Chapter 18. Mitosis would not be appropriate for this because it would produce sperm or ova with a cell's usual 46 molecules of DNA. Fertilization would then produce a zygote with 92 (i.e. 46+46) molecules of DNA, and hence an embryo with this number in its cells. In the succeeding generation, this would become 184 molecules of DNA, and so on. Clearly, the 46 molecules of DNA must be reduced to 23 in the ovum and sperm, so that the usual 46 will be restored in the zygote. This is why cell division by meiosis is sometimes referred to as 'reduction division'.

The reduction in chromosome number is through a carefully regulated process. An important principle operates here: meiosis involves the separation of the members of the chromosome pairs to leave just one member of each pair within the gamete (Figure 20.13):

1 As with mitosis, meiosis commences with duplication of the germ cell's DNA to form the characteristic 'X'-shaped chromosomes.

2 The nuclear membrane breaks down, and the chromosomes align themselves at the centre of the cell and

attach to the spindle by their centromeres. At this point, meiosis and mitosis begin to differ.

3 The chromosomes align in their pairs. The two chromosomes in each pair are bound together for a while by proteins, during which time they may exchange genetic material: the significance of this mixing is explained later in relation to the inheritance of genes.

4 The binding proteins break, and the pairs of chromosomes separate. In this way, entire chromosomes pass along the spindle fibres, with members of each pair moving to opposite poles of the cell. The chromosome pairs have thus been separated, and there will be just one copy of each pair at each pole of the cell (Figure 20.13).

5 An intervening cell membrane forms. At this point, the original cell is said to have completed the first part of meiosis, referred to as 'meiosis I'. Each chromosome still has the characteristic shape, since they are still comprised of their chromatids.

6 Each 'group' of chromosomes becomes attached to new spindles (Figure 20.13), and the chromatids immediately separate.

7 The chromatids pass to the poles of the newly formed cells.

8 New nuclear membranes and further intervening cell membranes form. The second part of meiosis, 'meiosis II', has now been completed.

9 As a result, four 'daughter' cells have been formed from the original parent cell (mitosis only produces two), but each has only 23 molecules of DNA. The cells are said to be *haploid*.

As in mitosis, each stage of the division process has a characteristic name (Table 20.3); again, however, it is the behaviour of the chromosomes that is important here. Whereas mitosis conserves genetic information in the new cells, the separation of the pairs of chromosomes during meiosis means that gametes contain only half of the total genetic make-up of the germ cells. Thus, when an ovum is fertilized, half of the genetic material of the resultant embryo will be of maternal origin, and the other half will be paternal. This genetic mixing has important implications for the inheritance of characteristics and for congenital disorder, as we shall see in the next section.

Meiosis and formation of the early embryo

Meiosis in women is completed, and the ovum formed, in the early phases of the menstrual cycle before ovulation. However, the process commences much earlier, around the time of birth, when the chromosome pairs collect at

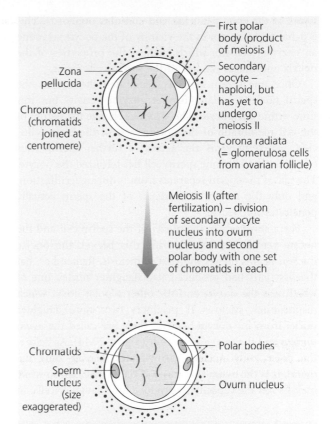

Figure 20.14 Changes in the secondary oocyte at fertilization. For clarity, only four chromosomes are shown. The ovum and sperm nuclei soon fuse, and the polar bodies disintegrate.

Q. When does a secondary oocyte become an ovum, and an ovum a zygote?

the equator of the cells before their separation. Thus, ovulation releases from an ovary a cell that has already undergone the first part of the meiotic division, but has yet to complete the second phase in which the chromatids are separated and the division process is completed. Recall that meiosis I produces two daughter cells from a single germ cell. This first division produces a cell called the *secondary oocyte* and a nucleus (rather than a whole cell) called the *first polar body* (Figure 20.14). The secondary oocyte is the cell that will be shed by the ovary; the polar body plays no further role and disintegrates.

When released, the oocyte is surrounded by a protective layer of glycoprotein called the *zona pellucida*, and a cloud of granulated cells called the *cumulus oophorus* (from the ovarian follicle). These layers help to protect the oocyte as it passes along the Fallopian tube; at this point, the oocyte is very vulnerable and its wellbeing will be affected by any adverse changes in the fluid composition within the tube.

Fertilization normally takes place within the Fallopian tube. Of the millions of spermatozoa ejaculated during intercourse, only a few hundred will arrive in the vicinity of the oocyte, and only one will penetrate and fertilize it. To do this, a sperm cell must penetrate the protective layers of the zona pellucida and cumulus oophorus. This is achieved by sperm in the vicinity of the oocyte secreting an enzyme, acrosin, which changes the properties of the matrix and makes passage of the sperm cells easier.

Once one sperm cell has penetrated the oocyte, the sperm nucleus initiates further enzyme activity but this time within the oocyte. The enzymes change the nature of the cell membrane of the oocyte, and of the zona pellucida, which prevents the access of further sperm, thus ensuring that only one sperm cell has fertilized the oocyte. The tail of the sperm separates from it during fertilization, and only the head (i.e. nucleus) of the sperm actually penetrates the oocyte.

For a short while, the nuclei of the sperm cell and the oocyte remain separate. During this period, the oocyte nucleus begins the second part of meiosis. Remember that the first part had produced two daughter nuclei, one of which was the oocyte and the other a polar body, which disintegrates. Meiosis II produces two more daughter nuclei from the oocyte nucleus: these are called the *ovum nucleus* and the *second polar body* (Figure 20.14). As before, the polar body nucleus disintegrates, leaving only the ovum. It is the ovum that forms a viable new cell, so while meiosis has the capacity to produce four daughter cells, in females only one of these may survive to contribute to reproduction in men, all four daughter cells may form viable sperm cells, a factor that facilitates the production of very large numbers of them.

The ovum nucleus now combines with the sperm nucleus, thus restoring the normal (diploid) quota of 46 DNA molecules. If the chromosome pairs do not separate normally during the meiosis division, this has implications for the number of chromosomes present after fertilization, and hence in the resultant embryo. This is known as *non-dysjunction*, and is considered later as a cause of congenital disorder.

Meiosis and inheritance

If meiosis occurs normally, then sex cells will be formed with half the usual number of chromosomes. Since we inherit half of our DNA from one parent and half from the other, then logic suggests that it ought to be possible for someone to inherit a set of chromosomes from, say, the mother that are identical in genetic code as the set that she inherited from her mother, and so on. However, although we all know people who look very similar to a parent or

---

BOX 20.8 TWINS

Monozygotic twins

Monozygotic (literally 'one zygote') twins arise because, for unknown reasons, the zygote formed at fertilization divides into two before development of the morula stage. Thus, two morulae and hence two embryos are produced, and both may implant. Since they are derived from the same zygote, they are genetically identical.

Siamese twins are monozygotic twins in whom the division of the zygote produced two new nuclei but the separation of the new cells was not completed. Each product of the incomplete division continues to develop to form an embryo. The incomplete separation means that the fetuses will be joined at a point subsequent to tissue differentiation. For example, the embryo may share

development at the head end, so the fetuses will be joined at that point. The extent of the separation at the zygote stage also determines the extent of organ sharing. This can be profound. Surgery may be used to separate the twins, although this is not always the case, and there are numerous instances of Siamese twins who remain joined as adults. If surgery is used, the outcome will be influenced by the level of organ sharing in the infants.

Dizygotic twins

Although the ovary normally releases only one oocyte per month, it occasionally releases two (or more); alternatively, an oocyte may be released from each ovary. Separate fertilization of these oocytes produces genetically distinct zygotes (since each oocyte and sperm will be genetically unique).

BOX 20.9 CLONING

Cloning is a technique in which individual organisms are produced that have an identical genetic make-up to that of another living (or dead) organism. The method entails removing the nucleus from an oocyte, then taking the nucleus of a cell from, perhaps, an adult animal (the donor of the oocyte or another one) and transferring it into the enucleated oocyte. This newly constituted cell is then transferred to a uterus where, if successful, it will implant and form a new individual genetically identical to the donor of the nucleus. From a purely scientific perspective, demonstrating that cloning is possible highlights that the activation of development genes is feasible, even in DNA taken from an adult cell. However, the success of cloning

experiments has also raised serious ethical and moral issues (Sanchez-Sweatman, 2000).

The technique has been performed successfully only recently. 'Dolly' the sheep is credited with being the first cloned animal (in 1996). The method has since been extended to other animals and and is considered feasible in humans. On a positive side, the method is considered to have potential beneficial applications in agriculture, in helping infertile couples, and in the development of tissue for transplantation. On the negative side, there is concern that there is enormous potential for abuse, e.g. by enabling an individual to clone him/herself either whilst still alive or after death.

perhaps a grandparent, they are never identical. This is because meiosis promotes gene mixing, achieved in three ways: segregation of alleles, independent assortment of alleles, and cross-over of alleles between chromosomes.

Segregation of alleles

This has been the focus of much of the discussion on inheritance so far. To recap, when the homologous chromosome pairs separate during the formation of the gametes, meiosis separates (or segregates) the pairs of alleles. This means that for a given gene, an individual will inherit only one allele from each parent, thus raising the likelihood of a different pairing in the offspring. Thus, in the heterozygous state, an individual may not be affected by an allele because of its recessive nature but by separating it from its dominant counterpart, meiosis raises the possibility that it will be paired with another recessive allele in the offspring. If this happens, then the recessive alleles will be operative.

Independent assortment of alleles

We noted earlier how characteristics may result from the expression of more than one gene. It is likely that the genes that make up this 'group' are located on more than one pair of chromosomes. For these alleles, the inheritance of the characteristic will also depend upon which members of the chromosome pairs pass into the gamete. This, in turn, depends on how the different chromosomes assort themselves when they line up during meiosis.

Figure 20.15 illustrates a possible arrangement of three pairs of homologous chromosomes during meiosis. It can

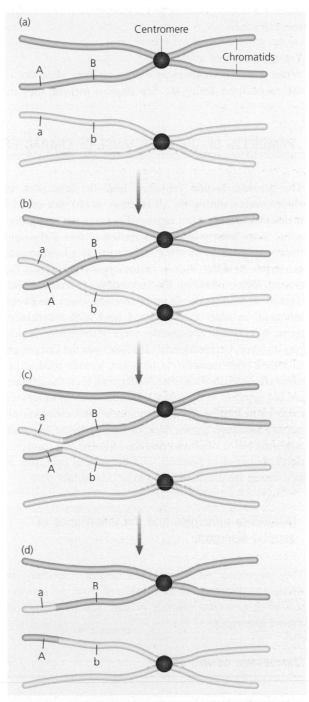

Figure 20.16 Allelic mixing produced by exchange of DNA (cross-over) between chromosomal pairs during meiosis. (a) Chromosome pair aligns at metaphase stage of meiosis. (b) Arms of the two chromosomes interact. (c) Cross-over of DNA from one chromosome to another complete chromosome. (d) Chromosome pair ready to separate during the next stage of meiosis. Note the different allelic pairing on each chromosome, compared with (a).

Q. What is cross-over?

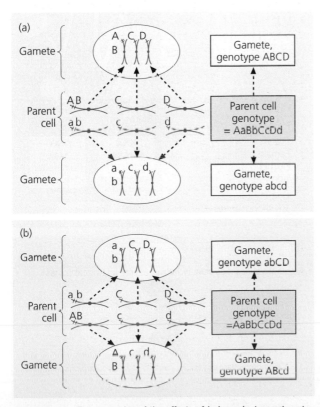

Figure 20.15 Two examples of the effects of independent assortment of three chromosome pairs on the genotypes of gametes produced by meiosis. The genotype of the parent cell is the same in each case, but that of the gametes is very different.

be seen that the combination of alleles passed into the gametes varies according to how these chromosomes are assorted before they separate. In this way, meiosis once again ensures that alleles are mixed in the next generation. Note, however, that the assortment of the pairs during meiosis is entirely random and is independent of the alignment of others.

Translocation of alleles

When a pair of homologous chromosomes align before their separation during the first stage of meiosis, they are briefly bound together by proteins. At this point, some of the DNA may be exchanged between the chromosomes, taking with it the constituent alleles (Figure 20.16). This is called 'crossing over' or, more technically, 'translocation'; it causes the composition of the chromosomes concerned to be altered. If a number of alleles on a single chromosome contribute to a particular phenotype, then translocation mixes these and can potentially alter the phenotype. As a point of interest, the enzymes that facilitate this exchange of DNA are used by scientists to 'clip out' or 'paste in' pieces of DNA in genetic engineering.

PRINCIPLES OF THE INHERITANCE OF CHARACTERISTICS

The previous section explained how the separation of chromosomes during the production of the sex cells by meiosis ensures there is a mixing of genes in the next generation. Since most genes are comprised of two alleles, and these may either be identical (referred to as a homozygous genotype) or differ slightly (heterozygous genotype), the characteristics inherited by succeeding generations will depend on whether dominant or recessive alleles have been inherited. In order to understand how such inheritances occur, it is necessary to consider some of the general principles involved. Gregor Mendel (1822–84) was the first person to record how 'recessive' (a term not actually used in his time) characteristics can arise in offspring, even though they are not apparent in the parents. Mendel went on to identify many of the features of the inheritance of characteristics, but he was restricted by the lack of knowledge at the time regarding DNA, chromosomes, etc. However, his contribution is recorded in posterity, and the general principles of inheritance are usually referred to as 'Mendelian'.

Mendelian principles and the inheritance of genetic disorders

The inheritance of altered phenotypes, especially in relation to disorder, can be considered from the perspective of chromosome number or size, and inheritance of altered genotypes.

Chromosome number or size

Non-dysjunction

As we have seen, cells other than the gametes normally contain two copies of each autosome and two sex chromosomes. The inheritance of a numerical disturbance will arise either if a chromosome pair failed to separate at meiosis when the gametes were formed, or if the chromatids of a chromosome in the second stage of meiosis failed to separate (Figure 20.17). This is referred to

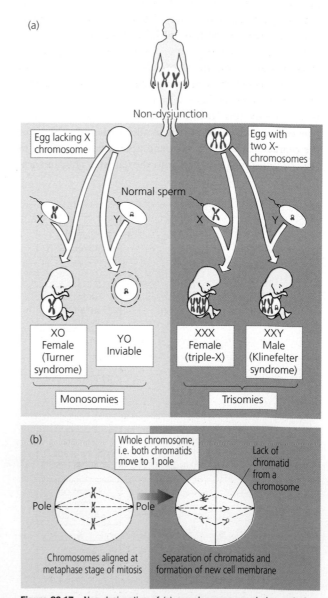

Figure 20.17 Non-dysjunction of (a) sex chromosomes during meiosis and (b) chromatids during mitosis. The non-dysjunction in (b) may also occur in the second meiotic division.

Q. What is Down's syndrome?

as non-dysjunction. Whichever stage of meiosis it occurs in, non-dysjunction will result in a gamete that contains two of the same chromosome (similarly, there must also be a gamete lacking it). Fertilization will therefore produce a zygote with either three copies of the chromosome (two from one partner, and one as normal from the other; known as *trisomy*), or just one copy (from just one partner; known as *monosomy*). Examples of inherited trisomies and monosomies are given in Box 20.10.

Non-dysjunction arises most often during the formation of the oocyte. This is because meiosis commences in women around the time of birth, and the oocytes then go into stasis until triggered after puberty. The stage at which development is suspended is when the homologous pairs of chromosomes have aligned in meiosis I; at this point, the chromosomes are bound together and they therefore remain bound for many years. Failure to break the bonds relates to maternal age, presumably because of ageing of the primary oocytes in the ovary. For example, the incidence of trisomy 21 in Down's syndrome is about 1 in 700 births overall, but if the mother is over 45 years old, then the risk is 1 in 50.

Occasionally, non-dysjunction arises in both meiosis I and meiosis II. This can lead to gametes that have up to four copies of a chromosome. Such excessive copies are only viable in relation to sex chromosomes (see Box 20.10).

Mosaicism is a very unusual form of non-dysjunction that results in a proportion of cells within the individual having chromosomal defects while the rest are normal. Within the embryo, such an occurrence could not be explained by the inheritance of an extra chromosome from the parents, as all cells would be expected to have the same karyotype as the zygote. The condition arises because of incomplete separation of chromatids during mitosis of cells in the embryo itself, especially in the early stages of tissue differentiation. It is a form of non-dysjunction that may produce developmental disorders, but these cannot be considered inherited (although they will be congenital, since this term covers both inherited influences and those that occur in utero). In mosaicism in Down's syndrome (see Box 20.10), new cells formed by mitosis may then contain:

- the normal 2 chromatids from chromosomes 21;

- the whole of a chromosome 21 (two chromatids) together with the usual one chromatid from the other member of the chromosome pair, i.e. three copies instead of two of the DNA molecules that comprises chromosome pair 21;

- one copy of the DNA molecule that comprises chromosome 21, rather than the usual two.

Subsequent successful cell divisions will then increase the numbers of cells that have the trisomy, hence the symptoms of Down's syndrome.

BOX 20.10 INHERITED TRISOMIES AND MONOSOMIES

Trisomy and polysomy of the sex chromosomes (See also Figure 20.17(a))

Klinefelter's syndrome is observed in males who have an extra X chromosome (i.e. these people are XXY). The consequences are small testes and low secretion of androgens. Sperm may be absent, though some people with the syndrome have fathered children (note that the presence of the Y chromosome makes these people male). Cognitive functions may be affected, but only slightly.

Trisomy of the X chromosome is called *triple X syndrome*. This is frequently found within a population, but individuals usually do not have distinctive phenotypic characteristics. In the absence of a Y chromosome, triple-X people are always female. Although some of these women have menstrual difficulties, many are fertile.

Non-dysjunction during both meiosis I and meiosis II may also lead to the inheritance of multiple sex chromosomes (i.e. polysomy). Even the pentasomy XXXXX ('penta-' = 5) has been observed, although the consequences are more severe than for trisomy, and it is associated with learning disabilities.

Trisomy of the autosomes

Trisomy of chromosome 21 is the only viable autosomal trisomy, although even with this form, the majority of fetuses do not go to term. Trisomy 21 is usually known as *Down's syndrome* (after the clinician who first described it). Other trisomies are known, e.g. Patau's syndrome (chromosome 13) and Edwards' syndrome (chromosome 18), but these babies are so profoundly affected that the pregnancy rarely goes to term, and those infants that are born have a very short period of survival.

Trisomy 21 produces a number of developmental anomalies:

- learning disability: this may be profound, but it varies between individuals because the trisomy may only be partial (see below);
- distinctive facial characteristics, especially of the forehead and eyes;
- an open mouth with a protruding tongue;
- cardiovascular anomalies, especially of heart structure;
- a third fontanelle of the skull;
- a single palmar crease.

Not all cases of Down's syndrome represent complete trisomy 21, although about 95% do. Partial trisomy 21 is possible (see *Chromosomal fragmentation* in the text), and is observed in about 3–4% of cases. The remaining cases occur through 'mosaicism', involving chromosome 21 (see text).

Monosomy

Cells usually require at least two copies of each chromosome, so monosomic fetuses might not be expected to be viable. The exception is of the X chromosome, i.e. *Turner's syndrome* in which individuals are XO (i.e. X nought). Of these fetuses, 98% abort spontaneously; the 2% who are born are female, as no Y chromosome is present. Development of the gonads and body growth are slowed.

If a zygote inherits just a Y chromosome (i.e. YO), it will not develop. Apparently, at least one copy of an X chromosome is a minimum requirement.

Approximately 1% of cases of Down's syndrome arise through mosaicism, i.e. many cells are trisomic for chromosome 21, while many other cells are derived from embryonic cells that divided normally and therefore have the usual two copies. The consequences for development will depend on the extent of the mosaicism, which relates to the period of embryo/fetal development when the non-dysjunction occurred. If it occurred early in development, then most cells in the later embryo will be trisomic; if it occurred later in development, then a lot of cells and tissues will have a normal number of chromosomes.

Chromosomal fragmentation

Fragmentation leads to the inheritance of a chromosome with extra DNA or deficient in DNA, and may occur if there is an error in cross-over (translocation) during meiosis. Thus, a chromosome may receive DNA from its homologous partner as normal, but in doing so may not release its own DNA. The chromosome with the additional fragment will therefore contain some duplicated alleles; when the chromosome is paired up with its chromatid counterpart in the zygote after fertilization, these alleles will be present in triplicate. Alternatively, the detached fragment may attach to a totally different chromosome. The net effect may be the same, however, with the zygote having two copies of the chromosome, as usual, plus a fragment of it. The effects on the health of the infant will depend on the additional alleles gained.

Down's syndrome may occur through fragmentation that results in translocation of a fragment of chromosome 21. Approximately 3–4% of cases arise because a piece of chromosome 21 breaks off during the cross-over stage of meiosis, and translocates to become attached to another chromosome, often number 14. The zygote then may inherit a copy of chromosome 21 from each parent, and also the additional fragment attached to another chromosome. This results in a partial trisomy 21, and causes many of the symptoms associated with Down's syndrome, although they are usually milder than the full trisomy.

Failure to swap DNA normally can also mean that a piece is lost from a chromosome. Since there are usually two pairs of alleles, the loss of one set of alleles may not necessarily be detrimental. In the case of the sex chromosomes, however, the X chromosome contains alleles that in males will be the only copies present. *Fragile X syndrome* results from fragmentation of the X chromosome, and is a frequent cause of learning disability. In this case, the error is due to a 'fragile' section of DNA that tends to break during meiosis, with the result that a whole piece of chromosome is lost. As a consequence, the resultant zygote will be deficient in the alleles found on the lost fragment. The presence of only one X chromosome in males means that the effects will be more pronounced than in females, and this condition is considered to be sex linked. The cause of the breakage of the chromosome is not understood fully, but there is evidence for a 'fragile' gene at the location.

Inheritance of altered genotypes

The likelihood of progeny inheriting alleles that cause cell dysfunction depends on whether the alleles concerned are recessive or dominant, and whether they are found on the autosomes or sex chromosomes.

Autosomal recessive inheritance

We have seen how meiosis separates homologous chromosomes and in doing so separates the gene alleles. If the individual is heterozygous for a given pair of alleles, then half of the gametes will contain the 'normal' (i.e. dominant) allele and half the recessive form. Should his or her partner also be heterozygous, there is a one in four chance that a zygote formed will be homozygous for the recessive allele (Figure 20.18(a)).

In contrast, there is no possibility of a recessive homozygous offspring when one parent is heterozygous and the other is homozygous for the 'normal' (i.e. dominant) alleles. There is, however, a on in two chance that the child will be heterozygous (Figure 20.18(b)). In this case, any disorder associated with the recessive allele will 'skip' that generation, but there remains the possibility that the homozygous form will appear in the next generation. For this reason, the heterozygous individual is frequently referred to as a *carrier* of the recessive allele.

There are many examples of recessive disorders that result from a single gene defect. The genes responsible for some of the commoner disorders have now been identified, and the defective cell process studied. Some of the commoner disorders are discussed in Box 20.11.

Sex-linked recessive inheritance

The discrepancy between the sizes of the X and Y chromosomes has important implications for conditions arising from gene mutations on the X chromosome. This is because there are some 200–300 alleles on the X chromosome but only a handful on the Y chromosome, hence not all of the alleles on the X will have counterparts on the Y (also, the Y chromosome appears to be functionally 'quiet' after birth). In females, the expression of recessive alleles on the X chromosome will be observed only if both chromosomes have a copy of the allele, much like the case for recessive alleles on the autosomes. In males, however, a recessive allele on the X chromosome will usually be expressed, as there is no dominant 'normal' allele on the Y chromosome (Figure 20.19). For example, red–green colour-blindness arises because of a gene mutation on the X chromosome, so colour-blindness is more likely to be found in males than in females.

Some gene mutations on the X chromosome produce much more severe problems. Examples of sex-linked inheritance are given in Box 20.12.

Considering autosomal gene A, possible genotypes are:

AA   Homozygous for dominant alleles
Aa   Heterozygous
aa   Homozygous for recessive alleles

Figure 20.18 Autosomal inheritance. Influence of parental genotype on the phenotype of offspring. In each case the phenotype outcome is shown if the recessive allele, a, or the dominant allele f is a gene mutation that potential could induce change.

Q. What would be the genotypes and phenotypes of offspring with the following genetic crosses of parental ABO blood groupings: (i) AO X BO; (ii) AA X OB; and (iii) AB X AD?

(a) Parental genotypes Aa × Aa

Possible offspring genotypes:

Gametes		
	A	a
A	AA	Aa
a	Aa	aa

	Phenotype			
	If a = mutation	Ratio	If A = mutation	Ratio
AA	Normal	1:4	Affected	
Aa	Normal/carrier		Affected	
Aa	Normal/carrier	2:4	Affected	3:4
aa	Affected	1:4	Normal	1:4

(b) Parental genotypes Aa × aa

Possible offspring genotypes:

Gametes		
	A	a
a	Aa	aa
a	Aa	aa

	Phenotype			
	If a = mutation	Ratio	If A = mutation	Ratio
Aa	Normal/carrier	2:4	Affected	2:4
Aa	Normal/carrier		Affected	
aa	Affected	2:4	Normal	2:4
aa	Affected		Normal	

(c) Parental genotypes AA × Aa

Possible offspring genotypes:

Gametes		
	A	A
A	AA	AA
a	Aa	Aa

	Phenotype			
	If a = mutation	Ratio	If A = mutation	Ratio
AA	Normal	2:4	Affected	
AA	Normal		Affected	4:4
Aa	Normal/carrier	2:4	Affected	
Aa	Normal/carrier		Affected	

BOX 20.11 AUTOSOMAL RECESSIVE CONDITIONS

Cystic fibrosis

This is the most common inherited condition in the UK. It is characterized by the secretion of viscous mucus in the lungs and gastrointestinal tract that may obstruct airways and the pancreatic duct. The disorder arises because of a defect in chloride transport, and hence water movement, across the cell membranes of mucosal cells as a consequence of a failure of the recessive gene to cause the synthesis of the appropriate protein. The gene is found on chromosome 7. Care is aimed at removing secretions with physiotherapy, and preventing infection in the obstructed tissues (Steen, 1997). Severe pancreatic obstruction may compromise digestion, and pancreatic enzymes or simple foodstuffs may then have to be administered directly into the small intestine.

Phenylketonuria

Phenylketonuria (PKU) is characterized by an accumulation of the essential amino acid phenylalanine in tissues. The amino acid is obtained from dietary protein, and some is converted in the liver to tyrosine, which is used by the body to synthesize proteins, the pigment melanin and catecholamine hormones. Tyrosine synthesis is catalysed by the enzyme phenylalanine hydroxylase; it is the absence of this enzyme that promotes the disorder. Young children in particular are at risk of the consequences of this problem (phenylalanine accumulation slows brain development), but the condition is controllable by reducing the dietary intake as compensation for the decreased utilization. Analysis of a blood sample (the neonatal screening test previously called the Guthrie test) will show clearly whether excessive phenylalanine is present. The gene for this condition is found on chromosome 12. See also Case 4: Chapter 27.

Familial hyperlipidaemia

In familial hyperlipidaemia (hypercholesterolaemia), there is an excessively high lipid concentration in the blood, which promotes the development of atheromatous deposits in vessels. The elevated lipid results from a defect in the uptake mechanism in liver cells. The gene for this condition is found on chromosome 19. Care is aimed at encouraging patients to have a low (saturated) fat diet, and at using cholesterol-lowering drugs.

Consider gene A present on the X chromosome but absent on the Y:

Possible genotypes

Female (XX)   AA   Homozygous for dominant alleles
               Aa   Heterozygous

Male (XY)   AO   Where O indicates lack of homologous
               aO   allele on Y-chromosome

Parental genotypes Aa × AO

i.e. the female is a carrier (heterozygous) for the recessive allele, the male has the normal allele

Possible offspring genotypes:

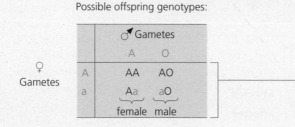

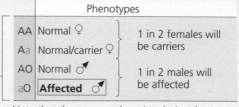

Note that there cannot be a 'carrier' male

Figure 20.19   Sex-linked inheritance of a recessive characteristic.
Q. Describe what is meant by sex-linked inheritance.

BOX 20.12 EXAMPLES OF SEX-LINKED INHERITED CONDITIONS

Duchenne's muscular dystrophy

This condition is characterized by loss of the muscle protein dystrophin, which has a role in the maintenance of the sarcolemma. Loss of the protein results in progressive wastage of muscle. The example of inheritance given in Figure 20.19 assumes a 'normal' father and a heterozygous 'carrier' mother, and is the most likely pattern of inheritance for this condition. This is because a woman who had the condition would have to be homozygous for the gene and so would have to have inherited an affected X chromosome from her father (who would have had this progressive condition himself, and so would be unlikely to have children). Thus, a woman might have one copy and so be a carrier of the muscular dystrophy allele, but is unlikely to have two copies and hence have the condition. Nevertheless, a handful of cases of women with Duchenne's muscular dystrophy are known worldwide.

Haemophilia A

This condition results from a loss of the liver enzyme necessary for the synthesis of clotting factor VIII. The condition has been known for many years to be primarily a condition of boys, although a few incidences in girls have been documented. Unlike Duchenne's muscular dystrophy, haemophilia is now controllable (through administration of extrinsic factor VIII) and so does not now place a reproductive restriction on the inherited genotype (Susman-Shaw and Harrington, 1999). Thus, it should be feasible for a man with haemophilia to father a daughter who, if she also inherited an affected X chromosome from her carrier mother, would be homozygous for the condition. The sex linkage of this condition therefore seems likely to be weaker than it is for Duchenne's muscular dystrophy. However, the mutated allele has a low frequency within the population; this means that the partner of the (affected) father is unlikely to be also carrying the gene, so the condition remains predominantly a problem in males.

Autosomal dominant inheritance

A mutated allele will occasionally (rarely) behave in a dominant fashion. This means that the influences of that allele will be observed even in the heterozygous condition, because the 'normal' allele will now be recessive to it. Thus, with two heterozygous parents there is a three in four (75%) chance that the offspring will have the phenotype associated with the allele because of a two in four chance that the progeny will be heterozygous, and a one in four chance that a child will be homozygous for the dominant allele (Figure 20.18(a)).

If only one parent is heterozygous, and the other is homozygous for the 'normal' (now recessive) allele, then there is still a 50% chance that the dominant phenotype will be inherited (Figure 20.18(b)). Clearly, if a parent is homozygous for that gene, then all children will inherit the phenotype (Figure 20.18(c)).

Conditions associated with a dominant allele might be expected to be apparent from birth, but this is not always the case, as some genes seem to be screened in a way that remains unclear. Examples of autosomal dominant conditions are given in Box 20.13.

Huntington's disease

Huntington's disease (Huntington's chorea) is a neurological disorder. The expression of the disorder typically does not occur until well into adulthood. The condition is characterized by a deficiency of the neurotransmitter gamma-aminobutyric acid (GABA) from neurological areas involved in the control of movement. It is unclear why there is a delay in expression of the disorder. The gene is found on chromosome 4 (see Chapter 17: Box 17.14 for further information).

Retinoblastoma

This is a rare eye tumour that originates in the retina of one or both eyes. In approximately half of cases, the condition is acquired in the early years, but it can be expressed as an inherited condition. The reason for this variation is that the gene can exhibit incomplete penetrance, i.e. in some cases, the gene is not expressed; the mechanism is unclear. The gene is located on chromosome 13.

Incomplete dominance

Sickle-cell anaemia arises because one of the polypeptide chains in the haemoglobin molecule contains a single amino acid substitution when compared with 'normal' haemoglobin. This small change alters the properties of the pigment, causing it to distort after releasing oxygen, and so causing the 'sickling' of the erythrocyte. The cell membrane is more fragile in the sickled state, resulting in haemolysis, and hence anaemia. The cells also become 'sticky' and clump together. Most tissues are affected as a consequence (see Chapter). As might be anticipated, the disorder is seen in the homozygous condition. However, blood samples from heterozygous people will also show numbers of sickled erythrocytes, in addition to normal ones, as both 'normal' and 'sickle' alleles are expressed. Thus, this condition represents an example of one produced by alleles that exhibit incomplete dominance (or incomplete recessiveness, depending on the perspective). The degree of sickling in the heterozygous state may not be sufficient to produce severe symptoms of the condition; the state is actually advantageous in certain countries, because the sickled cells convey resistance to infection by malarial parasites. The gene is located on chromosome 11.

Polygenic inheritance

Polygenic characteristics are produced by the actions of several genes located on a number of different chromosomes. When several genes are involved, pronounced changes in cell function will arise only if a 'vital' gene within the sequence is mutated, or if a number of the genes within the group are mutated (Figure 20.11). It is not surprising that the frequency of congenital disturbances arising from such mutations is small.

It is now considered likely, however, that the inheritance of homozygous recessive and heterozygous genotypes within the functional 'group' of genes may provide a predisposition to a condition that may arise later in life should further mutation of the remaining genes occur. This influence of environmental factors to cause further genetic mutation throughout the lifespan helps to explain why, for some individuals at least, many diseases of adulthood seem to have a weak familial linkage (e.g. some cancers, heart disease, Alzheimer's disease and insulin-independent diabetes mellitus; see Box 20.14).

Introduction to population genetics

The above sections consider the likelihood of gene mutations carried by the parents being inherited in the offspring. The chances of the gene mutation being present in the parents will relate to the frequency of the gene within the population, since this influences the chance of someone meeting another carrier. The alleles present within a population comprise the gene pool. The frequency of a gene within this is determined by various factors: natural selection, inbreeding, population drift, and spontaneous or acquired mutations.

Natural selection

'Gene mixing' during reproduction produces offspring with genotypes that will differ to those of the parents. This variation may prove beneficial when compared with the

Colorectal cancer is an example of an inherited predisposition. In this condition, familial linkage is recognized but is lower than might be anticipated from Mendelian principles. The cancer exhibits a benign precancerous phase as polyps within the colon or rectum; the presence of polyps shows a much higher genetic concordance (the gene for familial polyposis coli is found on chromosome 5). As with other cancers, it is thought that the polyps arise because of inherited alleles or the occurrence of mutation through the actions of initiator factors, and progress to cancerous lesions because of

further mutations to genes by promotor factors (further genes involved in the genesis of colorectal cancer have been identified on chromosome 5, 12, 17 and 18). This multiple 'hit' approach to gene mutation means that lifestyle factors are likely to figure prominently in the genesis of cancer (and disorders of other polygenic characteristics, such as heart disease). Research is targeting the genes involved in an attempt to understand the factors concerned, and to raise the possibility of new therapeutic approaches.

population as a whole, and so over many generations the success of such offspring should increase the incidence of the advantageous alleles. Similarly, any gene mutation that is detrimental to life should tend to reduce in frequency in the gene pool. This is the basis of the proposals forwarded by Charles Darwin in the nineteenth century in his theory of evolution. Darwin called the process 'natural selection' (see Box 20.15).

For many conditions, however, medical advances in recent years have ensured survival at least until adulthood and, to some degree, have negated selection processes.

Inbreeding

Inbreeding within a family line increases the likelihood that both parents are carriers of a particular allele. The effect is not confined simply to inbreeding between close relatives: if a population is small and stable with little immigration or emigration, then the likelihood increases of people being related, perhaps from several generations earlier. This is a factor in the incidence of clusters of inherited conditions in some districts, when compared with national figures.

Population drift

The immigration or emigration of people into or out of a population will respectively add to or remove genes from that population. The process can alter the incidence of a particular gene mutation within a gene pool, and may even result in the introduction of novel mutations. We see this in the physical characteristics of people in parts of the world where cultures have integrated. In another example, Huntington's disease seems likely to have been introduced into North America by European settlers.

Spontaneous or acquired mutation

Cells can often self-repair any alterations to the genetic code that have occurred spontaneously, but some of these may persist and therefore be inherited. This means that inherited conditions are unlikely to be eradicated from a population, as new mutations will continuously occur within the gene pool. The cause of spontaneous mutation is unclear. Cosmic radiation is one factor, but it may be that there are other as-yet-unidentified environmental factors. The acquisition of gene mutations produced by environmental factors may also help to explain the occurrence of local clusters of disorders, e.g. leukaemia induced by radon gas emission from granite rocks.

BOX 20.15 NATURAL SELECTION AND ALLELE FREQUENCY IN THE GENE POOL

Natural selection might be expected to reduce the incidence of severe genetic disorders, and this undoubtedly is a factor in the rarity of most such conditions. Exceptions are the high frequency of the allele for sickle cell anaemia in Afro-Caribbean cultures (a carrier rate of one in ten), and the allele for cystic fibrosis alleles in Caucasian cultures (a carrier rate of 1 in 25). The implication of these two examples is that natural selection has actually favoured the occurrence of the allele within the population, even though having two copies produces the inherited disorder, because having one copy conveys a survival advantage.

A person who has just one copy of the sickle cell allele has a degree of protection against malaria, because the parasite involved finds it difficult to live inside the red blood cells. The person may experience mild symptoms of sickle cell anaemia, but the protection against malaria is thought to be so advantageous to survival in some parts of the world that natural selection increased the frequency of the allele in the population.

An advantage to the frequency of the cystic fibrosis allele is less clear. The same ion transport mechanism is affected in both cystic fibrosis and cholera, so perhaps it was advantageous to be a carrier of the allele when cholera was once rife. The link is tenuous, however, and remains to be determined.

GENES AND AGEING

This chapter has provided an overview of why genes and their actions are so important to cell activity and health. The focus has been very much on genes and basic tissue functions, in particular to explain the occurrence of congenital disorder. This final section considers how the acquisition of gene changes are also involved in ageing and conditions associated with increasing age.

Ageing and declining homeostatic efficiency

The functions of individual organs and tissues in healthy people are at a premium during the mid- to late-20s, when the conditions necessary for 'normal' cell function are maintained optimally via finely controlled and efficient

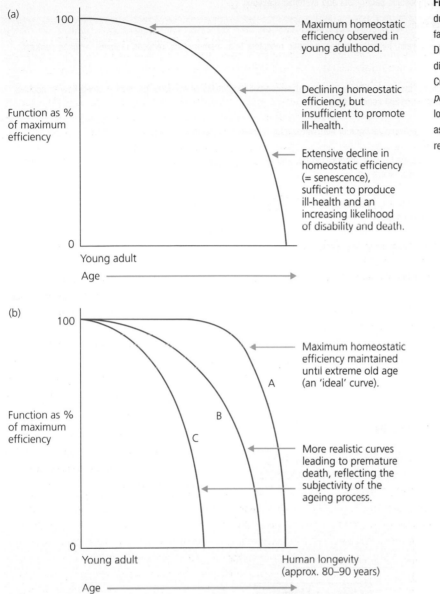

(a)

Maximum homeostatic efficiency observed in young adulthood.

Declining homeostatic efficiency, but insufficient to promote ill-health.

Extensive decline in homeostatic efficiency (= senescence), sufficient to produce ill-health and an increasing likelihood of disability and death.

(b)

Maximum homeostatic efficiency maintained until extreme old age (an 'ideal' curve).

More realistic curves leading to premature death, reflecting the subjectivity of the ageing process.

Figure 20.20 Survival curves. (a) Survival during ageing is depicted in terms of the failing capacity to maintain homeostasis. (b) Different shaped curves indicate relative differences in the consequences of ageing. Curve A indicates maximal survival of a *population* (i.e. health maintained to maximal longevity). Curve B indicates a situation much as today. Curve C indicates a situation more representative of the early twentieth century.

homeostatic processes. Adaptive mechanisms are also in place, so the capacity to change organ function to perform exercise will also be at a peak. The integrated, homeostatic efficiency of the adult means that the individual is considered to have a maximal functional capacity.

Ageing per se does not necessarily mean a complete loss of homeostatic control, but the effectiveness of that control in response to physical challenge declines (Figure 20.20). Problems become apparent at all stages of the control process. Thus, receptor density decreases and the threshold rises at which stimulation occurs, i.e. a greater change in a parameter is required to stimulate a response. The afferent and efferent signalling becomes less precise because hormone release or neural function declines. Further loss of efficiency occurs because the effector tissues respond more slowly due to age-related changes in the cells of tissues, e.g. tissue atrophy, disruption of cell architecture, loss of

membrane receptors, decreased contractility of muscle cells, and decreased secretory activity of glandular cells (Table 20.4). The picture is one of increasingly profound alterations in cell functions.

Functional decline generally commences after about the late 20s, and leads to an increased susceptibility to disease and an increased probability of death (collectively referred to as *senescent* changes). The considerable physiological 'reserve' that people possess means that functional decline causes little serious hardship for many people until the 'reserve' is reduced significantly. Thus, a capacity to compete in physical events may be diminished by early middle age, but day-to-day functioning is generally adequate. For most people, therefore, senescence does not produce notable physical difficulties until late adulthood/elderly years (and even then, many do not experience major difficulties). With improvements in the

Table 20.4 Selected age-related changes in homeostatic parameters and systemic functions

System	Change and/or consequence
Nervous	Loss of neurons, myelin, neurotransmitter, synaptic receptors (e.g. memory loss, reduced reflexes, reduced postural control)
Senses	Decreased receptor density/sensitivity, decreased accommodating ability of eye lens, decreased blood flow to cochlea (e.g. loss of hearing, visual acuity, taste)
Endocrine	Decreased synthesis/release/actions of hormones (poor regulation of parameters, e.g. blood glucose)
Cardiovascular	Effects of autonomic inadequacy, atherosclerosis, and reduced peripheral circulation (e.g. hypotension, hypertension, coronary heart disease, ulceration)
Skeletal	Decreased bone density (e.g. osteoporosis), decreased vertebral column length (i.e. decreased height), fissures of joint cartilage (e.g. osteoarthrosis)
Gastrointestinal tract	Effects of autonomic inadequacy (e.g. decreased motility, decreased secretions)
Lungs	Loss of elastin (reduced vital capacity)
Kidneys	Loss of nephrons (decreased glomerular filtration rate)
Immune system	Decreased immunity, increased autoimmunity

Q. Why are the above changes associated with ageing?

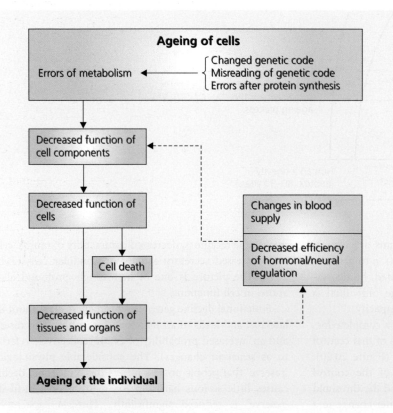

Figure 20.21 Cellular ageing and ageing of the individual. Note the role of genes/gene expression within cells (see also Figure 20.22), and the positive feedback effect of deterioration in circulatory, hormonal and neural functioning.

treatment of infectious disease, and a growing understanding of the nature of many inherited disorders, senescent processes are increasingly viewed as the major challenge to health in the developed world.

Humans have a finite lifespan and the effects of age on the functioning of physiological systems exhibit many similarities between individuals. However, the rate at which function declines with time varies considerably.

Reasons for this are not understood entirely, and the completion of the Human Genome Project (see Box 20.1) is expected to provide opportunity for further research into the genetic components. There is also an association of certain disorders of, for example, the circulatory system, the digestive and respiratory tracts, and the skeletomuscular system with environmental influences, such as diet, employment and lifestyle; such extrinsic links have prompted vigorous health education and promotion programmes in recent years. As the genome is increasingly better understood, it is likely that new health education recommendations will evolve that will reduce the risk of accumulating genetic changes that might also lead to ill-health (see *Polygenic inheritance* earlier). In other words, senescence may not be considered inevitable, or at least its progress might be slowed.

Theories of biological ageing

Various theories have been proposed during the last 50 years to explain physiological decline during adulthood. Some researchers have looked for evidence of the presence of a 'central clock', or controlling tissue, which might be responsible for triggering ageing. For example, the thymus gland involutes towards the end of adolescence, and then atrophies. The incidence of autoimmune disorders also increases with age; this, together with thymus changes, could implicate the immune system as an ageing clock. It is also feasible, however, that autoimmune responses are a consequence rather than a cause of the ageing process. Other research has centred on the pineal gland. This gland produces melatonin (involved in circadian rhythmicity; see Chapter 23) and calcifies during adulthood, hence its putative link with ageing. Interestingly, melatonin is a potent antioxidant, and so may provide a degree of protection against cellular changes with age (see below), and its secretion is decreased with age (Reister, 1995). The possibility of a central clock mechanism cannot be discounted entirely, but most age research today focuses on processes that are occurring within individual cells.

In the 1960s, Hayflick and co-workers demonstrated that cultured human cells could only undergo about 50 cell divisions before the culture declined and died (Hayflick and Moorhead, 1961), and that this was independent of factors such as nutrient supply. Findings that the maximum possible number of divisions (the 'Hayflick limit') is considerably reduced in cultured cells from individuals with inherited forms of accelerated ageing (progeria), and in normally aged individuals, strongly suggest that ageing is an intracellular phenomenon. Although unrepresentative of cells that do not undergo cell division through life, the Hayflick number is considered by most researchers to reflect the ageing process (see Box 20.16).

Recent studies therefore have tended to concentrate on cellular processes and ageing (Figure 20.21). Many suggest that cumulative disturbances of enzymatic processes in cells are the causes of senescence, and that therefore senescence could one day be slowed by clinical intervention. Generally, the metabolic disturbances may result from cumulative genetic mutation – or the activation of 'ageing' genes – or errors in protein synthesis (Figure 20.22).

Genetic influences

The *programme theory of ageing* suggests that there are specific genes that promote metabolic decline once they are activated or deactivated. These would act as a genetic 'clock'. The inherited syndromes of accelerated ageing (progeria) provide strong evidence for the presence of such genes. In addition, molecular biologists have also identified genes that may be activated during the normal ageing process. The role of 'ageing genes' is debatable, however, and some researchers consider that such genes probably determine the maximal longevity of species and that there are other mechanisms that promote senescence, the rate of which varies considerably between individuals (See Box 20.17.).

The *somatic mutation theory of ageing* (Morley, 1995) suggests that DNA mutations accumulate throughout life, with consequences for cell functions. There is a degree of evidence for this, but the extent of nuclear DNA mutation that has been observed is debatably insufficient to account for the functional disturbances associated with ageing.

Recent studies have extended this theory by showing that mitochondrial DNA and mitochondrial membranes are damaged during life. Mitochondrial DNA is extranuclear DNA that contains only a small number of genes particularly involved in controlling mitochondrial

BOX 20.15 TELOMERES

Telomeres are pieces of DNA found at the tips of the chromosomes. The integrity of these stretches is maintained through the activity of an enzyme called telomerase. The Hayflick limit to cell divisions (see text) is related to the loss of telomere length, caused by declining activity of telomerase. These are interesting findings, because the process provides insight into the declining ability of cells to divide as we age (Goyns and Lavery,

2000). Finding a means of manipulating telomerase is an avenue of current research into the biology of ageing.

Of further interest is the way in which cancer cells are able to maintain telomerase and their telomere length. In doing so, they are able to 'escape' the Hayflick limit, and so become 'immortal' (Klingelhutz, 1999). Preventing cancer cells from behaving this way is another area of research activity.

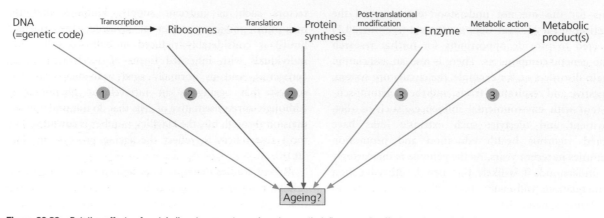

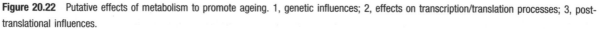

Figure 20.22 Putative effects of metabolism to promote ageing. 1, genetic influences; 2, effects on transcription/translation processes; 3, post-translational influences.

Q. What effect does ageing have on metabolism?

function. Mutation of these genes will have consequences for cellular respiratory processes, and evidence indicates that oxidative metabolism does indeed decline with age (Wei, 1998).

Superoxidant chemicals – 'free radicals' – have been implicated as the cause of mitochondrial damage. These are produced by normal respiratory reactions, but are so reactive that they are rapidly catabolized. Although existing only transiently, their continued production means that they are always present, albeit in small quantities, and will exert some activities. The *free-radical theory* (proposed by Harman, 1956) is not new, but recent advances in the study of molecular biology have only recently made it possible to investigate its implications. This is now the major theory in the biology of ageing (Ashok and Ali, 1999)

Errors in protein synthesis

The *error catastrophe theory* (Orgel, 1963) proposes that errors in transcribing the genetic code, or in ribosomal translation of that code, result in the loss of vital enzymes,

or perhaps the production of novel ones. This theory is supported by findings that substances do, indeed, accumulate in cells with age, e.g. lipofuscin (age pigment) observable as brown patches in the skin. Lipofuscin does not appear to be detrimental to cell function, although it is possible that other substances may be. The theory is 'catastrophic' because it implies that the loss of enzymes, or the production of novel substances, could disturb the activities of other enzymatic processes, which in turn causes further disruption, and so on.

Recent studies have found that there is an accumulation of aberrant proteins during ageing, e.g. proteins that have been glycated (collectively called Maillard products). Glycation is the spontaneous but inappropriate combination of glucose with proteins, and occurs as a consequence of the continuous presence of glucose within the cell. It is distinct from the process in which certain proteins are combined metabolically with glucose to produce glycoproteins that are vital for cell function. Glycated enzymes will not be effective. The theory suggests that the resultant accumulation of Maillard products disturbs cell function. Readers interested in this topic might like to consult Gallant *et al.* (1997) for further information.

BOX 20.17 LONGEVITY OR SENESCENCE?

'Longevity' is a term used in connection with the maximal lifespan of a species. In humans, this is of the order of 90 years or so (longevity does not equate with statistics of average life expectancy). Some people do live longer than this, but they are exceptional. Longevity varies between species and undoubtedly has a genetic basis, and some of the genes involved have now been identified, leading to speculation that gene manipulation might in the future extend human longevity to 120 years or even more.

'Senescence' covers the processes of chronic decline in biological function that contributes to species longevity but also determines the individual's actual lifespan. It is these processes

that social change and medical science have influenced during the last 150 years (Figure 20.20(b)), but they have led to concerns of demographic change in which the numbers of elderly people in the population are increasing. The problem is largely one of dependency: if senescence can be understood better so that late adulthood is still a period of health and/or economic activity, then the demographic change becomes less of a concern. Extending human longevity, therefore, may not be desirable unless the rate of senescence can be reduced. This means understanding more of the cellular mechanisms of ageing, but also the environmental factors that contribute to functional decline.

The *cross-linkage theory* (Bjorksten, 1968) proposes that proteins synthesized by cells increasingly link together during life, with resultant disruption of protein structure and function. For example, the loss of intermolecular cross-linkage of collagen is largely responsible for the loss of tissue elasticity, including skin wrinkling. This might be considered as an aberrant protein, and the older we are the greater will be its accumulation.

A unified theory?

In terms of their basic proposals, the theories that suggest post-translational changes in proteins are responsible for senescence overlap with theories of genetic mutation and transcriptional/translational errors. A growing view is that age-related changes in cell functions arise through an integration of effects arising from increasing amounts of inactive proteins, a rise in the functional 'half-life' of proteins, increased damage to mitochondria, and a drop in energy generation per mitochondrion. This unification of many of the major biological theories has produced a *network theory of ageing* (Kowald and Kirkwood, 1996).

When does ageing begin?

Metabolic theories of ageing imply an accumulation of errors in cell functioning. This could mean that the ageing process is initiated much earlier in life, perhaps even before birth. The emphasis currently placed on preconceptual and antenatal care, and the possible link between maternal environment and the lifespan of progeny (Scrimshaw 1997), might support this notion. For many people, however, biological ageing is synonymous with physiological decline during adulthood. The involution of the thymus gland in late adolescence, and the possibility that 'ageing genes' are activated at some time during the life-cycle, could support the triggering of ageing as an event in early/middle adulthood. Senescence is sometimes explained in terms of a 'disposable soma', i.e. genes and hence cell functions are maintained during the peak reproductive years, but then errors are 'allowed' to accumulate and so cell functions begin to decline.

In functional terms, the years between conception and adolescence mark a period of increasing physiological efficiency, which also argues against the view that age-related cellular homeostasis decline occurs throughout life. It could, of course, be that the dynamic changes induced by developmental responses, prompted by altered genetic activity and resultant hormonal changes, exceed any negative effects of the ageing process.

Clearly, this is a debatable area, but it is one that is important in the context of producing health promotion and health education programmes, e.g. in the possible use of antioxidant vitamin supplements to counteract free-radical activity (Vendemiale *et al.*, 1999).

IMPLICATIONS OF ADVANCES IN GENETICS FOR HEALTHCARE

Genetic disorders have proved extremely resistant to curative methods. Therapies have generally been directed at the maintenance of health for as long as possible, rather than cure. However, large leaps in the identification of genes, and understanding how they operate, have been made during the last 20 years as part of the Human Genome Project and related research. Recent advances in molecular biology have also furthered knowledge and understanding of genetic disease, and advances in the treatment of such disorders are on the horizon. Developments to existing clinical processes, such as screening techniques, and the development of new ones, e.g. genetic engineering, are likely to have a significant impact in the near future. New therapies, including gene therapy and pharmaceutical preparations that will modulate gene actions or actions of gene products, are beginning to appear or enter trials. Alongside these developments are studies that are increasing the understanding of how environmental factors influence gene and gene expression; the findings from these are likely to impact on health education and health promotion activities in much the same way as recognition of the effects of smoking and exercise on the cardiovascular system has done during the last 30 years.

In other words, advances in gene technologies and in understanding how genes work seem likely to have a major impact on future health and healthcare delivery, not to mention social factors (e.g. the controversy surrounding genetically modified foods, and even the use of gene scanning for approval for life insurance policies). This section outlines some of the processes that will underpin future health developments based on genes and their activities.

Screening

The identification of fetuses at risk is not new. Techniques such as amniocentesis and chorionic villus sampling have, for a long time, enabled clinicians to obtain samples of fetal cells for chromosomal analysis. In this way, the sex of the fetus is readily identified, and any chromosomal abnormalities determined. Screening of the karyotype allows the prospective parents to be aware before birth of the likelihood of certain neonatal abnormalities.

The likelihood of genetic disorders in offspring has traditionally been established by pedigree analysis of family history. Thus, familial incidences of a disorder, going back through a number of generations, can identify the presence of a mutated allele within the family line. Such analyses, however, can only highlight the possibility, not probability, that an individual is a carrier of the allele, and likewise if his or her partner might also be a carrier. Family histories are also usually incomplete, or extend back only one or two generations, so people are often unaware of any genetic disorders within the family line. Thus, often a couple become aware that they are carriers of a recessive allele only at the birth of an affected (homozygous recessive) child. Counselling may then be initiated should the parents plan further pregnancies.

This situation is changing rapidly as techniques are now available that can identify the presence of certain mutated genes in cells, although this might only be looked for if there is a known risk. This extends possibilities to include embryo selection based on the presence or absence of affected genes. The screening of early embryos is possible in vitro because cells can be removed from the morula embryological stage without affecting later development of that embryo. Chromosomal and gene analysis of the extracted cell can then identify which embryos will be affected; unaffected embryos might then be chosen for implantation.

In adults, gene-screening techniques could also identify the risk of developing a polygenic condition since the predisposition can be assessed. This could provide a means of enabling people to predict risk, e.g. a gene scan might one day enable assessment of the risk of developing insulin-dependent diabetes mellitus (the group of genes involved are now known). The advantage is that if there are any environmental risk factors in the progression from predisposition to the actual condition, then these could perhaps be minimized or avoided. However, if there is access to the information, then this could also have implications if the individual wishes to obtain life insurance or perhaps even long-term employment. Individuals also may not wish to be aware of the propensity, or perhaps may not be able to afford a scan. There are important moral and ethical questions to be asked, but these situations are increasingly possible and likely. Gene analysis may seem extraordinarily high tech, but the cost of gene analysis is falling rapidly as technology improves, and there has even been speculation that self-testing might be a possibility in the near future.

Genetic engineering and gene therapies

Genetic engineering utilizes recombinant DNA technology that was developed during the 1970s and 1980s as a means of producing large quantities of a particular gene or gene product so that enough of it was available for research purposes. It involves either (i) incorporating a fragment of DNA into a host cell (usually a bacterium), which, by multiple cell division, then produces multiple copies of the DNA fragment and its genes, which can then be extracted; or (ii) utilizing the enzyme DNA polymerase to directly produce multiple copies of the DNA fragment. Modern genetic engineering has extended these techniques to the incorporation of DNA fragments into cells of higher, more complex organisms, including humans, with the intention of altering cell functioning.

Gene transplantation (transgenics) involves incorporating a piece of DNA that contains the required allele into a vector, such as a modified virus or a microscopic lipid droplet (called a liposome), and allowing the vector to penetrate the target cells. The DNA becomes incorporated into the genome of the recipient cell. If the transplanted allele is a dominant form, then this will influence cell function. The expansion of technologies to facilitate this can be seen in the increasing developments of genetically modified foods. To be effective in correcting an established recessive disorder, a normal allele must be transplanted into the majority of the affected cells in extensive, already differentiated tissues. One way is to transplant the gene into stem or germinative cells, from which new tissue cells will be derived; another way is to use a method that provides access to large areas of tissue, perhaps using viruses that specifically infect those tissues. In humans, the method has been used, with apparent success, to treat leukaemia in young babies; attempts are currently being made to introduce sufficient genes to produce significant health improvements in people with conditions such as cystic fibrosis. Transgenics therefore is a development that, for the first time, could aid the prevention or correction of genetic disorders.

The transplantation of genes into embryos involves much the same techniques, and so is technologically feasible. The manipulation of genes within embryos is restricted, however, and such work has been confined to animal studies. It understandably raises concern regarding the legal and ethical position of embryo manipulation, and the prevention of abuse of these techniques to enable parents to select 'desirable' characteristics for their offspring.

Designer drugs

A spin-off from gene research is that drugs can be designed to target inappropriately functioning genes, or the actions of those genes. For example, some areas of cancer research are currently investigating this approach by using antibody–drug complexes to target abnormal antigens on tumour cells, or by using drugs that will act to modify or replace the actions of those altered proteins involved in the cell cycle.

Cloning

Box 20.9 identified some of the issues in relation to cloning. A major potential benefit is the use of such techniques to produce tissue for transplantation. If (when?) developmental genes can be modulated, then cloning techniques could generate tissues that have been triggered to form specific cell types for implantation into recipients. In this way, functioning tissues could be transplanted to replace dysfunctional ones, leading to new repair technologies in disorders, such as Parkinson's disease, that currently have no known cure (see Box 20.18).

Genetic fingerprinting

The ability of scientists to replicate a DNA sample many times over, and hence to determine the genetic coding of the sample, has enabled the analysis of minute traces of DNA. This has facilitated crime investigations (hence the term 'DNA fingerprinting') and the identification of related species of plant or animal (both extant and extinct), and plays a role in the debate regarding the evolutionary links of human cultures. In addition, the human genome contains within it sequences that mutate little and that will be almost constant between closely related individuals. The family link can also be assessed by comparing mitochondrial DNA (i.e. DNA found within the cell mitochondria rather than in the nucleus). This DNA is only inherited through the female line, as the mitochondria of sperm are jettisoned with the tail at fertilization.

BOX 20.18 STEM CELLS

Gene therapy has potential for the development of transplantation tissue from stem cells. These are cells found in most, if not all, tissues, even in adults. They are undifferentiated or only partially differentiated cells that might be triggered to develop further and differentiate into cells of a particular tissue type. This may occur within a damaged tissue. Recent research has begun to identify the chemical factors produced by tissues that trigger this, and that also might be used by medicine to manipulate the differentiation. Coupled with cloning techniques, this raises the possibility of producing large numbers of activated stem cells in vitro for transplantation, e.g. into neural tissue. Such cells could regenerate new tissue in disorders such as Parkinson's disease, or where there has been tissue trauma.

Large numbers of stem cells are required to raise the confidence of success and the level of functional improvement, should the transplantation be accepted. Young cells (i.e. embryological cells) are also likely to be most effective. These two aspects have led to suggestions that the government should allow the cultivation of early human embryos to provide the stem cells. This is clearly an emotive area fraught with moral and ethical issues.

Summary

1 Genes are sections of DNA and a sequence of constituent bases that provides the information necessary for a cell to synthesize a specific polypeptide, and hence determine that cell's characteristics.

2 The DNA of a cell is packaged before cell division as chromosomes. There are 23 pairs of chromosomes in each body cell, i.e. 23 chromosomes inherited from each parent. There is thus a duplication of genes (except on the sex chromosomes of males, where the Y chromosome is considerably smaller than the X chromosome). Each member of a pair of genes is called an allele. The pairs of alleles separate in meiosis during the formation of the gametes, and the alleles on either chromosome can potentially be inherited by offspring.

3 Fertilization of an oocyte by a sperm cell produces a zygote, which undergoes a number of changes before implantation into the uterus. Selective gene activation is first apparent in the blastocyst phase. Tissue differentiation continues, and increases in complexity, following implantation. Differentiation is further evidence of selective gene activation, and most tissues are basically formed by 7–8 weeks after fertilization. The embryo is now considered to be a fetus.

4 Fetal development is primarily one of growth and functional maturation. Nutrient exchange with the mother is facilitated by the development of the placenta, although this also has numerous other functions.

5 Embryo differentiation and fetal development are influenced by the gene mix that has been inherited from the parents, and by environmental factors that impact on the uterine environment and/or maternal wellbeing.

6 Mutation or alteration of the genetic code in one of a pair of alleles is possible, in which case the person is said to be heterozygous. Such a mutation may be of no consequence if the mutated allele is recessive to the normal dominant one on the homologous chromosome, since the normal protein associated with the gene will be synthesized. If the mutation is dominant, however, then the cell will synthesize the protein determined by that allele, with possible damaging effects.

7 Although recessive alleles may remain 'hidden' in heterozygous people, there is always a possibility that a child may inherit copies of the allele from each parent. With no dominant counterpart to suppress it, the mutated allele will now contribute to protein synthesis and cell function. The potential effects of losing a normal protein, or of producing the novel protein, can be devastating; this is the basis of most recognized genetic diseases.

8 Mutated alleles on the X chromosome are unlikely to have corresponding alleles on the smaller Y chromosome. Thus, male offspring will always be affected, even if the mutation is recessive to the normal form. This means that males cannot be 'carriers' of a recessive allele in the usual sense, and some

Summary (Continued)

disorders typically are observed more frequently in boys than girls.

9 Characteristics produced by the net effects of multiple genes are less sensitive to the effects of mutation of an individual allele within the group, but the more mutations that are inherited, the greater the likelihood will be that mutation of the remainder of the 'group' will occur during life. Thus, a propensity to a disorder can be inherited with consequences later in life.

10 Functional changes during adulthood are mainly those of declining homeostatic efficiency, with an increasing susceptibility to ill-health.

11 Theories abound as to how the ageing process affects tissues. Most focus on interference with the synthesis of functional proteins, especially enzymes. Recent advances have pinpointed specific metabolic effects, primarily in relation to cell respiration, but the influence of extrinsic factors on the ageing process is still unclear.

12 Pedigree analysis can identify people at risk of genetic disorder, and so pregnancies can be avoided (depriving a couple of children) or couples prepared for the outcome. Traditional therapies for inherited disorder have been aimed at maintaining as high a standard of life as possible – cures have not been possible. Alternatively, affected fetuses may be aborted. The development of in vitro fertilization techniques, coupled with recent advances in the identification of mutated genes, has meant that the implantation of embryos known to be lacking certain mutations is possible and will result in an unaffected child.

13 Advances in genetic engineering are beginning to make the treatment of certain genetic disorders appear possible, and such genetic therapies could represent a major breakthrough in medicine. However, gene therapy and related genetic technologies evoke powerful moral and ethical debate, the outcomes of which have, in many instances, still to be resolved.

References

Agustines, L.A., Lin, Y.G., Rumney, P.J., Lu, M.C., Bonebrake,R., Asrat, T. *et al.* (2000) Outcomes of extremely low weight infants between 500 and 750 g. *American Journal of Obstetrics and Gynaecology* **182**(5): 1113–6.

Ashok, B.T. and Ali, R. (1999) The aging paradox: free-radical theory. *Experimental Gerontology* **34**(3): 293–303.

Bjorksten, J. (1968) The cross-linkage theory of aging. *Journal of the American Geriatric Society* **16**: 408–27.

Gallant, J., Kurland, C., Parker, J., Holliday, R. and Rosenberger, R. (1997) The error catastrophe theory of aging. Point counterpoint. *Experimental Gerontology* **32**(3): 333–46.

Goyns, M.H. and Lavery, W.L. (2000) Telomerase and mammalian ageing: a critical appraisal. *Mechanisms of Ageing and Development* **114**(2): 69–77.

Harman, D. (1956) Aging: a theory based on free-radical and radiation chemistry. *Journal of Gerontology* **11**: 298–300.

Hayflick, L. and Moorhead, P.S. (1961) The serial subcultivation of human cell strains. *Experimental Cell Research* **25**: 585–621.

Klingelhutz, A.J. (1999) The roles of telomeres and telomerase in cellular immortalisation and the development of cancer. *Anticancer Research* **19**(6A): 4823–30.

Kowald, A. and Kirkwood, T.B. (1996) A network theory of ageing: the interaction of defective mitochondria, aberrant proteins, free radicals and scavengers in the ageing process. *Mutation Research* **316**(5–6): 209–36.

Kubas, C. (1999) Noninvasive means of identifying fetuses with possible Down syndrome: a review. *Journal of Perinatal and Neonatal Nursing* **13**(2): 27–46.

Lemaire, L. and Kessel, M. (1997) Gastrulation and homeobox genes in chick embryos. *Mechanisms of Development* **67**(1): 3–16.

Mark, M., Rijli, F.M. and Chambon, P. (1997) Homeobox genes in embryogenesis and pathogenesis. *Paediatric Research* **42**(4): 421–9.

Morley, A. (1995) The somatic mutation theory of aging. *Mutation Research* **338**(1–6): 19–23.

Orgel, L.E. (1963) The maintenance of accuracy of protein synthesis and its relevance to aging. *Proceedings of the National Academy of Sciences, USA* **49**: 5117–21.

Reister, R.J. (1995) The pineal gland and melatonin in relation to ageing: a summary of the theories and of the data. *Experimental Gerontology* **30**(3–4): 199–212.

Sanchez-Sweatman, L.R. (2000) Reproductive cloning and human health: an ethical, international, and nursing perspective. *International Nursing Review* **47**(1): 28–37.

Stables, D (1999a) Physiology in Childbearing. Bailliere Tindall; London. Chapter 48: Adaptations to extrauterine life 1. Respiration and cardiovascular function. p565.

Stables, D (1999b) Physiology in Childbearing. Bailliere Tindall; London. Chapter 51: Neonatal cardiovascular and respiratory disorders. p601

Scrimshaw, N.S. (1997) The relation between fetal malnutrition and chronic disease in later life. *British Medical Journal* **3115**: 825–6.

Steen, C.D. (1997) Cystic fibrosis: inheritance, genetics and treatment. *British Journal of Nursing* **6**(4): 192–9.

Stranc, L.C., Evans, J.A. and Hamerton, J.L. (1997) Seminar. Chorionic villus sampling and amniocentesis for prenatal diagnosis. *Lancet* **349**(9053): 711-14.

Suddaby, E.H., & Grenier, M.A. (1999) The embryology of congenital heart defects. Paediatric Nursing, **25**(5): 499–504.

Susman-Shaw, A. and Harrington, C. (1999) Haemophilia: the facts. *Nursing Standard* **14**(3): 39–47.

Vendemiale,G., Grattagliano, I. And Altomare, E. (1999) An update on the role of free radicals and antioxidant defense in human disease. *International Journal of Clinical and Laboratory Research* **29**(2): 49–55.

Wald, N. (1991) Prevention of neural tube defects: results of the Medical Research Council Vitamin Study. *Lancet* **338** (8760): 131–7.

Wald, N.J. Watt, H.C. and Hackshaw, A.K. (1999) Integrated screening for Down's syndrome based on tests performed during the first and second trimesters. *New England Journal of Medicine* **341**(7): 461–7.

Wei, Y.H. (1998) Oxidative stress and mitochondrial DNA mutations in human ageing. *Proceedings of the Society for Experimental Biology and Medicine* **217**(1): 53–63.

Chapter 21

Pain

INTRODUCTION

Most people think they know what pain is, yet from a scientific point of view, much still has to be discovered. It is difficult for researchers to agree upon a definition, and further difficulties arise in developing a suitable theory to account for all the different observations that have been made (Melzack and Wall, 1996). An person's personality, culture, anxiety level, perception of the painful situation, mood and social influence have all been suggested to affect the perception and expression of pain (Horn and Munafo, 1997). Although pain perception can be considered to be a 'sense', to understand how pain can be subjective needs more discussion than was possible when the senses were described in Chapter 7.

The chapter begins with a definition of pain. It then investigates the functions of pain, and the types of pain a person may perceive. The neurophysiology associated with Melzack and Wall's gate control theory of pain perception will also be discussed. An integrated scientific perspective using the nature–nurture interactions as a template will be used to understand the gate control theory. This involves linking the sociopsychology with the neurophysiology associated with pain perception. Various assessment tools will be also reviewed, and those factors that must be taken into consideration during objective assessment of pain will be discussed. Finally, the gate's underpinning analgesic site of action of pharmacological and non-pharmacological agents employed by the healthcare professional will be mentioned.

Definition of pain

The word 'pain' is derived from the Greek word 'poine' for 'penalty', and thus suggests the concept of punishment and retribution. Any credible definition because of its importance in medicine, nursing and allied healthcare professions must include the subjective nature of pain, as emphasized by McCaffery's (1983) famous definition that 'Pain is whatever the experiencing person says it is, existing whenever he says it does.'

Pain thresholds

Pain threshold refers to the level of stimulation at which the person just begins to perceive pain. There is considerable debate over the existence of an absolute pain threshold for each individual, since the threshold is affected by sociopsychological and 'physical' factors, such as anxiety, hospitalization, and the pain relief technique used. Thus, individual thresholds fluctuate within the individual, as well as being subjective to individuals within the population. Some of the factors that account for this subjectivity are highlighted later in the chapter. Thresholds can be divided into those of:

- pain perception, when the perception of stimuli, e.g. temperature change or pressure, reaches a level when the person begins to feel pain for the first time;

- severe pain, i.e. the point when the pain becomes unbearable for the person if stimulus strength is increased further. This is sometimes referred to as pain tolerance.

There is little difference between the values obtained for pain perception thresholds across different social and ethnic groups (Davidhizar *et al.*, 1997). However, values for the severe pain threshold differ markedly, and this may be explained by cultural and psychophysiological variations.

Functions of pain

Pain has survival and protective values. For instance, the pain sensation that occurs before serious injury, such as when a person picks up a hot plate, produces immediate withdrawals in order to prevent further damage. Subsequently, through conditioned learning and socialization, the person avoids future injurious objects.

Pain associated with injuries may be considered a homeostatic imbalance, since damaged cells are involved in the release of pain-producing substances. Injuries set limits on activity by enforcing inactivity and rest, which itself aids faster recovery. In this sense, rest and inactivity could be considered as crude homeostatic adaptive mechanisms. Injury pain therefore serves useful purposes. However, on occasions, pain seems to have no useful value, e.g. some amputees suffer excruciating phantom limb pain for years (Ehde *et al.*, 2000).

Exercise

Discuss what you understand by the statement that 'pain is an homeostatic imbalance'.

Varieties of pain

Classifying the type of pain aids the selection of appropriate assessment tools and therapies to suit the individual needs of the patient. Clinically, pain is classified as acute or chronic.

Acute pain

Acute pain is usually dealt with adequately, and is relatively short lived: a beginning and an end are often identifiable (Melzack and Wall, 1996). It is viewed positively as a warning signal, which draws attention to injury or illness, and is experienced by everyone at some stage in their lives. Acute pain can range from a relatively minor acute pain, such as toothache, to a relatively major pain, such as postoperative pain. The characteristics of acute pain are usually those associated with tissue damage and anxiety-led features exhibited in the psychophysiological 'fight and flight' reactions (see Chapter 22). Accompanying these reactions is a preoccupation with the cause of the pain and its consequences.

Chronic pain

In contrast to acute pain, chronic (intractable) pain has no biological value. It is disabling and is easily recognizable, but it is poorly understood. The pain overwhelms the patient, and is often associated with anxiety, depression and insomnia.

Exercise

Read the articles by Redeker *et al.* (1998), Fitzsimons *et al.* (2000), and Chen and Chang (2000).

A qualitative difference between acute and chronic pain exists since it affects the person differently, whether psychologically, physiologically, emotionally or spiritually. It is impossible to predict when chronic pain will end, it often gets worse rather than better, it is poorly controlled, and therapies are generally ineffective. Examples include arthritic and cancer pains (Cunningham, 2000). Chronic

---

BOX 21.1 PERIOPERATIVE ACUTE PAIN

Surgical nurses are certain to encounter patients in pain during perioperative care. In acute situations, the surgical patient is often admitted in pain; postoperative pain is also a normal occurrence of surgery itself. A considerable number of patients discharged from hospital are in pain. The problem of inadequate pain control may be enhanced further, since there are increasing numbers of patients undergoing day-case or short-stay surgery (Dobson, 1997). Thus, there is a need for better education of hospital staff in postoperative pain control (Mann and Redwood, 2000). In support of this, we would argue that surgical nurses must have a sound knowledge of the neurophysiology associated with the subjective nature of this phenomenon, since this would be helpful in the understanding of:

- the different types of pain expressed by the surgical patient;
- the variation that exists between patients in their expression of differing pain intensities, and duration and qualities of pain;
- the site of action of pharmacological and non-pharmacological methods of pain control.

Such an understanding is paramount in assisting the decision-making processes that underpin effective individualized perioperative pain management.

pain can be so terrible and detrimental to one's life that some people would rather die than continue living with it.

Pain perception: an overview

Pain perception is a function of the whole nervous system (Wright, 1999). It involves five components (Figure 21.1):

- *Specialized pain receptors.* It is unclear what constitutes a pain receptor (nociceptor). Some nociceptors are probably free nerve endings, which are only sensitive to chemicals (e.g. bradykinin, lactic acid, prostaglandins) perhaps released from damaged cells in the vicinity. These are classified as a type of chemoreceptor. Other nociceptors are complex encapsulated structures sensitive to pronounced mechanical deformation (e.g. stretching, crushing, tearing, cutting) and extreme temperature change (e.g. scalding, burning, freezing). These are classified as types of mechanoreceptors and thermoreceptors, respectively. Some nociceptors respond to only one type of stimulus, while others are capable of responding to chemical, mechanical and thermal stimuli – known as polymodal nociceptors.

Nociceptors are attached to distal ends of primary afferent pain fibres.

- *Primary afferent pain fibres.* These are sensory fibres that transmit the pain message as an electrical impulse towards the central nervous system. Other primary afferents function to inhibit the passage of pain impulses.

- *Ascending nociceptive nerve fibre tracts.* These are stimulated by a pain neurotransmitter released from the primary afferent pain fibres at synapses throughout the dorsal horn of grey matter spinal cord (and certain brain sites). They conduct the pain impulse to the higher pain centres of the brain.

- *Higher pain centres of the brain.* These interpret the electro-chemical impulse conducted in pain fibres, originally derived from the noxious stimuli, as a perception of pain.

- *Descending nerve fibre tracts.* The descending nerve fibre systems from the brain to the spinal cord are involved in modulating the perception of pain.

Once pain has been perceived, the body responds in a variety of ways. Responses to pain are categorized as either behavioural or manifested by sympathetic activity. The former responses include vocal responses (e.g. moaning,), verbal statements (e.g. 'Ouch, that hurts'), facial expression (e.g. grimacing), restricting movement and/or adopting a guarding behaviour ('protective rigidity'). Sympathetic responses include nausea, vomiting, gastric stasis, decreased gut motility, and impaired renal activity.

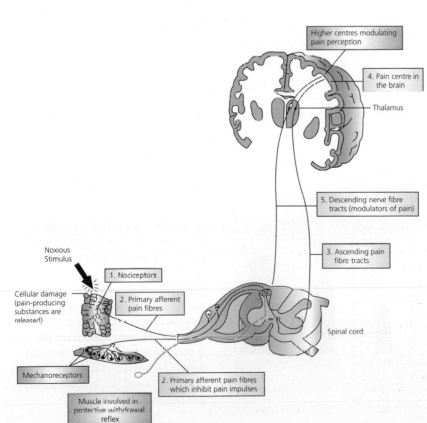

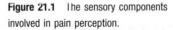

Figure 21.1 The sensory components involved in pain perception.

Q. What is the relative distribution of sodium and potassium ions on either side of the cell membrane of neurons/muscle cells required to establish the resting membrane potential? What movement of these ions is necessary to produce the (i) depolarized, (ii) repolarized and (iii) hyperpolarized phases of the action potential? Refer to chapter 8 if you are having difficulty.

Neurophysiology associated with pain perception

In order to generate pain, there is usually cellular damage. This may arise as a result of a surgical incision, traumatic injury, tumours compressing surrounding soft tissues, myocardial infarction, etc. Tissue damage promotes the appearance of the classic signs of inflammation. Accompanying inflammation are a variety of chemicals secreted from nerve endings, blood vessels, phagocytes, lymphocytes and tissues cells as a number of homeostatic reflexes go into operation to promote the healing of the damaged tissue (Clancy and McVicar, 1997). These chemicals are responsible for promoting the familiar localized signs (swelling/oedema, redness/erythema, heat/vasodilation, and pain) of the inflammatory process. This chapter is concerned only with the chemicals that induce pain and those that enhance responses to painful stimuli.

NEUROPHYSIOLOGY OF PAIN PERCEPTION

Pain-producing substances

Pain-producing substances released from damaged tissue include histamine, prostaglandins and kinin-like compounds, such as bradykinin. These substances combine with receptor binding sites on nociceptors, the initiators of the neural transmission associated with the perception of pain. In order to initiate a neural impulse, the interaction between pain-producing substances and nociceptors must reach the person's pain threshold. The brain interprets the intensity of pain according to the number of pain impulses it receives within a set period of time, i.e. the more impulses it receives, the greater the intensity of the pain (Figure 21.2).

Prostaglandins are among the most important initiators of pain. These chemicals are synthesized from arachidonic acid aided by the enzyme prostaglandin synthetase. Prostaglandins sensitize nociceptors, thereby enhancing the effects of other pain-producing substances. Accordingly, these chemicals may be considered the most important pain-producing substances in the human body (Clancy and McVicar, 1998). They also enhance pain fibre response to non-noxious stimuli in polymodal nociceptors.

Kinins (e.g. bradykinin) sensitize polymodal nociceptors to heat and mechanical stimuli.

The secretion of histamine from basophils (mast cells) is instigated by a number of chemical mediators, including interleukin 1 and nerve growth factor, released in the vicinity of damaged tissue. At low concentrations, histamine stimulates sensory neurons to produce an itching sensation; at high concentrations, these chemicals evoke a painful sensation.

Nociceptors are located extensively in the dermal layer of the skin, periosteum (layer of fibrous tissue surrounding bones), articular surfaces of joints, walls of arteries, and the dura mater (outer membrane covering of the spinal cord and brain). Deeper tissues, particularly the walls of the viscera (internal organs) are supplied less extensively. Cutaneous pain receptors have a relatively high threshold. Thus, a strong stimulus is required to generate an electrical signal that initiates the train of events resulting in pain perception.

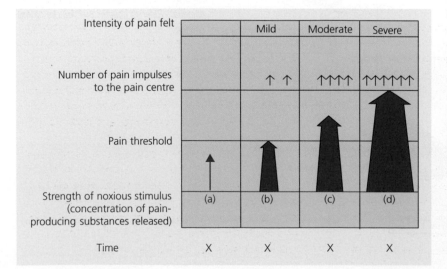

Figure 21.2 Pain threshold and the intensity of pain perception. (a) Minimal tissue damage, threshold not met, no pain impulse, no pain felt. (b) More tissue damage, threshold reached, few pain impulses sent to the pain centre, 'mild' pain felt. (c) Further tissue damage, threshold superseded, more pain impulses sent to the pain centre, 'moderate' pain felt. (d) Severe tissue damage, threshold superseded further, many more pain impulses sent to the pain centre, 'severe' pain felt. *Q. Using the text and this figure, distinguish between the following: (i) pain perception threshold, (ii) severe pain threshold, and (iii) pain tolerance.*

Anatomical location of nociceptors

Nociceptors are located at the distal end of afferent pain neurons. These neurons are small-diameter, myelinated A-delta fibres and smaller, unmyelinated C fibres. These are classified as the 'fast' and 'slow' pain fibres, respectively, since faster transmission is associated with thicker fibres and the presence of a myelin sheath. The A-delta fibres conduct messages at a speed of 5–25 m/s; C fibres conduct messages at 0.5 2 m/s. Nociceptors for fast pain fibres are located only in the skin and mucous membranes; nociceptors for slow pain fibres are found in the skin and most other body tissues, except the brain's nervous tissue, which is insensitive to pain.

The gate control theory

Melzack and Wall in 1965 proposed a gating mechanism within the dorsal horn of grey matter of the spinal cord. These gates were the layer of cells called the substantia gelatinosa, through which sensory (afferent) pain impulses have to pass before they are relayed to, and perceived in, the pain centre(s) of the brain. It is now generally accepted that every neuron is a 'gate'. The gates are symbolic of synapses between afferent neurons and various ascending and descending tract neurons. The gate control theory suggests that information can only pass through when the gate is 'open', and not when the gate is 'closed'. The opening of the gate is caused by the release at the synapse of excitatory neurotransmitter chemicals. The closing of the gate is brought about by the release of inhibitory neurotransmitters and neuromodulators (Figure 21.3).

Exercise

Before continuing, review the relevant sections in Chapter 8 for a discussion on excitatory and inhibitory neurotransmitters involved in synaptic conduction. It will help your understanding if you also look at Figures 21.3 and 21.4 while reading the following section.

The gating mechanism depends upon two modifying factors:

- the balance of activity of primary afferent (sensory) neurons;
- the modulator control of pain provided by descending fibres from the brain's higher centres.

Primary afferent fibre input

The afferent neurons, which provide input to the gate, are:

- the nociceptors containing A-delta and C pain fibres. These neurons release substance P, an excitatory neurotransmitter, at synapses (i.e. 'gates') within the central nervous system;
- the mechanoreceptors containing thick myelinated faster transmitting A-beta neurons. These fibres release inhibitory neurotransmitters (e.g. serotonin) at synapses within the central nervous system.

If the dominant input to the gate is via the faster transmitting A-beta fibres, then the gate will close due to the release and action of the inhibitory neurotransmitters.

BOX 21.2 SHARP AND DULL PAINS AND REFLEXES: AIDS TO DIAGNOSING

If the patient describes their pain as sharp and prickling, this informs the practitioner that the pain fibres involved are mainly of the A-delta type. This type of pain can be located precisely by the patient, because A-delta fibre nociceptors send pain signals along discrete pathways to the somatosensory cortex of the brain, which enables the pain to be established to within a few centimetres of the source (Bennett, 2000).

See Figure 8.8 to identify the location of the somatosensory areas of the brain.

Fast pain is often accompanied by withdrawal reflexes, activated via flexor motor neurons in the anterior horns of the spinal cord that activate the effector organ, usually a muscle, to instigate a protective withdrawal contraction in an attempt to avoid any further damage (Bennett, 2000). This reflex exhibits itself when a person stands on a sharp object or touches a hot surface. To the

trained practitioner, protective withdrawal reflexes may be used to establish the origin of the damage, and thus may be considered an aid to diagnosis. For example, when a patient instinctively covers the right lower quadrant of the abdomen or the left side of the chest, the practitioner may suspect the pain/damage is of appendix or cardiac origin, respectively. This knowledge, together with other signs and symptoms, may aid a diagnosis of appendicitis and angina, respectively.

If the assessment indicates that the pain is of a characteristically dull, burning, troublesome, aching, poorly localized and persistent nature, and is somatic in origin, it informs the practitioner that the pain fibres involved are C-type fibres (Wright, 1999). Torrance and Sirens (1997) proposed that the immediate pain of a surgical incision is mediated by A-delta fibres, but within a few seconds, the pain becomes more widespread due to C-fibre activation.

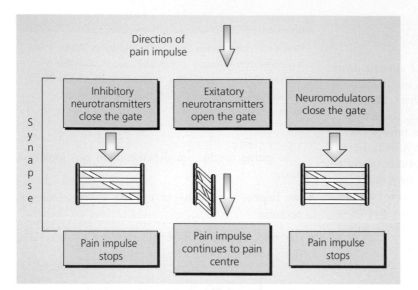

Figure 21.3 The chemicals involved in opening and closing the gateway of pain.

Q. *Name the pain-producing substances mentioned in this chapter.*

Exercise

Using Figure 8.22 and Table 8.3, review the conduction properties of myelinated A-delta and A-beta fibres (i.e. saltatory transmission) and unmyelinated C fibres (i.e. local circuitry, non-saltatory transmission).

There are many possible modes of action of these inhibitory neurotransmitters (Clancy and McVicar, 1998). These are summarized in Figure 21.4. Inhibitory neurotransmitters may be operative presynaptically via:

- repressing the gene activity necessary for the enzyme synthesis involved in substance P production;

- blocking the 'active site' of the enzyme, thus inhibiting the production of substance P;

- destroying the presynaptic fibres stores of substance P;

- preventing substance P release by decreasing the presynaptic membrane permeability, or by inducing its hyperpolarization.

Inhibitory neurotransmitters may be operative synaptically by destroying substance P within the synapse (although this seems unlikely). Inhibitory neurotransmitters may be operative post-synaptically by competing for substance P's post-synaptic membrane receptor binding sites, hence inhibiting the impulse from travelling in post-synaptic pain fibres.

In contrast, if the dominant input to the gate is from the afferent A-delta and/or C pain fibres, the gate may be open (see later section on additional influences from descending modulator control), owing to the release and the post-synaptic action of the excitatory neurotransmitter substance P (Figure 21.4). The pain impulse passes from the dorsal horn of the grey matter in ascending pathways, which, in the main, cross to the opposite side's (lateral) anterior commissure of the spinal cord before relaying upwards to the thalamus of the brain. These pathways are logically called the anterolateral spinothalamic ascending pain tracts. Some ascending pain fibre tracts (referred to as ipsilateral spinothalamic tracts; 'ips-' = same) relay upwards to the thalamus, while remaining on the same side of the cord.

Most A-delta fibres terminate in the thalamus, where they synapse with further neurons that transmit the signals to other basal areas of the brain and to the somatosensory cortex. Up to one-quarter of the C pain fibres terminate in the thalamus; the rest terminate in three distinct areas of the brainstem. Melzack and Wall (1996) stated that the cerebral cortex may not contain specific pain centres, and may just process the information it receives before transmitting it deeper into the brain tissue. It is generally believed that pain is felt in the midbrain, but the appreciation of its unpleasant qualities depends on the cerebral cortex. Specific pain centre(s) have not yet been located.

Note that pain perception will only occur if there is no or insufficient interference via descending fibre input to the gate from higher centres of the brain.

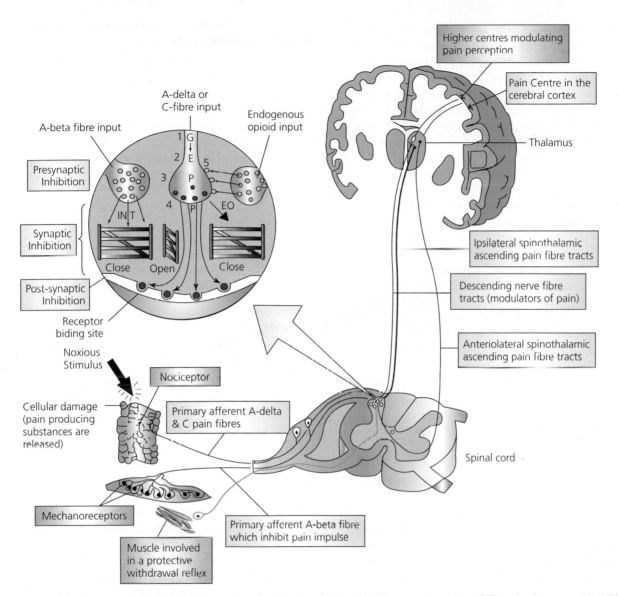

Figure 21.4 The gate control theory of pain perception. Possible sites of action of inhibitory neurotransmitters (INTs) and endogenous opiates (EOs). ***Presynaptic inhibition***: 1 INTs repress the gene necessary for the synthesis of substance P's enzyme. 2 INTs block enzyme activity, thus inhibiting the production of substance P. 3 INTs destroy vacuolated substance P. 4/5 INTs and EOs prevent substance P release by decreasing the presynaptic membrane permeability. ***Synaptic inhibition***: INTs destroy substance P within the synapse. ***Post-synaptic inhibition***: INTs compete for substance P's receptor binding sites.

Q. *Differentiate between the following: (i) nociceptor and polymodal nociceptors; and (ii) inhibitory neurotransmitters and excitatory neurotransmitters.*

EO, endogenous opiates (neuromodulators); INT, inhibitory neurotransmitters; P, substance P; PPS, pain-producing substances.

Descending modulator control from higher centres of the brain

The gate theory proposes that even if pain A-delta and C fibre input into the central nervous system dominates over the mechanoreceptor A-beta fibre input, the gate may still be closed. This is because areas of the brainstem, such as the reticular formation, raphe nuclei, trigeminal nuclei, vestibular nuclei, and various nuclei of the hypothalamus and cerebral cortex, can modify the gating process via descending neural mechanisms (Figure 21.5). These are termed pain inhibitory complexes in the dorsal horns of

the spinal cord (Bennett, 1999). The neurons of this descending fibre system release a variety of endogenous opiates (enkephalins, endorphins, dynorphins). These neuromodulators bind to opiate receptor sites on the presynaptic membrane of the pain fibres, and 'close the gate' by inhibiting the release of the pain neurotransmitter, substance P (Figure 21.4). Because of their function, these opiates have been referred to as the body's own natural painkillers (Clancy and McVicar, 1998). The distribution of opioid binding sites has been found to be uneven, with the highest concentration in the limbic system, thalamus, hypothalamus, midbrain and spinal cord (Thomas, 1996).

The reticular formation projections from the brainstem exert a powerful inhibitory control over the spinal gating mechanism. These projections are also influenced via somatic (body) input, and input from auditory and visual centres. In addition, cortical projections, particular from the frontal cortex (this area subserves cognitive processes, such as past experience), also pass to the reticular formation to mediate the control over the spinal gating mechanism. Cognitive processes can also influence gating mechanisms directly via their large fast-conducting corticospinal (pyramidal) fibre tracts (Figure 21.5). Melzack and Wall (1965) proposed the idea of a 'central trigger' that activates particular brain processes, such as past experience and memories. Psychological processes have an extremely important role in pain perception, and research has shown that psychological factors, such as anxiety and helplessness, can intensify the pain experienced. Thus, interventions that reduce anxiety or helplessness can reduce the pain experienced and enhance coping (Thomas *et al.*, 1995).

Exercise

Use Figure 21.4 and the interim summary below to revise your understanding of the operational workings of the gate control theory of pain perception.

Interim summary

If the combined effect of pain modifiers (i.e. inhibitory neurotransmitters and endogenous neuromodulators) does not exceed the pain fibre input to the gate, the gate is opened, and afferent neurons transmit activity via the anterolateral spinothalamic tracts from the spinal cord to the thalamus. Within the thalamus, they synapse with other neurons, which transmit the impulses to the pain centre(s) of the brain (wherever they are!). Therefore, the 'closing of the gate' is the basis of pain relief and is thus achieved via the inhibition of:

- the synthesis and/or the secretion of pain-producing substances;

- nociceptor activation;

- the electrical events associated with depolarization of pain fibre membranes;

- substance P synthesis or release;

- the actions of substance P.

In short, for the person to perceive pain, the afferent pain fibre input to the gate must dominate. To provide analgesic relief, this domination must be removed via increasing the mechanoreceptors afferent input and/or the descending neuron input to the gate. The concept of individualized pain relief is therefore based on a knowledge of the patient's background, the progress of the illness, the type and magnitude of the injury (e.g. surgical procedure employed), the area undergoing damage, and the durability/delicateness of the surrounding tissues. These are all relevant factors that need to be considered if perioperative pain management is going to be successful.

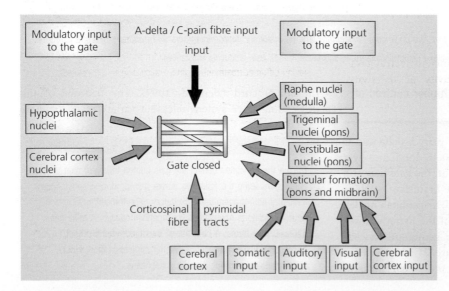

Figure 21.5 Higher centre descending fibres modulating control of pain. This shows that the higher centre input to the gate dominates over the pain fibre input so pain is not felt; however, this is not always the case.
Q. Name the endogenous opioids mentioned in this chapter.

The subjectivity of pain

Pain is a subjective experience, since each individual has a unique range of anatomical, physiological, social and psychological identities. These identities, using the nature–nurture interactions template, can be applied to the gate control theory to help explain the subjective nature of pain perception. The concept of individualized pain relief is based upon this template to the gate theory.

Anatomical subjectivity

The size and shape of the human body is controlled genetically and modified environmentally. Thus, a tremendous variation in human body shapes and sizes exists, and it is therefore not surprising that the distribution of nociceptors varies between individuals. This could be expected to produce regional variations of anatomical subjectivity in sensitivity to stimuli.

Biochemical and physiological subjectivity

Individuals have different production capacities of the biochemicals involved in the transmission of pain. A person's genome is responsible for the production of physiologically active enzymes necessary for the biochemical synthesis of pain-producing substances, substance P, inhibitory endogenous opiates, and inhibitory neurotransmitters. If the genes responsible for the synthesis of pain-producing substances or substance P are changed (i.e. mutated) or repressed, or the nociceptors become desensitized to pain-producing substances, then it would be possible to experience tissue injury without perceiving pain. Alternatively, people may not report pain, despite tissue damage, if the genes necessary for the production of the endogenous opioids or inhibitory neurotransmitters are repeatedly expressed, since their high levels would close the gate. Conversely, high levels of pain-producing substances (and consequently substance P), or low levels of endogenous opioids and/or inhibitory neurotransmitters as a consequence of gene activity or inactivity,

respectively, would lead to pain hypersensitivity. Congenital disorders of pain perception exist; some people are born insensitive to pain, while others feel pain without any detectable injury (Melzack and Wall, 1996).

Exercise

Review your understanding of the Operon theory in Chapter 2.

Sociopsychological subjectivity

Sociopsychological factors affect physiological processes and may be responsible indirectly for either opening or closing the gate. Social factors influence the development of the brain; these higher cortical centres may conceivably influence the physiological, neuronal and synaptic activity of the gate by influencing the descending control.

Anxiety is a state that may be determined genetically and/or socialized environmentally. In nursing literature, it is well documented that elevated anxiety levels are associated with a patient's increased pain perception. The gate control theory would attribute this to depressed endogenous opiate levels, or to an increased substance P level; the former is most likely, according to descending control theory.

Cultural differences in the perception of pain are also observed, and therefore need to be taken into consideration when assessing pain. This could suggest that past socializing experiences and individual conditioning have important influences on the subjective elements of pain. Socialization determines psychological behaviour, which could conceivably affect the output of endogenous opiates.

The importance or meaning of a situation can affect one's perception of pain.

BOX 21.5 CARING FOR ALL CULTURES

Practitioners should be concerned with management of a particular type of pain by using constant patient monitoring, rather than having different treatment regimens according to the patient's perception of their pain. Healthcare professionals should be familiar with cultural differences when reducing the patient's anxiety before assessing the appropriate care to be implemented (Davidhizar et al., 1997).

Exercise

What do you understand by the following statement. 'Pain is a subjective experience depending on an individual's characteristics'? Think about your answer using the nature–nurture template described in this book.

BOX 21.4 CARE AND ANXIETY

A patient's anxiety level is heightened with admission to hospital, the thought of the impending diagnostic procedures and, if applicable. surgery itself. These features influence the person's perception of pain, and are often associated with pre-hospitalization sleep loss. (Desjardins 2000). Nursing care should aim to reduce the patient's anxiety levels before attempting to quantify the pain that the patient perceives.

Pain management: a gate control perspective

The different characteristics associated with acute, chronic benign, chronic malignant, phantom, bone and muscle pains necessitates different therapeutic approaches emphasizing the subjectivity of pain perception and consequently of pain management. Nurses adopt a psychological approach in assisting the patient to understand and to cope with their pain, while perhaps it could be argued that doctors are more concerned with the physiological role of

diagnosing pain and instigating treatment. However, a considerable degree of overlap exists, depending on the philosophy of the ward staff, a factor itself that demonstrates subjectivity. On the whole, we would argue that the nurse must have a sound knowledge of the neurophysiology associated with this subjective phenomenon, since such an understanding is paramount in assisting the decision-making process that underpins effective individualized pain management.

You are advised to re-familiarize yourself with the content of the previous pages before continuing. In theory,

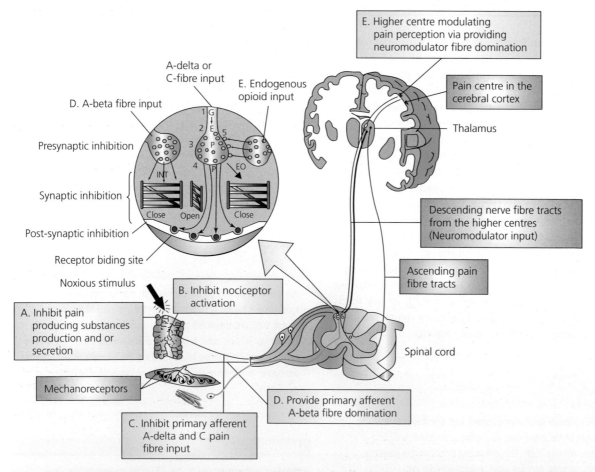

Figure 21.6 Perioperative pain management. A gate control perspective. Analgesia action is provided by: (Box A) inhibiting the production and/or secretion of pain-producing substances; (Box B) inhibiting nociceptor activation; (Box C) inhibiting afferent pain fibre input; (Box D) replacing afferent pain fibre input domination by promoting mechanoreceptors afferent fibre input; and (Box E) replacing afferent pain fibre input domination by promoting neuromodulator descending fibre input domination.

pain can be prevented or relieved by pharmacologically blocking the initiation and/or the transfer of nerve impulses anywhere from the site of damage to the pain centres in the brain. In practice, this is so (Figure 21.6). Thus, the inhibition or modulation of:

- the stimulatory effects of pain-producing substances and the blockade of nociceptive binding sites can be achieved pharmacologically with local mild oral analgesics;

- the electrical transmission along afferent pain fibres can be achieved via the administration of local anaesthetics;

- the secretion of the pain neurotransmitter, substance P, through synapses ('gates') can be achieved by the administration of the opioid analgesics.

Non-pharmacological approaches to pain management basically operate via increasing the patient's production of endogenous inhibitory transmitters and neuromodulators (Figure 21.6, pathways D and E).

We will now review the specific analgesic qualities of pharmacological and non-pharmacological agents. Before this discussion, however, it must be stressed that a good rapport and verbal communication with the patient (if conscious) are essential aspects of caring, so that the patient feels confident in the practitioner's ability to reduce or abolish their pain. Perhaps this operates via a placebo effect, whereby it is working by increasing the body's natural opiates. (A placebo is any inactive substance resembling medicine given during controlled experiments or to satisfy a patient.)

PHARMACOLOGICAL PAIN MANAGEMENT

The use of analgesic drugs is the mainstay of immediate pain management. The important aspects of pharmacological therapies are to provide the patient with sufficient pain relief to allow rest, relaxation, pain-free sleep and mobilization, and to avoid the toxic effects of the drugs and the occurrence of breakthrough of pain (Zeppetella *et al.*, 2000). The administration of regular, adequate doses will prevent the latter (Figure 21.7(a)). If breakthrough pain occurs, higher dosages may be deemed necessary by the nurse, rendering the possibility of the appearance of drug toxicity (Figure 21.7(b)). Analgesic drug administration can be via a variety of routes, namely oral, sublingual, rectal, inhalation, intramuscular, intravenous, subcutaneous, transdermal, spinal and epidural. Intravenous drugs may also be administered using patient-controlled administration systems.

Pain may be controlled using non-opioid and/or opioid analgesics. If pain persists, then the principles of the 'analgesic staircase' are employed in an attempt to improve pain control (Figure 21.8). The choice of drug depends on:

- the location, type and severity of pain experienced. In general, non-opioid simple analgesics are given to relieve mild to moderate pain. Nonsteroidal anti-inflammatory drugs (NSAIDs) are used for generalized pains or local inflammation. Some weak opioids are used to relieve mild to moderate pain, and others are used to relive

moderate to severe somatic pain. Stronger opioids are used for severe somatic pain;

- its pharmacological mode and site of action;

- its potential toxic effects.

Non-opioid analgesics

Since NSAIDs do not have the side effects of opioid drugs (e.g. respiratory depression, inhibition of gastrointestinal motility), they are useful alternatives in the management of, for example, postoperative pain, although they may be inadequate for relief of severe pain. The non-opioids that are used frequently in clinical pain management are paracetamol and the NSAIDs diclofenac, ketoprofen, naproxen and ibuprofen (administered for mild to moderate pain relief) and ketorolac (administered for moderate to severe pain relief). Intravenous infusion of diclofenac is also used to prevent the occurrence of postoperative pain (Omoigui, 1995).

Analgesic action

Analgesically, some non-opioids act outside the central nervous system in the periphery at the site of injury. For

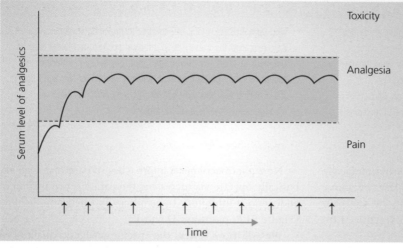

(a)

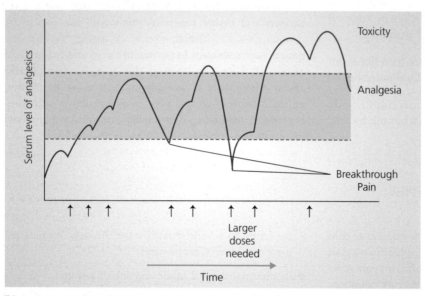

(b)

Figure 21.7 (a) Drug administration in successful analgesia. Regular, adequate doses of analgesia are required to alleviate pain. (b) Drug administration in breakthrough pain. Analgesics given at irregular intervals may result in breakthrough pain. Higher doses may then be deemed necessary, rendering the possibility of drug toxicity.

Q. How is breakthrough pain prevented?

↑ – doses of analgesia

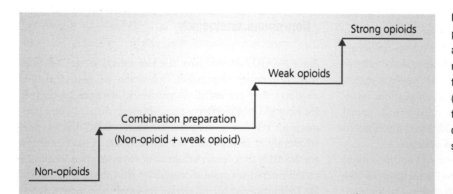

Figure 21.8 The analgesic staircase. This pathway may be used in order to reduce or abolish a patient's pain. If the pain is not removed using non-opioids (e.g. paracetamol), then a combined preparation may be given (e.g. paracetamol plus codeine phosphate). If the pain is still not removed, then weak opioids are given. If pain still persists, then a strong opioid is given.

example, paracetamol (e.g. Panadol®) inhibits the formation of prostaglandins by inhibiting the enzyme prostaglandin synthetase (Figure 21.6, pathway A). Prostaglandins sensitize nociceptors (attached to the distal ends of afferent pain A-delta and C fibres) to mechanical stimulation, and enhance the effects of other pain-producing substances.

Diclofenac and aspirin are thought to inhibit prostaglandin secretion from cells in the damaged area. Ibuprofen, ketoprofen and naproxen (and also aspirin) provide analgesic relief by inhibiting the secretion of other chemical initiators (e.g. bradykinin, histamine) of pain (Omoigui, 1995).

Table 21.1 Analgesic potency values of commonly used potent opioids

Drug	Potency value (compared with morphine)
Buprenorphine	30 times greater
Fentanyl	75–125 times greater
Meperidine	1/10 times greater
Nalbuphine	Equal potency
Penatzocine	1/3 times greater

Opioid analgesics

Narcotics or weaker substitutes are classified as opioids because of their chemical resemblance to the body's endogenous neuromodulator opioids (i.e. the endorphins, enkephalins and dynorphins). Thus, their analgesic sites of action are the specialized opioid receptors located on the presynaptic membrane of the afferent pain fibres (Figure 21.6, pathway E). Aspirin may also operate centrally on these opioid receptor sites, thus inhibiting pain transmission (Omoigui, 1995).

Thomas (1996) stated that opioids provide analgesic relief in a patient by:

- depressing the appreciation of pain at the spinal cord level in the dorsal horn region;
- stimulating activity in descending inhibitory pathways in the brainstem;
- exerting mood-elevating effects, acting through the limbic system;
- allaying anxiety.

Weak opioid analgesics

The weak opioid analgesics frequently used for the treatment of mild to moderate pain include codeine phosphate, co-dydramol, co-proxamol, and co-codamol. These opioids are classified as narcotic agonists, i.e. their analgesic site of action is at the endogenous opiate receptor binding site. Codeine phosphate is often used in combination with non-narcotic analgesics, such as paracetamol, for symptomatic treatment of mild to moderate pain.

Potent narcotic opioid analgesics

Potent opioid narcotics are the most effective analgesics. The potency value of commonly used narcotics is expressed in Table 21.1. These drugs are particularly suitable for treating moderate to severe pain of somatic origin. Administration may be via intravenous, intramuscular, epidural or spinal routes. The advantages of epidural administration, according to Omoigui (1995), are:

- lower dosages are needed;
- the effects are longer lasting;
- mobilization is improved;
- the effects are limited to the immediate area;
- respiratory depression resulting form the effects of the analgesics on the brainstem is minimized.

Narcotics produce other effects, even in normal analgesic dosages. All narcotics produce powerful depression of the respiratory centres in the medulla oblongata, and acute poisoning is always associated with slow, inadequate respiration, which can endanger the life of these patients (naloxone is administered to reverse respiratory depression). All the drugs of this type are liable to induce nausea and vomiting because they have a stimulant action on the vomiting centre in the brain postoperatively; this may necessitate giving anti-emetics (e.g. metoclopramide, cyclizine) at the same time. Many of them produce characteristic stimulation of the parasympathetic nervous system, which results in constipation (British National Formulary, 2000).

The analgesic qualities and side effects of opioids are a result of the opioid system being comprised of four distinct types of receptors: mu (μ), kappa (κ), delta (δ) and sigma (θ). There are two types of mu receptor: mu-1 and mu-2; the former are believed to mediate analgesia, and the latter mediate the side effects of respiratory depression, nausea, vomiting and constipation (Dobson, 1997). According to Case and Case (1994), exogenous opioid stimulation of kappa receptors results in spinal analgesia, respiratory depressions and sedation. Opioid stimulation of sigma receptors results in dysphoria, depression, hallucinations and vasomotor stimulation. Delta receptors are only stimulated by endogenous opioids. The opioids have different affinities for these receptors, e.g. morphine's affinity for mu receptors is 100 times greater than its affinity for kappa receptors.

The dangers (particularly of respiratory depression) of the opioids have stimulated research into discovering analgesic compounds that minimize this side effect. A number of such compounds exist, e.g. codeine phosphate and dihydrocodeine (DF118) are weak analgesics but are very good cough suppressants. They are, however, constipating.

Analgesic actions

Opioid drugs may act as narcotic agonists (e.g. morphine, diamorphine), partial narcotic agonists (e.g. buprenorphine) and agonist–antagonists (e.g. nalbuphine) at any or all of the opioids receptors mentioned above (Figure 21.6, pathway E). All of these drugs are used for the symptomatic treatment of acute severe pain, such as that imposed by surgery. However, penatzocine (an agonist–antagonist) is administered for the management of mild to moderate pain (Omoigui, 1995).

The primary effects of morphine and diamorphine are on the central nervous system and organs containing smooth muscle. Administration for analgesic purposes causes binding to opioid presynaptic membrane receptors (mu-1 receptors) on the pain fibres in the substantia gelatinosa of the spinal cord, thus inhibiting substance P release in the dorsal horn of grey matter and dopamine release in the basal ganglia. The side effects of morphine are due to its indiscriminate activity at other opioid receptor sites, i.e. mu-2 and kappa receptors (Dobson, 1997).

The use of other narcotic agonists such as fentanyl and pethidine is also very common. Fentanyl enhances the peripheral nerve block analgesic action of local anaesthetics, since this opioid drug also has weak local anaesthetic properties. High doses suppress nerve conduction (by energizing the sodium/potassium ATPase pump) and have effects on opioid receptors in peripheral nerve terminals. Low dosages of fentanyl prevent pain by blocking nociceptor input and processing in the spinal cord.

Local anaesthetics

Local anaesthetics provide regional anaesthesia by stabilizing afferent pain fibre membranes, by inhibiting the ionic fluxes required for the initiation and conduction of electrical impulses. In short, they cause a reversible block to conduction along the pain afferent nerve fibres (Figure 21.6, pathway C).

The local anaesthetics used vary widely in their potency, toxicity, length of effects, solubility, stability, and ability to permeate mucous membranes. These variations determine their suitability of administration route, e.g. infiltration, plexus, topical (surface), epidural or spinal block (Omoigui, 1995). Epidural analgesia is commonly used during surgery, often combined with general anaesthesia, because of its protective effects against the stress response of surgery. It is often used when good postoperative pain is essential, e.g. in aortic aneurysms or major gut surgery (British National Formulary, 2000).

It is common practice to give several drugs with different actions to produce a state of surgical anaesthesia with a minimal risk of toxic side effects. An intravenous anaesthetic is usually administered for induction, followed by maintenance with inhalation anaesthetics, perhaps supplemented by other drugs administered intravenously. Specific drugs are used to produce muscle relaxation. For certain procedures, controlled hypotension may be required, thus labetalol may be used. Beta-blockers may be used to control arrhythmia during anaesthesia. Glyceryl trinitrate is used to control hypertension, particularly postoperatively.

Local anaesthetics that are used frequently include bupivacaine, chloroprocaine, etidocaine, lignocaine and procaine. Lignocaine is the most widely used anaesthetic drug. It acts more rapidly and is more stable than other local anaesthetics. The duration of block (with adrenaline) is about 1.5 h.

BOX 21.8 PATIENT-CONTROLLED ANALGESIA

Patient-controlled analgesia (PCA) is an essential part of the healthcare professional's role in ensuring patient compliance. PCA allows patients to give themselves their own analgesia by activating a syringe pump. It provides a flexible form of pain control. Thomas *et al.* (1995) acknowledged that the more the patient feels in control of their own pain management, the lower the requirement for analgesia. These researchers also claim that PCA reduces pain dramatically postoperatively, and therefore promotes earlier discharge – hence the advocacy of PCA.

Other reported advantages of PCA include:

- its apparent safe method of analgesic delivery (Thomas, 1996);
- it bypasses the delays and deficiencies of the more conventional intramuscular injection method (Parsons, 2000);

- it reduces anxiety (Schwender, 1998). However, we would dispute this generalization, since not all patients feel comfortable being in control of their own analgesic relief.

The most frequently used route and drug for the control of acute postoperative pain, particularly following major surgery, is intravenous injection of morphine, although epidural and subcutaneous routes of administration are also used. The use of morphine is, however, dictated by the intensity of pain, and therefore should be given only when weaker analgesics fail to give relief. The use of diamorphine, pethidine and fentanyl is also very common. Other opioid analgesics either have too long or too short a duration of action for them to be utilized with PCA.

Bupivacaine's onset of action is fairly rapid, and the duration of anaesthesia is significantly longer than with any other commonly used local anaesthetic, which is a great advantage of this local anaesthetic. It is often used in lumbar epidural blockade. Epidural administration provides long-acting neural blockade. Transmission is blocked at the nerve root and dorsal root ganglia. Bupivacaine is the principle drug for spinal anaesthesia in the UK (British National Formulary, 2000).

Intravenous administrations of chloroprocaine may also produce central analgesia perhaps due to inhibition of substance P secretion from afferent C pain fibres, and central sympathetic blockade with a decrease in pain-induced reflex vasoconstriction.

Procaine has a similar potency value to lignocaine, but has a shorter duration of effect. It is now seldom used. Etidocaine provides a significant motor blockade and abdominal muscle relaxation when used for peridural analgesia.

NON-PHARMACOLOGICAL TECHNIQUES OF PAIN MANAGEMENT

Non-pharmacological techniques are frequently more within the direct control of the healthcare practitioner. They may be used in isolation or combination with medically prescribed analgesics, and may be utilized as a useful adjunct to analgesia in the immediate postoperative period in lessening the side effects of drugs (Torrance and Serginson, 1997).

A variety of non-pharmacological approaches to pain management exist. These include the giving information and verbal support to the patient, and the therapies of touch, relaxation, distraction, imagery, biofeedback, and transcutaneous nerve stimulation. While some of these fall naturally to the role of the nurse, others require specialized therapists.

Non-pharmacological therapies provide analgesic relief by replacing the dominance of the afferent pain fibre to the pain gates needed to evoke a sensation of pain with inhibitory neurotransmitter domination (Figure 21.6, pathway D) and/or neuromodulator dominance (Figure 21.6, pathway E). The next section discusses these methods in more detail.

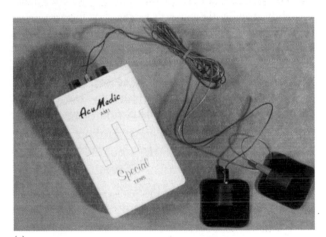

(a)

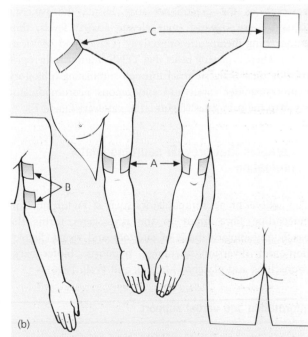

(b)

> ### Exercise
>
> Review Figures 21.3–21.6 to gain maximum benefit from the following discussion

Therapies that provide inhibitory neurotransmitter domination

Transcutaneous electrical nerve stimulation

The technique in administering transcutaneous electrical nerve stimulation (TENS) requires very little training. It involves the electrical stimulation of the nervous system using a pulse generator, an amplifier and a system of electrodes (Figure 21.9). The mode of action is controversial. Gadsby and Flowerdew (2001) suggest TENS stimulates the release of endogenous neuromodulator opioids, while Melzack and Wall (1996) suggest that it provides continuous analgesic relief by ensuring the domination of A-beta

Figure 21.9 (a) TENS machine with electrodes attached. (Photo kindly supplied by the Acumedic Centre, London.) (b) Electrode placement for brachial plexus lesion: A, complete anaesthesia below the elbow and pain in the whole hand; B, complete anaesthesia below the elbow and pain in the little and ring fingers; C, complete anaesthesia below the shoulder. *Q. How does the application of TENS relieve pain?*

afferent fibre input to the pain gates, and thus reduces the need for narcotics. The place of TENS in today's management of postoperative pain is of great doubt: some health authorities have abandoned its use since it has been tried and found to be ineffective in many cases.

Touch

Touch therapies include massage, aromatherapy, acupressure and reflexology. Their analgesic qualities stem from encouraging domination of the A-beta afferent fibres (with the mechanoreceptors at their distal ends) input to the pain gates. It may even simply involve holding a patient's hand, or lightly stroking the patient's forehead or forearm.

Reflexology – the art of foot and hand massage – brings relief from some stress while encouraging the homeostatic reflexes associated with wound healing (Clancy and McVicar, 1997). Aromatherapy is the use of essential oils that have been extracted from plants to treat problems such as dyspepsia, nausea or flatulence; the oils may be used as relaxing agents (Torrance and Serginson, 1997).

Touch therapies are designed to comfort and relax patients, and thus promote pain relief perhaps by enhancing the release of endogenous opioids. Touch promotes hypothalamic stimulation of the parasympathetic nervous system; used correctly, it can also relieve anxiety and reassure the patient that someone cares and understands (Torrance and Serginson, 1997). One must be careful with this therapy, however, as the practitioner may invade the patient's 'personal space', which may elevate anxiety levels, thus emphasizing therapeutic subjectivity (Clancy and McVicar, 1998). There is general belief that TENS and touch therapies provide dual analgesic relief through stimulating inhibitory neurotransmitter input and endogenous neuromodulator input to the pain gates (Figure 21.6, pathways D and E).

Therapies that provide neuromodulator domination

The actions of neuromodulators such as endorphins on descending fibre input to the pain gates forms the psychophysiological basis of auditory and visual distraction and diversion therapies, hypnosis, biofeedback, counselling and placebo (Melzack and Wall, 1996).

Information and verbal support

Melzack and Wall (1996) stated that anxiety could produce a physiological response similar to acute pain. Thus, the criteria that should be part of any pain management plan are based on establishing a good patient–nurse relationship, so as to reduce the patient's anxiety and fears regarding:

- their impending stay in hospital
- progression of their disease state
- different pain relief techniques
- potential complications.

The authors emphasize, however, that this information is to be provided in a manner that the patient can understand, so as to individualize care.

Anxiety promotes behavioural responses, including muscle spasms and increased sympathetic activity. The former response compromises blood flow to tissues, causing ischaemia, thus increasing pain perception via the release of pain-producing substances, such as lactic acid (a by-product of anaerobic metabolism). The latter response can lead to pulmonary problems, increased cardiovascular work, altered muscle metabolism, increased oxygen consumption, and even death. Such behavioural responses can be minimized by the nurse using appropriate communications skills to reduce the patient's anxiety and pain (Torrance and Serginson, 1997). Perhaps, then, an appropriate nursing action might be just to empathize, sit and support the patient in pain, since this physical assurance may have analgesic qualities (Clancy and McVicar, 1998). This is because of the pain–anxiety linkage. Perhaps nursing care should aim to reduce the patient's anxiety levels before attempting to quantify the pain that the patient perceives.

The reassurance and communication skills used by nurses during the patient's stay in hospital probably enhance the neuromodulator descending fibre input to the pain gates.

Relaxation, distraction and imagery techniques

Relaxation is thought to remove or reduce pain by allaying a patient's anxiety. Relaxation and distraction techniques may act on both the higher centres involved in pain perception and the pain gating mechanism (Figure 21.6).

Distraction draws attention away from the pain, focusing it to a pleasant sensory stimulus. The use of appropriate music can help the patient to relax, and simple deep breathing exercises enhance this effect (Biley, 2000; McCaffery and Good, 2000). It could be argued, however, that the music must be pleasing to the patient to be beneficial, otherwise it may be a source of irritation, raising anxiety levels and thus the patient's perception of pain.

Imagery involves the patient focusing on a situation that is completely incompatible with pain. It may include one or a combination of all senses, incorporating a pleasurable sensation. This ranges from a simple sensation, such as getting the patient to describe a favourite pastime, to a complex mental visualization, which involves deep concentration on detailed tasks. Imagery promotes relaxation, which in turn alleviates or eliminates anxiety

(Ackerman and Turkiski, 2000). The effectiveness of this therapy depends on the image used and the imagery ability of the individual patient.

Neurosurgery

Today, neurosurgeons abandon the use of such techniques in favour of non-destructive methods, such as devices that electrically stimulate nerves, the spinal cord, and discrete but accessible areas of the brain.

According to Melzack and Wall (1996), neurosurgery is regarded as being fully justified to improve the quality of life of patients who have a limited time to live, e.g. in the later stages of terminal cancer as a short-term analgesic control. However, long-term analgesia is rarely achieved and this method may be associated with additional unpleasant sensations. For example, surgical section of peripheral nerves permanently disturbs 'normal' input patterning, but may also produce 'abnormal' inputs from scar tissue.

Interim summary

Many pain therapies exist, and numerous texts are available for further details. The aetiology and management of perioperative pain is varied and sometimes complex. Management of pain requires adequate planning and skill on the part of the nurse in terms of both assessment and implementation of care. Therapies used fall into two categories: pharmacological and non-pharmacological. Analgesic drugs have actions that can be related directly to the neurophysiology of pain, especially in relation to the gating mechanisms put forward by Melzack and Wall in 1965. Non-pharmacological therapies have actions that remain debatable, although many can be related to the known neurophysiology. These alternative or complementary therapies provide potentially useful additional methods for pain relief, and can reduce the amount of analgesia used. The use of such methods emphasizes how psychosocial aspects can influence physiological processes and serve to highlight the subjective nature of pain. Therefore, any approach employed is effective only if it is adapted to the patient's individual needs. If the patient is dissatisfied, then care must be reassessed and be adapted to ensure that the patient's comfort is achieved as soon as possible.

The complexity of pain demands a multifaceted and multidisciplinary approach if the patient is to achieve effective pain relief. A prerequisite to good patient care is that the practitioner actually believes the patient. Unless this happens, one cannot get much further with pain assessment, and consequently its management. We suggest that a good understanding of the individualistic nature of the patient's pain, underpinned by a sound knowledge of the neurophysiology of pain, is essential before practitioners attempt to plan and rationalize a patient's care.

Table 21.2 The site of action of pharmacological and non-pharmacological analgesics. Essentially, successful pain management blocks the electrochemical impulses of the pain pathway at different locations en route to the brain's pain centre. Using this information, place a tick in the appropriate boxes of this table to show the proposed operational activity of the listed therapeutic interventions. Note that there may be more than one tick required for each intervention

Therapeutic interventions	Site of action						
	A	B	C	D	E	F	G
Non-opioid analgesics							
Paracetamol							
Diclofenac							
Ketoprofen							
Ketorolac							
Ibuprofen							
Naproxen							
Local anaesthetics							
Lignocaine							
Chloroprocaine							
Bupivacaine							
Etidocaine							
Procaine							
Weak opioid analgesics							
Codeine phosphate							
Co-dyaramol							
Co-proxamol							
Co-codamol							
Narcotic opioid analgesics							
Morphine							
Diamorphine							
Alfentanil							
Fentanyl							
Pethidine							
Distraction and relaxation therapies							
Transcutaneous nerve stimulation							
Verbal support							
Imagery							
Touch therapies							

A, inhibits prostaglandin synthetase; B, inhibits secretion of prostaglandin; C, inhibits secretion of bradykinin and histamine; D, activates the sodium/potassium ATPase pump; E, dominates the A-beta fibre input to the pain gates; F, blocks the secretion of substance P; G, dominates the descending neuromodulator fibre input to the pain gates

BOX 21.9 PAIN RELIEF DURING CHILDBIRTH

A broad spectrum of analgesics is used in maternity care during both normal childbirth and operative procedures. All methods of pain relief offered are to provide the optimum level of pain relief without compromising the health of the woman or fetus.

Woman today are turning increasingly to non-drug forms of pain relief for labour and childbirth, including relaxation techniques, breathing exercises to cope with the waves of labour pains, the adoption of positions that maximize comfort, aromatherapy, acupuncture, reflexology and TENS. None of these techniques, if administered by appropriately qualified professionals, has an effect on the fetus.

Hospitals now offer routine administration of Entonox® (50% oxygen, 50% nitrous oxide) via a face mask or mouthpiece. This method is very popular, as it is controlled by the woman and has the added benefit of aiding fetal oxygenation.

Also available is the narcotic pethidine, a powerful analgesic with sedative and antispasmodic effects. The dosage ranges from 50 to 200 mg, and may be prescribed and administered by a midwife for a woman in labour. Unfortunately, pethidine is not strong enough to completely remove labour pain, but it does enable most women to cope with labour. There are a number of side effects, including nausea and vomiting, for which an anti-emetic is provided, loss of self-control, and reduction in blood pressure. The drug passes through the placental barrier and affects the fetus: if the baby is delivered within 2–3 h of administration, pethidine may cause drowsiness and delay in the onset of respiration or respiratory depression, requiring the antagonist naloxone hydrochloride 0.01 mg/kg to reverse the effects.

Regional epidural analgesia is now available in most maternity units; this is performed by an experienced anaesthetist. Improvements in local anaesthetics have improved the effects of the block provided, and women are now more able to move freely after administration; a 'mobile epidural' allows the woman to bear weight and even to walk/mobilize. An epidural may be topped up with stronger anaesthetics in cases where operative vaginal or abdominal delivery is required.

In the event of elective or emergency Caesarean section, spinal (subarachnoid) analgesia is used, in which local anaesthetic is introduced into the subarachnoid space between L2 and L5 (see Figure 8.4) Spinal analgesia has a rapid effect, and is quicker to perform than an epidural. Postoperative pain management is usually in the form of narcotics, with epidural top-up from narcotics or bupivacaine.

ASSESSMENT OF PAIN

Pain and nursing are linked inextricably, because assessment and management of the pain process is one of the most common roles of the nurse. The measurement of pain, however, is a contentious and controversial issue with debate from two schools of thought. One school of thought believes that pain measurement is necessary and feasible. Certainly, communication is an essential step towards measurement and relief of pain. Therefore, problems in communication and poor understanding of the complexity of pain can result in its poor management. However, it must be stated that the ward environment influences the success of communication. For example, critical care patients are often vulnerable to communication barriers, such as the presence of highly technical equipment and the sight of other critically ill patients. Technical equipment may increase or decrease anxiety levels, since its presence may or may not aid the patient's understanding of their condition and may or may alleviate the fear of the unknown. The presence of other critically ill patients also may or may not increase anxiety, according to individual experience.

A second school of thought believes that pain experiences can never be measured because of the subjective nature of pain. In support of this, there are numerous pain assessment studies, which have demonstrated that nurses tend to underestimate the patient's pain, and that if assessment of pain is judged simply on a patient's behaviour (such as restlessness, groaning or grimacing), it can be misleading. In addition, classical signs such as an increased heart rate and lowered blood pressure may also be absent in some patients experiencing pain, thus exposing the dangers of using generalizations.

Both schools of thought emphasize that there is no easy way of understanding what a patient is suffering, or of conveying information from one person to another, although doctors, nurses and other healthcare practitioners need to do so.

In short, many factors affect pain assessment, and these are often interrelated. They all stem from the complex nature of pain, and one cannot expect a certain stimulus to produce a predictable outcome, as other factors may intervene. Melzack and Wall (1996), who stated that pain could not be measured directly so one cannot be sure how much pain someone is suffering, support this. It could also be argued, however, that accurate pain assessment and measurement are essential if the sufferer is to obtain appropriate and successful pain relief.

Clinicians treating patients need to know how the pain changes throughout the day, the descriptive quality of pain, and whether there are any aggravating or relieving factors. Perhaps such information will make clinical diagnosis more accurate and allow easier evaluation of treatments.

An individualized approach to the assessment and control of pain is the obvious solution. This is easier said than done, because in order to assess pain, one must take into account individuality with respect to those who have the pain (patients) and those who are trying to assess it (practitioners).

Patient factors

Patient factors affect the patient's expression of pain, rather than the amount of pain perceived, and consequently assessment must also be affected. This is complicated further by the fact that patients have difficulty in describing the pain and in expressing its location.

Cultural backgrounds

Different cultures have different socialization attitudes and behaviours, thus the cultural background of the patient may be responsible for some aspects of inadequate pain assessment and management. It is important to recognize how cultural bias can influence patient care.

Personality typing

Anxiety is heightened by hospitalization and surgery, and therefore exacerbates the patient's interpretation of pain. Personality and anxiety can be interrelated; this is supported by the historical findings of Friedman and Rosenmann, who, in 1974, correlated personality types A, B, and C with the incidence of anxiety-provoked myocardial infarctions.

Social class

Social class is an instrumental factor in pain assessment. If the nurse's and patient's social classes are comparable, then more sympathy and better management of pain ensues. Patients from higher social classes are usually more effective in expressing their pain, and thus are more likely to receive better pain management. Language, therefore, is another significant factor, and impairment of communication (e.g. impaired hearing or sight, or foreign languages) makes pain assessment, and hence management, more difficult (Melzack and Wall, 1996).

Past experience

The patient's past experiences are significant, since attitudes to pain and suffering are, in part, socially learned responses and hence affect one's judgement of pain and what the pain means to the patient. For example, a lay person having an electrocardiogram (ECG) for the first time may suffer psychosomatic pain if the practitioner does not clarify that the electrodes do not produce painful electric currents when they are applied to the chest and limbs. However, on

---

BOX 21.10 PRACTITIONER FACTORS IN THE ASSESSMENT OF PAIN

The factors that affect the patient's experience and interpretation of pain are equally likely to affect that of the practitioner, since individual differences are evident according to nature–nurture interactions. In addition, a number of other factors are important. Some authorities believe that training has placed the responsibility of pain control with the doctors; consequently, nurses are unaware of their importance in pain control. Nursing training affects attitudes to painkillers, and misplaced concerns, such as opioid analgesic addiction and dependency, may cause the nurse to give less than the prescribed analgesia, both in terms of frequency and amount (Bell, 2000). Therefore, a more realistic training in pharmacology would help reduce such fears and would benefit patient care (McQuillan et al., 1996).

The practitioner has to infer the amount of pain and suffering a patient is experiencing, since it cannot be assessed directly. Although complex, it is our view that knowledge of the nature–nurture interactions associated with the subjective nature of pain is therefore essential to improving the practitioner's assessment and management of pain. The nurse's own beliefs and values might influence their assessment of pain, and they must be aware of this in order to be objective.

Pain relief may be affected further by busy ward routines, staff shortages and frequent staff changes, all of which increase the difficulties in establishing a good practitioner–patient relationship. Frequent patient changeover in a ward also affects patient–patient relationships, which can affect the expression of pain by the patient. Thus, ward policy may influence assessment, and hence pain management. Current cost-cutting changes to the skill mix in nursing may well compound the problem.

It will always be difficult to assess adequately an individual's perception of pain, because of the complexity in understanding subjectivity. The concept of 'holistic' care attempts to close this gap and minimize the differences between practitioner and patient assessments, which still exist. Superficially, pain assessment seems easy, and nurses may underestimate the difficulties associated with pain perception/assessment. In addition, communication skills need time and training to develop, and may cause inaccuracies in assessment (Davies and McVicar, 2000): some patients assume that the practitioner knows when they are in pain, and some nurses assume that patients will report their pain. It is not surprising that the pain then goes unchecked, and is controlled inadequately. Thus, there needs to be a good working relationship between the patient and the practitioner in which both parties must have mutual trust in each another.

subsequent visits, when the person has had time to reflect on the method, socially learned responses result in the individual not experiencing psychosomatic pain.

Location of the pain

The location of the pain is important, since some areas of the body are more acceptable discussion topics than others. For example, rectal pain may be an 'unacceptable' topic for discussion, and needs to be assessed differently from pain associated with a sore finger.

Gender differences

Gender differences need to be taken into consideration when assessing a patient's pain, since in westernized societies males tend to be socialized into being courageous, and females into expressing their emotions. McCaffery and Ferrel (1992) demonstrated that generally there are differences in how a nurse thinks men and women respond to pain. They observed that, of 362 nurses, approximately one-third argued that there were gender differences in pain expression. Regarding the patient's pain tolerance, approximately 50% of the nurses thought that females tolerated pain better than males, while only 15% thought men had a better tolerance. Pain and distress trends seemed to be reversed: 41% believed men showed greater distress when in pain, while only 18% believed women exhibited more distress. Fifty-three per cent,

compared with 27%, believed that men rather than women were likely to under-report their pain. However, the practitioner must not sexually stereotype the relationship, since this would not be treating the patient as an individual.

Interim summary

The experience of pain is so complex, being influenced by many variables (subjective to the patient and practitioner), that the practitioner may or may not be able to predict them. It must be stressed, however, that at all times it is important not to stereotype the factors mentioned above. For example, when caring for patients from different cultures, the practitioner must be aware not only that cultural difference exists in pain expression, but also that those individual differences occur within each culture. That is, if the practitioner expects a Caucasian patient to be stoic and they are not, then there may be a danger that they could be labelled as attention seeking or even malingering. Thus, it is still the patient who is the only one who knows how much pain he/she has. The patient must be involved, whenever possible, in any assessment of pain. An individualized approach in assessing and controlling pain is the obvious solution. To conclude, nurses who operate on the basis of stereotyping (cultural, gender, social class, etc.) are in danger of ignoring the individuality of pain perception, and consequently pain assessment and management become unsatisfactory.

BOX 21.11 THE CLINICAL MEASUREMENT OF PAIN

An accurate assessment of pain is essential for adequate therapy. The subjective nature of pain, both in the sufferer and in the observations made by the health practitioner, makes assessment difficult. This section highlights the strengths and shortcomings of frequently used clinical assessment methods.

Measurements of pain involve informal and formal observations. The informal observations are made when the patient is unaware that he/she is being assessed, since this is when the most natural reactions occur. These involve monitoring facial expression, difficulties in performing physical movement, and mood. Formal observations encourage a more accurate assessment, and are important in providing continuity of care. They stress the objective measurements performed by doctors and nurses, and are based on the patient's experiences and comments, and the observer's own experience of pain and/or traditional/cultural beliefs about pain and the level to be expressed in a given illness, etc. Verbal report is of obvious significance: we hope this chapter has implied that, owing to nature–nurture interactions, pain occurs when the patient says it does.

A 'word' scale could be used in the clinical measurement of pain, but these are open to distortion and observer bias. More attention is thus currently being paid to pain involving the patient's own estimate of pain as a basis for treatment. Such measures include the scales and charts detailed below. The article by Stephenson and Herman (2000) compares different pain scales.

Simple verbal rating scales

For example: No pain. Mild pain. Moderate pain. Severe pain. Unbearable pain.

Verbal rating scales (descriptive scales) are crude, and give only a rough approximation of the pain experienced. In addition, individuals cannot be compared readily. Although these scales are easy to use, they can have a limited usefulness in that there may be:

- misinterpretation of words by the patient/practitioner;
- a limit to the number of words one uses;
- different assumptions made by the practitioner or patient that the intervals between the words are of equal value.

Descriptive scales also are too complicated for use in acute pain.

Visual analogue scale

Visual analogue scales (VASs), also known as graphic rating scales, have been used in an attempt to overcome the problem of expressing 'pain language'. The analogue scale might consist of a line 100 cm long:

No pain   Worst possible pain

————————————————100 cm————————————————

The patient marks the line, and this represents the level of pain at that moment. The distance of the mark from the left end is measured and is called the 'pain score'. This may be repeated several times each day to form the basis of a pain profile for the patient. This type of scale avoids the use of gradation, reduces the misinterpretation of language, is user friendly, and may be modified to assess pain relief by having 'no pain relief' and 'complete pain relief' at opposite ends of the scale.

Shortcomings of the scale are that it is an abstract concept that can be difficult to understand, most answers cluster around the extremes of the scale with little use of the midpoints, and the relevance to patients experiencing acute pain is questionable.

Both the verbal and visual scales view pain one-dimensionally, since they do not take into account other variables that may have an impact on the amount of pain experienced.

Numerical scales

Numerical scales use a continuum comprising a numerical rating scale of either 0–10 or 0–100, with 0 signifying no pain and 10 or 100 signifying unbearable pain. These scales allow greater sensitivity and avoid misinterpretation of the meanings of words. Such scales are used commonly in assessing pain associated with acute myocardial infarction patients, relating pain scores with morphine requirements.

The pain thermometer

The pain thermometer ('painmeter'), designed by the Burford Nursing Development Unit at Oxford, UK (Figure 21.10), acts as a visual aid for the patient to describe their pain experience. It has been used extensively in the care of the elderly, because patients find it easy to understand. The practitioner and the patient decide how often the painmeter is to be used, and analgesia can be administered accordingly. Although limited in range, it may be helpful in assisting the nurse to improve the control of pain relief.

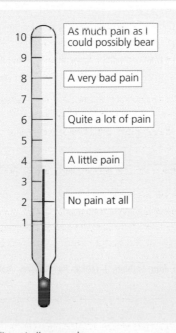

Figure 21.10   The pain thermometer.

The London Hospital pain observation chart

The London Hospital pain chart (Figure 21.11) improves communication between the practitioner and the patient by making the recording of pain more systematic. It makes the information that is useful when making decisions about the management of pain readily available in one place. The chart focuses attention on the mechanisms of different pains by recording each site of pain separately, and is a means of communication to be used with the patient, not on the patient. Occasionally, the patient keeps one chart and the staff keeps another.

The McGill–Melzack pain questionnaire

Rather than viewing pain as a specific sensory experience, this questionnaire attempts to measure pain on a broader level by categorizing it into dimensions of pain experience: the sensory, affective and evaluative levels (Figure 21.12). From the list presented, the patient selects the words that best describes their pain; from these measurements, the pain is assessed quantifiably and quantitatively (the higher the total score, the greater the pain).

The questionnaire is used frequently in clinical practice, mainly for work in pain clinics with chronic pain sufferers. However, difficulties arise in the interpretation of the words into the dimension of pain experienced, and it appears difficult to adapt its bulky format to the acute pain setting. Possibly the questionnaire benefits from being used with other assessment tools, and is in need of some refinement before it can become widely applicable.

Home diaries

Home diaries are useful in combining measurements with the patient's description of the pain (Figure 21.13). These include how the pain changes with respect to time, the precipitating factors of pain, and the success of the analgesic method used to alleviate the pain.

Indirect clinical measures of pain

Such techniques depend on the effect that pain has on bodily functions, or on the amount of analgesia required to bring pain relief. Specific measures have been developed for use in specific clinical environments, e.g. the following questions could be used in the coronary care setting:

1 How do you feel? Describe the sensation.
2 Where does it hurt?
3 Does the sensation travel anywhere?
4 Did anything trigger it off?
5 How long did it last?
6 Has anything made it worse or better?
7 Are there any other relevant signs or symptoms?

This has the advantage of being a quick procedure with the questions overlapping with each other in the scope of the answers, and allowing a place for physical signs and symptoms that may be relevant. The disadvantages of the method are that the replies cannot be standardized, and the assessment is still subjected to the practitioner's interpretation of the patient's reply.

This chart records where a patient's pain is and how bad it is, by the nurse asking the patient at regular intervals. If analgesics are being given regularly, make an observation with each dose and another half-way between each dose. If analgesics are given only 'as required', observe two-hourly. When the observations are stable and the patient is comfortable, any regular time interval between observations may be chosen.

To use this chart, ask the patient to mark all his or her pains on the body diagram below. Label each site of pain with a letter (i.e. A, B, C, etc).

Then at each observation time ask the patient to assess:

1. The pain in each separate site since the last observation.
   Use the scale above the body diagram, and enter the number or letter in the appropriate column.

2. The pain overall since the last observation. Use the same scale and enter in column marked overall.

Next, record what has been done to relieve pain. In particular:

3. Note any analgesic given since the last observation, stating name, dose, route and time given.

4. Tick any other nursing care or action taken to ease pain.

Finally note any comment on pain from patient or nurse (use the back of the chart as well, if necessary) and initial the record.

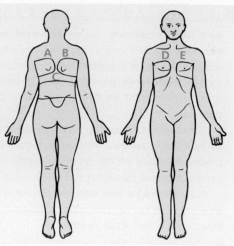

| Date _____ | Sheet number _____ | Patient identification label |

Time	Pain rating By sites								Overall	Measures to relieve pain (specify where starred)								Comments from patients and/or staff	Initials
	A	B	C	D	E	F	G	H		Analgesic given (Name, dose, route, time)	Lifting	Turning	Massage	Distracting activities	Position change*	Additional aids*	Other*		

The complete Pain Observation Chart.
Adapted from the London Hospital Pain Observation Chart

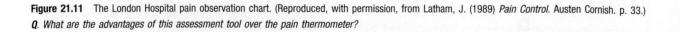

Figure 21.11 The London Hospital pain observation chart. (Reproduced, with permission, from Latham, J. (1989) *Pain Control.* Austen Cornish. p. 33.)

Q. What are the advantages of this assessment tool over the pain thermometer?

Figure 21.12 The McGill—Melzack pain questionnaire.

1	8	16
Flickering	Tingling	Annoying
Quivering	Itchy	Troublesome
Pulsing	Smarting	Miserable
Throbbing	Stinging	Intense
Beating	**9**	Unbearable
Pounding	Dull	**17**
2	Sore	Spreading
Jumping	Hurting	Radiating
Flashing	Aching	Penetrating
Shooting	Heavy	Piercing
3	**10**	**18**
Pricking	Tender	Tight
Boring	Taut	Numb
Drilling	Rasping	Drawing
Stabbing	Splitting	Squeezing
Lancinating	**11**	Tearing
4	Tiring	**19**
Sharp	Exhausting	Cool
Cutting	**12**	Cold
Lacerating	Sickening	Freezing
5	Suffocating	**20**
Pinching	**13**	Nagging
Pressing	Fearful	Nauseating
Gnawing	Frightful	Agonizing
Cramping	Terrifying	Dreadful
Crushing	**14**	Torturing
6	Punishing	**PPI**
Tugging	Gruelling	0 No pain
Pulling	Cruel	1 Mild
Wrenching	Vicious	2 Discomforting
7	Killing	3 Distressing
Hot	**15**	4 Horrible
Burning	Wretched	5 Excruciating
Scalding	Binding	
Searing		Constant
		Periodic
		Brief

This questionnaire enables researchers to compare to some extent people's level of pain. Each descriptive word carries its own score – the lower down in its group, the higher its value. The sum of the scores gives what is termed a person's "pain rating index" – in other words, their overall pain intensity. The final "present pain intensity" (PPI) section gives an idea of the pain level at the moment the questionnaire is completed.

Interim summary

The use of pain assessment tools has been shown to improve pain control and aid care. The tools, however, are still not in common practice. Introducing a pain system of measurement would improve the practitioner's awareness of pain, which would inevitably result in improved patient care. However, the tool that is chosen depends on the type of pain, the clinical setting, and the patient group, among other factors. Measurement tools are essential to avoid possible difficulties in practitioner–patient communication, and therefore to avoid unnecessary patient suffering. However, it could be argued that the assessment of pain barely considers the patient's social, psychological and neurophysiological factors, all of which must be considered if assessment is to be accurate. The development of appropriate assessment tools specific to certain clinical settings must be considered of vital importance in the practitioner's bid to improve the quality of patient care.

Exercise

What factors should be taken into consideration when assessing pain? List the clinical tools used to assess pain, and comment on the usefulness and drawbacks of the tools mentioned in this chapter.

	Notes of any different pain, symptom or problem, and any unusual activity or exercise during each day	Any other comments
Day 1		
Day 2		
Day 3		
Day 4		
Day 5		
Day 6		
Day 7		

HOME DIARY

NAME...............................

DATE STARTED ....

How to fill in the home diary

1 *Sleep:* In this column, fill in hours slept, then ring word that best describes how much your pain disturbed your rest.

2 *Pain:* In the column for each part of the day, write the number of doses of painkiller (tablets, spoonfuls) taken. Then choose the best word to describe your pain for that part of the day. Put in the chart the *pain number* next to the word you chose.

3 On the back of the diary, make a note of any different pains, symptoms or problems, and note any unusual activities or exercise that day.

4 Add any other comments of your own.

Excruciating	5
Very severe	4
Severe	3
Moderate	2
Just noticeable	1
No pain at all	0

	Sleep	Morning (to 12 noon)	Afternoon (noon to 4pm)	Early evening (4 – 8 pm)	Late evening (from 8 pm)
Day 1	Hours of sleep Pain disturbed sleep never/a bit/often/a lot	No. of painkillers Pain number	No. of painkillers Pain number	No. of painkillers Pain number	No. of painkillers Pain number
Day 2	Hours of sleep Pain disturbed sleep never/a bit/often/a lot	No. of painkillers Pain number	No. of painkillers Pain number	No. of painkillers Pain number	No. of painkillers Pain number
Day 3	Hours of sleep Pain disturbed sleep never/a bit/often/a lot	No. of painkillers Pain number	No. of painkillers Pain number	No. of painkillers Pain number	No. of painkillers Pain number
Day 4	Hours of sleep Pain disturbed sleep never/a bit/often/a lot	No. of painkillers Pain number	No. of painkillers Pain number	No. of painkillers Pain number	No. of painkillers Pain number
Day 5	Hours of sleep Pain disturbed sleep never/a bit/often/a lot	No. of painkillers Pain number	No. of painkillers Pain number	No. of painkillers Pain number	No. of painkillers Pain number
Day 6	Hours of sleep Pain disturbed sleep never/a bit/often/a lot	No. of painkillers Pain number	No. of painkillers Pain number	No. of painkillers Pain number	No. of painkillers Pain number
Day 7	Hours of sleep Pain disturbed sleep never/a bit/often/a lot	No. of painkillers Pain number	No. of painkillers Pain number	No. of painkillers Pain number	No. of painkillers Pain number

Figure 21.13 Home diary.

Summary

1 Melzack and Wall's gate control theory of pain perception is a credible model that explains pain perception and control.

2 Pain perception is dependent on the balance of afferent neuron input to the gating mechanisms, and, the descending neuron input to the gating mechanisms. If the afferent pain fibre input dominates, the gate is 'open' and one perceives pain. If the mechanoreceptors afferent input and/or the descending neuron input dominate, then the gate is 'closed' and pain is not perceived.

3 Pain is a subjective experience that depends on the nature–nurture interactions that determine the characteristics of the individual. Subjectivity is determined by the individual's unique blend of genes and his/her unique environmental experiences.

4 The subjective nature of pain has wide implications for assessing, evaluating, planning and monitoring the care of people in pain. Thus, the complexity of pain states demands a multifaceted and multidisciplinary approach if the patient is to achieve effective pain relief.

5 Assessment of pain is multifactorial. It is affected by factors attributed to the patient, the practitioner, ward policy and hospital environments, and it must be questioned whether it can really be assessed adequately.

6 Pain assessment tools, it could be argued, are of limited use in measuring pain. Their usefulness is largely in monitoring the effectiveness/appropriateness of the analgesic method used, and the effectiveness of the practitioner in managing the patient's pain.

7 A prerequisite to good patient care is that the practitioner actually believes the patient. Unless this happens one cannot get much further with pain assessment, and consequently its management. We suggest that a good understanding of the individualistic nature of the patient's pain is essential before practitioners attempt to plan and rationalize a patient's care.

8 Biomedical and physiological research have provided great understanding of some dimensions associated with pain, and psychological research has increased knowledge of the relationships between stress, anxiety and pain. Psychometric studies have generated various methods of measuring pain. However, because of the complexity of the phenomenon we call 'pain', there are many unanswered questions; continued research into the interrelations of these disciplines is the only way forward to unfold some of these mysteries.

Review questions

1 Pain seems to be an unnecessary and distressing nuisance for patients and nurses creating discomfort and anxiety. What are the purposes of pain?

2 What is a nociceptor?

3 What role do histamine and prostaglandins play in our experience of pain? Bear in mind that some drugs act to reduce prostaglandin synthesis, e.g. aspirin.

4 Pain is conveyed to the brain via sensory A-delta and C fibres. Which fibres are myelinated?

5 What effect does myelination have on impulse transmission?

6 What do you understand by the term 'pain threshold'?

7 What factors may lessen a persons' pain threshold?

8 Why might a marathon runner who has sprained an ankle during a race only feel pain after he/she has finished the race?

9 Make short notes on the gate control theory to explain why rubbing a site of injury will reduce the feeling of pain from that area.

10 Using your knowledge gained from Melzack and Wall's gate control theory of pain suggest: (i) why pain is regarded as an individualized perception; and (ii) how a knowledge of integrated science helps in the understanding of pain control.

11 How can a knowledge of integrated science help a nurse contribute more effectively to the assessment of pain in patients?

REFERENCES

Ackerman, C.J. and Turkiski, B. (2000) Using guided imagery to reduce pain and anxiety. *Home Healthcare Nurse* **18**(8): 524–30.

Biley, F.C. (2000) The effects on patient well-being of music listening as a nursing intervention: a review of the literature. *Journal of Clinical Nursing* (5): 668–77.

Bell, F. (2000) A review of the literature on the attitudes of nurses to acute pain management. *Journal of Orthopaedic Nursing* **4**(2): 64–70.

Bennett, G.J. (2000) Update on the neurophysiology of pain transmission and modulation: focus on the NMDA-receptor ... NMDA-receptor antagonists: evolving role in analgesia, proceedings of a meeting sponsored by Algos Pharmaceutical Corporation, New York City, *Journal of Pain and Symptom Management* **19**(1S suppl): S2–6.

British National Formulary (2000) London: British Medical Association and Royal Pharmaceutical Society for Great Britain.

Carr, E. (1997) Overcoming barriers to effective pain control. *Professional Nurse* **12**(6): 13–20.

Chen, B. and Chang, M (2000) Anxiety and depression in Taiwanese cancer patients with and without pain. *Journal of Advanced Nursing* **32**(4): 944–51.

Clancy, J. and McVicar, A.J. (1997) Wound Healing: a series of homeostatic responses. *British Journal of Theatre Nursing* **7**(4): 25–33.

Clancy, J. and McVicar, A.J. (1998) Neurophysiology of pain. *British Journal of Theatre Nursing* **7**(10): 15–24.

Cosentino, B.W. (2000) Guided visualization and imagery for chronic pain. *Nursing Spectrum* (New York/New Jersey Metro edn) **12A**(10): 8–9.

Cunningham, M. (2000) Chronic pain: potential sequel of cancer and cancer treatment ... reprinted with permission from Mary Cunningham, MS, RN, AOCN. *Missouri Nurse* **69**(6): 8–9.

Davidhizar, R., Dowd, S. and Giger, J.N. (1997) Cultural differences in pain management. *Technology* **64**(4): 345–8.

Davies, J. and McVicar, A.J. (2000) Clinical practice. Issues in effective pain control 1: assessment and education. *International Journal of Palliative Nursing* **6**(2): 58, 60–5.

Desjardins, P.J. (2000) Patient pain and anxiety: the medical and psychological challenges facing oral and maxillofacial surgery. *Journal of Oral and Maxillofacial Surgery* **58**(10 Suppl 2): 1–3, 2000.

Dobson, F. (1997) Anatomy and physiology of pain. *British Journal of Community Nursing* **2**(6): 283–91.

Ehde, D.M., Czerniecki, J.M., Smith, D.G., Campbell, K.M., Edwards, W.T., Jenson, M.P. and Robinson, L.R. (2000) Chronic phantom sensations, phantom pain, residual limb pain, and other regional pain after lower limb amputation. *Archives of Physical Medicine and Rehabilitation* **81**(8): 1039–44.

Field, L. (1996) Are nurses still underestimating patient's pain postoperatively? *British Journal of Nursing* (bd>5,bd>)(13): 778–84.

Fitzsimons, D., Parahoo, K. and Stringer, M. (2000) Waiting for coronary artery bypass surgery: a qualitative analysis. *Journal of Advanced Nursing* **32**(5): 1243–52.

Friedman, H. and Rosenmann, R.H. (1974) *Type A Behaviour and Your Heart*. London: Wildwood.

Horn, S. and Munafo, M. (1997) *Pain: theory, research and intervention*. Buckingham, UK: Open University press.

Gadsby, J.G. and Flowerdew, M.W. (2001) Transcutaneous electrical nerve stimulation and acupuncture-like transcutaneous electrical nerve stimulation for chronic low back pain. The Cochrane Library. Oxford: Update Software.

Johnson, M.I. (2000) The clinical effectiveness of TENS in pain management. *Critical Reviews in Physical and Rehabilitation Medicine* **12**(2): 131–49.

Mann, E. and Redwood, S. (2000) Clinical. Improving pain management: breaking down the invisible barrier. *British Journal of Nursing* **9**(19): 2067–72.

McCaffery, M. (1983) Nursing the Patient in Pain. London: Harper Row.

McCaffery, M. and Ferrell, B.R. (1992) Does the gender gap affect your pain control? *Nursing* **22**(8): 48–51.

McCaffrey, R.G. and Good, M. (2000) The lived experience of listening to music while recovering from surgery. *Journal of Holistic Nursing* **18**(4): 378–90.

McQuillan, R., Finlay, I., Branch, C., Roberts, D. and Spencer, M. (1996) Improving analgesic prescribing in a general teaching hospital. *Journal of Pain and Symptom Management* **11**(3): 172–80.

Melzack, R. and Wall, P.D. (1965) Cited in Melzack and Wall (1996).

Melzack, R. and Wall, P.D. (1996). *The Challenge of Pain*, updated 2nd edn. London: Penguin.

Omoigui, S. (1995) *The Pain Drugs Handbook*. London: Mosby.

Parsons, G. (2000) Patient controlled analgesia was more effective than nurse controlled analgesia after cardiac surgery. *Evidence-Based Nursing* **3**(2): 53.

Redeker, N.S., Tamburri, L. and Howland, C.L. (1998) Prehospital correlates of sleep in patients hospitalized with cardiac disease. *Research in Nursing and Health* **21**(1): 27–37.

Reilly, M.P. (2000) Clinical applications of acupuncture in anesthesia practice. *CRNA – the Clinical Forum for Nurse Anesthetists* **11**(4): 173–9.

Schofield, P. and Davis, B. (2000) Sensory stimulation (snoezelen) versus relaxation: a potential strategy for the management of chronic pain. *Disability and Rehabilitation* **22**(15): 675–82.

Stephenson, N.L. and Herman, J. (2000) Research brief. Pain measurement: a comparison using horizontal and vertical analogue scales. *Applied Nursing Research* **13**(3): 157–8.

Szirony, G.M. (2000) A psychophysiological view of pain: mind-body interaction in the rehabilitation of injury and illness. *Work: a Journal of Prevention, Assessment and Rehabilitation* **15**(1): 55–60.

Thomas, V.J., Heath, M.L., Rose, D. and Flory, P. (1995) Psychological characteristics and the effectiveness of patient controlled analgesia. *British Journal of Anaesthesia* **74**: 271–6.

Thomas, N. (1996) Patient controlled analgesia. *Nursing Standard* **14**(47): 49–53.

Torrance, C. and Serginson, E. (1997) *Surgical Nursing*. London: Baillière Tindall.

Wright, A. (1999) Recent concepts in the neurophysiology of pain. *Manual Therapy* **4**(4): 196–202.

Zeppetella, G., O'Doherty, C.A. and Collins, S. (2000) Prevalence and characteristics of breakthrough pain in cancer patients admitted to a hospice. *Journal of Pain and Symptom Management* **20**(2): 87–92.

FURTHER READING

Wiffen, P., Collins, S., McQuay, H., Carroll, D., Jadad, J. and Moore, A. (2001). Anticonvulsant drugs for acute and chronic pain. The Cochrane Library. Oxford: Update Software.

Williams, J. (2000) Clinical management. Critical appraisal of invasive therapies used to treat chronic pain and cancer pain. *European Journal of Palliative Care* **7**(4): 121–5.

Stress

INTRODUCTION

Stress is an inextricable part of life, according to the physiologist Selye (1976), 'essentially reflected by the rate of all the wear and tear caused by life.' Stress is evident to most people, since it manifests itself with obvious, often visible physiological and psychological body responses. Responses to particular stressful situations are highly individualistic, hence there is a strong subjective element. An understanding of stress has contributed considerably to the present understanding of health and illness. The existence of a link between stress and illness has grown to near-acceptance in the scientific world. According to Clancy and McVicar (1998a), few people now doubt that physiological and psychological factors play an important role in mental health and physical disease.

The multi-definitional aspects of stress will be explored briefly in this chapter. We suggest that stress is a psychophysiological response (since mind–body interactions are inseparable) caused by environmental stressors. Nature–nurture interactions will be the main focus in describing the subjective nature of stressors, the stress response and coping methods. Stress-related illnesses will also be discussed with this nature–nurture template in mind. The stress models used in reviewing this subjectivity are the transactional theory of Cox and McKay, a physiological theory called the general adaptation syndrome (GAS) described by Selye, and a modified GAS or psychophysiological model put forward by Selye and Lazarus.

Definitions of stress

Various attempts have been made to find a suitable definition of stress. We can conclude that stress has different connotations for different people.

Stimulus-based definition

A layperson often views stress as an environmental incident (stimulus) that causes strain within the body in the form of fatigue and/or distress (Figure 22.1(a)). These environmental stresses for the person could be, for example, a situation or conditions at work, the formalities of a divorce process, the highly technical equipment used

> **BOX 22.1 NURSES NEED TO UNDERSTAND STRESS**
>
> It essential that nurses have a clear understanding of the subjectivity of stress in everyday life, in relation to illness, and in the process of hospitalization. Because of their contact with patients and their relatives and loved ones, nurses are in an ideal position to take action to prevent unnecessary stress and to minimize and alleviate prolonged stress. Nurses with this insight will be able to cope effectively with their own stress and that of their peers, colleagues and patients and their relatives (see Box 22.3).

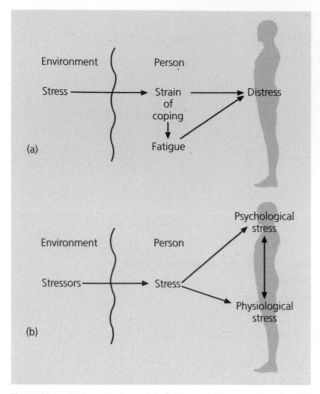

Figure 22.1 (a) Layperson's model of stress. (b) Response-based model of stress.

Q. Differentiate between stressors and stress.

in the intensive care setting, or lifestyle problems created after being diagnosed HIV positive.

Such stimulus-based definitions are incomplete, since any situation may or may not be stressful, depending on the individual and the meaning of the situation for that person.

Response-based definition

Although there is no generally accepted definition of 'a state of stress' in biological or social systems, biologists and behavioural scientists continue to use the term. Biologists and medical scientists tend to be concerned with the sources of stress that are concrete and observable, and can otherwise be considered as 'causes' of illness and injury. The response-based definition views stress as a person's bodily physiological and/or psychological responses to environmental stressors. What is not explained satisfactorily is the uniqueness of these stressors to individuals, and the individual responses, presumably because the complexity of humans always makes it impossible to comprehend fully the interrelationships of psychological and physiological (mind–body) processes that arise due to environmental influences. Thus, the layperson's environmental stresses are recognized as stressors to the biomedical scientist, and it is the accumulation of these that produces stress within

the body. This can be identified as physiological stress or psychological stress. However, these two disciplines are inseparable from each another (Figure 22.1(b)) and from the environment. For example, in anxiety provoked by an environmental threat, one may become consciously aware of a faster and more powerful heart beat (a physiological stress indicator), which in turn may increase the person's perception of their anxiety state (a psychological stress indicator). We may never know which indicator is the starting trigger. Thus, in reality, anxiety is described better as a psychophysiological bodily state induced by environmental stressors.

Social and behavioural scientists tend to be concerned with sources of stress that represent information arising from outside the person, and responses are mediated by higher centres of the brain. It is clear that such psychological stresses can lead to alterations of internal functions, even at the biochemical level, and that these are potential causes of disease. Equally, psychological responses are a consequence of biochemical (enzymatic) changes induced by gene expression. These are not, however, independent of other mechanisms, including environmental stressors, which ultimately are of a sociocultural origin. In other words, the sources of stress are environmental/social stressors outside (exogenous) and/or inside (endogenous) the body that may produce a psychophysiological stress response.

Selye (1956) defined stress as 'the non-specific response of the body and that freedom from stress is death.' This definition views stress as being the nonspecific (i.e. common) result of any mental or somatic demand placed upon the body. That is, stress is the response to a 'threat' (i.e. a change in the environment), and its integrity is based on evaluating the information received.

The authors view perceptional stress as being a disturbed homeostasis, which manifests itself by many psychophysiological indicators (Table 22.1). Thus, although historically stress has been viewed in terms of physiological, psychological and sociological phenomena, the authors feel that theorists need to integrate the scientific disciplines in order to appreciate the subjective nature of stress.

A generally accepted historical definition of stress is 'a state which arises from an actual or perceived demand–capability imbalance in the organism's vital adjustment actions which is partially manifested by a nonspecific response' (Lazarus and Folkman, 1984).

This definition emphasizes the continuity between physiological and psychological theory. However, the authors feel the need for a wider definition in order to integrate the three disciplines, and view stress as being a psychophysiological homeostatic imbalance that arises when there is an actual and/or perceived demand–capability mismatch between the individual and his/her environment. In other words, what was referred to briefly in the introduction as the interactionist or transactional model of stress.

Table 22.1 Some psychophysiological indicators of the stress response

Physical indicators	Behavioural indicators	Emotional indicators
▲ High blood pressure	● Poor work performance	● Emotional outbursts/crying
● Increased heart rate	● Accidents at work and home	● Irritability with people
● Increased respiratory rate	● Overindulgence in smoking, alcohol and drugs	▲ Depression
▲ Increased muscle tension	● Loss of interest	● Tendency to blame others
▲ Increased restlessness	● Daydreaming	● Hostile and insulting behaviour
▲ Upset stomach	● Diminished attention to detail	● Tiredness
● Sweaty palms	● Forgetfulness	● Anxiety
● Loss of appetite	● Mental blocking	
▲ Indigestion or heartburn	▲ Social isolation	
● Change in sleep patterns	▲ Marital and family breakdowns	
▲ Tension headaches		
▲ Cold hands and feet		
▲ Nausea		
▲ Nail biting		
▲ Constipation or diarrhoea		
▲ Backache		

Note: The above are termed psychophysiological indicators because physical, behavioural and emotional indicators are inseparable, being both cause and effect, i.e.

Physical ⟷ Behavioural
Emotional

Q. Distinguish between exogenous and endogenous stressors.

● Usually short-term effects. ▲ Usually long-term effects.

Stress is generally thought of and expressed in a negative sense, with a view that stress is potentially harmful when the stress threshold is reached or super-

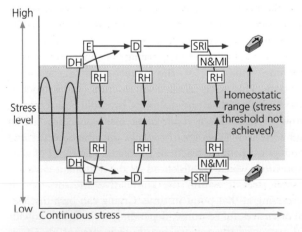

Figure 22.2 Perceptual stress: a disturbed homeostasis.
Q. Define the concept of stress threshold.

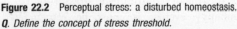

D, distress; DH, disturbed homeostasis (stress threshold reached or superseded); E, eustress; N&MI, nursing and medical intervention; RH, re-established homeostasis; SRI, stress-related illness, death.

seded. The threshold is the minimum cumulative stressor value necessary to evoke a stress response. However, as Selye (1976) stated, stress can be related to positive and pleasurable experiences, such as playing competitive sports. He referred to this as 'the ecstasy of fulfilment' or the 'spice of life' that contributes to the wear and tear of life. Thus, stress can be associated with both positive and negative experiences. Selye referred to 'eustress' and 'distress' to distinguish between the two. Eustress is the amount of stress necessary for an active, healthy life. Our focus in this chapter will be on maladaptive stress, since it is this form of stress that produces most distress and disease.

Figure 22.2 illustrates homeostasis as a dynamic concept. Note that the parameters fluctuate either within the homeostatic range (i.e. stress threshold is not achieved when one is not consciously aware of the response to stressors), or outside the homeostatic range (i.e. threshold is reached or superseded when one may become aware of the response to stressors). This is responsible for producing psychophysiological imbalances, as indicated in Table 22.1. These imbalances depend on the cumulative effects of the stressors. These include everyday and long-term stressors.

Eustressors

Eustressors (everyday stressors) are positive experiences perceived as beneficial stressors, such as playing competitive sport or reviving an unconscious patient. Eustress is the amount of stress necessary for an active life, therefore it promotes the 'healthy' stress response. Eustress triggers homeostatic controls to remove, adapt or cope with the initiating stressor(s) and so restore homeostasis.

Extreme, long-lasting or unusual stressors

Distressors produce distress, i.e. the negative or 'unhealthy' stress response. If homeostasis is restored, it is at a cost to the body (i.e. the person's resistance to stress is reduced). If homeostatic mechanisms are not re-established, then a stress-related illness or even death may occur.

Figure 22.2 illustrates that eustress is time-dependent. When homeostasis is not restored within a certain time (which is individually subjective, depending on the causes of the imbalance and the homeostatic control efficiency), then eustress becomes distress. As a result a different psychological perception of the stressors occurs producing the disturbed homeostasis. Accompanying eustress is a sense of 'psychological' well being, whereas distress is associated with many negative feelings such as those emotional and behavioural indicators illustrated by Table 22.2.

Table 22.2 Psychological classification of the stress response

Eustress	Distress
Increased mental acuity	Diminished attention to detail, forgetfulness, poor work performance
Pleasure, happiness	Emotional outbursts, sadness
Euphoria	Lethargy, apathy

Q. List some potential eustressors associated with the occupation of nursing.

An example of the transition of eustress into distress can be found in competitive sports, such as boxing. At the commencement of a fight, a boxer usually believes he is going to beat his opponent, and so experiences eustressful responses on the first bell. The perception extends until the boxer gets tired or is hurt; then he doubts winning, and eustress is transformed into distress.

Exercise

Identify three situations you may come across in your day-to-day nursing of a patient when a eustressful experience is transformed into a distressful one, and vice versa.

Interim summary

Stress is the psychophysiological response of the body to environmental (exogenous and endogenous) stimuli called stressors (eustressors or distressors). The perceptions of stressors differ quantitatively and qualitatively between individuals, as do the stress thresholds. Psychophysiological responses to stressors are also subjective, since individuals experience either eustress or distress, depending upon their perception of the stressors. In addition, as Table 22.1 demonstrates, there is a range of physical, emotional and behavioural indicators that occur when people are stressed (the main emphasis is on indicators when one is distressed), and it is unlikely that two people will display the same indicators. The psychophysiological response is also time dependent. For example, eustress may be converted to distress, and perceptions of the response vary daily, and even within the same day, since humans are social beings who display circadian rhythmicity (see Chapter 23).

The individual nature of the psychophysiological stress response can be explained using the nature–nurture interaction template, i.e.

$$\text{Genotype} \rightarrow \text{Phenotype}$$
$$\uparrow$$
$$\text{Environment}$$

The unique blend of genes (the genotype) that a person possesses partly determines the measurable psychophysiological indicators (phenotypes) of the stress response. Genes are expressed or suppressed when the necessary environmental factors (stressors) prevail. For example, everyone has a genetic potential for developing an intellect, but the necessary environmental factors must be present for that potential to be achieved: primary, secondary and tertiary socialization. These are associated with the necessary environmental triggers such as books, intellectual peers, etc. Hence, the environment modifies the expression of the genotype.

As a further example, crying (a phenotype) is a common indicator of the psychophysiological stress response. This act is labelled an emotion, and as such is usually dealt with in the realms of psychological teaching. However, crying is a result of excessive tear production and secretion. Tears are chemicals, and thus are the end product of chemical reactions produced as a result of gene expression, which is influenced by the dominant environmental stressor within the cumulative stressors one is perceiving at that point in time. Crying can be a distressful or eustressful response, depending on how the individual perceives the major contributory stressor(s), i.e. as joyful or unhappy events. It must be remembered, however, that psychological perception of environmental stressors is a consequence of physiological processes (nerve impulses), thus giving credibility to the interactionist or transactional model of stress.

THE SUBJECTIVITY OF STRESS

Human beings react to stress in different ways because of the different societies they live in, the way they live their lives within that society, the type and dynamic fluctuations of societal stressors, and genetic variation. Individualism, therefore, is a combination of our own unique blend of genes and how we react to the individualized environment in which we live. Even identical twins differ in their biochemistry, due to their genetic uniqueness (genetic mutations will occur during uterine development and with age) and in their family experiences. Although parents like to think that they treat their children the same, in reality they do not. Different experiences occur even in the womb, depending on how the mother is living her life in different gestatory periods; even the position and the degree of placentation influences development, even with identical twins.

Before we become aware of the bodily stress response, the cumulative stressors one perceives at that point must have reached or superseded the stress threshold. These stressors, and the threshold, are dynamic and subjective, fluctuating with night–day activities (broadly defined as circadian rhythms) in the individual and between individuals as they proceed through the developmental stages of life. For example, consider the liking for loud music of some young people; while this may be included in your own list of stressors now, it may not have always done so.

The subjectivity of stressors

People are constantly exposed to stressors, and are either consciously or unconsciously aware of their existence. Stressors are classified as being social, physical, psychological, environmental and developmental.

Social stressors

Social readjustment rating scale
An historical publication by Holmes and Rahe (1967) identified 43 common stressful life events by examining the case histories of about 5000 people and identifying the life events that regularly preceded the onset of illness (Table 22.3(a)). Holmes and Rahe argued that there is an increase in the incidence of stress-related illnesses following stressful life events because of the extent of coping activities such 'adaptive' changes require. 'Negative' and 'positive' perceived events, such as divorce and marriage, respectively, are stressful since they necessitate adjustments by the person to a new lifestyle. Using their rating scale, the person reports any change in lifestyle, and each change is assigned a life change unit (LCU) score; a total LCU score is then calculated. Holmes and Rahe ranked people

as experiencing mild, moderate or severe stress (according to their LCU score; Table 22.3(b)).

Life events operate as stressors to the extent that they tax or exceed the adaptive resources of the person. They may be divided into major and minor. The former include events such as divorce, unemployment, serious illness and death of a loved one; the latter include daily stressors such as noise, job dissatisfaction and enjoyment.

Daily hassles of life
In 1981, Lazarus developed the Daily Hassles Scale, comprising 117 items that people may find frustrating or irritating, e.g. silly practical mistakes, losing one's purse, or having an argument with a loved one or workmate (Lazarus and Folkman, 1984). Participants of the study were required to distinguish which hassles they had come across during the preceding month, and then rate each entry on a three-point scale to indicate how severe the hassle had been during that period. Lazarus and Folkman stated that 'daily hassles are experiences and conditions of daily living that have been appraised as salient and harmful to the person's wellbeing.' Lazarus is working within a transactional model of stress where stress is influenced by a person's appraisal of a situation and their perceived ability to cope with it.

When quantifying stress within this conceptual framework, subjective elements such as personal beliefs and

Table 22.3(a) The Holmes and Rahe social readjustment rating scale

Event	Life crisis score (points)
Death of spouse	100
Divorce	73
Marital separation	65
Personal injury or illness	53
Marriage	50
Pregnancy	40
Sexual problems	39
Change in responsibilities at work	29
Outstanding personal achievement	28
Trouble with the boss	23
Change in working hours or conditions	20
Change in social activity	18
Vacation	13
Christmas	12

Q. What are the main criticisms of this scale?

Table 22.3(b) Magnitude of life crisis

Magnitude of life crisis	LCU score
Mild	150–199
Moderate	200–299
Severe	300+

appraisal have to be included, since the perception of stress is more important than the event itself. These workers argued that the influence of hassles might be reduced by 'uplifts' (i.e. desirable experiences, such as feeling healthy or working well with your colleagues). They then developed a 135-item Uplifts Scale. This scale was administered alongside the Hassles Scale, and the strength of each uplift was also rated on a three-point scale.

Major life events and daily hassles are almost certainly connected. For instance, a major life event such as death of a spouse may create a number of more minor hassles, such as sorting out financial arrangements, being a one-parent family, sorting out childcare facilities, and so on.

Further research is clearly needed to explore the complex relationship between major life events, minor frequent irritations, and the onset of illness, especially since individual variation has been reported in the way people react.

Physical stressors

Physical distressors involve overexertion as well as bodily change, which may affect one's mood. They result from malnutrition, hormonal/biochemical imbalances, illnesses, injuries caused, for example, by too much activity and strain on the skeletomuscular system, or from drug and alcohol abuse. An example of physical eustress is when exercise increases one's perception of fitness level.

Psychological stressors

Psychological stressors include innate and socialized 'fears' and 'fantasies' that, if provoked, will produce either distressed (anxiety) or eustressed responses.

Environmental stressors

Environmental distressors include:

● Societal pressures, such as overcrowding, antisocial behaviour, conforming to societal norms and values, and parental wishes.

● Work distressors associated with imposed conditions, such as levels of noise, glare, or restricted movement, 'work overload' in terms of too much work (quantitative overload) or too difficult work (qualitative overload) and, conversely, quantitative and qualitative 'underload'. Conditions of employment, such as low pay, low status, shift work, staff shortages, and lack of resources, are also included. Relationships at work are also important, and poor communication channels within these may be a source of distress. A lack of understanding of social support, and accountability levels, and other aspects, including career and promotion prospects, may all result in frustrations and distress, which may be associated with high absenteeism and work-related illnesses, and can result in the individual leaving that employment.

● Organizational stressors, such as work policy and procedures, could be restrictive and hence become distressful. Conversely, they may be viewed as being helpful in the day-to-day management of an individual's workload, and hence are potentially eustressful. Lack of positive feedback on performance or acceptance of new ideas could be perceived as a source of frustration and distress.

● The individual's organizational role could be a source of irritation, e.g. there may be a lack of defined authority, or no definite role specification. Interdepartmental conflicts with superiors or with colleagues/staff may occur. A difficulty in delegation, a lack of involvement in decision making, a lack of training for management, etc. are also perceived as sources of distress.

● Work–home interactions: two broad categories of stress for the person in work are occupational and private (domestic/personal). Stress, whether eustress or distress, in one part of life tends to spill over into other areas. Home and work conflicts may also arise with women's 'double shifts'. Their domestic labour, childcare, caring for dependants, etc. results in a lack of time for their choice of employment. Colleagues or spouse may relate this to the lack of recognition of work.

Physical eustress could be the perception of enjoyment one feels on a long-earned holiday or break from the distressors of work.

The 'stress' following birth is well documented. Holden (1992) identified that 50–70% of all mothers experience 'the blues' in the week following birth. 'The blues' are described as rapid mood fluctuations, where for no specific reason tears may follow elation. Although distressing for some women, these emotional mood swings usually resolve independently after a few days.

Exercise

Read the articles by Jones (1997), Moore (1997) and Al Rub (2000), which explore the stress associated with the nursing profession.

Read the article by Sawatzky (1998).

Read the article by Barber (1998), which identifies changing work patterns as a source of stress in midwifery.

BOX 22.2 SOCIAL READJUSTMENT RATING SCALE: ANY USE IN CLINICAL PRACTICE?

In support of such rating scales, it is possible to trace retrospectively from a patient's medical notes documented life events over a period of time preceding a stress-related illness. Figure 22.3, for example, highlights some common and most dominant (with regard to the LCU score) stressors a person who has had a coronary might perceive during a 10-year period.

The stressor scales are clinically useful in identifying potential distressors, so that the person can avoid them or learn how to cope with them, and in emphasizing the cumulative effects of multiple stressors in a person's life that cause the resultant signs of distress. However, theoretical and methodological weaknesses include:

- Some individuals undergo considerable life event changes without experiencing illness of any kind. Even Holmes and Rahe (1967) stated that 20% of scores bordering severe stress levels (LCU = 300) are not associated with a stress-related illness. Thus, individual differences in the ability to cope with stressful life events are overlooked.
- Attempts to quantify stressors in numerical order are crude and unscientific, since individuals rank life events differently according to their own perceptions. Thus, the transactional model of stress gives no consideration to the subjective appraisal of potential stressful situations. For example, when caring for a spouse during the terminal stage of cancer, death may not be the highest-ranked distressor in that person's life (at that particular moment in time), but it will depend on a number of factors, such as age, length and happiness of the relationship. Death of the partner may even bring relief to some, as it does not prolong the agony associated with seeing a loved one waste away.
- Some items appear ambiguous and vague, e.g. change in responsibilities at work.
- Self-reported stressful life events may also be unreliable because this is relying on an individual's ability to recall accurate perceptions. A person's state of mind is influential, e.g. a patient who is unwell may dwell and over-report negative events and under-report positive events.
- The meaning of specific events also changes with time, changing social, political and economic climates, and because

one's perception changes with experience. In fact, adult emotional distress relies upon personality characteristics formed early in life, but primary, secondary and tertiary socialization must also be taken into account. These include current experiences that take place with continuing changes (stressors) in one's life. Values, beliefs, ideologies, interactional patterns, interests and activities – indeed the entire range of dispositions and behaviours – are subject to modification as one proceeds through the lifespan. While exposure to stressful situations varies with the social circumstances of people, it is also true that identical circumstances have different effects on individuals within the group, depending on the social contexts. For example, retirement may be eustressful to a person who had an unstimulating job, or in a culture, such as Japan, that values its elders. Alternatively, retirement may lead to chronic distress and consequently depression in a person who thoroughly enjoyed their work and now does not have enough to occupy their mind, or in a culture, such as Britain, that views elderly people negatively. Societies influence individual change and adaptation. They are sources of hardship and challenges and, by providing contexts that give meaning to the consequences of these hardships, help people fend off the harmful emotional distress that may otherwise result. The strain among people of different ages is especially relevant to developmental concerns. They can be summarized simply because of their uniqueness to particular individuals, whether it is work related or the strains associated with being single, married or divorced. Temperamentally, however, everyone is different. Thus, how we respond to stressors is subjective. Personality, it could be argued, is largely determined socially, since the family is important in providing mental stability or instability in developing our attitudes to eustress/distress. The way in which we face a crisis or disaster is learned from those around us in our youth.

- The scales focus only on distressful events and omit eustressful experiences.

This variation demonstrates that subjectivity exists even in the perception of stress. We would argue that this is due to differences in the adaptability of individuals to cope with stressors.

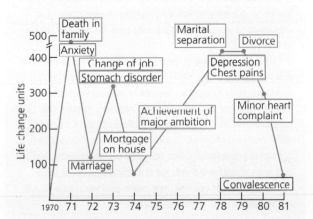

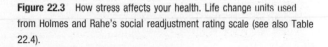

Figure 22.3 How stress affects your health. Life change units used from Holmes and Rahe's social readjustment rating scale (see also Table 22.4).

Table 22.4 Categories of stressors identified by Lees and Ellis (1990). For each stressor, the percentage of each group, and of the total group of 53 subjects, citing it as a stressor is given. (Reproduced with permission from the *Journal of Advanced Nursing*.)

Stressor	Trained	Student	Leaver	Total
Understaffing	75	25	23	43
Dealing with death and dying	25	55	46	41
Conflict with nurses	35	25	46	34
Overwork	25	30	ls	25
Conflict with doctors	40	15	8	23
Hours	10	10	39	17
Cardiac arrests	5	30	8	ls
Responsibility/accountability	25	5	8	13
Training junior staff	25	0	0	9
Dealing with relatives	is	5	8	9
Lack of resources (beds/equipment)	20	0	0	8
Aggressive patients	10	5	0	6
Study/exams	0	15	0	6
Carrying out certain nursing procedures	5	5	0	4
Feeling inadequate to carry out procedures	0	10	0	4
Seeing patients in distress	0	5	8	4
Staff rough to patients	0	0	ls	4
Conflict with others (porters/administration)	5	0	0	2
Child abuse	5	0	0	2
Dealing with overdose patients	5	0	0	2
Living in nurses' home	0	0	8	2
Open visiting	5	0	0	2
Doing the off-duty rota	5	0	0	2
Disorganization of workload on the wards	0	0	8	2
Being in a new situation for the first time	0	5	0	2
Heat in hospital	0	0	8	2

BOX 22.3 THE STRESS OF NURSING AND MIDWIFERY

Historically, nursing has always been thought of as a stressful profession. Lees and Ellis (1990) identified a wide array of stressors associated with the occupation of nursing. Twenty-six categories emerged in their study of 53 participants, comprising of 20 post-qualified (trained) staff, 20 pre-registration (students) and 13 ex-students (leavers) who had left their training programmes before the end. A number of the stressors (e.g. dealing with death and dying, conflict with doctors; see Table 22.4(a)) were highlighted in the three groups, while others were found to affect some groups more than others, and some were limited to one group only. The stressors that affected only one group were associated specifically with that group's role (e.g. only trained staff allocate the off-duty roster).

These researchers also asked respondents to quantify which incidents and/or situations they found to be the major stressors. For the trained staff, these were understaffing (*n* = 75% of trained staff), followed by conflict with doctors (*n* = 40%). For the students and the leavers, the major stressor was dealing with death and dying (*n* = 55% and 46%, respectively).

Perhaps it could be concluded that the levels of distress demonstrated by this study might be partly responsible for the high attrition rate from pre-registration education programmes. Interestingly, since the introduction of Project 2000 in the UK in 1989, interest has focused on comparisons between the two forms of preparation, and on the levels of stress associated with the revised form of pre-registration education.

Rhead (1995) found that in general, RGN students were considerably less stressed than the Diploma (Project 2000) students. The RGN students found the practical elements of their preparation to be more stressful than the academic elements, while the Diploma students were equally stressed by both the practical and academic elements.

Other studies have focused on specialist clinical areas. It has been found that some areas, e.g. critical care settings (Norrie, 1995) and accident and emergency departments (Sowney, 1996), are more stressful than others (e.g. care of the elderly, outpatients). However, it must be stated that stress is subjective, and one nurse may experience stimulation working in a critical care area, while another may be overstimulated and feel under pressure, which subsequently causes stress. The experience of stress also differs with time (time of day, phase of life, etc).

There is a shortage of literature regarding stress in midwives (but see Carlisle *et al.*, 1994). Cavanagh and Snape's (1997) qualitative study focused on sources of stress encountered by student midwives (*n* = 127, from 12 midwifery centres). The most common stressor among the participants were concerns about finding employment following qualification. There were a number of professional issues raised by the respondents, who felt they were disenchanted with the profession because of their perceptions of poor practice, long hours, poor job prospects and low wages.

Postnatal depression is a more severe and longer lasting disorder, that occurs in 10–16% of mothers (Cox *et al.*, 1992). These studies identify that women experience psychological problems for several months – sometimes years – following birth. Women who experience postnatal depression are at increased risk of further depression particularly after subsequent births.

The most serious form of postnatal depression is puerperal psychosis, which is rare and affects 2–3 in 1000 women. Symptoms include depression, mania, delusions and delirium, which resemble schizophrenia. The main concern is that the woman may be at risk of unintentionally harming herself or her baby as a result of her symptoms. The onset is sudden, and urgent treatment is required, usually in a psychiatric mother-and-baby unit on an in-patient basis. The disorder has an excellent prognosis, with a 2–3-month recovery period in most cases.

Developmental stressors

In an attempt to make sense of the 'meaning of life', science has always tried to classify objects, living matter, etc. Human development is no exception. Various stages of development have been attributed labels, so we can distinguish one developmental stage from another in order to aid advances in specialist knowledge in these areas. Thus, we have arguably the 'beginnings of life' stage, known as the zygote. This stage progresses into the morula, the blastocyst, the embryo, the fetus, the neonate, the infant, the child, the pubertal adolescent, the adult, the stage we equate with old age, retirement and beyond, and finally the terminal stage of 'death', which, according to Selye, is when we are free from stress.

Each stage is identifiable from the others by differential psychophysiological characteristics. For example, the emotional and physical characteristics of the adolescent and adult are obviously different. Each psychophysiological characteristic arises through enzymatically controlled reactions, which are ultimately controlled by gene expression. Environmental factors (stressors) and the timing of exposure to such factors influence this gene expression, and these are responsible for the range of onset of developmental stages. For example, the onset of puberty is between 10 and 12 years for girls and between 12 and 14 years for boys; this results from the production of adequate quantities of the male and female steroid hormones, which promote the development of the secondary sexual characteristics. Genes must be expressed to produce the enzymes necessary for hormone synthesis. Most people have the genetic potential for pubertal onset, and the age range given above demonstrates subjectivity. Perhaps premature or delayed pubertal onset may be a result of premature or delayed exposure to those environmental factors necessary for gene expression.

Therefore, psychophysiological subjectivity exists across the lifespan. Society also has positive and negative effects on development, e.g. technological advancement is usually centred on young people, who are more adaptable to changes; this may lead to the elderly feeling depersonalized and helpless.

Exercise

List the potential social, physical, psychological, developmental and environmental distressors that a nurse may encounter with
(i) his/her patients, and (ii) the occupational hazards of nursing.

Interim summary

So far, this discussion has focused on the subjectivity of how people perceive stressors. The cumulative effect on an individual of such stressors (social, developmental, physical, environmental and psychological) also demonstrates subjectivity. Thus, stressors may or may not be perceived consciously as such by different individuals, because no two people are alike. It is also unlikely that any two people will experience identical stressors. Furthermore, the perceived stressors must reach or supersede the stress threshold of the individual. Stress thresholds are dynamic and are not fixed entities. They are subjective to individuals, according to the individual's resistance to stressors, their available coping mechanisms or 'adaptation energy', and to the stress-related conditions they have experienced throughout their lives.

Subjectivity is based upon at least five factors:

1 The person's genotype.

2 The person's upbringing.

3 The person's environment.

4 The person's personality (which depends on factors 1 and 2).

5 Circadian rhythm fluctuations.

Once the cumulative effect of the stressors has reached or superseded the stress threshold, then individuality of the psychophysiological bodily response is observed, and the person experiences either distress or eustress, depending on the cognitive interpretation of the stressors.

THE SUBJECTIVITY OF STRESS RESPONSES

Transactional model of stress

Cox and McKay (1976) described the stress response as occurring when there is a mismatch between the perceived environmental demands and the person's perceived capabilities (Figure 22.4(a)). An important aspect of this model is that it is the individual's *perception* of demands (and not actual demands) placed upon him/her that may produce the stress response. That is, if the person's perception of demands exceeds their perceived capabilities to cope with them, then too much stress (hyperstress) becomes apparent. Conversely, if perceived capabilities of coping exceed the perceived demands, then too little stress (hypostress) is evident. When capabilities and demands are matched, then, we would argue that the individual experiences eustress. Thus, coping or adapting to hyperstress or hypostress situations involves changing one's perceptions of demands according to one's capabilities and vice versa (Figure 22.4(b)). Yerkes-Dodson (1982) stated that optimum stress provides maximum performance, and from this one may then potentially experience eustress. Stress levels below or above these optima result in deteriorating performance and can be a potential source of distress (Figure 22.5). See the case studies of a man with occupational hyperstress and a woman with occupation hypostress in Section 6.

Exercise

'Stress is a subjective perception.' Discuss this statement using the principles of Cox and McKay's transactional model of stress.

The general adaptation syndrome

The demand–capability model could be linked with the earlier work of Selye (1956), who described the general adaptation syndrome (GAS). This attempted to explain the physiological responses to stress. Selye labelled this a nonspecific (i.e. stereotypic) response – 'the sick syndrome' – as he realized that patients with a variety of diseases had similar signs and symptoms, including weight loss, appetite loss, decreased muscular strength, and no ambition. His animal studies demonstrated that three changes occurred during exposure to continued or extreme stress:

1 The adrenal cortex enlarges or hypertrophies, and therefore becomes hypersecretive.

2 The thymus, spleen and lymph nodes decrease in size or atrophy.

3 Bleeding ulcers appeared in the gastrointestinal tract.

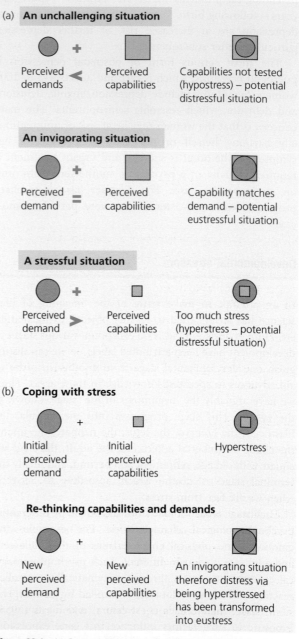

Figure 22.4 (a) Cox and McKay's transactional model of stress. (b) Coping with stress.

Q. Distinguish between perceived demands and perceived capability regarding a nurse (i) coping and (ii) not coping with her role.

Selye argued that a variety of dissimilar situations, such as arousal, grief, pain, fear, unexpected success ad loss of blood, are all capable of producing similar physiological stress responses. Thus, although people may face quite different stressors, in some respects their bodies respond in a stereotypical pattern. According to Selye, this involved

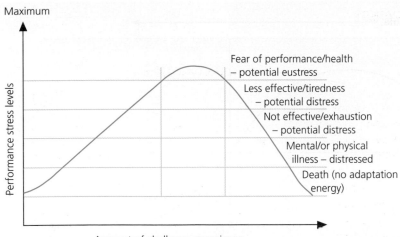

Maximum

Performance stress levels

Fear of performance/health
– potential eustress

Less effective/tiredness
– potential distress

Not effective/exhaustion
– potential distress

Mental/or physical
illness – distressed

Death (no adaptation
energy)

Amount of challenge experience

Figure 22.5 Yerkes-Dodson's law on human performance and stress.
Q. Distinguish between hypostress and hyperstress with reference to the workload of different occupations.

identical biochemical changes that enabled them to cope with any type of increased demand on the body. Thus, Selye believed that stress was the nonspecific adaptive response of the body to any demand placed upon it. Later, he argued that stress, whether pleasurable (eustress) or threatening (distress), produces physiological changes to restore the body's homeostasis, which was disrupted by the stressors. Selye also suggested that continued exposure to stressors results in three distinct phases of alarm, resistance (adaptation) and exhaustion.

The alarm stage

Alarm is predominantly initiated and controlled by the sympathetic nervous system, and affects visceral effector organs such as the brain, heart and skeletal muscles (Figure 22.6). These initial sympathetic effects are prolonged by the simultaneous release of the catecholamines (adrenaline and noradrenaline) from the adrenal medulla, which function at the sympathetic neuromuscular and neurosecretory effector sites. Selye viewed this as being anticipatory of a threat, and the necessity of taking action. The alarm stage, therefore, is equivalent to Cannon's (1935) famous 'fright, fight, flight' statement when describing the effects of adrenaline and noradrenaline. The effects of this stage can be viewed as short-term homeostatic controls operating, hopefully, to enable us to cope with, or adapt to, the dominant stressor(s), which contributed to the person reaching the stress threshold. If these controls are successful, or the dominant stressor is perceived to have fallen below threshold level, then visceral organ functions return to their 'normal' baselines (i.e. within their homeostatic ranges). However, if the stressors remain at or above threshold level, and/or additional stressors occur, then Selye argued that the individual goes into the second stage of resistance or dies. Progress depends on the person's perception of the intensity and duration of the demand.

Resistance or adaptation stage

Resistance is controlled predominantly by the endocrine system, and is mediated by the hypothalamus. Such events are analogous to intermediate and long-term homeostatic controls, which act to re-establish homeostasis. This stage is maintained by the hormone cortisol, the main glucocorticoid hormone produced by the adrenal glands. Growth hormone is also released from the pituitary gland; the actions of cortisol and growth hormone are highlighted in Figures 22.6 and 22.8. Notice in particular the actions of the two hormones to mobilize metabolic fuels. Cortisol is sometimes referred to as the 'hormone of stress', since people who are unable to produce it in sufficient quantities adapt very poorly to stressful situations.

The alarm and resistance phases facilitate our ability to cope with stressors. In other words, although it may seem that hormonal homeostasis in these phases has failed, the responses do promote the conditions necessary for survival and so are examples of homeostatic adaptation.

The majority of hormones released are hyperglycaemic agents (i.e. chemicals that raise the blood sugar levels) that provide cells with energy to cope with the effects of the stressors. Selye (1956) referred to the concept of 'adaptation energy'. He stated that our amount of adaptation energy might be compared with our inherited bank

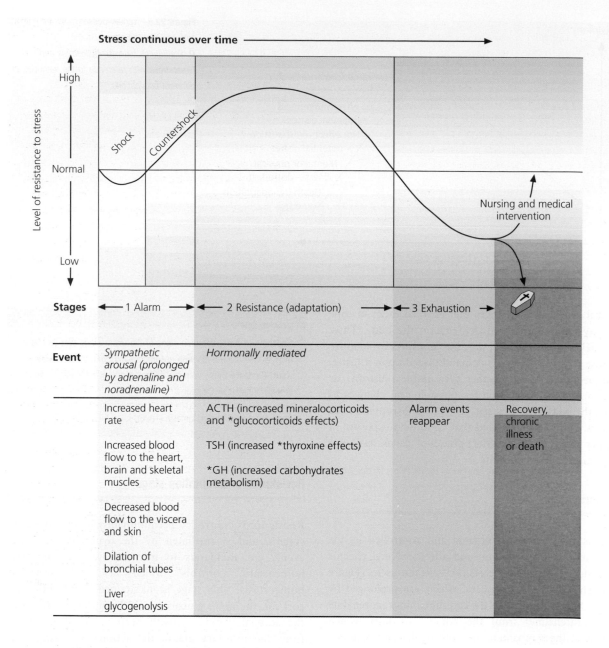

Figure 22.6 Selye's general adaptation syndrome.

ACTH, adrenocorticotropic hormone; GH, growth hormone; TSH, thyroid-stimulating hormone.

*Increased glucose availability for catabolism (possibly provides a source of adaptation energy).

Q. Describe the events associated with the triphasic stages of the general adaptation syndrome.

account, determined by our individualistic genotype, from which we can make withdrawals, but into which we apparently cannot make deposits. Every stressor causes wear and tear, leaving some irreversible scars, which accumulate and contribute to the signs of ageing (see Chapter 20). If this is the case, then adaptation energy should be used wisely rather than squandered. It is still not understood what is lost, except that it is unlikely to be simply calorific energy. If there is no adaptation (or resistance), or if attempts to reduce the cumulative effects of the stressors below thresh-

old level are unsuccessful, then, Selye argued, we would go into the final stage of exhaustion.

Exhaustion

In exhaustion, the signs of the alarm stage reappear, which is an indication that the body's homeostatic controls have failed. Consequently stress-related illnesses appear – Selye called these 'diseases of adaptation' – or death results.

BOX 22.4 BURNOUT AND DISEASE OF ADAPTATION

Burnout

To burn out is 'to fail, wear out or become exhausted by making excessive demands on energy, strength or resources' (Howells-Johnson, 1998). Some of the signs of burnout include feelings of exhaustion and fatigue, not being able to shake off a cold, feeling worn out, frequent headaches and gastrointestinal tract disturbances, loss of weight and depression. Burnout is sometime viewed as progressive stress divided into four stages:

1 The idealistic enthusiasm is demonstrated by a high degree of personal motivation to achieve goals (some of which may be unrealistic). This stage may last up to a year, e.g. within a new job.
2 The individual realizes that the goals are unrealistic and cannot be achieved. Personal energy levels begin to fade, and motivation declines progressively. Disappointments may be experienced. Outside interests begin to take precedence over work.
3 Frustrations become evident, e.g. the nurse cannot achieve unrealistically set goals, and often feels thwarted. In this case, the frustrations arise from not satisfying the needs of patients.
4 Signs of apathy appear, e.g. the nurses tends to see the job as a job. Typically, the nurse arrives late at work, leaves early and become mechanical in his/her tasks. Often, this stage is associated with the nurse complaining and bickering about being dissatisfied with the occupation.

Managers and nurses should be aware of these stages, since the teaching of stress management will reduce the risk of burnout.

Diseases of adaptation

In the context of this book, 'diseases of adaptation' are when clinical intervention is required to restore the person's homeostatic processes. First, there is a need to assess or identify the major stressors associated with the illness. Then care must be planned and implemented so as to minimize, remove or treat these stressors. For example, bacteria or social problems would be treated with antibiotics or controlled by teaching stress management techniques, respectively. We argue that serious conditions that are not commonly recognized as being stress related, such as terminal cancers and acquired immune deficiency syndrome (AIDS), are in fact just that, and that the agents that instigate these conditions (carcinogens and HIV, respectively) are stressors. These conditions are fatal, as the person cannot adapt. Perhaps this could be due to depleted adaptation energy. Arguably, depleted adaptation energy as a consequence of ageing reduces our capacity to cope with disease.

Only the most severe stress leads rapidly to the exhaustion stage and maybe death. Most physical and/or psychological exertion, infection and other stressors act upon us for a limited period of time and produce changes corresponding only to the first and second stages. At first, the stressors of the alarm stage upset us, i.e. we are distressed, but then we adapt, either consciously because alarm signs cause us to employ stress management techniques, or unconsciously in the resistance stage via our hormonally mediated homeostatic controls. Thus, throughout life,

we go through these first two stages many times in order to adapt to all the demands within our environment.

The triphasic nature of the GAS indicates that the body's adaptation energy is finite, since continuous distress eventually produces exhaustion, and the person succumbs to a stress-related condition. The type and severity of these conditions reflect, yet again, subjective elements. Selye (1976) classified GAS responses as synotoxic and catatoxic reactions of the body's defence against potential internal and/or external aggressors (stressors). Synotoxic reactions help us put up with the aggressor, and catatoxic reaction help us to destroy it. Synotoxic stimuli act as tissue tranquillizers, permitting a peaceful co-existence with the aggressors, whereas catatoxic agents mainly involve the induction of destructive enzymes, which generate an attack on the pathogen, usually by accelerating its metabolic degradation.

Corticoids are among the most effective synotoxic hormones. This hormonal group inhibits inflammation and promotes other defence mechanisms, such as transplant rejection. The main purpose of inflammation is to prevent irritants from entering the circulation by localizing them. However, once the foreign agent is rendered harmless, the suppression of inflammation becomes advantageous. Clinically, anti-inflammatory corticoids are given in such cases, and have proven to be effective in treating diseases in which the major complaint is inflammation of the eyes, joints or respiratory passageways.

Alternatively, when the aggressor is dangerous, the defence reaction should be increased above the normal level. This is achieved by catatoxic substances, such as antibodies, lysozymes and pain-producing substances, which carry messages to fight the 'invaders' (stressors) even more actively than normal.

The major physiological response of the body to excessive stress is vascular collapse. The body may overcome this by neural/endocrine changes that re-establish vascular homeostasis. This response is potentially life saving in acute situations, but if stressors are prolonged or intense, it can lead to organ system failure, resulting in, for example, cardiovascular and gastrointestinal disease. The interdependency of organ systems and their component parts means that if one system is affected, then others will also be affected. A good example of this is in maturity-onset diabetes mellitus, which demonstrates that a failure at cellular level results in multiple organ system failure. This condition is exacerbated by the prolonged effects of carbohydrate-rich (distressor) diets, which promote the hyperglycaemia (= excessively high glucose concentration in blood) as the insulin target receptor sites become 'desensitized' to the hormone insulin. The hyperglycaemia (now a distressor) must be corrected. Glucose is excreted in the urine (glycosuria), which helps to moderate the hyperglycaemia, but there are no endogenous agents, other than insulin, that will reverse it. In addition, diabetes is also associated with fat breakdown, which produces hyperlipidaemia (another distressor) with an atherosclerotic effect. Atherosclerosis is another distressor in diabetes; it diminishes the functions of the blood vessels of multiple organs, and partly explains why a diabetic person's eyes, heart, blood pressure and kidneys may all be affected. Although diabetic people exhibit the same biochemical and response mechanisms, the degree of change is individual, so the organs that are affected, and how much they are affected, varies. Perhaps the host of factors that form the basis of nature–nurture interaction subjectivity also explains this variation.

A severely stressed person also presents a clinical picture that results from of the cumulative effects of various stress hormones.

For example, hypertension could be due to the vasoconstrictory actions of adrenaline, noradrenaline and angiotensin II, or to the circulatory volume-expanding effects of aldosterone and antidiuretic hormone, or to an increased cardiac output caused by adrenaline and noradrenaline (see Chapter 12). The latter hormones may also cause tachycardia, hyperventilation, bowel dysfunction, and other fight and flight responses (alarm reactions). Again, however, there is individual variability.

Exercise

Examine your own behaviour and that of colleagues for signs of burnout. Read the articles by Farrington (1997), Simoni and Paterson (1997) and Rausch (1996), which explore the concept of burnout in the nursing profession.

Analysis of the general adaptation syndrome

Although on the whole we agree with Selye's ideas, looking at Table 22.1 we could argue that stressed people do not have consistent physiological, behavioural and emotional response indicators. In addition, when stressed, individuality is again observed according to whether the person perceives the stress response as distress or eustress, and whether the person is consciously aware of this stress response.

The pituitary-adrenocortical activity in response to stress is also not as broad and consistent as Selye suggested. He found that some physically harmful stressors, such as fasting, did not increase corticosteroid levels when the stressors were weak. However, when fasting was strengthened by psychological factors (e.g. an unhealthy desire to be thin), the nonspecific response occurred. Thus, it is only demands that tax the person's capabilities that are stressful, i.e. those that reach or exceed the person's stress threshold. The extent of the stress response depends on the individual's evaluation of the consequences of unfulfilled demands. The stress response is not stereotypical, and stress is not manifested as a single syndrome, such as the GAS. Multiple factors governed by situational and individualistic variables are involved.

The disadvantages of Selye's GAS are that it fails to clarify what conditions cause stress or what constitutes a demanding stressor capable of initiating it, and it does not take into account situational and individualistic variables involved in the activation of this stress response. Consequently, it really describes a theory of adaptation to stress rather than a stress theory.

Selye's work, however, can be defended easily using the stress threshold concept. If stressor strength is below threshold level ('subconscious' stress), then the reactions of the GAS do not appear; it is only when the threshold is met or superseded that the reactions of the GAS come into operation.

The influence of Lazarus (1966) marked a change in the stress research field, which previously had been dominated by Selye. Lazarus identified three important aspects of stress:

1 Stress is determined by the perception of a stressful situation rather than by the situation itself.

2 Individuals differ in their reactivity to stress.

3 The extent of stress depends partly on the capabilities of the individual to cope.

Therefore, according to Lazarus (1966), 'Stress occurs when there are demands on the person which tax or exceed his adaptive resources.' This definition views stress as involving a cognitive appraisal of a demand–capability imbalance. Factors important in the perception of environmental stressors involve:

● *perception of control:* if one is not in control then distress is more likely;

● *predictability of the outcome:* if one cannot predict the outcome, then distress is more likely;

● *past experiences:* if one has no past experience with potential distressors, then one is more likely to experience distress until a coping strategy can be developed.

Exercise

Identify clinical situations in which healthcare professionals utilize perception of control, predicting the outcome and past experiences to minimize distress in patients.

In contrast to Selye's biological theory, the emphasis of 'psychological' stress is on the input side, in particular on the kind of situation and the individual interaction that evokes a stress state. Both approaches are complementary. Lazarus's psychological theory outlines the conditions that determine the evocation of stress, while Selye's physiological theory describes its form (Figure

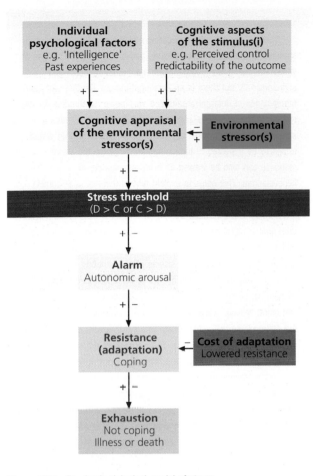

Figure 22.7 Psychophysiological model of stress.

C, capabilities; D, demands; +, continue; —, removal.

Q. Stress is said to be a psychophysiological bodily response arising through environmental stressors. What do you understand by this statement?

22.7). This integrated approach provides Selye's formulations with the breadth needed to encompass the stress of living.

The psychological effects of stress are subjective and multiple. They may result in depression, lack of personal accomplishment, avoidance of decisions, depersonalization or a feeling of emotional emptiness. The effects of these stressors can result in a shift from a positive to a negative view, which can lead to an uncaring disposition. Absenteeism, guilt, error and helplessness can follow.

BOX 22.5 STRESS REDUCTION: A CLINICAL PERSPECTIVE

Scientific breakthroughs include the use of tranquillizers in combating 'mental' illnesses, and the use of anti-ulcer drugs. Most of these agents are directed not against stress, but against some of its manifestations. Increasing attention is being given to psychological and behavioural techniques that anyone can use to avoid producing the stress response. Relaxation techniques, such as transcendental meditation, must be given the respect they deserve as they do work on some of those people who try them

Exercise

'Stress is a subjective phenomenon.' Discuss this statement in relation to the individualistic nature of the following: (i) stressors; (ii) stress threshold; (iii) stress response; and (iv) stress-related illnesses.

Suggest why it is difficult to measure or assess subjective experiences such as stress.

BOX 22.6 THE METABOLIC STRESS RESPONSE TO SURGERY

Surgical trauma promotes metabolic responses, which can be divided into various phases. Following surgery, the patient rapidly enters the 'ebb' phase, in which there is reduced metabolism and the concentration of metabolic fuels within the blood increases. This phase is usually quite short, and actually may start before injury due to responses associated with the 'alarm' phase of stress responses, as identified by Selye. After several hours, the patient enters the 'flow' phase, which is characterized by tissue catabolism and an increased metabolic rate: these responses may be substantial, especially after severe trauma. In the longer term, anabolic phases can also be identified, during which the metabolic status of the patient returns to normal. This box is concerned largely with the flow phase, since this phase covers the immediate week or so after surgery, and it is within this period that the major adaptive responses for recovery are observed.

Although the GAS can be criticized for various reasons (see earlier), the hormonal responses it describes are identifiable in the patient undergoing physical trauma, such as surgery. In this

context, stress responses would be eustressful if the patient recovered from surgery, but could potentially be distressful if the hormonal responses were excessive or persistent. The principles of the GAS therefore provide a useful means of introducing these responses, but you should bear in mind that the hormonal changes it describes largely occur simultaneously following injury (Clancy and McVicar, 1998b).

Stress response in the postoperative period

The metabolic changes that are promoted in the alarm and resistance phases equate with the injury (i.e. ebb and flow) phase of surgical recovery. This section looks at how these responses enable the individual to cope with, and recover from, surgical stress.

The activity of the sympathetic nervous system, adrenaline and cortisol during the ebb phase stimulate breakdown of glycogen (glycogenolysis) and fat (lipolysis), and hence promote the mobilization of glucose and fatty acids. However, sympathetic activity to the pancreas inhibits insulin secretion, while growth hormone released from the pituitary gland reduces the capacity of cells to take up glucose (i.e. insulin resistance is promoted). The mobilization of glucose, coupled with an inhibited insulin release and elevated insulin resistance, leads to high blood sugar (hyperglycaemia). This favours the functioning of insulin-independent tissues, especially the brain, while tissues that are insulin sensitive will become more dependent on the generation of energy from fatty acids, thus resulting in the consequential accumulation of ketone bodies.

Despite these changes, basal metabolism does not increase overall during the ebb phase; in fact, it often decreases, suggesting that there are additional biochemical adaptations. However, the ebb phase is usually quite short, and the patient soon enters the flow phase, when the metabolic responses facilitate an increased metabolic rate.

As the flow phase becomes established, fatty acid metabolism will still be the most important energy store for the body as a whole, although glucose supply to insulin-independent tissues continues to be supported by hyperglycaemia. The latter is maintained by further glucose synthesis prompted by the actions of cortisol to induce protein breakdown and the release of amino acids. Protein catabolism also results in the increased synthesis and excretion of urea (a 'waste' product of amino acid metabolism). Protein synthesis is also decreased, exacerbating the reduction in protein. Muscle provides the main source of protein in the body, but the increased protein catabolism may also decrease the concentration of some plasma proteins, although fibrinogen and those involved in immunity may even increase, perhaps as haemostatic and anti-infection mechanisms. The flow phase responses are summarized in Figure 22.8.

The elevated metabolism observed during the flow phase causes an increase in body temperature, an elevation in heart rate (to promote effective circulation), and an elevation in lung ventilation (to promote oxygen uptake and carbon dioxide excretion). The significance of increased mobilization of metabolic fuels is that cell division and tissue growth and repair are facilitated. A further action of an elevated release of cortisol is to reduce immune responses. Although at first this might seem detrimental to recovery from surgery, the response is probably important later in the flow phase when the persistence of inflammation and fibrosis will hinder wound healing. The anti-inflammatory actions of steroids are well known and they are used widely in clinical practice; the effects of cortisol released during stress are also of interest to researchers studying incidences of infection following lifestyle stress. Chronic use of steroids has depressive actions on the immune system.

Circulatory responses

The cardiovascular actions of sympathetic nerves, backed up by catecholamines, represent part of the stress response to surgery. They are worth reviewing here because they reinforce the advantages that stress responses facilitate during and after trauma. The roles of sympathetic activation can be related to the circulation and to haemostasis.

A significant loss of blood during surgery could be expected to stimulate sympathetic nerve activity, and to promote the release of vasoactive hormones (especially adrenaline, vasopressin and angiotensin II), but there is an additional aspect. Contact with, and manipulation of, internal organs is a very powerful stimulus for the release of the hormones, regardless of fluid loss. In a 'natural' sense, such contact would represent a severe trauma that would ordinarily be expected to induce haemorrhage, so the alarm response can also be viewed as being anticipatory of hypovolaemia. This helps to explain why abdominal and thoracic surgery is a particularly powerful stimulus for hormone release.

Surgery is a controlled trauma, in that blood loss is minimized. With limited blood loss, a powerful release of vasoactive hormones might be expected to elevate arterial blood pressure, but their actions are offset against the effects of anaesthetics, some of which depress the brainstem control of the autonomic nervous system, hence cause a decline in sympathetic output to the heart and blood vessels. However, the release of vasoactive hormones in the alarm phase will actually help to control arterial blood pressure in the presence of anaesthesia. The permissive actions of cortisol on the catecholamines provide additional support following trauma.

Further actions of adrenaline, vasopressin and angiotensin II include the promotion of blood clotting (adrenaline) and the initiation of water and electrolyte conservation (all three hormones, but especially vasopressin and angiotensin). These actions again are of obvious benefit should blood loss have occurred, but they will also have implications for the patient's water balance in the post-surgical period (Clancy and McVicar, 1997a).

Implications of metabolic responses to surgery

The metabolic responses to surgery represent a resetting of homeostatic means, and so promote the functional changes necessary for recovery. As such, according to stress theory, they are adaptive, eustressful mechanisms that promote the health (or a return to health) of the patient. The release of the hormones supporting the changes declines gradually as the flow phase progresses, so homeostatic means eventually return to normal. However, there is a metabolic 'cost' of the flow phase, particularly in relation to protein synthesis: the catabolism of muscle proteins produced by growth hormone and cortisol during the flow phase induces a loss of muscle tissue. The resultant increase in urea production from amino acid metabolism promotes a negative nitrogen balance, since urea has incorporated into it the nitrogen found in amino acid molecules. Persistence of protein depletion may hinder long-term wound healing, and also has implications for the general welfare of the patient.

Selye's GAS would relate these implications to a transition from resistance into exhaustion and distress, i.e. the metabolic cost of recovery places the patient at risk of ill health. Wound healing can be enhanced, and protein depletion reduced, by ensuring that the patient has adequate protein nutrition during the flow phase. The amino acids arginine and glutamine are especially important in this respect, as they stimulate collagen production, fibroblast activity and immune functions, all of which are central to the wound healing process (Clancy and McVicar, 1997b). A good-quality diet

BOX 22.6 CONTINUED

should be available to patients, although commercially available supplements may also be used (Wallace, 1994), and will help to minimize protein depletion before the patient enters the anabolic phase of recovery.

See the case study of a man with a surgical wound in Section 6.

Diabetes mellitus and surgery

The discussion so far has centred on the responses of patients who do not have an underlying metabolic problem on admission for surgery (although malnourishment is not rare). Diabetic patients are faced with additional hazards, which are related to chronic complications of the disorder, e.g. nephropathy, angiopathy and neuropathy, and that result from the imposition of metabolic responses to surgery upon the person's disturbed metabolism. Under these circumstances, responses that are ordinarily adaptive

can become maladaptive, and so have immediate implications for health (Marshall 1996).

In diabetes, the shortage of insulin or the presence of insulin resistance intensifies the metabolic response to surgery. The risks associated with this are:

● enhanced hyperglycaemia, with the associated risk of coma. Polyuria and polydipsia would also be expected;
● increased fatty acid mobilization and ketone body formation, to the extent that the risk of ketoacidosis is increased.

Such risks mean that monitoring blood glucose concentration accurately, and paying particular attention to maintaining the patient's metabolic control, will be important aspects for perioperative care of people with diabetes mellitus (Marshall, 1996).

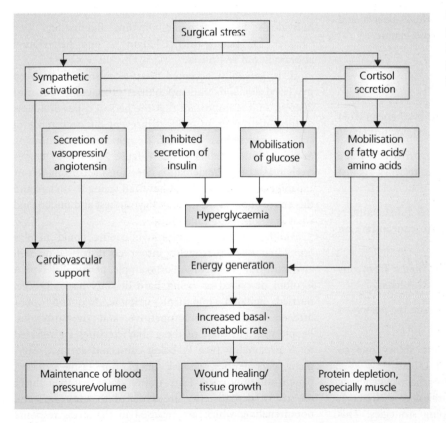

Figure 22.8 Summary of the main events in the flow phase of recovery from surgery. Note how the net effect of the responses is generally one of facilitating recovery, apart from the metabolic 'cost' of protein depletion.

Exercise

Remind yourself of what the term 'basal metabolic rate' means, and its significance to clinical practice, and identify the factors that might influence it during the postoperative period.

Using Chapter 9, review how the control of cortisol is normally controlled.

Review your understanding of the two main types of diabetes mellitus, and consider how metabolic control might be achieved with each type after surgery. Reference to Marshall (1996) might help.

How might the presence of nephropathy, angiopathy and neuropathy in the diabetic patient affect processes involved in wound healing?

COPING MECHANISMS AND FEATURES OF FAILURE

Stress management attempts to reduce or prevent distress and its harmful effects. There are three classes of management: to change one's environment and/or lifestyle, to change one's personality and/or one's perceptions, and to change the biological response to stress.

In general, the term 'coping' is usually reserved for behavioural (psychological) responses, and 'adaptation' is applied to the physiological responses. Thus, as stress is viewed by the authors as a psychophysiological bodily response, then we prefer the use of the term 'adaptive coping', as stress-management techniques are employed to alleviate the negative consequences of the whole-body stress response. It is obviously outside the scope of this chapter to describe stress-management techniques in any detail; however, some methods are illustrated in Table 22.5. The important point to note is that the usefulness of each technique is subjective to an individual's beliefs, and that these beliefs are time dependent and dynamic.

Coping

Everybody possesses strategies or defence mechanisms that they often do not recognize they have used, including:

- *denial:* e.g. a practitioner who refuses to concede the existence of stress (the nurse continues to work against all odds);

- *escape:* e.g. taking time out to avoid stressful encounters or avoiding the demands of the job to concentrate on trivial tasks;

- *displacement:* transferring feelings or blame from one person to another, often easier to use scapegoat;

- *intellectualization:* distancing oneself from the person or situation causing stress.

An awareness of these mechanisms allows one to observe signs of stress in oneself and in others.

This section is concerned with how people generally cope with stress using cognitive appraisal of distressors, but does not discuss individual coping strategies. This book has demonstrated that stressors are necessary to perform the 'characteristics of life', and that it is how a person copes or fails to adapt to distressors that is important in determining whether he or she succumbs to stress-related conditions, or progresses through developmental stages of the lifespan.

Cognitive coping

A cognitive approach to coping involves transferring distress into eustress, or removing distressors to below the stress threshold level by reducing perceived or actual demands on the body. The success of coping methods is subjective, since individuals differ in respect of their cognitive and behavioural efforts to manage, reduce or tolerate the internal and external demands of the person–environment transactions. Success is also time dependent, since individuals have circadian rhythm fluctuations (see Chapter 23) that influence cognitive and behavioural appraisals and responses.

It is generally accepted that a mismatch between perceived demands and capabilities produces a source of distress, so it is important that the person copes or adapts to these distressors in order to prevent the occurrence of stress-related illness. This can be achieved by rethinking our capabilities and demands (Figure 22.4(b)) by cognitively reassessing the demands (stressors) according to our capabilities. For example, rather than trying to understand this entire book, you can only do your best and understand what is within your capabilities.

Another method of cognitive coping could involve 'moulding' one's personality into a less distressed or even an eustressful personality. For example, personality type A is often described as being hard-driving, hasty, hostile, hurried, agitated, impatient, irritable, frequently poor listeners, rushed, overcompetitive and overambitious. People who have few of these characteristics are referred to as personality type B, being calm and content, easy-going personalities, good-listeners, not easily irritated, patient and unhurried. Type A often claim that they 'thrive on stress' (perhaps they are addicted to adrenaline and noradrenaline, which are released in the stress response alarm and exhaustion stages). Excessive, frequent and prolonged release of these catecholamines is thought to

Table 22.5 Some stress management techniques

Environmental/lifestyle	Personality/perception	Biological response
Time management	Assertiveness training	Progressive relaxation
Proper nutrition	Thought stopping	Relaxation response
Exercise	Refuting irrational ideas	Meditation
Finding alternatives to frustrated goals, e.g. stopping smoking or drinking.	Stress inoculation modifying type A behaviour	Breathing exercises, biofeedback autogenics

increase one's susceptibility to stress-related conditions, such as heart disease, hypertension, migraines and ulcers. However, not all type A personalities succumb to the ill effects of stress. Perhaps if a type A person consciously recognizes what is happening, they can actually become more resistant to stress, i.e. he or she becomes type C (sometimes referred to as type H or hardy personality). These people now look upon situations as challenges rather than threats, and convert the distressful life events of type A into opportunities or possibilities (eustressful life events) for personal growth and benefit, i.e. they have rethought their demands and capabilities.

In order to be 'stress-wise', it is important, therefore, to identify type A behaviour in ourselves by recognizing attitudes and expectations that engage us in a constant struggle to gain control over our environment. For example, when a type A personality perceives emotional threats or challenges, the stress response is triggered automatically, even when there is no real danger, e.g. when waiting in a traffic jam, queuing in the bank, etc. As a result, much unnecessary 'stress' (and loss of adaptation energy) is created, which keeps the person frequently outside the normal range of the stress balance and in the distressed area. The difficulty is in appraising our behaviour and altering our responses to stressors. Lazarus (1966) put forward a stress appraisal model based on coping with mental illnesses. According to Lazarus, primary appraisal of the initiating situation involved three possibilities:

1 A stressor is considered irrelevant.

2 A stressor is seen as being positive with respect to wellbeing, having positive and pleasant emotions.

3 The stressors are regarded as damaging and threatening, with negative emotions such as anxiety.

These three possibilities can therefore be equated to being unconsciously aware of the psychophysiological indicators of the stress response, eustress and distress. The outcome of these possibilities determines the emotions experienced. This experience promotes the necessary action to be taken, and results in a secondary appraisal that involves planning and evaluating possible coping methods: to change the stressors or situation, to modify the meaning of the situation, or to regulate the experienced emotions. In other words, distress may be transferred into eustress, the person may flee the situation, one's perceptions of demands and capabilities may be altered, or distressful emotions may be minimized.

The term 'coping', like 'stress', has acquired many meanings. It may refer to efforts to master conditions of harm or threat of challenge, when a routine or automatic response is not readily available. Here, environmental demands must be met with new behavioural solutions, or old ones must be adapted to meet the current stress. There are two sources of coping: problem-focused and emotion-focused coping.

BOX 22.7 TYPE A PERSONALITY NURSES

According to Howells-Johnson (1998), there is an increased prevalence of type A behaviour among nurses. Whether a type A person becomes nurse, or whether nursing changes people into type A personalities, is difficult to assess.

Ask yourself these questions. How often as a nurse do you:

- engage in races against the clock trying to squeeze more and more patient care into each shift?
- perform two or more jobs at any one time?
- view peers as competitors?
- interpret an offer of help as a slur on your competence?
- work double shifts, denying time for restful periods?

Problem-focused coping

Problem-focused coping deals directly with the problem. After appraising the situation, the person either changes the distressors (i.e. problems) or avoids them in order to cope with the troubled person–environment relationship. This involves an ergonomic approach. First, the person identifies the potential distressors, such as a quantitative work overload as experienced with time pressures and staff shortages. An ergonomic approach to stress management might reduce workload, because it cannot increase staff numbers. This approach operates on the principle of optimizing efficiency levels, and so reduces the time spent on specific tasks. This can be achieved by keeping abreast of professional developments, perhaps with the aid of advanced technology. For example, centralizing information can reduce the time spent in unnecessary meetings, and the 'freed' time can be used in other ways, including easing the burden of time-pressurizing tasks. If the problem or distress is caused by a lack of involvement in decision making, then restructuring gives more emphasis to a team approach. If the distress is a result of desynchronizing circadian rhythms by the removal of the natural light and dark cues, as occurs with night work or during periods of hospitalization (see Chapter 23), then the ergonomic approach coping could involve the use of solar spectrum artificial lighting to reduce the extent of desynchronization.

Emotion-focused coping

Emotion-focused coping is a more indirect means of coping. Such methods do not alter the damaging conditions, but are used to make the person feel better. Emotion-focused coping is concerned more with reducing anxiety than with dealing with the situation responsible for producing anxiety. Traditionally, emotion-focused coping can become pathological or maladaptive. For example, denial defence mechanisms may be used to deny that a suspicious lump may be cancerous. Such coping strategies can become dangerous when they prevent essential direct action, but they are considered beneficial in providing the person with a sense of 'psychological' wellbeing.

Voluntary behaviour habits, such as the use of alcohol, cigarettes, tranquillizers, sedatives and excessive caffeine, act as distressors themselves, and have long-term pathological consequences and thus may be detrimental to health. In addition, there are involuntary reactions in a stressed person, such as decreased appetite and disturbed

sleeping patterns (see Chapter 23), which are also potential distressors and thus can affect one's resistance to disease.

People usually employ a combination of these coping mechanisms, either consciously or unconsciously, in an attempt to counteract stress. Some coping methods are more successful than others, not only from the person's point of view but also within one of the domains of physiology, psychology or sociology. However, coping affects all three domains since they are inseparable entities.

BOX 22.8 COPING FAILURE: PSEUDO-ORGANIC AND ORGANIC DISEASE

Pseudo-organic disease

Some people with coping failure present symptoms that suggest the presence of an organic disease, e.g. pseudo-angina, which upon consultation and examination show no evidence of the actual disorder. Frequently, such patients are treated with mild analgesics; if these prove ineffective, then more powerful analgesics may be administered. The patient may be very anxious and complain that it is the pain that is the stressor, and that this is causing a lack of sleep. Consequently, the patient may be prescribed antidepressants; after taking a few months to recover, the patient then rarely complains of the 'angina' again. It may be speculated that the reason for an increased pain perception is that there is a decrease in arousal levels in the depressed state. That is, the depression is a failure of adaptation, and is a sign that may be attributed to the exhaustion stage of the GAS, when the levels of endogenous painkillers such as endorphins might be expected to be low. Guillemin was awarded the Nobel Prize in 1977 for discovering endorphins, which have anti-stress effects by acting as painkillers. They may be amongst the first mediators in the alarm stress response.

Organic disease

There are possibly two pathways in which stress is related to the onset of disease. First, stress may have direct psychophysiological effects that affect health via disturbed homeostatic controls within cells influenced by the neuroendocrine responses to stress. Second, stress may lead to health-impairing habits (e.g. smoking, alcohol abuse) and altered behaviours (e.g. biting nails). These are referred to as palliative coping methods.

These two pathways explain the relationship between stress and the onset of disease. For example, hormonal changes and immune system decline are thought to reduce the host's resistance, thereby increasing the risk of disease. Once an illness occurs, then one may be

subjected to illness behaviour, which influences the course of the disease, and so would form a third pathway. For example, in the case of bereavement, a clear link exists between the increased incidence of mortality and an increased likelihood of illness among widows and widowers who have suffered a recent bereavement of their spouse. One may argue that the evidence is suggestive but not conclusive. However, what is important is that the dominant stressor (death of the spouse) demonstrates individuality with respect to the differing illnesses acquired, and even death in those who seem unable to cope with the bereavement. As far as cardiovascular diseases are concerned, there are a number of well-designed retrospective studies that provide evidence in favour of the hypothesis that factors such as personality type may be important in the aetiology of disease.

Some may question whether ischaemic heart disease is a disease of stress. In a 'biological' sense it is, however, since 90% of myocardial infarctions are due to atherosclerosis, a contributory factor (stressor) to this process is a constant and heavy intake of saturated fat as a source of 'stress' for the person. In this case, the liver responds to the hyperlipidaemia by synthesizing large amounts of cholesterol from circulatory fats. As time passes, more and more cholesterol is deposited in blood vessels, including the coronary arteries, which may be sufficient to restrict blood flow to the organs they supply. At first, this may be transient or partial (e.g. at times of high oxygen demand, angina pectoris may be induced), and later, total and permanent (e.g. in myocardial infarction). The stress response observed will vary according to the nature–nurture interaction subjectivity associated with the resultant ischaemic pain (see Chapter 21). Myocardial oxygen demands are not within the affected person's capabilities, but the degree of angina or the extent of the myocardial infarction emphasizes the subjectivity of this process. Following the classic formulation of Selye, people with ischaemic heart disease either

BOX 22.8 CONTINUED

adapt partially – angina – or do not adapt at all – myocardial infarction.

In our opinion, diseases are not due solely to one predisposing factor (stressor), but are due to the cumulative affects of multiple stressors. Using the example above, the stressors include all the risk factors associated with cardiovascular disease. These can generally be classified as being:

● within the body, e.g. a genetic predisposition (endogenous stressor) to hypercholesterolaemia. A gene was identified in 1992 that predisposes the individual to a myocardial infarction;
● outside the body, e.g. cigarette smoking, high dietary fat, and distressful life events (exogenous stressors), all of which are hypercholesterolaemic agents. This again demonstrates stressor subjectivity with relation to an individual's exposure to such a diverse range of stressors.

It is the cumulative effect of all coronary risk factors that is responsible for the resultant cardiac problem. The common view of stress is that it results from difficulties associated with lifestyle and professional or personal relationships. We believe, however, that every illness can be viewed ultimately as a stress-related illness (a disturbed homeostasis), whereby the individual's homeostatic controls have failed to cope with the imbalance, or 'adaptation energy' has been depleted. This applies regardless of whether it is:

● a commonly referred to stress-related condition, such as coronary heart disease or an infection. Then, all the risk factors could be referred to as stressors, which may be linked to environmental influences on gene expression;
● a serious condition not commonly labelled as being stress related, e.g. AIDS. The stressors associated with AIDS are HIV and the pathogenic stressors of the opportunistic infections that have led to the person being diagnosed with AIDS. Perhaps the disease can be regarded as a phenomenon that occurs when an agent or condition threatens to destroy the dynamic state (i.e. homeostatic mechanisms) upon which the integrity of the organism depends, and the manifestations of disease appear to be, in large measure, manifestations of the organism's efforts to adapt to and contain threats to its integrity. In this sense, all diseases are, to some extent, disorders of adaptation, as Selye suggested in 1956.

Exercise

What do you understand by the statement, 'all illnesses are stress related'?

Summary

1 Stress is a disturbed homeostasis that manifests itself via certain psychophysiological bodily responses (imbalances).

2 Stress occurs only when the cumulative effects of stressors reach or supersede the stress threshold, which varies between individuals and within the individual with time, since it may be influenced by circadian fluctuations and as the individual goes through the different developmental stages.

3 The stress experienced is either eustress or distress. The former is regarded as a healthy bodily response, the latter an unhealthy response.

4 A person's perception of stressors, stress thresholds, their resistance or adaptation to stress, their coping strategies, the stress-related illnesses people experience in their lives, and their eventual outcome are all subjective.

5 The basis of subjectivity depends on an individual's genotype (i.e. nature) and the unique environmental perceptions (nurture) they are exposed to throughout their lives.

6 Although the general adaptation syndrome (GAS) has been criticized, it is accepted as a description of the physiological responses observed when the body is subjected to stress. Stress induces changes that involve the sympathetic nervous system and various hormones and, superficially, would appear to represent a significant failure of the homeostatic process. However, as this book has illustrated, homeostasis is not about constancy or even balance, but is about the provision of optimal conditions. Thus, physiological processes in general have to be adaptable. Stress responses help to maintain the circulatory system and facilitate wound healing, and so should be viewed as being of benefit (i.e. eustressful) to the recovery, for example, from trauma and surgery. However, they are influenced by factors such as sensitivity and an altered metabolic baseline; under these circumstances, optimal conditions may not prevail, or the adaptive responses themselves promote a metabolic 'deficit', so the responses become distressful with consequences for general wellbeing and recovery. Nutritional support and the use of fluid therapies are therefore important considerations in the postoperative care of the surgical patient, especially if there is a pre-existing metabolic disturbance, such as diabetes mellitus. In this case, even normal adaptive responses can be distressful.

7 Integration of sociology, psychology and physiology is required to investigate stress from a nature–nurture perspective. This would involve focusing attention on the multiple cumulative stressors that are responsible for each stress-related condition, since it is our opinion that all diseases are a result of cumulative stressors (including physical, psychological, environmental, social and developmental). Some disorders are easily identifiable, while others are difficult to pinpoint.

8 Since stress is acquired via nature–nurture interactions, it follows that stress management must involve a multidimensional approach. Organizations and individuals must work together for their mutual self-interests. It is important for everyone to become educated in this area of research, in order to identify distress in oneself and then to take appropriate action via individualized coping methods so as to transfer distress into eustress, or to remove or adapt to distressors. It may be a matter of 'life and death' – *yours!*

Review questions

1 Stress involves interaction of the autonomic nervous system and the endocrine system. Communication throughout the body occurs via nervous and chemical messages. Why do we need two different methods of communication?

2 The adrenal gland has the potential to help us overcome potentially harmful situations. Look up the anatomical layout of this endocrine organ and locate the cortex and medullary regions.

3 The adrenal cortex produces aldosterone, a mineralocorticoid. Find out how this hormone helps to regulate the concentration of the extra cellular fluid.

4 Glucocorticoids are also produced by the adrenal cortex. An example is cortisol. What are the functions of this hormone.

5 What is the third type of hormone produced by the adrenal cortex?

6 The adrenal medulla secretes catecholamines. Name these hormones.

7 Catecholamines are sympathomimetic, which means they initiate the fright/fight/flight response. Imagine you are confronted with an angry dog running towards you. Describe the changes to your breathing, heart rate and energy levels.

8 The changes discussed in your answer to question 7 are the first stage of the general adaptation syndrome, adapted homeostatic responses designed to deal with the immediate emergency. What happens in the second and third stages of this response?

9 'Stress is a subjective experience.' Discuss this statement with reference to (i) patients' illnesses; (ii) how it may help a nurse to recognize and relieve distress in patients; and (iii) the occupation of nursing from a student's perspective.

REFERENCES

Al Rub, R.A. (2000) Legal aspects of work related stress in nursing: exploring the issues. *AAOHN Journal* **48**(3): 131–5.

Barber, T. (1998) Stress and the management of change. *RCM Midwives Journal* **1**(1): 26–7.

Cannon, W.B. (1935) Stressses and strains of homeostasis. *American Journal of Medical Sciences* **189**: 1.

Carlisle, C., Baker, G.A., Riley, M., and Dewey, M. (1994) Stress in midwifery: a comparison of midwives and nurse using work environmental scale. *International Journal of Nursing Studies* **31**(1): 13–22.

Cavanagh, S.J. and Snape, J. (1997) Stress in student midwives: an occupational perspective. *British Journal of Midwifery* **5**(9): 528–32.

Clancy, J. and McVicar, A.J. (1997a) Homeostasis – the key concept to physiological control: perioperative influences on water and electrolyte homeostasis. *British Journal of Theatre Nursing* **7**(8): 27–32.

Clancy J. and McVicar, A.J. (1997b) Homeostasis – the key concept to physiological control: wound healing – a series of homeostatic responses. *British Journal of Theatre Nursing* **7**(4): 25–34.

Clancy, J. and McVicar, A.J. (1998a) Homeostasis and nature–nurture interactions: a framework for integrating the life sciences. In Hinchliff, S.M., Norman, S.E. and Schober, J.E. *Nursing Practice and Health*, 3rd edn. London: Arnold.

Clancy, J. and McVicar, A.J. (1998b) The metabolic response to surgery. *British Journal of Theatre Nursing* **8**(3): 12–18.

Cox. T. and McKay, C.J. (1976) Psychological model of occupational stress. Paper presented to the Medical Research Council Meeting – Mental Health in Industry, London.

Cox, J.L., Connor, Y. and Kendell, R.E. (1992) Prospective study of the psychiatric disorders of childbirth. *British Journal of Psychiatry* **140**: 111–17.

Farrington, A. (1997) Clinical management. Strategies for reducing stress and burnout in nursing. *British Journal of Nursing* **6**(1): 44–50.

Holden, J.M. (1992) Emotional problems associated with childbirth. In Alexander, J., Levy, V. and Roch, S. *Midwifery Practice. Postnatal Care. A Research-based Approach.*

Holmes, T.H. and Rahe, R.H. (1967) The social adjustment rating scale. *Journal of Psychosomatic Research* **11**: 213–18.

Howells-Johnson, J. (1998) Manifestations and management of stress in health-care workers. *British Journal of Nursing* **8**(3): 25–30.

Jones, E. (1997) Creating healthy work: stress in the nursing workplace. *Revolution* **7**(2): 56–8.

Lazarus, R.S. (1966) *Psychological Stress and Coping Process*. New York: McGraw-Hill.

Lazarus, R.S. and Folkman, S. (1984) *Stress: Appraisal and Coping*. New York: Springer.

Lees, S. and Ellis, N. (1990) The design of a stress management programme for nursing personnel. *Journal of Advanced Nursing* **15**: 946–61.

Lepore, J.S., Palsane, M.N. and Evans, G.W. (1991) Daily hassles and chronic strains: a hierarchy of stressors. *Social Science and Medicine* **33**(9): 1029–36.

Marshall, S.M. (1996) The perioperative management of diabetes. *Care of the Critically Ill* **12**(2): 64–7.

Moore, E. (1997) Occupational and dysfunctional stress in nursing. *British Journal of Theatre Nursing* **7**(6): 23–4.

Norrie, P. (1995) Do intensive care staff suffer more stress than other staff in other care environments? A discussion. *Intensive Care Nursing* **11**(5): 293–7.

Rausch, D.T. (1996) Providing care for the caregiver ... roles of the infertility nurse ... understanding of stress and burnout in the nursing profession. *Infertility and Reproductive Medicine Clinics of North America* **7**(3): 623–36.

Rhead, M.M. (1995) Stress among student nurses: is it practical and academic? *Journal of Clinical Nursing* **4**(6): 369–76.

Santamaria, N. (1996) The difficult patient stress scale: a new instrument to measure interpersonal stress in nursing. *Australian Journal of Advanced Nursing* **13**(2): 22–9.

Sawatzky, J.V. (1998) Understanding nursing students' stress: a proposed framework. *Nurse Education Today* **18**(2): 108–15.

Selye, H. (1956) The general adaptation syndrome and diseases of adaptation. *Journal of Clinical Endocrinology* **6**: 117–18.

Selye, H. (1976) *The Stress of Life*. New York: McGraw-Hill.

Simoni, P.S. and Paterson, J.J. (1997) Hardiness, coping, and burnout in the nursing workplace. *Journal of Professional Nursing* **13**(3): 178–85.

Sowney, R. (1996) Stress debriefing: reality or myth? *Accident and Emergency Nursing* **4**(91): 38–9.

Wallace, E. (1994) Feeding the wound: nutrition and wound care. *British Journal of Nursing* **3**(13): 662–7.

Yerkes-Dodson, P. (1982) Cited in Dodson, C.R. (1982) *Stress. The hidden adversary*. Lancaster: MTP Press. pp. 29–30.

FURTHER READING

Admi, H. (1997) Nursing students' stress during the initial clinical experience. *Journal of Nursing Education* **36**(7): 323–7.

Boey, K.W. (1999) Distressed and stress resistant nurses. *Issues in Mental Health Nursing* **20**(1): 33–54.

Circadian rhythms

INTRODUCTION: RELATION OF RHYTHMS TO HUMANS

The term 'circadian' stems from the Latin words 'circa' meaning 'about', and 'dies' meaning 'one day'. A rhythm refers to a sequence of events that repeat themselves through time in the same order and at the same interval. Thus, human circadian rhythms refer to the physiological, biochemical and behavioural (or psychological) events that are repeated in the body every 24 h. Some human rhythms, however, are persistent and are of shorter duration, i.e. not circadian. For example, the adult heart rate, with approximately 70 beats/min. Luce (1977) reported that it was Ogle in 1866 who first identified human circadian rhythm (of body temperature) and Simpson and Galbraith in 1906 who established that the monkey's temperature rhythm was harmonized (or synchronized) according to the light and dark cycle.

Most human studies came much later. In 1959, Halberg stated that physical, psychological and biochemical parameters are intrinsic to individuals with a day and night periodicity of 20–30 h, i.e. the intrinsic rhythm must be entrained to one of 24-h periodicity.

Rhythms, though not necessarily circadian, are associated with all forms of life. Because organisms are a part of the physical environment they live in, they are responsive to natural rhythmical changes within that environment.

Circannual rhythms are of a yearly periodicity and are very important in plant and animal species as they control breeding and hibernation. Humans are not obviously a rhythmic or cyclical species, as they have no breeding season, migration, hibernation, etc. Thus, it is debatable whether these rhythms are present in humans, although they may be responsible for mood swings at certain times of the year. That is, some people feel good and are at their happiest during the spring and summer months, which may explain in part why suicide rates are at their lowest at this time of the year. In contrast, some people feel low and depressed in winter months (this corresponds with seasonal affected disorder, SAD), which may be linked to the higher suicide rates during this time of the year. The mood swings may be related to the amount of natural daylight, since light is arguably one of the most important environmental stimuli that control human rhythms.

Exercise

Distinguish between circadian, circannual and persistent rhythms.

CONTROL OF CIRCADIAN RHYTHMS

It is obviously outside the scope of this book to discuss 'psychological' circadian rhythms; these will be omitted owing to the nature of this textbook. Biochemical rhythms will be limited to just a few common examples associated with physiological rhythms. The reader should be aware, however, that these three parameters of bodily function are inseparable and are interdependent entities. Although physiological rhythms such as body temperature will be described, the reader should bear in mind that heat is produced as a consequence of metabolic reactions, which are dependent on cellular biochemistry. In addition, physiological parameters can be influenced by one's psychological functions (or vice versa); for example, the majority of 'psychological' performance peaks are associated with peaks in body temperature. The purpose of this chapter is to emphasize that if we were to 'look inside' our bodies, we would see a number of repetitive psychophysiological patterns. Some cells would be more active in the morning when the body is in an awake state, while others will be more pronounced at night when we are asleep. These 'normal' patterns become disturbed in illness, or when we change our natural timing of sleep–wake patterns, such as in staying up late at weekends, admission to hospital, doing shift work, or travelling across different time zones.

Technical advances now mean that non-invasive assessment of physiological variables can be performed, and that measurements can be made on very small samples of fluids, including plasma, urine and saliva. Thus, sequential measurements can be carried out during the circadian period.

Body temperature

The body temperature of circadian rhythm does not markedly differ in 'normal' healthy people, and thus is one of the most reliable indicators of 'time' inside the body. Body temperature is an indicator of the level of a person's metabolism: an increased body temperature is associated with a high rate of metabolism, which necessitates quicker heart and respiratory rates in order to deliver more nutrients and oxygen to the active cells. A high rate of metabolism requires more energy (ATP) to drive the metabolic reactions. Consequently, the metabolic pathways of cellular respiration are faster, with the result that more heat energy is produced, thus increasing the body temperature.

Figure 23.1 illustrates the expected circadian rhythmicity of oral temperature. The pattern of change is:

1 A steep rise in the morning, becoming maximal during late morning (or early afternoon in some people).

2 A slight decline from the maximum, followed by a return to the maximum or a value close to it later in the afternoon; this is called the 'post-lunch dip'.

3 A decline in the afternoon or early evening, continuing through the night.

4 The minimum value (or nadir) in the early hours of the morning.

One would expect such rhythmicity, since the increase in body temperature, hence metabolism, begins just before awakening, preparing the body for the waking process and subsequent events. The rise continues during the morning and early afternoon, which are the times when we require a higher rate of metabolism to deal with daily activities. The fall-off during late afternoon and the declining levels in the evening are a consequence of our activities slowing down and getting ready for sleep. Upon sleeping, such parameters are at their lowest (body temperature falls at night by about half a degree Celsius, which represents a considerable change in metabolic activity), since a function of sleep is to replenish energy levels in preparation for the following daily activities. The temperature reflects changes in thyroxine, since this hormone controls the metabolic rate during the 24-h period. Only people who are very sick, e.g. with cancer, fevers (pyrexias) or encephalitis, show distortions of this rhythm.

Body temperature is actually related more closely to changes in skin temperature than it is to metabolism. Constriction of superficial skin (cutaneous) blood vessels reduces heat loss, and so promotes a rise in body temperature. The change in skin temperature occurs before the body temperature is elevated, so body core temperature changes seem also to be a consequence of rhythmic vasomotor changes in the skin vessels, in addition to a change in metabolic rate.

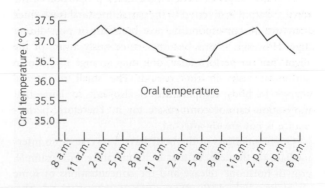

Figure 23.1 Oral temperature over 36 h.

The diurnal rhythm of performance and arousal seem to parallel that of body temperature. The most consistent improvement in efficiency occurs during the first 3 h, when the temperature rise is most noticeable. On a general note, peak performance corresponds to the peak temperature and arousal levels, occurring between midday and 6 p.m., which is also the period of quickest reaction times and best psychomotor coordination. The poorest performance coincides with the intervals of lowest temperature and arousal; this is between 3 a.m. and 6 a.m. This is generally referred to as the 'dead spot', and it is not surprising since, between 2 a.m. and 7 a.m. there is a natural urge to sleep.

Subjectivity of circadian rhythmicity

The timing or duration of maximum temperature and 'post-lunch dips' (PLDs) may vary between people, but the rhythmicity tends to be consistent in the same individual. 'Morning people', in whom temperature shows a faster rise and peaks earlier in the morning (i.e. the peak in Figure 23.1 would move to the left), claim that they perform physical and mental tasks better in the morning. In 'evening people', the day temperature rises more slowly and peaks later (i.e. the peak in Figure 23.1 moves to the right). The steepness of the rise, the timing and duration of the peaks of temperatures (morning and evening people), PLD variations, the steepness of the decline, dead spot times, etc. all demonstrate that there is subjectivity of circadian rhythmicity variation within the population.

The PLD phenomenon has not been explained satisfactorily, as it occurs irrespective of whether we have lunch or not. The PLD does not affect one's performance during this period simply because an increased proportion of the cardiac output is diverted to the gastrointestinal tract, since there are no corresponding post-breakfast or post-dinner dips. However, if one becomes consciously aware of the slight 'lull' in performance, one may arrange to perform automatic tasks in this period. The small rhythmical change in body temperature is also not so large that motivation cannot compensate for it. Therefore, performance is not greatly affected.

Other functions of the body have a reverse or an intermediate rhythmicity to that of temperature. For example, growth hormone release and the concentrations of some electrolytes in body fluids tend to have their maximal value nocturnally.

Urination

Figure 23.2 demonstrates a rhythm in urinary excretion, which involves the production of a large volume of urine in the morning and midday and lower volumes at night. The urinary circadian rhythm may result from the influence of bodily rhythms in parameters such as glomerular filtration rate (GFR), tubular reabsorption, antidiuretic hormone (ADH) secretion, or from fluid intake. The rise in urine flow is dependent on the switchover from dark to light. A decreased recognition of light cues in elderly people and blind people, therefore, may result in abnormal rhythms.

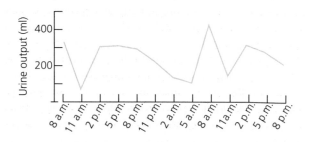

Figure 23.2 Urine output over 36 h.
Q. How is the urinary output circadian pattern associated with the sleep—wake cycle?

Urinary excretory products, e.g. sodium (Na^+) and potassium (K^+), demonstrate separate activities (Figure 23.3). Potassium excretion changes are pronounced. Generally, for a person who goes to bed at 11 p.m. and rises at 7 a.m., most potassium excretion would be between 10.30 p.m. and 2.30 a.m. Variations in these are explained by individual differences in diets and routines.

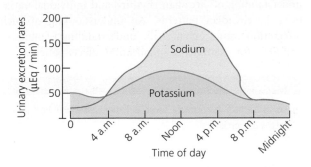

Figure 23.3 Urinary excretion of potassium (K⁺) and sodium (Na⁺).

Blood components

Figure 23.4 illustrates individual variation with reference to the timing of peaks and nadirs, and the duration of troughs and plateaux of the concentrations of certain plasma components. The rhythms of iron, phosphate and corticosteroid hormones demonstrate considerable consistency, and thus can be of practical importance. For example, corticosteroids are released from the adrenal gland in a series of discrete episodes, including an increase in release early in the morning, and a declining frequency as the day proceeds, although throughout this broad pattern there is a series of small sharp peaks. Figure 23.5 illustrates a typical circadian pattern in a 'normal' healthy subject. A steep rise from low nocturnal values to a maximum about 1 h before waking is observed, and the peak is just before the end of the dark phase at a time when we are usually awakening. Perhaps this may promote central nervous system arousal, which causes waking up.

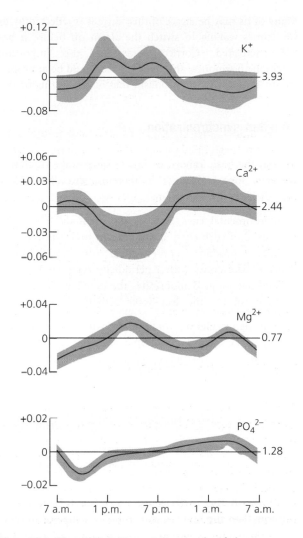

Figure 23.4 Mean (indicated by zero) diurnal cycles of plasma concentrations of potassium (K⁺), calcium (Ca^{2+}), magnesium (Mg^{2+}) and phosphate (PO_4^{2-}). Shaded areas indicate the subjectivity of individual circadian parameters.

Q. Discuss what circadian pattern variation or subjectivity means.

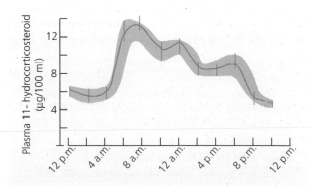

Figure 23.5 Circadian rhythm of plasma 11-hydrocorticosteroid concentrations. The shaded area represents subjectivity in the population studied.

Q. Describe the 'normal' circadian pattern of hydrocorticosteroid, and relate it to performance of physical and mental tasks and arousal levels during a 24-h period.

Many of us may be aware of this, since it is reflected by us sometimes waking to switch the alarm off before it has been activated. Corticosteroids are also important metabolic hormones, and their release would be appropriate for the move in metabolism that occurs at this time.

Rhythm synchronization

At rest, the basic inborn or innate sleep–wake rhythm is generally longer than 24 h, therefore circadian (24-h) periodicity is dependent on:

- environmental cues, such as the night–day cues. The removal of such cues, as observed in underground cave studies, produces non-circadian (or 'free-running') sleep–wake cycles with a periodicity range of 16–50 h. The huge range demonstrates the individual's variation in control over the sleep–wake 'activity' cycles;

- levels of circulating compounds, which influence the sleep–wake cycle. For example, waking may be associated with the stimulatory effects of corticosteroids on the brainstem, including the respiratory and cardiac areas.

> **Exercise**
>
> Identify the location and functions of the cardiac and respiratory centres. If you are having difficulty, refer to Chapters 12 and 14.

When all the rhythms are following their expected patterns then the body is said to be in a state of internal synchronization. It is now considered unusual to find a 'physiological' variable without a rhythm. The authors suggest that since mind–body functions are interdependent, this synchronization can be achieved only by integrating psychophysiological rhythms and observing how the environment affects each rhythm. In this way, nature–nurture interactions become instrumental in our understanding of circadian rhythms and individual variations in circadian patterns. An understanding of such integration would enhance the understanding of illnesses and how, for example, hospitalization affects patients.

> **Exercise**
>
> How is the body temperature circadian pattern associated with the sleep–wake cycle?

Control of circadian rhythms

It is generally accepted that there is a genetic (endogenous) basis of control, with environmental (exogenous) modification of the circadian rhythms.

Endogenous rhythms are 'free-running' (i.e. shorter or longer than 24 h), being modified exogenously to give a 24-h rhythmicity; this is the process of entrainment or synchronization. These modifying exogenous cues (called 'zeitgebers' or synchronizers') include light/dark, clocks, radio, television, and a regular lifestyle involving work, leisure and mealtimes.

Rhythms vary in the relative influence of their endogenous and exogenous components. For example, body temperature has a large endogenous component, which is why its circadian variation is minimal, but the release of some hormones has large exogenous components, e.g. adrenaline surges occur whenever the individual is stressed.

> **Exercise**
>
> Using Chapter 22, list other hormones that are released in the adaptation stage of the Selye's general adaptation syndrome.

Light and dark cues are generally considered to be the most important exogenous cues to which species synchronize their bodily rhythms. In humans, the importance of light as an exogenous zeitgeber is supported by isolation studies, studies involving blind people and studies of Eskimos.

> ## BOX 23.3 POOR SLEEPERS
>
> Body temperature curves strongly suggest that poor sleepers might be out of synchrony with the 24-h day. Their temperature declines less when compared with good sleepers, and is still declining when they rise in the morning. Poor sleepers may wish that they could go to bed later and rise later than is socially convenient, for the body time actually may lag behind the clock time (i.e. showing a longer period than 24 h). These free-running periods are common in response to distress, and may help to explain the insomnia that accompanies many illnesses, particularly in mentally ill patients. Thus, during this free-running period, the individual is performing their waking tasks with a 'sleeping' body, and subsequently may develop psychosomatic and emotional symptoms as a result of this imbalance or desynchronization.

> ## BOX 23.4 THE HUMAN GENOME PROJECT TO IDENTIFY CIRCADIAN GENES?
>
> One of the objectives of the Human Genome Project is to identify the endogenous location(s) of circadian rhythms in humans. Once this is identified, scientists may then identify the link between the gene(s) and seasonal affective disorders. Furthermore, an understanding of the clock's molecular working might suggest therapies for these conditions, as well as means of alleviating the problems associated with insomnia, jet lag and shift work (See later.).

Isolation studies

Mills (1973) studied a young man who wore a wristwatch throughout a 3-month stay in a cave. Although the subject resolved to sustain a 24-h routine, Mills demonstrated that the subject got out of bed later, slept when tired, and generally lived on an activity–rest cycle that was longer than 24 h. In other words, free-running rhythms were exhibited because of the removal of exogenous cues. Other studies have demonstrated sleep–wake (endogenous) rhythms to be of a greater periodicity than 24 h, although the range documented for this cycle has been between 16- and 50-hourly rhythms. The difference in the free-running periods demonstrates individual variation in the control of the sleep–wake cycle. Subjectivity is not surprising, as each individual is comprised of their own unique blend of genes and their unique environmental perceptions. Although the environment is controlled to a certain extent in isolation studies by the removal of exogenous cues, we would argue that we cannot control the individual's perceptions of that removal.

In contrast to the sleep–wake cycle, rhythms such as body temperature are controlled more genetically and are less dependent on environmental modification, as they exhibit a 25-h rhythmicity in isolation studies. Thus there are two classes of circadian oscillations:

- poorly entrained and easily modified patterns, e.g. sleep–wake cycle;

- strongly sustained rhythms, e.g. body temperature, hormone secretion, enzyme production and urine excretion.

Studies involving blind people

The endogenous control and exogenous modification of circadian rhythms is evident in studies involving people who are born blind. These people still exhibit rhythmicity, although the rhythms are a little disorganized and low in amplitude; consequently, these are often referred to as 'flattened' rhythms. However, such people still show some degree of periodicity that approximates to about 25 h. Perhaps this rhythmicity is brought about by blind people putting a greater emphasis (compared with sighted people) on exogenous cues, such as televisions and clocks, in order to entrain their rhythmicity. These changes have also been demonstrated in elderly people who have a decreased sensitivity to light (see later).

Studies involving Eskimos

The Eskimo year includes 6 months of continuous light and 6 months of continuous dark (twilight). Eskimos are therefore devoid of night–day circadian rhythms, and their rhythms are free running. To date, short-duration studies have demonstrated no adverse effects of this, so it could be questioned as to why we have circadian rhythms. However, researchers involved in longitudinal studies may identify adverse effects – only time will tell.

Whether or not light is the most important zeitgeber in humans remains unresolved. What is certain is that human circadian rhythms are a result of the cumulative zeitgebers, such as choice of mealtimes, sleep times, time to be sociable, lifestyle, etc. that enable us to co-operate as a social group. Thus, cultural differences, and differences within the same culture, produce individual variation.

Exercise

Explain the meaning of the German name for synchronizers.

Location of circadian control

The occurrence of free-running rhythms in the absence of synchronizers supports an innate location of rhythm generation. Early suggestions of a 'biological clock' within the hypothalamus were put forward as the 'inherited clock theory'. That is, a group of hypothalamic cells were suggested to be responsible for the inherent rhythmicity, which control the activity of the rest of the body, probably through pituitary endocrine activity, and so the rhythm may be 'born, not made'. In 1994, the so-called 'clock' gene on chromosome 5 was identified; whether this is activated only in the hypothalamic cells remains to be seen.

There is almost certainly more than one clock, perhaps all operating at once. These may, however, be controlled or synchronized to a 24-h rhythm by a 'master' clock. The clocks may be the homeostatic control centres of the brain, such as the medullary cardiac, respiratory and vasomotor centres, which in turn would be responsible for free-running patterns. Considerable research has tried to establish the location(s) of the clock(s) and the neuroendocrine communicating channels between them. The suprachiasmatic nucleus (SCN) of the hypothalamus has been strongly advocated as being the link between the clocks, and hence could be the 'master' clock. This is a plausible theory, since the hypothalamus is the centre of many activities, e.g. satiety, hunger and temperature control. A direct retinohypothalamic link also terminates in the SCN, which may explain why light is an important exogenous cue.

If the hypothalamus is the master clock, then damage to it will result in damage to other circadian functions. Evidence suggests that damage to the hypothalamic temperature control area (as occurs when one is subjected to recurrent fever) results in other interrelated bodily rhythms being affected, e.g. those of heart rate and respiratory rates. The circadian rhythms that become desynchronized presumably depend on which area of the hypothalamus is damaged.

The pineal gland has also been suggested to be the 'master' clock, since it is this gland that responds to light and dark, and it is an important link between light and dark reception and central nervous system function. The anatomical pathway that links the gland with the eye is as follows:

Retina
↓
Nucleus of Bochenek (in the cerebral peduncles)
↓
Medulla (in the brainstem)
↓
Superior cervical ganglia (a pair of sympathetic ganglia)
↓
Pineal gland

In this way, light incident on the retina will stimulate the pineal gland. Noradrenaline acts as an inhibitory neurotransmitter for the release of the pineal hormone melatonin. Thus, light stimulates noradrenaline at the neuropineal synapse, and so suppresses melatonin secretion. Figure 23.6 shows that melatonin secretion is 20 times higher in the dark than during the light phase. The functions of melatonin seem to be to induce sleep, and increase endocrine secretions from the pituitary, gonads and adrenal glands.

The fact is that we still don't know where the clock is, or even if there are many clocks controlled by a 'master' clock. Although the inherited clock theory receives most support, other theories do exist. For example, the basis of the 'imprint theory' is that initially an animal is arrhythmic (without rhythms), and it then learns from environmental conditions and parental behaviour what 24 h constitutes. This theory does not receive much support, as some rhythms appear in uterine development. It cannot

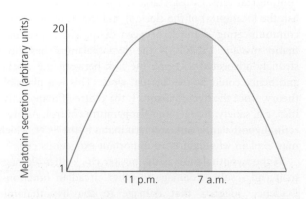

Figure 23.6 Melatonin secretion during the night.
Q. 'Circadian rhythms are controlled endogenously and modified exogenously.' What do you understand by this statement?

be demonstrated, however, that these rhythms are inherent in the fetus or result from changes in the mother, but it is likely that the fetus does respond to maternal rhythms, and that we are born with some form of rhythmicity. Neonatal rhythms are low in amplitude (flattened). As the body adapts to the light–dark activity, the rhythm becomes more mature, and eventually full maturity is developed in a light and dark environment. The rate of maturation varies between individuals with respect to the different rhythms. For example, the sleep–wake cycle must develop before there is a capability to entrain to light–dark cues. At approximately 20 weeks of age, some infants begin to synchronize with parents, but in others it takes more time (up to a few years) before synchronization is fully mature. Bladder control, which normally occurs within 2 years, can take up to several years; this late control is thought to be a result of a lack of light and dark cue modification of endogenous control of urine volume early on in the developmental processes. Further support comes from studies of children in nurseries in which artificial light predominates, which is thought to delay bladder control in some children. Other evidence includes studies involving jaundiced newborns; these babies are put into high-intensity light to reduce the jaundice, but the light prolongs the time for maturation of circadian rhythms.

Exercise

Suggest why elderly people are more reliant upon exogenous time-givers for circadian rhythmicity.

Discuss the suggested roles of the hypothalamus and the pineal gland in the entrainment of circadian rhythms.

ROLE OF CIRCADIAN RHYTHMS IN HOMEOSTASIS

Cells are the 'basic units of life', and therefore must ultimately control each circadian rhythm, and hence homeostatic function, via:

Genotype   Phenotype
(controller of   →   (circadian parameters)
endogenous rhythms)
                           ↑
                    Environment
                (exogenous modulators)

Phenotypes include all the measurable circadian parameters within the body, e.g. body temperature, levels of biochemicals such as neurotransmitters (e.g. acetylcholine, adrenaline), hormones (e.g. growth hormone, insulin), chemicals such as glucose, amino acids and electrolytes, and others such as pain-producing substances (e.g. kinins, prostaglandins), and pain-relieving substances

(e.g. endorphins, enkephalins). Owing to the interdependency of mind–body functions, factors such as mood, sleep and cognition will also be affected.

All circadian parameters are influenced by cellular metabolism and thus ultimately are mediated enzymatically. The production of enzymes is determined genetically (endogenously) and influenced environmentally (exogenously) by social modulators. For example, noise disturbances (exogenous modulator) may lead to less sleep because 'stress' hormones are increased, which affects the activity–rest (wake–sleep) cycle, which in turn can alter neural metabolism and affect one's mood. So is it the genetic, biochemical, physiological and psychological homeostatic disturbances that affect circadian rhythmicity, or is it circadian rhythm disturbances that lead to psychophysiological disturbances? Your guess is as good as ours!

CIRCADIAN RHYTHM DESYNCHRONIZATION: A HOMEOSTATIC IMBALANCE

It can be argued that health occurs only when the body has normal synchronized psychophysiological circadian rhythms. Once these rhythms are acquired, then their disturbance or desynchronization must be due to unnatural or 'abnormal' exogenous cues, such as shift work, travelling across time zones, illness, staying up late at weekends, or hospitalization. These cues can modify the expression of a person's genotype to produce psychophysiological imbalances by changing the body's pronounced daily rhythms of eating, sleeping, body temperature, performance, etc. This disturbance requires the body to

resynchronize, or re-establish homeostasis; otherwise, if desynchronization is chronically imposed, it can be detrimental to health. Such disturbances are referred to as 'phase shifts', because rhythms persist but the peaks and nadirs occur at times out of phase with periods of activity and inactivity (Figure 23.7).

Exercise

Look up the World Health Organization definition of 'health'. Now incorporate circadian rhythms with this definition.

Figure 23.7 Circadian rhythms: a homeostatic function. (a) Homeostasis = synchronized psychophysiological circadian rhythmicity = health. Range is dynamic, reflecting individual variation of parameter rhythmicity within the population based on the individual's unique genotype and perceptions of environmental cues. (b) Disturbed homeostasis = desynchronized psychophysiological 'circadian' rhythms = phase shifts due to (i) extreme, unusual or abnormal exogenous cues (stressors, zeitgebers, etc.), e.g. shift work, travelling across time zones, potential pathogens, and hospitalization; and (ii) a deviation in genotypes, e.g. congenital malformation, cancer, etc. (c) Homeostatic control systems re-establishing the balance = circadian rhythm resynchronization, as occurs following the removal of extreme, unusual or abnormal exogenous cues, e.g. shift-work patterns, cease chronic travelling across time zones, body's successful defence against potential pathogens, and community care. (d) Homeostatic imbalances as a result of control failure = free-running psychophysiological rhythms = ill-health/illness. (e) Clinical intervention, e.g. health

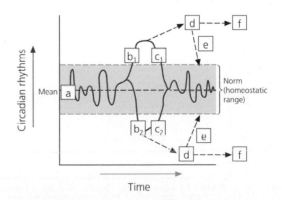

Time

education, community care, etc. (f) Untreatable clinical imbalances, e.g. terminal illness.

Q. Describe why illness and hospitalization are said to cause circadian rhythm desynchronization.

Q. Give an example of a rhythm that has a strong endogenous component, and a rhythm that is easily disrupted by exogenous cues.

The following sections discuss the consequences of such phase shifts as experienced by shift workers and by patients through their illness and hospital admission.

Shift work

Health consequences of shift work

A significant percentage of the working populations of industrialized countries are shift workers. Continuous shift work is necessary for a variety of reasons:

- *Economic gains.* Shift work is a high priority for the country's gross national profit.

- *Technological reasons.* Some industries, e.g. petroleum and steel, need to operate on a 24-h basis.

- *Human services.* The population requires public services throughout 24 h for security (police, military, etc.) and health reasons (healthcare workers).

- *Job security.* Workers may have to choose between shift work and redundancy.

- *Economic necessity for the workers.* Shift work brings financial bonuses that may be needed in order to maintain standards of living.

Various shift patterns exist, but studies are few and controversial. Shifts are classified according to the number of hours worked. Generally, 8 h constitutes a shift, and

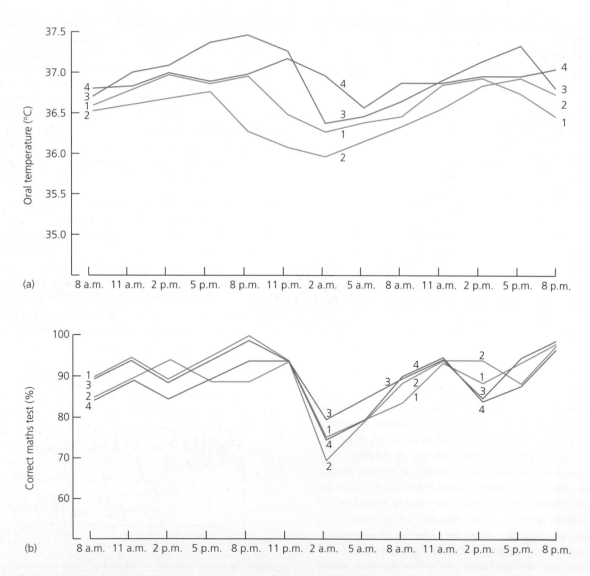

Figure 23.8 (a) Relationship between oral temperature and time over 36 h. (b) Relationship between mathematical testing efficiency (%) and time over 36 h. (c) Times of peak temperature values in non-shift workers and shift workers over a 7-day period. (d) Times of peak performance levels in mathematical testing between non-shift workers and shift workers over a 7-day period. 1 and 2: control subjects (non-shift workers); 3 and 4: experimental subjects (shift workers before commencing the shift) (Clancy and McVicar, 1995).

Q. Suggest why shift work researchers use the phrase 'maladaptation syndrome'.

shifts are split into mornings ('earlies'), afternoons ('lates') and nights. Twelve-hour shifts may also be used; this usually involves reducing the number of working days from five down to four or three.

Shifts in healthcare, especially nursing, depend on regional and hospital policies. Work patterns of nurses and midwives are either two shifts (earlies and lates) in association with permanent nights, or three shifts (mornings, e.g. 7 a.m.–3 p.m.; afternoons, e.g. 2 p.m.–10 p.m.; and nights, e.g. 9.30 p.m.–7.30 a.m.). The latter pattern is described as rotational, as workers rotate their shifts between afternoons, nights and earlies. Shifts produce a chronic alteration in environmental time (i.e. exogenous cues) (Figure 23.8). As a result, such shift work has important implications for both the personal wellbeing of the

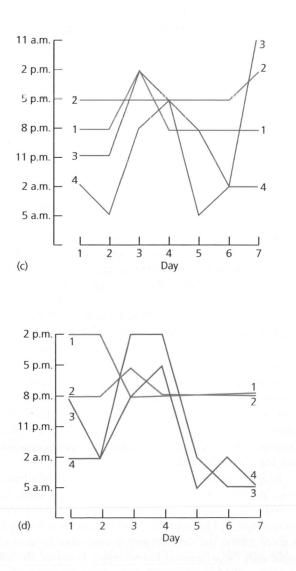

(c)

(d)

workers and the safety of the general public, both in and out of the work place.

There are many potential implications for the unsynchronized (unadapted) shift worker. 'Social' problems may exist as a result of a lack of qualitative and quantitative time spent with family and friends, and a lack of regular leisure time. Perhaps this may explain in part the high divorce rate see in shift workers. These social stressors can lead to a sense of isolation and helplessness in the shift worker, which have been linked by research to an increased incidence of psychophysiological imbalances, including:

- neurosis;

- depression (more common in night workers);

- some cases of schizophrenia;

- disorganized and poor eating patterns, which leads to a significantly higher incidence of gastrointestinal tract disorders. Common complaints are peptic and duodenal ulcers; shift workers are eight times more likely to get stomach disease and ulcers. An increased incidence of gastroduodenitis and other gastrointestinal-associated problems, such as anorexia and constipation, are also common. It may be that shifts promote the eating of more 'junk food', and increased caffeine consumption and smoking, which are responsible for, or contribute to, the gut disorders;

- disorganized sleep patterns: some workers have difficulty falling asleep because their sleep–wake pattern is affected. This is not surprising, because in night workers, the cycle of sleep and wakefulness is reversed completely and is initially at odds with other rhythms. Sleep disturbances are more common in the evening shift, while fatigue is associated with the night shift because day sleep is shorter. On average, night workers get 1.5 h less sleep than day workers (i.e. 6 h versus 7.5 h). The quality of sleep is reduced, even when daily noises are absent, i.e. rapid eye movement (REM) sleep is of low amplitude. There is also less REM sleep, and sleep is of shorter periods. Changing sleep patterns can have dramatic effects: sleep is one of the most important circadian rhythms, and its desynchronization has multiple effects on other circadian rhythms. Sleep disturbance may also be a contributing factor to the higher consumption of alcohol, cigarettes, sleeping pills and tranquillizers in shift workers. Performance is affected because night workers are working when bodily rhythms are geared up to sleep, and they sleep when the rhythms are geared for activity. For example, low levels of corticosteroids and adrenaline at night when night workers must function at their best cause them to be less efficient, and vice versa. It is not surprising, therefore, that sleep is of a poor quality and quantity.

- cardiovascular problems: shift work is associated with an increased risk of myocardial infarction (MI) when the shift pattern lasted between 11 and 15 years, although the incidence appears to decrease if the shift is continued for more than 20 years. A greater incidence of hypercholesterolaemia occurs in shift workers, the link being that 90% of MIs are a result of atherosclerosis;

- nervousness, tension and fatigue.

Shifts and work performance

The imbalances listed above (which may be considered as distressors) are likely to affect work performance. Research has demonstrated that general accidents in factories and cars are greater at 1 a.m., most industrial accidents occur between 2 a.m. and 4 a.m., and doctors and nurses are less efficient at night. Sweden's meter readers recorded most errors at night, and telephone operators identified 3 a.m.–4 a.m. as their 'dead spot', since more errors were recorded. In addition, impaired retention, decreased factual recall, poorer manual dexterity, slow information processing, slow problem solving, increased anxiety, hyperirritability, less social affection, depersonalization and divorce problems are also frequently quoted as consequences of shift work. These stressors may cause stress-related conditions, such as ulcers, hypertension, cardiac complaints, depression, neurosis, and even an increase in suicidal tendencies.

Night shifts, in particular, are associated with a high rate of absenteeism because of reported 'stress-related' conditions. The question is whether these conditions are due to the night work itself or are a consequence of the person's daily activities. Whichever is the case, we can safely say that night work is less efficient from the employers' and employees' points of view.

Afternoon (late) shifts are the most popular among shift workers, followed by morning (early) shifts, and then nights. Factors contributing to the popularity of late shifts are the lesser effects on social life, less susceptibility to digestive disorders, and less fatigue.

The scheduling of nursing shifts was cited most often as a reason for resignation. Thus, we can only assume that financial gain, job security, and devotion to patients are a few reasons why they remain.

Adaptation to shift work

Adaptation is a problem, since it takes several days to completely readjust to just a 1-h phase shift. It is not surprising that when a person works on night shift, their entire body enters a state of transition for many days. Although the individual responds to 'resetting' or synchronizing sleep and activity cycles, the problem is that our numerous rhythms do not reset at once. Blood pressure takes about 2 days to adapt, but body temperature takes

more than 5 days, in response to a 1-h time change in shifts; other rhythms (e.g. serum potassium) may take up to 2 weeks to reset to a new schedule of sleep and rest.

Research has identified there is a significant increase in road traffic accidents in the week after a change of shift work pattern, and suggests that this may be caused by the rhythms being desynchronized (maladapted). The positive correlation between shift workers and disorders also indicates maladaptation. But the 'adaptability' of some people suggests that some are more able to do shift work than others. This is difficult to analyse, because shift workers tend to be self-selected groups. The nature of this transitional vulnerability arising through phase shifting, perhaps due to a desynchronization of internal rhythms, remains one of the interesting questions of work–rest scheduling.

Longitudinal studies, which investigate the desynchronizing effects on the human lifespan, are not forthcoming. However, we would argue that the cumulative effects of shift-induced imbalances (stressors) would result in decreasing one's adaptation resistance to stress at a greater rate in shift workers. Also, a removal of shift work may actually decrease or diminish the stressors associated with the shift worker's situation.

Shifts probably affect people differently, since people's tolerance varies depending on their genotype and their perceived environmental (socializing) experiences. In addition, the rate and direction of shift change varies as a result of social, societal, organizational and public requirements, which is very important in one's perception of adaptation. The problem is that the individual may think that they are in control and adapted, but most people are unaware of the damaging effects of shift work on their bodies and their relationships. This was supported by the Rhone Valley survey of 1000 industrial workers, 45% of whom could not adjust to a 7-day shift rotation, and 34% could not adjust to a 2-day rotation. Thus, 55% and 66% respectively thought they were adapted. Interestingly, body temperature did not adapt in either group. The phrase 'shift maladaptation syndrome' is used in shift work research since it describes a condition affecting people who cannot adapt to shifts. The survey argued that this was characterized by a higher incidence of sleep–wake problems and gastrointestinal and cardiovascular pathology.

Body temperature is often used as an index of adaptation; in shift work involving consecutive night work for periods of 1–3 weeks, a phase shifting of the minimal body temperature will be observed. The temperature will shift to a point within the new sleeping period after 7+ days of night shift, i.e. adaptation has occurred. However, in shift systems with a single night shift, the natural circadian rhythm of body temperature is not altered significantly; linking this with performance, fewer errors will be recorded. Perhaps this is why certain health authorities employ a rapid-rotation shift system for their nursing staff.

BOX 23.6 SHIFT WORK IN NURSING

Health authorities argue that the reasons for rotational shift work in nursing are:

- slow rotation results in slow adaptation, so efficiency of work declines for up to 1 week. Thus, in a month of shifts there will be three efficient weeks and one inefficient week. However, improved safety measures for the nurse and the patient are needed at lower efficiency levels, and, as mentioned above, the nurses' body clocks are tending to revert back to their normal

circadian patterns during the days off. In our opinion, three efficient weeks is a misconception;

- rapid rotation (the majority of nurse shifts) produces very little adaptation of circadian rhythms, and workers just feel tired and fatigued. It is generally considered that rapidly rotating shifts do not affect efficiency. However, substantive longitudinal data that look at the cumulative effects of rapidly rotating shifts on the wellbeing of the nurse, and on efficiency levels, which are going to affect the wellbeing of the patients, are required

Plasma potassium (K^+) concentration can also be used, as it is a good indicator of how quickly a person is adjusting to phase shifts and living to non-circadian schedules. For a reversal of the patterns, the shift worker must work 14 nights to achieve adaptation, i.e. 14 consecutive nights before the K^+ concentrations have been inverted from their daily pattern of change.

Most night shifts are approximately 5 nights' duration, therefore some rhythmic patterns will be adapted and others will not. For example, body temperature takes a week to adapt, but then reverts back to normal during subsequent rest days. Because of the body's attempt to resynchronize during rest days, there can be no shift pattern with totally synchronized circadian rhythms, with the exception of the 'normal' synchronized daily shift, i.e. between 8 a.m. and 6 p.m.

Hypothetically, an ideal shift pattern would be one that takes into account the adaptation of all the rhythms. Thus, since 14 nights are necessary for adaptations of some rhythms, such as K^+, then one would have to be constantly at work, as days off would result in the individual trying to resynchronize to the 'normal' circadian pattern. Even constant working (without time off) would not help, however, since the worker would become easily fatigued and exhausted, which consequently would enhance the likelihood of illness (which itself also desynchronizes rhythms) and absenteeism. During absence from work, the person would then revert back to the 'innate' rhythms associated with a daily work routine.

Three major strategies have been used to address the problem of adaptation to shifts:

1 Schedule workers on straight shifts without rotation. The problem would be staffing the night shift.

2 Use a rapid rotation of shifts in order to escape the consequences of partial adaptation. The problem is that the circadian rhythms may still be affected, otherwise why would we feel tired and fatigued if the rest–activity cycle was within its homeostatic parameters?

3 Select people who seem to have the best tolerance to shift work or have abnormal sleeping rhythms, i.e. those with rhythms of low amplitude.

Wild (1992) replaced her 'normally' revised 2-week rota with a repeating rota shift system in nursing. This new system involved a work pattern of 5 days off and 9 days on over a fortnightly period. It also incorporated the following elements: days off before night duty, early shifts before days off, late shifts following time on the ward, as far as possible no single days off, alternate weekends off, and a 'scallywag' system. The scallywag staff varied their shifts according to the needs of the ward, i.e. cover for sickness, doubling up during busy times, etc. The benefits of such a system after a 3-monthly trial noted by Wild's staff were:

- being able to predict shifts in advance meant that staff could plan their social lives better;

- swapping shifts accommodated individual requests for time off;

- alternate weekends off were seen as an advantage, even to staff who worked weekends, as it provided time to do other things;

- from a managerial point of view it was much easier to organize.

In summary, shift work will always be a necessity because of its importance to the country's economy. This will become more of a problem to health as more and more of the world becomes industrialized and trends to run continuous around-the-clock operations increase. Since it is the authors' view that no shift can provide totally synchronized circadian rhythms (except 'normal' day work), then one must seek compensatory behaviours to reduce the desynchronizing effect of shift work. Such interventions include napping and exercise.

Napping

Napping can be used as a sleep supplement; many Japanese companies offer their workers rest rooms for this 'activity' during their shifts. They believe that this results in decreased fatigue and reinstated arousal, which increases the performance of their workforce. However, to the individual napper, this can reduce the quality and duration of the subsequent night's sleep, and research has shown that naps need to be controlled with reference to the individual's shift pattern if the person is to benefit. For example, if the next main sleep is on the following night, it is better not to take a nap in order to ensure that the sleep is of good, restorable quality. However, if the following night is a working night, then an afternoon nap is advisable to reduce the inevitable fatigue that accompanies night work.

Exercise

Regular, moderate exercise increases one's fitness and, as a result, decreases skeletomuscular signs of fatigue. There is also an increased alertness. Perhaps exercise increases resynchronization efficiency, resulting in quicker adaptation rates.

> **Exercise**
>
> Suggest what interventionary schemes may be used to compensate for desynchronized rhythms associated with shift work.

Interim summary

Further research is needed in this area to minimize the disadvantageous effects of shift work. This is being addressed in North America, where chronobiological departments have been developed to study circadian rhythms in an attempt to improve schedules. Chronobiologists (scientists who study time; 'chrono-' = time) believe that the best shift is the one that takes account of the natural circadian patterns. They also believe that night workers are able to accommodate their sleep disruption more satisfactorily if they go to sleep as soon as they finish their night shift, rather than staying up for a few hours following their night shift and going to sleep before normal sleep time. Chronobiologists have demonstrated that improved shift change patterns are those that rotate clockwise, i.e. mornings to afternoons to evening, and back to morning. In most shifts, this is usually at a frequency of 1 or 2 days, but if this period is extended, then it also improves circadian effects. Rotational shift patterns are a source of debate, as rhythms are constantly being disrupted and adaptation depends on the speed of rotation. The time interval between each shift in a slow rotation is generally only long enough for the rhythms to adapt partially; this partial resynchronization is potentially harmful to rhythms that do not adapt fully. Rapid rotation avoids the problems of continued partial resynchronization, and so is considered more satisfactory. The major problems associated with rapid rotation are the greater disruptions they cause to domestic and social life, which is why many people prefer slow rotation. With regard to rapid rotation, it is not known what cumulative effects will result over a long period of time. Some

German companies provide optional medical check-ups for their employees, and provide special hospital admission arrangements for them to normalize their desynchronized rhythms in an attempt to avoid long-term problems for their employees.

> **Exercise**
>
> Distinguish between the following terms: synchronization, desynchronization and resynchronization.

Travelling across time zones

When crossing time zones, a person becomes desynchronized as the body time is not in phase with the external cues. Body temperature adjustment times vary from 5 to 21 days according to different studies, demonstrating individual variation. This is hardly surprising when we consider that if we fly west from the UK to the USA, there is a time difference of between 5 and 8 h (east and west coasts, respectively). Thus, the phases of Americans are approximately 5–8 h behind, and consequently their peaks and troughs occur earlier than those of Europeans (Figure 23.9). People find it hard to adjust, and most (if not all) travellers are aware of the fatigue associated with 'jet lag'. Furthermore, continued exposure to this causes the 'jet syndrome', with symptoms of general malaise, sleep disruptions, feelings of disorientation, headaches, burning

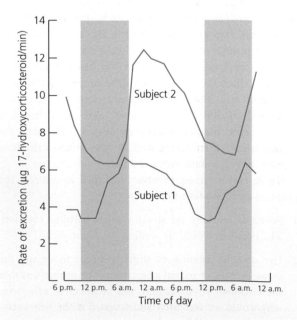

Figure 23.9 Excretion rates of 17-hydroxycorticosteroids in adults at different times of the day. Subject 1: Americans. Subject 2: Europeans. *Q. Describe why travelling across different time zones is said to cause circadian rhythm desynchronization.*

or unfocused eyes, gastrointestinal tract problems, sweating and shortness of breath. These are similar problems to those experienced by shift workers. Research has demonstrated that life expectancy of persistent flyers is reduced by 10%; however, this is not irreversible, and the symptoms disappear with time when persistent flyers stop flying.

The components responsible for travel fatigue are:

● *external desynchronization:*the weak time cues on arrival lead to slow adjustment;

● *internal desynchronization:* leads to a decrease in psychomotor skills.

When we invert our sleep pattern by east–west travel, or vice versa, we expose our bodies to potential pathogens, viruses and infection during the very phase when production of antibodies is at its lowest. Perhaps this may account for the high incidences of colds and infections that many travellers, students studying for exams, and people doing shift work experience. Melatonin is given in the USA to decrease the incidence of jet lag, aid quicker recovery in sufferers of jet lag, and increase alertness in shift workers. This supports the evidence that the light and dark cycle is one of the most important circadian rhythms, and that the pineal and other light and dark centres may be the master synchronizer(s) of other circadian rhythms.

BOX 23.7 CIRCADIAN RHYTHMS, ILLNESS AND HOSPITALIZATION

Some illnesses produce specific changes in normal circadian rhythms. For example, variations and desynchronized patterns of blood glucose occur in diabetic patients. Liver-diseased patients show urination and temperature peaks at night instead of in the morning.

The authors suspect that desynchronization of circadian rhythms could eventually explain recurrent symptoms; perhaps all illnesses need to be studied for disturbed circadian rhythms so as to contribute to the understanding of the associated signs and symptoms. Constant exposure to distressors (in this case desynchronized rhythms) leads to a deterioration of the adaptive system, and consequently one succumbs to an illness (stress-related illness). It is possible, perhaps, that this deterioration may even be caused by one or more circadian rhythm(s) moving out of phase.

Observations of circadian patterns have demonstrated that there are times in the day–night cycle that correlate with specific illnesses. For example, the peak frequency for the onset of myocardial infarctions is between 8 a.m. and 10 a.m. Peripheral circulation in the arms and legs reaches a low point between midnight and 4 a.m. Tissues receive less oxygen during this period, and therefore it is not surprising that some people with peripheral arterial disease are awakened with acute pain from their sleep at this time.

There also appears to be a peak time for births and deaths. Most labours begin around midnight, and births are more frequent in the early hours of the morning. Induced births, however, are opposite to natural labour, since from an economic point of view more staff are available during the day. Interestingly, the number of stillbirths follow the induced curves, and it is tempting to speculate, therefore, that the timing of the induction may be a contributory factor to the number of stillbirths, since it is not the natural time for delivery. Deaths are more likely to occur at night, but this is not surprising, since metabolism is at its lowest and so we are more at risk.

All illnesses are associated with desynchronized circadian rhythms. The rhythms that are most disturbed depend on the illness. For example, feverish illness produces pronounced desynchronized body temperature rhythms (and associated rhythms, e.g. heart, respiratory and metabolic rates).

Hospitalization

This chapter has already provided evidence that alterations in exogenous cues as experienced by shift work produce illness; these cues are markedly altered by hospitalization.

As mentioned previously, illnesses induce desynchronized circadian rhythms. These may be disturbed further and other unaffected rhythms may become desynchronized upon admission to hospital, since exogenous synchronizers are replaced partly by those cues determined by the ward policy and new environment. In addition, admission can potentially produce a greater desynchronization in people (e.g. blind people, elderly people) who have a greater dependency upon set exogenous cues for their circadian rhythmicity. Furthermore, not only are elderly people desynchronized to a greater extent following hospital admission, but they also find it more difficult to adapt to the imposed hospital zeitgebers.

All patients upon admission lose some of their exogenous synchronizers. Some wards still wake their 'geriatric' patients during the night to commode, which further disrupts the sleep–wake and associated rhythms; the nurse may report this as confusion. However, the authors would argue that any person may appear temporarily confused and distressed when awakened at these times, especially if they are awakened when in stage IV (deep) sleep. When labelled confused, the patient may be sedated, thus disrupting the sleep–wake and associated circadian rhythms further. Awakening policies are not restricted to care-of-the-elderly wards, since research has shown that patients are disrupted during sleep by nursing staff and noises and lights on the ward.

The hospitalized patient, whether elderly or not, has many additional routines or zeitgebers. For example, the last drug round is at about 10 p.m., with lights out soon after this. The patient is awakened at 6.30 a.m.–7 a.m., and there are specific meal times (breakfast at 8.30 a.m., lunch at midday, and dinner at 5.30 p.m.). Patients must also adapt to the presence of complicated and unfamiliar machinery in specialized ward areas. During this period of adaptation, the patient may appear to be confused. Increasing social interaction may be the way to reduce or remove this confusion. Research as highlighted the importance of face-to-face therapy at the patient's level of understanding, since a potential

BOX 23.7 CONTINUED

desynchronizer to patients comes from communication between nurses and staff.

The removal of wall-to-wall seating, which is still found in many hospital rest rooms, may improve social contact and so help remove the appearance of 'confusion' in patients and abolish unnecessary sedation. Perhaps it may also decrease the amplitude of circadian rhythm disturbances and reduce the adaptation period, thus improving the quality of care.

The study of circadian rhythms thus may aid the assessment of the individual needs of patients. Thus, forcing patients (and in particularly elderly patients) into a rigidly conforming pattern of care is not only going to potentially make them worse, but also

may make them confused and disoriented, thus increasing the level of dependency on the nurse. Conversely, it could be argued that rhythmicity might be promoted by adopting a highly regularized living routine, even if different from the one followed previously, since some improvement is noted in some elderly patients following an initial post-admission period of confusion. Perhaps this may be due in part to mundane routine rather than medical intervention. It remains controversial whether imposing environmental rhythms that do not coincide with a patient's own internal rhythms fosters the wellbeing of older patients.

See the case study of a man with a learning disability leaving a long-stay institution in Section 6.

BOX 23.8 CIRCADIAN RHYTHMS AND VULNERABILITY TO DRUGS

Chronopharmacology and chronopharmacokinetics are comparatively 'new' areas of research, and little is known. However, there is much evidence to suggest that a lower pharmacological tolerance exists at night, thus if the same dosages are given at night then they have greater pharmacological effects. For example, digitalis is 40 times more effective at night than during the day – but it is common ward practice to administer digitalis in the morning. This is 'normal' practice with drugs that are administered once daily, and depressed tolerance levels are not, on the whole, taken into account for drugs that are needed two, three or four times a day, as the same dosage is given at night as during the day.

Tolerance depends on the absorption rates of drugs, their distribution rates, their metabolism by the liver, and their excretory rates. All of these are depressed at night. Drug tolerance variation is even more pronounced in older people, since absorption rates are potentially much slower. However, the main problem is that older people are more likely to be affected by drug combinations, since many older people are taking multiple drugs. Thus, there is an increased drug distribution, resulting in a longer half-life of the drugs. This arises because older people have lower plasma albumin (which binds to certain drugs) concentrations, leaving more 'free' drug, therefore increased pharmacological activity occurs.

There is also a decreased activity of drug-metabolizing enzymes in the livers of elderly people. Depressed drug metabolism may also be due to a decrease in hepatic blood flow, therefore reduced dosages are required, and dosage intervals need to be less frequent in elderly people. Kidney clearance of drugs by the elderly is also reduced, which supports the need for decreased dosages and less frequent intervals.

A misunderstanding of drug dosages and drug intervals could conceivably lead to further desynchronization of circadian rhythms, and, as a result, hospitalization. A proportion of hospital admissions is due solely or partly to adverse drug reactions.

Older people seem to be a particular vulnerable group. Adverse drug reactions in them stem from the fact that a high proportion are taking some form of drug medication, and many are taking multiple drugs. Many older people are given repeat prescriptions without regular medical check-ups. In addition, self-medication is also a problem in older people, because they self-administered certain drugs before the introduction of the National Health Service. As a result, older people may exhibit drug-induced diseases. For example, overindulgence in laxatives (drugs to counteract constipation) has been demonstrated to have a strong link with the incidence of colonic cancers. It must also be remembered that sedatives and opiates also alter a patient's perception and ability to respond to environmental cues, and these classes of drugs are common in older people.

BOX 23.9 IMPLICATIONS FOR CARE

There is a need for the healthcare professions to study patients' circadian rhythms, and their disturbances, as rhythm desynchronization is an important diagnostic tool. For example, a continued increase in plasma calcium ion concentration beyond its normal circadian parameters could represent a gradual decalcification of bone, which is known to accompany continuous recumbency, and a fall in blood nitrogen is typical of the effects of starvation. Deviation in patterns can be indicative of disturbed homeostatic functions, e.g. in Addison's disease and Cushing's syndrome, the normal variation in cortisol release is largely or

entirely absent. In Addison's disease, cortisol concentrations are lower, but may not be any lower than is observed in normal subjects at night. Conversely, with Cushing's syndrome, elevated cortisol levels may be no higher than those shown in a healthy subject when rising in the morning. Diagnosis is thus aided by taking a morning and evening serum sample. If only single samples are permitted by hospital policy, then a morning sample would be better to detect Addison's disease, and an evening sample would be better to detect Cushing's syndrome. The timing of samples, however, is complicated if the patient is a shift worker,

BOX 23.9 CONTINUED

as there is no guarantee of their 'adapted' rhythmicity. In addition, the patient's nationality may have to be taken into consideration, e.g. an unadapted (resynchronizing) American visitor would have rhythms 5–8 h (depending on which coast they came from) ahead of Europeans (Figure 23.9). All these variations demonstrate the importance of individualized care for patients.

Where possible circadian rhythms should be applied routinely to all aspects of care. The following should become a matter of routine in order to improve the quality of care administered:

- Clinical staff could investigate optimal times (i.e. increased responsiveness) for chemotherapeutic administration, especially for medications that commonly cause allergic responses. Allergy testing should be investigated in the evening, when allergic responses are at their highest.
- Clinical staff could investigate optimal times for laboratory specimens. Since variations in the peaks of leucocyte counts, electrolyte concentrations, haematocrit, blood gas composition, temperature, urinary output, etc. all exist, it makes the common practice for collection of samples questionable. The 'typical' sample should be collected closest to the mean for that person, rather than at the time when it would be at its highest or lowest values. In addition, daily comparative sampling will be of maximal value only if it is performed at the same time of day every time to take into account circadian fluctuations. Presently, samples are usually drawn at 6 a.m. so that they are ready for when the physician arrives at the unit, a time when some of the rhythmic values are at their minimum. If regular samples (e.g. every 4 h) were taken, then a circadian pattern for the patient could be plotted after a few days (a process called 'circadian mapping'). Once established, circadian patterns can be used to avoid:
  - reactionary responses, e.g. decreased urinary output at night should not be controlled diuretically;
  - increased stressors or exercise at the patient's lowest resource point, e.g. the lowest pain response is between midnight and 4 a.m., so intravenous catheterization and other painful procedures could be started early in the rest cycle in order to minimize the pain response. The optimal time for treatment and surgery scheduling is thought to be in the early morning hours when the patient's metabolism is low, despite the practitioner's metabolism also being low and consequently risking error and accident. Also, care may be improved by monitoring patients closely at more susceptible times. For example, exaggerated bronchoconstrictory rhythm occurs in asthmatics at about 6 a.m., and special alertness is required at this time.
- A knowledge of circadian patterns can be of value from a health education point of view, since the body temperature peak is associated with a better performance in relation to both teaching (practitioner) and learning (patient). We would argue that the most important teaching time ideally would coincide with the patient's peak temperatures, in order to gain maximum benefit from the teaching. However, body temperature cannot always be used as a reliable indicator of the person's

performance, since illness and hospital admission may be associated with rhythm desynchronization in the patient.
- Research needs to investigate the circadian timing of 'stress-related' events, in order to avoid 'stressors', which can potentially affect the circadian rhythms of the patient.
- One could minimize circadian problems for patients by maintaining the patient's natural social synchronizers, e.g. emphasizing community care, particularly for the elderly. Night admission wards could be introduced to cater for insomniacs, people who are nocturnally disturbed, and people who are frightened of being alone at night. In addition to providing an extra element of care, this would also remove the 'burden' from families who obviously have their sleep patterns disturbed by the nocturnal activities within their homes.

The patient is in a period of desynchronization and/or resynchronization because of the illness itself, the admission process, and the stressors associated with being a patient. Therefore, care should support previous circadian rhythms where possible, and should not be associated with ward conformity. For example, sleep is usually influenced by social and occupational pressure, and removal of these pressures, e.g. with retirement or hospital admission, may result in a 'polycyclic' sleep pattern, i.e. 'cat naps' during the day. Napping reduces the quality and quantity of night-time sleeping; if the patient (particularly the elderly), either in the community or on the ward, complains of sleep disturbances, then this may result in narcotic prescription. We would argue that the best treatment would be to detect the stressors (e.g. boredom) that cause the naps, and remove (e.g. increase social interaction) or replace (e.g. face-to-face therapy) the stressors. The need for narcotics may be diminished, or better still abolished, thus benefiting the patient by removing the effects of the drugs, and also giving a sense of time.

If polycyclic sleep is evident on the wards, then one must question whether it is imposed or whether it is a normal routine for the patient. The nurse must try to remove it only if it is not the patient's normal routine, since a disturbed rest–activity cycle can lead to desynchronization of other rhythms. Providing a stimulating environment specific to each patient can prevent it. If polycyclic sleep is a normal occurrence for the patient, then we would argue that this should be encouraged in hospitals.

Patients are often overloaded with many additional stressors, and nurses should minimize these potential desynchronizers by various means. Interviews should be conducted as a series of short meetings rather than one long-winded interview, in order to develop a care plan. This should be by the same nurse if possible. The interviews should coincide with the patient's most receptive time, borne out by the body temperature peak. The patient should be involved in the decision-making process. Also, subsequent to discussions with the nurse, the patient should be allowed to 'sleep on it' before coming to a final decision. The patient should also be involved in rehabilitation, since increasing sensory input can transform distress into eustress. Finally, the patient's individuality should be considered. For example, the nurse could investigate whether the patient is a 'morning' or an 'evening' person, a shift

BOX 23.9 CONTINUED

worker, or an unacclimatized traveller, as this could influence assessing, planning, implementing and evaluating care.

Care of unconscious or comatose patients necessitates clinical intervention to maintain physiological equilibrium, so that the endogenous rhythm approximates to its innate time minus the zeitgebers. The nurse has to assume, therefore, that the rhythms are free running. If the patient is unconscious for a long period of time, or if there is brain injury, then desynchronization must be assumed. In such cases, it is essential that the nurse supports the previous circadian rhythms. In order to do this, the nurse must maintain the patient's physiological equilibrium. The patient must also be helped to reorient the brain to previous temporal and life experiences. This may involve playing favourite music or a relative talking about the past, for example.

Exercise

What is the possible link between community care and circadian rhythm resynchronization?

Summary

1 Human circadian rhythms are bodily processes that are repeated every 24 h.

2 The genetic (endogenous) component of such rhythms (demonstrated by studies of isolation, elderly people, congenitally blind people, and Eskimos) is responsible for producing innate rhythms that are free running, i.e. outside the 24-h periodicity.

3 The free-running rhythms are synchronized (entrained) by environmental cues (zeitgebers or synchronizers) to give the 24-h (circadian) periodicity.

4 Most circadian patterns (e.g. body temperature) show a rise and general peak (or plateau) during the waking hours, and a fall and nadir during the sleeping hours, although some (e.g. the release of growth hormone) display a reversal of this pattern.

5 Individual variation or subjectivity of circadian parameters occurs with relation to the timing of peaks and troughs, the degree of inclines and declines, and the timing of post-lunch dips and dead spots, according to an individual's genotype and their perception of environmental cues.

6 The hypothalamus appears to be the master clock synchronizing the free-running rhythms of the homeostatic control centres. There may also be a link with the pineal gland, since this is responsive to light–dark cues, which are very important zeitgebers.

7 Health is associated with internal synchronization, i.e. all the circadian rhythm parameters being within their homeostatic ranges.

8 Desynchronization occurs when the circadian rhythms are outside their homeostatic range; such a disturbance is known as a phase shift.

9 Phase shifts have been demonstrated in shift workers, people who travel across different time zones, during illness and upon hospitalization.

10 Chronobiologists suggest compensatory changes are necessary to minimize the circadian disturbances. For example, in shift work, shifts should be changed clockwise (i.e. morning to afternoon to evening, etc.). Longer intervals between changes must be introduced so workers have time to 'normalize' their patterns. In the healthcare setting, chronopharmacology removes some adverse drug interactions and decreases the need for hospitalization, and consequently the person's exogenous cues are maintained. This involves dosages and timing of dosages being calculated using the circadian changes that are associated with the illness and the process of hospitalization. Finally, if the nurse is hoping to meet the total needs of the patient, they must take into account the effects of circadian rhythmicity on temporal, physiological and psychological co-ordination when planning, assessing, implementing and evaluating care, and use this knowledge to aid a more speedy recovery.

Review questions

1 Discoveries from the Human Genome Project will undoubtedly substantiate the statement that bodily rhythms are controlled endogenously and modified exogenously to give a circadian periodicity. Discuss.

2 Shift work can seriously damage your health. Discuss this statement with relation to shifts associated with nursing

3 In health, all bodily processes display circadian rhythmicity. Discuss the long-term and short-term implications of hospitalization on this rhythmicity, and discuss how this knowledge may improve the quality (standards) of patient care.

REFERENCES

Halberg, F. (1959) Chronobiology. *Annual Review of Physiology* **31**: 675–725.

Luce, G.G. (1977) *Body Time*. St Albans, UK: Paldin.

Mills, J.N. (1973) *Biological Aspects of Circadian Rhythms*. New York: Plenum Press.

Wild, W. (1992) Changing times. *Nursing Times* **88**(29): 34-5.

FURTHER READING

Aschoff, J. (1966) Adaptive cycles. *International Journal of Biometeorology* **10**: 305–24.

Baxendale, S., Clancy, J. and McVicar, A.J. (1997) Circadian rhythms: the application to patient care. *British Journal of Nursing* **5**(26): 303–9.

Clancy, J. and McVicar, A.J. (1994) Circadian rhythms 1: physiology. *British Journal of Nursing* **3**(13): 657–61.

Clancy, J. and McVicar, A.J. (1994) Circadian rhythms 2: shift work and health. *British Journal of Nursing* **3**(14): 712–17.

Dobree, L. (1993) How do we keep time? *Professional Nurse* **8**: 444–9.

Fossey, E. (1990) Shiftwork can seriously damage your health. *Professional Nurse* **5**: 476–80.

Harker, J.E. (1964) *The Physiology of Diurnal Rhythms*. Cambridge: Cambridge University Press.

Klietman, N. (1967) *Sleep and Wakefulness*. Chicago: University of Chicago Press.

Minors, D.S. (1988) Practical Applications of Circadian Rhythms to Shift Work. The biological clock – current approaches. Southampton: Inprint (litho) Limited.

Mestel, R. (1994) Mouse gene could help master rhythm. *New Scientist* **7**: 15.

Minors, D.S. and Waterhouse, J.M. (1985) Circadian rhythms in deep body temperature, urinary excretion and alertness in nurses on night work. *Ergonomics* **28**(11): 523–30.

Moore-Ede, M.C. and Richardson, G.S. (1982) Medical implications of shift work. *Annual Reviews of Medicine* **36**: 607–17.

Petrie, K., Conagelen, J.V., Thompson, L. and Chamberlain, K. (1989) Effects of melatonin on jet lag after long haul flights. *British Medical Journal* **298**: 705–7.

Rutenfranz, E. (1982) Occupational health measures for night and day shift workers. *Journal of Human Ergology* **11**(suppl): 17.

Simpson, H.W. (1965) Transatlantic differences in circadian rhythms. *Journal of Endocrinology* **32**: 179–81.

Tureck, F.W. (1981) Are the suprachiasmic nuclei the location of the biological clock in mammals? *Nature* **220**: 280 00.

Section Six

Homeostasis in action: case studies

Adult care case studies
Childcare case studies
Mental healthcare case studies
Learning difficulties case studies

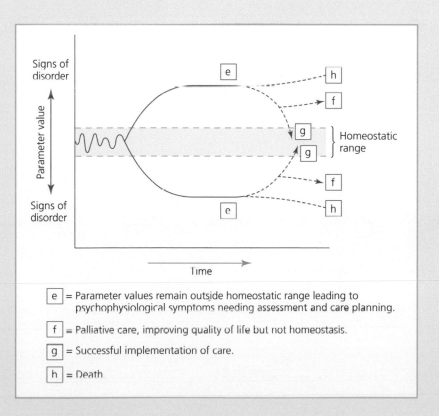

e = Parameter values remain outside homeostatic range leading to psychophysiological symptoms needing assessment and care planning.

f = Palliative care, improving quality of life but not homeostasis.

g = Successful implementation of care.

h = Death

The central theme of this book is human biological functioning. The concept of homeostasis has been used to illustrate and emphasize how parameters within the internal environment are regulated through appropriate responses of cells and tissues. In this way, an optimal environment is maintained in health, and cell needs are met.

Ill-health represents the consequences of an inability to maintain the internal environment. Section 5 of this book illustrated how this failure to maintain homeostasis arises through both intrinsic processes (i.e. genetic change and/or ageing) and extrinsic processes (i.e. through interaction with our external environment). These latter processes help to identify why homeostatic mechanisms must be dynamic, since interaction continually presents the body with challenges to its internal parameters.

Exercise

Before reading Section 6, you are recommended to re-read Chapter 1 and ensure that you are familiar with the principles of homeostasis, and the notion that clinical care represents extrinsic homeostatic mechanisms that replace those that have failed in patients.

If ill-health represents a failure to maintain homeostasis, then the care for a sick person logically must help to reduce the impact of such failure, or may even replace the failed mechanism. This notion that care provides an extrinsic homeostatic mechanism (to use the terminology, an extrinsic 'effector') was identified in Chapter 1, where we illustrated how the planning of care follows a process analogous to that of homeostasis. Section 6 relates this theme to common examples of disorders. Thus, the chapters of this section provide examples of case studies in the four branches of nursing care (adult, child, mental health and learning disabilities). In doing so, each case study notes the homeostatic failure that has produced the disorder, and the rationale and implementation of care that provides the extrinsic processes that help to improve or restore homeostasis. In each case, a version of the graph that has been utilized at points throughout this book (see Chapter 1 for full explanation of its basis) is provided as a means of aiding understanding.

In providing examples from each branch of nursing, this book notes the application of homeostasis principles to these very different areas of care. While the concept was developed to explain physical control, the need to maintain optimal neurological functioning also makes it applicable to cognitive and behavioural functions.

Each case considers the problem as a homeostatic disturbance, and is presented in the following format:

1   The case scenario.

2   The case as a homeostatic imbalance: background and presentation.

3   Restoring (or improving) homeostasis: aims of care, and implementation of care.

The cases are taken and modified from Clancy and McVicar (1998). The authors acknowledge the help of various people, identified at the beginning of the book, in preparing the cases. Please note that the cases presented are intended not to be comprehensive but to provide common examples that illustrate homeostatic principles in their pathology and in the care delivered.

Reference

Clancy, J. and McVicar, A.J. (eds) (1998) *Nursing Care: a homeostatic approach*. London: Arnold.

Adult care case studies

Case 1: a woman with breast cancer
Case 2: a man with chronic bronchitis
Case 3: a man with myocardial infarction

Case 4: a man with benign prostatic hyperplasia
Case 5: a young woman with secondary (renal vascular) hypertension
Case 6: a woman with rheumatoid arthritis

CASE 1: A WOMAN WITH BREAST CANCER

Scenario:

Janet is a 44-year-old married woman who recently discovered a painless lump in her right breast. Her GP referred her to a breast care surgeon, who performed a needle biopsy and subsequently diagnosed an adenocarcinoma ('adeno-' = of glandular tissue; 'carcinoma' = cancerous tumour). Janet was subsequently admitted to hospital for an operation to remove the lump (a lumpectomy) and also for an excision of axillary lymph glands. She was then referred to an oncologist for further treatment, including radiotherapy and cytotoxic chemotherapy.

Breast cancer as a homeostatic disturbance

Background

Breast cancer represents a disorder of the mechanisms that regulate cell division and proliferation, and arises from a profound change in the genetic composition of the cells (see Chapter 20, Box 20.14). As a consequence, breast cancer cells lose many of the characteristics of normal cells.

The most common types of breast cancer are infiltrating ductal adenocarcinoma (75%) and infiltrating lobular adenocarcinoma (5-10%). Breast cancer is the most common form of cancer that occurs in women. Currently, the UK has the highest mortality rate in Europe for this disease. The cause of breast cancer is unknown. Recently, a gene (BRA1) has been identified that is implicated in familial breast cancer. However, only a small percentage of breast cancers show this inherited component and, furthermore, not all women with the gene actually develop the disease. This is because cancer is a polygenic condition, and one gene alone will not induce its formation (see Box 20.14). Several cancer-promoting genes (oncogenes) have been discovered that play a role in the development of breast cancer.

Hormones play an important role in the development of breast cancer, although their exact role is as yet unclear. Some studies have linked long-term use of high-dose oral contraceptives with an increased incidence, while others suggest that breastfeeding and early age of first pregnancy offer some protection.

Presentation

Cells dividing at an accelerated rate eventually give rise to a palpable mass (tumour). Apart from invading local tissue areas, cancer cells are also capable of migrating (metastasizing) from their sites of origin to develop secondary tumours elsewhere. The most common sites of metastatic spread from breast cancer are bone and liver, diagnosed by bone and liver scans, respectively. These investigations are not performed routinely, but Janet may undergo them at a later date, or if problems arise. Bone metastases usually present with pain in the affected area. Liver metastases are often asymptomatic until late in the course of the disease, but may present with pain, liver enlargement (hepatomegaly) and/or jaundice.

Restoring homeostasis

See Figure 24.1.

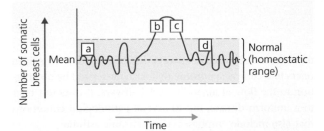

Figure 24.1 Breast cancer. (a) Numbers of somatic breast cells within homeostatic range, i.e. balance between production and action of cell growth factors and growth inhibitors. (b) Abnormal breast tissue growth as a consequence of excessive oncogene (cell growth) genes and/or decreased suppressor gene (growth inhibition) expression. (c) Intervention to reduce the number of abnormal cells (radiotherapy and/or chemotherapy or hormonal therapy to suppress tumour growth). (d) Successful reduction of somatic breast cells. This is difficult to assess accurately; a person is said to be in remission if there are no visible signs.

Aims of care

Treatment is aimed at surgical removal of the primary tumour, eradication of any remaining abnormal cells that may lead to the development of metastases, and suppression of tumour growth from any remnant cells. Care will also involve considerable psychosocial support. The outcome of breast cancer treatment depends largely on the stage of the disease at diagnosis.

Implementation of care

Surgery

The term 'cancer' (= crab) is well made: tumours are not bounded firmly (unlike cysts or nodal tissue) and cells extend out into surrounding tissue. Surgery therefore removes adjoining tissue in an attempt to remove the whole tumour. Cells may also drain from the tumour into lymph, so lymph nodes in the area (i.e. axillary nodes in the case of breast cancer) may also be excised.

Eradication of remaining cells using radiotherapy and chemotherapy

Radiotherapy is a local treatment, aimed at destruction of any abnormal cells that may remain in the breast after excision of the tumour. Radiation restores intracellular homeostasis by causing the breakdown of genetic material, thus preventing the accelerated cell division of tumour cells. A number of normal cells in the treatment area will also be affected, but unlike damaged tumour cells, normal cells can repair/reproduce themselves.

Radiotherapy causes extreme fatigue and skin sensitivity, therefore the treatment is given in divided doses and careful observation of the treatment area is required. Although radiotherapy treatment is completely painless, it often produces anxiety. Patients may find the physical environment of the radiotherapy unit overwhelming, particularly the technical equipment. In addition, for the duration of the treatment, the patient has to remain very still on the treatment couch and is alone, although staff will always be visible behind protective lead screens (that do not permit passage of radiation). Ideally, the patient should visit the department before treatment is started to enable them to meet the staff and become familiar with the surroundings.

Chemotherapy is also aimed at the destruction of abnormal cells. Because it is a systemic treatment, given intravenously, its side effects are prevalent. Chemotherapeutic drugs have a variety of actions, but all in some way disrupt cellular growth, either by damaging DNA directly or by interfering with aspects of the cell cycle. Chemotherapy therefore targets normally dividing cells as well as malignant cells. Leucocytes are particularly at risk, so Janet's blood will be monitored at regular intervals for the duration of treatment to enable early diagnosis of leucocyte imbalances.

Cytotoxic chemotherapy is highly toxic, and often induces nausea and vomiting. These side effects can now be controlled effectively with anti-emetic drugs.

Suppression of further tumour growth: anti-hormonal therapy

Hormonal therapy manipulates the hormonal environment of breast tissue cells to suppress cell growth. Oestrogens are important factors in breast cell activity. The drug tamoxifen is an oestrogen antagonist: it binds to oestrogen receptors of cells and thereby inhibits the growth-stimulating effects of oestrogen and impedes the growth of malignant cells. Not all breast tumours are oestrogen-receptor positive, however. Although early trials suggest that tamoxifen therapy is likely to be beneficial in terms of increased survival, the degree of efficacy and optimal treatment regimens remain unclear, particularly in relation to women who develop breast cancer before the menopause.

Support

Janet will require skilled nursing care to enable her to cope with the demands of her treatment. Patient support and education are an essential part of treatment. Not only will Janet be coming to terms with the diagnosis of a life-threatening disease, but she will also be recovering from surgery and facing several weeks of unpleasant treatment. Janet's family will also require support. Most hospitals now offer the services of specialist breast care nurses, and there are also a number of charitable organizations and self-help groups that provide care and support for those with breast cancer. The British Association of Cancer United Patients (BACUP) for example, provides booklets and videos, and has a telephone help-line for patients and their relatives.

Further reading

Smedira, H.J. (2000) Practical issues in counseling healthy women about their breast cancer risk and use of tamoxifen citrate. *Archives of Internal Medicine* **160**(20): 3034–42.

Zack, E. (2001) Mammography and reduced breast cancer mortality rates. *Medical Surgical Nursing* **10**(1): 17–21.

CASE 2: A MAN WITH CHRONIC BRONCHITIS

Scenario:

George is 72 years old and suffers from chronic bronchitis. He lives alone in a one-bedroom, ground-floor flat. George smoked all his life, until 2 years ago when he finally gave it up. His mobility is moderately limited due to shortness of breath, but he still manages to live relatively independently.

Over the past few days, he has experienced increased shortness of breath at rest and increased cough with production of yellow purulent sputum, and has become bedridden from generalized malaise. His GP has been called to visit him at home.

On examination, the GP notes immediately that George has great difficulty in holding a conversation due to severe shortness of breath. Assessment of vital signs yields the following results:

Pulse: 110 beats/min (normal = 60–100 beats/min).

Blood pressure: 170/95 mm Hg (normal = 160/90 at age 70 years).

Respiratory rate: 32 breaths/min (normal = 12–15 breaths/min).

Temperature: 37.8°C (normal = 36.9–37.2°C).

In addition, George has a continuous cough with purulent sputum expectoration. Exaggerated breathing movements with the use of accessory muscles are apparent, and George complains of exhaustion. His best peak expiratory flow recording is well below that predicted for his age and height. He has been unable to eat properly for some days.

The GP decides that George requires hospital admission and calls for an ambulance. Further assessment is made using:

● pulse oximetry, to assess the saturation of haemoglobin with oxygen from moment to moment;

● arterial blood gas analysis, to provide an accurate assessment of blood oxygenation, and to identify the severity of carbon dioxide retention and pH change;

● clinical examination and chest X-ray interpretation, to identify the site and extent of infection.

Assessment identifies an oxygen saturation of 87% and a mild acidosis.

Chronic bronchitis as a homeostatic disturbance

Background

In the UK, chronic bronchitis occurs in approximately 15% of men and 5% of women. Chronic bronchitis is an example of a chronic obstructive airways disease (COAD). This term refers to a clinical syndrome that is characterized by obstruction to the flow of air in the distal airways. It does not refer to a uniform disease, but to several pathological conditions that also include emphysema and chronic asthma.

Cigarette smoking is overwhelmingly the most important factor in the genesis of chronic bronchitis. Tobacco smoke irritates the bronchial tissue, initiating the inflammatory response that brings about an increase in glandular activity, oedema and congestion. At a cellular level, smoking causes loss of cilia and increased production of mucus. Large quantities of viscid secretions are produced that are difficult to expectorate. The tendency to retain secretions encourages bacterial growth, which provokes further attacks of acute inflammation, and airway obstruction is commonly present. Severe chronic exacerbations lead to obliteration of some alveoli and bronchioles. Atmospheric pollution and poor socioeconomic status are also linked to the aetiology of chronic bronchitis.

The loss in time of alveoli and bronchioles exacerbates the problem, and even lead to emphysema, an even more debilitating condition.

Presentation

Chronic bronchitis by definition is based on the presence of a productive cough on most days, for at least 3 months in the year, over a period of at least 2 years. The term actually refers to the symptoms of cough and sputum, and the colour and consistency of George's sputum would suggest infection.

The presence of mucus makes expiration difficult, and may even exacerbate it if the airflow causes plugging of the airways. The effect of obstruction is to reduce the efficiency of alveolar ventilation, thus causing the composition of alveolar gases to move away from normal (becoming richer in carbon dioxide and deficient in oxygen). Poor oxygenation of blood, and the retention of carbon dioxide, then become problematic:

● There is a stimulation to breathe, including the use of active expiration. This accounts for George's increased breathing rate and respiratory effort.

● The increased respiratory effort will cause anxiety, resulting in further effort and a worsening of the airway plugging.

● The poor oxygenation of George's blood will produce tissue hypoxia, resulting in cardiovascular responses that will help to provide more oxygen to the tissues. This is observed as the rise in pulse rate and blood pressure.

● The inflammatory response to the presence of infection explains George's slight rise in body temperature.

Restoring homeostasis

See Figure 24.2.

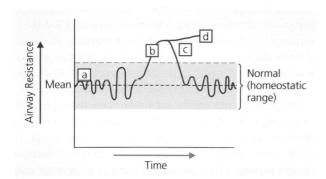

Figure 24.2 Chronic obstructive airway disease. (a) Normal airway resistance (b) increase resistance caused by excessive mucus production, airway hypertrophy and/or inflammation. (c) Intervention to reduce airway resistance by using bronchodilator and expectorant therapy, relieving anxiety, etc. (d) Failure of intervention to correct an increased airway resistance, leading to further deterioration of alveolar ventilation and gas exchange.

Aims of care

George's symptoms relate to the occurrence of poor alveolar gas composition as a consequence of airway obstruction, and to the presence of infection. The aim of care will therefore be to improve blood oxygenation and remove carbon dioxide, and to remove the infection that has provoked the episode. A further aim is to encourage long-term management and so reduce the likelihood of repeat episodes.

Implementation of care

Improving alveolar gas composition

George will receive bronchodilator drugs, even before the ambulance arrives. These are adrenergic agonists; they stimulate beta-2 receptors on bronchial smooth muscle cells, and so relax the muscle and facilitate alveolar ventilation. George's anxiety will also be reduced by reassuring him that his hospital admission is temporary until he is back on his feet again. The nurse and physician will provide reassurance through close supervision and effective communication skills.

During transportation to the hospital, the paramedic will administer 28% oxygen via a facemask (normal air composition is 21% oxygen) and monitor haemoglobin saturation with oxygen using pulse oximetry (acceptable saturation (>90%). Oxygen therapy increases the proportion of oxygen in the inspired air, thereby increasing the alveolar partial pressure of oxygen. A higher percentage of oxygen is inadvisable in George's case because the 'drive' for George's breathing is the hypoxia (see Box 14.29), and complete oxygenation will remove the drive for breathing and lead to hypoventilation or even apnoea.

George will be nursed in an upright position that he finds comfortable. Such positioning reduces the weight of abdominal organs pressing on the diaphragm, and so facilitates breathing movements.

Removing the infection

It will be explained to George that he has developed a severe chest infection and must be treated with antibiotics. Intravenous administration will normally be used; administration of antibiotics via the intravenous route is indicated in those patients with severe respiratory distress since it provides rapid therapeutic plasma levels in a controlled environment.

Sputum collection pots will be made available and George will be actively encouraged to expectorate. It is the role of the nurse and physiotherapist to encourage effective sputum expectoration. This is essential to clear airway obstruction, minimize hypoxia, and prevent further infection. Sputum culture identifies the specific invading bacterial organism and confirms sensitivity to antibiotic therapy. Before culture results are returned, which may take several days, most infections are assumed to be *Haemophilus influenzae* and are treated as such to instigate antibiotic therapy at the earliest opportunity.

Long-term management

Chronic bronchitis is recurrent, and George will need advice and help to ensure that the impact of incidences is minimized. A comprehensive dietary assessment will identify George's nutritional status. This is because an inadequate dietary intake may suppress the immune system and so decrease his ability to fight infection.

All patients suffering from chronic respiratory disease should have their inhaler technique checked regularly and be given information regarding the status of their condition. Long-term effective management relies heavily on appropriate self-management that can be achieved only through education and efficient communication.

Further reading

Ball, P. (1995) Epidemiology and treatment of chronic bronchitis and its exacerbations. *Chest* **108**(2 suppl): 43S–52S.

CASE 3: A MAN WITH MYOCARDIAL INFARCTION

Scenario:

Paul is 54 years old. He is a slightly overweight builder who smokes 20 cigarettes a day and takes little recreational exercise. Today, Paul was admitted to the local coronary care unit, having experienced a central crushing chest pain that radiated to his left arm and jaw. The pain occurred at rest, and was accompanied by breathlessness, nausea and vomiting. On examination, Paul was also found to be cold and clammy to the touch; he was tachycardic and hypotensive.

After a rapid physical examination, Paul's electrocardiogram (ECG) was recorded. This demonstrated ST segment elevation over the anterior chest leads (V1–V6). As these ECG changes are indicative of an acute anterior myocardial infarction, blood tests for the cardiac specific enzymes were taken to confirm the diagnosis.

Myocardial infarction as a homeostatic imbalance

Background

The risk of suffering a myocardial infarction in a given individual or community reflects the interplay between genetic susceptibility to the disease and environmental factors, such as smoking, elevated cholesterol levels, and lack of physical exercise. In addition, there are gender differences in relation to heart disease, with the incidence being highest in men and postmenopausal women.

Myocardial infarction is a homeostatic imbalance that reflects myocardial oxygen insufficiency, usually arising from a partially or totally occluded coronary artery (generally referred to as myocardial ischaemia; Chapter 12). Blood flow to the tissue beyond the occluded site ceases; if the occlusion is complete, the affected myocardial tissue dies.

The diagnosis of acute myocardial infarction is made in three steps: the patient's history, the ECG, and enzyme studies. In many ways, the patient's story of their illness is the prime factor in reaching the diagnosis. However, the history, regardless of how typical it may be, is not diagnostic in its own right, and other steps must be taken to prove that the acute infarction has actually occurred.

The ECG is the single most valuable immediate diagnostic tool. Paul's ECG typically demonstrates that the problem is in the ventricle (primarily the left ventricle). However, additional confirmation of the diagnosis can be made by detecting raised plasma activities of cardiac enzymes (intracellular enzymes that leak from injured myocardial cells into the blood stream). The more extensive the damage, the greater the release of these enzymes. Particular attention is paid to the enzymes CK-MB (a variant of creatinine kinase, CK) and tropinin-T. Retrospective diagnosis can also be made from aspartate aminotransferase (AST) and lactic dehydrogenase (LDH1 and LDH2); however, these enzymes are not cardiac specific.

Prognosis in myocardial infarction is related principally to the age of the patient and the residual left ventricular function. A major myocardial infarction may result in death from cardiogenic shock, cardiac dysrhythmias or cardiac rupture. If the person recovers, their lifestyle may be restricted by chronic left ventricular failure or by intermittent myocardial ischaemia, particularly when active (angina pectoris).

Presentation

Occlusion of the coronary vessels is usually due to the presence of atheroma and subsequent thrombosis formation. The disorder reinforces the need for cells to receive adequate oxygen (see Chapter 4). Insufficient oxygen supply to the myocardium inhibits the complete metabolism of glucose for energy; as a result, anaerobic metabolism occurs and lactic acid accumulates. Lactic acid is known to stimulate pain fibres found within the myocardium, so myocardial infarction is commonly associated with severe chest pain. The occurrence of pain at rest is indicative of advanced disease, distinct from more moderate forms that produce pain when the heart is stimulated during activity or excitement.

Sensory impulses travel from the myocardium via sympathetic nerve fibres to the thoracic sympathetic ganglia and then to nerve roots T1–T5 (see Chapter 8). These spinal nerves supply the anterior chest wall but also the inner aspect of the arm and head. For this reason, pain is felt in the region bounded by these nerves, including the left arm.

The poorly functional myocardium prevents a normal ejection of blood during systole, and so will usually promote a low blood pressure (hypotension). The presence of hypotension can be gauged from the patient's cognitive functions/awareness, and this will form part of the initial assessment. The cardiovascular response to hypotension is to increase heart rate (producing tachycardia) and to promote vasoconstriction in peripheral tissues (and so raise peripheral resistance). These responses were described in Chapter 12. The latter actions explain the pale, cool appearance of Paul's skin. Vasoconstriction is mediated by sympathetic nerve stimulation, which also causes the skin to sweat, producing clamminess.

Restoring homeostasis

See Figure 24.3.

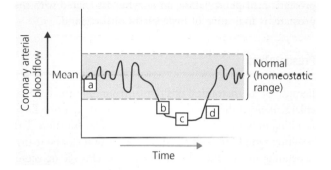

Figure 24.3 Myocardial infarction. (a) 'Normal' blood flow in coronary arteries. (b) Coronary arterial insufficiency caused by stenosis or vasospasm, and resultant myocardial ischaemia. (c) Partial or complete arterial occlusion, and subsequent myocardial infarction. (d) Restoration of near-normal cardiac function following reperfusion with vasodilator or thrombolytic therapy, arterioplasty, etc.

Aims of care

In the first instance, Paul's treatment will be to ensure survival by improving coronary blood supply and to remove pain. The first 48 h are the most critical time for Paul. Necrosis can advance for several hours after the infarction (and possibly for a number of days), as does the risk of shock, so continuous cardiac monitoring is essential in this early phase. Subsequent care will be directed at rehabilitation.

Implementation of care

Teatment for acute myocardial infarction focuses on re-canalization of the occluded artery to limit the size of the infarction (i.e. of the necrotic area). Immediately following admission, Paul may have an intravenous cannula inserted, and a powerful analgesic such as diamorphine administered for pain relief. Diamorphine acts quickly, and has the added benefits of reducing anxiety, ensuring rest and reducing myocardial preload due to venous pooling. An anti-emetic may be used to counteract consequential nausea.

Other drugs may also be administered:

- Sublingual or intravenous nitrates (e.g. glyceryl trinitrate) will induce dilation of coronary arteries.

- Thrombolytics, such as streptokinase, may be used to reduce blood clots (Chapter 11). Thrombolysis reduces mortality in patients with acute myocardial infarction. The best results in terms of preserving ventricular function and improving survival are obtained by starting thrombolytic therapy as soon as possible after the onset of the symptoms. Aspirin has also been proven to enhance the benefit of thrombolysis. Conversely, the potential benefit of thrombolytic therapy in a patient with a small myocardial infarction who is pain free and haemodynamically stable has to be weighed against the risk of a major bleeding complication and sensitization to streptokinase.

- Beta-blockers may be used to reduce cardiac contractility (and hence the work being done) and to encourage normal cardiac rhythm.

During the acute phase, Paul would be nursed in bed in a semi-recumbent position and attached to continuous cardiac monitoring for constant observation of his heart rate and rhythm. Throughout this time, a nurse would remain with him to monitor his blood pressure and observe for signs of anaphylaxis.

Rehabilitation

After 48 h without ischaemic chest pain, Paul will be transferred to a medical ward for mobilization and rehabilitation. During the rehabilitation phase of hospitalization, particular attention is paid to modifying the patient's cardiac risk factors in the hope of preventing recurrent infarction. In Paul's case, he would need advice on stopping smoking, diet and weight loss, and the importance of exercise.

Further reading

Docherty, B. (2001) Education campaigns in coronary heart disease. *Professional Nurse* **16**(4): 1048–51.

Doering, L.V. (1999) Pathophysiology of acute coronary syndromes leading to acute myocardial infarction. *Journal of Cardiovascular Nursing* **13**(3): 1–20, 119–20.

Fleury, J. and Moore, S.M. (1999) Family-centered care after acute myocardial infarction. *Journal of Cardiovascular Nursing* **13**(3): 73–82.

Lockhart, L., McMeeken, K., Mark, J., Cross, S., Tait, G. and Isles, C. (2000) Secondary prevention after myocardial infarction: reduction the risk of further cardiovascular events. *Coronary Health Care* **4**(2): 82–91.

CASE 4: A MAN WITH BENIGN PROSTATIC HYPERPLASIA

Scenario:

Bill is 72 years old, and retired from the civil service 7 years ago. He had enjoyed good health, but had suffered from nocturia (passing urine two to three times each night) for several years, without consulting his GP, believing it to be a normal phenomenon one suffers as one grows older.

About 8 months ago, Bill had suffered a bout of urinary retention. He had a hot bath, which resolved it. The next morning, he consulted his GP. On examination, nothing abnormal was detected in the urine or kidneys. There was no bladder distension, but the GP found a large soft prostate on rectal examination. As Bill had suffered an episode of retention, the GP decided to refer him to a consultant. In the meantime, a blood specimen was obtained to check urea, electrolytes and prostatic acid phosphatase (PSA) concentrations. Urea and electrolytes were normal, but PSA was raised. This enzyme is a marker for prostatic tumour, and its elevated blood concentration is indicative of hyperplasia.

A biopsy under general anaesthetic found no evidence for malignancy, and Bill was diagnosed as suffering from benign nodular hyperplasia of the prostate. Because of his symptoms, he was placed on the waiting list for a transurethral resection of prostate (TUR).

While waiting for his operation, Bill suffered a series of urinary tract infections, which were treated with the appropriate antibiotics. At one stage, Bill had to be catheterized as he had another episode of urinary retention.

Bill eventually had his TUR, but his problems did not end. He suffered from further episodes of urinary tract infections, with frequency of micturition and nocturia. A rectal examination by the GP confirmed a still-sizeable prostate remnant. He was therefore referred back to the consultant. In the meantime, Bill lost weight and generally felt unwell.

A cystoscopy carried out under general anaesthesia showed a grossly trabeculated bladder, and a residual volume of urine of 950 ml. A further TUR was then carried out. This was successful; Bill has had no problems since and has gained weight.

Prostatic hyperplasia as a homeostatic imbalance

Background

As middle age approaches, the prostate gland gradually hypertrophies. The reason for the hypertrophy is unclear, but it may be related to changes in the balance of androgen and oestrogen production. The presence in blood of prostatic acid phosphatase, an enzyme associated with the prostate, is indicative of hyperplasia of the gland.

Presentation

Because of its anatomical position surrounding the urethra, enlargement of the prostate is likely to obstruct urine flow, resulting in homeostatic imbalance of bladder function. The resulting symptoms from urethral obstruction can be many, depending on whether the obstruction is chronic or acute. In chronic obstruction, frequency, dribbling, urgency, nocturia, incontinence, hesitancy, and stream and intensity decrease can be experienced. In acute obstruction, anuria, pain and a distended palpable bladder usually present as an emergency episode, and the man will have to be catheterized.

Urethral obstruction may also lead to problems with the urethras and kidneys (see Chapter 15):

- The urethra may become distorted and displaced, so urine flow is impeded further.

- If urine is not excreted sufficiently, dilation of the renal pelvis and calyces, and the collecting ducts, will occur, leading to renal failure if left untreated. The excretion of waste products is essential for the homeostatic maintenance of all systems in the body.

- If renal failure does occur, a gross disturbance of body fluid composition arises, which would eventually be fatal if uncorrected.

- If the bladder wall is affected, there is incomplete emptying with urinary stasis. This predisposes to the formation of stones (calculi) and infection, as stagnant urine serves as a culture for bacterial growth.

The presence of urinary retention and calculi are detectable by palpation, while renal failure or depressed renal function could be expected to produce retention of urea (and hence its elevation in blood plasma). This is why Bill's GP suggested the investigations. The conclusion was that his problem was prostate enlargement, rather than secondary to other problems.

Restoring homeostasis

See Figure 24.4.

Aims of care

Bill's treatment would be aimed at restoring the normal flow of urine. This in turn will restore normal fluid and

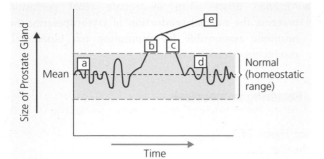

Figure 24.4 Prostatic hypertrophy. (a) Prostate gland size appropriate to the age of the person. (b) Prostatic hypertrophy. This typically occurs in late adulthood for as yet unidentified reasons. If excessive, the hypertrophy will cause urethral obstruction and will require intervention. Hypertrophy may also be indicative of prostatic cancer. (c) Correction of prostatic hypertrophy by surgery and pharmacological therapy. (d) Restoration of prostate size to within normal limits. (e) Persistent hypertrophy leading to risk of renal failure secondary to urethral obstruction and infection.

electrolyte balance, which may have been disrupted by the obstructive process. Happily for Bill, the prostate enlargement was not malignant, but surgery is still implicated. Had malignancy been present, then he would also receive treatment for the tumour, which may or may not be removed.

Implementation of care

Treatment for benign prostatic hypertrophy might entail both medical and surgical procedures. Medical interven-

tions aim to relax smooth muscle surrounding the prostate gland and urethra, and so promote urinary flow:

- Before the prostate hypertrophy was advanced, Bill's first bout of urinary retention was reversed by a hot bath. The bath probably caused muscle relaxation.

- Although not used in Bill's case, selective alpha-blocking drugs (see Chapter 8), e.g. prazosin, may also be used to block the actions of sympathetic nerves in the area and so relax smooth muscle.

- The sex steroid activities that might have precipitated the hypertrophy may also be modified pharmacologically. For example, the 5-alpha reductase inhibitor, finasteride, blocks the formation of dihydrotesterosterone and induces shrinkage of hyperplastic tissue in the prostate.

- As hypertrophy advances, hot baths or drugs will not resolve the retention. Consequently, Bill's urinary retention became more pronounced and catheterization was necessary.

Eventually, surgical reduction of the prostate (i.e. prostatectomy) will be necessary. Benign prostatic hypertrophy normally results from enlargement of the inner tissue of the gland. The surgical procedure used therefore is normally via the urethra and is called 'transurethral resection'.

While it is a commonly applied surgical procedure, the position of the prostate in relation to the urethra and bladder can make it difficult to sufficiently reduce the gland without causing extensive damage to the urethra. A risk of this method is that the ejaculatory ducts may be damaged where they exit into the urethra (see Chapter 18), thus making ejaculation impossible. Hyperplasia of remnant tissue is possible, and a second operation may be required — as in Bill's case.

CASE 5: A YOUNG WOMAN WITH SECONDARY (RENAL VASCULAR) HYPERTENSION

Scenario:

Jean, aged 28 years, has been to her doctor with symptoms of tiredness, anorexia, nausea and headaches. Her blood pressure was found to be 160/110 mm Hg (normal 120/80 mm Hg), and a blood sample showed raised urea concentration, raised creatinine concentration (collectively referred to as uraemia), and lowered haemoglobin concentration (i.e. anaemia).

The concentration of the hormone angiotensin II was found to be elevated in her blood. Further tests of renal function were performed. Jean was subsequently diagnosed with renal vascular hypertension due to renal artery stenosis.

Renal vascular hypertension as a homeostatic imbalance

Background

Stenosis of an artery is often caused by hyperplasia (i.e. excessive growth) of the arterial wall, leading to narrowing of the lumen of the arteries. Its cause is frequently unknown. Renal artery stenosis is a condition found more frequently in young women; it rarely occurs in men.

The increased vascular resistance produced by the stenosis will cause a decrease in blood pressure within the kidneys, a reduced blood flow distal to the narrowing, and a decrease in glomerular filtration rate (Chapter 15). The consequence is that the kidney responds as though systemic blood pressure has decreased. Adaptive responses occur that ordinarily would increase systemic blood pressure and hence restore renal blood flow, but in renal arterial stenosis such responses are not appropriate:

- The reduced blood pressure is detected by the stretch receptors in the afferent arteriole that leads into the glomerulus, which causes the juxtaglomerular cells in the vicinity to secrete the enzyme renin. The macula densa cells in the walls of the distal convoluted tubule of the nephron may also detect a fall in the amount of filtered sodium, which promotes the release of renin.

- Renin acts on the plasma peptide, angiotensinogen, and converts it to angiotensin I (Chapter 9 and 12). Angiotensin I is further converted by angiotensin-converting enzyme in the pulmonary endothelial surfaces to angiotensin II.

- Angiotensin II is a powerful vasoconstrictor that acts to increase peripheral resistance and systemic blood pressure.

- Angiotensin II also stimulates the adrenal cortex to release aldosterone, a hormone that causes reabsorption of sodium, and consequently water, by the distal convoluted tubule, resulting in an increased extracellular fluid and hence blood volume (Chapter 9). This will tend to increase systemic blood pressure.

The complications are severe because the hypertension it induces has serious long-term consequences as it can damage small arterioles and lead to further hyperplastic arteriosclerosis. The complications include cardiac disorder, cerebral thrombosis and/or haemorrhage, or nephrosclerosis and renal failure.

Presentation

The responses to renal stenosis act to increase systemic arterial blood pressure beyond normal values. If the kidney continues to be poorly perfused, then the renin–angiotensin system continues to cause vasoconstriction and salt and water reabsorption, so maintaining hypertension and promoting fluid overload.

Diminished glomerular filtration has other consequences:

- There will be a disturbance in body fluid composition, with symptoms such as nausea and anorexia.

- Body fluid disturbances are detected readily as being of renal origin by monitoring the blood plasma concentrations of substances that rely especially on a high glomerular filtration rate for their excretion (i.e. creatinine and urea) (see Chapter 15).

- Anaemia arises when inadequate renal perfusion prevents the normal production of erythropoietin, the hormone responsible for promoting red blood cell production (see Chapter 11).

Restoring homeostasis

See Figure 24.5.

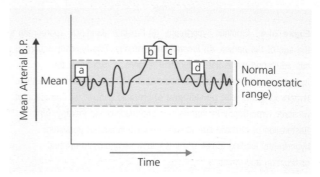

Figure 24.5 Secondary hypertension. (a) Mean blood pressure in a healthy person (appropriate for age). (b) Secondary hypertension: blood pressure elevated as a result of the activation of the renin—angiotensin system arising from poor renal blood flow. (c) Decreased blood pressure caused by preventing the generation of angiotensin II using an angiotensin-converting enzyme (ACE) inhibitor, e.g. captopril and by use of diuretics to reduce blood volume. (d) Blood pressure restored to normal via good pharmacological control.

Aims of care

Hypertension itself is often idiopathic, i.e. of unknown cause. In Jean's case, the hypertension is clearly secondary to a renal disorder and subsequent production of a vasoactive hormone, angiotensin II. The main aims of care in this case, therefore, are to pharmacologically control the hypertension, to reduce the disturbances in body fluid composition, and to slow renal deterioration.

Implementation of care

Reducing the hypertension

The use of inhibitors of angiotensin-converting enzyme (i.e. ACE inhibitors, e.g. captopril) may be particularly useful here, because they prevent the conversion of angiotensin I to the active angiotensin II. Other antihypertensives, such as calcium channel blockers (e.g. nifedipine), may also be useful.

Diuretics such as frusemide may be useful because they increase the excretion of sodium and water and so help to correct the imbalance in body fluid volume. A further aim is to control blood volume through regulating dietary sodium chloride and fluid intake.

Jean would also be advised to avoid other risk factors: if overweight, she is likely to be put onto a low-calorie diet, and if she is a smoker, she would be advised to stop or at least reduce her smoking.

Reducing disturbances in body fluid composition

Extrinsic regulation of body fluid sodium chloride content is just one aspect of dietary control recommended for patients with secondary renal hypertension. People with kidney disease must also restrict the amount of potassium in their diets, because poor kidney function can promote hyperkalaemia with consequences for cardiac and neural functions (see Chapters 6 and 8). The amount of protein in the diet must also be controlled to lower the potential of retaining urea (from protein metabolism; see Chapter 15).

Reducing the stenosis

This is difficult. Arterial stenosis can be corrected surgically, but renal damage may already have occurred by the time diagnosis is made.

Further reading

Little, C. (2000) Renovascular hypertension. *American Journal of Nursing* **100**(2): 46–52.

CASE 6: A WOMAN WITH RHEUMATOID ARTHRITIS

Scenario:

Mary is a 50-year-old married woman who works as a shop assistant. She visited her GP complaining of extreme tiredness together with painful, stiff, swollen hands and knees, particularly first thing in the morning. She has become limited in her mobility.

Examination confirmed inflammation of the joints of both wrists, the metacarpophalangeal joints (i.e. the joints between the metacarpal bones of the hands and the phalanges of the fingers), and the proximal interphalangeal joints (i.e. between the finger bones). Joint effusion (excess synovial fluid) restricted Mary's knee and shoulder movements.

Routine blood tests revealed that she was anaemic. Her haemoglobin was 9.8 g/dl (normal 12–16 g/dl), but the erythrocytes were of normal size and had normal haemoglobin content (i.e. the anaemia was apparently due to too few cells rather than any defect of cell structure). Mary also had an elevated erythrocyte sedimentary rate (ESR) at 90 mm/h (normal 5–15 mm/h in women; 1–5 mm/h in men) and a positive rheumatoid factor test. She was referred to the rheumatology department of her local hospital.

On questioning, Mary said she had lost 3 kg in weight, and complained of early-morning joint stiffness that lasted 4–6 h. A diagnosis of rheumatoid arthritis was made.

Rheumatoid arthritis as a homeostatic disturbance

Rheumatoid arthritis is a chronic, debilitating, inflammatory arthritis for which there is no cure. The Arthritis and Rheumatism Council literature suggests that 30% of people who develop rheumatoid arthritis will recover completely within 1–2 years but 60% will continue to have problems intermittently with slowly progressing disease, and 5–10% will become severely disabled.

The disorder is more common in females than males (ratio 3 : 1). Its cause is unknown cause, but it is an autoimmune problem characterized by the production of autoantibodies that attack synovial tissue. It is likely to be due to a combination of genetic and environmental factors. Individuals may have a predisposition to developing rheumatoid arthritis, but it is not inherited directly. As rheumatoid arthritis is much more common in young women than young men under the age of 40 years, it is considered that this suggests a possible role of the female sex hormones.

The condition causes inflammation of the synovial membrane (see Chapter 3) that lines movable joints and tendon sheaths. The inflammation causes pain, stiffness and swelling, which in the long term may result in joint damage and malformation, and hence decreased mobility. It is characterized by periods of remission and flares, and may produce tiredness, anaemia and weight loss. Additional features include nodules of vesicular tissue over bony prominences, and possible inflammation of the sclera (scleritis), arteries (arteritis) and pericardium (pericarditis).

Investigations demonstrate a number of features:

- Skeletal changes evidenced by X-rays are used in the diagnosis of rheumatoid arthritis, and to monitor the severity and to assess the progression of the disease. Changes are seen early in the disease, particularly in the hands and feet.

- Occurrence of anaemia: rheumatoid arthritis is associated with decreased production of erythrocytes. The problem is one of rate of production rather than defective cells. Typically, the cells appear normal and have a normal haemoglobin content.

- Presence of rheumatoid factor: this is an autoantibody (in fact, a number are involved) raised against self-antigens, usually of the IgM or IgG types. The presence of rheumatoid factor is diagnostic, and its concentration (titre) appears to relate to the severity of the condition.

● Elevated erythrocyte sedimentation rate (ESR): the ESR is measured simply by allowing a column of blood to separate into cell and plasma components through the effects of gravity. As the cells sediment out, a column of plasma forms; the ESR is a measure of the rate of formation of this column (the higher the ESR, the faster the red cells sediment out). Mary's elevated ESR is typical of autoimmune conditions. The faster rate of sedimentation probably relates to changes in plasma protein consistency, but also to the 'stacking' of red cells.

The disease has psychosocial implications and, in particular, can have wide-ranging effects on the family and relationships between loved ones.

Improving homeostasis

See Figure 24.6.

Aims of care

Rheumatoid arthritis requires a multidisciplinary approach from healthcare practitioners. The aims of care are to use disease management to suppress the inflammatory process, relieve pain and promote optimum function, and to reduce the psychological and social consequences of the condition.

Implementation of care

Promoting optimal function
Mary would have both knees aspirated and injected with a long-acting corticosteroid to counteract the inflammation. Intra-articular steroid injections are very effective for flares, and when only one or two joints are troublesome. They can significantly reduce pain and swelling in a joint for several months.

In advanced conditions that are unresponsive to conventional corticosteroid therapy, second-line drugs such as methotrexate may be prescribed. Second-line drugs are used as disease-modifying agents, with the aim of inducing and maintaining remission. They are potentially toxic, so patients need to be monitored carefully. Regular blood and urine tests, together with direct questioning of the patient, are normally carried out to detect possible side effects.

Nonsteroidal anti-inflammatory drugs such as ibuprofen help relieve the pain, stiffness and inflammation, but they have no effect on the disease progression.

Physiotherapy and occupational therapy are of particular relevance. The physiotherapist aims to maintain physical function and to teach the patient how to exercise their

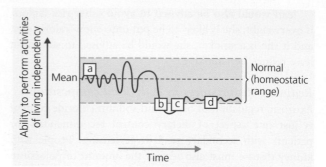

Figure 24.6 Rheumatoid arthritis. (a) Physical independence. The ability of the self to perform the activities of living. (b) Imbalance. In rheumatoid arthritis, this is caused by flare, or slowly progressing disease, with particular consequences for mobility. (c) Effects of intervention — medical/surgical/nursing/physiotherapy/occupational therapy/self-help — to improve mobility and to facilitate the meeting of needs. (d) Successful return to physical independence. There is, however, no cure for rheumatoid arthritis, and only partial restoration of mobility may be achieved.

joints. Treatments such as heat, cold and hydrotherapy are administered in the physiotherapy department. The occupational therapist assesses the activities of daily living and teaches joint protection and energy conservation. Aids and appliances can be provided to make carrying out the activities of daily living easier.

Orthotics and prosthetic departments and orthopaedic surgeons may also become involved to enable the patient to remain as independent as possible.

Psychosocial care
Social workers may be involved in community care of people with rheumatoid arthritis, but nurses have a particular role here, both to provide psychosocial support and as a resource in relation to the aspects highlighted above. The role of the nurse is to:

● assess the patient, identify their needs and co-ordinate their care;

● provide education regarding the disease, and to give patients and their family the opportunity to discuss issues with the nurse;

● monitor some of the disease-modifying drugs, and to provide access to specialist knowledge and advice through a telephone help-line;

● act as a liaison between the community, hospital and patient.

Further reading

Grossman, J.M. and Brahn, E. (1997) Rheumatoid arthritis: current clinical and research directions. *Journal of Women's Health* **6**(6): 627–38.

Ramsburg, K.L. (2000) Rheumatoid arthritis. *American Journal of Nursing* **100**(11): 40–43.

Childcare case studies

The cases presented here are intended not to be comprehensive, but to provide common examples that illustrate homeostatic principles in their pathology and in the care delivered.

CASE 1: A BOY WITH ASTHMA

Scenario:

Thomas is 4 years old. He has a long-standing history of recurrent chest infections and persistent cough. More recently, he has developed a noticeable wheeze that gets worse at night and continues during the morning 'at nursery school. These nocturnal episodes have been causing interruptions to his sleep, and he has had to miss school on several occasions because of a persistent cough.

The family GP has taken a full clinical history from Thomas' mother. The history shows that in addition to the symptoms of persistent cough and nocturnal wheeze, Thomas also has a history of mild eczema and allergies to certain foods, such as eggs and peanuts. His father has a history of asthma from the age of 12 years.

Following a physical examination, the GP referred Thomas for further investigations:

● Allergy skin (Heaf) tests demonstrated a positive skin test to airborne allergens.

● Peak expiratory flow recordings were significantly below the predicted values for age and height, indicating increased airway resistance.

● Forced expired volume in 1 s (FEV_1) was reduced in comparison to predicted values for age and height, indicating increased airway resistance.

The tests confirmed that Thomas has asthma.

Asthma as a homeostatic imbalance

Background

Asthma is the most common chronic illness in childhood. It represents hypersensitivity reactions to an antigen (i.e. to an allergen) following previous exposure. The resulting antigen–antibody reaction induces the release of large quantities of chemicals, enzymes and cell stimulators. The consequence is a disease of the airways characterized by chronic inflammation with infiltration of lymphocytes, eosinophils and mast cells (see Chapter 13), together with epithelial desquamation, thickening and disorganization of the tissues of the airway wall, and mucus plugging of the airways.

Inhaled allergens are the most common route for precipitating allergic (or atopic) asthma, especially in children. Inhaled allergens include pollens from grass, trees and weeds, fungi, the house-dust mite, and animal dander. Pollens and fungal allergens tend to cause seasonal symptoms of allergic rhinitis and/or conjunctivitis. Allergy to house-dust mites is extremely common, causing IgE-mediated hypersensitivity reactions (see Chapter 13) in asthma especially in children. Asthma triggered by animal dander is most commonly associated with cats.

A strong family history of atopic asthma is often found in children who develop persistent asthma. Allergies to foods and/or the presence of allergic dermatitis at an early age indicate the presence of an atopic immune system. Later sensitivity to airborne allergens is implicated in the development of asthma.

Presentation

Such pathology presents as variable airflow obstruction associated with the inflammation of the airways, and symptoms of cough, wheeze, chest tightness and paroxysms of dyspnoea. The excessive airway narrowing occurs in response to a variety of provoking stimuli, such as allergens, environmental pollutants, exercise, infections, drugs, and psychological factors.

The narrowing of the airway is detectable by investigations in which Thomas exhaled forcibly either through a peak flow meter or a spirometer. Increased airway resistance will impede the maximal flow rate that he should be capable of achieving, and will also mean that he is unable to expel at least 80% of his vital capacity in 1 s (referred to as the FEV%; see Chapter 14).

Restoring homeostasis

See Figure 25.1.

Aims of care

Once asthma has been recognized and diagnosed, the aims of care are to abolish symptoms and restore normal or best possible airway function. In addition, the risk of severe attacks must be reduced; in children, normal growth and minimizing absence from school are priorities. A combination of pharmacological and educational interventions should result in effective long-term management of asthma.

Implementation of care

The means of treating asthma are to control the airways either by preventing the onset of a severe attack, and by maintaining the airway should an attack occur. The drugs are usually administered via an inhaler or large-volume spacer. Large-volume spacers are devices that assist the patient (particularly children) to administer their inhaled drugs effectively, as the synchronization of intake of breath with the operation of an inhaler device is not required. The lung deposition of the inhaled drug is increased, and for smaller children spacers are easier to use than some inhalers. Thomas would be placed on a therapeutic trial undertaken aggressively for 3–4 weeks, since most childhood asthma would be expected to show some response to pharmacological therapy within that time.

Preventing inflammation and bronchoconstriction
Drug therapy includes:

- a short-acting beta-2 adrenoceptor agonist, such as salbutamol, to be used as required. These drugs act to promote the bronchodilator actions of the sympathetic nervous system on airways.

- regular sodium cromoglycate. This can reduce the incidence of asthma attacks, and is useful in children as it may prevent the need for steroid therapy. The mode of action of sodium cromoglycate is not completely understood, but it is known to reduce the inflammatory response (i.e. histamine release) to irritants, and as such is an important preventive drug.

- a short course of steroid, such as prednisolone, to reduce inflammation may be required as a trial for 1 month if Thomas' asthma is not stabilized using sodium cromoglycate.

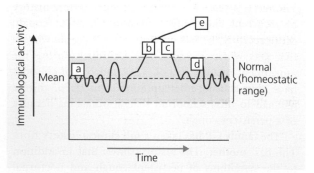

Figure 25.1 Asthma. (a) Normal homeostatic sensitivity and functioning of the immune system. (b) Hypersensitive reaction. In asthma, this is in response to a frequent exposure to an irritant and is referred to as a type 1 response. (c) Intervention to reduce the reaction. In the short term, this will involve pharmacological therapy. In the long term, it will also involve avoidance of the suspected irritant. (d) Restoration of normal immune activity. (e) Uncontrolled hypersensitive reaction. This is potentially life threatening, as there will be pronounced lung hypoventilation and resultant hypoxia.

Indicators of assessing the outcome of asthma treatment include:

- number of days off school;

- amount of daytime and night-time cough and wheeze;

- limitation of activity;

- frequency of relief medication;

- understanding by parents or child that medications must be varied according to symptoms or peak flow recordings, or both.

Health education and support

Health education will provide Thomas and his parents with information about the disease process, causes, treatment and self-management programme. Continuing support for the family will be provided via a nurse-led asthma clinic or GP.

The family will also be encouraged to monitor Thomas's peak flow rate to ascertain severity and progression of changes in airway resistance, so they will be provided with instruction on technique/recording. They will also be encouraged to maintain a symptom diary card to monitor the frequency of episodes and allergen types.

Successful management in children involves participation from both the parents and the child in partnership with the health professional. Education is the foundation for long-term successful management, as it fosters understanding and effective skills. Appropriate changes in behaviour are more likely to occur if the child and family are given adequate opportunity to express any fears or concerns, and expectations of both the condition and its treatment.

Further reading

Conway, A. (1999) Adherence and compliance in the management of asthma. *British Journal of Nursing* 7: 1374–6.

CASE 2: A CHILD WITH INSULIN-DEPENDENT DIABETES MELLITUS

Scenario:

James is 8 years old and has recently started drinking large amounts of sweetened drinks. James now complains of being too tired for football with his friends, and his mother describes him as listless. His grandmother suggested the symptoms were similar to those of James's aunt Sylvia, when she had diabetes mellitus diagnosed as a child.

James and his mother visit the doctor's surgery. The doctor listens to the story; knowing that diabetes may occur in families, the doctor checks James's blood glucose using a glucometer, which reveals he has a blood glucose level of 12 mmol/l. He explains to James and his mum that grandma may be right, as the level is higher than normal, and that he is going to contact the paediatric diabetic nurse attached to the local paediatric department.

In later visits, the diabetic nurse educates James and his parents about diabetes in greater depth. She would show them the location of the pancreas, perhaps by using a flip book of the body, and explain that insulin is a hormone, released into the blood when necessary, to control blood glucose. The need for insulin injections and their timing will be explained.

carbohydrate-rich meal. In health, insulin is secreted from the beta cells of the islets of Langerhans in the pancreas, which stimulates the uptake of glucose in the target tissues, mainly liver and skeletal muscle cells (Chapter 9).

In patients with insulin-dependent diabetes mellitus (IDDM), there is poor or no production of insulin. Many tissues are unable to utilize glucose in the absence of insulin. This apparent deficiency of glucose results in the body recognizing its need for carbohydrates, and creates a craving for sweet things. If profound, diabetes causes an increased metabolism of fats and proteins, yielding fatty acids and amino acids for energy but also producing ketone bodies (see Chapter 4). These latter may induce ketoacidosis.

Presentation

The main symptoms of insulin-dependent diabetes mellitus are:

- hyperglycaemia;

- hyposecretion of insulin;

- glycosuria, as blood glucose rises above the concentration of the renal threshold for glucose appearing in urine;

- urinary tract infection, arising from the presence of glucose;

- increased urine production due to the osmotic effects of the glucose in the forming urine;

Diabetes mellitus as a homeostatic imbalance

Background

Blood glucose has a homeostatic range of 3.5–5.5 mmol/l (fasting), but naturally rises post-absorption of a

- thirst and excessive drinking, due to the dehydrating effects of the excessive urine production;

- behavioural changes, if blood glucose reverts rapidly to hypoglycaemia (the paradox of diabetes is that eating may induce hyperglycaemia whilst not eating, or undertaking a bout of exercise, may precipitate the opposite). Such episodes may even induce coma and may be life threatening;

- weight loss due to fat and protein protein metabolism.

There is a need to control the hyperglycaemia partly because doing so will reverse the other symptoms, and partly because persistent hyperglycaemia has long-term consequences for nerve cells and small blood vessels. Uncontrolled diabetes raises the risk of peripheral neuropathy and problems arising from poor circulation, such as blindness, renal failure, skin ulcers and peripheral necrosis. There is also an elevated risk of coronary heart disease because of the effects of hyperglycaemia and atheroma arising from the excessive release of fatty acids. These long-term effects are irreversible.

Restoring homeostasis

See Figure 25.2.

Aims of care

Children with diabetes are not 'ill' in the conventional sense, and are not admitted to hospital with suspected diabetes, unless it is absolutely necessary. This is to maintain a 'normal' lifestyle for the child and family.

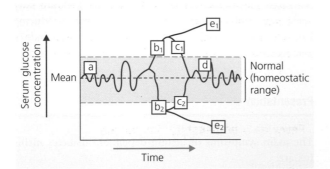

Figure 25.2 Insulin-dependent diabetes mellitus. (a) Normal serum glucose concentration within a child with diabetes as a result of good extrinsic control. (b₁) Hyperglycaemia caused by excessive intake of carbohydrate. (b₂) Hypoglycaemia caused by poor carbohydrate intake or increased utilization, e.g. in exercise. (c₁) Effect of administered insulin to restore normal serum glucose concentration. (c₂) Ingestion of biscuits or dextrosol to increase serum glucose concentration. (d) Normal serum glucose concentration restored by extrinsic control. (e₁) Persistent hyperglycaemia resulting from poor control, leading to long-term complications. (e₂) Persistent reduced hypoglycaemia, leading to behavioural change or coma.

In this case, there are three main aims of treatment: blood glucose regulation, for James and his parents to be in control of the condition, and to enable James to lead a normal life.

Implementation of care

Blood glucose regulation

The management of diabetes is a balancing act between meeting energy requirements with a healthy diet and providing enough exogenous insulin so that the cells can use the glucose provided.

Insulin is given by injection because it is inactive given by mouth. Using modern, long-acting types of insulin, most people need to inject only twice a day. To check how well insulin is controlling the blood glucose, equipment supplied by the nurse is used to assess a small blood sample obtained by pricking James's finger. Good control means giving the correct dose of insulin to keep the blood glucose within normal range for as much as possible. James will need to inject insulin about half an hour before his breakfast and evening meal to give the insulin time to take effect. It is then important to ensure that he does eat, otherwise the insulin injection will promote hypoglycaemia.

James will also be placed onto a controlled diet, so that the likelihood of episodes of severe hyperglycaemia (and possible hypoglycaemia) can be avoided. A 'diabetic diet' is a normal healthy diet and special foods are not required, but a few simple rules have to be followed. These include:

- eating at regular intervals;

- ensuring meals consist of some long-acting carbohydrate, such as bread and cereals, which are broken down slowly, so that glucose is released slowly and maintains blood glucose levels within the homeostatic range for longer. Short-acting carbohydrates like sweets cause a short burst of glucose and should be restricted;

● eating extra carbohydrate before taking part in any strenuous exercise.

The nurse explains that if James needs more glucose, his body will let him know. Signs may include feeling dizzy, having blurred vision or trembling/tingling of his hands, and starting to sweat. These signs are indicative that hypoglycaemia is developing. It is useful to have a source of glucose available, as hypoglycaemia can develop quickly. Dextrosol® tablets may be kept at hand, but sugar lumps or a sweet drink will also work. These foods raise blood glucose quickly, and soon reverse the symptoms of hypoglycaemia. Once James feels better, he should be given something containing long-acting carbohydrate to help stabilize his blood glucose concentration.

Being in control of the diabetes

James's parents will need to be fully informed regarding the condition, how to use the blood tests, and the need for James to be careful. The nurse facilitates this by arranging an appointment for them at the children's diabetic clinic, where they will meet the consultant who specializes in children with diabetes, and a dietician who can give further advice on meals, tailored to James's preferences. By knowing about diabetes and who is available to support them, James and his parents can regain control of their lives.

Enabling James to lead a normal life

It is important for James to participate fully in all aspects of childhood, play, education and social activities. The nurse might contact his school so James can return to school knowing that his teachers understand the modern management of diabetes, and so they can express any individual concerns. The nurse may also offer information about the British Diabetic Association local branch, and will arrange for James and his parents to meet other families for mutual support if they wish.

Further reading

Richmond, A. (1998) Childhood diabetes: dietary aspects. *Paediatric Nursing* **10**(2): 29–35.

Taylor, J. (2000) Partnership in the community and hospital: a comparison. *Paediatric Nursing* **12**(5): 28–30.

CASE 3: A FEBRILE TODDLER

Scenario:

Joe has had a febrile convulsion and has been brought to the hospital by ambulance. Joe is 18 months old, and has, to date, been a healthy baby reaching all his normal milestones of development. Over the last 24 h, he has become irritable, pulling at his ear, and he is off his food. Alison, his mother, was concerned by this, and took Joe to see their doctor, who diagnosed a middle ear infection and prescribed antibiotics. While Alison was at the chemist waiting for the prescription, Joe had a fit.

On admission to the accident and emergency (A&E) department of the local hospital, Joe was no longer fitting and was assessed rapidly using airway, breathing and circulation (ABC) procedures. Some secretions were suctioned from his mouth and nose, and a set of baseline observations were taken, including weight, temperature, pulse and respiration. The nurse would have liked to check his blood pressure, but Joe became so distressed that the attempt was abandoned. A child who is distressed will have a raised blood pressure, and in these circumstances its measurement does not provide useful clinical information.

Joe's temperature is taken with a tympanic membrane sensor and a value of 40°C is noted; this is higher than normal. The tympanic method is a very accurate method of recording a child's temperature in seconds, rather than with other methods that take 4–6 min and require a great deal of co-operation from the child. Joe's pulse and respiration are both elevated.

Joe is stripped to his nappy and a thin T-shirt with Alison's help. The doctor prescribes rectal paracetamol and an antibiotic. These are administered in the A&E department, and Alison is encouraged to get Joe to drink some squash before his transfer to the ward for overnight observation.

The nurse explains to Alison about febrile convulsions, and gives Alison a hand-out that reinforces the main points made.

Fever as a homeostatic imbalance

Background

Febrile convulsions affect 3–5% of all children, and tend to occur between the ages of 6 months and 3 years. They will usually accompany intercurrent infections, typically viral illness, tonsillitis, pharyngitis and otitis media. They are unusual after the age of 5 years. Otitis media is very common in early childhood, and may often be the precipitating factor in febrile convulsions. This is due to the shortness of the auditory tube, which links the back of the nasopharynx with the middle ear, and provides a route for infecting agents to access the middle ear (Chapter 7). The distance becomes greater as the length of the tube grows with the child, and middle ear infections become less frequent.

The normal set point for core temperature in a toddler is 36.7–37.7°C, but with infection pyrogens produced by the bacteria and some of Joe's white blood cells cause an increase in the set point. Joe's core temperature of 40°C results from this resetting, so fever (pyrexia) is actually an adaptive response achieved by resetting homeostatic parameters (Chapter 16). The elevated (aerobic) metabolism that generates the extra heat in pyrexia will also generate extra carbon dioxide, which will trigger a response in the peripheral chemoreceptors (see Chapter 14). This explains Joe's increased respiratory rate. His increased pulse rate is also associated with the increased metabolic rate; tissues have a greater oxygen demand, and the circulation increases accordingly.

Presentation

A young child's hypothalamus is immature, which means that the new set point is likely to be higher than might be anticipated with the extent of the infection, making the child more susceptible to extreme temperature changes. Neural tissue is especially susceptible to a change in core temperature, and the high core temperature excites a group of cells known as the epileptogenic focus. This explains Joe's fit at the onset of his fever. Febrile seizures or fits are generalized, being of a tonic/clonic nature, with the tonic phase lasting for 10–20 s and the clonic phase lasting for about 30 s (but varying from a few seconds to 30 min).

Restoring homeostasis

See Figure 25.3.

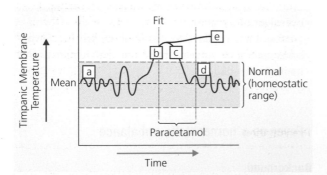

Figure 25.3 Febrile toddler. (a) Body temperature before febrile episode within homeostatic range for age group (36.7—37.7°C): balance between heat loss and heat gain. (b) Rising temperature as heat gain exceeds heat loss because a new set point has been fixed. If the set point is too high for normal neural function, then a fit may ensue. (c) Effect of antipyretic drug, plus other interventions (e.g. removal of clothing) to reduce temperature. (d) Following antibiotic therapy, the body temperature returns to normal range. Over the next 24 h, the set point will return to normal. (e) Worst-case scenario: no intervention takes place and the toddler is unable to rectify heat gain with heat loss. Temperature remains at the new set point, potentially causing neural damage.

Aims of care

Upon arrival in the A&E department, Joe underwent a series of initial investigations, first to ensure that his vital functions were satisfactory, and second to establish changes from baseline. Following this, the aims of care are to reverse his pyrexia to make him more comfortable, and to make it unlikely that he will fit again. Care will also include supporting his parents at this time.

Implementation of care

Initial investigations

Joe underwent a rapid assessment using the ABC process in order to check for respiratory or circulatory distress. His mouth and nose were suctioned to remove any collection of secretions. Infants and toddlers tend to nose breathe, so secretions will raise airway resistance and cause an increased respiratory effort.

Baseline observations of temperature, pulse and breathing rate were taken to facilitate continued monitoring for changes that may indicate that he is in danger of having a further fit.

Joe would be encouraged to drink – squash is usually more palatable than water. His increased metabolic rate can easily lead to dehydration; this problem may be exacerbated in toddlers by their large surface area relative to their body size (roughly twice that of an adult), from which perspiration can take place (Chapter 15). Joe may suffer from physical fatigue following the fit, making him reluctant to drink.

Reducing the pyrexia

Joe will be weighed, and the weight recorded on his drug chart, so that drug doses can be prescribed accurately. An antipyretic drug, such as paracetamol, would be administered rectally. The rectal mucosa is thin, so rectal administration is a very efficient way to administer drugs as they are absorbed very quickly, if the rectum is empty. In addition, Joe's distress makes it likely that he would resist attempts to make him swallow a strange liquid in an unknown environment, so rectal administration can be less distressing. It is also more likely that the child will receive the full dose by this route. Antibiotics would be given to assist Joe's immune system to remove the bacteria.

A persistently raised temperature following the administration of an antipyretic means that further fits may occur if other steps are not taken to cool the child. Removing Joe's clothes to a minimum will reduce trapped air and lessen any insulating effect that the clothes produce. In this way, conductive heat loss to the environment is enhanced (Chapter 16). Regular monitoring of vital signs will take place overnight, usually 2-hourly when oral paracetamol is used, as it reaches its maximum effect in 2.5 h. The nurse will also use close observation of Joe's behaviour and the general condition of his skin to assess changes.

Parental support

Joe's parents, who have undergone a very frightening experience, will receive considerable support and reassurance. Reassurance is based on the fact that for many families the child will only have one episode of febrile fit. The likely occurrence of other febrile fits is linked to the age of the child (the younger the child, the more they are likely to reoccur), as is a family history of febrile fits. Time will also be spent in educating the parents in the steps they can take to lessen the chances of another febrile fit. Education is centred on giving the parents the skills to recognize when the child is becoming pyrexial, and the appropriate steps to take to minimize the risk of a febrile convulsion:

1 If the child appears hot when a hand is placed on the nape of the neck or abdomen, it is advisable to remove outer layers of clothes to enable cooling to take place.

2 This should be closely followed by observing the child for signs of pyrexia, such as red face, flushed skin and general lethargy.

3 Administer an antipyretic such as oral soluble paracetamol in the recommended dose for the child's age if the temperature appears to be increasing.

4 Encourage a high fluid intake.

5 Seek medical advice if fever persists.

Further reading

McGreal, P.A. (1997) Pediatric management problems ... febrile convulsions. *Pediatric Nursing* **23**(2): 192–3.

Hawksworth, D.L. (2000) Simple febrile convulsions: evidence for best practice. *Journal of Child Health Care* **4**(4): 149–53.

Purssell, E. (2000) The use of antipyretic medications in the prevention of febrile convulsions in children. *Journal of Clinical Nursing* **9**(4): 473–80.

CASE 4: A BOY WITH LEUKAEMIA

Scenario:

William is 5 years old. He had been a healthy 'normal' boy, but recently he has been experiencing painful, swollen joints. He has also shown signs of general malaise, including pallor, fatigue and fever. Frequent nosebleeds have also proved troublesome, and William's mother has noticed small blood spots (petechiae) in his skin. His GP referred him for further examination.

Blood analysis showed that William was anaemic and that his platelet count was only 100 000/mm³ ('normal' is around 250 000/mm³). His total white blood cell count was 10 000/mm³, only slightly above normal, but a differential count showed an excess of lymphocytes, especially B-lymphocytes. Also, many of the white cells in the sample appeared immature, or had morphological or chromosomal abnormalities. Subsequent aspiration of a bone marrow sample showed a preponderance of lymphocytic stem cells (lymphoblasts), and confirmed that William had acute lymphoblastic leukaemia.

Leukaemia as a homeostatic imbalance

Background

Acute lymphoblastic leukaemia is the most common form of leukaemia that occurs in children. As with all cancers, leukaemia arises because of profound genetic disturbances, especially in stem cells. The cause of the genetic mutation is unknown, but is speculated to involve environmental agents. The typical early onset, the predisposition of children with Down's syndrome to this type of leukaemia, and the high concordance between affected identical twins suggests that there may also be an inherited component.

In this type of leukaemia, there is a change in the behaviour of lymphocyte stem cells within the bone marrow. Other cells are crowded out by these rapidly dividing cells, so production of red blood cells, platelets and white blood cell types is decreased. The white cells that are produced also appear abnormal and immature.

Presentation

The symptoms shown by William reflect the effects of the changes described above:

● Decreased red blood cell synthesis produces anaemia, and hence pallor and fatigue.

● The platelet deficiency reduces the capacity for blood clotting, leading to episodes of bleeding.

● The abnormal white cells are generally more mobile than normal cells, and may infiltrate tissues. Infiltration of skeletal joint capsules and subsequent inflammation are responsible for joint swelling and pain.

- The rapid turnover of marrow cells in leukaemia results in the release of excessive amounts of uric acid (a product of nucleic acid catabolism); deposition of uric acid crystals in joints will exacerbate joint pain.

- White blood cells, particularly lymphocytes, are central to the body's defence against microorganisms (Chapter 11 and 13). The abnormal cells observed in acute lymphoblastic leukaemia mean that William will be more susceptible to infection.

The main risk to life in leukaemia is internal haemorrhage, especially in the brain, and uncontrolled infection.

Restoring homeostasis

See Figure 25.4.

Aims of care

The aim of care is to use chemotherapy to disrupt the rapid division of the leukaemic cells, and to destroy them. William and his parents will also require a lot of support.

Implementation of care

Chemotherapy

William would be placed on a regime of chemotherapy using anti-leukaemic drugs. A cocktail of drugs is normally given. The aims of chemotherapy are to remove the abnormal white cells, and to destroy the leukaemia stem cells (the lymphoblasts) in bone marrow. In doing so, the crowding-out effect is removed, and red cell and platelet counts in the blood are restored. Thus, white blood cells will become 'normal', and the differential cell count will return to those observed in health. The actions of the drugs are indiscriminate, however, and so are very toxic, especially at the high doses used. They will therefore also affect healthy cells, so side effects of the treatment are wide ranging.

Hair loss during chemotherapy is extensive. Observations will include watching for signs of neuropathy (e.g. personality change, weakness of hand grip, ptosis of eyelids), gastrointestinal disorder (e.g. gastric ulcer, abdominal pain), cardiovascular disturbance (e.g. hypertension, ECG abnormalities) and fluid retention. Temperature, blood pressure, pulse and respiratory movements are monitored during drug administration, and signs of local irritation at the infusion site are looked for.

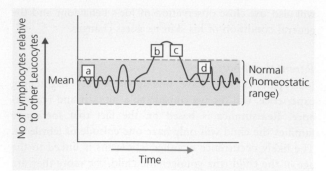

Figure 25.4 Leukaemia. (a) Normal differential blood cell count: numbers of lymphocytes relative to other blood cells appropriate for health. (b) Excessive number of lymphocytes. Slight elevations could indicate infection. Pronounced increases as observed in lymphocytic leukaemia result from an excessive activity of lymphoblasts in bone marrow. (c) Influence of therapies (chemotherapy and/or radiotherapy) to reduce lymphoblastic activity. (d) Successful effects of therapies to restore the differential cell count to normal. The person is now in remission.

Should the platelet count fall sharply, William will also be infused with pooled platelets.

Acute lymphoblastic leukaemia responds well to treatment and has a high remission rate. The success of chemotherapy depends partly on the aetiology of the leukaemia. The profound genetic disturbances noted in cancer cells can initially occur in a small number of cells as a result of a localized environmental 'insult' (cells produced from this focus will then dominate, and chemotherapy is directed at these cells). The alternative is that a genetic mutation could have been inherited or occurred in utero, in which case most of the stem cells will be affected. In this case, ionizing radiation may also be used to eradicate the stem cells, and new, healthy cells introduced via a bone marrow transplant.

Support

William will require considerable support because of the unpleasant effects of the drugs, the hair loss induced by chemotherapy, and the treatment regime. The parents will also require support from the healthcare team, hence the emphasis on the management of side effects and emotional support. Parental education will be an important part of this therapy.

Further reading

Taylor, B. (1999) Parental autonomy and consent to treatment. *Journal of Advanced Nursing* **29**(3): 570–6.

CASE 5: A BABY BOY WITH NECROTIZING ENTEROCOLITIS

Scenario:

Sean was born early at 28 weeks gestation, weighing 1.24 kg to a primiparous mother. The pregnancy had been reasonably uncomplicated until a small antepartum haemorrhage progressed to preterm labour. Sean was in excellent condition at birth, but as a precaution he was intubated and maintained on minimal ventilatory support for 12 h.

At 24 h of age, he developed pyrexia and his neutrophil count was raised, indicating bacterial invasion. His abdomen was becoming distended, and an X-ray revealed pneumoperitoneum (i.e. free gas under the diaphragm) and pneumotosis intestinalis (i.e. intramural bubbles). Intramural gas is mainly hydrogen produced as a product of carbohydrate metabolism by anaerobic bacteria in the bowel. Bowel sounds were absent. A few hours later, Sean was in obvious pain, and the distended abdomen was splinting his diaphragm, causing respiratory distress with deteriorating blood gases (hypercapnia, hypoxia and acidosis).

In spite of the absence of bloody stools and only minimal bilious aspirate, a diagnosis of perforated necrotizing enterocolitis (NEC) was eventually made.

Necrotizing enterocolitis as a homeostatic imbalance

Background

The pathogenesis of necrotizing enterocolitis is multifactorial, but it is an acquired neonatal disorder following a combination of vascular, mucosal and toxic insults to an immature gut. Epidemiological studies indicate that most associated factors describe events in a population of high-risk neonates, and that no maternal or neonatal factors, other than prematurity, exist. One possible factor is the lack of immunoprotective factors in formula milk, but antibiotics and giving only breast milk do not prevent the disease; however, the slow introduction of feeds, minimizing episodes of hypotension, hypoxia and hypothermia, and the use of umbilical catheters appear to have some relevance. Sean's NEC was most probably the result of his premature birth, although it was unusual to develop so early and without enteral feeding.

The incidence is 0.3–15/1000 live births, and is more common in boys. The majority of babies affected are less than 1500 g at birth. NEC has become a major problem in the last 30 years, with higher survival rates due to improved clinical expertise producing an ever-enlarging group of increasingly premature and low-birth-weight infants. It is the most serious surgical disorder among infants who have endured intensive care intervention, and is a significant cause of morbidity and mortality.

Presentation

The condition involves ischaemia of the gut mucosa, followed by infection with gas-forming organisms. Toxins produced cause further cell damage. The presence of infection is indicated by Sean's pyrexia, which is a physiological response to the presence of pyrogens released by pathogens (see Chapters 13 and 16).

There are five stages of NEC, ranging from mild abdominal distension without systemic symptoms to a fulminant course of sepsis due to endotoxin release, disseminated intravascular coagulation, collapse and death (Table 25.1). Sean has the severest form – advanced necrotizing enterocolitis – and presented with deteriorating vital signs and electrolyte imbalance with shock syndrome. There was evidence of perforation and generalized peritonitis and pneumoperitoneum.

Restoring homeostasis

See Figure 25.5.

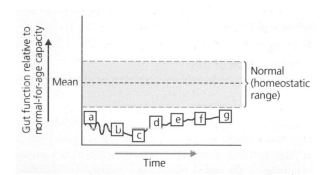

Figure 25.5 Necrotizing enteritis. (a) Compromised bowel function caused by prematurity at birth. (b) Ischaemic episodes soon after birth. (c) Necrotizing enterocolitis with infection. (d) Clinical stabilization using antibiotics, respiratory support, and analgesia/sedation. (e) Resection of the bowel and formation of a stoma. (f) Intestinal continuity restored. Oral feeding resumed. (g) Bowel function almost fully recovered.

Aims of care

Depending on the severity of NEC, the means of management may entail simple medical intervention or may

Table 25.1 The stages of, and specific treatment for, necrotizing enterocolitis

Stage	I (pre-NEC)	IIA (mild NEC)	IIB (moderate NEC)	IIIA (advanced NEC)	IIIB (advanced NEC)
Signs and symptoms	Nonspecific Apnoea, bradycardia, lethargy, unstable temperature, gastric aspirate, occult blood in stools, nonspecific ileus	As stage I, plus prominent abdominal distension ± tenderness, absent bowel sounds, gross blood in stools, ileus and dilated loops of bowel with focal areas of inflated intestine (pneumotosis) on X-ray	Mild acidosis and thrombocytopoenia, abdominal wall tenderness ± palpable mass, extensive pneumotosis and early ascites and intrahepatic venous gas	Respiratory and metabolic acidosis requiring ventilation for apnoea, hypotension and decreased urine output, spreading oedema, erythema, prominent ascites, no perforation	Deteriorating vital signs and lab indices, shock syndrome and electrolyte imbalance, evidence of perforation with peritonitis and pneumoperitoneum
Treatment	Nil by mouth, continuous nasogastric drainage, 2–4-hourly observations of vital signs, removal of umbilical catheters, antibiotics, monitor fluid balance, septic screen and blood picture, serial X-rays If cultures negative after 3 days, stop antibiotics and recommence feeds	As stage I, but continue antibiotics for 10 days, give total perenteral nutrition, withhold enteral feeds for at least 7–10 days after X-ray shows clearing of pneumotosis, supplemental oxygen if hypoxic, platelet transfusion if thrombocytopoenic, treat acidosis, ?surgical option	As stage IIa	As stage IIb and respiratory support as dictated by blood gas levels and clinical status, blood pressure support/volume expansion – inotropes, colloid to replace ongoing fluid losses, blood and platelet transfusions	As stage IIa, then surgery when as clinically stable as possible Peritoneal drainage can be done on ward or laparotomy with resection ± stoma or anastomosis

require aggressive multisystem medical support and surgery. In Sean's case, the aim would be to provide clinical stabilization, followed by surgical intervention to prevent rapid deterioration and possible death. The seriousness of the problem is such that Jamie's parents will be distressed, so care will also aim to provide them with substantial psychological support.

Implementation of care

Clinical stabilization

Medically, the main homeostatic imbalances relate to the infection/septicaemia, poor blood gas composition because of hypoventilation arising as a consequence of pain on breathing, a distended bowel, and nutritional/hydration disturbance due to the disorder. Care therefore addresses these disturbances.

When Sean first became ill, he would be prescribed triple antibiotics – broad-spectrum penicillin and gentamicin, plus metronidazole, which has specific activity against anaerobic bacteria found in the gut.

Gaseous exchange would be facilitated by Sean's re-intubation and ventilation. Morphine infusion to provide analgesia and sedation would also be commenced so that breathing could be more efficient. Placement of a nasogastric tube would permit free drainage to decompress the bowel. Hydration and nutrition would be achieved parenterally.

Surgery

Sean required urgent surgery. The ileum would be examined in order to confirm the diagnosis. In advanced NEC, the ileum is likely to be perforated and meconium (intestinal secretions formed when Sean was a fetus) found in the peritoneal cavity. The diseased bowel would be removed, and a dysfunctioning double-barrelled ileostomy (i.e. a stoma is formed by exteriorization of the two cut ends) formed to allow the bowel to heal, if resection and anastomosis was not possible.

Postoperatively:

● Jamie would be ventilated for 48 h, or until blood gases had normalized;

● antibiotics would be continued for 10 days;

● analgesia would be provided using perhaps bupivacaine via an epidural catheter (causing less respiratory depression than systemic opioids);

● stoma care, overseen by a nurse specialist, would be meticulous (it is crucial to preserve the integrity of preterm skin);

● total parenteral nutrition (TPN) would be commenced after 2 days to deliver substrates directly into the circulation, while allowing the bowel to heal;

● enteral feeds to supplement TPN would normally be introduced cautiously at 2 weeks, once the bowel had recovered and gastric aspirates were clear. Once Sean's intestinal continuity is restored, he should thrive.

Parental support

Sean's parents require empathetic emotional and psychological support, and should be given every encouragement to be involved in Sean's care. His recovery may be long and difficult, with several relapses and complications requiring perhaps months of hospitalization. Readmission after discharge for emergency surgery is a risk if his stoma prolapses. Infants with stages 1 or IIA NEC are likely to recover completely with few, if any, complications.

Further reading

Buonomo, C. (1999) The radiology of necrotising enterocolitis. *Radiology Clinics of North America* **37**: 1187–98.

McCormack, K. (2000) Necrotizing colitis: part 1. Predisposing risk factors. *Journal of Neonatal Nursing* **6**(3): 75–8.

McCormack, K. (2000) Necrotizing enterocolitis: part 2. Diagnosis and treatment. *Journal of Neonatal Nursing* **6**(4): 127–31.

CASE 6: A CHILD WITH HYPERTROPHIC PYLORIC STENOSIS

Scenario:

Charlie is 7 weeks old, and was born following an uneventful pregnancy. During the last week, he began vomiting between breastfeeds but otherwise he appeared well. The vomiting has now settled into a regular pattern following most feeds, and although initially ravenous following these episodes, Charlie has become increasingly listless. His mother reports that his nappies have not been as wet as usual, and his stools have become more formed.

On examination, Charlie does not object to being handled, and he remains quiet and lethargic. His eyeballs appear sunken and his anterior fontanelle is depressed. There is also loss of skin elasticity and his abdomen appears distended.

Charlie is given a 'test feed', during which his abdomen is palpated. An olive-shaped mass is felt in the epigastric region, and visible peristaltic waves are observed moving across the abdomen from left to right. Following the test feed, Charlie proceeds to have a projectile vomit. His history and current signs and symptoms lead to a diagnosis of hypertrophic pyloric stenosis.

Pyloric stenosis as a homeostatic imbalance

Background

Hypertrophic pyloric stenosis is one of the most common surgical disorders of infancy. It is five times more common in male than female infants, affecting approximately 5 in 1000 males and only 1 in 1000 females. The cause is unknown, but there is thought to be some hereditary involvement.

The pyloric sphincter guards the exit from the stomach. It is normally in a semi-permanent state of contraction; consequently, although it allows some gastric fluid to pass rapidly into the intestine, it prevents solid and semi-solid food leaving until gastric digestion is completed (see Chapter 10). Pyloric stenosis is an obstructive disorder arising from hypertrophy (excessive growth) of the circular smooth muscle of the pyloric sphincter. This results in the narrowing of the lumen, which partially/completely impedes the passage of chyme from the stomach.

Presentation

If the problem present at birth, the infant initially appears well because the sphincter is able to relax sufficiently to allow the passage of partially digested milk. As the condition progresses, delayed emptying of the stomach eventually leads to an increase in gastric pressure. Vomiting ensues; the vomitus may be foul-smelling, containing undigested milk, mucus and curds of stale, insoluble milk protein. Small flecks of fresh and digested blood (which have the appearance of coffee grounds) may also be seen in later stages as a result of chronic inflammation of the gastric mucosa.

As hypertrophy of the pylorus continues, obstruction becomes more severe. Episodes of vomiting are more frequent, and projectile vomiting usually develops, with vomitus being forcefully ejected a metre or so from the sitting infant. During test feeding, the abdomen is palpated gently to detect the enlarged pyloric sphincter. The term 'pyloric tumour' refers to the hypertrophied pyloric muscle, and does not in any way infer a malignant (cancerous) condition. Therefore, caution must be exercised when using such terminology with Charlie's parents and the general public.

The peristaltic waves visible on Charlie's abdomen, moving from left to right, are evidence of powerful peristaltic action, as the muscular stomach wall attempts to overcome the obstruction. Assessment of pain in infants is difficult, but it is to be expected that Charlie would experience some degree of colicky pain from such exaggerated peristalsis.

Apart from pain, nausea and abdominal distension, Charlie will experience the consequences of being unable to adequately pass food from his stomach to his intestines:

- Differences in body and organ size, and the immaturity of the physiological processes concerned with fluid balance, leave infants with minimal reserves of body fluid when intake is increasingly impaired, such as in Charlie's case (see Chapter 6). Protracted vomiting soon leads to dehydration.

- If fluid balance is not maintained, fluid rapidly becomes lost from both extra- and intracellular compartments. Loss of skin elasticity, sunken eyeballs and a depressed fontanelle are all signs of increasing dehydration.

- Charlie's listlessness could be attributable directly to such dehydration and to malnourishment.

- Homeostatic mechanisms aimed at water conservation will therefore be activated. Charlie's urine output will diminish as antidiuretic hormone, released by the posterior pituitary gland, results in renal salt and water retention.

- Fluid will also be increasingly absorbed from the colon, accounting for the semi-formed stools of a breastfed infant becoming more solid and less frequent.

Restoring homeostasis

See Figure 25.6.

Aims of care

Care is directed initially at reducing the likelihood of vomiting, removing abdominal distension and pain, and improving nourishment. Surgical correction of the stenosis will then be performed.

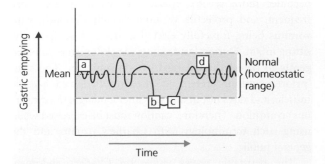

Figure 25.6 Pyloric stenosis. (a) Gastric emptying appropriate to feeding pattern, and age of the infant. (b) Inadequate gastric emptying. In this case, the result of a hypertrophied pyloric sphincter. (c) Surgical reduction of the hypertrophied sphincter (pyloromyotomy). (d) Normal gastric emptying restored following healing.

Implementation of care

Reducing vomiting, and removing abdominal distension and pain

It is usual for the stomach to be decompressed following diagnosis. This is achieved by passing a nasogastric tube, which may be aspirated (artificial removal of gastric contents) and/or left on free drainage. This facilitates the removal of residues of partially digested milk curds, and helps prevent the accumulation of gases that may be causing Charlie's abdominal distension. Occasionally, normal saline lavages (fluid introduced slowly into the stomach via a nasogastric tube and then aspirated) are prescribed, which fully empty and cleanse the stomach. Normal saline is isotonic with body fluids, therefore no water absorption will take place across the gastric mucosa. Charlie will not be allowed oral fluids, so arrangements will be made for his mother to express her breast milk.

Improving nourishment

The primary focus of preoperative care is to restore fluid and electrolyte balance, and to prepare the child and family for surgery. Where there are no obvious signs of dehydration, surgery is performed without delay. In Charlie's case, his fluid balance and general condition were assessed and monitored closely. Surgery would be postponed for 24 h to allow rehydration to take place.

Charlie will be weighed, an assessment made for fluid replacement, and an intravenous infusion commenced. Frequent assessment of fluid and serum electrolyte levels will be undertaken during the rehydration process. A glucose and saline solution will initially be administered to correct water depletion and prevent further malnutrition. Blood glucose may drop rapidly as vomiting and imposed starvation deplete stores of glycogen.

Hyponatraemia (low serum sodium; see Chapters 6 and 15) and reduced chloride levels invariably accompany prolonged periods of vomiting and nasogastric aspiration. Potassium is also lost in the same way as sodium, but management with potassium infusion will normally be delayed. This is because during dehydration, potassium is withdrawn from dehydrated (hyperosmotic) cells, creating a state of hyperkalaemia (high serum potassium). Renal function is restricted during dehydration and as a result, excretion of this excess potassium is impaired. During rehydration, extracellular potassium moves back into the intracellular compartment. Correction of potassium depletion via the intravenous infusion will therefore only take place once normal renal function has been restored. Care must be taken to ensure that the required infusion rate is adhered to as too rapid administration may lead to heart block and cardiac arrest (Chapter 6).

Hydrogen ions are also lost from vomit and gastric aspirate (due to loss of hydrochloric acid). This may lead rapidly to metabolic alkalosis (Chapter 6). Accurate monitoring of electrolyte balance is essential during rehydration to detect imbalances and allow prompt adjustment of intravenous therapy.

Vital signs of pulse, respiration, temperature, urine output and weight will be monitored to evaluate the effectiveness of rehydration therapy. Accurate records will be made of all fluid input and output (See Chapter 15), including any episodes of vomiting and bowel actions. General hygiene for a dehydrated infant is important, particularly of the skin and mouth. Charlie's mouth will be kept moist with boiled water as he will not be taking oral fluids, and his skin will be checked for integrity and signs of pressure. He will be monitored for infection, since dehydration and malnutrition may increase his susceptibility. Pain will be assessed using an age-appropriate tool, and analgesia administered accordingly.

Surgery to restore pyloric function

Once his hydration and ions/electrolytes have been stabilized, Charlie will be prepared for surgery according to the local hospital policy. Pyloromyotomy is the standard surgical technique; it consists of a longitudinal incision being made through the circular muscle fibres of the pylorus down to, but not including, the submucosa. This has the effect of enlarging the lumen of the sphincter, thereby overcoming the intestinal obstruction.

Postoperatively, normal feeding patterns are usually established within 24 h, but this may vary according to local practice. The success rate of pyloromyotomy is high where correction of fluid and electrolyte imbalance has been achieved preoperatively. Vomiting may persist in the immediate postoperative period, but it will gradually diminish as the pylorus adjusts to its normal size and function. Intravenous therapy is discontinued when adequate fluid levels are being taken orally. Using dissolvable sutures negates the need for removal of stitches. Recovery is usually unremarkable. Charlie will be discharged from hospital on the second to sixth postoperative day, depending on his progress.

Further reading

Davenport, M. (1996) Paediatric fluid balance. *Care of the Critically Ill* **12**(1): 26–31.

Fisher S. Postoperative pain management in paediatrics. *British Journal of Perioperative Nursing* **10**(2): 80–84.

Chapter 26

Mental healthcare case studies

Case 1: a man with Alzheimer's disease
Case 2: an adolescent girl with anorexia nervosa
Case 3: a man with depression

Case 4: a woman with Huntington's disease
Case 5: a young man with schizophrenia
Case 6: distress

The cases presented here are intended not to be comprehensive, but to provide common examples that illustrate homeostatic principles in their pathology and in the care delivered.

CASE 1: A MAN WITH ALZHEIMER'S DISEASE

Scenario:

Steven Harris is a retired schoolteacher aged 68 years. He is married, and has three children and two grandsons. Over the past 2 years, his memory for recent events has deteriorated, and his previous, rather pleasant outlook on life has changed to that of an irritable and sometimes aggressive person. Following a disagreement with his wife about his judgement in handling family finances, he became very upset and stormed out of the house, into the path of a passing car. Fortunately, Steven suffered only a few minor bruises, but accident unit staff were concerned about his mental state and he was kept in hospital overnight.

The following morning, he was noticed to be rather more confused than might be expected in the circumstances. When his wife described the changes she had seen in him over the previous 2 years, medical staff began to suspect that, in the absence of any head injury, a disease process affecting brain function may lie behind his altered behaviour. The history given by Mrs Harris pointed quite firmly towards the presence of a developing form of dementia known as Alzheimer's disease.

Alzheimer's disease as a homeostatic imbalance

Background

Dementia arises when significant parts of the brain deteriorate, leading to a reduction in cognitive (i.e. intellectual) functioning. There are various forms of dementia, classified according to aetiology (e.g. brain trauma or tumour), and to clinical and laboratory signs.

Common pathological changes in Alzheimer's disease are loss of neurons in certain areas of the brain, neurofibrillary tangles (abnormal changes in the cytoplasm of brain cells) and neuritic plaques (clusters of degenerating nerve endings). The presence of proteinaceous deposits inside and outside the cell is evidence of a change in the synthesis and/or structure of proteins normally present as part of neuronal structure. In particular, the production and modification of amyloid precursor protein, and the structure of apolipoprotein E, are affected. The cause of these pathological changes is unknown, but theories of inheritance and environmental influence are under investigation.

Unfortunately, the disease is very difficult to diagnose with certainty during life, so much evidence has to be gained post mortem.

Presentation

Alzheimer's disease is a form of dementia that impairs higher mental functions, such as memory, problem solving, judgement and emotional reactions. This disturbance occurs without clouding the consciousness of the person, and follows a progressive course that can continue for a period of years. The memory disturbance is usually for recent events, and is very often the most noticeable feature in the early stages of the disease. A further and related problem is an associated deterioration in language ability.

Improving homeostasis

See Figure 26.1.

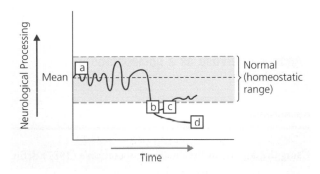

Figure 26.1 Alzheimer's disease. (a) Balance between the neurological pathways involved in neural processing appropriate for cognitive functioning. (b) Imbalance of neural pathways arising from presence of a brain tumour, cerebral vascular accident, or slow onset of neuronal loss, e.g. ageing or Alzheimer's disease. (c) Partial restoration of neural functioning by reinforcement therapy or by using drugs to modify neurochemistry. (d) Persistent deterioration in neural functioning observed in Alzheimer's disease as a result of progressive loss of neurons.

Aims of care

Alzheimer's disease is progressive and, currently, irreversible. The care of people with the disease is therefore aimed mainly at compensating for, and limiting, the negative consequences of dementia. Drugs may be used to reduce the symptoms of the disease, but cognitive support for Steven and his family will be the main focus.

The level of Steven's malfunction, and the management of his disease, would be assessed by physicians, psychiatrists and psychologists. Nurses, occupational therapists and physiotherapists will have a very significant part to play in his care, but a large burden may also be placed on his family and their relationships with him and with one another.

Implementation of care

Drug therapy

Drug treatment is, as yet, relatively ineffective in either halting or improving the disease process. However, some drugs such as the anticholinergic agent selegiline, have been observed to help in redressing neurochemical imbalance associated with the disease. Other drugs may be used to lessen the effects of confusion so commonly seen in Alzheimer's disease.

Cognitive management

Specific nursing care involves activities such as reality orientation, risk assessment and protection, and help with maintaining the activities of living while encouraging optimum independence.

The disease is progressive, so the care of Steven over what may be some years may take a toll on his family. Although healthcare professionals can ease this pressure by providing caring and sensitive support, they can never compensate for the loss of the husband and father his family knew. Families can easily become dysfunctional because of these pressures, and professional carers must work closely with them in order to help them maintain equilibrium. Steven is likely to develop more disturbing and unpleasant symptoms and, whilst medical and nursing care can relieve much of his discomfort, his family will need to know that help is also available to them.

In particular, it is vital to help Steven's wife feel a valued and significant contributor to her husband's care. As Steven's disease is at a relatively early stage, his wife is likely to find there is much she can do to help him maintain as much of his normal functioning as possible. In the past, early hospitalization has been shown to lead to problems of institutionalization and more rapid decline, whereas professionally supported home care can help sufferers and relatives maintain comparative normality for significantly longer. As far as is practicable, effective homeostasis in Steven's case can be encouraged through ensuring the availability of professional care and ongoing assessment that is supportive of the loving input of his own family.

Further reading

Caron, W. and Goetz, D.R.(1998) A biopsychosocial perspective on behavior problems in Alzheimer's disease. *Geriatrics* **53**(suppl 1): S56–60.

Kane, M.N. (1999) Mental health issues and Alzheimer's disease. *American Journal of Alzheimer's Disease* **14**(2): 102–10.

Mayeux, R. and Sano, M. (1999) Drug therapy: treatment of Alzheimer's disease. *New England Journal of Medicine* **341**(22): 1670-79.

Salib, E. (2000) Risk factors for Alzheimer's disease. *Elderly Care* **11**(10): 12–15.

Shah, Y., Tangalos, E.G. and Petersen, R.C. (2000) Mild cognitive impairment: when is it a precursor to Alzheimer's disease? *Geriatrics* **55**(9): 62–8.

CASE 2: AN ADOLESCENT GIRL WITH ANOREXIA NERVOSA

Scenario:

Jane is a 17-year-old young lady who was admitted, at the request of her GP, to the acute ward of a large psychiatric hospital. On admission to the ward, Jane was noted to have a pale complexion, and looked emaciated and thin. In addition, there was an apparent lack of subcutaneous fat, and parts of her skin – especially her face – were covered with very fine hair. She reported that she had difficulty in getting to sleep, and when sleep did occur it was only for short periods of up to an hour. She also tended to awaken earlier.

During the nursing assessment, Jane denied that she was experiencing any medical problems. She appeared aloof and was restless, and was always in motion during the interview. On further questioning, Jane reported that she had not menstruated for the last 6 months, but denied any possibility of being pregnant. Although Jane expressed feelings of sadness and depression, she did not express any desire to commit suicide. Jane felt that, although to others she may appear thin, she was fat and needed to lose more weight so as to appear attractive. Jane occasionally felt hungry but managed to suppress the desire for food by diverting her thoughts to images of the fashion models featured on television. Throughout the assessment, Jane continued to appear disinterested and gave the impression that the person being discussed was someone else and not her.

Jane's mother, who accompanied her to the ward and was present during the interview, said that Jane had been very careful with her dietary intake for a long time. Jane used to eat only very small amounts and occasionally missed entire meals. Jane was always aware of the amount she had eaten during the course of the day. Mrs Smith reported that if comments were made of Jane's dietary habits, Jane was likely to become hostile, and if anyone encouraged Jane to eat more, she would burst into floods of tears and leave the room abruptly. Although Jane was not interested in her own food consumption, she helped to prepare meals for the rest of her family and took pride in ensuring that the meals she prepared were well presented and were enjoyed by all those who ate them.

Jane's mother commented that until Jane began to become very concerned with her food consumption,

Jane had been a happy girl and was always striving for perfection in everything that she did. She took part in games and enjoyed dancing, and for a short period of time had ballet lessons. Even after she began dieting, Jane constantly did physical exercise, and it was only in the last 3 weeks that her exercise levels were reduced.

Jane had always enjoyed school until comments were made of her body shape by some of her contemporaries. Her mother said that, on reflection, changes in Jane's behaviour and her marked obsession with dietary habits appeared to coincide with the time that these comments were made. Jane had changed from a lively girl to become withdrawn and sad.

Anorexia nervosa as a homeostatic disturbance

Background

Using the American Psychiatric Association's (1987) definition, anorexia nervosa is diagnosed using four criteria:

- presenting weight below 85% that would be expected for the person's weight and height;

- behaviours directed to maintaining this weight are present or reported;

- a phobia or dislike for the normal body weight and shape;

- amenorrhoea for at least 3 months.

Jane's weight of 39 kg was much lower than that of the matched population, being approximately 70% of the expected weight. According to UK Department of Health guidelines (Chapter 5), Jane would require a dietary intake that would produce 2100–2200 kcal/day (8800–9200 kJ/day). This means that Jane would have to consume approximately 500 g of carbohydrate or 200 g of fat a day. Her intake clearly does not approach these values. In anorexia nervosa, the intake of carbohydrates and fats is very much reduced, although the protein intake is usually adequate. Her behaviour, attitude to her own weight, and the absence of menstruation for 6 months places her within the diagnosis of anorexia nervosa.

There are two main methods by which a person tries to achieve and maintain a weight that is below the expected norm; this helps to classify anorexia nervosa into its two types:

- *Restricting type:* during episodes of dieting, there is no binge eating.

- *Binge eating/purging type:* binge eating and laxative abuse occur during episodes of anorexia nervosa.

Jane's diagnosis is of the restrictive type.

Although at one time it was believed that anorexia nervosa was present only in Western and modern societies, there have been cases in developing countries. Furthermore, recent media interest in anorexia nervosa may have given the impression that it is a modern day phenomenon with an increasing incidence and prevalence, yet the term 'anorexia nervosa' was coined in the nineteenth century. Anorexia nervosa remains fairly uncommon. It is more common in females than in males, and the age of onset is commonly between 14 and 17 years. The prevalence is approximately 1% of adolescent girls.

Anorexia nervosa may be induced by social/cultural, psychological, physiological and genetic factors. The onset of anorexia nervosa may be associated with certain physiological processes, e.g. puberty and the associated changes in body shape (i.e. the redistribution of body fat, and the development of breasts), and events such as leaving home, divorce of parents, preparing for school examinations, and being teased at school.

Presentation

During the initial stages, Jane's carbohydrate (glycogen) stores are used. When these are diminished, fatty acids are used as the source of energy (Chapter 1). This would explain Jane's lack of subcutaneous fat. With progression to protein breakdown, her thinness will become very apparent.

As the episodes of enforced starvation progress in duration and severity, it is common to see the effects of this starvation on other body systems, including the endocrine failure responsible for Jane's amenorrhoea. Other systems (and symptoms) that may be affected include:

- cardiovascular system (bradycardia and hypotension, anaemia and thrombocytopoenia);

- gastrointestinal system (erosion of the teeth, oesophageal and intestinal erosion);

- renal system (decreased glomerular filtration rate, resulting in altered blood composition).

In addition to these complications, Jane's ability to regulate body temperature will also be altered because of energy deficits, lack of subcutaneous fat, lethargy, and diminished cardiovascular responses. People with anorexia nervosa may require interventions to ensure that an ideal body temperature is maintained. Dermatological changes are also observed, which explains Jane's fine downy hair, called lugano hair, on her face and back.

As well as physical effects, anorexia nervosa may also produce social and psychological disturbances. These may be exhibited as social isolation from friends, peers and family, restlessness in behaviour, and irritability with others. There is a preoccupation with self rather than others, and feelings of loss of control over one's life are also exhibited. This is an important element, because of the close association between puberty and anorexia nervosa.

Restoring homeostasis

See Figure 26.2.

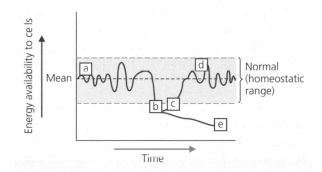

Figure 26.2 Anorexia nervosa. (a) Availability of energy within the range necessary for optimal cell function, i.e. nutrient intake, digestion, delivery to tissues, assimilation appropriate for health. (b) Reduced availability of energy. In anorexia, the problem is one of inadequate intake. (c) Therapies to increase energy availability. In anorexia, this would entail psychotherapeutic intervention, and dietary advice (d) Restoration of nutrient availability to within optimal range. (e) Persistent malnourishment, as observed in anorexia nervosa. Cell functioning will gradually deteriorate and may even become life threatening.

Aims of care

Anorexia nervosa is a disease that may become chronic, and some people may die as a direct result of it. Although there are many modes of treatment of the disease, there is no one method that is superior to others. The development of a long-term therapeutic relationship between the patient and the health professional requires time at the beginning of the relationship for the development of a rapport and trust.

Although the person may present with complex symptoms, the presenting problem is essentially one of inadequate food intake arising, in Jane's case, from poor body image. However, the cause of the problem is likely to be psychological. The aims of care, therefore, are to restore Jane's nutritional and metabolic homeostasis, and to restore her psychosocial equilibrium.

Implementation of care

Restoration of nutritional and metabolic homeostasis

The dietary programme established for Jane should restore her weight to that which is similar to the mean-matched population weight. Other systemic malfunctions will then diminish as optimal conditions are restored. Dietary change will involve a degree of negotiation between Jane, her named nurse and a dietician. The amount of food eaten at both meal times and between meals will be recorded, and Jane's weight will be measured and recorded daily.

Although it would be tempting to restore Jane's weight as quickly as possible, a certain degree of caution is necessary:

- the person with anorexia nervosa may have developed the ability to tolerate and cope with periods of starvation and electrolyte imbalances;
- any attempt at rapid weight gain may result in a degree of morbidity and even mortality.

As weight gain progresses, Jane may be discharged home and the care continued on a day-patient basis.

Restoration of psychosocial equilibrium

This is achieved through gaining Jane's recognition of her altered perception of her body using individual therapy, and the restoration of her social interactions using group therapy. Individual, group and family psychotherapy sessions would be planned; however, Jane's initial involvement in these may be minimal, since she would be unable to recognize the severity of her condition and may feel that it was the people around her who were experiencing the problem. After the first few individual therapy sessions, Jane would hopefully begin to make some progress.

Reference

American Psychiatric Association (1987) *Diagnostic and Statistical Manual of Mental Disorders (DSM-II-R)* Washington, DC: American Psychiatric Press.

Further reading

Serpell, L., Treasure, J., Teasdale, J. and Sullivan, V. (1999) Anorexia nervosa: friend or foe? *International Journal of Eating Disorders* **25**(2): 577–86.

Thomas, D. (1999) An unhealthy obsession with body image. *Practice Nurse* **17**(4): 252–55.

CASE 3: A MAN WITH DEPRESSION

Scenario:

William is a 30-year-old man who is married with one child aged 5 years. He has worked for 12 years as a miner in a colliery near to his home. He has now been made redundant, and after seeking employment for 6 months he has still not found an alternative job. He received redundancy pay, but the amount was small in comparison with the outstanding mortgage on his home. His wife has a part-time job and feels that she would like to expand the number of hours she works because of financial and social reasons. William is resistant to this development because he feels he should provide for his family, which emphasizes his feelings of inadequacy and worthlessness.

Their present circumstances have been the source of many arguments between William and his wife. Both parties are becoming increasingly distanced by the frustration that they feel at the intransigence of their spouse. William has loss interest in his daughter with whom he previously interacted and played regularly. He is described as being withdrawn and lethargic by family friends. He eats without enthusiasm and has lost weight, which is remarked upon by people who know him well. He previously liked to read extensively, but

he now finds it difficult to concentrate beyond short periods of time. He suffers from insomnia and feels tired and fatigued during most of his waking hours.

Depression as a homeostatic disturbance

Background

Generally, depression is more prevalent among women than men, and evidence implies that this may be because more women than men experience a relapse. Controversy surrounds the long-standing idea that depression can be ascribed to 'endogenous' or 'reactive' influences. Originally, this distinction attempted to differentiate between people whose depression arose from biochemical interaction within the brain and those who were depressed in reaction to external stresses.

Biochemically, depression appears to be associated with a deficiency in certain parts of the brain of the excitatory transmitters noradrenaline and serotonin. As a consequence, there is excessive expression of inhibitory pathways (see Chapter 8).

Psychological and sociological perspectives of depression have spanned a range of possible formulations that influence the development of the condition. Some theories that have been proposed as leaving people vulnerable to and maintaining the depressive state have been behavioural in emphasis, involving notions such as reduced social reinforcement, the inability of the person to reinforce their own behaviour, and learned helplessness. Cognitive theories of depression have embraced three main ideas:

● the concept of negative thoughts spontaneously arising in the person;

● the component of systematic logical errors in the thinking of depressed people;

● the notion of the presence of depressogenic schema's, which are long-standing attitudes or assumptions about the world that people use to organize their past and present experiences.

Depressive illness is now considered to result from a combination of physiological, psychological and social factors. What remains unclear is whether biochemical changes cause alterations of mood and affect, whether they are the results of alterations of mood or affect, or whether both factors interact in reciprocal ways.

Presentation

The term 'depression' is used frequently in everyday language to describe normal downswings in mood, thus many people in any population are affected at a given moment in time. These downswings are normally of short duration, and may serve to highlight a specific loss and activate the person to establish links with people who may be able to help. However, at other times, the depression may deepen to such an extent that it serves to attract more symptoms that are more problematic than helpful.

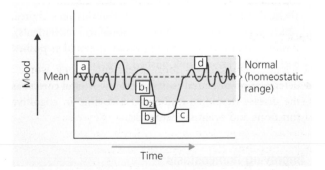

Figure 26.3 Depression. (a) Emotional state within normal 'mood swings'. (b₁) Genetic predisposition to depression, tending to move state towards lower end of homeostatic range. (b₂) Influence of life events to exacerbate change in mood. (b₃) Imbalance in excitatory neurotransmitters disrupts neurological functions, resulting in depressive illness. (c) Use of cognitive therapies and antidepressants drugs to promote neurological functioning. (d) Return of emotional state to normal range.

Restoring homeostasis

See Figure 26.3.

Aims of care

The aim of care in William's case is to restore the balance between excitatory and inhibitory pathways. This will be achieved by taking measures to restore his psychological equilibrium, and to intervene acutely with medication to help restore the balance to his brain chemistry. Both interventions will act on the same neurological pathways, and opinion is divided as to which method is most effective. A combination of the two may be used.

Implementation of care

Pharmacological intervention
The aim of medication (see Chapters 8 and 19) is to:

● improve the release of the excitatory neurotransmitter such as noradrenaline or serotonin; or

● prevent the reuptake of excitatory neurotransmitter from the synaptic cleft, so prolonging the activation of post-synaptic receptors; or

● provide agonistic actions similar to those of the deficient neurotransmitter.

One aspect to consider is that the neurotransmitters will also have roles elsewhere in the nervous system. As William commences a course of these drugs, nurses should monitor his response in order to respond to any side effects.

Psychological intervention
William is experiencing a major depressive episode. The main emphasis of the care adopts a cognitive-behavioural approach. The underlying assumption of this strategy is that the patient's depression follows on from distortions in thinking. Treatment therefore seeks to change the patterns of thinking, and so bring about a long-lasting resolution of the problem. Some general characteristics of cognitive therapy give structure to the approach:

● The therapist reviews with the patient the subjects that are to be discussed during the session.

● The therapist structures the therapy time so that a balance is achieved between the central and peripheral issues.

● The therapist summarizes periodically during the session, and invites the patient's reaction to the summary.

- The session is dominated by a questioning approach by the therapist. Statements of fact or offering of advice are avoided.

- The therapist agrees with the patient that they will reflect in time outside the sessions on areas that proved problematic. Also, the therapist asks the patient to sum up what has happened during the session and indicate what they feel has been helpful, inappropriate or hurtful about the session. The patient is also asked to explain what they think is required of them during the further reflection time.

Nurses working with William will encourage him to articulate the emotional pain that he is experiencing following the loss of his job in both individual and group situations. He will be encouraged to discuss his feelings with his wife and daughter. This should promote increased communication between the parties who have increasingly become estranged from each other. It therefore serves the function of enabling William to increase feelings of support and decrease his feelings of isolation.

Further reading

Ambrosini, P.J. (2000) A review of pharmacotherapy of major depression in children and adolescents. *Psychiatric Services* **51**(5): 627–33.

Beck, D.A., Koenig, H.G. and Beck, J.S. (1998) Depression. *Clinics in Geriatric Medicine* **14**(4): 765–86.

Kaye, J., Morton, J., Bowcutt, M. and Maupin, D. (2000) Stress, depression, and psychoneuroimmunology. *Journal of Neuroscience Nursing* **32**(2): 93–100.

CASE 4: A WOMAN WITH HUNTINGTON'S DISEASE

Scenario:

Sarah is 38 years old. On a recent visit to her GP for a routine check-up, her doctor was concerned to see that Sarah frequently, and apparently unintentionally, smacked her lips and grimaced slightly. She was also irritable and fidgety. The doctor was aware of Sarah's family history – her father had died several years earlier of Huntington's disease – so he referred her to a neurologist for a further examination.

In view of her age, family history and symptoms, the diagnosis was that Sarah was exhibiting the early signs of Huntington's disease.

Huntington's disease as a homeostatic imbalance

Background

Huntington's disease is an autosomal genetic condition (see Chapter 20), and so affects both sexes equally. It is caused by a dominant gene mutation. Spontaneous mutation of the gene within the early embryo is a very rare occurrence, so the condition is usually inherited. Being a dominant gene, this means that a parent would also be affected since the gene cannot be 'carried' in the way that a recessive gene may be. Although the gene is dominant, however, the condition does not usually have its onset until the individual is 30–45 years old. The late onset of the disease is not understood.

Presentation

It is also poorly understood how the Huntington gene operates, but neurological changes are observed that typically include a disturbance of the functioning of the basal ganglia of the forebrain and the substantia nigra of the midbrain. These brain nuclei are involved in the control of posture and movement (see Chapter 17), particularly the control of the muscles of the face and of the manipulative ability of limbs.

The gene responsible causes:

- a progressive loss of the inhibitory neurons that utilize the neurotransmitter gamma-aminobutyric acid (GABA). This disturbance of neurochemical homeostasis is responsible for the initial symptoms of the condition;

- a progressive decline and eventual atrophy of the brain nuclei, leading to a worsening of symptoms. Involuntary jerky movements of the head, arms and legs occur (the alternative name for the disease is Huntington's chorea, which relates to the dance-like or choreiform movements). Postural abnormalities develop, with the shoulders pushed back and the lower trunk pushed forward;

- deterioration of neural pathways to the frontal cortex, as the disease develops, leading to a decline in cognitive functions and eventual dementia.

Improving homeostasis

See Figure 26.4.

Aims of care

Huntington's disease is irreversible and its progression cannot be prevented. Aims of care, therefore, are to manage

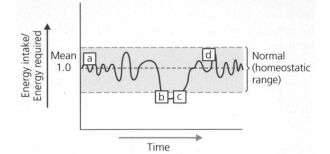

Figure 26.4 Metabolism in Huntington's disease. (a) Energy balance occurs (requirement = intake). (b) Disturbance in energy demands because energy requirement exceeds that available from diet as a result of increasing (involuntary) muscle activity. Emaciation will result if dietary intake is not increased, as in (c). (d) Good control re-established with complete compensation of energy demands. Neurological deficits will continue to worsen, however.

the condition as effectively as possible, to enable Sarah to maintain self-care, and to provide psychological support for her and her family. Therapy is directed at delaying admission to residential care for as long as possible.

Implementation of care

The rationale for most aspects of the care provided in Huntington's disease is self-evident, bearing in mind the increasing supervision that Sarah will require as the disorder progresses. In the early stages, mild tranquillizers may reduce the muscle contractions, but these actions become progressively weaker. Then care will:

- help Sarah to communicate effectively;
- prevent Sarah from becoming isolated. Education of friends and relatives is important in this respect. Nurses must also contain their reactions to sudden abnormal movements;
- ensure Sarah's food intake is appropriate. In relation to the dietary needs, it should be remembered that muscle

contraction is an efficient means of generating energy. Dietary energy content must be increased accordingly. Also, since feeding can become difficult and messy as the condition progresses, it is important to ensure that food is in manageable pieces. A drinking straw may also help;

- maintain Sarah's personal hygiene as self-care diminishes;
- maintain Sarah's personal safety;
- provide Sarah with psychological support to facilitate acceptance of the changing self, frustration and terminal nature of the disease. Day-centre care, voluntary visitor schemes and means of entertainment are important means of reducing depression and the risk of suicide risk arising as a consequence;
- support Sarah's family;
- provide genetic counselling for Sarah's children. With one affected (heterozygous) parent, there is a 50% risk that offspring will inherit the gene (see Chapter 20). Sarah's children, therefore, will have to consider the possibility that they too might eventually develop the disease, and one day may also pass on the gene to their children. The Huntington gene has been identified (on chromosome 4), and predictive gene testing may eventually become widely available. This still presents a dilemma for children of an affected person, as 'knowing' can be worse than 'not knowing'.

Further reading

Diederich, N.J. and Goetz, C.G. (2000) Neuropsychological and behavioral aspects of transplants in Parkinson's disease and Huntington's disease. *Brain and Cognition* **42**(2): 294–306.

Hofmann, N. (1999) Understanding the neuropsychiatric symptoms of Huntington's disease. *Journal of Neuroscience Nursing* **31**(5): 309–13.

Sobel, S. and Cowan, D.B. (2000) The process of family reconstruction after DNA testing for Huntington disease. *Journal of Genetic Counselling* **9**(3): 237–51.

CASE 5: A YOUNG MAN WITH SCHIZOPHRENIA

Scenario:

Paul is 17 years old. He is single and lives at home with his mother. He is employed as a store person in a large furniture warehouse. Until recently, Paul had no previous significant medical history, although he has been described as 'quiet'.

On her return from a holiday Paul's mother found him to be withdrawn, uncommunicative, anxious and exhibiting what she described as 'bizarre behaviour'. He believed he was receiving messages from the televi-

sion set and his favourite records. Over a period of 2–3 weeks, he increasingly became difficult to manage, refusing to eat meals as he believed they were poisoned. He would stay awake for long periods during the night, and occasionally would be verbally aggressive towards his mother. Paul refused to leave the house and attend work, and eventually he shared his fear with her that the house was being watched and 'they' were spying on him. At this point, his mother contacted their GP.

Schizophrenia as a homeostatic imbalance

Background

'Schizophrenia' is a term used frequently to describe a group of disorders. There are some indications that biological disposition to schizophrenia is caused by an excess of the neurotransmitter dopamine within the hippocampus of the brain (see Chapter 8). This may result from the presence of certain dopamine receptors or producing the dopamine in excessive amounts. This would raise the possibility that a disposition to schizophrenia may be inherited. Some research has provided strong evidence that there are greater risks of developing schizophrenia the closer the blood relationship is to the sufferer, but there is insufficient evidence to state that schizophrenia is unequivocally a genetic disorder.

Psychological and social perspectives on schizophrenia have become much more popular in research over the last three decades. These theories offer a greater recognition of the multifactorial models that seek to explore the interactions of biological, social and psychological factors that influence the potential physical and mental health problems for the sufferer. Vulnerability models (Birchwood and Tarrier, 1995) help the practitioner to understand the interactions between the environment and the person's responses to these factors. Environmental factors can affect the person, and stress and tension make the symptoms worse, possibly triggering exacerbation of the illness. Such factors range from problems at birth, peer group problems, social stressors, relationships within the family or life events.

While there are many diverse research explanations as to the origins of schizophrenia, a common factor is that there is an imbalance of neurological functioning (i.e. of neurochemistry). The issues are what causes that imbalance, and how best to restore it.

Presentation

Schizophrenia is manifested by characteristic disturbances of mood and behaviour. Symptoms of schizophrenia include delusions (false beliefs) and hallucinations (false perceptions); the most common types take the form of hearing voices and visualizing. Also, there are difficulties in thinking and feeling, and in expressions of behaviour.

Improving homeostasis

See Figure 26.5.

Aims of care

The aim of Paul's care is to restore his psychophysiological equilibrium through extrinsic intervention. His care will

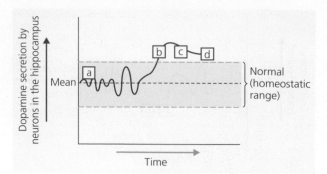

Figure 26.5 Dopamine model of schizophrenia. (a) Secretion of neurotransmitter within dopaminergic pathways appropriate for normal emotional and behavioural responses. (b) Hypersecretion of dopamine, leading to an imbalance of activity in neurological pathways. The causes and levels of secretion may be indicative of the severity of signs and symptoms. (c) Reduced dopamine secretion. In health, this would be a physiological response to maintain cognition within norms (a negative feedback response). In schizophrenia, there seems to be a failure of such processes, requiring medication and cognitive therapies to facilitate change. (d) Incomplete return to the homeostatic range. Symptoms will persist but with less severity.

centre on two approaches. First, pharmacological treatment will be used to try to normalize Paul's neurochemistry. Second, a cognitive approach will then be used to encourage Paul to appraise his situation and behaviour in an attempt to improve the circumstances that precipitated the schizophrenia. This second approach recognizes the multifactorial causes of schizophrenia and raises the possibility of long-term re-establishment of neurochemical balance.

Implementation of care

Drug therapy
Paul would be likely commenced on the neuroleptic drug chlorpromazine. This is often used, as it can help with anxiety symptoms and the behavioural disturbances that Paul sometimes exhibits. A by-product of chlorpromazine is that it also has a sedative effect, which would help to reduce Paul's anxiety and improve his sleep pattern.

A community psychiatric nurse would visit Paul. Initially, visits would be twice a week to monitor the effect of the medication, and to initiate and develop a therapeutic relationship with both Paul and his mother. Visits would subsequently be reduced to once a week.

Cognitive therapy
Paul would be encouraged to express his feelings initially to the nurse and then in joint sessions with his mother. Relatives often do not understand the problems their loved ones are experiencing, and at times may be intolerant of the sufferer's behaviour. The nurse would explore

the family dynamics using a pragmatic and flexible approach.

A cognitive behavioural model would be adopted to encourage Paul to change his thinking pattern and to increase his self-esteem. In this way, the 'bizarre behaviour' observed by his mother should lessen.

Goals would be negotiated and agreed with Paul. These may be to:

- ensure Paul has an adequate dietary intake;

- add some structure into his day to avoid sleeping or withdrawing. Various options might be suggested, e.g. Paul might be encouraged to join a local group run as a social support by the community psychiatric nurse and volunteers;

- gradually socialize with his close friends and take up his previous leisure pursuits;

- remain on present medication and be monitored by his community psychiatric nurse or GP on a regular basis.

Reference

Birchwood, M. and Tarrier, N. (1995) *Innovations in the Psychological Management of Schizophrenia.* Chichester, UK: J. Wiley & Sons.

Further reading

Adams, C., Wilson, P., Gilbody, S., Bagnall, A. and Lewis, R. (2000) Drug treatments for schizophrenia. *Quality in Health Care* **9**(1): 73–9.

Fox, J.C. and Kane, C.F. (1998) Schizophrenia. *Annual Review of Nursing Research* **16**: 287–322.

CASE 6: DISTRESS

Two cases are presented: hyperstress and hypostress.

Case: a young woman with occupational hyperstress

Scenario: 1

Polly is a 23-year-old paediatric nurse. Previously enthusiastic, sensitive and compassionate, during the past 6 months Polly has become cool and detached towards her patients, uncommunicative with them, and aloof and distant from her colleagues. Her delivery of care has remained competent, but she feels beset by doubts as to her own ability, constantly checking and rechecking procedures and equipment with which she has been involved. There never seems time to complete everything expected of her, and the increasing difficulty that she finds in expressing herself in the nursing care plans means that this aspect of her work is left to the last possible moment. She has begun to dread returning to work following her time off duty, and has missed several days suffering from migraine.

Polly lives with her boyfriend, Tom, who has little patience with her current moods, and feels that if she no longer likes children then she should change her job.

Case: a man with occupational hypostress

Scenario: 2

Gordon is 43 years old and has recently lost his job as manager of a farm when the owner sold it to a large co-operative with its own management structure. He has been applying for similar positions without success, a factor he attributes to his age and to his reluctance to move out of the area and disrupt his children's secondary schooling. He has had to leave the tied house that went with his old post, and has moved into rented council accommodation. To continue to support his family, Gordon has reluctantly accepted a position as a tractor driver on a neighbouring farm.

The reality of the situation is that he has moved from a position of considerable responsibility and great variety (managing a team of men and a substantial budget on a large farm with mixed arable enterprises and a pedigree breeding stock of pigs, sheep and cattle). His current role is subordinate; his salary, status and standard of living are reduced, and he finds the work repetitive, boring and lacking in any stimulation or challenge.

Gordon visits his GP, and complains of tiredness, poor sleep and indigestion.

Hyperstress and hypostress as homeostatic imbalances

Background

Although the concept of stress is relatively modern, its study has attracted an immense amount of interest, and a variety of definitions and models have emerged (see Chapter 22). Stress has been identified as causing (i.e. as a stimulus) or as constituting a response to potentially damaging internal or external demands upon the person. This focus produced a preoccupation with the causative components of stress that has dominated research in this field. Subsequent work has developed the concept of negative stressors, and sought to identify these in relation to significant life events. The results of negative stress have been seen in terms of occupational dissatisfaction, disengagement and 'burnout'.

While the traditional approach has concentrated on the negative effects of stress, the contemporary stance, in defining stress in terms of homeostatic balance, admits to the concept of deleterious and beneficial stress, respectively 'distress' and 'eustress'. Furthermore, a normal individual range is established, beyond the bounds of which (i.e. of the stress threshold) that person can be said to be experiencing hyperstress or hypostress (Figures 26.6 and 26.7). To date, research has concentrated on hyperstress, with only a comparatively recent recognition of the potentially, equally injurious situation in which sustained hypostress occurs. Occupational areas that make low demands on the workers but provide little support (or actual constraint) in fulfilling those demands are potentially more stressful than highly demanding areas that give a good level of support.

Presentation

Given the situations as they are presented, it seems probable that Polly is suffering from occupational hyperstress. It seems likely that the principal cause of her hyperstress is occupationally based, as she is showing the characteristic symptoms of 'burnout' (an extreme reaction to unrelieved stress that has long been associated with those engaged in the 'caring professions'). These can be summarized as disaffection and withdrawal of involvement with those for whom they care.

However, Tom's recent lack of sympathy, while it may be purely a response to the change he sees in Polly, could be indicative of deeper problems within the relationship that may have impacted on Polly's ability to cope with the demands of her job.

Gordon's description of boredom and frustration in his work, and the feeling of 'being tired doing nothing', support his hypostress. He demonstrates increased psycho-

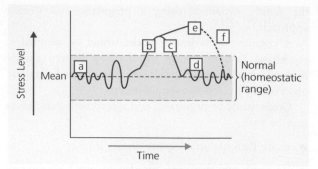

Figure 26.6 Occupational hyperstress. (a) Stress level maintained within homeostatic norms (perceived capabilities = perceived demands). (b) Distress: stress threshold superseded, leading to hyperstress (perceived capabilities less than perceived demands). Stress-related signs and symptoms may be observed. (c) Reduction in stress by identification of stressors and by stress management (capability—demand mismatch is reduced). (d) Stress level returns to homeostatic norm. (e) Failure of individual coping mechanisms leading to exacerbation of stress-related signs and symptoms, and stress-related disorders. (f) Intervention: provision of healthcare support to control symptoms and facilitate coping.

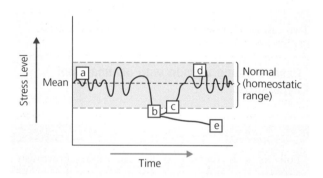

Figure 26.7 Occupational hypostress. (a) Stress level maintained within homeostatic norms (perceived capabilities = perceived demands). (b) Distress: hypostress (perceived capabilities greater than perceived demands). Signs and symptoms may be observed. (c) Use of alternative stimuli to promote eustress. This may be prompted by clinical intervention. (d) Stress level returns to homeostatic norm. (e) Failure to restore capability—demand balance. Prolonged hypostress with exacerbation of signs and symptoms, leading to stress-related disorders.

logical and physiological morbidity, including boredom, lethargy and chronic tiredness. He is disaffected, and shows lack of motivation and a range of psychosomatic disorders, leading to increased incidence of sickness and absenteeism. He is showing signs of depression. Severe depression may arise, with the risk of suicide.

However, Gordon has recently experienced significant trauma in losing a responsible job and an established home, and these events cause distress. This emphasizes the difficulty in determining a rigid 'diagnosis' of hyperstress or hypostress, and endorses the concept of constantly fluctuating levels of stress.

Restoring homeostasis

See Figures 26.6 and 26.7.

Aims of care

These cases relate to people who are currently experiencing distress thought to be principally occupational in origin. Current thinking favours an eclectic approach that recognizes the complex interrelationship between mind and body, and cause and effect (see Chapter 22). Stress may be viewed, therefore, as a homeostatic imbalance that arises when there is actual or perceived demand–capability mismatch between the person and their environment.

In the context of assisting the person to return to a level of stress within the normal homeostatic range defined by their stress thresholds, the model of clinical supervision that is advocated is one of support and development, rather than the more narrow regulation and standard setting.

Implementation of care

Hyperstress

Appropriate support for Polly will be identified only once the predominant source of her distress is recognized. It may be that Polly's stress is not isolated but indicative of job dissatisfaction among her colleagues. Any recent changes in practice (e.g. altered shift patterns) and any undue pressures should be identified and, where possible, measures taken to address these. As Polly's stress appears to be occupationally founded, support must be provided in the workplace. This will operate at two levels, i.e. individual support for Polly through involvement of the occupational health department and awareness of her manager, and an assessment of the current environment within the paediatric unit where she works.

Support will entail the following:

- Those caring for her, and Polly herself, must recognize that the level of stress she is experiencing is outside the usual limits within which her previous homeostatic norm has naturally fluctuated. During this time, the demands made upon her were balanced by her individual capability.

- Care for Polly will need to restore the homeostatic balance by reducing stress levels to below the upper threshold. Specialist psychological intervention may be indicated, with the appropriate medical treatment for her presenting physiological problems, e.g. her migraine.

- An individual programme of stress reduction should be instituted, incorporating techniques whereby Polly will be able to recognize and use the beneficial effects of everyday stressors (eustressors) to counteract the adverse effects of her current hyperstress.

- Medical, nursing or specialist counselling intervention will need to address the occupational focus of her distress, probably by providing career guidance. Has her original ambition in joining the paediatric unit been realized? If so, does she still feel that this is appropriate, or can she be developed in the role, and what will facilitate her career development? If not, what alternatives are there, and how can she access them? (Note that in either eventuality, it is important to concentrate on Polly's strengths and aspects about which she feels positive and less distressed.)

The importance of a non-judgemental approach is paramount. Hyperstress and 'burnout' are known to affect those who are caring and conscientious. Above all, a level of care should be instituted that effectively restores the state of balance between demands and capabilities, irrespective of Polly's ultimate decisions about her work and her relationships.

Hypostress

Although Gordon's problems seem to be related to hypostress, there is a possibility that some of his symptoms arise from other causes. Gordon will therefore require medical investigation in case there is a non-occupational cause for his symptoms. His GP will wish to exclude other physiological causes for his tiredness (e.g. possible anaemia), and establish the reason for his indigestion (e.g. ulcer, hiatus hernia, etc.). The sleep problem will need to be investigated thoroughly, as a history of disturbed rest and early-morning waking may indicate a level of clinical depression that will require immediate intervention to prevent suicidal behaviour.

While these investigations are being conducted, and treatment and, where necessary, specialist referral, is being undertaken, Gordon will need help in restoring his presenting homeostatic imbalance:

- Gordon needs to be able to utilize everyday beneficial stressors ('eustressors') that will help to restore this balance. Measures to promote the beneficial effects of eustressors that will provide an alternative source of stimulation and a necessary 'healthy' stress response might include working with Gordon to get him to recognize remaining areas of challenge in his life.

- Gordon has suffered an inevitable loss of self-esteem, and the lack of challenge and respect in his current work endorse this. He may be experiencing a sense of shame where his family and wider circle of friends are concerned, tension in his relationships, and feelings of profound isolation.

● The fact that Gordon has sought medical opinion is encouraging, as it shows a recognition on his part of the need for action to restore his equilibrium. Support for Gordon will need to capitalize and develop this self-awareness, to promote alternative strategies for him to adopt in relation to his work. It may be that he can be encouraged to find some unrealized potential in the job, or he may be able to find this fulfilment in other interests, family, hobbies or organizations. Given his former level of responsibility and involvement, the challenges he needs to develop to establish a pattern of healthy stressors in his life are more likely to be found in social/community activities, where he can use his former expertise and regain his self-respect.

Further reading

Read Chapter 22 of this book.

Jones, M.C. and Johnston, D.W. (2000) Reducing distress in first level and student nurses: a review of the applied stress management literature. *Journal of Advanced Nursing* **32**(1): 66–74.

Edwards, D., Burnard, P., Coyle, D., Fothergill, A. and Hannigan, B. (2000) Stress and burnout in community mental health nursing: a review of the literature. *Journal of Psychiatric and Mental Health Nursing* **7**(1): 7–14.

Sawatzky, J.V. (1998) Understanding nursing students' stress: a proposed framework. *Nurse Education Today* **18**(2): 108–15.

Learning disability care case studies

The cases presented here are intended not to be comprehensive, but to provide common examples that illustrate homeostatic principles in their pathology and in the care delivered.

CASE 1: A MAN WITH DOWN'S SYNDROME

Scenario:

Tony is 50 years old. He lives at home with his parents, who are both elderly. Shortly after his birth, Tony was discovered to have Down's syndrome. As a baby, he exhibited hypotonia and his parents remember him as a 'floppy' baby who was quiet and passive throughout most of his early childhood. His IQ, measured at 12 years of age using the Wechsler Adult Intelligence Scale (WAIS), was found to be 60: lower than normal. He received little formal education during his childhood, and has attended a day centre since his late adolescence.

Tony has poor eyesight and commonly experiences conjunctivitis and blepharitis. His visual disability is exacerbated by his frequent refusal to wear spectacles that have been prescribed for his visual impairment. Tony also has hearing difficulties. The combination of sight and hearing difficulties often have an adverse impact on Tony's attempts to communicate with other people, particularly acute when he attempts to converse with strangers. Throughout his childhood and adult life, Tony has been mildly obese.

Recently, Tony has become withdrawn and is described as apathetic by his parents and people who know him well. Although previously he could undertake self-help skills, such as bathing independently, he now requires a considerable amount of assistance to perform these skills successfully. Tony also appears to be confused by situations that he previously understood well, such as hobbies he used to enjoy. His parents are particularly frightened by a recent incident during the night in which Tony appeared to be confused by the darkened staircase leading to the ground floor when his parents were sleeping. Tony fell down several of the steps but suffered no serious ill effects.

Down syndrome as a homeostatic disturbance

Background

Down's syndrome occurs as a consequence of an additional chromosome 21 (see Chapter 20), and so may be observed in both males and females. The most common occurrence is an inherited trisomy, in which non-dysjunction of this chromosome pair during meiosis leaves a gamete (usually the oocyte; non-dysjunction is more frequent in the mother) with both of the usual copies of chromosome 21. Fertilization then produces the trisomy. Less frequently, the disorder arises because the gamete has one full copy of the chromosome but also another fragment of chromosome that is attached to another chromosome. This error again usually occurs during meiosis, and so is inherited. A rare form of the condition arises when non-dysjunction occurs during mitosis within the early embryo; this means that some embryological cells will be trisomic but others will not. The variety of causes of the disorder means that the syndrome has a spectrum of severity.

The overall incidence of Down's syndrome is often quoted as 1 in 600 live births, but this is based on recorded incidence across several decades of a mother's life, and the incidence of inherited Down's syndrome varies with maternal age.

Presentation

Down's syndrome is the most common chromosomal disorder that causes learning disabilities. Although a number of common anatomical and functional irregularities are found, they may vary greatly in their manifestation in each individual sufferer. Some of the more common features are:

- brachycephalia, with reduced cranial capacity. This largely accounts for the learning difficulties observed in Down's syndrome;

- an epicanthic fold on the inner aspect of the upper eyelid. Strabismus, nystagmus and cataracts are common. Brushfield's spots are flecked through the iris, which may be poorly developed. There is often reduced production of the enzyme lysozyme, which has antiseptic qualities, in tear secretion. These changes account for Tony's visual problems;

- the bridge of the nose is often small with a high narrow palate. The tongue is large, with horizontal fissures, which leads to tongue protrusion with subsequent mouth breathing. Such features contribute to the communication difficulties observed;

- heart problems, which affect approximately half of all babies with Down's syndrome; historically, this has led to many their early deaths;

- thyroid deficiency (much more common in people with Down's syndrome), responsible for a slowed metabolic rate.

Tony's more recent lapses are indicative of the onset of Alzheimer's disease. Links between Alzheimer's disease and Down's syndrome are generally accepted as substantial (both involve chromosome 21), but the full extent of the association between the conditions is not understood fully. It is generally accepted that Alzheimer's disease occurs more commonly in people with Down's syndrome than in the general population, and that onset is at an earlier age.

Improving homeostasis

See Figure 27.1.

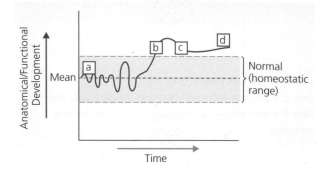

Figure 27.1 Down's syndrome. (a) Anatomical/functional development of embryological tissues appropriate to norms for embryological age. (b) An accumulation of anatomical and functional abnormalities in the embryo as a result of genetic or environmental influences. In Down's syndrome, such changes arise from a surplus of genes provided by an additional chromosome. (c) Limited correction of developmental change after birth, e.g. surgical realignment of the blood vessels of the heart. (d) Persistence of abnormalities that cannot be corrected.

Aims of care

Although chromosome 21 is one of the smallest chromosomes, it clearly produces profound anatomical and functional abnormalities. Some of these, e.g. disorders of cardiac anatomy, might be correctable with surgery, and visual problems can be improved with aids, but many of Tony's physical problems are uncorrectable. This means that Tony's care is directed mainly at enabling him to have a higher quality of life by maintaining his current wellbeing, and by improving his functional capacity, where possible.

Implementation of care

Maintaining or improving cognitive functions
Tony is likely to be referred to a community learning disability nurse who will aim to enable Tony to cope more completely with his psychological deficits, such as failing memory and confusion. The aim will be to change the environment in which Tony functions so that it better fits his diminishing cognitive capacities. Alongside these

objectives, the nurse recognizes the need to work with Tony's parents to minimize their anxiety and to co-opt them as partners in working to meet their son's needs.

The community nurse also begins strategies with Tony that aim to maintain his capacity to retain information via long-term memory. This has taken the form of using imagery and reality orientation in conjunction with Tony's parents. Thus, at every possible opportunity, Tony's parents reinforce with him notions such as the time of day, Tony's and their own names. and subjects such as forth-coming holidays. The community nurse will also give careful consideration to the apathy that Tony appears to display. For example, it might be agreed that Tony's father will encourage him to participate in activities that they can enjoy together, such as gardening. The impact of inter-ventions such as these on cognitive functions illustrates the partial plasticity of brain function.

Providing a safe environment

With regard to restructuring the environment, Tony's bedroom within the family home will be moved to the ground floor of the house so as to avoid risk associated with the stairs.

Further reading

Kubas, C. (1999) Noninvasive means of identifying fetuses with possible Down syndrome: a review. *Journal of Perinatal and Neonatal Nursing* **13**(2): 27–46.

Ryder, I.H. (1999) Prenatal screening for Down syndrome: a dilemma for the unsupported midwife? *Midwifery* **15**(1): 16–23.

Scott, H. (2000) Are people with Down's syndrome denied care? *British Journal of Nursing* **9**(18): editorial.

CASE 2: A GIRL BORN WITH CYTOMEGALOVIRUS INCLUSIVE BODY DISEASE

Scenario:

Maria was born after a relatively uneventful first pregnancy. Generally, her mother Cassandra was well, although she recalls feeling 'a little under the weather' at the end of the first trimester of pregnancy. She did not find this remarkable as she frequently compared notes with other pregnant women, who also complained of fatigue.

Maria was diagnosed as having jaundice in the first 24 h, and later was observed to have infantile spasms. Her development was monitored frequently during her preschool years, as her head measurements showed that she was microcephalic and her infantile spasms had developed into tonic clonic epileptic seizures.

Maria received full-time education until she was 19 years old in a school for children with special needs, as she was assessed as having severe learning disabilities. Owing to her hyperactivity, lack of concentration, and poor eyesight, Maria places herself at great risk by wandering out of buildings and stepping out into the road without any recognition of danger.

Maria is now 22 years old. Caring for Maria placed Cassandra's marriage under great strain, and eventually Maria's parents separated with animosity. Now alone, Cassandra is exhausted from caring for all of Maria's needs and from constantly watching her to ensure her wanderings don't put her in danger.

As a result of her high levels of activity and severe learning disabilities, it was hard to find full-time day care for Maria. After 3 years, the social services department has offered Maria 2 days a week in a special care unit attached to a day centre. Finding appropriate respite care has also been difficult, as small care units were unpre-pared to lock all their clients into the building and compromise their freedom for the sake of Maria.

Maria has undergone a number of treatments for her epilepsy. Currently, she is prescribed sodium valproate, which controls the seizures reasonably well.

Cytomegalovirus inclusive body disease as a homeostatic imbalance

Background

The cytomegalovirus is one of the herpes family of viruses. The virus is widespread in the environment, and there is suggestion that 80% of adults may have suffered an infec-tion: the symptoms of cytomegalovirus infection may be slight and often go unnoticed. It is found worldwide, and is particularly prevalent in developing countries and people in lower socioeconomic groups. The virus may be present in semen, cervical secretions, urine, blood, saliva, breast milk and stools, and is therefore generally transmit-ted by close contact or by direct transfer of cells or fluids. When present, typical symptoms may resemble glandular fever, including malaise, fever, swollen lymph glands and abnormal liver function. Diagnosis can be made by cell culture.

People with cytomegalovirus are also at risk from superinfection from bacteria and fungi. People with reduced or compromised immunity, such as babies, elderly people, people with HIV infection and AIDS, and people being treated with immunosuppressive drugs, are at a higher risk of suffering more serious complications, including life-threatening illnesses such as pneumonia.

The developing fetus is also at risk from maternal infection via the placenta, particularly when the mother is suffering from a primary infection. As with maternal rubella, the fetus is at greatest risk of damage during the period of organ differentiation during the first trimester (see Chapter 20). However, unlike maternal rubella, the infection of the fetus may also occur much later in the pregnancy.

It is thought that 10–20% of babies who are infected by maternal transmission become learning disabled. Indeed, the virus is now thought to be responsible for more cases of amentia than maternal rubella.

Presentation

The presence of the virus in the fetus has a number of consequences, particularly for the development of the central nervous system:

- birth weight is low;
- there is microcephaly (small head, severe damage to the nervous system);
- the eyes are abnormally small (microphthalmos), and vision is usually poor;
- epilepsy is often present, often presenting first as infantile spasms (West's syndrome);
- there is cerebral palsy;
- there is deafness;
- the child will be hyperactive;
- a wide range of learning disabilities, from mild to severe, may be present;
- there will be enlargement of the spleen and liver for the first few months, resulting characteristically in jaundice.

Improving homeostasis

See Figure 27.2.

Aims of care

There is currently no known treatment for the cytomegalovirus condition. Health and social carers can only respond to service users like Maria in a sympathetic and humane way. The aims of care are to divert Maria's energy into more rewarding pursuits, to encourage relaxation, and to control her epilepsy.

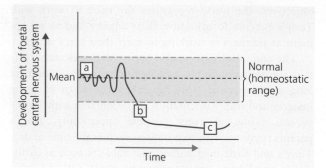

Figure 27.2 Cytomegalovirus. (a) Development of the fetal central nervous system at rates within the normal range appropriate for age. (b) Diminished development arising from the presence of a teratogen, such as cytomegalovirus, leading to learning difficulty. (c) Permanent microcephaly as a consequence of cytomegalovirus infection. Although some functional improvement can be promoted by using, for example, relaxation therapies, the effect of intervention is limited.

Implementation of care

Care plans must involve extensive programmes that aim to increase concentration span and to make constructive and meaningful use of the person's energy and hyperactivity by recognized, valued and enjoyable exercise and activity. Maria will also need to be encouraged to relax. Therapeutic areas such as (snoezelens) snoozelams (see *Case 6: a young man with sensory deprivation* in this chapter) may be beneficial in encouraging interest, concentration and relaxation.

Maria's epilepsy will be monitored regularly. A vigilant awareness of the side effects of anti-seizure drugs such as sodium valproate must be maintained. Side effects include abdominal pain, hair loss, weight gain and rashes. Particularly relevant in Maria's case is that prolonged use of sodium valproate may cause liver damage, so regular liver function tests are important.

Equally important is caring for the carer who may be looking after a highly active individual. In Maria's case, her mother is now caring for her virtually alone. Care of difficult-to-manage people may result in social isolation, as others may find the behaviour of service users such as Maria difficult to understand, and find their constant fidgeting and unpredictable activity stressful and embarrassing.

Further reading

Lazzarotto, T., Varani, S., Guerra, B., Nicolosi, A., Lanari, M. and Landini M.P. (2000) Prenatal indicators of congenital cytomegalovirus infection. *Journal of Pediatrics* **137**(1): 90–95.

CASE 3: A MAN WITH LEARNING DISABILITIES LEAVING A LONG-STAY INSTITUTION

Scenario:

Simon is a 50-year old man with a moderate learning disability as established by assessment using adaptive behaviour scales (Nihira *et al.*, 1974). He has lived in a hospital for people with learning disabilities for the last 40 years. During his stay in the hospital, he has lived in a variety of settings. For the past 5 years, he has shared accommodation with 14 other men who have various learning disabilities. In the last 2 weeks, Simon has left the hospital in order to live in an ordinary dwelling with four other people who have learning disabilities.

With the goal of Simon's complete independence in mind, staff have been working with him to determine what his wants and needs are associated with his future life. Following discussion, Simon has revealed that he is experiencing a number of problems following his move from the hospital environment. The problems are principally connected with disturbed sleep, lack of appetite and general tiredness.

Leaving a long-stay institution as a homeostatic imbalance

Background

A substantial number of people with learning disabilities have spent the majority of their lives in hospital wards. It has been recognized for some time, however, that many people with learning disabilities do not require care that necessitates their stay in a hospital setting, since they are not subject to an ongoing acute illness of any kind.

For many people, resettlement means giving up routines and a way of life that have been theirs for most of their childhood and adult life. In many cases, this traditional regime of care will have involved practices that have perpetuated the dependence of clients upon carers, and led to the erosion of their ability to indulge in decision making. Simon's symptoms are indicative of this and probably result from a desynchronization of his circadian rhythms.

Circadian rhythms refer to events that are repeated in the body every 24 h (See Chapter 23). Humans are not obviously rhythmic or cyclical, as they have no breeding season, migration or hibernation, but some stable rhythms can be observed, e.g. temperature, heart activity and metabolic rates. When these rhythms follow the expected patterns, the body is said to be in a state of internal synchronization, i.e. parameters such as eating, sleeping, body temperature and performance are synchronized with

the person's activity–rest cycles (Chapter 23). However, a disturbance in lifestyle can desynchronize these rhythms.

Presentation

The potential for desynchronization is greater in people such as Simon, because he has been subjected to institutional practices and so has experienced regular exogenous cues that will have helped him to maintain the synchronization of his circadian rhythms. This helps to explain the tiredness and lack of appetite he demonstrates in his new lifestyle and environment. The situation is probably exacerbated by his learning disability, since this reduces his capacity to interpret and react to the changes in his lifestyle.

Restoring homeostasis

See Figure 27.3.

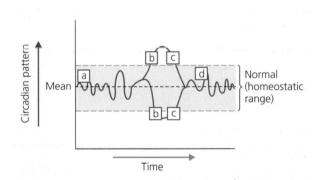

Figure 27.3 Circadian rhythm desynchronization. (a) Parameters fluctuating within range established by circadian entrainment within the hospital. (b) Circadian pattern desynchronized by the loss of (institutionally imposed) cues, and incorporation of new cues (from the community). (c) Nursing intervention to re-establish resynchronization, i.e. short-term to encourage sleep—wake and mealtime patterns as they were in hospital, and long term to encourage the establishment of rhythms based on new cues. (d) Parameters fluctuating within range now established by cues provided by the community environment.

Aims of care

The main thrust of the care is aimed at transferring the locus of power away from its traditional location in the hands of carers to the prerogative of clients. Much of the creation of power is associated with the possession of information and the subsequent decision making that takes place. Institutions have reinforced tendencies in which clients are acted upon by carers, rather than with carers, leading to institutionalized practices. Community care emphasizes the client's rights as having the same human value as other members of the community. The small scale of the home in which Simon now lives makes privacy and dignity more possible, and avoids the distress and dehumanization that may accompany overcrowding.

The two main aims of care for someone in Simon's position will therefore be to reduce the impact of the changes associated with his move from hospital to community, and to facilitate the resynchronization of his circadian rhythms once the move has occurred.

Implementation of care

Reducing the impact of Simon's move

The move should be gradual. With this in mind, a number of occasions on which Simon can stay in the new home might be arranged for a number of months, with the duration of the stay being increased gradually. Thus, in the first instance Simon might attend the home in order to have a meal with some of the clients who already live there. Following this, he might stay overnight in the home. With time, he might extend his stay to a whole weekend.

Facilitating resynchronization of Simon's circadian rhythms

Simon's symptoms should be discussed with him to clarify that his problems are associated with the differences between his present lifestyle and his previous residence in the hospital environment. For example, it might be identified that previously he was woken in the morning by carers at an early hour because of the necessity to eat breakfast and leave the home area to attend day care. He now has responsibility for

this activity himself and is free to remain in bed longer if he so wishes. It is likely that Simon will find that he is unable to sleep beyond the time dictated by his previous routine. Similarly, if he ate meals according to a schedule devised for the convenience of the hospital kitchen, then he would be free in his new environment to have meals when he wants or in co-operation with other residents in the home.

In order to compensate for the desynchronizing effect of the shift between the long-established routines and those that are new, staff would agree with Simon to effect a number of changes to enable him to achieve homeostasis once more. For example, Simon's sleep pattern should adapt over a longer exposure time, but short-term strategies might involve him having a short nap around lunchtime in the day care service that he attends. This would enable him to avoid the fatigue due to lack of sleep that he had been experiencing.

Another strategy that might be used is to encourage Simon to adopt an activity programme that involves cycling to improve his level of all-round fitness. The benefits of this are an increased resistance to fatigue, and a raising of Simon's feeling of wellbeing.

Reference

Nihira, K., Foster, R., Shellhaas, M. and Leland, H. (1974) *AAMD Adaptive Behaviour Scale, 1974 Revision*. Washington, DC: American Association on Mental Deficiency.

Further reading

Parrish, A. (1998) Community care for people with a learning disability. *British Journal of Community Nursing* **3**(7): 352–5.

CASE 4: A MAN WITH PHENYLKETONURIA

Scenario:

Jim is 36 years old. His birth was uneventful and normal. Unlike his parents, Jim has light blonde hair, blue eyes and a pale complexion. As a child, he was described as being irritable, immature and overdependent; he was 'hyperactive', and rocking back and forth, waving his arms and grinding his teeth were not uncommon. His skin and urine are often described as having a 'musty' or 'mousy' odour.

When he was 16 years old, Jim was diagnosed as having severe learning disability. At times, he suffers from epileptic seizures, dystonia and dysphagia. His behaviours have become too trying for his parents, and consequently he has been received into care at a local residential home. Neither parent exhibits the disorder, nor does his sister.

Jim was subsequently diagnosed as having phenylketonuria (PKU).

Phenylketonuria as a homeostatic disturbance

Background

PKU is an inherited metabolic disorder. Its absence in both of Jim's parents, and in his sister, indicates that it is autosomal recessive in nature, so Jim must be homozygous for the condition, while both parents are heterozygous and therefore 'carriers' (see Chapter 20). The worldwide incidence of PKU is 1 in 10 000 live births, although geographic and/or cultural factors will influence these figures.

PKU results from an inability of the person to convert the amino acid phenylalanine to tyrosine as a consequence of a deficiency of the enzyme phenylalanine hydroxylase. Phenylalanine concentration in the blood then becomes elevated. PKU is irreversible, but it can be controlled if diagnosed early, and babies born in Britain today are tested routinely. As a consequence, the occurrence of people with problems such as those experienced by Jim has diminished in recent years.

Presentation

The signs and symptoms exhibited by Jim arise because:

● excess phenylalanine interferes with the entry of other amino acids into the brain across the blood–brain barrier. A full range of amino acids is required for normal protein synthesis, so amino acid deficiency interferes with brain development in PKU;

● tyrosine deficiency in the brain prevents the normal production of adrenergic neurotransmitters, such as noradrenaline, and so affects synapse development (see Chapter 8);

● some of the excess phenylalanine is broken down to produce phenylpyruvic acid (also known as phenylpyruvate), which is responsible for the 'musty' or 'mousy' odour of Jim's sweat and urine;

● tyrosine is a precursor for the skin pigment melanin and its deficiency, therefore, produces fair hair, blue eyes and a pale complexion.

Note how the severe disturbances especially relate to neurological functioning – PKU will cause learning disability if uncorrected.

Improving homeostasis

See Figure 27.4.

Aims of care

The disorder is irreversible, so the prospects for returning Jim to health are poor. Care for him is therefore directed at maintaining and promoting as much self-care as possible.

Implementation of care

Jim's placement in a residential home is indicative of the profound difficulties PKU produces. He will require a high level of care to manage his dysphagia and to manage or reduce his epilepsy.

Although the condition is irreversible, normalizing phenylalanine and tyrosine concentrations in Jim's body fluids may improve his general wellbeing (but not his learning difficulty). The homeostatic balance between

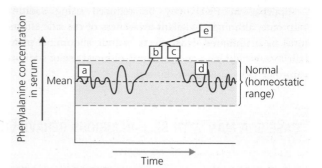

Figure 27.4 Phenylketonuria. (a) Serum phenylalanine concentration within its normal range, i.e. dietary intake and utilization of the amino acid are in balance. (b) Rising phenylalanine concentration as a result of inadequate utilization. (c) Intervention to reduce phenylalanine imbalance by reducing dietary intake, as in (d), i.e. intake is now in balance with the decreased utilization. (e) Persistently elevated phenylalanine concentration in serum, resulting in signs of phenylketonuria caused by inadequate dietary control. The neurological damage that may occur in a child is irreversible.

phenylalanine utilization by tissues and its addition to body fluids from the diet (phenylalanine is an essential amino acid and so cannot be synthesized by the liver) can be restored. Increased utilization of phenylalanine cannot be promoted, so therapy is directed primarily at reducing the dietary intake of the amino acid.

FURTHER INFORMATION

We noted earlier that PKU can be controlled if it is identified early in infancy (Box 20.11). A simple blood test (the neonatal screening test, once known as the Guthrie test) taken up to 7–10 days after birth will detect whether the phenylalanine concentration is elevated. Antenatal gene testing is increasingly available, and will enable earlier recognition of the problem. The problem is observed in about 1 in 10 000 births in the UK. If phenylalanine is elevated, the baby will be placed on a low-phenylalanine, or phenylalanine-free, diet. Regular blood testing is required, and appropriate alterations will be made to the diet. Dietary control will be important until the child is about 10 years old, although mental faculties may still be impaired in older children and adults if phenylalanine is allowed to rise too much.

If severe tyrosine deficiency occurs, then dietary tyrosine supplements may be required. Maintaining adequate tyrosine will help to protect against adverse changes in neuronal development.

Both aspects of care will require education of the parents, and the child when he/she is old enough to understand, of the necessity of controlling the diet.

The irreversibility of the damage caused by the condition means that control must commence at an early age before brain development has progressed to an advanced stage. Phenylalanine is abundant in natural food proteins. Dietary control of phenylketonuria is therefore highly restrictive.

Epilepsy in PKU may be reduced using sodium valproate, although a vigilant awareness of the side effects must be maintained. Side effects include abdominal pain, hair loss, weight gain and rashes. Prolonged use of sodium valproate may cause liver damage.

Further reading

De Freitas, O., Izumi, C., Lara, M.G. and Greene, L.J. (1999) New approaches to the treatment of phenylketonuria. *Nutrition Reviews* **57**(3): 65–70.

CASE 5: A MAN WITH SELF-INJURIOUS BEHAVIOUR

Scenario:

Danny is 45 years old. He has lived for more than 20 years in various home areas in several different hospitals for people with learning disabilities. During most of that time, he has shared accommodation with other people who have self-injurious behaviours (SIB). He has limited verbal language. Assessments using adaptive behaviour scales (Nihira *et al.*, 1974) indicate that he has severe learning disabilities. Danny has a long history of challenging behaviour, including aggressive tendencies towards staff and other clients, destructive behaviour related to his clothing, and SIB, which includes head banging.

During the day, Danny generally avoids the company of others and sits in a chair in the home area that he regards as only his to use. In the past, he has frequently hit staff who have tried to communicate with him and many now avoid him as much as possible.

Self-injurious behaviour as a homeostatic imbalance

Background

Some people with learning disabilities indulge in repetitive acts directed toward themselves that result in physical harm or tissue damage. This is usually referred to as self-injurious behaviour. It is generally agreed that SIB is more prevalent among people who have profound learning disabilities. This link with severe cerebral dysfunction has also led to some discussion that the existence of SIB arises because of reduced sensitivity to pain. This suggestion is supported by the observation that SIB can occur at high levels over long periods of time and result in severe injury. The idea is supported further by the observation that the person, while oblivious to pain caused by the SIB, may be sensitive to pain associated with peripheral stimulation. This has led to the assumption that the disorder is of a central nature associated with parts of the brain such as the thalamus, reticular formation, and areas of the limbic system (see Chapter 8). However, the link between SIB and reduced sensitivity to pain has not been established

conclusively, and is complicated further by the multifactorial nature of the perception of pain (see Chapter 21).

Speculation about the organic cause of SIB is fuelled further by evidence related to some rare conditions in which SIB often occurs. An example is Lesch–Nyhan syndrome. In this disorder, it is thought that the distribution of neurotransmitters in the brain may be the cause of SIB. The area of the brain most implicated is the limbic system. However, evidence to support hypotheses that SIB arises from the biological constitution of the person has yet to yield the exact mechanism, and it is thought that organic causation is not the only determinant. The appearance of SIB in normal infants has fuelled the suggestion that this is the persistence of developmentally normal behaviour. Some possible flaws in this argument are related to the differences in which the behaviour is manifest. For example, normal infants exhibit head banging usually in only one situation, which rarely produces major injuries and does not persist to the same extent as similar behaviour in some disabled infants.

A possible explanation of SIB is that it serves to provide sensory stimulation that is rewarding. The main thrust of this argument is that SIB is essentially stereotypical in nature. Thus, when confronted by an environment that is bleak in sensory experience, the SIB serves to heighten stimulation. Other theories of stereotypes suggest that the behaviour helps to reduce the person's level of tension or arousal.

The learned behaviour hypothesis suggests that SIB may have originated from any one of a variety of factors. The SIB is then perpetuated because it is reinforced or rewarded by some influence, usually a social response. Following reinforcement or reward, the same behaviour is more likely to occur in the future.

Presentation

It is difficult for observers to pinpoint the exact moment when a person's SIB originated, but the factors that first produce the SIB may not be the same as those that lead to its perseverance. For example, head banging that originated in response to pain, e.g. a headache, may persist because of the social response to the behaviour. The likelihood is that SIB is motivated and maintained by a range of permutations of such motivating factors that is unique to each individual.

Commonly observed behaviours are head banging, self-biting and self-scratching. Behaviour is pushed or pulled by factors within the biological constitution or environment surrounding the person. By their response to these influences, a person with SIB is communicating a refusal to conform to the socially acceptable norms and values of the world in which they live. Thus, the behaviour is purposeful to the person in various ways:

● to obtain something tangible that they want;

● to escape from a situation that they want to avoid;

● to obtain attention from other people;

● to increase the sensory stimulation levels in the environment.

Improving homeostasis

See Figure 27.5.

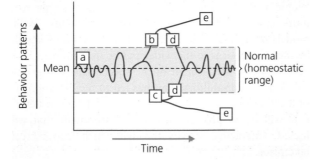

Figure 27.5 Self-injurious behaviour. (a) Behaviour within socially accepted norms. (b) Self-injurious behaviour as a result of biological, operant or environmental factors, leading to penalized behaviour, including possible loss of liberty. (c) Institutionalized behaviour, leading to learned helplessness, perpetuated by labelling and sanctioning of activities by staff. (d) Skilled nursing intervention, e.g. the positive reinforcement of appropriate behaviours to reduce inappropriate behaviour patterns. (e) Continued self-injurious behaviour following unsuccessful interventions.

Aims of care

With the lack of consensus on the type of organic change that might be involved in SIB, Danny's care would focus on his perceptions of the situation and his relationships with others. The aims of the intervention would be to increase Danny's independence by promoting skills that are socially acceptable to others but that allow him to retain individuality. Danny's perceptions of being in control will be important. Much of nursing intervention is based upon the value base of the practitioner, so the individuality of clients might be suppressed. Nurses, therefore, should admit to these tendencies and implement systems that seek to diminish them and so promote an objective view of the care delivered.

Implementation of care

An assessment of Danny's behaviour would be carried out to establish whether his SIB served any useful functions for him. For example, it might be discovered that the SIB was most likely to be exhibited when Danny wanted to obtain something, such as fruit that he seemed to enjoy, and to avoid some activities that he did not seem to relish, e.g. bathing. A number of strategies would then be employed with Danny to reduce the incidence of SIB:

● Staff would begin to develop his communication skills primarily by beginning to teach him Makaton sign language.

● Patterns of staff avoidance of Danny would be acknowledged and reversed, thus his overall sensory stimulation would be increased and the attention he receives will not focus exclusively on his episodes of SIB. This activity also serves to give Danny alternative skills with which to express himself.

● Staff would review the conditions surrounding bathing if Danny disliked it. The process of bathing would be made more leisurely by allowing Danny to have more control over when he bathed and how long the activity took to complete. The activity might be made more fun by the use of water play.

● Danny would be given greater access to the food that he enjoys, e.g. fruit. Previously, staff might have had exclusive control of access.

Reference

Nihira, K., Foster, R., Shellhaas, M. and Leland, H. (1974) *AAMD Adaptive Behaviour Scale, 1974 Revision*. Washington, DC: American Association on Mental Deficiency.

Further reading

Gates, B. (2000) Self-injurious behaviour: reviewing evidence for best practice. *British Journal of Nursing* 9(2): 96–102.

CASE 6: A YOUNG MAN WITH SENSORY DEPRIVATION

Scenario:

Peter is 30 years old and lives at home with his parents. Assessment of his adaptive behaviour reveals that he has a severe learning disability and has no verbal language. He receives day care through a healthcare trust; nurses working with him have observed that he has an affinity to the multisensory environment that they have developed. Since Peter has no spoken language, nurses involved in his care have based their approach on careful observation of his behaviour assisted by the trust and rapport that has been established over several months of relationship building.

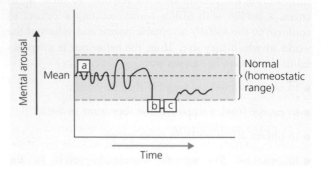

Figure 27.6 Sensory deprivation. (a) Normal level of arousal in people without learning difficulty. (b) Reduced level of arousal promoted by learning difficulty. (c) Exposure of a person with learning difficulties to a sensory stimulus, e.g. visual, olfactory, auditory or gustatory, to increase arousal to as near normal as possible. Stimuli may be provided within a multisensory environment that provides the full range of stimulation.

Sensory deprivation as a homeostatic imbalance

Background

There is a tendency to consider homeostasis as being a physical concept, with processes requiring the sensing of a change to the internal environment. However, an inability to understand our external environment will also have an impact on wellbeing (Chapter 7); Peter's case is an example of the disequilibrium or imbalance that arises when the body cannot interpret sensory information adequately.

Presentation

The problem relates essentially to the neurological disturbance that has contributed to Peter's severe learning difficulties. In such cases, the person finds it difficult to perceive the environment; most importantly, this will influence the ability of the person to respond to the environment.

Improving homeostasis

See Figure 27.6.

Aims of care

Nurses working with people who have learning disabilities have recognized the importance of enabling the development of learning via the construction of opportunities for the people to use their senses to interpret the environment that surrounds them. With this in mind, services for

people with learning disabilities have increasingly paid more attention to the leisure needs of clients. While models of normalization dictate that these needs should be met via services in the wider public domain, there has been an acknowledgement of the special needs of people with learning disabilities. This has led to the development of multisensory environments. The aim of care in Peter's case will be to provide such an environment that will include interactive activity through which learning can take place.

Implementation of care

The origins of the multisensory environment can be traced back to the use of 'snoezelen' in the Netherlands. This word is a combination of two Dutch words, the English equivalents being 'to sniff' and 'to doze'. Thus, a snoezelen environment provides a means of promoting both stimulation and relaxation. The multisensory environment offers a number of advantages as a learning platform for Peter. It gives him a range of opportunities to develop discriminatory skills, and the heightened arousal of his senses should then ensure an increase in the likelihood of learning taking place.

A number of other issues associated with the development of his independence are implicit in this style of care:

● He can exercise control over his own activities, thus developing decision-making and choice skills. This is an important issue for people with learning disabilities, because they may be particularly vulnerable to exposure to institutional practices because of their perceived incapacity to articulate their needs and aspirations.

- The multisensory environment can be used as a vehicle for discovery at the individual pace of Peter.

- Peter can control the level of sensory arousal, so that they can determine the levels of 'heating up' and 'chilling out' with regard to duration, frequency and pitch.

Another consideration is that Peter will have a poorly developed sense of danger. All the exploratory activity within the multisensory environment can remain loosely supervised, thus ensuring maximum independence, but can also be checked regularly for safety.

The multisensory environment that Peter uses contains a number of different areas constructed so each stimulates primarily a single sense while affecting others at a lower level. The intention is to provide a range of experiences that Peter can use to construct sensory images that will facilitate his cognition and learning, thus removing the imbalances associated with this aspect of his learning disability. The areas used are as follows:

- Room one has dimmed lighting and soft furnishings, including a water bed, which encourage relaxation. Soft music is played, which accentuates the calming effect of the room. This room is intended to provide an environment in which environmental stressors are relatively few. Thus, the person is encouraged to assume a physiological, psychological and sociological condition whereby the learning opportunities of this and other rooms are more likely to be accessed.

- Room two contains a floor surface with areas that activate sounds when they are stepped on. Other aspects of this room include wall-mounted panels that emit light when activated by sounds such as the human voice. This room gives Peter the opportunity to develop skills associated with discrimination of tone, pitch and frequency.

- Room three has soft furnishings and windows with coloured glass that makes the exterior appear unusual and illuminates the interior with a warm glow. In this room, visual impact is provided by the use of tall transparent tubes filled with water, through which coloured bubbles percolate. The walls have a number of collages, and a projector can be used to illuminate the room with interesting patterns and designs. A fibre-optic tail in the room undergoes a succession of changes of colour. Other effects are possible via the use of mirrors and lighting set within the walls. Within this environment, Peter is likely to experience a variety of stimuli. The environment encourages the use of discriminatory skills, such as the appreciation of light and shade. This is possible because the receptor cells devoted to detection of visible colour (the cones) and those sensitive to low light intensities (the rods) will be influenced by the differing conditions within the room.

- Room four is filled with materials that provide interesting tactile experiences, including materials with soft, smooth and rough properties. Some of the materials are ordinary materials, such as pasta shells and spirals. These have the advantage of being safe if Peter explores their properties by putting them in his mouth. The materials chosen for this activity could be selected so as to provide the taster with an opportunity to experience the four basic tastes of sweet, sour, bitter and salt. In addition, the room also includes a ball pool, which gives the possibility for the user to enjoy safe movement through an unusual medium. In this room, Peter is able to gain experience of mass, density, texture, temperature and dimensions of objects.

- Room five contains a number of means for the user to experience different sensations associated with smell. A number of tubes attached to the walls contain harmless substances that convey a range of smells. By using this equipment, Peter can refine his discriminatory skills associated with the sensation of sweet or acrid smells, and also the difference between subtle or pungent smells.

Further reading

Gammon, J. (1999) The psychological consequences of source isolation: a review of the literature. *Journal of Clinical Nursing* **8**(1): 13–21.

Schofield, P.A., Davis, B.D. and Hutchinson, R. (1998) Snoezelen and chronic pain: developing a study to evaluate its use (part I). *Complementary Therapies in Nursing and Midwifery* **4**(3): 66–72.

Appendices

Appendices

Appendix A

UNITS OF MEASUREMENT

International system of units

The International System of Units (Système Internationale, or SI units) is a system of standard units used by the scientific, medical, and technical fraternity throughout most of the world. Most units used in this country are now SI units (e.g. grams, litres) but some imperial units (e.g. pounds, stones, pints, and gallons) are still in everyday usage.

The following are SI units for various parameters. Note that the basic SI unit for temperature is the Kelvin but the use of a Celsius scale is more practical for most measurements, since 0 Kelvin is –273°C!

Measurement	SI unit and symbol
Mass	gram (g)
Length	metre (m)
Volume	litre (l)
Temperature	degrees Kelvin (K) (or Celsius, °C)
Time	second (s)
Amount of substance	mole (mol)
Pressure	pascal (Pa)
Frequency	hertz (Hz)
Energy/heat	joule (J)
Radioactivity	becquerel (Bq)
Force	newton (N)
Electrical potential	volt (V)
Electric current	ampere (A)
Power	watt (W)

The following are some useful conversions from Imperial into SI units.

Lengths

Length	Metric equivalent
1 yard (yd)	0.9144 metre (m)
1 foot (ft)	0.31 metre (m)
1 inch (in)	2.54 centimetres (cm)
	25.4 millimetres (mm)

Metric length	Equivalent
1 metre (m)	100 centimetres (cm)
	1000 millimetres (mm)
	39.37 inches (in)
1 centimetre (cm)	10 millimetres (mm)
	0.39 inches (in)
1 millimetre (mm)	0.1 centimetre (cm)
	1000 micrometres (μm)
1 micrometre (μm)	1000 nanometres (nm)

Weights

Weights	Metric equivalent
1 pound (lb)	373 grams (g)
	373 000 milligrams (mg)
1 ounce (oz)	31.1 grams (g)
	31 000 milligrams (mg)

Metric weight	Equivalent
1 kilogram (kg)	1000 grams (g)
	1000 000 milligrams (mg)
	1000 000 000 micrograms (μg)
	32 ounces (oz)
	2.7 pounds (lb)
1 gram (g)	1000 milligrams (mg)
	1000 000 micrograms (μg)
1 milligram (mg)	1000 micrograms (μg)

Volumes

Volume	Metric equivalent
1 fluid ounce (fl oz)	29.6 millilitres (ml)
	29.6 cubic centimetres (cm³)
1 pint (pt)	473 millilitres (ml)
	473 cubic centimetres (cm³)

Metric volume	Equivalent
1 litre (l)	1000 millilitres (ml)
	1000 cubic centimetres (cm³)
	2.1 pints (pt)
1 millilitre (ml)	1 cubic centimetre (cm³)

Factors, prefixes and symbols for decimal multiples

Factor	Prefix	Symbol
10^6	mega	M
10^3	kilo	k
10^2	hecto	h
10^1	deca	da
10^{-1}	deci	d
10^{-2}	centi	c
10^{-3}	milli	m
10^{-6}	micro	μ
10^{-9}	nano	n
10^{-12}	pico	p

Units of concentration, pressure and osmotic pressure

Substance concentration, the pressure of a gas or fluid, and the osmotic pressure of a fluid, are important measurements in physiology and it is worthwhile considering the units used in more detail.

Units of concentration

The concentrations of substances in body fluids and urine may be expressed as grams or milligrams per unit volume, for example grams per litre (written as g/1). Although widely used, such units are of limited use in considering chemical activities because they give no indication of the concentration of atoms or molecules present. Atoms of different elements are of different size and mass and so the number of atoms in, say, a milligram will vary between substances. The SI unit of concentration is called the mole, and 1 mole of an element will contain 6.02×10^{23} atoms (called Avogadro's number); if the substance consists of

molecules then a mole of the substance will contain that number of molecules. A mole of atoms or molecules is also equal to the atomic, or molecular, weight of the substance.

Consider glucose (chemical formula $C_6H_{12}O_6$):

$$\begin{array}{ccc} 1\ \text{mole} & & 180\ \text{g} \\ \text{of} & = & \text{of} \\ \text{glucose} & & \text{glucose} \end{array} \quad (= \text{its molecular weight})$$

made up of 6 moles of carbon atoms

$6 \times$ atomic weight of carbon	$= (6 \times 12 = 72\ \text{g})$
12 moles of hydrogen atoms	$(12 \times 1 = 12\ \text{g})$
and 6 moles of oxygen atoms	$(6 \times 16 = 96\ \text{g})$
	180 g

(Note that hydrogen is the atomic 'standard', i.e. 1 mole weighs 1 g.)

A molar solution of a substance contains 1 mole of it per litre of solution (usually dissolved in water). A molar solution of glucose, therefore, will contain 180 g of glucose per litre. This is actually a very high concentration, far higher than is found in body fluids. The concentrations of substances in physiological fluids are usually given in millimoles (1 mmol = 1 mole $\times 10^{-3}$) or micromole (1 μmol = 1 mole $\times 10^{-6}$). Some biochemicals are of even lower concentrations and are measured in nanomoles (1 nmol = 1 mole $\times 10^{-9}$) or even picomoles (1 pmol = 1 mole $\times 10^{-12}$).

Sometimes the concentration of a hormone or an enzyme is recorded in Units or milliUnits per millilitre. In this case, the unit relates to the biological activity of the substance, with 1 milliUnit producing a known, quantified physiological response.

Units of pressure

Fluids are non-compressible. Gases, however, can be compressed into a smaller volume or expanded into a larger one. Such compressions and expansions alter the concentration of gas molecules as the same number of molecules are now contained in different volumes. Pressure is a measure of the interactions made between gas molecules and the surface of its container or chamber – the greater the concentration of a gas, the more interactions there will be per unit time. Traditionally, pressure was measured by observing how high mercury would rise up a thin tube as a consequence of collisions between gas molecules and the surface of the pool of mercury in which the tube stood. At sea level, standard air pressure is 760 mm of mercury (written as 760 mmHg; the symbol for mercury is Hg).

The SI unit for pressure is the pascal (Pa) although mmHg (or even mmH$_2$O for low pressure; water has a lower density than mercury) is still used for many parameters, such as blood pressure (note that pressure also applies to fluids within enclosed chambers, such as blood vessels). The pressures of respiratory gases are usually given in kilopascals (kPa) and 1 kPa approximates to 7.6 mmHg. For example, the pressure of oxygen in the alveoli after inspiration is 13.3 kPa (equivalent to about 100 mmHg).

Units of osmotic pressure (osmolarity)

The direct measurement of osmotic pressure of a solution is difficult when dealing with small samples of body fluid. However, osmotic pressure is directly related to the concentration of solute in the solution. A convenient means of measuring the total concentration of solute, and therefore its osmotic potential, is to measure how much the freezing point of the solvent (i.e. water) has been depressed by the solute. Body fluids contain a variety of substances and the unit of concentration of solute used is the osmole, to distinguish it from the mole unit for the concentrations of individual substances present. Physiological fluids are normally in the milliosmole range, for example plasma has an osmolarity of about 285 mosmol per litre. The higher the osmolar concentration, the greater the osmotic potential of the fluid.

Appendix B

BLOOD, PLASMA, OR SERUM VALUES

Test	Normal values*	Significance of change
Bicarbonate	22–26 mmol/l	↑in metabolic alkalosis ↑in respiratory alkalosis ↓in metabolic acidosis
Blood urea nitrogen (BUN)	5–25 mg/dl	↑with increased protein intake ↓in kidney failure
Blood volume	*Women*: 65 ml/kg body weight *Men*: 69 ml/kg body weight	↓during a haemorrhage
Calcium	8.4–10.5 mg/dl	↑in hypervitaminosis D ↑in hyperparathyroidism ↑in bone cancer and other bone diseases ↓in severe diarrhoea ↓in hypoparathyroidism ↓in avitaminosis D (rickets and osteomalacia)
Chloride	96–107 mmol/l	↑in hyperventilation ↑in kidney disease ↑in Cushing's syndrome ↓in diabetic acidosis ↓in severe diarrhoea ↓in severe burns ↓in Addison's disease
Clotting time	5–10 minutes	↓in haemophilia ↓(occasionally) in other clotting disorders
Creatine phosphokinase (CPK)	*Women*: 0–14 IU/l *Men*: 0–20 IU/l	↑in Duchenne muscular dystrophy ↑during myocardial infarction ↑in muscle trauma
Glucose	70–110 mg/dl (fasting) (4–6 mmol/l approx.)	↑in diabetes mellitus ↑in liver disease ↑during pregnancy ↑in hyperthyroidism ↓in hypothyroidism ↓in Addison's disease ↓in hyperinsulinism

Test	Normal values*	Significance of change
Haematocrit (packed cell volume)	*Women*: 38–47% *Men*: 40–54%	↑in polycythaemia ↑in severe dehydration ↓in anaemia ↓in leukaemia ↓in hyperthyroidism ↓in cirrhosis of liver
Haemoglobin	*Women*: 12–16 g/dl *Men*: 13–18 g/dl *Newborn*: 14–20 g/dl	↑in polycythaemia ↑in chronic obstructive pulmonary disease ↑in congestive heart failure ↓in anaemia ↓in hyperthyroidism ↓in cirrhosis of liver
Iron	50–150 µg/dl (can be higher in male)	↑in liver disease ↑in anaemia (some forms) ↓in iron-deficiency anaemia
Lactate dehydrogenase isoenzymes (LDH_{1-5})	60–120 u/ml	↑during myocardial infarction ↑in anaemia (several forms) ↑in liver disease ↑in acute leukaemia and other cancers
Lipids – total Cholesterol – total High-density lipoprotein (HDL) Low-density lipoprotein (LDL)	450–1000 mg/dl 120–220 mg/dl >40 mg/dl <180 mg/dl	↑(total) in diabetes mellitus ↑(total) in kidney disease ↑(total) in hypothyroidism ↓(total) in hyperthyroidism ↑in inherited hypercholesterolaemia ↑(cholesterol) in chronic hepatitis ↓(cholesterol) in acute hepatitis ↑(HDL) with regular exercise
Mean corpuscular volume	82–98 µl	↑or↓in various forms of anaemia
Osmolality	285–295 mosmol/l	↑or↓in fluid and electrolyte imbalances
PCO_2	35–43 mmHg (4.6–5.7 kPa)	↑in severe vomiting ↑in respiratory disorders ↑in obstruction of intestines ↓in acidosis ↓in severe diarrhoea ↓in kidney disease
pH	7.35–7.45	↑during hyperventilation ↑in Cushing's syndrome ↓during hypoventilation ↓in acidosis ↓in Addison's disease
Plasma volume	*Women*: 40 ml/kg body weight *Men*: 39 ml/kg body weight	↑or↓in fluid and electrolyte imbalances ↓during haemorrhage
Platelet count	150 000–400 000/mm³	↑in heart disease ↑in cancer ↑in cirrhosis of liver ↑after trauma ↓in anaemia (some forms) ↓during chemotherapy ↓in some allergies
PO_2	75–100 mmHg (breathing standard air) (10–13.3 kPa)	↑in polycythaemia ↓in anaemia ↓in chronic obstructive pulmonary disease

Test	Normal values*	Significance of change
Potassium	3.8–5.1 mmol/l	↑in hypoaldosteronism ↑in acute kidney failure ↓in vomiting or diarrhoea ↓in starvation

Protein – total
  Albumin
  Globulin
	6–8.4 g/dl
	3.5–5 g/dl
	2.3–3.5 g/dl
		↑(total) in severe dehydration
		↓(total) during haemorrhage
		↓(total) in starvation

Red blood cell count	*Women:* 4.2–5.4 million/mm³ *Men:* 4.5–6.2 million/mm³	↑in polycythaemia ↑in dehydration ↓in anaemia (several forms) ↓in Addison's disease ↓in systemic lupus erythematosus
Reticulocyte count	25 000–75 000/mm³ (0.5–1.5% of RBC count)	↑in haemolytic anaemia ↑in leukaemia and metastatic carcinoma ↓in pernicious anaemia ↓in iron-deficiency anaemia ↓during radiation therapy
Sodium	136–145 mmol/l	↑in dehydration ↑in trauma or disease of the central nervous system ↑or↓in kidney disorders ↓in excessive sweating, vomiting, diarrhoea ↓in burns (sodium shift into cells)
Transaminase	10–40 u/ml	↑during myocardial infarction ↑in liver disease
Viscosity	1.4–1.8 times the viscosity of water	↑in polycythaemia ↑in dehydration

White blood cell count
  Total
  Neutrophils
  Eosinophils
  Basophils
  Lymphocytes
  Monocytes
	
	4500–11 000/mm³
	60–70% of total
	2–4% of total
	0.5–1% of total
	20–25% of total
	3–8% of total
		↑(total) in acute infections
		↑(total) in trauma
		↑(total) some cancers
		↓(total) in anaemia (some forms)
		↓(total) during chemotherapy
		↑(neutrophils) in acute infection
		↑(eosinophils) in allergies
		↓(basophil) in severe allergies
		↑(lymphocyte) during antibody reactions
		↑(monocyte) in chronic infections

*Values vary with the analysis method used and between individuals.
1 dl = 100 ml.

URINE COMPONENTS

Test	Normal values*	Significance of change
Routine urinalysis		
Acetone and acetoacetate	None	↑during fasting ↑in diabetic acidosis
Albumin	None to trace	↑in hypertension ↑in kidney disease ↑after strenuous exercise (temporary)
Calcium	<150 mg/day	↑in hyperparathyroidism ↓in hypoparathyroidism
Colour	Transparent yellow, straw-coloured, or amber	Abnormal colour or cloudiness may indicate: blood in urine, bile, bacteria, drugs, food pigments, or high solute concentration
Odour	Characteristics slight odour	Acetone odour in diabetes mellitus (diabetic ketosis)
Osmolality	500–800 mosmol/l	↑in dehydration ↑in heart failure ↓in diabetes insipidus ↓in aldosteronism
pH	4.6–8.0	↑in alkalosis ↑during urinary infections ↓in dehydration ↓in emphysema
Potassium	25–100 mmol/l	↑dehydration ↑in chronic kidney failure ↓in diarrhoea or vomiting ↓in adrenal insufficiency
Sodium	75–200 mg/day	↑in starvation ↑in dehydration ↓acute kidney failure ↓in Cushing's syndrome
Creatinine clearance	100–140 ml/min	↑in kidney disease
Glucose	0	↑in diabetes mellitus ↑in hyperthyroidism ↑in hypersecretion of adrenal cortex
Urea clearance	>40 ml blood cleared per min	↑in some kidney diseases
Urea	25–35 g/day	↑in some liver diseases ↑in haemolytic anaemia ↓during obstruction of bile ducts ↓in severe diarrhoea
Microscopic examination		
Bacteria	<10 000/ml	↑during urinary infections
Blood cells (RBC)	0–trace	↑in pyelonephritis ↑from damage by calculi ↑in infection ↑in cancer
Blood cells (WBC)	0–trace	↑in infections

Appendix C

WORD PARTS COMMONLY USED AS PREFIXES

Word part	Meaning	Example	Meaning of example
a-	Without, not	Apnoea	Cessation of breathing
af-	Toward	Afferent	Carrying toward
an-	Without, not	Anuria	Absence of urination
ante-	Before	Antenatal	Before birth
anti-	Against, resisting	Antibody	Unit that resists foreign substances
auto-	Self	Autoimmunity	Self-immunity
bi-	Two; double	Bicuspid	Two-pointed
circum-	Around	Circumcision	Cutting around
co-, con-	With; together	Congenital	Born with
contra-	Against	Contraceptive	Against conception
de-	Down from, undoing	Defibrillation	Stop fibrillation
dia-	Across, through	Diarrhoea	Flow through (intestine)
dipl-	Twofold, double	Diploid	Two sets of chromosomes
dys-	Bad; disordered; difficult	Dysplasia	Disordered growth
ectop-	Displaced	Ectopic pregnancy	Displaced pregnancy
ef-	Away from	Efferent	Carrying away from
endo-	Within	Endocarditis	Inflammation of heart lining
epi-	Upon	Epimysium	Covering of a muscle
ex-, exo-	Out of, out from	Exophthalmos	Protruding eyes
extra-	Outside of	Extraperitoneal	Outside of peritoneum
eu-	Good	Eupnoea	Good (normal) breathing
hapl-	Single	Haploid	Single set of chromosomes
Haem-, haemat-	Blood	Haematuria	Bloody urine
hemi-	Half	Hemiplegia	Paralysis in half the body
Hom(e)o-	Same; equal	Homeostasis	Standing the same
hyper-	Over; above	Hyperplasia	Excessive growth
hypo-	Under; below	Hypodermic	Below the skin
infra-	Below, beneath	Infraorbital	Below the (eye) orbit
inter-	Between	Intervertebral	between vertebrae
intra-	Within	Intracranial	Within the skull
iso-	Same, equal	Isometric	Same length
macro-	Large	Macrophage	Large eater (phagocyte)
mes-	Middle	Mesentery	Middle of intestine
micro-	Small; millionth	Microcytic	Small-celled
milli-	Thousandth	Millilitre	Thousandth of a litre
mono-	One (single)	Monosomy	Single chromosome
non-	Not	Non-dysjunction	Not disjoined
para-	By the side of; near	Parathyroid	Near the thyroid
per-	Through	Permeable	Able to go through
peri-	Around; surrounding	Pericardium	Covering of the heart
poly-	Many	Polycythaemia	Condition of many blood cells

post-	After	Postmortem	After death
pre-	Before	Premenstrual	Before menstruation
pro-	First; promoting	Progesterone	Hormone that promotes pregnancy
quadr-	Four	Quadriplegia	Paralysis in four limbs
re-	Back again	Reflux	Backflow
retro-	Behind	Retroperitoneal	Behind the peritoneum
semi-	Half	Semilunar	Half-moon
sub-	Under	Subcutaneous	Under the skin
super-, supra-	Over, above, excessive	Superior	Above
trans-	Across; through	Transcutaneous	Through the skin
tri-	Three; triple	Triplegia	Paralysis of three limbs

WORD PARTS COMMONLY USED AS SUFFIXES

Word part	Meaning	Example	Meaning of example
-aemia	Refers to blood condition	Hypercholesterolaemia	High blood cholesterol level
-al, -ac	Pertaining to	Intestinal	Pertaining to the intestines
-algia	Pain	Neuralgia	Nerve pain
-aps, -apt	Fit; fasten	Synapse	Fasten together
-arche	Beginning; origin	Menarche	First menstruation
-ase	Signifies an enzyme	Lipase	Enzyme that acts on lipids
-blast	Sprout; make	Osteoblast	Bone maker
-centesis	A piercing	Amniocentesis	Piercing the amniotic sac
-cide	To kill	Fungicide	Fungus killer
-clast	Break; destroy	Osteoclast	Bone breaker
-crine	Release; secrete	Endocrine	Secrete within
-ectomy	A cutting out	Appendectomy	Removal of the appendix
-emesis	Vomiting	Haematemesis	Vomiting blood
-gen	Creates; forms	Lactogen	Milk producer
-genesis	Creation, production	Oogenesis	Egg production
-graph(y)	To write, draw	Electrocardiograph	Apparatus that records heart's electrical activity
-hydrate	Containing H_2O (water)	Dehydration	Loss of water
-ia, -sia	Condition; process	Arthralgia	Condition of joint pain
-iasis	Abnormal condition	Giardiasis	*Giardia* infestation
-ic, -ac	Pertaining to	Cardiac	Pertaining to the heart
-in	Signifies a protein	Renin	Kidney protein
-ism	Signifies 'condition of'	Gigantism	Condition of gigantic size
-itis	Signifies 'inflammation of'	Gastritis	Stomach inflammation
-lepsy	Seizure	Epilepsy	Seizure upon seizure
-logy	Study of	Cardiology	Study of the heart
-lunar	Moon; moon-like	Semilunar	Half-moon
-malacia	Softening	Osteomalacia	Bone softening
-megaly	Enlargement	Splenomegaly	Spleen enlargement
-metric, -metry	Measurement, length	Isometric	Same length
-oma	Tumour	Lipoma	Fatty tumour
-opia	Vision, vision condition	Myopia	Nearsightedness
-ose	Signifies a carbohydrate (especially sugar)	Lactose	Milk sugar
-osis	Condition, process	Dermatosis	Skin condition
-oscopy	Viewing	Laparoscopy	Viewing the abdominal cavity
-ostomy	Formation of an opening	Tracheostomy	Forming an opening in the trachea
-otomy	Cut	Lobotomy	Cut of a lobe
-philic	Loving	Hydrophilic	Water-loving
-penia	Lack	Leucopenia	Lack of white (cells)
-phobic	Fearing	Hydrophobic	Water-fearing
-plasia	Growth, formation	Hyperplasia	Excessive growth
-plasm	Substance, matter	Neoplasm	New matter
-plegia	Paralysis	Triplegia	Paralysis in three limbs
-pnoea	Breath, breathing	Apnoea	Cessation of breathing
-(r)rhage, -(r)rhagia	Breaking out, discharge	Haemorrhage	Blood discharge
-(r)rhoea	Flow	Diarrhoea	Flow through (intestines)

-some	Body	Chromosome	Stained body
-tensin, -tension	Pressure	Hypertension	High pressure
-tonic	Pressure, tension	Isotonic	Same pressure
-uria	Refers to urine condition	Proteinuria	Protein in the urine

WORD PARTS COMMONLY USED AS ROOTS

Word part	Meaning	Example	Meaning of example
acro-	Extremity	Acromegaly	Enlargement of extremities
aden-	Gland	Adenoma	Tumour of glandular tissue
aesthe-	Sensation	Anaesthesia	Condition of no sensation
alveol-	Small, hollow, cavity	Alveolus	Small air sac in the lung
angi-	Vessel	Angioplasty	Reshaping a vessel
arthr-	Joint	Arthritis	Joint inflammation
bar-	Pressure	Baroreceptor	Pressure receptor
bili-	Bile	Bilirubin	Orange-yellow bile pigment
brachi-	Arm	Brachial	Pertaining to the arm
brady-	Slow	Bradycardia	Slow heart rate
bronch-	Air passage	Bronchitis	Inflammation of pulmonary passages (bronchi)
calc-	Calcium; limestone	Hypocalcaemia	Low blood calcium level
carcin-	Cancer	Carcinogen	Cancer-producer
card-	Heart	Cardiology	Study of the heart
cephal-	Head, brain	Encephalitis	Brain inflammation
cerv-	Neck	Cervicitis	Inflammation of (uterine) cervix
chem-	Chemical	Chemotherapy	Chemical treatment
chol-	Bile	Cholecystectomy	Removal of bile (gall) bladder
chondr-	Cartilage	Chondroma	Tumour of cartilage tissue
chrom-	Colour	Chromosome	Stained body
corp-	Body	Corpus luteum	Yellow body
cortico-	Pertaining to cortex	Corticosteroid	Steroid secreted by (adrenal) cortex
crani-	Skull	Intracranial	Within the skull
crypt-	Hidden	Cryptorchidism	Undescended testis
cusp-	Point	Tricuspid	Three-pointed
cut(an)-	Skin	Transcutaneous	Through the skin
cyan-	Blue	Cyanosis	Condition of blueness
cyst-	Bladder	Cystitis	Bladder inflammation
cyt-	Cell	Cytotoxin	Cell poison
dactyl-	Fingers, toes (digits)	Syndactyly	Joined digits
dendr-	Tree; branched	Oligodendrocyte	Branched nervous tissue cell
derm-	Skin	Dermatitis	Skin inflammation
diastol-	Relax; stand apart	Diastole	Relaxation phase of heart beat
ejacul-	To throw out	Ejaculation	Expulsion (of semen)
electr-	Electrical	Electrocardiogram	Record of electrical activity of heart
enter-	Intestine	Enteritis	Intestinal inflammation
eryth(r)-	Red	Erythrocyte	Red (blood) cell
gastr-	Stomach	Gastritis	Stomach inflammation
gest-	To bear, carry	Gestation	Pregnancy
gingiv-	Gums	Gingivitis	Gum inflammation
glomer-	Wound into a ball	Glomerulus	Rounded tuft of vessels
gloss-	Tongue	Hypoglossal	Under the tongue
gluc-	Glucose, sugar	Glucosuria	Glucose in urine
glyc-	Sugar (carbohydrate); glucose	Glycolipid	Carbohydrate–lipid combination
hepat-	Liver	Hepatitis	Liver inflammation
hist-	Tissue	Histology	Study of tissues
hydro-	Water	Hydrocephalus	Water on the brain
hyster-	Uterus	Hysterectomy	Removal of the uterus
kal-	Potassium	Hyperkalaemia	Elevated blood potassium level
kary-	Nucleus	Karyotype	Array of chromosomes from nucleus
lact-	Milk; milk production	Lactose	Milk sugar
leuc-	White	Leucorrhoea	White flow (discharge)
lig-	To tie, bind	Ligament	Tissue that binds bones

Word part	Meaning	Example	Meaning of example
lip-	Lipid (fat)	Lipoma	Fatty tumour
lys-	Break apart	Haemolysis	Breaking of blood cells
mal-	Bad	Malabsorption	Improper absorption
melan-	Black	Melanin	Black protein
men-, mens-, (menstru-)	Month (monthly)	Amenorrhoea	Absence of monthly flow
metr-	Uterus	Endometrium	Uterine lining
muta-	Change	Mutagen	Change-maker
my-, myo-	Muscle	Myopathy	Muscle disease
myel-	Marrow	Myeloma	(Bone) marrow tumour
myx-	Mucus	Myxoedema	Mucous oedema
nat-	Birth	Neonatal	Pertaining to newborns (infants)
natr-	Sodium	Natriuresis	Elevated sodium in urine
nephr-	Nephron, kidney	Nephritis	Kidney inflammation
neur-	Nerve	Neuralgia	Nerve pain
noct-, nyct-	Night	Nocturia	Urination at night
ocul-	Eye	Binocular	Two-eyed
odont-	Tooth	Periodonitis	Inflammation (of tissue) around the teeth
onco-	Cancer	Oncogene	Cancer gene
ophthalm-	Eye	Ophthalmology	Study of the eye
osteo-	Bone	Osteoma	Bone tumour
oto-	Ear	Otosclerosis	Hardening of ear tissue
ov-, oo-	Egg	Oogenesis	Egg production
oxy-	Oxygen	Oxyhaemoglobin	Oxygen–haemoglobin combination
path-	Disease	Neuropathy	Nerve disease
phag-	Eat	Phagocytosis	cell eating
pharm-	drug	Pharmacology	Study of drugs
photo-	Light	Photopigment	Light-sensitive pigment
physio-	Nature (function) of	Physiology	Study of biological function
pino-	Drink	Pinocytosis	Cell drinking
plex-	Twisted; woven	Nerve plexus	Complex of interwoven nerve fibres
pneumo-	Air, breath	Pneumothorax	Air in the thorax
pneumon-	Lung	Pneumonia	Lung condition
pod-	Foot	Podocyte	Cell with feet
poie-	Make; produce	Haemopoiesis	Blood cell production
presby-	Old	Presbyopia	Old vision
proct-	Rectum	Proctoscope	Instrument for viewing the rectum
pseud-	False	Pseudopodia	False feet
psych-	Mind	Psychiatry	Treatment of the mind
pyel-	Pelvis	Pyelogram	Image of the kidney pelvis
pyro-	Heat; fever	Pyrogen	Fever producer
ren-	Kidney	Renocortical	Referring to the cortex of the kidney
sarco-	Flesh; muscle	Sarcolemma	Muscle fibre membrane
semen-, semin-	Seed; sperm	Seminiferous tubule	Sperm-bearing tubule
sept-	Contamination	Septicaemia	Contamination of the blood
sigm-	Greek Σ or Roman S	Sigmoid colon	S-shaped colon
son-	Sound	Sonography	Imaging using sound
spiro-, -spire	Breathe	Spirometry	Measurement of breathing
stat-, stas-	A standing, stopping	Homeostasis	Staying the same
syn-	Together	Syndrome	Sings appearing together
systol-	Contract; stand together	Systole	Contraction phase of the heart beat
tachy-	Fast	Tachycardia	Rapid heart rate
therm-	Heat	Thermoreceptor	Heat receptor
thromb-	Clot	Thrombosis	Condition of abnormal blood clotting
tox-	Poison	Cytotoxin	Cell poison
troph-	Grow; nourish	Hypertrophy	Excessive growth
tympan-	Drum	Tympanum	Eardrum
varic-	Enlarged vessel	Varicose vein	Enlarged vein
vas-	Vessel, duct	Vasoconstriction	Vessel narrowing
vol-	Volume	Hypovolaemic	Characterized by low volume

* Tables in Appendix C are reproduced, with permission from Thibeaudeau, G.A. and Patton, K.T. (1992). *The human body in health and disease*. St Louis: Mosby.
* A term ending in *-graph* refers to apparatus that results in a visual and/or recorded representation of biological phenomena, whereas a term ending in *-graphy* is the technique or process of using the apparatus. A term ending in *-gram* is the record itself. Example: In electrocardio*graphy*, an electrocardio*graph* is used in producing an electrocardio*gram*.

Appendix D

SYMBOLS AND ABBREVIATIONS

Many medical terms are commonly expressed in abbreviated form. The following list is designed to familiarize you with some of these abbreviations. Most of the terms have been used in the book, however, some are included because they are frequently used.

Symbols

♀, O	female
♂,	male
∞	infinity
α	alpha
β	beta
γ	gamma

Abbreviations

Ab	antibody; abortion		CO	cardiac output; carbon monoxide
ACTH	adrenocorticotropic hormone		COAD	chronic obstructive airways disease
ADH	antidiuretic hormone		CSF	cerebrospinal fluid
Ag	antigen		CVA	cerebrovascular accident
AIDS	acquired immune deficiency syndrome		CVD	cardiovascular disease
ANS	autonomic nervous system		CVS	chorionic villus sampling
ARD	acute respiratory system		DBP	diastolic blood pressure
ARF	acute renal failure		DNA	deoxyribonucleic acid
ATP	adenosine triphosphate		DVT	deep venous thrombosis
AV	atrioventricular		ECF	extracellular fluid
BBB	blood–brain barrier; bundle branch block		ECG	electrocardiogram
BBT	basal body temperature		EEG	electroencephalogram
BMR	basal metabolic rate		EM	electron micrograph
BP	blood pressure		EMG	electromyogram
BPM	beats per minute		EPSP	excitatory post-synaptic potential
BS	blood sugar		ER	endoplasmic reticulum
C	Celsius		ESR	erythrocyte sedimentation rate
CABG	coronary artery bypass grafting		ESV	end-systolic volume
CAD	coronary artery disease		F	Fahrenheit
CCU	cardiac care unit; coronary care unit		FAS	fetal alcohol syndrome
CF	cystic fibrosis; cardiac failure		FSH	follicle-stimulating hormone
CH	cholesterol		GAS	general adaptation syndrome
CHF	congestive heart failure		GFR	glomerular filtration rate
CNS	central nervous system		GI	gastrointestinal

GIFT	gamete intrafallopian transfer	pH	hydrogen ion concentration
Hb	haemoglobin	PKU	phenylketonuria
hCG	human chorionic gonadotropin	PMS	premenstrual syndrome
Hct	haematocrit	PNS	peripheral nervous system
HDL	high-density lipoprotein	PRL	prolactin
HDN	haemolytic disease of newborn	PROG	progesterone
HF	heart failure	PTH	parathyroid hormone
hGH	human growth hormone	RBC	red blood cell; red blood count
HR	heart rate	RDS	respiratory distress syndrome
HSV	herpes simplex virus	REM	rapid eye movement
ICF	intracellular fluid	Rh	rhesus
Ig	immunoglobin	RNA	ribonucleic acid
IPSP	inhibitory post-synaptic potential	RR	respiratory rate
IUD	intrauterine device	RRR	regular rate and rhythm (heart)
i.v.	intravenous	SA	sinoatrial
IVC	inferior vena cava	SBP	systolic blood pressure
IVF	*in vitro* fertilization	SCA	sickle cell anaemia
KS	Kaposi's sarcoma	SCD	sudden cardiac death
kPa	kilopascal	SCID	severe combined immunodeficiency syndrome
LDL	low-density lipoprotein	SIDS	sudden infant death syndrome
LH	luteinizing hormone	SNS	somatic nervous system
mEq/l	milliequivalents per litre	STD	sexually transmitted disease
MI	myocardial infarction	SV	stroke volume
mm³	cubic millimetre	SVC	superior vena cava
mmHg	millimetres of mercury	T	temperature
MS	multiple sclerosis	TB	tuberculosis
MSH	melanocyte-stimulating hormone	TIA	transient ischaemic attack
NSAID	non-steroidal anti-inflammatory drug	TPR	temperature, pulse, and respiration
NTP	normal temperature and pressure	TSH	thyroid-stimulating hormone
OD	overdose	URI	upper respiratory infection
OT	oxytocin	UTI	urinary tract infection
P	pressure	UV	ultraviolet
PCP	*Pneumocystis carinii* pneumonia	VF	ventricular fibrillation
PCV	packed cell volume	VS	vital signs
PG	prostaglandin	WBC	white blood cell; white blood count

Index